S0-BNX-894

3rd edition

comprehensive pharmacy review

3rd edition

comprehensive pharmacy review

EDITORS

Leon Shargel, Ph.D., R.Ph.
Alan H. Mutnick, Pharm.D., R.Ph.
Paul F. Souney, M.S., R.Ph.
Larry N. Swanson, Pharm.D., R.Ph.
Lawrence H. Block, Ph.D., R.Ph.

Williams & Wilkins

A WAVERLY COMPANY

BALTIMORE • PHILADELPHIA • LONDON • PARIS • BANGKOK
BUENOS AIRES • HONG KONG • MUNICH • SYDNEY • TOKYO • WROCLAW

Editor: Elizabeth A. Nieginski
Managing Editor: Alethea H. Elkins, Amy G. Dinkel
Production Coordinator: Felecia R. Weber
Cover Designer: Maria Karkucinski
Typesetter: Graphic World
Printer: Victor Graphics
Binder: Victor Graphics

Copyright © 1997 Williams & Wilkins

351 West Camden Street
Baltimore, Maryland 21201-2436 USA

Rose Tree Corporate Center
1400 North Providence Road
Building II, Suite 5025
Media, Pennsylvania 19063-2043 USA

All rights reserved. This book is protected by copyright. No part of this book may be reproduced in any form or by any means, including photocopying, or utilized by any information storage and retrieval system without written permission from the copyright owner.

Accurate indications, adverse reactions and dosage schedules for drugs are provided in this book, but it is possible that they may change. The reader is urged to review the package information data of the manufacturers of the medications mentioned.
Printed in the United States of America

NABPLEX® and NABP® are federally registered trademarks owned by the National Association of Boards of Pharmacy. This book is in no way authorized or sponsored by the NABP®.

Library of Congress Cataloging-in-Publication Data

Comprehensive pharmacy review/editor, Leon Shargel; associate editors, Alan H. Mutnick . . . [et al.] — 3rd ed.
p. cm.
Includes index.
ISBN 0-683-07681-7
1. Pharmacy—Examinations, questions, etc. 2. Pharmacy—Outlines, syllabi, etc.
I. Shargel, Leon, 1941– . II. Mutnick, Alan H.
[DNLM: 1. Pharmacy—examination questions. 2. Pharmacy—outlines.
QV 18.2 C737 1997]
RS97.P49 1997
615'.1'076—dc20
DNLM/DLC
for Library of Congress 96-34127
CIP

The publishers have made every effort to trace the copyright holders for borrowed material. If they have inadvertently overlooked any, they will be pleased to make the necessary arrangements at the first opportunity.

To purchase additional copies of this book, call our customer service department at **(800) 638-0672** or fax orders to **(800) 447-8438.** For other book services, including chapter reprints and large quantity sales, ask for the Special Sales department.

Canadian customers should call **(800) 268-4178,** or fax **(905) 470-6780.** For all other calls originating outside of the United States, please call **(410) 528-4223** or fax us at **(410) 528-8550.**

Visit Williams & Wilkins on the Internet: **http://www.wwilkins.com** or contact our customer service department at **custserv@wwilkins.com.** Williams & Wilkins customer service representatives are available from 8:30 am to 6:00 pm, EST, Monday through Friday, for telephone access.

97 98 99
1 2 3 4 5 6 7 8 9 10

Contents

Contributors

Loyd V. Allen, Jr., Ph.D., R.Ph.
Professor and Chair
Department of Medicinal Chemistry and Pharmaceutics
College of Pharmacy
The University of Oklahoma
Oklahoma City, Oklahoma

Anton H. Amann, Ph.D.
Senior Vice President
Scientific Operations
Apotex USA, Inc.
New York, New York

Ernest R. Anderson, Jr., M.S.
Director of Pharmacy Services
Lahey Clinic
Burlington, Massachusetts

Connie Lee Barnes, Pharm.D.
Assistant Professor of Pharmacy Practice
Director Drug Information Center
Campbell University School of Pharmacy
Buies Creek, North Carolina

Amy J. Becker, Pharm.D., R.Ph.
Clinical Pharmacy Specialist/Hematology-Oncology
The University of Iowa Hospitals and Clinics
Adjunct Assistant Professor
University of Iowa, College of Pharmacy
Division of Clinical and Administrative Pharmacy
Iowa City, Iowa

Lawrence H. Block, Ph.D., R.Ph.
Professor of Pharmaceutics
Chair, Department of Medicinal Chemistry and Pharmaceutics
Mylan School of Pharmacy
Duquesne University
Pittsburgh, Pennsylvania

Ralph N. Blomster, Ph.D.
Professor Emeritus
University of Maryland School of Pharmacy
Baltimore, Maryland

Riccardo L. Boni, Ph.D.
Assistant Professor of Pharmaceutical Chemistry
Mylan School of Pharmacy
Duquesne University
Pittsburgh, Pennsylvania

Lyndon Braun, R.Ph., Pharm.D., MBA
Manager, Product Development
Wellpoint Pharmacy Management
Calabasas Hills, California

Todd A. Brown, R.Ph.
Assistant Clinical Specialist
Bouve College of Pharmacy and Health Sciences
Northeastern University
Boston, Massachusetts

Ronald J. Callahan, Ph.D., B.C.N.P.
Assistant Professor of Radiology
Harvard Medical School
Adjunct Associate Professor of Radiopharmaceutics
Massachusetts College of Pharmacy and Allied Health Sciences
Director of Nuclear Pharmacy
Massachusetts General Hospital
Boston, Massachusetts

Charles C. Collins, Ph.D., R.Ph.
Associate Professor of Pharmaceutics
Mylan School of Pharmacy
Duquesne University
Pittsburgh, Pennsylvania

Stephen C. Dragotakes, R.Ph., B.C.N.P.
Instructor in Radiopharmaceutics
Massachusetts College of Pharmacy and Allied Health Sciences
Division of Nuclear Medicine
Department of Radiology
Massachusetts General Hospital
Boston, Massachusetts

James K. Drennen, III, Ph.D.
Associate Professor of Pharmaceutics
Mylan School of Pharmacy
Duquesne University
Pittsburgh, Pennsylvania

Mary Ann R. Dzurec, Pharm.D.
Clinical Information Specialist
Kaiser Permanente, Ohio Region
Parma, Ohio

Helen L. Figge, Pharm.D., R.Ph.
Research Associate, Department of Pathology
Albany Medical College
Albany, New York

Godwin W. Fong, Ph.D.
Director of Quality Control and Quality Assurance
Innovir Laboratories, Inc.
New York, New York

Stephen H. Fuller, Pharm.D.
Associate Professor of Pharmacy Practice
Campbell University School of Pharmacy
Buies Creek, North Carolina
Kaiser Permanente
Cary, North Carolina

Marc W. Harrold, Ph.D., R.Ph.
Associate Professor of Medicinal Chemistry
Mylan School of Pharmacy
Duquesne University
Pittsburgh, Pennsylvania

John E. Janosik, R.Ph., Pharm.D.
Clinical Pharmacist
Lexi-Comp, Inc.
Hudson, Ohio

Kevin P. Keating, M.D.
Assistant Professor of Surgery
Associate Director
Surgery Critical Care
Director
Nutritional Support Services
Hartford Hospital
Hartford, Connecticut

David C. Kosegarten, Ph.D., R.Ph.
Associate Professor of Pharmacology and Toxicology
Massachusetts College of Pharmacy and Allied Health Sciences
Boston, Massachusetts

Edward F. LaSala, Ph.D., R.Ph.
Emeritus Professor of Chemistry (retired)
Massachusetts College of Pharmacy and Allied Health Sciences
Boston, Massachusetts

John D. Leary, Ph.D., R.Ph.
Professor of Biochemistry
Massachusetts College of Pharmacy and Allied Health Sciences
Boston, Massachusetts

Pui-Kai Li, Ph.D., R.Ph.
Associate Professor of Medicinal Chemistry
Mylan School of Pharmacy
Duquesne University
Pittsburgh, Pennsylvania

Scott F. Long, Ph.D., R.Ph.
Assistant Professor of Pharmacology
Mylan School of Pharmacy
Duquesne University
Pittsburgh, Pennsylvania

Vincent C. LoPresti, Ph.D.
Goffstown, New Hampshire

D. Byron May, Pharm.D., BCPS
Associate Professor of Pharmacy Practice
Campbell University School of Pharmacy
Buies Creek, North Carolina
Clinical Pharmacy Specialist
Director Pharmacy Practice Residency Program
Duke University Medical Center
Durham, North Carolina

H. William McGhee, Pharm.D., R.Ph.
Clinical Pharmacy Coordinator
Children's Hospital of Pittsburgh
Pittsburgh, Pennsylvania

Constance A. McKenzie, Pharm.D.
Associate Professor of Pharmacy Practice
Director of Experiential Programs
Campbell University School of Pharmacy
Buies Creek, North Carolina

David I. Min, M.S., Pharm.D., R.Ph.
Assistant Professor
University of Iowa, College of Pharmacy
Division of Clinical and Administrative Pharmacy
Iowa City, Iowa

J. Edward Moreton, Ph.D.
Professor
University of Maryland School of Pharmacy
Department of Pharmaceutical Sciences
Program in Pharmacology & Toxicology
Baltimore, Maryland

Alan H. Mutnick, Pharm.D., F.A.S.H.P., R.Ph.
Senior Assistant Director, Clinical Practice
The University of Iowa Hospitals and Clinics
Adjunct Associate Professor
University of Iowa, College of Pharmacy
Division of Clinical and Administrative Pharmacy
Iowa City, Iowa

Robert C. Pavlan, Jr., B.S., Pharm., J.D.
Principal, Pavlan & Associates
Attorneys at Law
Clinical Assistant Professor
Bouve College of Pharmacy and Health Sciences
Northeastern University
Attending Pharmacist
Massachusetts General Hospital
Boston, Massachusetts

Julianne B. Pinson, Pharm.D.
Assistant Professor of Pharmacy Practice
Campbell University School of Pharmacy
Buies Creek, North Carolina
Clinical Pharmacist
Reynolds Health Center
Winston-Salem, North Carolina

David Platt, Pharm.D.
Associate Director
Department of Pharmacy Services
Hartford Hospital
Hartford, Connecticut
Assistant Clinical Professor
University of Connecticut School of Pharmacy
Storrs, Connecticut

John J. Ponzillo, Pharm.D., R.Ph.
Critical Care Pharmacist
Departments of Pharmacy and Critical Care Medicine
St. John's Mercy Medical Center
Assistant Professor
Department of Surgery
Saint Louis University, School of Medicine
St. Louis, Missouri

Robert A. Quercia, M.S., BCNSP
Associate Clinical Professor
University of Connecticut School of Pharmacy
Storrs, Connecticut
Supervisor
Drug Information Service
Director
Total Parenteral Nutrition Service
Department of Pharmacy
Hartford Hospital
Hartford, Connecticut

Azita Razzaghi, R.Ph., Pharm.D.
Clinical Pharmacist
St. Elizabeth's Medical Center
Brighton, Massachusetts

Gerald E. Schumacher, Pharm.D., Ph.D.
Professor of Pharmacy
Bouve College of Pharmacy and Health Sciences
Northeastern University
Boston, Massachusetts

Leon Shargel, Ph.D., R.Ph.
Senior Research Pharmacist
Johns Hopkins Bayview Medical Center
National Institutes of Health/National Institute of Drug Abuse
Division of Intramural Research
Adjunct Associate Professor of Pharmacy
School of Pharmacy
University of Maryland
Baltimore, Maryland
Visiting Associate Professor of Pharmacy
College of Pharmacy & Pharmaceutical Sciences
Howard University
Washington, DC

Gail Snitkoff, Ph.D.
Associate Professor
Department of Biological Sciences
Albany College of Pharmacy
Albany, New York

Paul F. Souney, R.Ph., M.S.
Medical Information Scientist
Astra Merck, Inc.
Providence, Rhode Island
Adjunct Professor of Clinical Pharmacy
Massachusetts College of Pharmacy and Allied Health Sciences
Boston, Massachusetts

Marilyn K. Speedie, Ph.D.
Dean
College of Pharmacy
University of Minnesota
Minneapolis, Minnesota

Cheryl A. Stoukides, R.Ph., Pharm.D., BCPS
Pharmacotherapy Consultant
Medical Outcomes Management, Inc.
Foxborough, Massachusetts

Larry N. Swanson, Pharm.D.
Professor and Chairman
Department of Pharmacy Practice
Campbell University School of Pharmacy
Buies Creek, North Carolina

Barbara Szymusiak-Mutnick, M.H.P., R.Ph.
Clinical Pharmacist
The University of Iowa Hospitals and Clinics
Iowa City, Iowa

Andrew L. Wilson, Pharm.D., R.Ph.
Director, Pharmacy Services
SLUCare/St. Louis University Health Sciences Center
Associate Professor of Internal Medicine
St. Louis University, College of Medicine
Editor, Pharmacy Practice Management Quarterly
St. Louis, Missouri

Laura A. Wilson, Pharm.D.
Clinical Information Specialist
Kaiser Permanente, Ohio Region
Parma, Ohio

Margaret C. (Peggy) Yarborough, MS Pharm.D., CDE, FAPP
Associate Professor of Pharmacy Practice
Campbell University School of Pharmacy
Associate Director of Pharmacy Education and Practice
Area L AHEC
Rocky Mount, North Carolina
Pharmacist Clinician and Director of Diabetes Outcomes Management Program
Wilson Community Health Center
Wilson, North Carolina

Nelson S. Yee, M.D., Ph.D., R.Ph.
Resident Physician
Department of Medicine
Hospital of the University of Pennsylvania
Philadelphia, Pennsylvania

Andrew B.C. Yu, Ph.D., R.Ph.
Associate Professor of Pharmaceutics
Albany College of Pharmacy
Union University
Albany, New York

Preface

Pharmacy practice and education are continually evolving. More colleges and schools of pharmacy are now offering only the Doctor of Pharmacy (Pharm.D) degree. Pharmaceutical care, which has always been an important component of pharmacy practice, is being emphasized more strongly. Pharmacy students and practitioners must be more knowledgeable of primary care, interdisciplinary practice, health promotion, and disease management to improve patient care outcomes economically. Pharmaceutical education, including pharmaceutical science and practice, must prepare pharmacy practitioners for the future. This new edition of *Comprehensive Pharmacy Review* has been revised to reflect the current progress of pharmacy education and practice.

Our initial plan for *Comprehensive Pharmacy Review* was modest enough—to produce a comprehensive study guide for pharmacy students who are preparing for the NAPLEX®. Accordingly, we set out to develop outlines and practice questions for the subjects in the pharmacy school curriculum. These, along with the separate booklet of simulated NAPLEX® exams that supplements this review, would provide both guidance and test practice for NAPLEX® candidates.

What actually materialized is something more ambitious. While the principal market for *Comprehensive Pharmacy Review* remains NAPLEX® candidates, the book is also intended for a broader audience of pharmacy undergraduates and professionals who seek detailed summaries of pharmacy subjects. Encompassed by the review is a range of topics central to the study of pharmacy—chemistry, pharmaceutics, pharmacology, pharmacy practice, drug therapy—organized to parallel the pharmacy curriculum and presented in outline form for easy use. It can therefore be used as a quick review (or preview) of essential topics by a diverse group of readers, including:

- Matriculating pharmacy students. The organization and topical coverage of *Comprehensive Pharmacy Review* are such that many pharmacy students will want to purchase it in their freshman year and use it throughout their undergraduate training to prepare for course examinations.

- Instructors and preceptors. *Comprehensive Pharmacy Review* also functions as an instructor's manual and a reference for teachers and tutors in pharmacy schools. Chapter outlines can be used to organize courses and to plan specific lectures.

- Professional pharmacists. *Comprehensive Pharmacy Review* offers practitioners a convenient handbook of pharmacy facts. It can be used as a course refresher and as a source of recent information on pharmacy practice. The appendices include prescription dispensing information, common prescription drugs, and general pharmacy references.

The organization of the third edition has been revised to reflect the current changes in the undergraduate pharmacy curriculum. Part I, *Pharmaceutical Sciences,* contains subject matter pertaining to the basic science of pharmacy. Part II, *Pharmacy Practice,* contains subject matter for the practice of pharmacy with emphasis on pharmaceutical care.

This volume represents the contributions of more than two dozen specialists, each delivering a current summary of his or her field to a review guide that is not only accurate and up-to-date, but also comprehensible to students, teachers, and practitioners alike. If you have any suggestions on how we might improve *Comprehensive Pharmacy Review,* please write us at Williams & Wilkins, Rose Tree Corporate Center, Bldg. 2, 1400 N. Providence Road, Ste. 5025, Media, PA 19063.

Introduction to the NAPLEX®

In 1975, the Study Commission on Pharmacy presented its report to the American Association of Colleges of Pharmacy.* This study commission, chaired by John S. Millis, evaluated the state of pharmacy practice and pharmaceutical education of pharmacists, recognizing the changes that have occurred in medical knowledge and public expectation of health care. The study commission's report stimulated changes in the scope of pharmaceutical education and pharmacy practice.

According to the Study Commission report, pharmacy should be conceived as a "knowledge system" in which the pharmacist generates knowledge about drugs; acquires relevant knowledge from the biological, chemical, physical, and behavioral sciences; and tests, organizes, and applies that knowledge. Included in the report was a suggestion that the curricula of the schools of pharmacy should be based on competencies desired for their graduates rather than on the basis of knowledge available in the several relevant sciences.

After graduating from an accredited pharmacy program, the prospective pharmacist must demonstrate that he or she has the competency to practice pharmacy. Currently, every state and the District of Columbia require that the graduate pass an examination for licensure to practice pharmacy. All states except California use the North American Pharmacy Licensing Examination (NAPLEX®), which is available for administration in 1997 in March, June, July, and October by the National Association of Boards of Pharmacy (NABP®).

The standards of competence for the practice of pharmacy are set by each state board. The NAPLEX® is not a competitive examination; however, it is the principal instrument used by the state boards of pharmacy to assess the knowledge and proficiency necessary for a candidate to practice pharmacy. All NAPLEX® questions are based on competency statements, which are reviewed and revised periodically. The competency statements summarize the knowledge that the candidate is expected to have acquired and should be able to demonstrate.

The original NABPLEX® (National Association of Boards of Pharmacy Licensing Examination) was introduced to state boards in 1976 and was composed of five subtexts: pharmacy, mathematics, chemistry, pharmacology, and pharmacy practice. These tests examined basic skills and knowledge without regard to geographic or practice setting. Because of the evolution of pharmacy practice, the current NAPLEX® has an integrated format, focusing on patient profiles and practice situations. According to NABP®, the intent of the test is to approximate practice conditions as closely as possible and to examine the basic skills and knowledge that a pharmacist needs.

---

*Study Commission on Pharmacy: *Pharmacists for the Future.* Ann Arbor, Health Administration Press, 1975.

NAPLEX® Competency Statements

The questions in the NAPLEX® are based on the NAPLEX® Competency Statements and are published annually.* According to the National Association of Boards of Pharmacy (NABP®), the competency statements were "developed to reflect the skills and knowledge important to an entry-level pharmacist and to form the foundation of the NAPLEX® examination." Those candidates planning to take the NAPLEX® should review the competency statements published in the latest edition of the *NAPLEX® Candidates Review Guide.*

Essentially, the NAPLEX® Competency Statements cover three major areas of pharmacy practice, and a percentage of the test covers the practice component. In addition, for each major competency statement, a subset of statements details individual competencies.

The revised competency statements effective March 1997 focus on drug therapy, with three overall competency areas:

1. Manage Drug Therapy to Optimize Patient Outcomes
2. Assure the Safe and Accurate Preparation and Dispensing of Medications
3. Provide Drug Information and Promote Public Health

**NAPLEX® Candidates Review Guide.* National Association of Boards of Pharmacy, 700 Busse Highway, Park Ridge, IL 60068.

PART I

PHARMACEUTICAL SCIENCES

1 Drug Product Development in the Pharmaceutical Industry

Anton H. Amann
Leon Shargel

I. INTRODUCTION

A. Drug substance

1. A **drug substance** is the active ingredient or component that produces pharmacologic activity.
2. The drug substance may be **produced by** chemical synthesis, recovery from a natural product, enzymatic reaction, recombinant DNA technology, fermentation, or a combination of these processes. Further purification of the drug substance may be needed before it can be used in a drug product.
3. A **new chemical entity (NCE)** is a drug substance with unknown clinical, toxicologic, physical, and chemical properties.

B. Drug product

1. A **drug product** is the finished dosage form (e.g., capsule, tablet, ointment) that contains the drug substance, generally in association with other excipients, or inert substances.
2. Different **approaches** are generally used to produce drug products that contain NCEs, product line extensions, generic drug products, and specialty drug products.

C. Drug products containing new chemical entities.

The following phases of product development proceed sequentially.

1. **Preclinical stage.** Animal pharmacology and toxicology data are obtained to determine the safety and efficacy of the drug. An **investigational new drug (IND) application** for human testing is submitted to the Food and Drug Administration (FDA). Because it is highly probable that the product will not reach the marketplace at this stage, no attempt is made to develop a final formulation.
2. **Phase I**
   a. Clinical testing takes place after the IND application is submitted.
   b. Healthy volunteers are used in phase I clinical studies to determine drug tolerance and toxicity.
3. **Phase II**
   a. A limited number of patients with the disease or condition for which the drug was developed are treated under close supervision.
   b. Dose–response studies are performed to determine the optimum dosage regimen for treating the disease.
   c. Safety is measured by attempting to determine the **therapeutic index** (ratio of toxic dose to effective dose).

d. A final drug formulation is developed. This formulation is bioequivalent to the dosage form used in the initial clinical studies.

4. **Phase III**

   a. Large-scale, multicenter **studies** are performed with the final dosage form developed in phase II. These studies are done to determine the safety and efficacy of the drug product in a large patient population with the disease or condition for which the drug was developed.

   b. **Side effects** are monitored. In a large population, new toxic effects may occur that were not evident in previous clinical trials.

5. **Submission of a new drug application (NDA).** When the clinical trials are completed to the satisfaction of the medical community and the drug product is found to be effective by all parameters, an NDA is submitted to the FDA for review and approval.

6. **Phase IV**

   a. After the NDA is submitted, and before approval to market the product is obtained from the FDA, manufacturing **scale-up** activities occur. Scale-up is the increase in the batch size from the clinical batch, the pilot batch, or both, up to several hundred thousand dose units to the full-scale production batch size, using the finished, marketed product.

   b. The **drug formulation** may be modified slightly as a result of data obtained during the manufacturing scale-up and validation process.

7. **Phase V**

   a. After the FDA grants market approval of the drug, product development may continue.

   b. The drug product may be improved as a result of equipment, regulatory, supply, or market demands.

D. **Product line extensions** are dosage forms in which the physical form or strength, but not the use or indication, of the product changes. Product line extension is usually performed during phase III, IV, or V.

E. Generic drug products

1. After **patent expiration** of the brand drug product, a generic drug product may be developed. A generic product contains the same amount of the drug in the same type of dosage form (e.g., tablets, liquids, injectables).

2. A generic drug product must be **bioequivalent** (i.e., have the same rate and extent of drug absorption) to the brand drug product. Therefore, a generic drug product is expected to give the same clinical response (see Chapter 6). These studies are normally performed with healthy human volunteers.

3. The generic drug product may differ from the brand product in **physical appearance** (i.e., size, color, shape) or in the amount and type of excipients.

4. Before a drug product is marketed, the manufacturer must submit an **abbreviated new drug application (ANDA)** to the FDA for approval. Because preclinical safety and efficacy studies have already been performed for the NDA-approved brand product, only bioequivalence studies are required for the ANDA.

F. **Specialty drug products** are existing products that are developed in a new delivery system or for a new therapeutic indication. The safety and efficacy of the drug have been established in an NDA-approved dosage form. For example, the nitroglycerin transdermal delivery system (patch) was developed after experience with nitroglycerin sublingual tablets.

II. PRODUCT DEVELOPMENT. For each drug, various activities and information are required to develop a safe, effective, and stable dosage form.

A. New chemical entities

1. **Preformulation** is the characterization of the physical and chemical properties of the active drug substance, such as the therapeutic use of the drug, the type of drug delivery system

(e.g., immediate release, controlled release, suppository), and the route of administration (e.g., oral, parenteral, transdermal).

a. **Preformulation** activities are usually performed during the preclinical stage. However, these activities may continue into phases I and II.

b. The following information is obtained during preformulation:

(1) **General characteristics,** including particle size and shape, crystalline features, density, surface area, hygroscopicity (ability to take up and retain moisture), and powder flow

(2) **Solubility characteristics,** including intrinsic dissolution, pH solubility profile, and general solubility characteristics in various solvents

(3) **Chemical characteristics,** including surface energy, pH stability profile, pK_a, temperature stability (dry or under various humidity conditions), and excipient interactions

(4) **Analytic methods development,** including development of analytic, stability, and cleaning methods, and identification of impurities

2. **Formulation development** is a continuing process. Initial drug formulations are developed for early clinical studies. When the submission of an NDA is considered, the manufacturer attempts to develop the final dosage form. The route of administration is important in determining the modifications needed.

a. **Injectable drug product**

(1) A final injectable drug product is usually developed in the preclinical phase.

(2) A major concern is the stability of the drug in solution.

(3) Because few excipients are allowed in injectable products, the formulator must choose a final product early in the development process.

(4) If the formulation is changed, bioavailability studies are not required for intravenous injections because the product is injected directly into the body.

(5) Formulation changes may require acute toxicity studies.

b. **Topical drug products for local application** include antibacterials, antifungals, corticosteroids, and local anesthetics.

(1) The final dosage form for a topical drug product is usually developed during phase I because any major formulation changes may require further clinical trials.

(2) The release of the drug from the matrix is measured in vitro with various diffusion cell models.

(3) Significant problems include local irritation and systemic drug absorption.

c. **Topical drug products for systemic drug absorption** include drug delivery through the skin (transdermal), mucous membranes (intranasal), and rectal mucosa.

(1) A prototype formulation is developed for phase I.

(2) A final topical drug product is developed during phase III after the available technology and desired systemic levels are considered.

d. **Oral drug products**

(1) Prototype dosage forms are often developed during the **preclinical phase** to assure that the drug is optimally available and that the product dissolves in the gastrointestinal tract.

(2) In the early stages of product development, capsule dosage forms are often developed for **phase I** clinical trials. If the drug shows efficacy, the same drug formulation may be used in phase II studies.

(3) Final product development begins when the drug proceeds to phase III clinical studies.

3. **Final drug product.** Considerations in the development of a final dosage form include:

a. Color, shape, size, taste, viscosity, sensitivity, skin feel, and physical appearance of the dosage form

b. Size and shape of the package or container

c. Production equipment

d. Production site

e. Country of origin

f. Country in which to market the drug

B. **Product line extensions** are drug products containing an NDA-approved drug in a different dosage strength or in a different dosage form (e.g., modified release).

1. **Solid oral product line extensions**

a. The simplest dosage form to develop is a different **dosage strength** of a drug in a tablet or capsule. Only bioequivalence studies are needed.

b. It is more difficult to develop a **modified-release** dosage form when only an instant-release dosage form exists. Clinical trials are normally required.

c. **Considerations** in developing these dosage forms are similar to those for the final drug product (see II A 3).

d. **Marketing** has a role in the choice of the dosage form.

e. Because the original brand drug product information contributes to the body of knowledge about the drug, no preformulation is needed. All other factors considered for the original product are similar. If the relation between **in vitro dissolution** and **in vivo bioavailability** is known, the innovator can progress to a finished dosage form relatively quickly.

f. **Regulatory approval** is based on the following:

(1) Stability information

(2) Analytic and manufacturing controls

(3) Bioequivalence studies

(4) Clinical trials (in the case of modified-release dosage forms)

g. A new therapeutic indication for a drug requires new **efficacy studies** and a new NDA.

2. Liquid product line extensions

a. If the current marketed product is a liquid preparation, then the same factors as for the **solid oral dosage** forms are considered (see II B 1 a–g).

b. If the marketed product is a solid oral dosage form and the product line extension is a liquid, product **development** must proceed with **caution** because the rate and extent of absorption for liquid and solid dosage forms may not be the same.

c. **Regulatory approval** requires:

(1) Bioequivalence studies

(2) Stability information

(3) Analytic and manufacturing controls

(4) Safety studies (e.g., depending on the drug substance, local irritation)

III. PREAPPROVAL INSPECTIONS (PAIs)

A. The **manufacturing facility** is inspected after an NDA, abbreviated antibiotic drug application (AADA), or ANDA is submitted, and before the application is approved.

B. A PAI may be initiated if a **major change** is reported in a supplemental application to an NDA, AADA, or ANDA.

C. During the PAI, the investigator:

1. **Performs** a general cGMP inspection relating specifically to the drug product intended for the market

2. **Reviews** the development report to verify that the drug product has enough supporting documentation to assure a validated product and a rationale for the manufacturing directions

3. **Consults** the chemistry, manufacturing, and control (CMC) section of the NDA, AADA, or ANDA and determines the capability of the manufacturer to produce the drug product as described

4. **Verifies** the traceability of the information submitted in the CMC section to the original laboratory notebooks

5. **Recommends** whether to approve the manufacture of the drug product after the PAI

IV. SCALE-UP AND POSTAPPROVAL CHANGES (SUPAC)

A. Definition. These guidelines, published in the *Federal Register* on November 30, 1995, apply only to immediate-release solid oral dosage forms. The guidelines do not apply to any other dosage form.

B. Purpose. These guidelines are intended to reduce the number of manufacturing changes that require preapproval by the FDA.

C. Function. These guidelines provide recommendations to sponsors of NDAs, AADAs, and ANDAs during the following changes in the postapproval period:

1. To change the **components** or **composition** of the formulation, which may include a change in the raw materials, a change in the excipients, or both
2. To change the **site** of manufacture
3. To **scale-up** (increase) or **scale-down** (decrease) the batch size of the formulation
4. To change the manufacturing **process** or **equipment**

D. The FDA must be notified about a proposed change to a drug product through different **regulatory documentation,** depending on the type of change proposed.

1. **Annual report.** Changes that are unlikely to have any detectable effect on formulation quality and performance can be instituted without approval by the FDA, and reported annually. Examples of these changes include:
   a. **Compliance** with an official compendium
   b. **Label description** of the drug product or how it is supplied (not involving dosage strength or dosage form)
   c. Deletion of an **ingredient** that effects only the color of the product
   d. Extension of the expiration date based upon full shelf-life data obtained from a protocol approved in the application
   e. **Container** and **closure system** for the drug product (except a change in container size for nonsolid dosage forms) based on equivalency to the approved system under a protocol approved in the application or published in an official compendium
   f. Addition or deletion of an **alternate analytical method**
2. **Changes being effected supplement.** Changes that probably would not have any detectable effect, but require some validation efforts, require specific documentation, depending on the change. A supplement is submitted, and the change can be implemented without previous approval by the FDA. However, the FDA may reject this supplement. Some examples of reasons for submitting a supplement include:
   a. Addition of a **new specification** or test method or changes in methods, facilities, or controls
   b. **Label change** to add or strengthen a contraindication, warning, precaution, or adverse reaction
   c. Use of a **different facility** to manufacture the drug substance and drug product (the manufacturing process in the new facility does not differ materially from that in the former facility, and the new facility has received a satisfactory current good manufacturing practice inspection within the previous 2 years covering that manufacturing process)
3. **Preapproval supplement.** Changes that could have a significant effect on formulation quality and performance require specific documentation. This supplement must be approved before the proposed change is initiated. Some appropriate examples for preapproval supplement are:
   a. Addition or deletion of an **ingredient**
   b. Relaxing of the limits for a **specification**
   c. Establishment of a new **regulatory analytical method**
   d. Deletion of a **specification** or regulatory analytical method
   e. Change in the method of **manufacture** of the drug product, including changing or relaxing an in-process control
   f. Change in **container** size (except for solid dosage forms) without a change in the container and closure system
   g. Extension of the **expiration date** of the drug product based on data obtained under a new or revised stability testing protocol that has not been approved in the application

E. When any change to a drug product is proposed, the manufacturer must show that the resultant drug product is **bioequivalent** and **therapeutically equivalent** to the original approved drug product.

1. If the proposed change is considered **minor** by the FDA, bioequivalence may be demonstrated by comparative dissolution profiles for the original and new formulations.

2. If the proposed change is considered **major** by the FDA, bioequivalence must be demonstrated by an in vivo bioequivalence study comparing the original and new formulations.

V. GOOD MANUFACTURING PRACTICES (GMPs) are regulations developed by the FDA. GMPs are minimum requirements that the industry must meet when manufacturing, processing, packing, or holding human and veterinary drugs. These regulations, also known as current good manufacturing practices, establish criteria for personnel, facilities, and manufacturing processes to assure that the finished drug product has the correct identity, strength, quality, and purity characteristics.

A. **Quality control** is the section within the manufacturer that is responsible for establishing process and product **specifications.** Once these specifications are established, the quality control department **tests** the product and verifies that the specifications are met. Included in this testing is the **acceptance** or **rejection** of the incoming raw materials, packaging components, drug products, water system, and environmental conditions (e.g., heating, ventilation, and air-conditioning; air quality; microbial load) that exist during the manufacturing process.

B. **Quality assurance** is the group within the manufacturer that determines that the systems and facilities are adequate, and that the **written procedures** are followed to assure that the finished drug product meets the applicable specifications for quality.

STUDY QUESTIONS

Directions: Each item below contains three suggested answers of which **one or more** is correct. Choose the answer

A if **I only** is correct
B if **III only** is correct
C if **I and II** are correct
D if **II and III** are correct
E if **I, II, and III** are correct

1. Healthy human volunteers are used in drug development for

I. phase I testing after the submission of an investigational new drug (IND) application
II. generic drug development for an abbreviated new drug application (ANDA) submission
III. phase III testing just before the submission of a new drug application (NDA)

2. The required information contained in a new drug application (NDA) that is NOT included in the abbreviated new drug application (ANDA) consists of

I. preclinical animal toxicity studies
II. clinical efficacy studies
III. human safety and tolerance studies

3. A product line extension contains the new drug application (NDA)-approved drug in a

I. new dosage form
II. new dosage strength
III. new therapeutic indication

Directions: The item below is followed by a completion of the statement. Select the **one** lettered answer that **best** completes the statement.

4. The regulations developed by the FDA for the pharmaceutical industry in meeting the minimum requirements in the manufacturing, processing, packing, or holding of human and veterinary drugs are known as

(A) good manufacturing practices (GMPs)
(B) quality assurance
(C) quality control
(D) preapproval inspection (PAI)
(E) scale-up and postapproval changes

ANSWERS AND EXPLANATIONS

1. The answer is C (I, II) *[I C 2 b, 4 a].*
Phase I testing is the first set of human studies performed during new drug development. Phase I studies establish the tolerance and toxicity of the drug in humans. Clinical studies for generic drug development are most often performed in healthy human volunteers. These studies establish the bioequivalence of the generic drug product against the brand drug product. Phase III testing entails large-scale, multicenter clinical studies performed in patients with the disease or condition to be treated. Phase III studies determine the safety and efficacy of the drug in a large patient population.

2. The answer is E (I, II, and III) *[I C 5, E 4].*
The development of a new drug requires extensive toxicity and efficacy testing in animals and humans. The new drug application (NDA) documents all studies performed on the drug. The abbreviated new drug application (ANDA) is used for generic drug product submissions. The generic drug product is similar to the original brand drug product that has already been marketed. Because the efficacy, safety, and toxicity of this drug product have been studied and documented, further studies of this nature are unnecessary.

3. The answer is C (I, II) *[I D].*
Product line extensions are developed after further studies with the original new drug application (NDA)-approved drug product. From these studies, the manufacturer may develop a new dosage form (e.g., controlled-release product) or a new dosage strength. A new therapeutic indication requires an NDA.

4. The answer is A *[V].*
Quality control and quality assurance follow good manufacturing practice (GMP) regulations in assuring that the finished product meets all applicable specifications for quality. The Food and Drug Administration (FDA) may inspect a manufacturing site [preapproval inspection (PAI)] before the drug application is approved. Additionally, the FDA must be notified about any proposed changes to an approved drug product.

2
Pharmaceutical Calculations and Statistics

James K. Drennen, III
Riccardo Boni

I. FUNDAMENTALS OF MEASUREMENT AND CALCULATION

A. Ratio and proportion

1. **Ratio.** The relative magnitude of two like quantities is a ratio, which is expressed as a fraction. Certain basic principles apply to the ratio, as they do to all fractions.
   a. When the two terms of a ratio are multiplied or divided by the same number, the value of the ratio is unchanged.

$$1/3 \times 2/2 = 2/6 = 1/3$$

   b. Two ratios with the same value are equivalent. Equivalent ratios have equal cross products and equal reciprocals. As an example,

$$1/3 = 2/6$$

and

$$1 \times 6 = 3 \times 2 = 6$$

If two ratios are equal, then their reciprocals are equal.

$$\text{if } 1/3 = 2/6, \text{ then } 3/1 = 6/2$$

2. **Proportion.** The expression of the equality of two ratios is a proportion. The product of the extremes is equal to the product of the means for any proportion. Furthermore, the numerator of the one fraction equals the product of its denominator and the other fraction, i.e., one missing term can always be found given the other three terms.
   a. Most pharmaceutical calculations can be performed by use of proportion. Several examples follow.
      (1) If 240 ml of a cough syrup contains 480 mg of dextromethorphan hydrobromide, then what mass of drug is contained in a child's dose (5 ml) of syrup?

$$\frac{240 \text{ ml}}{5 \text{ ml}} = \frac{480 \text{ mg}}{X \text{ mg}}$$

$$X = \frac{480 \times 5}{240} = 10 \text{ mg}$$

      (2) If a child's dose (5 ml) of a cough syrup contains 10 mg of dextromethorphan hydrobromide, what mass of drug is contained in 240 ml?

$$\frac{240 \text{ ml}}{5 \text{ ml}} = \frac{X \text{ mg}}{10 \text{ mg}}$$

$$X = \frac{240 \times 10}{5} = 480 \text{ ml}$$

      (3) If the amount of dextromethorphan hydrobromide in 240 ml of cough syrup is 480 mg, what would be the volume required for a child's dose of 10 mg?

$$\frac{X \text{ ml}}{240 \text{ ml}} = \frac{10 \text{ mg}}{480 \text{ mg}}$$

$$X = \frac{10 \times 240}{480} = 5 \text{ ml}$$

b. Mixed ratios. Some pharmacists use mixed ratios (where dissimilar units are used in the numerator and denominator of each ratio) in their proportion calculations. Such computations generally give correct answers, providing the conditions where mixed ratios cannot be used are known. A later example shows mixed ratios leading to failure in the case of dilution, where inverse proportions are required. For **inverse proportions,** similar units must be used in the numerator and denominator of each ratio. Following is an example of a mixed ratio calculation using the previous example problem.

$$\frac{X \text{ ml}}{10 \text{ mg}} = \frac{240 \text{ ml}}{480 \text{ mg}}$$

$$X = \frac{240 \times 10}{480} = 5 \text{ ml}$$

The **same answer** is obtained in this example whether we use proper ratios, with similar units in numerator and denominator, or mixed ratios. This is not the case when dealing with inverse proportions.

3. **Inverse proportion.** The most common example of the need for inverse proportion for the pharmacist is the case of **dilution.** Whereas in the previous examples of proportion the relationships involved direct proportion, the case of dilution calls for an inverse proportion (i.e., as volume increases concentration decreases). The necessity of using inverse proportions for dilution problems is shown in this example:

If 120 ml of a 10% stock solution are diluted to 240 ml, what is the final concentration? Using inverse proportion,

$$\frac{120 \text{ ml}}{240 \text{ ml}} = \frac{X\%}{10\%}$$

$$\frac{120 \times 10}{240} = 5\%$$

As expected, the final concentration is one half the original concentration because the volume is doubled. However, if the pharmacist attempts to use direct proportion and neglects to estimate an appropriate answer, the resulting calculation would provide an answer of 20%, which is twice the actual concentration.

$$\frac{120 \text{ ml}}{240 \text{ ml}} = \frac{10\%}{X\%}$$

$$\frac{240 \times 10}{120} = 20\% \text{ (incorrect answer)}$$

Likewise, the pharmacist using mixed ratios fails in this case.

$$\frac{120 \text{ ml}}{10\%} = \frac{240 \text{ ml}}{X\%}$$

and

$$\frac{10 \times 240}{120} = 20\% \text{ (again, an incorrect answer)}$$

B. Aliquot. A pharmacist requires the aliquot method of measurement when the **precision** of his measuring device is not great enough for the required measurement. Aliquot calculations can be used for measurement of solids or liquids, allowing the pharmacist to realize the required precision through a process of measuring a multiple of the desired amount followed by dilution and finally selection and measurement of an aliquot part that contains the desired amount of material. This example problem involves weighing by the aliquot method, using a prescription balance.

A prescription balance has a sensitivity requirement of 6 mg. How would you weigh 10 mg drug with an accuracy of ± 5%, using a suitable diluent?

1. First, calculate the least weighable quantity for the balance with a sensitivity requirement of 6 mg, assuming ± 5% accuracy is required.

$$\frac{100 \times 6 \text{ mg}}{5} = 120 \text{ mg (least weighable quantity for our balance)}$$

2. Now, it is obvious that an aliquot calculation is required because 10 mg of drug are required, whereas the least weighable quantity is 120 mg in order to achieve the required percentage of error. Using the least weighable quantity method of aliquot measurement, use the smallest quantity weighable on the balance at each step in order to preserve materials.
   - **a.** Weigh 12 × 10 mg = 120 mg of drug.
   - **b.** Dilute the 120 mg of drug (from step **a**) with a suitable diluent to achieve a mixture that will provide 10 mg of drug in each 120 mg aliquot. The amount of diluent to be used can be determined through **proportion.**

$$\frac{120 \text{ mg drug}}{10 \text{ mg drug}} = \frac{X \text{ mg total mixture}}{120 \text{ mg aliquot mixture}}$$

$$X = 1440 \text{ mg total mixture}$$

$$1440 \text{ mg total} - 120 \text{ mg drug} = 1320 \text{ mg diluent}$$

   - **c.** Weigh 120 mg (1/12) of the total mixture, which will contain the required 10 mg of drug.

II. SYSTEMS OF MEASURE.

The pharmacist must be familiar with **three systems** of measure, including the **metric system** and two "common systems" of measure (the **avoirdupois** and **apothecaries'** systems). The primary system of measure in pharmacy and medicine is the metric system. Most students find it easiest to convert measurements in the common systems to metric units. A table of conversion equivalents is provided and should be memorized by the pharmacist (see Appendix A). The metric system, because of its universal acceptance and broad use, will not be reviewed here.

A. Apothecaries' system of fluid measure. The apothecaries' system of fluid measure is summarized in Appendix A.

B. Apothecaries' system for measuring weight. The apothecaries' system for measuring weight includes units of grains, scruples, drams, ounces, and pounds (see Appendix A).

C. Avoirdupois system of measuring weight. The avoirdupois (AV) system of measuring weight includes the grain, ounce, and pound. The grain is a unit common with the apothecaries' system and allows for easy conversion between the systems. The avoirdupois pound, however, is 16 AV ounces in contrast to the apothecaries' pound, which is 12 apothecaries' ounces (see Appendix A).

D. Conversion equivalents (see Appendix A)

III. REDUCING AND ENLARGING FORMULAS.

The pharmacist is often required to reduce or enlarge a recipe. Problems of this type are solved through proportion, or by multiplication or division by the appropriate factor to obtain the required amount of each ingredient that will give the desired total mass or volume of the formula. Formulas can be provided in amounts or in parts.

A. Formulas that indicate parts. When dealing with formulas that specify parts, parts by weight will require the determination of weights of ingredients, whereas parts by volume warrant the calculation of volumes of ingredients. Always find the total number of parts indicated in the formula and equate that total with the total mass or volume of the desired formula in order to set up a proportion. Such a proportion will allow calculation of the mass or volume of each ingredient in units common to the total mass or volume.

What quantities should be used to prepare 100 g of camphorated parachlorophenol?

R_x	Parachlorophenol	7 parts
	Camphor	13 parts

$$7 \text{ parts} + 13 \text{ parts} = 20 \text{ parts total}$$

$$\frac{7 \text{ parts}}{20 \text{ parts}} = \frac{X \text{ g}}{100 \text{ g}}, \; X = 35 \text{ g of parachlorophenol}$$

$$\frac{13 \text{ parts}}{20 \text{ parts}} = \frac{X \text{ g}}{100 \text{ g}}, \ X = 65 \text{ g of camphor}$$

B. Formulas that indicate quantities

The previous prescription for cold cream provides a 100 g quantity. What mass of each ingredient is required to provide one pound (AV) of cream?

R_x	White wax	12.5 g
	Mineral oil	60.0 g
	Lanolin	2.5 g
	Sodium borate	1.0 g
	Rose water	24.0 g

454/100 = 4.54, a factor to use in calculating the quantities of each ingredient.

$$12.5 \text{ g} \times 4.54 = 56.8 \text{ g of white wax}$$
$$60.0 \text{ g} \times 4.54 = 272 \text{ g of mineral oil}$$
$$2.5 \text{ g} \times 4.54 = 11.4 \text{ g of lanolin}$$
$$1.0 \text{ g} \times 4.54 = 4.54 \text{ g of sodium borate}$$
$$24 \text{ g} \times 4.54 = 109 \text{ g of rose water}$$

IV. CALCULATING DOSES. Calculation of doses generally can be performed with dimensional analysis. **Problems** encountered in the pharmacy include calculation of the number of doses, quantities in a dose or total mass/volume, amount of active or inactive ingredients, and size of dose. Calculation of **children's doses** is commonly performed by the pharmacist. Dosage is optimally calculated by using the child's body weight or mass and the appropriate dose in mg/kg. Without this data, the following formulas based on an adult dose can be used.

A. Fried's rule for infants:

$$\frac{\text{age (in months)} \times \text{adult dose}}{150} = \text{dose for infant}$$

B. Clark's rule:

$$\frac{\text{weight (in lb)} \times \text{adult dose}}{\text{150 lb (ave. wt. of adult)}} = \text{dose for child}$$

C. Child's dosage based on body surface area (BSA):

$$\frac{\text{BSA of child (in m}^2\text{)} \times \text{adult dose}}{1.73 \text{ m}^2 \text{ (ave. adult BSA)}} = \text{approximate child's dose}$$

V. PERCENTAGE, RATIO STRENGTH, AND OTHER CONCENTRATION EXPRESSIONS

A. Percentage weight-in-volume (w/v)

1. **Definition.** Percentage, indicating parts per hundred, is an important means of expressing concentration in pharmacy practice. Percentage w/v indicates the number of grams of a constituent per 100 ml of solution or liquid formulation. The pharmacist may be required to perform **three types** of calculations: determine the **weight** of active ingredient in a certain volume when given the percentage strength, determine the **percentage w/v** when the weight of substance and volume of liquid formulation are known, and determine the **volume** of liquid mixture when the percentage strength and amount of substance are known.

2. **Tolu balsam syrup.** Tolu balsam tincture contains 20% w/v tolu balsam.

   What is the percentage concentration of tolu balsam in the syrup?

Tolu balsam tincture	50 ml
Magnesium carbonate	10 g
Sucrose	820 g
Purified water, qs ad	1000 ml

a. First, determine what the amount of tolu balsam is in the 50 ml quantity of tincture used for the syrup. Then, by proportion, calculate the concentration of tolu balsam in the syrup.

$$\text{tolu balsam tincture} = 50 \text{ ml} \times \frac{20 \text{ g}}{100 \text{ ml}} = 10 \text{ g tolu balsam},$$

$$\frac{10 \text{ g}}{1000 \text{ ml}} = \frac{X \text{ g}}{100 \text{ ml}}, X = 1 \text{ g}/100 \text{ ml} = 1\% \text{ tolu balsam in the syrup}$$

In answering this one question, the first two types of problems listed above have been solved, while exhibiting two methods of solving percentage problems, namely, by **dimensional analysis** and **proportion.**

b. For an example of the **third type** of percentage w/v problem, determine what volume of syrup could be prepared if we had only 8 g of magnesium carbonate.

(1) First, calculate the percentage strength w/v of magnesium carbonate.

$$\frac{10 \text{ g}}{1000 \text{ ml}} = \frac{X \text{ g}}{100 \text{ ml}}, X = 1 \text{ g}/100 \text{ ml} = 1\% \text{ magnesium carbonate}$$

(2) Now, use proportion again to find the total volume of syrup that can be made using only 8 g of magnesium carbonate.

$$\frac{10 \text{ g}}{1000 \text{ ml}} = \frac{8 \text{ g}}{X \text{ ml}}, X = 800 \text{ ml}$$

B. Percentage volume-in-volume (v/v). Percentage v/v indicates the number of milliliters of a constituent in 100 ml of liquid formulation. The percentage strength of mixtures of liquids in liquids are indicated by % v/v, which indicates the parts by volume of a substance in 100 parts of the liquid preparation. The **three types** of problems that are encountered involve calculating **percentage strength,** calculating **volume of ingredient,** or calculating **volume of the liquid preparation.** Using the same tolu balsam syrup formula from above, we'll now work a % v/v problem.

What is the percentage strength v/v of the tolu balsam tincture in the syrup preparation? By proportion, we can solve the problem in one step.

$$\frac{50 \text{ ml tolu balsam tincture}}{X \text{ ml tolu balsam tincture}} = \frac{1000 \text{ ml syrup}}{100 \text{ ml syrup}}, X = 5\%$$

C. Percentage weight-in-weight (w/w). Percentage w/w indicates the number of grams of a constituent per 100 g of formulation (solid or liquid). Solution of problems involving percentage w/w is straightforward when the total mass of the mixture is available or if the total mass can be determined from the available data. In calculations similar to those for percentage w/v or v/v, the pharmacist might need to solve several types of problems, including determination of the weight of a constituent, the total weight of a mixture, or the percentage w/w.

1. How many grams of drug substance should be used to prepare 240 g of a 5% w/w solution in water?

a. The first step in any percentage w/w problem is to attempt identification of the total mass of the mixture. In this problem the total mass is obviously provided (240 g).

b. The problem can be solved easily through **dimensional analysis.**

$$240 \text{ g mixture} \times \frac{0.05 \text{ g drug}}{100 \text{ g mixture}} = 12 \text{ g}$$

2. When the total mass of the mixture is unavailable or can not be determined, an **extra step** is required in the calculations. Because it is usually impossible to know how much volume is displaced by a solid material, the pharmacist is unable to prepare a specified volume of a solution given the percentage w/w.

How much drug should be added to 30 ml of water to make a 10% w/w solution? The volume of water that is displaced by the drug is unknown, so the final volume is unknown. Likewise, even though the mass of solvent is known (30 ml × 1 g/ml = 30 g), it is not known how much drug is needed, so the total mass is unknown. The water represents

100% − 10% = 90% of the total mixture. Then, by proportion, the mass of drug to be used can be identified.

$$\frac{30 \text{ g of mixture (water)}}{X \text{ g of mixture (drug)}} = \frac{90\%}{10\%}, X = 3.33 \text{ g of drug required to make a solution}$$

The **common error** that many students make in solving problems of this type is to assume that 30 g is the total mass of the mixture. Solving the problem with that assumption gives the following incorrect answer.

$$\frac{X \text{ g drug}}{10 \text{ g drug}} = \frac{30 \text{ g mixture}}{100 \text{ g mixture}}, X = 3 \text{ g of drug (incorrect answer)}$$

D. Ratio strength. Solid or liquid formulations that contain low concentrations of active ingredients will often have concentration expressed in **ratio strength.** Ratio strength, as the name implies, is the expression of concentration by means of a ratio. The numerator and denominator of the ratio indicate g or ml of a solid or liquid constituent in the total mass (g) or volume (ml) of a solid or liquid preparation. Because **percentage strength** is essentially a ratio of parts per hundred, conversion between ratio strength and percentage strength is easily accomplished by proportion.

1. **Express 0.1 percent w/v as a ratio strength.**
   a. Ratio strengths are by convention expressed in reduced form, so in setting up our proportion to solve for ratio strength, use the number 1 in the numerator of the right hand ratio as shown below:

$$\frac{0.1 \text{ g}}{100 \text{ ml}} = \frac{1 \text{ part}}{X \text{ parts}}, X = 1000 \text{ parts, for a ratio strength of } 1{:}1000$$

   b. Likewise, conversion from ratio strength to percentage strength by proportion is easy, as seen in the following example. Keep in mind the definition of percentage strength (parts-per-hundred) when setting up the proportion.

2. **Express 1:2500 as a percentage strength.**

$$\frac{1 \text{ part}}{2500 \text{ parts}} = \frac{X \text{ parts}}{100 \text{ parts}}, X = 0.04, \text{ indicating } 0.04\%$$

E. Other concentration expressions

1. **Molarity** (M) is the expression of the number of moles of solute dissolved per liter of solution. It is calculated by dividing the moles of solute by the volume of solution in liters.

$$M_A = \frac{n_A}{V_{\text{solin, liters}}}$$

2. **Normality.** A convenient way of dealing with acids, bases, and electrolytes involves the use of equivalents. One equivalent of an acid is the quantity of that acid that supplies or donates one mole of H^+ ions. One equivalent of a base is the quantity that furnishes one mole of OH^- ions. One equivalent of acid reacts with one equivalent of base. Equivalent weight can be calculated for atoms or molecules.

$$\text{Equivalent weight} = \frac{\text{atomic weight or molecular weight}}{\text{valence}}$$

The **Normality** (N) of a solution is the number of gram-equivalent weights (equivalents) of solute per liter of solution. Normality is analogous to molarity, however, it is defined in terms of equivalents rather than moles.

$$\text{Normality} = \frac{\text{\# equivalents of solute}}{\text{\# liters of solution}}$$

3. **Molality** (m) is the moles of solute dissolved per kilogram of solvent. Molality is calculated by dividing the number of moles of solute by the number of kilograms of solvent. Molality offers the advantage over

$$m_A = \frac{n_A}{mass_{solvent,\ kg}}$$

4. **Mole fraction** (X) is the ratio of the number of moles of one component to the total moles of a mixture or solution.

$$X_A = \frac{n_A}{n_A + n_B + n_C + \ldots},\ \text{where } X_A + X_B + X_C + \ldots = 1$$

VI. DILUTION AND CONCENTRATION.

If the amount of drug remains constant in a dilution or concentration, then any change in the mass or volume of a mixture is inversely proportional to the concentration.

A. Dilution and concentration problems can be solved by:

1. Inverse proportion (as mentioned earlier)
2. The equation: $\text{quantity}_1 \times \text{concentration}_1 = \text{quantity}_2 \times \text{concentration}_2$
3. Determining the amount of active ingredient present in the initial mixture and, with the assumption that the initial quantity does not change, calculation of the final concentration of the new total mass or volume
4. **Alligation medial**—a method for calculating the average concentration of a mixture of two or more substances
5. **Alligation alternate**—a method for calculation of the number of parts of two or more components of known concentration to be mixed when the final desired concentration is known

B. Dilution of alcohols and acids

1. **Dilution of alcohols.** When alcohol and water are mixed, a contraction of volume occurs. As a result, the final volume of solution cannot be determined accurately. Nor can the volume of water needed to dilute to a certain percentage v/v be identified. Accordingly, percentage w/w is often used for solutions of alcohol.
2. The **percentage strength** of concentrated acids are expressed as percentage w/w. The concentration of diluted acids is expressed as percentage weight-in-volume. To determine the volume of concentrated acid to be used in preparing a diluted acid requires the specific gravity of the concentrated acid.

C. Dilution and concentration of liquids and solids. Dilution and concentration problems are often easily solved by identifying the amount of drug involved followed by use of an appropriate proportion.

1. **How many milliliters of a 1:50 stock solution of ephedrine sulfate should be used in compounding the following prescription?**

   ℞ Ephedrine sulfate 0.25%
   Rose water ad 30 ml

   0.25 g/100 ml × 30 ml = 0.075 g drug required

   $$\frac{50\text{ ml}}{1\text{ g}} = \frac{X\text{ ml}}{0.075\text{ g}},\ X = 3.75\text{ ml of stock solution required for the prescription}$$

2. **How many milliliters of a 15% w/v concentrate of benzalkonium chloride should be used in preparing 300 ml of a stock solution such that 15 ml diluted to 1 L will yield a 1 to 5000 solution?**

   a. First determine the amount of drug in 1 liter of 1 to 5000 solution.

   $$\frac{5000\text{ ml}}{1000\text{ ml}} = \frac{1\text{ g}}{X\text{ g}},\ X = 0.2\text{ g of benzalkonium chloride in the final solution}$$

   b. Now, because 15 ml of the stock solution is being diluted to 1 L, a stock solution is needed where 15 ml contain 0.2 g of drug. By proportion, the amount of drug required to make 300 ml of the stock solution is found.

stock $\frac{0.2\ g}{X\ g} = \frac{15\ ml}{300\ ml}$, and X = 4 g of drug required to make 300 ml of solution

c. Finally, to determine the amount of 15% concentrate required,

$\frac{15\ g}{4\ g} = \frac{100\ ml}{X\ ml}$, and X = 26.7 ml of 15% solution required to obtain necessary drug

3. When the relative amount of components must be determined for preparation of a mixture of a desired concentration, the problem is most easily solved using alligation alternate.

How many grams of 2.5% hydrocortisone cream should be mixed with 360 g of 0.25% cream to make a 1% hydrocortisone cream?

2.5%		0.75 parts of 2.5% cream	= 1 part	0.75/2.25 = 1/3
	1%			
0.25%		1.5 parts of 0.25% cream	= 2 parts	1.5/2.25 = 2/3
		2.25 parts total	= 3 parts	

The relative amounts of the 2.5% and 1% creams are 1 to 2, respectively. By proportion, the mass of 2.5% cream to use can be determined. If 2 parts of 0.25% cream is represented by 360 g, then the total mass (3 parts) is represented by what mass?

$$\frac{2\ parts}{3\ parts} = \frac{360\ g}{X\ g},\ X = 540\ g\ total$$

With the total mass known, the amount of 2.5% cream can be identified. If 3 parts represent the total mass of 540 g, then 1 part represents the mass of 2.5% cream (X g = 180 g).

$$\frac{1\ part}{3\ parts} = \frac{X\ g}{540\ g},\ X = 180\ g\ of\ 2.5\%\ cream$$

VII. ELECTROLYTE SOLUTIONS.

VII. ELECTROLYTE SOLUTIONS. Electrolyte solutions contain species (electrolytes) that dissociate into ions. The **milliequivalent** (mEq) is the unit used to express the concentration of electrolytes in solution. The following table exhibits some physiologically important ions and their properties (Table 2-1).

A. Milliequivalents. The milliequivalent is the amount, in milligrams, of a solute equal to 1/1000 of its gram equivalent weight. Conversion of concentrations in the form of milliequivalent to concentrations in percentage strength, mg/ml or any other terms, begins with calculation of number of milliequivalents of drug. The following examples exhibit the calculation of milliequivalents and manipulation of data from the table in order to perform the required calculations for preparing electrolyte solutions.

What is the concentration, in percent w/v, of a solution containing 2 mEq of potassium chloride per milliliter?
Calculations involving milliequivalents are easily solved if the practitioner follows a predefined procedure to determine the milliequivalent weight. This involves three steps.

1. Find the molecular weight.

Atomic wt K = 39
Atomic wt Cl = 35.5   39 + 35.5 = 74.5 g = mol wt of KCl

2. Calculate the equivalent weight of KCl.

Eq wt = mol wt/valence = 74.5/1 = 74.5 g

3. Determine the milliequivalent weight, which is 1/1000 of the equivalent weight.

mEq wt = 74.5 g/1000 = 0.0745 g or 74.5 mg

Now that we know the milliequivalent weight, we can calculate by dimensional analysis and proportion the concentration in percentage in a fourth step.

4. 0.0745 g/mEq × 2 mEq = 0.149 g of drug

Table 2-1. Valences, Atomic Weights, and Milliequivalent Weights of Selected Ions

Ion	Formula	Valence	Atomic/Formula Weight	Milliequivalent Weight (mg)
Aluminum	$A1^{+++}$	3	27	9
Ammonium	NH_4^+	1	18	18
Calcium	Ca^{++}	2	40	20
Ferric	Fe^{+++}	3	56	18.7
Ferrous	Fe^{++}	2	56	28
Lithium	Li^+	1	7	7
Magnesium	Mg^{++}	2	24	12
Bicarbonate	HCO_3^-	1	61	61
Carbonate	CO_3^-	1	60	30
Chloride	Cl^-	1	35.5	35.5
Citrate	$C_6H_5O_7^{---}$	3	189	63
Gluconate	$C_6H_{11}O_7^-$	1	195	195
Lactate	$C_3H5O_3^-$	1	89	89
Phosphate	$H_2PO_4^-$	1	97	97
Sulfate	SO_4^{--}	2	96	48
Potassium	K^+	1	29	39
Sodium	Na^+	1	23	23
Acetate	$C2H3O_2^-$	1	59	59

$$\frac{0.149 \text{ g drug}}{1 \text{ ml}} = \frac{X \text{ g drug}}{100 \text{ ml}}, \; X = 14.9 \text{ g/100 ml} = 14.9\%$$

How many milliequivalents of Na^+ would be contained in a 15 ml volume of the following buffer?

$Na_2HPO_4 \cdot 7H_2O$		180 g
$NaH_2PO_4 \cdot H_2O$		480 g
Purified water	ad	1000 ml

For each salt, the mass (and milliequivalents) must be found in a 15 ml dose.

mol wt $Na_2HPO_4 \cdot 7H_2O$ (disodium hydrogen phosphate) = 268 g

Eq wt = 268/2 = 134 g

1 mEq = 0.134 g or 134 mg

$$\frac{180 \text{ g}}{X \text{ g}} = \frac{1000 \text{ ml}}{15 \text{ ml}}, \; X = 2.7 \text{ g of disodium hydrogen phosphate in each 15 ml}$$

$$2.7 \text{ g} \times \frac{1 \text{ mEq}}{0.134 \text{ g}} = 20.1 \text{ mEq of disodium hydrogen phosphate}$$

mol wt $NaH_2PO_4 \cdot H_2O$ (sodium biphosphate) = 134 g

Eq wt = 134 g

1 mEq = 0.134 g

$$\frac{480 \text{ g}}{X \text{ g}} = \frac{1000 \text{ ml}}{15 \text{ ml}}, \; X = 7.2 \text{ g of sodium biphosphate in each 15 ml}$$

$$7.2 \text{ g} \times \frac{1 \text{ mEq}}{0.134 \text{ g}} = 53.7 \text{ mEq of sodium biphosphate}$$

20.1 mEq + 53.7 mEq = 73.8 mEq of sodium in each 15 ml of solution

B. Milliosmoles (mOsmol). Osmotic pressure is directly proportional to the total number of particles in solution. The milliosmol is the unit of measure for osmotic concentration. For nonelectrolytes, 1 millimole represents 1 milliosmole. However, for electrolytes, the total number of particles in solution is determined by the number of particles produced in solution and influenced by the degree of dissociation. Assuming complete dissociation, 1 millimole of KCl represents 2 milliosmoles of total particles, 1 millimole of $CaCl_2$ represents 3 milliosmoles of total particles, etc. The ideal osmolar concentration can be calculated with the following equation.

$$\text{mOsmol/L} = \frac{\text{wt. of substance in g/L}}{\text{molecular weight in g}} \times \text{number of species} \times 1000$$

The pharmacist should recognize the difference between **ideal** osmolar concentration and **actual** osmolarity. As the concentration of solute increases, interaction between dissolved particles increases, resulting in a reduction of the actual osmolar values.

C. Isotonic solutions. An **isotonic** solution is one that has the same osmotic pressure as body fluids. **Isosmotic** fluids are fluids with the same osmotic pressure. Solutions to be administered to patients should be isosmotic with body fluids. A **hypotonic** solution is one with a lower osmotic pressure than body fluids, whereas a **hypertonic** solution will have an osmotic pressure that is greater than body fluids.

1. **Preparation of isotonic solutions.** Colligative properties, including freezing point depression, are representative of the number of particles in solution and considered in preparation of isotonic solutions.
   a. When 1 g mol wt of any nonelectrolyte is dissolved in 1000 g of water, the freezing point of the solution is depressed by 1.86°C. By proportion, the weight of any nonelectrolyte needed to make the solution isotonic with body fluid can be calculated.
   b. Boric acid (H_3BO_3) has a mol wt of 61.8 g. This, 61.8 g of H_3BO_3 in 1000 g of water should produce a freezing point of −1.86°C. Therefore, knowing that the freezing point depression of body fluids is −0.52°C,

$$-1.86°C/-0.52°C = 61.8\ g/X\ g, \text{ and } X = 17.3\ g$$

   and 17.3 g of H_3BO_3 in 1000 g of water provide a solution that is **isotonic.**
   c. The degree of dissociation of electrolytes must be taken into account in such calculations. For example, NaCl is approximately 80% dissociated in weak solutions, yielding 180 particles in solution for each 100 molecules of NaCl. Therefore,

$$-1.86°C \times 1.8/-0.52°C = 58.5\ g/X\ g, \text{ and } X = 9.09\ g$$

   indicating that 9.09 g of NaCl in 1000 g of water (0.9% w/v) should make a solution isotonic. Lacking any information on the degree of dissociation of an electrolyte, the following **dissociation values** (*i*) may be used.
   (1) Substances that dissociate into 2 ions: 1.8
   (2) Substances that dissociate into 3 ions: 2.6
   (3) Substances that dissociate into 4 ions: 3.4
   (4) Substances that dissociate into 5 ions: 4.2

2. **Sodium chloride equivalents.** The pharmacist will often be required to prepare an isotonic solution by adding an appropriate amount of another substance (drug or inert electrolyte or nonelectrolyte). Considering that isotonic fluids contain the equivalent of 0.9% NaCl, the question arises: How much of the added ingredient is required to make the solution isotonic? A **common method** for computing the amount of added ingredient to use for reaching isotonicity involves the use of **sodium chloride equivalents.**
   a. **Definition.** The sodium chloride equivalent represents the amount of NaCl that is equivalent to the amount of particular drug in question. For every substance there is one quantity that should have a constant tonic effect when dissolved in 1000 g of water. This is 1 g mol wt of the substance divided by its *i*, or dissociation value.
   b. **Examples**
   (1) Considering H_3BO_3, from the last section, 17.3 g of H_3BO_3 are equivalent to 0.52 g of NaCl in tonicity. Therefore, the relative quantity of NaCl that is equivalent to H_3BO_3 in tonicity effects is determined as follows:

$$\frac{\text{mol wt of NaCl}/i \text{ value}}{\text{mol wt of } H_3BO_3/i \text{ value}} = \frac{58.5/1.8}{61.8/1.0}$$

   Applying this method to atropine sulfate, recall that the mol wt of NaCl and the mol wt of atropine sulfate are 58.5 and 695 g, respectively, and their *i* values are 1.8 and 2.6, respectively. Calculate the mass of NaCl represented by 1 g of atropine sulfate

(Table 2-2). 695 × 1.8/58.5 × 2.6 = 1 g/X g, and X = 0.12 g NaCl represented by 1 g of atropine sulfate.

(2) An example of the practical use of sodium chloride equivalents is seen in the following problem.

How many grams of boric acid should be used in compounding the following prescription?

℞ Phenacaine hydrochloride	1%
Chlorobutanol	0.5%
Boric acid	q.s.
Purified water ad	60.0 ml
Make isoton. sol.	

The prescription calls for 0.3 g of chlorobutanol and 0.6 g of phenacaine. How much boric acid is required to prepare this prescription? The question is best answered in four steps.

(a) Find the mass of sodium chloride represented by all ingredients.

0.20 × 0.6 = 0.120 g of sodium chloride represented by phenacaine hydrochloride

0.24 × 0.3 = 0.072 g of sodium chloride represented by chlorobutanol
0.192 g of sodium chloride represented by the two active ingredients

(b) Find the mass of sodium chloride required to prepare an equal volume of isotonic solution.

$$\frac{0.9 \text{ g NaCl}}{100 \text{ ml}} = \frac{X \text{ g NaCl}}{60 \text{ ml}},$$ X = 0.540 g of sodium chloride in 60 ml of an isotonic sodium chloride solution

(c) Calculate, by subtraction, the amount of NaCl required to make the solution isotonic.

0.540 g NaCl required for isotonicity
0.192 g NaCl represented by ingredients
0.348 g NaCl required to make isotonic solution

(d) Because the prescription calls for boric acid to be used, one last step is required. 0.348 g ÷ 0.52 (sodium chloride eq. for boric acid) = 0.669 g of boric acid to be used.

VIII. STATISTICS

A. Introduction. Statistics can be used to describe and compare data distributions. Such **frequency distributions** are constructed by classifying individual observations into categories corresponding to fixed numeric intervals and plotting the number of observations in each such category (i.e., **interval frequency**) versus the category descriptor (e.g., the interval mean or range). Because of random errors, repeated observations or measurements (of the same value) are not identical. These observations have a **"normal distribution."** Normally, distributed data are described by a **bell-shaped (Gaussian) curve** with a maximum, μ (**population mean**), corresponding to the central tendency of the population, and a spread characterized by σ (the **population standard deviation**). Statistics derived from a **sample** or subset of a population can be used as estimates of the population parameters.

Table 2-2. Sodium Chloride (NaCl) Equivalents

Substance	NaCl Equivalent
Atropine sulfate (H_2O)	0.12
Boric Acid	0.52
Chlorobutanol	0.24
Dextrose (anhydrous)	0.18
Ephedrine hydrochloride	0.29
Phenacaine hydrochloride	0.20
Potassium chloride	0.78

B. Frequency distribution

1. **Estimates of population mean**. The population mean, μ, is the best estimate of the "true" value.
   a. **The sample mean**. For a finite number of observations the arithmetic average or mean, $\overline{X}$, is the best estimate of the "true" value, μ.

$$\overline{X} = \frac{\sum x_i}{n}$$

   where $\sum x_i$ is the sum of all (n) observations.
   (1) **Accuracy** is the degree to which a measured value (X or $\overline{X}$) agrees with the "true" value (μ).
   (2) **Error** (or bias) is the difference between a measured value (X or $\overline{X}$) and the "true" value (μ).

   b. **Median.** The median is the "mid-most" value of a data distribution. When all the values are arranged in increasing (or decreasing order), the median is the middle value for an **odd** number of observations. For an **even** number of observations, the median is the arithmetic mean of the two middle values. For a **normal distribution, median equals mean.** The median is less affected by "outliers" or by a "skewed" distribution.
   c. **Mode.** The mode is the most frequently occurring value (or values) in a frequency distribution. The mode is useful for non-normal distributions especially **bimodal** distributions.

2. **Estimates of variability.** For an **infinite** number of observations, the **population variance**, σ^2, can be used to describe the variability or "spread" of observations in a data distribution. For a **finite** number of observations, the **sample variance**, s^2, can be used to describe the variability or spread of observations in a data distribution.
   a. **Sample variance, s^2,** is estimated by

$$s^2 = \frac{\sum(x_i - \overline{X})^2}{(n-1)}$$

or

$$s^2 = \frac{\sum x_i^{\,2} - \frac{(\sum x_i)^2}{n}}{(n-1)}$$

   where $\overline{X}$ is the mean and (n−1) is the number of degrees of freedom (df).
   b. **Range.** For a very small number of observations, the **range (w)** can be used to describe the variability in the data set:

$$w = |X_{largest} - X_{smallest}|$$

   c. The **standard deviation** (s; SD), one of the most commonly encountered estimates of variability, is equal to the square root of the variance.

$$s = \sqrt{s^2} = \sqrt{\frac{\sum(x_i - \overline{X})^2}{(n-1)}}$$

or

$$s = \sqrt{s^2} = \sqrt{\frac{\sum x_i^{\,2} - \frac{(\sum x_i)^2}{n}}{(n-1)}}$$

   d. **Precision** (reproducibility) is the degree to which replicate measurements "made in exactly the same way" agree with each other. **Precision** is often expressed as the **relative standard deviation (RSD, %RSD)**:

$$\%RSD = \left(\frac{s}{\overline{X}}\right) \times 100$$

3. The **standard deviation of the mean (S_m)**, or standard error of the mean (SEM), is an estimate of the **variability** or **error in the mean** obtained from *n* observations. It is often used to establish confidence intervals for describing the mean of a data set or in comparing the means of two data sets.

$$S_m = \frac{s}{\sqrt{n}}$$

STUDY QUESTIONS

Directions: Each of the numbered items or incomplete statements in this section is followed by answers or by completions of the statement. Select the **one** lettered answer or completion that is **best** in each case.

1. If a vitamin solution contains 0.5 mg of fluoride ion in each milliliter, then how many milligrams of fluoride ion would be provided by a dropper that delivers 0.6 ml?

(A) 0.3 mg
(B) 0.1 mg
(C) 1 mg
(D) 0.83 mg

2. How many chloramphenicol capsules, each containing 250 mg, are needed to provide 25 mg per kg per day for 7 days for a person weighing 200 pounds?

(A) 90 capsules
(B) 64 capsules
(C) 13 capsules
(D) 25 capsules

3. If 3.17 kg of a drug are used to make 50,000 tablets, how many milligrams will 30 tablets contain?

(A) 1.9
(B) 1900
(C) 0.0019
(D) 3.2

4. A capsule contains 1/8 gr of ephedrine sulfate, 1/4 gr of theophylline, and 1/16 gr of phenobarbital. What is the total mass of the active ingredients in milligrams?

(A) 20 mg
(B) 8 mg
(C) 28 mg
(D) 4 mg

5. If one fluidounce of a cough syrup contains 10 gr of sodium citrate, how many milligrams are contained in 10 ml?

(A) 650 mg
(B) 65 mg
(C) 217 mg
(D) 20 mg

6. How many capsules, each containing 1/4 gr of phenobarbital, can be manufactured if a bottle containing 2 avoirdupois ounces of phenobarbital is available?

(A) 771
(B) 350
(C) 3500
(D) 1250

7. Using the formula for calamine lotion, determine the amount of calamine necessary to prepare 240 ml of lotion.

Calamine	80 g
Zinc oxide	80 g
Glycerin	20 ml
Bentonite magma	250 ml

Calcium hydroxide topical solution, a sufficient quantity to make 1000 ml

(A) 19.2 g
(B) 140 g
(C) 100 g
(D) 24 g

8. From the following formula, calculate the amount of white wax required to make 1 lb of cold cream. Determine the mass in grams.

Cetyl esters wax	12.5 parts
White wax	12.0 parts
Mineral oil	56.0 parts
Sodium borate	0.5 parts
Purified water	19.0 parts

(A) 56.75 g
(B) 254.24 g
(C) 54.48 g
(D) 86.26 g

9. How many grams of aspirin should be used to prepare 1.255 kg of the powder?

ASA	6 parts
Phenacetin	3 parts
Caffeine	1 part

(A) 125
(B) 750
(C) 175
(D) 360

10. A solution contains 1.25 mg of a drug per milliliter. At what rate should the solution be infused (drops/min) if the drug is to be administered at a rate of 80 mg/hour? (1 ml = 30 drops)

(A) 64
(B) 1.06
(C) 32
(D) 20

11. The recommended maintenance dose of aminophylline for children is 1.0 mg/kg/hour by injection. If 10 ml of a 25 mg/ml solution of aminophylline is added to a 100 ml bottle for dextrose, what should be the rate of delivery in ml/hour for a 40-pound child?

(A) 2.30
(B) 8.00
(C) 18.9
(D) 18.2

12. For children, streptomycin is to be administered at a dose of 30 mg/kg of body weight daily in divided doses every 6 to 12 hours. The dry powder is dissolved by adding water for injection, USP in an amount to yield the desired concentration as indicated in the following table (for a 1 gram vial).

Approximate Concentration (mg/ml)	**Volume (ml)**
200	4.2
250	3.2
400	1.8

Reconstituting at the lowest possible concentration, what volume (ml) would be withdrawn to obtain one day's dose for a 50 pound child?

(A) 3.4
(B) 22.73
(C) 2.50
(D) 2.27

13. The atropine sulfate is available only in the form of 1/150 gr tablets. How many atropine sulfate tablets would you use to compound the prescription?

Atropine sulfate	gr. 1/200
Codeine phosphate	gr. 1/4
Aspirin	gr. 5
d.t.d.	#24 caps.
Sig: cap 1 prn.	

(A) 3
(B) 6
(C) 12
(D) 18

14. In 25.0 ml of a solution for injection, there are 4.00 mg of the drug. If the dose to be administered to a patient is 200 μg, what quantity of this solution should be used?

(A) 1.25 ml
(B) 125 ml
(C) 12.0 ml
(D) none of the above

15. How many milligrams of papaverine will the patient receive each day?

Rx	Papaverine hydrochloride	1.0 g
	Aqua	30.0 ml
	Syrup tolu qs ad	90.0 ml
	Sig: One tsp. t.i.d.	

(A) 56
(B) 5.6
(C) 166
(D) 2.5

16. Considering the following prescription, how many grams of sodium bromide should be used in filling this prescription?

R_x	Sodium bromide	1.2 g
	Syrup tolu	2.0 ml
	Syrup wild cherry qs ad	5.0 ml
	d.t.d. #24	

(A) 1.2
(B) 1200
(C) 28.8
(D) 220

17. How many milliliters of a 7.5% stock solution of $KMnO_4$ should be used to obtain the KMnO needed?

> $KmnO_4$ qs.
> Distilled water ad 1000
> Sig: Two teaspoons diluted to 500 ml yield a 1 to 5000 solution.

(A) 267 ml
(B) 133 ml
(C) 26.7 ml
(D) 13.3 ml

18. The formula for Ringer's solution follows. How much sodium chloride is needed to make 120 ml?

R_x	Sodium chloride	8.60 g
	Potassium chloride	0.30 g
	Calcium chloride	0.33 g
	Water for injection qs ad	1000 ml

(A) 120 g
(B) 1.03 g
(C) 0.12 g
(D) 103 g

19. How many grams of talc should be added to 1 lb of a powder containing 20 g of zinc undecylenate per 100 g to reduce the concentration of zinc undecylenate to 3%?

(A) 3026.7
(B) 2572.7
(C) 17
(D) 257

20. How many milliliters of a 0.9% aqueous solution can be made from 20.0 g of sodium chloride?

(A) 2222
(B) 100
(C) 222
(D) 122

21. The blood of a reckless driver contains 0.1% alcohol. Express the concentration of alcohol in parts per million.

(A) 100 ppm
(B) 1000 ppm
(C) 1 ppm
(D) 250 ppm

22. Syrup is an 85% w/v solution of sucrose in water. It has a density of 1.313 g/ml. How many milliliters of water should be used to make 125 ml of syrup?

(A) 106.25
(B) 164.1
(C) 57.85
(D) 25.0

23. How many grams of benzethonium chloride should be used in preparing 5 gallons of a 0.025% w/v solution?

(A) 189.25
(B) 18.9
(C) 4.73
(D) 35

24. How many grams of menthol should be used to prepare this prescription?

R_x	Menthol	0.8%
	Alcohol qs ad	60.0 ml

(A) 0.48
(B) 0.8
(C) 4.8
(D) 1.48

25. How many liters of a 1 to 1500 solution can be made by dissolving 4.8 g of cetylpyridinium chloride in water?

(A) 7200
(B) 7.2
(C) 48
(D) 4.8

26. The manufacturer specifies that one Domeboro tablet dissolved in a pint of water makes a modified Burow's solution approximately equivalent to a 1 to 40 dilution. How many tablets should be used in preparing a half gallon of a 1 to 10 dilution?

(A) 16
(B) 189
(C) 12
(D) 45

27. How many milliosmoles of calcium chloride ($CaCl_2 \cdot 2H_2O$ – mol wt = 147) are represented in 147 ml of a 10% w/v calcium chloride solution?

(A) 100
(B) 200
(C) 300
(D) 3

28. How many grams of boric acid should be used in compounding the following prescription?

Phenacaine HCl 1.0% (NaCl eq. = 0.17)
Chlorobutanol 0.5% (NaCl eq. = 0.18)
Boric Acid qs. (NaCl eq. = 0.52)
Purified H_2O ad 30 ml
Make isotonic solution
Sig: One drop in each eye

(A) 0.37 g
(B) 0.74 g
(C) 0.27 g
(D) 0.47 g

29. A pharmacist prepares 1 gallon of KCl solution by mixing 565 grams of KCl (valence = 1) in an appropriate vehicle. How many milliequivalents of K^+ are in 15 ml of this solution? (Atomic weights: K = 39, Cl = 35.5)

(A) 7.5
(B) 10
(C) 20
(D) 30
(E) 40

Questions 30–33

Five ibuprofen tablets were assayed for drug content and the following results obtained by HPLC analysis: 198.2, 199.7, 202.5, 201.3, 196.4 mg.

30. What is the mean ibuprofen content?

(A) 196.9 mg
(B) 200.2 mg
(C) 199.6 mg
(D) 249.5 mg
(E) 202.5 mg

31. What is the standard deviation of ibuprofen content in the analyzed tablets?

(A) 2.17 mg
(B) 3.35 mg
(C) 2.42 mg
(D) 3.00 mg
(E) − 2.17 mg

32. What is the percent relative standard deviation (%RSD) for this ibuprofen tablet analysis?

(A) 1.69%
(B) 1.21%
(C) 8.25%
(D) 3.35%
(E) 1.50 %

33. What is the standard deviation of the mean drug content of this sample?

(A) 0.480 mg
(B) 0.605 mg
(C) 1.21 mg
(D) 1.08 mg
(E) 0.825 mg

ANSWERS AND EXPLANATIONS

1. The answer is A *[V E].*

2. The answer is B *[II].*

3. The answer is B *[II].*

4. The answer is C *[1 A 2; III A].*

5. The answer is C *[I A 2].*

6. The answer is C *[II].*

7. The answer is A *[V].*

8. The answer is C *[V].*
The formula tells the pharmacist that white wax represents 12 parts out of the total 100 parts in the prescription. What we wish to determine is the mass of white wax required to prepare 454 g (1 lb) of the recipe. This can be easily solved by proportion:

$$\frac{12 \text{ parts W.W}}{100 \text{ parts total}} = \frac{X}{454 \text{ parts (grams)}}, \ X = 54.48 \text{ g}$$

9. The answer is B *[V].*

10. The answer is C *[VI].*

11. The answer is B *[IV].*

12. The answer is A *[IV].*

13. The answer is D *[V].*

14. The answer is A *[VI].*
Dimensional analysis is often useful for calculating doses. Considering that 4 mg of drug are present in each 25 ml of solution, we can easily calculate the number of ml to be used to give a dose of 0.200 mg (200 μg). Always include units in your calculations.

$$25 \text{ ml}/4 \text{ mg} \times 0.200 \text{ mg} = 1.25 \text{ ml}$$

15. The answer is C *[V A 1].*

16. The answer is C *[V A 1].*

17. The answer is B *[I A].*
First, determine the mass of drug in the final diluted solution.

$$\frac{1 \text{ part}}{5000 \text{ parts}} = \frac{X \text{ g}}{500 \text{ g}}, \ X = 0.1 \text{ g}$$

Now, if 0.1 g of drug is present in 500 ml of 1 to 5000 solution, two teaspoonfuls (10 ml) of the prescription contain the same amount of drug (0.1 g) before dilution. From this, the amount of drug in 1000 ml (the total volume) of the prescription can be determined:

$$\frac{0.1 \text{ g}}{10 \text{ ml}} = \frac{X \text{ g}}{1000 \text{ ml}}, \ X = 10 \text{ g}$$

Finally, to obtain the correct amount of drug to formulate the prescription (10 g) we are to use a 7.5% stock solution. Recalling the definition of percentage strength w/v:

$$100 \text{ ml}/7.5 \text{ g} \times 10 \text{ g} = 133.3 \text{ ml or } 133 \text{ ml}$$

18. The answer is B *[IV].*

19. The answer is B *[V].*

20. The answer is A *[I A 3].*
Using dimensional analysis: 20 g × 100 ml/0.9 g = 2222 ml

21. The answer is B *[V A].*

22. The answer is A *[I A; V A 1].*

23. The answer is C *[I; V].*

24. The answer is A *[I; V].*

25. The answer is A *[I; V].*
The problem is easily solved by proportion. The question to be answered is: If 1 g of drug is present in 1500 ml of solution, what volume can be made with 4.8 g of drug?

$$\frac{1\text{ g}}{4.8\text{ g}} = \frac{1500\text{ ml}}{X\text{ ml}},\ X = 7200\text{ ml}$$ (the volume of 1:1500 solution that can be prepared from 4.8 g of drug)

26. The answer is A *[I; V].*

27. The answer is C *[VII B].*
Recalling the expression for ideal osmolar concentration:

$$\text{mOsmol/L} = \frac{100\text{ g/L}}{147\text{ g/mole}} \times 3 \times 1000 = 2040\text{ mOsmol/L} \times 0.147\text{ L} = 300\text{ mOsmol}$$

28. The answer is A *[VII C].*

29. The answer is D *[VII A].*

30. The answer is C *[VIII B 1].*
The mean is calculated directly from the equation:

$$\overline{X} = \frac{\sum x_i}{n} = \frac{998.1}{5} = 199.6\text{ mg}$$

31. The answer is C *[VIII B 3].*
The standard deviation can be calculated with either of the two most commonly used equations:

x_i	$(x_i - \overline{X})$	$(x_i - \overline{X})^2$
198.2	−1.4	1.96*
199.7	0.1	0.01
202.5	2.9	8.41
201.3	1.7	2.89
196.4	−3.2	10.24
$\sum x_i = 998.1$		$\sum(x_i - \overline{X})^2 = 23.51$

$$s = \sqrt{s^2} = \sqrt{\frac{\sum(x_i - \overline{X})^2}{(n-1)}} = \sqrt{\frac{23.51}{(5-1)}} = 2.42\text{ mg}$$

or

x_i	x_i^2
198.2	39,283.24*
199.7	39,880.09
202.5	41,006.25
201.3	40,521.69
196.4	38,572.96
$\sum x_i = 998.1$	$\sum x_i^2 = 199{,}264.23$

$$s = \sqrt{s^2} = \sqrt{\frac{199{,}264.23 - \frac{(998.1)^2}{5}}{(5-1)}} = 2.42 \text{ mg}$$

*Note: It is important to carry enough significant figures through the calculation in order to minimize round-off error.

32. The answer is B *[VIII B 4]*.

$$\%RSD = \left(\frac{s}{\overline{X}}\right) \times 100 = \left(\frac{2.42}{199.6}\right) \times 100 = 1.21\%$$

33. The answer is D *[VIII C]*.

$$s_m = \frac{s}{\sqrt{n}} = \frac{2.42}{\sqrt{5}} = 1.08 \text{ mg}$$

3
Pharmaceutical Principles and Drug Dosage Forms

Lawrence H. Block
Andrew B. C. Yu

I. INTRODUCTION. Pharmaceutical principles comprise the underlying physicochemical principles that make it possible for a drug to be incorporated in a pharmaceutical **dosage form** (e.g., solution or capsule)—whether extemporaneously compounded by the pharmacist or manufactured for commercial distribution in the form of a **drug product.**

A. The finished **dosage form** contains the active drug ingredient in association with nondrug (usually inert) ingredients (**excipients**), which comprise the **vehicle** or **formulation matrix.**

B. The **drug delivery system** concept, which has evolved over the last two decades, is a more holistic concept, embracing not only the drug (or prodrug) and its formulation matrix, but the dynamic interactions among the drug, its formulation matrix, its container, and the physiologic milieux of the patient. These dynamic interactions are the subject of **biopharmaceutics** (see Chapter 4).

II. INTERMOLECULAR FORCES OF ATTRACTION

A. Introduction. The application of pharmaceutic principles to drug dosage forms can best be appreciated when drug dosage forms are **categorized** according to their **physical state, degree of heterogeneity,** and **chemical composition.** The usual relevant states of matter are **gases, liquids,** and **solids.** Intermolecular forces of attraction are weakest in gases and strongest in solids. Interconversions from one physical state to another can involve simply overcoming intermolecular forces of attraction by the addition of energy (heat). Chemical composition can have a dramatic effect on physicochemical properties and behavior: a distinction between **polymers** or **macromolecules** and more conventional (i.e., smaller) molecules **(micromolecules)** is necessary.

B. Intermolecular forces of attraction. Because atoms vary in their electronegativity, electron-sharing between different atoms is likely to be unequal. This asymmetric electron distribution results in a shift in the overall electron cloud in the molecule and the tendency of the molecule to behave as a **dipole** (i.e., as if it had a positive and a negative pole). The dipole associated with each covalent bond has a corresponding **dipole moment** (μ) defined as the product of the distance of charge separation (d) and the charge (q):

$$\mu = q \cdot d$$

The molecular dipole moment may be viewed as the vector sum of the individual bond moments.

1. Molecules with **perfect symmetry** [e.g., carbon tetrachloride (Figure 3-1)] have dipole moments of zero and are referred to as **nonpolar** molecules.
2. **Asymmetric** molecules have nonzero dipole moments and are considered **polar** molecules.
3. When **dipolar** molecules approach one another close enough "positive to positive" or "negative to negative" so that their electron clouds interpenetrate, **intermolecular repulsive**

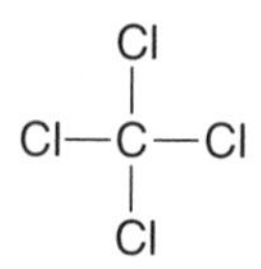

Figure 3-1.

forces arise. When these dipolar molecules approach one another with the positive pole of one close to the negative pole of the other, molecular **attraction** occurs **(dipole–dipole interaction).** If the identically charged poles of the two molecules are closer, then **repulsion** will occur.

C. Types of intermolecular forces of attraction include:

1. Nonpolar molecules do not have permanent dipoles. However, the instantaneous electron distribution in a molecule can be asymmetric, and the resultant transient dipole moment can induce a dipole in an adjacent molecule. This **induced dipole–induced dipole interaction (London dispersion forces),** with a force of about 0.5–1 kcal/mol, is sufficient to facilitate order in a molecular array. These relatively weak electrostatic forces are responsible for the liquefaction of nonpolar gases.

2. The transient dipole induced by a permanent dipole, or **dipole–induced dipole interaction (Debye induction forces)** is a stronger interaction, with a force of approximately 1–3 kcal/mol.

3. **Permanent dipole interactions (Keesom orientation forces),** with a force of about 1–7 kcal/mol, together with Debye and London forces, constitute **van der Waals forces** and, collectively, are responsible for the more substantive structure and molecular ordering in liquids.

4. **Hydrogen bonds.** Because of their small size and large electrostatic field, hydrogen atoms can approach highly electronegative atoms (e.g., fluorine, oxygen, nitrogen, chlorine, sulfur) and interact electrostatically to form a hydrogen bond. Depending on the electronegativity of the second atom and the molecular environment in which hydrogen bonding occurs, hydrogen bond energy can vary from approximately 1–8 kcal/mol.

5. **Ion–ion, ion–dipole, and ion–induced dipole forces. Positive–negative ion interactions** in the solid state involve forces of 100–200 kcal/mol. Ionic interactions tend to be reduced considerably in liquid systems in the presence of other electrolytes. **Ion–dipole** interaction or **dipole induction by an ion** also can affect molecular aggregation.

III. STATES OF MATTER

A. Gases. Molecules in the gaseous state can be pictured as moving along straight paths, in all directions, at high velocities (e.g., mean velocities for H_2O vapor, at 587 m/sec; for O_2, 440 m/sec), until collisions occur with other molecules. As a consequence of these random collisions, molecular velocities and paths change, leading to further collisions with other molecules and the boundaries of the system (e.g., the walls of a container holding the gas). This process, repeated incessantly, is responsible for the **pressure** exhibited within the confines of the system.

1. The interrelationship among **volume (V), pressure (P),** and the **absolute temperature (T)** is given by the **ideal gas law,** which is the equation of state for an ideal gas:

$$PV = nRT$$

and

$$PV = \left(\frac{g}{M}\right)RT,$$

where n is the number of moles of gas—equivalent to the number of grams (g) of gas divided by the molecular weight of the gas (M)—and R is the **molar gas constant** (0.08205 liter atm/mole deg).

2. Pharmaceutical gases include the **anesthetic gases,** such as nitrous oxide and halothane. **Compressed gases** include oxygen for therapy; nitrogen or carbon dioxide, and the **liquefiable gases** are used as propellants in **aerosol products (pressurized packaging).** The latter gases include certain **halohydrocarbons** and **hydrocarbons.** Ethylene oxide is a gas used for the sterilization and disinfection of heat-labile objects.

3. In general, as the temperature of a substance is increased, its **heat content** or **enthalpy** is increased.
   a. Substances can undergo a change of state or phase change from the solid to the liquid state **(melting)** or from the liquid to the gaseous state **(vaporization).**

b. Volatile liquids, such as ether, halothane, and methoxyflurane, are used as inhalation anesthetics. Amyl nitrite is a volatile liquid that has been inhaled for its vasodilating effect in acute angina.

c. In some instances, a solid can be heated directly to the gaseous or vapor state without passing through the liquid state. This is referred to as **sublimation** (e.g., camphor, iodine).

d. The reverse process (i.e., the direct transition from the vapor state to the solid state) has also been referred to as sublimation, although the preferred term is **deposition.** Some forms of sulfur and colloidal silicon dioxide are prepared in this manner.

4. The intermolecular forces of attraction in gases are virtually nonexistent at room temperature; gases display little or no ordering.

B. Liquids. The intermolecular forces of attraction in liquids **(van der Waals forces)** are sufficient to impose some ordering or regular arrangement among the molecules. **Hydrogen bonding,** when it occurs, increases the likelihood of cohesion in liquids and further affects their physicochemical behavior. However, these forces are much weaker than **covalent** or **ionic** forces. Thus, liquids, in general, tend to display short-range rather than long-range order. Hypothetically, although molecules of a liquid would tend to aggregate in localized clusters, no defined structuring would be evident.

1. Surface and interfacial tension

a. Molecules in the bulk phase of a liquid (A) are surrounded by other molecules of the same kind. Molecules at the surface of a liquid (B) are not completely surrounded by like molecules (Figure 3-2). As a result, molecules at or near the surface of a liquid experience a net inward pull from molecules in the interior of the liquid. This net inward intermolecular attraction results in the spontaneous tendency of the liquid surface to contract. Thus, liquids tend to assume a spherical shape (i.e., a volume with the minimum surface area), which represents the configuration with the minimum free energy.

b. Any expansion of the surface involves an increase in free energy of the system. **Surface free energy** can thus be defined by the work required to increase the surface area, A, of the liquid, by 1 area unit, which is expressed as the number of milli-Newtons (mN) needed to expand a meter-squared surface by one unit:

$$\text{work} = \gamma \cdot \Delta A$$

where ΔA is the increase in surface area and γ is the **surface tension** or **surface free energy,** in mN m^{-1} (equivalent to CGS units of dynes cm^{-1}). Water has a surface tension, at 20°C of 72 mN m^{-1}, whereas n-octanol has a surface tension of 27 mN m^{-1}. Thus, more work must be expended to expand the surface of water than to expand the surface of n-octanol (i.e., to proceed from a given bulk volume of bulk liquid to the corresponding volume of small droplets).

c. At the **boundary** or **interface** between two immiscible liquids in contact with one another, the corresponding **interfacial tension** (i.e., the free energy or work required to expand the interfacial area) is a reflection of the extent of intermolecular forces of attraction and repulsion at the interface between the two phases. At an interface between two liquids, there is substantial molecular interaction across the two phases, thereby reducing the imbalance in forces of attraction within each of the phases. The interfacial tension between n-octanol

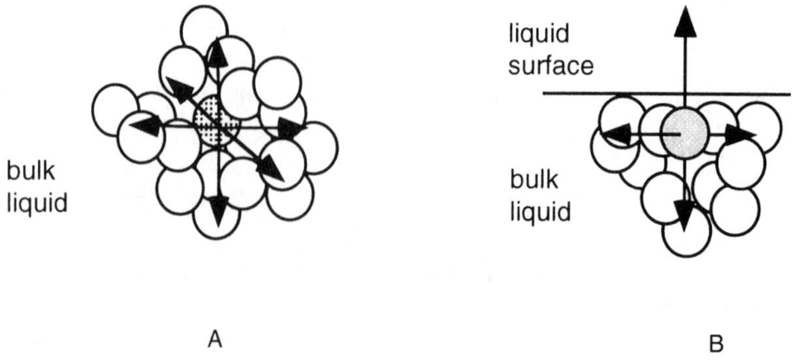

Figure 3-2.

and water is reduced to 8.5 mN m^{-1} from 72 mN m^{-1} (γ air/water), which is indicative, in part, of the interfacial interaction between n-octanol and water.

2. The flow of a liquid across a solid surface can be examined in terms of the liquid's **velocity** or rate of movement relative to the surface across which it flows. More insight can be gained by visualizing the liquid flow as involving the movement of numerous parallel layers of liquid between two flat plates with the uppermost plate movable and the lower plate fixed (Figure 3-3). The application of a constant force (F) to the uppermost plate causes it and the uppermost layer of liquid in contact with it to move with a velocity $\Delta y/\Delta x$. The interaction between the fixed bottom plate and the liquid layer closest to it prevents the movement of that bottom layer of liquid. The **velocity** (v) of the remaining layers of liquid between the two plates is proportional to their distance from the immovable plate (i.e., $\Delta y/\Delta x$). The **velocity gradient** leads to a deformation of the liquid with time, which is referred to as the **rate of shear,** dv/dx, or D. **Newton** defined flow in terms of the ratio of the force F applied to a plate of area A [**shear stress** (τ)] divided by the velocity gradient (D) induced by τ:

$$\frac{F}{A} = \eta \frac{dv}{dx},$$

or

$$\frac{\tau}{D} = \eta$$

The proportionality constant η is the (coefficient of) **viscosity** and is indicative of the resistance to flow of adjacent layers of fluid. The reciprocal of η is termed **fluidity.** Units of viscosity in the CGS system are dynes $cm^{-2}s^{-1}$, or poise; in the SI system, Newton $m^{-2}s^{-1}$, which corresponds to 10 poise. The viscosity of water at 20°C is about 0.01 poise, or 1 centipoise (cps), which corresponds to 1 mN $m^{-2}s^{-1}$.

a. Substances that flow in accordance with the above equation (Newton's law) are termed **Newtonian substances.** Liquids consisting of simple molecules and dilute dispersions tend to be **Newtonian.**

b. **Non-Newtonian substances** do not obey Newton's equation of flow. This may be manifested in a number of ways: non-Newtonians tend to exhibit **shear-dependent** or **time-dependent viscosity.** In either case, viscosity is more aptly termed **apparent viscosity** because Newton's law is not strictly obeyed. Heterogeneous liquids and solids are most likely non-Newtonians.

(1) **Shear-dependent viscosity.** This type of non-Newtonian behavior is displayed by suspensions of small, deflocculated particles with a high solids content (**shear thickening** or **dilatancy**) or by polymer solutions (**shear thinning** or **pseudoplastic** behavior), wherein the apparent viscosity increases or decreases, respectively, with an increase in the rate of shear. **Plastic** or **Bingham body** behavior is exemplified by flocculated particles in concentrated suspensions that show no apparent response to the imposition of low-level stress. Flow begins only after a limiting yield stress (the **yield value**) has been exceeded.

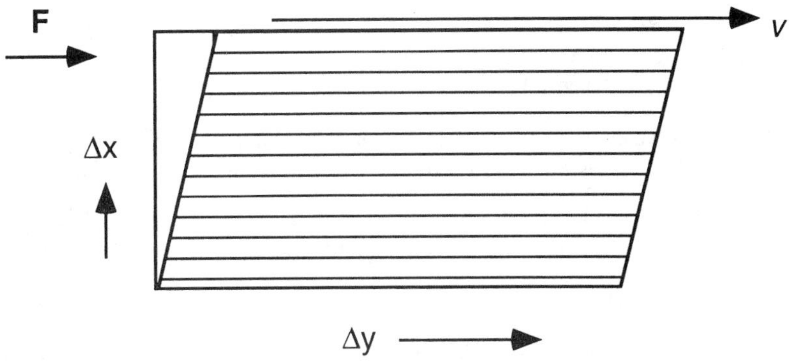

Figure 3-3.

(2) **Time-dependent viscosity**

(a) The yield value of **plastic** systems may be time-dependent (i.e., it might depend upon the timescale involved in the application of force. Systems that display shear-thinning behavior but do not immediately recover their higher apparent viscosity when the rate of shear is lowered, are **thixotropic** systems. Structural recovery in a thixotropic system is relatively slow in comparison to structural breakdown.

(b) **Thixotropy** is encountered with heterogeneous systems involving a three-dimensional structure or network. When such a system is at rest, it appears to have a relatively rigid consistency. Under shear, the structure breaks down and fluidity increases. This is a **gel-sol** transformation.

(c) **Negative thixotropy** or **antithixotropy** is observed when the apparent viscosity of the system continues to increase with continued application of shear up to some equilibrium value at a given shear rate. These systems display a sol-gel transformation. One explanation for antithixotropic behavior is that continued shear results in increased frequency of particle or macromolecule interactions, leading to increased structure in the system.

C. **Solids.** Intermolecular forces of attraction are strongest in solids in comparison to liquids or gases.

1. **Crystalline solids** have the following attributes:
   a. Fixed **molecular order** (i.e., molecules occupy set positions in a specific array)
   b. A distinct melting point
   c. **Anisotropicity** (i.e., their properties are not the same in all directions), with the exception of cubic crystals

2. Amorphous solids have these attributes:
   a. Randomly arranged molecules
   b. Nondistinct melting points
   c. **Isotropicity** (i.e., properties are the same in all directions)

3. **Polymorphism** is the condition wherein substances can exist in more than one crystalline form. These **polymorphs** differ from one another in their molecular arrangement or crystal lattice. As a result, the properties of these different polymorphs of a drug solid can vary. For example, melting points, solubilities, dissolution rates, density, and stability can differ considerably among the polymorphic forms of a drug. Many drugs exhibit polymorphic behavior: one drug class in which the incidence of polymorphism is especially high is **steroids.** Fatty (triglyceride) excipients such as theobroma oil (cocoa butter) have long been recognized for their polymorphic behavior.

4. **Melting point and heat of fusion.** The melting point of a solid is the temperature at which the solid is transformed to a liquid. When 1 g of a solid is heated and melts, the heat absorbed in the process is referred to as the **latent heat of fusion.**

IV. PHYSIOCHEMICAL BEHAVIOR

A. Homogeneous systems

1. **Solutions.** A solution is a homogeneous system in which a **solute** is molecularly dispersed (dissolved) in a **solvent,** the solvent being the predominant species. **Saturated solutions** are solutions which, at a given temperature and pressure, contain the maximum amount of solute that can be accommodated by the solvent. If the saturation (solubility) limit is exceeded, a fraction of the solute can separate from the solution and exist in equilibrium with it.
   a. **Solutes** can be gases, liquids, or solids; nonelectrolytes or electrolytes.

(1) **Nonelectrolytes** are substances that **do not form ions** when dissolved in water. Examples include estradiol, glycerin, urea, and sucrose. Their aqueous solutions do not conduct electric current.

(2) **Electrolytes** are substances that **do form ions** in solution. Examples include sodium chloride, hydrochloric acid, and atropine. As a consequence, their aqueous solutions do conduct electric current. Electrolytes can be characterized as **strong electrolytes** (e.g., sodium chloride, hydrochloric acid), which are **completely ionized** in

water at all concentrations, or as **weak electrolytes** (e.g., aspirin, atropine), which are **partially ionized** in water.

b. **Colligative properties of a solution** are those properties that are dependent upon the total **number of ionic and nonionic solute molecules in the solution.** They are dependent on ionization but **independent of other chemical properties of the solute.**

2. **Colligative properties** include the following:
   a. **Lowering of vapor pressure.** The **partial vapor pressure** of each volatile component in a solution is equal to the product of the mol fraction of the component in the solution and the vapor pressure of the pure component. This is **Raoult's law:**

$$p_A = p_A^0 \, x_A$$

where p_A is the partial vapor pressure, above a solution in which the mol fraction of the solute A is x_A and p_A^0 is the **vapor pressure** of the pure component A [i.e., the pressure at which an equilibrium is established between the molecules of A in the liquid state and the molecules of A in the gaseous (vapor) state in a closed, evacuated container]. The vapor pressure, while temperature dependent, is independent of the amount of the liquid and vapor. (Raoult's law holds for ideal solutions of nonelectrolytes.) For a **binary solution** (i.e., a solution of component B in component A)

$$\frac{\left(p_A^0 - p_A\right)}{p_A^0} = \left(1 - x_A\right) = x_B$$

The lowering of the vapor pressure of the solution relative to the vapor pressure of the pure solvent is proportional to the number of molecules of solute in the solution. The actual lowering of the solution's vapor pressure by the solute, Δp_A, is given by

$$\Delta p_A = \left(p_A^0 - p_A\right) = x_B p_A^0$$

   b. **Elevation of boiling point.** The **boiling point** is the temperature at which the vapor pressure of a liquid equals an external pressure of 760 millimeters of mercury (mm Hg). The boiling point of a solution of a nonvolatile solute is higher than that of the pure solvent because the solute lowers the vapor pressure of the solvent. The amount of elevation of the boiling point (ΔT_b) depends on the solute concentration:

$$\Delta T_b = \frac{RT_0^2 \, M_1 \, m}{1000 \cdot \Delta H_{vap}} = K_b m$$

where K_b is the molal boiling point elevation constant, R is the molar gas constant, T is absolute temperature (°K), M_1 is the molecular weight of the solute, m is the molality of the solution, and ΔH_{vap} is the molal enthalpy of vaporization of the solvent.

   c. **Depression of freezing point.** The **freezing point** (or melting point) of a pure compound is the temperature at which the solid and the liquid phases are in equilibrium under a pressure of 1 atmosphere (atm). The freezing point of a solution is the temperature at which the solid phase of the pure solvent and the liquid phase of the solution are in equilibrium under a pressure of 1 atm. The amount of depression of the freezing point (ΔT_f) depends on the molality of the solution:

$$\Delta T_f = \frac{RT_0^2 \, M_1 \, m}{1000 \cdot \Delta H_{fusion}} = K_f m$$

where K_f is the molal freezing point constant and ΔH_{fusion} is the molal heat of fusion.

   d. **Osmotic pressure. Osmosis** is the process by which solvent molecules pass through a semipermeable membrane (a barrier through which only solvent molecules may pass) from a region of dilute solution to one of more concentrated solution. Solvent molecules transfer because of the inequality in chemical potential on the two sides of the membrane. Solvent molecules in a concentrated solution have a lower chemical potential than solvent molecules in a more dilute solution.

   (1) The **pressure** that must be applied to the solution to prevent the flow of pure solvent into the concentrated solution is known as the **osmotic pressure.**

   (2) Solvent molecules move from a region where their **escaping tendency is high** to one where their **escaping tendency is low.** The presence of dissolved solute lowers the escaping tendency of the solvent in proportion to solute concentration.

(3) The **van't Hoff equation** defines the osmotic pressure π as a function of the number of moles of solute, n_2, in the solution of volume V:

$$\pi V = n_2 RT$$

3. Electrolyte solutions and ionic equilibria

a. Acid–base equilibria

(1) **Arrhenius dissociation theory.** According to this theory, an **acid** is a substance that liberates H^+ in aqueous solution, and a **base** is a substance that liberates hydroxyl ions (OH^-) in aqueous solution. This definition applies only under aqueous conditions, however.

(2) **Lowry-Brønsted theory.** This is a more powerful concept that applies to aqueous and nonaqueous systems; however, it is most commonly used for pharmaceutical and biologic systems because these are primarily aqueous systems.

(a) According to this definition, an **acid** is a substance (charged or uncharged) capable of donating a proton, and a **base** is a substance (charged or uncharged) capable of accepting a proton from an acid. The dissociation of an acid (HA) always produces a base (A^-) according to this formula:

$$HA \leftrightarrow H^+ + A^-$$

(b) HA and A^- are referred to as a **conjugate acid–base pair** (an acid and a base that differ in their structure by a proton and exist in equilibrium). The proton of an acid does not exist free in solution but combines with the solvent. [In water, this **hydrated proton** is known as a **hydronium ion** (H_3O^+).]

(c) The relative **strengths** of acids and bases are determined by their ability to donate or accept protons. For example, in water, HCl donates a proton more readily than does acetic acid. Thus, it is a stronger acid. Acid strength is also determined by the affinity of the solvent for protons. For example, HCl may dissociate completely in liquid ammonia but only very slightly in glacial acetic acid. Thus, HCl is a strong acid in liquid ammonia and a weak acid in glacial acetic acid.

(3) **Lewis theory.** This theory extends the acid–base concept to reactions in which protons are not involved. It defines an **acid** as a molecule or ion that accepts an electron pair from some other atom and a **base** as a substance that donates an electron pair to be shared with another atom.

b. H^+ concentration values are very small and, therefore, are expressed in **exponential notation as pH:** the pH is defined as the logarithm of the reciprocal of the H^+ concentration,

$$pH = \log \frac{1}{[H^+]}$$

where $[H^+]$ indicates the molar concentration of H^+. Because the logarithm of a reciprocal equals the **negative logarithm** of the number, this equation may be rewritten as:

$$pH = -\log[H^+], \text{ or } [H^+] = 10^{-pH}$$

Thus, the pH value may be defined as the negative logarithm of the $[H^+]$ value. For example, if the H^+ concentration of a solution is 5×10^{-6}, the pH value may be calculated as follows:

$$\begin{aligned} pH &= -\log [5 \times 10^{-6}] \\ \log 5 &= 0.669; \log 10^{-6} = -6.0 \\ pH &= -[-6 + 0.669] \\ &= -[-5.331] \\ &= 5.331 \end{aligned}$$

c. As pH decreases, **H^+ concentration increases exponentially:** When the pH decreases from 6 to 5, the H^+ concentration increases from 10^{-6} to 10^{-5}, or 10 times its original value. When the pH falls from 5 to 4.7, the H^+ concentration increases from 1×10^{-5} to 2×10^{-5}, or double its initial value.

d. Dissociation constants. Ionization refers to the complete separation of the ions in a crystal lattice when the salt is dissolved. **Dissociation** refers to the separation of ions in solution when the ions are associated by interionic attraction.

(1) For **weak electrolytes,** the dissociation is a reversible process. The equilibrium of this process can be expressed by the law of mass action, which states that the rate of the

chemical reaction is proportional to the product of the concentration of the reacting substances, each raised to a power of the number of moles of the substance in solution.

(2) For **weak acids,** dissociation in water is expressed as:

$$HA \leftrightarrow H^+ + A^-$$

The dynamic equilibrium between the simultaneous forward and reverse reactions is indicated by the arrows. By the law of mass action,

$$\text{rate of forward reaction} = K_1[HA]$$
$$\text{rate of reverse reaction} = K_2[H^+][A^-]$$

At equilibrium, the forward and reverse rates are equal. Therefore,

$$K_1[HA] = K_2[H^+][A^-]$$

Thus, the **equilibrium expression for the dissociation of a weak acid** is written as:

$$K_a = \frac{K_1}{K_2} = \frac{[H^+]\,[A^-]}{[HA]}$$

where K_a represents the acid dissociation constant. For a weak acid, the **acid dissociation constant** is conventionally expressed as **pK_a**, which is $-\log[K_a]$. For example, the K_a of acetic acid at 25°C is 1.75×10^{-5}. The pK_a is calculated as follows:

$$pK_a = -\log\,[1.75 \times 10^{-5}]$$
$$\log 5 = 0.243;\ \log 10^{-5} = -5$$
$$pH = -[0.243 + (-5)]$$
$$= -[-4.757]$$
$$= 4.76$$

(3) For **weak bases,** dissociation may also be expressed using the K_a expression for the **conjugate acid of the base** (the acid formed when a proton reacts with the base). For a base that does not contain a hydroxyl group,

$$BH^+ \leftrightarrow H^+ + B$$

The **dissociation constant** for this reaction is expressed as:

$$K_a = \frac{[H^+]\,[B]}{[BH^+]}$$

However, a **base dissociation constant** has traditionally been defined for a weak base, using this expression:

$$B + H_2O \leftrightarrow OH- + BH^+$$

$$K_b = \frac{[OH^-]\,[BH^+]}{[B]}$$

where K_b represents the dissociation constant of a weak base. This **dissociation constant** can be expressed as **pK_b**, as follows:

$$pK_b = -\log\,[K_b]$$

(4) **Certain compounds** (acids or bases) can accept or donate more than one proton and consequently have **more than one dissociation constant.**

e. Henderson-Hasselbalch equations describe the relationship between the ionized and nonionized species of a weak electrolyte.

(1) For **weak acids,** the Henderson-Hasselbalch equation is obtained from the equilibrium relationship described above [see II C]:

$$pH = pK_a + \log \frac{[\text{salt}]}{[\text{acid}]}$$

(2) Similarly, the Henderson-Hasselbalch equation for **weak bases** is as follows:

$$pH = pK_a + \log \frac{[B]}{[BH^+]}$$

where B is the unionized weak base and BH^+ is the protonated base.

f. **Degree of ionization (α),** the fraction of a weak electrolyte ionized in solution, is calculated from the following equation:

$$\alpha = \frac{[I]}{[I] + [U]}$$

where [I] and [U] represent the concentrations of the ionized and unionized species, respectively. The degree of ionization depends solely upon pH of the solution and pK_a of the weak electrolyte. **When pH = pK_a**, the Henderson-Hasselbalch equations are:

$$pH - pK_a = 0 = \log \frac{[B]}{[BH^+]}$$

$$\text{thus, } \frac{[B]}{[BH^+]} = 1$$

$$pH - pK_a = 0 = \log \frac{[A^-]}{[HA]}$$

$$\text{thus, } \frac{[A^-]}{[HA]} = 1$$

In effect, when the pH of the solution is numerically equivalent to the pK_a of the weak electrolyte, whether a weak base or a weak acid, [I] = [U] and the degree of ionization $\alpha = 0.5$ (i.e., 50% of the solute is ionized).

g. **Solubility of a weak electrolyte** varies as a function of pH.

(1) For a **weak acid,** the total solubility C_s is given by this expression:

$$C_s = [HA] + [A^-]$$

where [HA] is the intrinsic solubility of the nonionized weak acid and is denoted as C_0, whereas $[A^-]$ is the concentration of its anion. Because $[A^-]$ can be expressed in terms of C_0 and the dissociation constant K_a,

$$C_s = C_0 + \frac{K_a C_0}{[H^+]}$$

Thus, the **solubility of a weak acid increases with increasing pH** (i.e., with an increasing degree of ionization, as the anion is more polar and therefore more water soluble than the nonionized weak acid).

(2) Similarly, for **weak bases,**

$$C_s = C_0 + \frac{C_0[H^+]}{K_a}$$

solubility decreases with increasing pH because more of the weak base is in the unprotonated form, which is less polar, therefore, less water soluble.

h. **Buffers and buffer capacity**

(1) A **buffer** is a mixture of salt with acid or base that resists changes in pH upon addition of small quantities of acid or base. A buffer can be a **combination** of a weak acid and its conjugate base (salt) or a combination of a weak base and its conjugate acid (salt). However, buffer solutions are more **commonly prepared** from weak acids and their salts. They are not ordinarily prepared from weak bases and their salts because of the instability and volatility of weak bases.

(a) For a **weak acid and its salt,** the buffer equation below is satisfactory for calculations with a pH of 4–10 and is important in the preparation of buffered pharmaceutical solutions:

$$pH = pK_a + \log \frac{[salt]}{[acid]}$$

(b) For a **weak base and its salt,** the buffer equation is similar but also depends on the dissociation constant of water (pK_w). The equation becomes:

$$pH = pK_w - pK_b + \log \frac{[base]}{[salt]}$$

(2) **Buffer action** is the resistance to a change in pH.

(3) **Buffer capacity** is the ability of a buffer solution to resist changes in pH. The **smaller the pH change** caused by addition of a given amount of acid or base, the **greater the buffer capacity** of the solution.

(a) Buffer capacity may be defined as the number of gram equivalents in an acid or base that changes the pH of a liter of buffer solution by one unit.

(b) Buffer capacity is influenced by the concentration of the buffer constituents because a higher concentration of these provides a greater acid or base reserve. Buffer capacity (β) is related to the total concentration (C) as follows:

$$\beta = 2.3\ C\ \frac{K_a[H^+]}{[K_a + (H^+)]^2}$$

where C represents the molar concentrations of the acid and the salt.

(c) Thus, buffer capacity depends on the value of the ratio of the salt to the acid form. It increases as the ratio approaches unity; maximum buffer capacity occurs when $pH = pK_a$ and is represented by $\beta = 0.576\ C$.

B. Heterogeneous (disperse) systems

1. Introduction

a. A **suspension** is a two-phase system composed of a solid material dispersed in a liquid. The particle size of the dispersed solid is usually greater than 0.5 μm; the liquid can be oily or aqueous.

b. An **emulsion** is a heterogeneous system, consisting of at least one immiscible liquid intimately dispersed in another in the form of droplets (droplet diameter usually exceeds 0.1 μm). Emulsions are **inherently unstable** because the droplets of the dispersed liquid tend to coalesce to form large droplets until all of the dispersed droplets have coalesced. An **emulsifying agent,** the third component of the system, is used to prevent the coalescence and maintain the integrity of the individual droplets of dispersed liquid.

2. Dispersion stability. The dispersed particles in an **ideal dispersion** do not interact with one another, are uniform in size, and undergo no change in position other than the random movement resulting from Brownian motion. **Real** dispersions, on the other hand, are not usually uniformly sized (i.e., they are not **monodisperse**), are subject to particulate aggregation or clumping, and become more heterogeneous with time. The **rate of settling** (**separating** or **creaming**) of the dispersed phase in the dispersion medium is a function of the particle size, dispersion phase viscosity, and difference in density between the dispersed phase and the dispersion medium, in accordance with **Stokes' law:**

$$\text{Sedimentation rate} = \frac{d^2g(\rho_1 - \rho_2)}{18\ \eta}$$

where d is the particle diameter, g is the acceleration due to gravity, η is the viscosity of the dispersion medium, and $(\rho_1 - \rho_2)$ is the difference between the density of the particles (ρ_1) and the density of the dispersion medium (ρ_2). Although Stokes' law was derived for the settling or sedimentation of noninteracting spherical particles, it does provide guidance for dispersion stabilization:

a. Particle size should be as **small** as possible. Smaller particles yield slower sedimentation or flotation rates.

b. High particulate (dispersed phase) concentrations increase the rate of particle–particle collisions and interaction leading to partcle aggregation and increased instability as the aggregates behave as larger particles. In the case of liquid–liquid dispersions, particle–particle collisions can lead to coalescence (i.e., larger particles) and decreased dispersion stability. If the dispersed phase concentration is fixed, this might not be rectifiable.

c. Avoidance of particle–particle interactions

(1) Aggregation can be prevented if the particles have a similar electrical charge: particles in an aqueous system always have some electrical charge due to **ionization** of chemical groups on the particle surface or **adsorption** of molecules or ions at the interface. If the adsorbed species is an **ionic surfactant** (e.g., sodium lauryl sulfate), the charge associated with the surfactant ion (the lauryl sulfate anion, in this case) will accumulate at the interface; if a relatively non–surface-active electrolyte is adsorbed, however, the sign of the charge of the adsorbed ion is less readily predicted.

(2) The **magnitude of the charge** is the difference in electrical potential between the charged surface of the particle and the bulk of the dispersion medium and is approximated by the **electrokinetic** or **zeta potential** (ζ). The zeta potential is measured from the fixed, avidly bound layers of ions and solvent molecules on the particle surface. When ζ is high (e.g., 25 mV or more), interparticulate **repulsive forces** exceed the attractive forces and the dispersion is **deflocculated** and relatively stable to collision and subsequent aggregation **(flocculation)**. When ζ is sufficiently low that interparticulate **attractive forces** predominate, loose particle aggregates or **flocs** form (i.e., **flocculation** occurs).

d. **Density** can be manipulated to decrease the rate of dispersion instability: the settling rate decreases as $(\rho_1 - \rho_2)$ tends to zero. However, in few instances can the density of the dispersion medium be altered sufficiently to halt the settling (or flotation) process. Regarding the dispersed phase, solid particles' density is not readily altered, and liquid particles' density alteration would require the addition of a miscible liquid of higher (or lower) density. Also, composition alteration is problematic because most solid particles are denser than the dispersion medium; additives of higher (or lower) density might alter the biopharmaceutical characteristics of the formulation (e.g., drug-release rate; residence time at the administration or absorption site).

e. The sedimentation or **flotation rate** is inversely proportional to the **viscosity.** Thus, an **increase** in the **viscosity of the dispersion medium** will decrease the rate of settling or flotation. However, the rate of destabilization can be slowed down only by an increase in viscosity; it cannot be halted.

3. **Emulsion stability. Coalescence** is the phenomenon unique to emulsion systems whereby the liquid particles of the dispersed phase merge with each other to form larger particles. Coalescence is prevented, for the most part, by the **interfacial film** of surfactant around the droplets, which prevents direct contact of the liquid phase of the droplets. Droplet coalescence in o/w emulsions is also inhibited by the **electrostatic repulsion** of similarly charged particles. **Creaming** specifically refers to the **reversible** separation of a layer of emulsified particles. Mixing or shaking may be sufficient to reconstitute the emulsion system. Thus, creaming is not necessarily unacceptable. However, **cracking,** or **irreversible phase separation,** is never acceptable. **Phase inversion,** or emulsion-type reversal, involves the reversion of an emulsion from an o/w to a w/o form, or vice versa. The consequence of phase inversion can be a change in emulsion consistency or texture or a further deterioration in emulsion stability.

V. CHEMICAL KINETICS AND DRUG STABILITY

A. **Introduction.** The **stability** of a drug's **active component** is a major criterion in the rational design and evaluation of dosage forms for a drug. **Stability problems** can determine the acceptance or rejection of a given formulation.

1. Extensive chemical degradation of the active ingredient can cause **substantial loss** of active ingredient from the dosage form.
2. Chemical degradation can produce a **toxic product** with undesirable side effects.
3. Instability of the drug product can result in **decreased bioavailability,** which can lead to a substantial reduction in the therapeutic efficacy of the dosage form.

B. **Rates and orders of reactions**

1. **Rate of a reaction** (or degradation rate) is the velocity with which it occurs, expressed as dC/dt (the change in concentration, or C, within a given time interval, or dt).
   a. Reaction rates depend on conditions, such as **reactant concentration, temperature, pH,** and **presence of solvents or additives.** Radiation and catalytic agents, such as polyvalent cations, also have an effect.
   b. The effective study of reaction rates in the body requires application of **pharmacokinetic principles** (see Chapter 6).
2. **Order of a reaction** refers to the way in which the concentration of the drug or reactant in a chemical reaction influences the rate. The study of reaction orders is a crucial aspect of pharmacokinetics (see Chapter 6). Usually, **pharmaceutical degradation** can be treated

as a **zero-order,** a **first-order,** or **higher order reaction.** The first two are summarized below.

a. Zero-order reaction is one in which the **rate is independent of the concentration of the reactants** (see Chapter 6 V A 1 b for details). Other factors, such as absorption of light in certain photochemical reactions, determine the rate.

(1) A **zero-order reaction** can be expressed as:

$$C = -k_o t + C_o$$

where C is the drug concentration, k_o is the zero-order rate constant in units of concentration/time, t is the time, and C_o is the initial concentration.

(2) When this equation is plotted with C on the vertical axis (ordinate) against t on the horizontal axis (abcissa), the **slope of the line is equal to $-k_o$** (Figure 3-4). The negative sign indicates that the slope is decreasing.

b. First-order reaction is one in which the **rate depends on the first power of the concentration of a single reactant.**

(1) The **reaction rate** is directly proportional to the concentration of the reacting substance, according to this equation:

$$C = C_o e^{-kt}$$

where C is the concentration of the reacting material, C_o is the initial concentration, k is the first-order rate constant in units of reciprocal time, and t is time.

(2) In a first-order reaction, **drug concentration decreases exponentially with time.** A plot of the logarithm of concentration against time produces a straight line with a slope of $-k/2.303$ (Figure 3-5).

(3) The **half-life** of a reaction is the period of time required for the concentration of a drug to decrease by one-half ($t_{1/2}$). For a first-order reaction, this is expressed by:

$$t_{1/2} = \frac{0.693}{k}$$

(4) The **time required for 10% of a drug to degrade** ($t_{90\%}$) is also important, as it represents a reasonable limit of degradation for the active ingredients. The $t_{90\%}$ can be calculated as:

$$t_{10\%} = \frac{2.303}{k} \log \frac{100}{90} = \frac{0.104}{k}$$

(a) Because

$$k = \frac{0.693}{t_{1/2}}$$

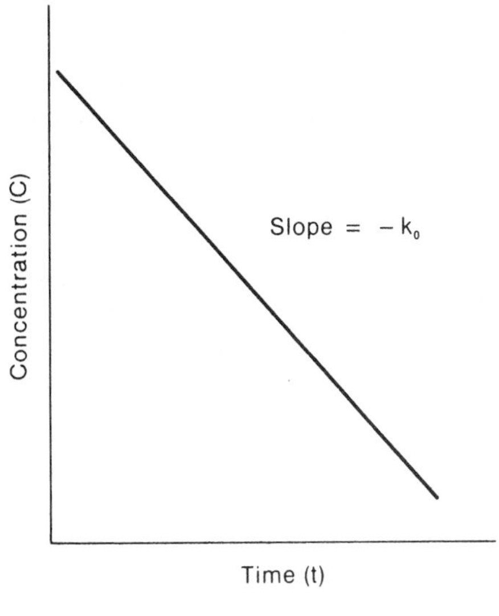

Figure 3-4. Linear plot of concentration *(C)* versus time *(t)* for a zero-order reaction. The slope of the line is equal to $-k_o$.
(Note: The slope of the line is **not** equal to the rate constant because it includes the minus sign.)

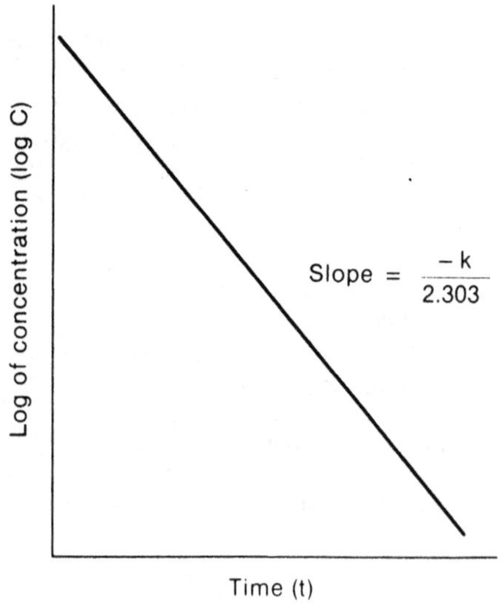

Figure 3-5. Linear plot of the logarithm of concentration *(log C)* versus time *(t)* for a first-order reaction. The slope of the line is equal to $^{-}k/2.303$.

(b) Then

$$t_{10\%} = \frac{0.104}{0.693/t_{1/2}} = 0.152t_{1/2}$$

(5) Both $t_{1/2}$ and $t_{90\%}$ are **concentration-independent;** that is, it takes the same amount of time to reduce the concentration of the drug from 100% to 50% as it does from 50% to 25%.

C. Factors affecting reaction rates. Factors other than concentration can affect a drug's reaction rate and stability. Among these are temperature, the presence of a solvent, pH, and the presence of additives.

1. Temperature. An **increase in temperature** causes an increase in reaction rate, as expressed in the equation first suggested by Arrhenius:

$$k = Ae^{-Ea/RT} \text{ or } \log k = \log A - \frac{Ea}{2.303} \times \frac{1}{RT}$$

where k is the specific reaction rate constant, A is a constant known as the frequency factor, Ea is the energy of activation, R is the gas constant (1.987 cal/degree x mole), and T is the absolute temperature.

a. The **constants A and Ea** may be obtained by determining k at several temperatures and then plotting log k against 1/T. The slope of the resulting line equals $-Ea/2.303R$, and the intercept on the vertical axis equals log A.

b. The activation energy (Ea) is the amount of energy required to put the molecules in an **activated state**—molecules must be activated to react. As **temperature increases,** more molecules are activated and the **reaction rate increases.**

2. Presence of solvent. Many dosage forms require the incorporation of a water-miscible solvent [low molecular-weight alcohols, such as the polyethylene glycols (PEGs)] to stabilize the drug.

a. In addition to **altering the activity coefficients** of the reactant molecules and the transition state, a change in the solvent system can bring about simultaneous changes in such physicochemical parameters as pK_a, surface tension, and viscosity, **indirectly affecting the reaction rate.**

b. In some cases, **additional reaction pathways** may also be generated. For example, with an increasing concentration of ethanol in the solvent, aspirin degrades by means of an extra route, forming the ethyl ester of acetylsalicylic acid. However, a **change in solvent also can stabilize the drug.**

3. Change in pH. The magnitude of the rate of a hydrolytic reaction catalyzed by H^+ and OH^- can vary considerably with pH.

a. **H^+ catalysis** predominates at **lower pH,** whereas **OH^- catalysis** operates at **higher pH.** At **intermediate pH,** the rate may be **pH-independent** or it may be catalyzed by **both H^+ and OH^-.** (Rate constants in the intermediate pH range are generally less than those at higher or lower pH values, however.)

b. To determine the **influence of pH on degradation kinetics,** decomposition is measured at several H^+ concentrations. The **pH of optimum stability** can be determined by plotting the logarithm of the rate constant (k) versus pH (Figure 3-6). The **point of inflection** of such a plot represents the pH of optimum stability, useful in the development of a stable dosage formulation.

4. **Presence of additives**

a. **Buffer salts** must be added to many drug solutions to maintain the formulation at optimum pH. These salts **can affect the rate of degradation,** primarily from salt increasing the ionic strength.

(1) Increasing salt concentrations (particularly from polyelectrolytes such as citrate and phosphate) can **substantially affect the magnitude of pK_a,** causing a change in the rate constant.

(2) Buffer salts can also **promote drug degradation** through general acid or base catalysis.

b. **Addition of surfactant agents** may accelerate or decelerate drug degradation.

(1) **Acceleration of degradation** is frequently observed due to micellar catalysis.

(2) **Stabilization of a drug** through addition of a surfactant is less frequently observed.

c. **Complexing agents** can improve drug stability. Aromatic esters such as benzocaine, procaine, hydrochloride, and tetracaine **increase in half-life** in the presence of caffeine. This increased stability appears to result from the formation of a less reactive complex between the aromatic ester and caffeine.

D. **Modes of pharmaceutical degradation.** The decomposition of active ingredients in a dosage form can occur through several pathways (e.g., hydrolysis, oxidation, photolysis). (For details, see Chapter 12, II A.)

1. **Hydrolysis** is the most frequent type of degradation because many medicinal compounds are esters, amides, or lactams.

a. **H^+ and OH^-** are the most common catalysts of hydrolytic degradation in solution.

b. **Esters** most frequently undergo hydrolytic reactions that result in drug instability. Because esters are rapidly degraded in aqueous solution, formulators are reluctant to incorporate drugs having ester functional groups into liquid dosage forms.

2. **Oxidation** is mediated usually through reaction with atmospheric oxygen under ambient conditions (auto-oxidation).

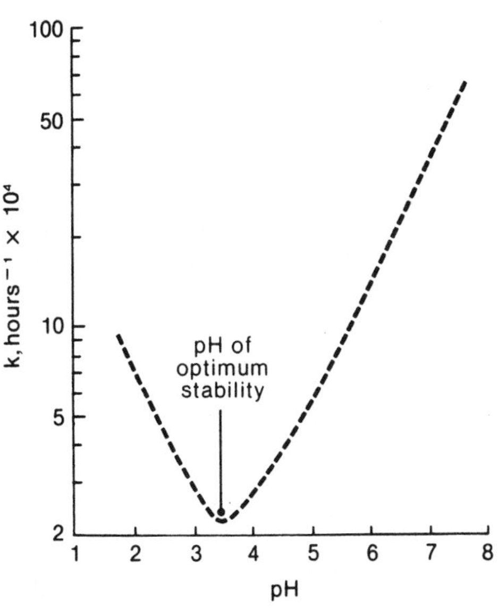

Figure 3-6. A plot of the logarithm of the rate constant *(k)* versus *pH,* used to determine the pH of optimum stability.

a. Medicinal compounds that undergo auto-oxidation at room temperature are affected by **oxygen dissolved in the solvent** and in the void space of their packages. These compounds should be packed under an **inert atmosphere** (e.g., nitrogen, carbon dioxide) to exclude air from their containers.

b. Most oxidation reactions involve a **free radical mechanism** and a **chain reaction.** (Free radicals tend to take electrons from other compounds.)

(1) **Antioxidants** in the formulation react with the free radicals by providing electrons and easily available hydrogen atoms, thus preventing the propagation of chain reactions.

(2) **Commonly used antioxidants** include ascorbic acid, butylated hydroxyanisole (BHA), butylated hydroxytoluene (BHT), propyl gallate, sodium bisulfite, sodium sulfite, and the tocopherols.

3. **Photolysis** is the degradation of drug molecules by normal sunlight or room light.

a. Molecules may absorb the proper wavelength of light and **acquire sufficient energy to undergo reaction.** Generally, photolytic degradation occurs upon exposure to light of wavelengths less than 40 μm.

b. An **amber glass bottle** or an **opaque container** acts as a barrier to this light, preventing or retarding photolysis. For example, sodium nitroprusside in aqueous solution has a shelf life of only 4 hours if exposed to normal room light. When protected from light, the solution is stable for at least 1 year.

E. **Determination of shelf life.** The shelf life of a drug preparation is the length of storage time before the preparation becomes unfit for use, through either chemical decomposition or physical deterioration.

1. **Storage temperature** affects shelf life and is generally understood to be ambient temperature unless special storage conditions are given.

2. **In general, a preparation is considered fit for use if it varies from the nominal concentration or dose by no more than ±5%,** provided the decomposition products are not more toxic or harmful than the original material.

3. **Shelf-life testing** aids in determining a formulation's standard shelf life.

a. Samples are stored at about 3°C–5°C and at room temperature (20°C–25°C). They are then analyzed at various time intervals to determine the **rate of decomposition,** from which shelf life can be calculated.

b. Because storage time at these temperatures can result in an extended testing time, **accelerated testing** is conducted as well, using a range of higher temperatures. The **rate constants** obtained from these samples are used to predict shelf life at ambient or refrigeration temperatures. **Temperature-accelerated stability testing** is not useful if temperature changes are accompanied by changes in the reaction mechanism or by physical changes in the system (e.g., solid to liquid phase change).

c. **Prediction of stability at room temperature** can be obtained from accelerated testing data by the Arrhenius equation:

$$\log \frac{k_2}{k_1} = \frac{Ea(T_2 - T_1)}{2.303\ RT_2T_1}$$

where k_2 and k_1 are the rate constants at the absolute temperatures T_2 and T_1, respectively, R is the gas constant, and Ea is the energy of activation.

d. As an **alternate method,** an expression of concentration can be plotted as a linear function of time. Rate constants (k) for degradation at several temperatures are obtained; the logarithm of the rate constant (log k) is then plotted against the reciprocal of absolute temperature (1/T) to obtain, by extrapolation, the rate constant for degradation at room temperature (Figure 3-7).

e. The **length of time the drug will maintain its required potency** can also be predicted by calculation of the drug's $t_{90\%}$ [see VI B]. This method applies to chemical reactions with activation energies in the range of 10–30 kcal/mol, which is the magnitude of the activation energy for many pharmaceutical degradations occurring in solution.

VI. DRUG DOSAGE FORMS

A. **Oral solutions. USP 23/NF 18** categorizes **oral solutions** as "liquid preparations, intended for oral administration, that contain one or more substances with or without flavoring, sweetening,

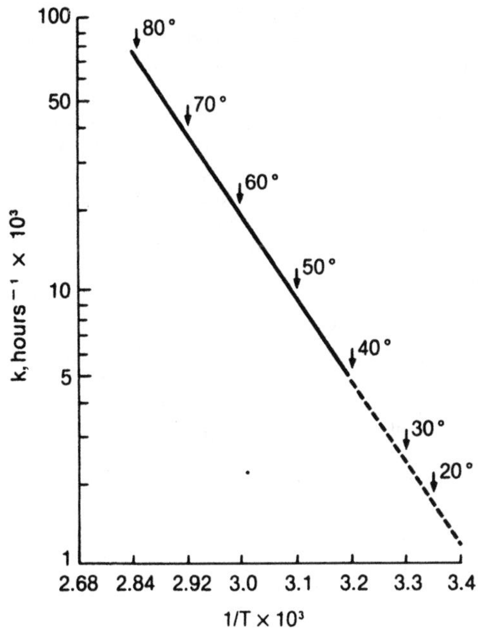

Figure 3-7. A plot of the logarithm of the rate constant *(k)* versus the reciprocal of absolute temperature *(1/T)*, showing the temperature dependency of degradation rates.

or coloring agents dissolved in water or cosolvent water mixtures." Oral solutions can contain certain polyols, such as sorbitol or glycerin, to inhibit crystallization and to modify solubility, taste, mouth feel, and other vehicle properties. They can be "formulated for direct oral administration to the patient or they may be dispensed in a more concentrated form that must be diluted prior to administration...." **Drugs in solution** are more homogeneous and easier to swallow than drugs in solid form. For drugs with a slow dissolution rate, onset of action and bioavailability are also improved. However, drugs in solution comprise bulkier dosage forms, degrade more rapidly, and are more likely to interact with constituents than those in solid form.

1. **Water** is the **most commonly used vehicle** for drug solutions. The **USP** recognizes six types of water for the preparation of dosage forms:
   a. **Purified water USP** is water obtained by distillation, ion exchange, reverse osmosis, or other suitable treatment. It cannot contain more than 10 parts per million (ppm) of total solid and should have a pH between 5 and 7. Purified water is used in prescriptions and finished manufactured products except parenteral and ophthalmic products.
   b. **Water for injection USP** conforms to the standards of purified water but is also free of pyrogen. It is used as a solvent for the preparation of parenteral solutions.
   c. **Sterile water for injection USP** is water for injection that has been sterilized and packaged in single-dose containers of type I and II glass that do not exceed a capacity of 1L. The limitations for total solids depend upon the size of the container.
   d. **Bacteriostatic water for injection USP** is sterile water for injection that contains one or more suitable bacteriostatic agents. It is also packaged in a single- or multiple-dose container of type I or II glass that does not exceed the capacity of 30 ml.
   e. **Sterile water for inhalation USP** is water purified by distillation or by reverse osmosis and rendered sterile. It contains no antimicrobial agents, except where used in humidifiers or other similar devices. It should not be used for parenteral administration or for other sterile dosage forms.
   f. **Sterile water for irrigation USP** is water for injection sterilized and suitably packaged. It contains no antimicrobial agent or other added substance.

2. **Oral drug solutions** include **syrups** and **elixirs** as well as other less widely prescribed classic (**Galenical**) formulations such as **aromatic waters, tinctures, fluidextracts,** and **spirits.**
   a. The term ***syrups*** traditionally has designated peroral solutions containing high concentrations of sucrose or other sugars. Through common usage, the term *syrup* has also come to include any other liquid dosage form prepared in a sweet, viscous vehicle; even peroral suspensions have been described as syrups.
      (1) **Syrup NF (simple syrup)** is a concentrated or nearly saturated aqueous solution of sugar (85% w/v).

(2) Syrups have a **low solvent capacity for water-soluble drugs** because the hydrogen bonding between sucrose and water is very strong. For this reason, it can be difficult or impossible to dissolve a drug in a syrup; often the drug is best dissolved in a small quantity of water to which the flavoring syrup is then added.

(3) The **sucrose concentration** of syrup plays a crucial role in the control of microbial growth. Dilute sucrose solutions are excellent media for microorganisms. As the concentration of sucrose approaches saturation, the syrup becomes self-preserving (i.e., it requires no additional preservative). However, a saturated solution is undesirable because the temperature fluctuations may cause crystallization. **Syrup USP** is a self-preserved solution with a minimal tendency to undergo crystallization.

b. The term ***elixirs*** traditionally has designated peroral solutions which contain alcohol as a cosolvent. Many peroral solutions are not described as elixirs but do, nonetheless, contain alcohol.

(1) To be termed an elixir, the solution **must contain alcohol.** Traditionally, the alcohol content of elixirs has varied from 5%–40%. Most elixirs become turbid when moderately diluted by aqueous liquids. Elixirs are not the preferred vehicle for salts as alcohol accentuates saline taste. Salts also have limited solubility in alcohol; therefore, the alcoholic content of salt-containing elixirs must be low.

(2) **Aromatic elixir NF,** prepared in part from syrup, contains about 22% alcohol. Its limited utility as a solvent for drugs was offset by the development of **iso-alcoholic elixir.** It consists of a low alcoholic elixir (8%–10% alcohol) and a high alcoholic elixir (75%–78% alcohol). By mixing appropriate volumes of the two elixirs, an alcoholic content sufficient to dissolve the drugs can be obtained.

B. Miscellaneous solutions

1. **Aromatic waters** are clear, **saturated aqueous solutions of volatile oils** or other aromatic or volatile substances. Aromatic waters may be used as pleasantly flavored vehicles for a water-soluble drug or as an aqueous phase in an emulsion or suspension. If a large amount of water-soluble drug is added to an aromatic water, an insoluble layer may form at the top. This **"salting out"** is a competitive process in which the molecules of water-soluble drugs have more attraction for the solvent molecules of water than the more volatile oil molecules. The associated water molecules are pulled away from the volatile oil molecules, which are no longer held in solution. Aromatic waters should be stored in tight, light-resistant bottles to reduce volatilization and degradation from sunlight. Aromatic waters are generally prepared by any of the following methods:

   a. Distillation—a universal method, but one which is not practical or economical for most products. It is the only method, however, for preparing strong rose water and orange flower water.

   b. Solution method—the volatile or aromatic substance is admixed with water, with or without the use of a dispersant such as talc.

2. **Spirits** (also called **essences**) are alcoholic or hydroalcoholic solutions of volatile substances containing 50%–90% alcohol. This **high alcoholic content** maintains the water-insoluble volatile oils in solution. If water is added to a spirit, the oils separate. Some spirits are **medicinal spirits** (e.g., aromatic ammonia spirit); many spirits (e.g., compound orange spirit, compound cardamom spirit) are used as flavoring agents. Spirits should be stored in tight containers to reduce loss by evaporation.

3. **Tinctures** are alcoholic or hydroalcoholic solutions of chemicals or soluble constituents of vegetable drugs. Although tinctures vary in drug concentration (up to 50%), those prepared from potent drugs are usually 10% in strength (i.e., 100 ml of the tincture has the activity of 10 g of the drug). Generally, tinctures are considered to be stable preparations. The alcohol content among the official tinctures varies from 17%–21% with opium tincture USP and from 74%–80% in compound benzoin tincture USP. Most tinctures are prepared by an **extraction process** of maceration or percolation. The selection of a **solvent** (also known as menstruum) is based on the solubility of the active and inert constituents of the crude drugs. Inactive constituents of tinctures can precipitate upon aging. Glycerin may be added to the hydroalcoholic solvent to increase the solubility of the active constituent and to reduce precipitation upon storage. Tinctures must be tightly stoppered and kept from excessive temperatures. Because many of the constituents found in tinctures undergo a photochemical change upon exposure to light, they must be stored in light-resistant containers.

4. **Fluidextracts** are liquid extracts of vegetable drugs containing alcohol as a solvent, preservative, or both. Fluidextracts are prepared by percolation so that each milliliter contains the therapeutic constituents of 1g of the standard drug. Due to their high alcohol content, fluidextracts are sometimes referred to as "100% tinctures." Fluidextracts of potent drugs are usually 10 times as concentrated (or potent) as the corresponding tincture (e.g., the usual dose of tincture belladonna is 0.6 ml; the equivalent dose of the more potent fluidextract would be 0.06 ml): many fluidextracts are considered too potent for self-administration by patients so they are almost never prescribed. In addition, many fluidextracts are simply too bitter. Today, therefore, most fluidextracts are modified by either flavoring or sweetening agents.

5. **Nasal, ophthalmic, otic,** and **parenteral solutions** are solutions; however, they are classified separately because of their specific use and method of preparation.

6. **Mouthwashes** are solutions used for cleansing the mouth or treating diseased conditions of the oral mucous membrane. They frequently contain alcohol or glycerin to aid in dissolving the volatile ingredients and are more often used cosmetically than therapeutically.

7. **Astringents** are locally applied solutions that precipitate protein, reducing cell permeability without injury. Astringents cause **constriction** with wrinkling of the skin and blanching. Because astringents **reduce secretions,** they can be used as antiperspirants.
   a. **Aluminum acetate** and **aluminum subacetate solutions** are used as wet dressings in contact dermatitis. The precipitation is minimized by the addition of boric acid.
   b. **Calcium hydroxide solution** is a mild astringent employed in lotions as a reactant and an alkalizer.

8. **Antibacterial topical solutions** (e.g., benzalkonium chloride, strong iodine, and povidone–iodine solutions) kill bacteria when applied to the skin or mucous membrane in the proper strength and under appropriate conditions.

C. Suspensions

1. **Lotions, magmas** (i.e., suspensions of finely divided material in a small amount of water), and **mixtures** are all suspensions that have had official formulas for some time (e.g., calamine lotion USP, kaolin mixture with pectin NF). Official formulas are given in the USP/NF.
   a. A **complete formula** and a **detailed method of preparation** are available for some official suspensions, whereas only the **concentration** for the active ingredients is given for others, allowing the manufacturer considerable latitude in the formulation.
   b. Some drugs are provided in a package in a **dry form** to circumvent the instability of aqueous dispersions. Water is added at the time of dispensing to complete the suspension.

2. **Purposes of suspension**
   a. **Sustaining effect.** For a sustained release preparation, suspension introduces a dissolution or diffusion step as the drug goes from solid form to solution form to final absorption.
   b. **Stability.** Drug degradation in suspension or solid dosage forms occurs much more slowly than degradation in solution form.
   c. **Taste.** A bad-tasting material can be converted into an insoluble form and then prepared as a suspension, obviating the taste problem.
   d. **Basic solubility.** When suitable solvents are not available, the suspension provides an alternative. For example, only water can be used as a solvent for ophthalmic preparations because of the possibility of corneal damage. Ophthalmic suspensions provide an alternative.

3. **Suspending agents** include hydrophilic colloids, clays, and a few other agents. Some of these are also used as **emulsifying agents** (see VI D).
   a. **Hydrophilic colloids** increase the viscosity of water by binding water molecules, thus limiting their mobility or fluidity. Viscosity is proportional to the concentration of the colloid. These agents **support the growth of microorganisms** and require a preservative. They are mostly **anionic** [with the exception of methyl cellulose (neutral) and chitosan (cationic)] and, thus, incompatible with quaternary antibacterial agents and other positively charged drugs. Most are **insoluble in alcoholic solutions.**
      (1) **Acacia** is usually used as the mucilage (35% dispersion in water). Viscosity is greatest between pH 5 and 9. It is susceptible to microbial decomposition.

(2) **Tragacanth** is usually used as a 6% dispersion in water (mucilage) and has an advantage over acacia in that less is needed. Also, tracanth does not contain the oxidase present in acacia, which catalyzes the decomposition of organic chemicals. Its viscosity is greatest at pH 5.

(3) **Methyl cellulose** is a polymer that is nonionic and stable to heat and light. It is available in several viscosity grades. Because it is soluble in cold water but not in hot water, dispersions are prepared by adding the material to boiling water and then cooling the preparation until the material dissolves.

(4) **Carboxymethylcellulose** is an anionic material that is soluble in water and available in three viscosity grades. Prolonged exposure to heat causes loss of viscosity.

b. **Clays** (e.g., bentonite, Veegum) are silicates that are anionic in aqueous dispersions. Strongly hydrated, they exhibit **thixotropy** (the property of forming a gel-like structure on standing and becoming fluid on agitation).

(1) **Bentonite's** official form is as the 5% magma.

(2) **Veegum** is hydrated to a greater degree than bentonite and, thus, is more viscous at the same concentration.

c. **Other agents** include agar, chondrus (carrageenan), gelatin, pectin, and gelatinized starch. The use of all these is limited by their susceptibility to bacterial attack, their incompatibilities, and their cost. Xanthan gum is used in many modern suspension formulations because of its stability and product excellence.

4. **Preparation**

a. **Solids are wetted initially** to separate individual particles and coat them with a layer of dispersion medium. Wetting is accomplished by **levigation** (i.e., the addition of a suitable nonsolvent, or **levigating agent,** to the solid material, followed by blending to form a paste), using a glass mortar and pestle; or a **surfactant** can be used.

b. **Suspending agents** are then added as dry powder along with the active ingredient. For best results, however, the suspending agent should be added in the form of its **aqueous dispersion.**

(1) This dispersion can be added to the solid (or the levigated solid) by way of **geometric dilution** to ensure proper dispersion.

(2) The preparation is then brought to the desired volume by stirring in the appropriate vehicle.

D. Emulsions

1. **Purposes of emulsions**

a. **Increased drug solubility.** Many drugs have limited aqueous solubility but have maximum solubility in the oil phase of an emulsion. Through partitioning of drug from the oil phase to the water phase, activity can be maintained or enhanced.

b. **Increased drug stability.** Many drugs are more stable when incorporated into an emulsion rather than an aqueous solution.

c. **Prolonged drug action.** Incorporation of a drug into an emulsion can prolong bioavailability, as with certain intramuscular injection preparations.

d. **Improved taste.** Objectionable medicinal agents are more palatable in emulsion form and, thus, more conveniently administered.

e. **Improved appearance.** Oleaginous materials intended for topical applications are more appealing in an emusified form.

2. **Phases of emulsions.** Most emulsions are considered to be **two-phase systems.**

a. The **liquid droplet** is known as the **dispersed phase,** the **internal phase,** or the **discontinuous phase.** The other liquid is known as the **dispersion medium,** the **external phase** or the **continuous phase.**

b. In pharmaceutical applications, one of the phases is usually an **aqueous solution,** and the other phase is usually **lipid** or **oily** in nature. The lipids range from vegetable or hydrocarbon oils to semisolid hydrocarbons and waxes. Emulsions are described conventionally in terms of water and oil, where oil represents the lipid or nonaqueous phase, regardless of its composition.

(1) If water is the **internal phase,** the emulsion is classified as a **water-in-oil (w/o)** type.

(2) If water is the **external phase,** the emulsion is classified as an **oil-in-water (o/w)** type.

c. The **type of emulsion** formed is primarily determined by the **relative phase volumes** and the **emulsifying agent** used.

(1) For an ideal emulsion, the maximum concentration of internal phase is 74% (i.e., an o/w emulsion can theoretically be prepared containing up to but not more than 74% oil).
(2) Choice of an emulsifying agent is perhaps more important in determining the final emulsion type. Most agents preferentially form one type of emulsion or the other if the phase volume permits.

3. **Emulsifying agents.** Any compound that lowers the interfacial tension and forms a film at the interface can potentially function as an emulsifying agent. The effectiveness of the emulsifying agent depends on its chemical structure, concentration, solubility, pH, physical properties, and electrostatic effect. **True emulsifying agents** (primary agents) are capable of forming and stabilizing emulsions by themselves. **Stabilizers** (auxiliary agents) do not form acceptable emulsions when used alone but do assist primary agents in stabilizing the product (e.g., they can increase viscosity). Emulsifying agents are **natural** or **synthetic.**

a. **Natural emulsifying agents:**

(1) **Acacia** forms a good stable emulsion of low viscosity that tends to cream easily, is acidic, and is stable at a pH range of 2–10. Like other gums, it is negatively charged, dehydrates easily, and generally requires a preservative. It is incompatible with Peruvian balsam, bismuth salts, and carbonates.
(2) **Tragacanth** forms a stable emulsion that is coarser than acacia emulsion. It is anionic, difficult to hydrate, and used mainly for its viscosity effects. Less than 1/10 of the amount used for acacia is needed.
(3) **Agar** is an anionic gum primarily used to increase viscosity. Its stability is affected by heating, dehydration, and destruction of charge. It is also susceptible to microbial degradation.
(4) **Pectin** is a quasi-emusifier that is used in the same proportion as tragacanth.
(5) **Gelatin** provides good emulsion stabilization in the concentration range of 0.5%–1.0%. It may be anionic or cationic, depending upon its isoelectric point. Type A gelatin (+) is used in acidic media; type B gelatin (−), in basic media.
(6) **Methyl cellulose** is nonionic and induces viscosity. It is used as a primary emulsifier with mineral oil and cod liver oil and yields an o/w emulsion. It is usually used in 2% concentration and forms a continuous film.
(7) **Carboxymethylcellulose** is anionic and usually used to increase viscosity. It tolerates alcohol up to 40%. It forms a basic solution and precipitates in the presence of free acids.

b. **Synthetic emulsifying agents** are anionic, catinic, or nonionic.

(1) **Anionic** synthetic agents include **sulfuric acid esters** (e.g., sodium lauryl sulfate), **sulfonic acid derivatives** (e.g., dioctyl sodium sulfosuccinate), and **soaps.** Soaps are for external use. They have a high pH and, therefore, are sensitive to the addition of acids and electrolytes.
 (a) **Alkali soaps** are hydrophilic and form o/w emulsion.
 (b) **Metallic soaps** are water insoluble and form w/o emulsion.
 (c) **Monovalent soaps** form w/o emulsion.
 (d) **Polyvalent soaps** form w/o emulsion.
(2) **Cationic** synthetic agents (e.g., benzalkonium chloride) are used as surface-active agents in 1% concentration. They are incompatible with soaps.
(3) **Nonionic** synthetic agents are resistant to the addition of acids and electrolytes (Table 3-1).
 (a) The **sorbitan esters** known as **Spans** are hydrophobic in nature and form w/o emulsions. They have low hydrophilic–lipophilic balance (HLB) values (1–9) [Table 3-2].

Table 3–1. Hydrophilic-Lipophilic Balance (HLB)

HLB Value Range	Surfactant Application
0–3	Antifoaming agents
4–6	Water-in-oil emulsifying agents
7–9	Wetting agents
8–18	Oil-in-water emulsifying agents
13–15	Detergents
10–18	Solubilizing agents

Table 3-2. Commonly Used Surfactants and Their Hydrophilic–Lipophilic Balance (HLB) Values

Agent	HLB Value
Sorbitan trioleate (span 85, Arlacel 85)	1.8
Sorbitan tristearate (span 65)	2.1
Propylene glycol monostearate (pure)	3.4
Sorbitan sesquioleate (Arlacel C)	3.7
Sorbitan monooleate (span 80y)	4.3
Sorbitan monostearate (Arlacel 60)	4.7
Sorbitan monopalmitate (span 40, Arlacel 40)	6.7
Sorbitan monolaurate (span 20, Arlacel 20)	8.6
Glyceryl monostearate (Aldo 28, Tegin)	5.5
Gelatin	9.8
Triethanolamine oleate (Trolamine)	12.0
Polyoxyethylene alkyl phenol (Igepal CA-630)	12.8
Tragacanth	13.2
Polyoxyethylene sorbitan monolaurate (Tween 21)	13.3
Polyoxyethylene castor oil (Atlas G-1794)	13.3
Polyoxyethylene sorbitan monooleate (Tween 80)	15.0
Polyoxyethylene sorbitan monopalmitate (Tween 40)	15.6
Polyoxyethylene sorbitan monolaurate (Tween 20)	16.7
Polyoxyethylene lauryl ether (Brij 35)	16.9
Polyoxyethylene monostearate (Myrj 52)	16.9
Sodium oleate	18
Sodium lauryl sulfate	40

(b) The **polysorbates** known as **Tweens** are hydrophilic in nature and tend to form o/w emulsions. They may form complexes with phenolic compounds. They have high HLB values (11–20).

4. Preparation. Emulsions are prepared by the following four methods:

a. Wet gum method (the **English method**). A primary emulsion of fixed oil, water, and acacia (in a 4 to 2 to 1 ratio) is prepared as follows:

(1) Two parts of water are added all at once to one part of acacia, and the mixture is triturated until a smooth mucilage is formed.

(2) Then, oil is added in small increments (1–5 ml) with continuous trituration until the primary emulsion is formed.

(3) The mixture (an o/w emulsion) is triturated for another 5 minutes.

(4) The mixture (o/w) can be brought to volume with water and mixing.

b. Dry gum method (also called the **Continental method**). A primary emulsion of the fixed oil, water, and acacia (in a 4 to 2 to 1 ratio) is prepared as follows:

(1) Oil is added to the acacia, and the mixture is triturated until the powder is distributed uniformly throughout the oil. Water is added all at once, followed by rapid trituration to form the primary emulsion.

(2) Any remaining water and other ingredients are added to finish the product.

(a) Electrolytes in high concentration tend to crack an emulsion; thus, they should be added last in as dilute a form as possible.

(b) Alcoholic solutions, which tend to dehydrate and precipitate hydrocolloids, should be added in as dilute a concentration as possible.

c. Bottle method (a variation of dry gum method used for volatile oils). Oil is added to the acacia in a bottle. The ratio of oil, water, and acacia should be 3 to 2 to 1 or 2 to 1 to 1, as the low viscosity of the volatile oil requires a higher proportion of acacia.

d. Nascent soap method. A soap is formed by mixing relatively equal volumes of an oil and an aqueous solution containing a sufficient amount of alkali. The soap thus formed acts as an emulsifying agent.

(1) This method can be used for forming an o/w or w/o emulsion, depending on the soap formed. For example, olive oil, which contains oleic acid, and lime water are mixed during the preparation of calamine lotion to calcium oleate, an emulsifying agent.

(2) A 50 to 50 ratio of oil to water ensures sufficient emulsifying agent, provided the oil contains an adequate amount of free fatty acid. (Olive oil usually does; cottonseed oil, peanut oil, and some other vegetable oils do not.)

(3) The addition of an acid destroys the emulsifying soap, causing separation of the emulsion.

5. **Incorporation of medicinal agents.** Medicinal agents can be incorporated into an emulsion either during the formation of the emulsion or after the emulsion is formed.
   a. **Addition of a drug during emulsion formation.** Generally, it is best to incorporate a drug into a vehicle during emulsion formation when it can be incorporated in molecular form. Soluble drugs should be dissolved in the appropriate phase (e.g., drugs soluble in the external phase of the emulsion should be added as a solution to the primary emulsion).
   b. **Addition of a drug to a preformed emulsion** can present some difficulty, which is overcome by keeping in mind the type of emulsion and nature of the emulsifier (Table 3-3).
      (1) **Addition of oleagenous materials to a w/o emulsion** presents no problem because of the miscibility of the additive with the external phase, but **addition of oleagenous materials to an o/w emulsion** can be difficult after emulsion formation.
         (a) Occasionally, a small amount of oily material is added, if some excess emulsifier was used in the original formation.
         (b) A small quantity of an oil-soluble drug can be added if it is dissolved in a very small quantity of oil by using geometric dilution techniques.
      (2) Addition of **water** or **an aqueous material** to a w/o emulsion is extremely difficult, unless enough emulsifier has been incorporated into the emulsion, but **addition of aqueous materials to an o/w emulsion** usually presents no problems if the added material does not interact with the emulsifying agent. Potential interactions should be expected with cationic compounds and salts of weak bases.
      (3) **Additions of small quantities of alcoholic solutions to an o/w emulsion** is possible, provided the solute is compatible or dispersible in the aqueous phase of the emulsion. If acacia or other gum is used as the emulsifying agent, the alcoholic solution should be diluted with water before addition. Some commercial emulsion bases and their general composition are given in Table 3-3.
      (4) **Addition of crystalline drugs to a w/o emulsion** occurs more easily if they are dissolved or dispersed in a small quantity of oil before addition.

E. Ointments

1. **Introduction. Ointments** are **semisolid preparations intended for external use.** They are easily spread; their plastic viscosity is controlled by modification of the formulation. Ointments are typically used as:
   a. **Emollients,** which make the skin more pliable
   b. **Protective barriers,** which prevent harmful substances from coming in contact with the skin
   c. **Vehicles** in which to incorporate medication

Table 3-3. Selected Commercial Emulsion Bases: Emulsion Type and Emulsifier Used

Commercial Base	Emulsion Type	Emulsifier Type
Allercreme Skin Lotion	o/w	Triethanolamine stearate
Almay Emulsion Base	o/w	Fatty acid glycol esters
Cetaphil	o/w	Sodium lauryl sulfate
Dermovan	o/w	Fatty acid amides
Eucerin	w/o	Wool wax alcohol
HEB Base	o/w	Sodium lauryl sulfate
Keri Lotion	o/w	Nonionic emulsifiers
Lubriderm	o/w	Triethanolamine stearate
Neobase	o/w	Polyhydric alcohol esters
Neutragena Lotion	o/w	Triethanolamine lactate
Nivea Cream	w/o	Wool wax alcohols
pHorsix	o/w	Polyoxyethylene emulsifiers
Polysorb Hydrate	w/o	Sodium sesquioleate
Velvachol	o/w	Sodium lauryl sulfate

w/o = water-in-oil
o/w = oil-in-water

2. **Ointment bases**

a. **Oleaginous bases** are anhydrous and insoluble in water; They cannot absorb or contain water and are not washable in water.

(1) **Petrolatum** is a good base for oil-insoluble ingredients. It forms an occlusive film on the skin, absorbs less than 5% water under normal conditions, and does not become rancid. Wax can be incorporated to stiffen the base.

(2) **Synthetic esters** are used as oleagenous base constituents, including glyceryl monostearate, isopropyl myristate, isopropyl palmitate, butyl stearate, and butyl palmitate. Long-chain alcohols, such as cetyl alcohol, stearyl alcohol, and polyethylene glycol (PEG), can be used also.

(3) **Lanolin derivatives** are commonly used in topical and cosmetic preparations. Examples include lanolin oil and hydrogenated lanolin.

b. **Absorption bases** are anhydrous, water-insoluble, and, therefore, not washable in water; however, these bases can absorb water. They permit the inclusion of water-soluble medicaments through prior solution and uptake of the solution as the internal phase.

(1) **Wool fat** (anhydrous lanolin) contains a high percentage of cholesterol as well as esters and alcohol containing fatty acids. It absorbs twice its weight in water and melts between 36°C and 42°C.

(2) **Hydrophilic petrolatum** is a white petrolatum combined with 8% beeswax, 3% stearyl alcohol, and 3% cholesterol, which are added to a w/o emulsifier. Prepared forms include Aquaphor, which employs wool alcohol to render white petrolatum emulsifiable. Aquaphor is superior in its ability to absorb water.

c. **Emulsion bases** may be w/o emulsions, which are water insoluble and not washable in water but can absorb because of their aqueous internal phase, or o/w emulsions, which are water insoluble but washable in water and able to absorb water in their aqueous external phase.

(1) **Hydrous wool fat** (lanolin) is a w/o emulsion containing about 25% water. It acts as an emollient and occlusive film on the skin, effectively preventing epidermal water loss.

(2) **Cold cream** is a w/o emulsion prepared by melting white wax, spermaceti, and expressed almond oil together, adding hot aqueous solution of sodium borate, and stirring until cool.

(a) Use of mineral oil rather than almond oil makes a more stable cold cream; however, cold cream prepared with almond oil makes a better emollient base.

(b) This ointment should be freshly prepared.

(3) **Hydrophilic ointment** is an o/w emulsion employing sodium lauryl sulfate as an emulsifying agent. It absorbs about 30%–50% w/w without losing consistency. It is readily miscible with water and, thus, can be removed from the skin easily.

(4) **Vanishing cream** is an o/w emulsion, which contains a large percentage of water as well as humectant (e.g., glycerin, propylene glycol), which retards surface evaporation of the product. An excess of stearic acid in the formula helps to form a thin film when the water evaporates.

(5) **Other emulsion bases** include Dermovan, a hypoallergenic, greaseless emulsion base, and Unibase, a nongreasy emulsion base that absorbs about 30% of its weight in water and has a pH close to that of the skin.

d. **Water-soluble bases** may be anhydrous or may contain some water. They are washable in water and absorb water to the point of solubility.

(1) **PEG ointment** consists of a blend of water-soluble polyethylene glycols that form a semisolid base capable of solubilizing water-soluble drugs and some water-insoluble drugs. It is compatible with a wide range of drugs.

(a) This base contains 40% PEG 4000 and 60% PEG 400 and is prepared by the fusion method (see VI E 3 b).

(b) Only a small amount of liquid (less than 5%) can be incorporated without loss of viscosity. This base can be made stiffer by increasing the amount of PEG 4000 up to 60%.

(2) **Propylene glycol** and **propylene glycol–ethanol** form a clear gel when mixed with 2% hydroxypropyl cellulose. This base has become popular as a dermatologic vehicle.

3. **Incorporation of medicinal agents.** Substances may be incorporated into an ointment base by **levigation** or by the **fusion method.** Insoluble substances should be first reduced to the

finest possible form and levigated before incorporation, with a small amount of compatible levigating agent or with the base itself.

a. **Levigation.** The substance is incorporated into the ointment by levigation on an ointment slab.
   (1) Stainless steel spatulas with long flexible broad blades should be used for levigating. If interaction with a metal spatula is possible (as when incorporating iodine and mercuric salts), a hard rubber spatula can be used.
   (2) Insoluble substances should be powdered finely in a mortar and then may be mixed with an equal quantity of base until a smooth grit-free mixture is obtained. The rest of the base is added in increments.
   (3) Levigation of powders into a small portion of base is facilitated by using a melted base or by using a small quantity of compatible levigation aid, such as mineral oil or glycerin.
   (4) Water-soluble salts are incorporated by dissolving them in the smallest possible amount of water and then incorporating the aqueous solution directly into the base, if the base is compatible.
      (a) Usually organic solvents such as ether, chloroform, or alcohol should not be used for dissolving the drug because the drug may crystallize as the solvent evaporates.
      (b) Solvents should be used as levigating aids only if the solid is going to become a fine powder, following the evaporation of the solvent.

b. **Fusion method.** This method is used when the base contains solids with higher melting points, such as waxes, cetyl alcohol, glyceryl monostearate. This method is also useful for solid medicaments, which are readily soluble in the melted base.
   (1) The oil phase should be melted separately, starting with materials with the highest melting point. All other oil-soluble ingredients are added in a decreasing order of melting point.
   (2) The ingredients in the water phase are combined and heated separately to a temperature equal to, or several degrees above, that of the melted oil phase.
   (3) The two phases are then combined. If a w/o system is desired, the hot aqueous phase is incorporated into the hot oil phase with agitation. If an o/w system is preferred, the hot oil phase is incorporated into the hot aqueous phase.
   (4) Volatile materials (e.g., menthol, camphor, iodine, alcohol, perfumes) should be added after the melted mixture has cooled to about 40°C or less.

F. Suppositories

1. **Introduction.** A suppository is a **solid or semisolid mass intended to be inserted into a body orifice** (e.g., the rectum, vagina, urethra) to provide either a local or systemic therapeutic effect. Once inserted, a suppository either melts at body temperature or dissolves (or disperses) into the cavity's aqueous secretions.
   a. Suppositories are frequently used for local effects, such as relief of hemorrhoids or infection in the rectum, vagina, or urethra.
   b. Suppositories can provide systemic medication when used rectally. The absorption of a drug from a suppository through the rectal mucosa into the circulation involves two steps:
      (1) Release of the drug from a vehicle is followed by diffusion of the drug through the mucosa.
      (2) The drug is then transported via veins or lymph vessels into systemic fluids or tissues. Because the rectal veins bypass the liver, the first pass effect is avoided.
   c. Rectal suppositories are useful when oral administration is inappropriate, as with infants, debilitated individuals, comatose patients, and patients with nausea, vomiting, and gastrointestinal disturbances. Some drugs can cause disturbances to the gastrointestinal tract.

2. **Types of suppositories**
   a. **Rectal suppositories** are usually cylindrical and tapered to a point, forming a bullet-like shape. Contraction of the rectum causes a suppository of this shape to move inward rather than outward. The adult suppository weighs about 2 g; suppositories for infants or children are smaller.
   b. **Vaginal suppositories** are oval and typically weigh about 5 g. Drugs administered by this route are intended to have a local effect, but systemic absorption can occur. Antiseptics, contraceptive agents, and drugs used to treat trichomonal, monilial, or bacterial infections are commonly formulated into suppositories.

c. **Urethral suppositories** are long and tapered, having a length of about 60 mm and a diameter of about 4–5 mm. Drugs administered by this route (usually anti-infectives) have local action only.

3. **Suppository bases**

a. **Criteria for satisfactory suppository bases.** Suppository bases should:

(1) Remain firm at room temperature for insertion. (Preferably, it should not soften below 30°C to avoid premature melting during storage)

(2) Have a narrow (or sharp) melting range

(3) Yield a clear melt just below body temperature or dissolve or disperse rapidly in the cavity fluid

(4) Be inert and compatible with a variety of drugs

(5) Be nonirritating and nonsensitizing

(6) Have wetting and emulsifying properties

(7) Have an acid value below 0.2, a saponification value in the range of 200–245, and an iodine value less than 7 if the base is fatty

b. **Selecting a suppository base.** Lipid–water solubility must be considered because of its relationship to the drug release rate.

(1) If an oil-soluble drug is incorporated into an oily base, the rate of absorption is somewhat less than that achieved with a water-soluble base. The lipid-soluble drug tends to remain dissolved in the oily pool from the suppository and has less tendency to escape into mucous secretions from which it is ultimately absorbed.

(2) Conversely, a water-soluble drug tends to pass more rapidly from the oil phase to the aqueous phase. Therefore, if rapid onset of action is desired, the water-soluble drug should be incorporated into the oily base.

c. **Bases that melt** include **cocoa butter,** other **combinations of fats and waxes,** the **Witepsol bases,** and **Wecobee bases** (Table 3-4).

(1) **Cocoa butter** (theobroma oil) is the most widely used suppository base. It is firm and solid up to a temperature of 32°C, at which point it begins to soften. At 34°C–35°C it melts to produce a thin, bland, oily, liquid.

(a) Cocoa butter is a good base for a **rectal suppository** but is less than ideal for a vaginal or urethral suppository.

(b) A mixture of triglycerides, cocoa butter exhibits polymorphism. Depending upon the fusion temperature, it can crystallize into any one of the four crystal forms.

(c) **Major limitations of cocoa butter.** Because of the following limitations, many combinations of fats and waxes are used as substitutes (see Table 3-4):

(i) An inability to absorb aqueous solutions. The addition of nonionic surfactants to the base ameliorates this problem to some extent; however, the resultant suppositories exhibit poor stability and may turn rancid rapidly.

Table 3-4. Composition, Melting Range, and Congealing Range of Selected Bases That Melt

Base	Composition	Melting Range (°C)	Congealing Range (°C)
Cocoa butter	Mixed triglycerides of oleic, palmitic, and stearic acids	34–35	28 or less
Cotmar	Partially hydrogenated cottonseed oil	34–75	. . .
Dehydag	Hydrogenated fatty alcohols and esters		
Base I		33–36	32–33
Base II		37–39	36–37
Base III		9 ranges	9 ranges
Wecobee R	Glycerides of saturated fatty acids C12–C18	33–35	31–32
Wecobee SS	Triglycerides derived from coconut oil	40–43	33–35
Witepsol	Triglycerides of saturated fatty acids C12–C18, with varied portions of the corresponding partial glycerides		
H-12		32–33	29–32
H-15		33–35	32–34
H-85		42–44	36–38

(ii) The lowering of the melting point produced by certain drugs (e.g., chloral hydrate)

(2) Witepsol bases contain natural saturated fatty acid chains between C_{12} and C_{18} with lauric acid being the major component. All 12 bases of this series are colorless and almost odorless. Witepsol H15 has drug-release characteristics similar to those of cocoa butter.

(a) Unlike cocoa butter, Witepsol bases do not exhibit polymorphism when heated and cooled.

(b) The interval between softening and melting temperature is very small. Because Witepsol bases solidify rapidly in the mold, lubrication of the mold is not necessary.

(3) Wecobee bases are derived from coconut oil and appear similar in action to Witepsol bases. Incorporation of glyceryl monostearate and propylene glycol monostearate makes these bases emulsifiable.

d. Bases that dissolve include **PEG** polymers with a molecular weight of 400–6000.

(1) At room temperature, PEG 4000 is a liquid, PEG 1000 is a semisolid, PEG 1500 and 1540 are fairly firm semisolids, and PEG 4000 and 6000 are firm, wax-like solids.

(2) These bases are water-soluble; however, the dissolution process is very slow. In the rectum and the vagina, where the amount of fluid is very small, they dissolve very slowly, but they soften and spread.

(3) Several drugs complex with PEG, which influences drug release and absorption.

(4) Mixtures of PEG polymers in varying proportions provide a base of different properties (Table 3-5).

4. Preparation. Suppositories may be prepared by the following three methods:

a. Hand-rolling involves molding the suppository with the fingers after the formation of a plastic mass.

(1) A finely powdered drug is mixed with the grated base in a mortar and pestle, using levigation and geometric dilution techniques. A small quantity of fixed oil may be added to facilitate the preparation of the mass.

(2) The uniformly mixed semiplastic mass is kneaded further, rolled into a cylinder, and divided into the requisite number of suppositories. Each small cylinder is then rolled by hand until a suppository shape is fashioned.

b. Compression is generally employed when cocoa butter is used as a base.

(1) A uniform mixture of drug and base is prepared as for the hand-rolling method.

(2) The mixture is then placed into a suppository compression device, pressure applied, and the mixture forced into lubricated compression mold cavities. The mold is then cooled and the suppositories ejected.

(3) This procedure generally produces a 2-g suppository; however, the volume of the active ingredients can affect the amount of cocoa butter required for an individual formula, if the active ingredient is present in a relatively large amount.

(a) The amount of cocoa butter needed is determined by calculating the total amount of active ingredient to be used, dividing this number by the cocoa butter density factor (Table 3-6) and subtracting the resulting number from the total amount of cocoa butter required for the desired number of suppositories.

Table 3-5. Mixtures of Polyethylene Glycol (PEG) Bases Providing Satisfactory Room Temperature Stability and Dissolution Characteristics

Base	Comments	Components	Proportion (%)
1	Provides a good general-purpose, water-soluble suppository base	PEG 6000 PEG 1540 PEG 400	50 30 20
2	Provides a good general-purpose base that is slightly softer than base 1 and dissolves more rapidly	PEG 4000 PEG 1000 PEG 400	60 30 10
3	Has a higher melting point than the other bases, which is usually sufficient to compensate for the melting-point lowering effect of such drugs as chloral hydrate and camphor	PEG 6000 PEG 1540	30 70

Table 3-6. Cocoa Butter Density Factors of Drugs Commonly Used in Suppositories

Drug	Cocoa Butter Density Factor	Drug	Cocoa Butter Density Factor
Aloin	1.3	Dimenhydrinate	1.3
Aminophylline	1.1	Diphenhydramine hydrochloride	1.3
Aminopyrine	1.3	Gallic acid	2.0
Aspirin	1.1	Morphine hydrochloride	1.6
Barbital sodium	1.2	Pentobarbital	1.2
Belladonna extract	1.3	Phenobarbital sodium	1.2
Bismuth subgallate	2.7	Salicylic acid	1.3
Chloral hydrate	1.3	Secobarbital sodium	1.2
Codeine phosphate	1.1	Tannic acid	1.6
Digitalis leaf	1.6		

(b) For example, suppose 12 suppositories, each containing 300 mg of aspirin, are required. Each mold cavity has a 2-g capacity. For 13 suppositories (calculated to provide one extra), 3.9 g of aspirin (13 x 0.3 g = 3.9 g) is required. This is divided by the density factor of aspirin (1.1) [see Table 3-6]. Thus, 3.9 g of aspirin replaces 3.55 g of cocoa butter. The total amount of cocoa butter needed for 13 suppositories of 2 g each equals 26 g; the amount of cocoa butter required is 26 g−3.55 g, or 22.45 g.

c. The **fusion method** is the principal way of making suppositories commercially and is used primarily when cocoa butter, PEG, and glycerin–gelatin bases are used. Molds made of aluminum, brass, or nickel–copper alloys are used and can make from 6–50 suppositories.

(1) Capacity of the molds is determined by melting a sufficient quantity of base over a steam bath, pouring it into the molds, and allowing it to congeal. The "blank" suppositories are then trimmed, removed, and weighed. Once the weight is known, the drug-containing suppositories can be prepared.

(a) To prepare suppositories, the drug is reduced to a fine powder, and a small amount of grated cocoa butter is liquefied in a suitable container placed in a water bath at 33°C or less.

(b) The finely powdered drug is mixed with melted cocoa butter with continuous stirring.

(c) The remainder of the grated cocoa butter is added with stirring, while maintaining the temperature at 33°C or below. The liquid should appear creamy rather than clear.

(d) The creamy melt is poured into the mold at room temperature. The mold must be very lightly lubricated with mineral oil; the melt should be poured continuously to avoid layering.

(e) The suppositories are allowed to congeal and then are placed in a refrigerator for 30 minutes to harden. Then they can be removed from the refrigerator, trimmed, and unmolded.

(2) The fusion process should be used carefully with **thermolabile drugs** and **insoluble powders.**

(a) Insoluble powders in the melt may settle or float during pouring, depending upon their density, or collect at one end of the suppository before the melt congeals, resulting in a nonuniform drug distribution.

(b) Hard crystalline materials (e.g., iodine, merbromin) can be incorporated by dissolving the crystals in a minimum volume of suitable solvent before incorporation into the base.

(c) Vegetable extracts can be incorporated by moistening with a few drops of alcohol and levigating with a small amount of melted cocoa butter.

G. Powders

1. Introduction. A pharmaceutical powder is a mixture of finely divided drugs or chemicals in dry form meant for internal or external use.

a. Advantages of powders

   (1) Flexibility of compounding
   (2) Good chemical stability
   (3) Rapid dispersion of ingredients (because of the small particle size)

b. **Disadvantages** of powders
   (1) Time-consuming preparation
   (2) Inaccuracy of dose
   (3) Unsuitability for many, unpleasant tasting, hygroscopic, and deliquescent drugs

c. **Milling** is the mechanical process of reducing the particle size of solids **(comminution)** before incorporation into a final product (Tables 3-7 and 3-8). The particle size of a given powder is related to the proportion of the powder that can pass through the opening of standard sieves of varying dimensions in a specified time period. (**Micromeritics** is the study of particles.) After milling, various substances are mixed as needed.
   (1) **Advantages** of milling
      (a) Increases the surface area, which may increase dissolution rate and bioavailability (e.g., griseofulvin)
      (b) Increases extraction or leaching from animal glands (such as the liver and pancreas) and from crude vegetable extracts
      (c) Facilitates drying of wet masses by increasing surface area and reducing the distance that moisture must travel to reach the outer surface; micronization and subsequent drying, in turn, increase stability as occluded solvent is removed
      (d) Improves mixing or blending of several solid ingredients if they are reduced to approximately the same size; minimizes segregation and provides greater dose uniformity
      (e) Permits uniform distribution of coloring agents in artificially colored solid pharmaceuticals
      (f) Improves the function of lubricants used in compressed tablets and capsules to coat the surface of the granulation or powder
      (g) Improves the texture, appearance, and physical stability of ointments, creams, and pastes
   (2) **Disadvantages** of milling
      (a) Can change the polymorphic form of the active ingredient, rendering it less active
      (b) Can degrade the drug as a result of heat buildup during milling, oxidation, or adsorption of unwanted moisture (due to increased surface area)
      (c) Decreases the bulk density of the active compound and excipients, causing flow problems and segregation
      (d) Decreases raw material particle size, possibly creating static charge problems that may cause particle aggregation and decreased dissolution rate
      (e) Increases surface area, which may promote air adsorption that may inhibit wettability of the drug

Table 3-7. *United States Pharmacopeia* (USP) Standards for Powders of Animal and Vegetable Drugs

Type of Powder	Sieve Size All Particles Pass Through	Sieve Size Percentage of Particles Pass Through
Very coarse (#8)	#20 sieve	20% through a #60 sieve
Coarse (#20)	#20 sieve	40% through a #60 sieve
Moderately coarse (#40)	#40 sieve	40% through a #80 sieve
Fine (#60)	#60 sieve	40% through a #100 sieve
Very fine (#80)	#80 sieve	No limit

Table 3-8. *United States Pharmacopeia* (USP) Standards for Powders of Chemicals

Type of Powder	Sieve Size All Particles Pass Through	Sieve Size Percentage of Particles Pass Through
Coarse (#20)	#20 sieve	60% through a #40 sieve
Moderately coarse (#40)	#40 sieve	60% through a #60 sieve
Fine (#80)	#80 sieve	No limit
Very fine (#120)	#120 sieve	No limit

(3) **Comminution techniques.** On a large scale, various mills and pulverizers (e.g., rotary cutter, hammer, roller, fluid energy mill) may be used during manufacturing. On a small scale, the pharmacist usually uses one of the following comminution techniques:

(a) **Trituration.** The substance is reduced to small particles by rubbing it in a mortar with a pestle. The term also is used to designate the process by which fine powders are intimately mixed in a mortar.

(b) **Pulverization by intervention.** Substances are reduced and subdivided with an additional material (i.e., solvent) that can be removed easily after pulverization is complete. The technique is often used with substances that are gummy and reagglomerate or resist grinding; for example, camphor can be reduced readily after the addition of a small amount of alcohol or other volatile solvent, which is then permitted to evaporate.

(c) **Levigation.** The substance is reduced in particle size by adding a suitable nonsolvent (levigating agent) to form a paste and then rubbing the paste in a mortar and pestle or using an ointment slab and spatula. This method is often used to incorporate solids into dermatologic or ophthalmic ointments and suspensions, to prevent a gritty feel. Mineral oil is a common levigating agent.

2. **Mixing powders.** Powders may be mixed (blended) by the following five methods:

a. **Spatulation.** Small amounts of powders are blended by the movement of a spatula through the powders on a sheet of paper or a pill tile.

(1) This method is not suitable for large quantities of powders or for powders containing one or more potent substances because homogeneous blending may not occur.

(2) It is particularly useful for solid substances that liquefy or form **eutectic mixtures** (mixtures that melt at a lower temperature than any of their ingredients) when in close and prolonged contact with one another since very little compression or compaction results.

(a) Such substances include phenol, camphor, menthol, thymol, aspirin, phenylsalicylate, phenacetin, and other similar chemicals.

(b) To diminish contact, powders prepared from such substances are commonly mixed in the presence of an inert diluent such as light magnesium oxide or magnesium carbonate, kaolin, starch, or bentonite.

(c) Silicic acid (about 20%) prevents eutexia with aspirin, phenylsalicylate, and other troublesome compounds.

b. **Trituration** is used both to comminute and to mix powders.

(1) If comminution is desired, a porcelain or a Wedgwood mortar with a rough inner surface is preferred to a glass mortar with a smooth working surface.

(2) A glass mortar is preferable for chemicals that stain a porcelain or Wedgwood surface and for simple admixture of substances without special need for comminution. A glass mortar cleans more readily after use.

c. **Geometric dilution** is employed when potent substances are to be mixed with a large amount of diluent.

(1) The potent drug is placed upon an approximately equal volume of diluent in a mortar, and the substances are thoroughly mixed by trituration.

(2) A second portion of diluent, equal in volume to the powder mixture in the mortar, is added, and the trituration is repeated. The process is continued, adding equal volumes of diluent to that powder present in the mortar until all the diluent is incorporated.

d. **Sifting.** Powders are mixed by passing them through sifters similar to those used to sift flour. This process results in a light, fluffy product and is generally not acceptable for incorporation of potent drugs into a diluent base.

e. **Tumbling** is the process of mixing powders in a large container rotated by a motorized process. These blenders are widely employed in industry, as are large-volume powder mixers, which use motorized blades to blend the powder contained in a large mixing vessel.

3. **Use and packaging of powders.** Depending upon their intended use, powders are packaged and dispensed by pharmacists as bulk powders or as divided powders.

a. Bulk powders are dispensed by the pharmacist in bulk containers: a **perforated** or **sifter can** for external dusting; an **aerosol container** for spraying onto skin; or a **widemouthed glass** that permits easy removal of a spoonful of powder.

(1) Powders commonly dispensed in bulk form
(a) **Antacid powders** and **laxative powders,** used by mixing the directed amount of powder (usually a teaspoonful or so) in a portion of liquid, which is then drunk
(b) **Douche powders,** dissolved in warm water and applied vaginally
(c) **Medicated or nonmedicated powders for external use,** usually dispensed in a sifter to aid convenient application to the skin
(d) **Dentifrices** or **dental cleansing powders,** used for oral hygiene
(e) Powders for **the ear, nose, throat, tooth sockets, vagina,** administered by means of insufflator (powder blower)

(2) **Nonpotent substances** are generally dispensed in bulk powder form. Those intended for external use should bear a label indicating this.

(3) **Hygroscopic, deliquescent,** or **volatile** powders should be packed in glass jars rather than pasteboard containers. Amber or green glass should be used if needed to prevent the light-sensitive components of the powder from decomposition. All powders should be stored in tightly closed containers.

b. **Divided powders** are dispensed in the form of individual doses, generally in properly folded **papers** (i.e., chartulae). However, they may also be dispensed in metal foil; small, heat-sealed or resealable **plastic bags;** or other containers.

(1) After weighing, comminuting, and mixing ingredients, the powders must be accurately **divided** into the prescribed number of doses.

(2) Depending upon the potency of the drug substance, the pharmacist decides whether to **weigh** each portion separately before packaging or to approximate portions by the **block-and-divide method.**

(3) **Powder papers** can be of any convenient size that fits the required dose. There are four basic types of powder papers:
(a) **Vegetable parchment,** a thin semiopaque moisture-resistant paper
(b) **White bond,** an opaque paper with no moisture-resistant properties
(c) **Glassine,** a glazed, transparent moisture-resistant paper
(d) **Waxed paper,** a transparent waterproof paper

(4) Hygroscopic drugs and volatile drugs can be protected best with waxed paper, double-wrapped with a bond paper to improve the appearance. Parchment and glassine papers are of limited use for these drugs.

4. **Special problems.** Volatile substances, eutectic mixtures, liquids, and hygroscopic or deliquescent substances present problems when mixing into powders that require special treatment.

a. **Volatile substances,** such as camphor, menthol, and essential oils, can be lost by volatilization after incorporation into powders. This process is prevented or retarded by use of heat-sealed plastic bags or by double wrapping with waxed or glassine paper inside white bond paper.

b. **Liquids** are incorporated into divided powders in small amounts.

(1) Magnesium carbonate, starch, or lactose can be added to increase the absorbability of the powders by increasing surface area.

(2) When the liquid is a solvent for a nonvolatile heat-stable compound, it is evaporated gently in a water bath. Some fluidextracts and tinctures may be treated in this way.

c. **Hygroscopic and deliquescent substances** that become moist because of an affinity for moisture in the air can be prepared as divided powders by adding inert diluents. Double-wrapping is desirable for further protection.

d. **Eutectic mixtures**

H. Capsules

1. **Introduction.** Capsules are solid dosage forms in which one or more medicinal or inert substances are enclosed within a small gelatin shell. Gelatin capsules may be hard or soft. Most capsules are intended to be swallowed whole, but occasionally the contents are removed from the gelatin shell and employed as a premeasured medicinal powder (e.g., Theo-Dur Sprinkle, an anhydrous theophylline preparation meant to be sprinkled on a small amount of soft food before ingestion).

2. **Hard gelatin capsules**

a. **Preparation of filled hard capsules** includes preparing the formulation, selecting the appropriate capsule, filling the capsule shells, and cleaning and polishing the filled capsules.

(1) Empty hard capsule shells are manufactured from a mixture of gelatin, colorants, and sometimes an opacifying agent such as titanium dioxide; the USP also permits the addition of 0.15% sulfur dioxide to prevent decomposition of gelatin during manufacture.

(2) Gelatin USP is obtained by the partial hydrolysis of collagen obtained from the skin, white connective tissue, and bones of animals. Type A and type B are obtained by acid and alkali processing, respectively.

(3) Capsule shells are cast by dipping cold metallic molds or pins into gelatin solutions maintained at a uniform temperature and an exact degree of fluidity.

(a) Variation in gelatin solution viscosity increases or decreases capsule wall thickness.

(b) Once the pins have been withdrawn from the gelatin solution, they are rotated while being dried in kilns through which a strong blast of filtered air with controlled humidity is forced. Each capsule is then mechanically stripped, trimmed, and joined.

b. **Storage.** Hard capsules should be stored in tightly closed glass containers, protected from dust and extremes of humidity and temperature.

(1) These capsules contain 12%–16% water, varying with the storage conditions. When humidity is low, the capsules become brittle; if humidity is high, the capsules become flaccid and shapeless.

(2) Storage in high-temperature areas also affects the quality of hard gelatin capsules.

c. **Sizes.** Hard capsules are available in a variety of sizes.

(1) Empty capsules are **numbered** from 000 (the largest size that can be swallowed) to 5 (the smallest size). Approximate capsule capacity ranges from 600 mg to 30 mg for capsules from 000 to 5, respectively; however, capacity varies because of varying densities of powdered drug materials and degree of pressure used in filling the capsules.

(2) Large sizes are available for **veterinary medicine.**

(3) **Selecting capsules.** Generally, hard gelatin capsules are used to encapsulate between 65 mg and 1 g of powdered material, including the drug and any diluents needed. Capsule size should be chosen carefully. A properly filled capsule should have its body filled with the drug mixture and its cap fully extended down the body. The cap is meant to enclose the powder, not to retain additional powder.

(a) If the drug dose for a single capsule is inadequate to fill the capsule, a diluent, such as lactose must be added.

(b) If the amount of drug representing a usual dose is too large to place in a single capsule, two or more capsules might be required to provide the particular dose.

(c) Lubricants such as magnesium stearate (frequently less than 1%) are added to facilitate the flow of the powder when an automatic capsule filling machine is used.

(d) Wetting agents such as lithium carbonate are added to capsule formulations to enhance drug dissolution.

d. **Filling capsules.** Capsules are usually filled by the punch method.

(1) The powder is placed on paper and flattened with a spatula so that the layer of powder is no more than about one-third the length of the capsule. The paper is held in the left hand, and the body of the capsule, held in the right hand, is pressed repeatedly into the powder until the body is filled. Then, the cap is replaced and the capsule weighed.

(2) **Granular** material that does not lend itself well to the punch method can be poured into each capsule from the powder paper on which it was weighed.

(3) **Crystalline** materials, especially materials consisting of a mass of filament-like crystals as with the quinine salts, will not fit into a capsule easily unless first powdered.

(4) Once filled, capsules must be cleaned and polished.

(a) On a **small scale,** capsules may be cleaned individually or in small numbers by rubbing them on a clean gauze or cloth.

(b) On a **large scale,** many capsule-filling machines have a cleaning vacuum that removes any extraneous material from the capsules as they leave the machine.

3. Soft gelatin capsules

a. Preparation

(1) Soft gelatin capsules are prepared from gelatin shells to which glycerin or a polyhydric alcohol (e.g., sorbitol) has been added, rendering the shells elastic or plastic-like.

(2) These shells contain preservatives (e.g., methyl and propyl parabens, sorbic acid) to prevent the growth of fungi.

b. **Uses.** Soft gelatin shells, which are oblong, elliptical, or spherical in shape, are used to contain liquids, suspensions, pasty materials, dry powders, or pelletized materials.

(1) Drugs commercially prepared in soft capsules include ethchlorvynol (Placidyl, Abbott), demeclocycline hydrochloride (Declomycin, Lederle), chlorotrianisene (TACE, Merrell Dow), chloral hydrate (Noctec, Bristol-Myer Squibb), digoxin (Lanoxicaps, Burroughs Wellcome) vitamin A, and vitamin E.

(2) Soft gelatin capsules are usually prepared by the plate process, using a rotary or reciprocating die.

4. Uniformity and disintegration

a. The **uniformity** of dosage forms can be demonstrated by either weight variation or content uniformity methods. The official compendia should be consulted for details of these procedures.

b. **Disintegration** tests are usually not required for capsules unless they have been treated to resist solution in gastric fluid (enteric-coated). In this case they must meet the requirements for disintegration of enteric-coated tablets.

I. Tablets

1. Introduction

a. The **oral route** is the most important method of administering drugs when systemic effects are desired. Oral drugs can be given as solids or liquids.

(1) **Advantages of solid dosage forms**

(a) Accurate dosage
(b) Easy shipping and handling
(c) Less shelf space needed per dose than for liquid
(d) No preservation requirements
(e) No taste-masking problem
(f) Generally more stable than liquids with longer expiration dates

(2) **Advantages of liquid dosage forms**

(a) The drug might be more effective in liquid than in solid form (e.g., adsorbents, antacids).
(b) They can be useful for patients who have trouble swallowing solid dosage forms (e.g., pediatric and geriatric dosage forms).

b. **Tablets** are the **most commonly used solid dosage forms.**

(1) **Advantages**

(a) Precision and low-content variability of the unit dose
(b) Low manufacturing cost
(c) Easy to package and ship
(d) Simple to identify
(e) Easy to swallow
(f) Lend themselves to special-release forms
(g) Best suited to large-scale production
(h) Most stable of all oral dosage forms
(i) Essentially tamperproof

(2) **Disadvantages**

(a) Some drugs resist compression into tablets.
(b) Some drugs (e.g., those with poor wetting, slow dissolution properties, intermediate to large doses, optimum absorption high in the gastrointestinal tract, or any combination of these features) may be difficult to formulate to provide adequate bioavailability.
(c) Some drugs (e.g., bitter-tasting drugs, drugs with an objectionable odor, those sensitive to oxygen or atmospheric moisture) require encapsulation or entrapment before compression. A capsule form might be a better approach.

2. Tablet design and formulation

a. **Characteristics of ideal tablets**

(1) Free of defects, such as chips, cracks, discoloration, and contamination
(2) Have the strength to withstand the mechanical stresses of production
(3) Chemically and physically stable over time
(4) Release the medicinal agents in a predictable and reproducible manner

b. Tablet excipients. Tablets are manufactured by **wet granulation, dry granulation,** or **direct compression.** Regardless of the method of manufacture, tablets for oral ingestion usually contain excipients, components added to the active ingredients that have special functions (Table 3-9).

(1) **Diluents** are fillers designed to make up the required bulk of the tablet when the drug dosage amount is inadequate. Diluents may also improve cohesion, permit use of direct compression, or promote flow.

(a) **Common diluents** include kaolin, lactose, mannitol, starch, powdered sugar, and calcium phosphate.

(b) **Selection of the diluent** is based partly on the experience of the manufacturer as well as on diluent cost and compatibility with the other tablet ingredients. For example, calcium salts cannot be employed as fillers for tetracycline products since calcium interferes with tetracycline's absorption from the gastrointestinal tract.

(2) **Binders and adhesives** are materials added in either dry or liquid form to promote the granulation process or to promote cohesive compacts during the direct compression process.

(a) **Common binding agents** include a 10%–20% aqueous preparation of cornstarch; a 25%–50% solution of glucose; molasses; various natural gums, such as acacia; cellulose derivatives, such as methylcellulose, carboxymethylcellulose, and microcrystalline cellulose; gelatins; and povidone. The natural gums are variable in composition and usually contaminated with bacteria.

(b) If the drug substance is adversely affected by an aqueous binder, a **nonaqueous binder** can be used, or the binder can be added dry. Generally, the binding action is more effective when the binder is mixed in liquid form.

(c) The **amount** of binder or adhesive used depends on the manufacturer's experience and on the other tablet ingredients. Overwetting usually results in granules

Table 3-9. Common Tablet Excipients

Diluents	**Disintegrants**
Calcium phosphate dihydrate NF (dibasic)	Alginates
Calcium sulfate dihydrate NF	Cellulose
Cellulose NF (microcrystalline)	Cellulose derivatives
Cellulose derivatives	Clays
Dextrose	PVP (cross-linked)
Lactose USP	Starch
Lactose USP (anhydrous)	Starch derivatives
Lactose USP (spray-dried)	**Lubricants**
Mannitol USP	PEGs
Starches (directly compressible)	Stearic acid
Starches (hydrolyzed)	Stearic acid salts
Sorbitol	Stearic acid derivatives
Sucrose USP (powder)	Surfactants
Sucrose-based materials	Talc
	Waxes
Binders and adhesives	**Glidants**
Acacia	Cornstarch
Cellulose derivatives	Silica derivatives
Gelatin	Talc
Glucose	**Colors, flavors, and sweeteners**
PVP	FD&C and D&C dyes and lakes
Sodium alginate and alginate derivatives	Flavors are available in two forms: spray-dried and oils
Sorbitol	Artificial sweeteners
Starch (paste)	Natural sweeteners
Starch (pregelatinized)	
Tragacanth	

D&C = drugs and cosmetics; *FD&C* = food, drugs, and cosmetics; *NF* = National Formulary; *PEG* = polyethylene glycol; *PVP* = polyvinylpyrrolidone, more commonly called povidone.

that are too hard for proper tableting; underwetting usually r
ration of tablets that are too soft and tend to crumble.

(3) **Disintegrants** are added to tablet formulations to facilitate tablet c
it contacts water in the gastrointestinal tract. Disintegrants app
drawing water into the tablet, swelling, and causing the tablet to
   - **(a)** Tablet disintegration may be critical to the subsequent dissolution of the drug and satisfactory drug bioavailability.
   - **(b)** **Common disintegrants** include cornstarch and potato starch; starch derivatives, such as sodium starch glycolate; cellulose derivatives, such as sodium carboxymethylcellulose; clays, such as Veegum and bentonite; cation exchange resins; and others.
   - **(c)** The total **amount of disintegrant** is not always added to the drug–diluent mixture. A portion can be added (with the lubricant) to the prepared granulation of the drug, causing double disintegration of the tablet. The portion of disintegrant added last causes the breakup of the tablets into small pieces or chunks; the portion added first breaks the pieces of tablet into fine particles.

(4) **Lubricants, antiadherents, and glidants** have overlapping function.
   - **(a)** **Lubricants** are intended to reduce the friction during tablet ejection between the walls of the tablet and the walls of the die cavity in which the tablet was formed. Talc, magnesium stearate, and calcium stearate are among those commonly used.
   - **(b)** **Antiadherents** reduce sticking or adhesion of the tablet granulation or powder to the faces of the punches or to the die walls.
   - **(c)** **Glidants** promote the flow of the tablet granulation or powder materials by reducing friction among particles.

(5) **Colors and dyes** serve to disguise off-color drugs, to provide product identification, and to produce a more elegant product. **Food, drug,** and **cosmetic dyes** are applied as solutions; **lakes** (dyes that have been absorbed on a hydrous oxide) are usually employed as dry powders.

(6) **Flavoring agents** are usually limited to chewable tablets or tablets intended to dissolve in the mouth.
   - **(a)** Generally, water-soluble flavors have poor stability; hence, flavor oils or dry powders usually are used.
   - **(b)** Flavor oils may be added to tablet granulations in solvents, dispersed on clays and other adsorbents, or emulsified in aqueous granulating agents. Usually, the maximum amount of oil that can be added to a granulation without influencing its tablet characteristics is 0.5%–0.75%.

(7) **Artificial sweeteners,** like flavors, are usually used only with chewable tablets or tablets intended to dissolve in the mouth.
   - **(a)** Some **sweetness** may come from the diluent (e.g., mannitol, lactose); agents, such as saccharin and aspartame, can also be added.
   - **(b)** **Saccharin** has an unpleasant aftertaste.
   - **(c)** **Aspartame** is not stable in the presence of moisture.

(8) **Adsorbents** (e.g., magnesium oxide, magnesium carbonate, bentonite, silicon dioxide) are substances capable of holding quantities of fluid in an apparently dry state.

3. **Tablet types and classes.** Tablets are classified by their route of administration, drug delivery system, and form and method of manufacture (Table 3-10).

   a. **Tablets for oral ingestion** are designed to be swallowed intact with the exception of chewable tablets. They can be coated to mask the drug's taste, color, or odor; to control drug release; to protect the drug from the stomach's acid environment; to incorporate another drug, providing sequential release or avoiding incompatibilities; or to improve appearance.

   (1) **Compressed tablets** are formed by compression and have no special coating. They are made from powdered, crystalline, or granular materials, alone or in combination with such excipients as binders, disintegrants, diluents, and colorants.

   (2) **Multiple compressed tablets** are layered or compression-coated.
   - **(a)** **Layered tablets** are prepared by compressing an additional tablet granulation around a previously compressed granulation. The operation is repeated to produce multiple layers.
   - **(b)** **Compression-coated tablets** (also called **dry-coated tablets**) are prepared by feeding previously compressed tablets into a special tableting machine and

ble 3-10. Tablet Types and Classes

Tablets for oral ingestion	**Tablets used in the oral cavity**
Compressed tablets	Buccal tablets
Multiple compressed tablets	Sublingual tablets
Layered tablets	Troches, lozenges, and dental cones
Compression-coated tablets	**Tablets used to prepare solutions**
Repeat-action tablets	Effervescent tablets
Delayed-action and enteric-coated tablets	Dispensing tablets
Sugar- and chocolate-coated tablets	Hypodermic tablets
Film-coated tablets	Tablet triturates
Air suspension-coated tablets	
Chewable tablets	

compressing an outer shell around them. This process applies a thinner, more uniform coating than sugar-coating and can be used safely with drugs sensitive to moisture. It can be used to separate incompatible materials, to produce repeat-action or prolonged-action products, or to provide a multilayered appearance.

(3) **Repeat-action tablets** are layered or compression-coated tablets in which the outer layer or shell provides an initial drug dose that rapidly disintegrates in the stomach [e.g., Repetabs (Schering) and Extentabs (Robins)]. The inner layer (or inner tablet) is comprised of components that are insoluble in gastric media but soluble in intestinal media.

(4) **Delayed-action** and **enteric-coated tablets** delay the release of a drug from a dosage form to prevent drug destruction by gastric juices, to prevent stomach lining irritation by the drug, or to promote absorption, which is better in the intestine than in the stomach.

(a) Tablets that are coated and remain intact in the stomach but yield their ingredients in the intestines are said to be **enteric-coated** [e.g., Enseals (Lilly) and Ecotrin (Smith Kline Beecham)]. Enteric-coated tablets are a form of delayed-action tablet, but not all delayed-action tablets are enteric or intended to produce an enteric effect.

(b) Among the agents used to enteric-coat tablets are fats, fatty acids, waxes, shellac, and cellulose acetate phthalate.

(5) **Sugar-** and **chocolate-coated tablets** are compressed tablets coated to protect the drug from air and humidity, to provide a barrier to the drug's objectionable taste or smell, or to improve the tablet's appearance. Chocolate-coated tablets are rare today.

(a) Sugar-coated tablets may be coated with a colored or an uncolored sugar. The process includes **seal coating** (waterproofing), **subcoating, syrup coating** (for smoothing and coloring), and **polishing,** all of which take place in a series of mechanically operated coating pans.

(b) **Disadvantages** of sugar-coating include the time and expertise required for the process and the increase in tablet size and weight. Sugar-coated tablets may be 50% larger and heavier than the original tablets.

(6) **Film-coated tablets** are compressed tablets coated with a thin layer of a water-insoluble or water-soluble polymer (e.g., hydroxypropyl methylcellulose, ethylcellulose, povidone, PEG).

(a) The film is generally colored, and it is more durable, less bulky, and less time-consuming to apply than sugar-coating. It typically increases tablet weight by only 2%–3% and provides increased formulation efficiency, increased resistance to chipping, and increased output.

(b) Film-coating solutions generally contain a film former, an alloying substance, a plasticizer, a surfactant, opacifiers, sweeteners, flavors, colors, glossants, and a volatile solvent.

(c) The volatile solvents used in these solutions are expensive and potentially toxic when released into the atmosphere. Hence, manufacturers are exploring the development and use of **aqueous-based solutions.**

(7) **Air suspension-coated tablets** are fed into a vertical cylinder and supported by a column of air that enters from the bottom of the cylinder. As the coating solution enters

the system, it is rapidly applied to the suspended, rotating solids **(Wurster process)**. Rounding coats can be applied in less than 1 hour with the assistance of warm air blasts released in the chamber.

(8) Chewable tablets disintegrate smoothly and rapidly when chewed or allowed to dissolve in the mouth, yielding a creamy base (from specially colored and flavored mannitol).

(a) These tablets are especially useful in formulations for children and are commonly used for multivitamin tablets.

(b) They are also used for some antacids and antibiotics.

b. Tablets used in the oral cavity are allowed to dissolve in the mouth.

(1) Buccal tablets and **sublingual tablets** allow absorption through the oral mucosa after dissolving in the buccal pouch (buccal tablets) or below the tongue (sublingual tablets). These forms are useful for drugs that are destroyed by gastric juice or poorly absorbed from the intestinal tract, such as sublingual nitroglycerin tablets, which dissolve very promptly to give rapid drug effects, and buccal progesterone tablets, which dissolve slowly.

(2) Troches, lozenges, and **dental cones** dissolve slowly in the mouth and provide primarily local effects.

c. Tablets used to prepare solutions are dissolved in water before administration.

(1) Effervescent tablets are prepared by compressing granular effervescent salts or other materials (e.g., citric acid, tartaric acid, sodium bicarbonate) that have the capacity to release carbon dioxide gas when in contact with water. Commercial alkalinizing analgesic tablets are frequently made to effervesce to encourage fast dissolution and absorption (e.g., Alka-Seltzer).

(2) Other tablets used to prepare solutions include dispensing tablets, hypodermic tablets, and tablet triturates.

4. Processing problems

a. Capping is the partial or complete separation of the top or bottom crowns of a tablet from the main body of the tablet. **Lamination** is separation of a tablet into two or more distinct layers. Both of these problems usually result from air entrapment during processing.

b. Picking is removal of a tablet's surface material by a punch. **Sticking** is adhesion of tablet material to a die wall. These problems result from excessive moisture or substances with low melting temperatures in the formulation.

c. Mottling is an unequal color distribution on a tablet, with light or dark areas standing out on an otherwise uniform surface. This results from use of a drug with a color different from that of the tablet excipients or from a drug with colored degradation products. Colorants solve the problem but can create other problems.

5. Tablet evaluation and control

a. General appearance of tablets is important for consumer acceptance, lot-to-lot uniformity, tablet-to-tablet uniformity, and monitoring of the manufacturing process. Tablet appearance includes visual identity and overall appearance. **Control of appearance** includes measurement of such attributes as size, shape, color, odor, taste, surface, texture, physical flaws, consistency, and legibility of any markings.

b. Hardness and **resistance** to friability are necessary for tablets to withstand the mechanical shocks of manufacture, packaging, and shipping, and to ensure consumer acceptance. Hardness relates to both tablet disintegration and to drug dissolution. Certain tablets intended to dissolve slowly are made hard, whereas others intended to dissolve rapidly are made soft. Friability relates to the tablet's tendency to crumble.

(1) Tablet hardness testers measure the degree of force required to break a tablet.

(2) Friabilators determine friability by allowing the tablet to roll and fall within a rotating tumbling apparatus. The tablets are weighed before and after a specified number of rotations, and the weight loss is determined.

(a) Resistance to weight loss indicates the tablet's ability to withstand abrasion during handling, packaging, and shipping. Compressed tablets that lose less than 0.5%–1% of their weight are generally considered acceptable.

(b) Some chewable tablets and most effervescent tablets are **highly friable** and require special unit packaging.

c. Weight of tablets is routinely measured to ensure that the tablet contains the proper amount of drug.

(1) The USP defines a **weight variation standard** to which tablets must conform.

(2) These standards are applicable for tablets containing 50 mg or more of drug substance in which the drug substance represents 50% or more (by weight) of the dosage form unit.

d. Content uniformity is evaluated to ensure that each tablet contains the amount of drug substance desired with little variation among contents within a batch. The USP defines content uniformity tests for tablets containing 50 mg or less of drug substance.

e. Disintegration is evaluated to ensure that the tablet's drug substance is fully available for dissolution and absorption from the gastrointestinal tract.

(1) All USP tablets must pass an **official disintegration test** conducted in vitro with special equipment.

(a) **Uncoated USP tablets** have disintegration times as low as 2 minutes (nitroglycerin) to 5 minutes (aspirin); the majority have a maximum disintegration time of less than 30 minutes.

(b) **Buccal tablets** must disintegrate within 4 hours.

(c) **Enteric-coated tablets** must show no evidence of disintegration after 1 hour in simulated gastric fluid. In simulated intestinal fluid, they should disintegrate in 2 hours plus the time specified.

(2) **Dissolution requirements** in the USP have replaced earlier disintegration requirements for many drugs.

f. Dissolution characteristics are tested to determine drug absorption and physiologic availability, which depend on the drug in its dissolved state.

(1) The USP gives **standards for tablet dissolution.**

(2) An increased emphasis on dissolution testing and determination of bioavailability has increased the use of sophisticated systems for the testing and analysis of tablet dissolution.

J. Controlled-release dosage forms

1. Introduction. Controlled-release dosage forms (also known as delayed-release, sustained-action, prolonged-action, sustained-release, prolonged-release, timed-release, slow-release, extended-action, and extended-release forms) are designed to **release drug substance slowly** for prolonged action in the body. Controlled-release forms have the following **advantages:**

a. Reduction of problems with patient compliance
b. Employment of less total drug
c. Minimization or elimination of local or systemic side effects
d. Minimization of drug accumulation (with chronic dosage)
e. Reduction of potentiation or loss of drug activity (with chronic use)
f. Improvement in treatment efficiency
g. Improvement in speed of control of condition
h. Reduction in drug level fluctuation
i. Improvement in bioavailability for some drugs
j. Improvement in ability to provide special effects (e.g., morning relief of arthritis by bedtime dosing)
k. Reduction in cost

2. Sustained-release forms. The variety of sustained-release forms available can be grouped by the pharmaceutical mechanism employed to provide controlled release.

a. Coated beads or granules [e.g., Theo-Dur Sprinkle (Key), Spansules (Smith Kline Beecham PLC), Sequels (Lederle)] produce a blood-level profile similar to that obtained with multiple dosing.

(1) A solution of the drug substance in a nonaqueous solvent (e.g., alcohol) is coated onto small, inert beads or granules made of a combination of sugar and starch. (When the drug dose is large, the starting granules can be composed of the drug itself.)

(2) Some of the beads or granules are left uncoated to provide an immediate release of the drug.

(3) Coats of a lipid material (such as beeswax) or a cellulosic material (e.g., ethylcellulose) are applied to the remainder of the granules, with some granules receiving few coats and some granules many. The various coating thicknesses produce a sustained-release effect.

b. Microencapsulation is a process by which solids, liquids, or even gases are encapsulated into microscopic capsules by formation of thin coatings of a "wall" material around the substance to be encapsulated. An **example** of a microencapsulated dosage form is Bayer time-release aspirin.

(1) **Coacervation,** which involves addition of a hydrophilic substance to a colloidal drug dispersion, causes layering and formation of microcapsules. This is the most common method of microencapsulation.

(2) **Film-forming substances,** which act as the coating material, are selected from a variety of natural and synthetic polymers, including shellacs, waxes, gelatin, starches, cellulose acetate phthalate, and ethylcellulose. Once the coating material dissolves, all the drug inside the microcapsule is immediately available for dissolution and absorption. Wall thickness can be varied from 1–200 μm by changing the amount of the coating material (3%–30% of total weight).

c. **Matrix tablets** employ insoluble plastics (e.g., polyethylene, polyvinyl acetate, polymethacrylate), hydrophilic polymers (e.g., methylcellulose, hydroxypropyl methylcellulose), or fatty compounds (e.g., various waxes, glyceryl tristearate). Examples include Gradumet (Abbott), Lonatabs (Geigy), Dospan (Merrell Dow), and Slow-K (Ciba).

(1) The most common method of preparation is **mixing of the drug with the matrix material** followed by **compression of the material into tablets.**

(2) The primary dose (the portion of the drug to be released immediately) is placed on the tablet as a layer or coat. The remainder of the dose is released slowly from the matrix.

d. **Osmotic systems** include the **Oros system (Alza),** an oral osmotic pump composed of a core tablet and a semipermeable coating with a 0.4-mm diameter hole (produced by a laser beam) for drug exit.

(1) This system requires only osmotic pressure to be effective and is essentially independent of pH changes in the environment.

(2) The drug-release rate can be changed by changing the surface area, the nature of the membrane, or the diameter of the drug-release aperture.

e. **Ion-exchange resins** can be complexed with drugs by passage of a cationic drug solution through a column containing the resin. The drug is complexed to the resin by replacement of hydrogen atoms. Examples include biphenamine capsules (Fisons; resin complexes of amphetamine and dextroamphetamine), Ionamin capsules (Fisons; resin complexes of phentermine), and the Pennkinetic system (Fisons), which incorporates a polymer barrier coating and bead technology in addition to the ion-exchange mechanism.

(1) After complexing, the **resin–drug complex** is washed and then tableted, encapsulated, or suspended in an aqueous vehicle.

(2) Drug release from the complex depends on the ionic environment within the gastrointestinal tract and on the resin's properties. Generally, release is greater in the highly acidic stomach than in the less acidic small intestine.

f. **Complex formation** is used for certain drug substances that combine chemically with other agents. For example, hydroxypropyl-β-cyclodextrin forms a chemical complex that can be only slowly soluble from body fluids, depending on the pH of the environment.

g. **Hydrocolloid systems** (e.g., Valrelease, a slow-release form of diazepam) include a unique, **hydrodynamically balanced drug delivery system (HBS)** developed by Roche.

(1) The HBS consists of a matrix designed so that the dosage form, on contact with gastric fluid, demonstrates a bulk density less than one and, thus, remains buoyant.

(2) When in contact with gastric fluid, the outermost hydrocolloids swell to form a boundary layer, which prevents immediate penetration of fluid into the formulation.

(3) This outer hydrocolloid layer slowly erodes with subsequent formation of a new boundary layer.

(4) The process is continuous, with each new outer layer eroding slowly. The drug is released gradually through each layer as fluid slowly penetrates the matrix.

STUDY QUESTIONS

Directions: Each of the numbered items or incomplete statements in this section is followed by answers or by completions of the statement. Select the **one** lettered answer or completion that is **best** in each case.

1. Which of the following substances is classified as a weak electrolyte?

(A) Glucose
(B) Urea
(C) Ephedrine
(D) Sodium chloride (NaCl)
(E) Sucrose

2. The pH value is calculated mathematically as the

(A) log of the hydroxyl ion (OH^-) concentration
(B) negative log of the OH^- concentration
(C) log of the hydrogen ion (H^+) concentration
(D) negative log of the H^+ concentration
(E) ratio of H^+/OH^- concentration

3. Which of the following properties is classified as a colligative property?

(A) Solubility of a solute
(B) Osmotic pressure
(C) Hydrogen ion (H^+) concentration
(D) Dissociation of a solute
(E) Miscibility of the liquids

4. The colligative properties of a solution are related to the

(A) pH of the solution
(B) number of ions in the solution
(C) total number of solute particles in the solution
(D) number of nonionized molecules in the solution
(E) pK_a of the solution

5. The pH of a buffer system can be calculated by using the

(A) Noyes-Whitney equation
(B) Henderson-Hasselbalch equation
(C) Michaelis-Menten equation
(D) Yong equation
(E) Stokes equation

6. Which of the following mechanisms is most frequently responsible for chemical degradation?

(A) Racemization
(B) Photolysis
(C) Hydrolysis
(D) Decarboxylation
(E) Oxidation

7. Which of the following equations is used to predict the stability of a drug product at room temperature from experiments at accelerated temperatures?

(A) Stokes equation
(B) Yong equation
(C) Arrhenius equation
(D) Michaelis-Menten equation
(E) Hixson-Crowell equation

8. Based on the relationship between the degree of ionization and the solubility of a weak acid, the drug aspirin (pK_a 3.49) will be most soluble at

(A) pH 1.0
(B) pH 2.0
(C) pH 3.0
(D) pH 4.0
(E) pH 6.0

9. Which of the following solutions is used as an astringent?

(A) Strong iodine solution USP
(B) Aluminum acetate topical solution USP
(C) Acetic acid NF
(D) Aromatic ammonia spirit USP
(E) Benzalkonium chloride solution NF

10. The particle size of the dispersed solid in a suspension is usually greater than

(A) 0.5 μm
(B) 0.4 μm
(C) 0.3 μm
(D) 0.2 μm
(E) 0.1 μm

11. In the extemporaneous preparation of a suspension, levigation is used to

(A) reduce zeta potential
(B) avoid bacterial growth
(C) reduce particle size
(D) enhance viscosity
(E) reduce viscosity

12. Which of the following compounds is a natural emulsifying agent?

(A) Acacia
(B) Lactose
(C) Polysorbate 20
(D) Polysorbate 80
(E) Sorbitan monopalmitate

13. Vanishing cream is an ointment that may be classified as

(A) a water-soluble base
(B) an oleaginous base
(C) an absorption base
(D) an emulsion base
(E) an oleic base

14. Rectal suppositories intended for adult use usually weigh approximately

(A) 1 g
(B) 2 g
(C) 3 g
(D) 4 g
(E) 5 g

15. In the fusion method of making cocoa butter suppositories, which of the following substances is most likely to be used for lubricating the mold?

(A) Mineral oil
(B) Propylene glycol
(C) Cetyl alcohol
(D) Stearic acid
(E) Magnesium silicate

16. A very fine powdered chemical is defined as one that will

(A) completely pass through a #80 sieve
(B) completely pass through a #120 sieve
(C) completely pass through a #20 sieve
(D) pass through a #60 sieve and not more than 40% through a #100 sieve
(E) pass through a #40 sieve and not more than 60% through a #60 sieve

17. Camphor is usually milled by which of the following techniques?

(A) Trituration
(B) Levigation
(C) Pulverization by intervention
(D) Geometric dilution
(E) Attrition

18. The dispensing pharmacist usually accomplishes the blending of potent powders with a large amount of diluent by

(A) spatulation
(B) sifting
(C) trituration
(D) geometric dilution
(E) levigation

19. Which type of paper will best protect a divided hygroscopic powder?

(A) Waxed paper
(B) Glassine
(C) White bond
(D) Blue bond
(E) Vegetable parchment

20. Which of the following capsule sizes has the smallest capacity?

(A) 5
(B) 4
(C) 1
(D) 0
(E) 000

21. The shells of soft gelatin capsules may be made elastic or plastic-like by the addition of

(A) sorbitol
(B) povidone
(C) polyethylene glycol (PEG)
(D) lactose
(E) hydroxypropyl methylcellulose (HPMC)

22. The *United States Pharmacopeia* (USP) content uniformity test for tablets is used to ensure which of the following qualities?

(A) Bioequivalency
(B) Dissolution
(C) Potency
(D) Purity
(E) Toxicity

23. All of the following statements concerning chemical degradation are true EXCEPT

(A) as temperature increases, degradation decreases
(B) most drugs degrade by a first-order process
(C) chemical degradation may produce a toxic product
(D) chemical degradation may result in a loss of active ingredients
(E) chemical degradation may affect the therapeutic activity of a drug

24. All of the following statements concerning zero-order degradation are true EXCEPT

(A) its rate is independent of the concentration
(B) a plot of concentration versus time yields a straight line on rectilinear paper
(C) its half-life is a changing parameter
(D) its concentration remains unchanged with respect to time
(E) the slope of a plot of concentration versus time yields a rate constant

25. All of the following statements concerning first-order degradation are true EXCEPT

(A) its rate is dependent on the concentration
(B) its half-life is a changing parameter
(C) a plot of the logarithm of concentration versus time yields a straight line
(D) its $t_{90\%}$ is independent of the concentration
(E) a plot of the logarithm of concentration versus time allows determination of the rate constant

26. A satisfactory suppository base must meet all of the following criteria EXCEPT

(A) it should have a narrow melting range
(B) it should be nonirritating and nonsensitizing
(C) it should dissolve or disintegrate rapidly in the body cavity
(D) it should melt below 30°C
(E) it should be inert

27. Cocoa butter (theobroma oil) exhibits all of the following properties EXCEPT

(A) it melts at temperatures between 33°C and 35° C
(B) it is a mixture of glycerides
(C) it is a polymorph
(D) it is useful in formulating rectal suppositories
(E) it is soluble in water

28. *United States Pharmacopeia* (USP) tests for ensuring the quality of drug products in tablet form include all of the following EXCEPT

(A) disintegration
(B) dissolution
(C) hardness and friability
(D) content uniformity
(E) weight variation

Directions: Each question below contains three suggested answers of which **one or more** is correct. Choose the answer

A if **I only** is correct
B if **III only** is correct
C if **I and II** are correct
D if **II and III** are correct
E if **I, II, and III** are correct

29. Forms of water that are suitable for use in parenteral preparations include which of the following?

I. Purified water USP
II. Water for injection USP
III. Sterile water for injection USP

30. The particles in an ideal suspension should satisfy which of the following criteria?

I. Their size should be uniform
II. They should be stationary or move randomly
III. They should remain discrete

31. The sedimentation of particles in a suspension can be minimized by

I. adding sodium benzoate
II. increasing the viscosity of the suspension
III. reducing the particle size of the active ingredient

32. Ingredients that may be used as suspending agents include

I. methylcellulose
II. acacia
III. talc

33. Mechanisms thought to provide stable emulsifications include the

I. formation of interfacial film
II. lowering of interfacial tension
III. presence of charge on the ions

34. Nonionic surface-active agents used as synthetic emulsifiers include

I. tragacanth
II. sodium lauryl sulfate
III. sorbitan esters (spans)

35. Advantages of systemic drug administration by rectal suppositories include

I. avoidance of first-pass effects
II. suitability when the oral route is not feasible
III. predictable drug release and absorption

36. True statements concerning the milling of powders include

I. a fine particle size is essential if the lubricant is to function properly
II. an increased surface area may enhance the dissolution rate
III. milling may cause degradation of thermolabile drugs

37. Substances that are used to insulate powder components that liquefy when mixed include

I. talc
II. kaolin
III. light magnesium oxide

38. A Wedgwood mortar may be preferable to a glass mortar when

I. a volatile oil is added to a powder mixture
II. colored substances (dyes) are mixed into a powder
III. comminution is desired in addition to mixing

39. Divided powders may be dispensed in

I. individual-dose packets
II. a bulk container
III. a perforated, sifter-type container

40. True statements about the function of excipients used in tablet formulations include

I. binders promote granulation during the wet granulation process
II. glidants help to promote the flow of the tablet granulation during manufacture
III. lubricants help the patient to swallow the tablets

41. Manufacturing variables that would be likely to affect the dissolution of a prednisone tablet in the body include

I. the amount and type of binder added
II. the amount and type of disintegrant added
III. the force of compression used during tableting

42. Agents that might be used to coat enteric-coated tablets include

I. hydroxypropyl methylcellulose (HPMC)
II. carboxymethylcellulose (CMC)
III. cellulose acetate phthalate (CAP)

43. The amount of nitroglycerin that a transdermal patch delivers within a 24-hour period depends on the

I. occlusive backing on the patch
II. diffusion rate of nitroglycerin from the patch
III. surface area of the patch

Directions: Each group of items in this section consists of lettered options followed by a set of numbered items. For each item, select the **one** lettered option that is most closely associated with it. Each lettered option may be selected once, more than once, or not at all.

Questions 44–47

For each of the tablet processing problems listed below, select the most likely reason for the condition.

(A) Excessive moisture in the granulation
(B) Entrapment of air
(C) Tablet friability
(D) Degraded drug
(E) Tablet hardness

44. Picking

45. Mottling

46. Capping

47. Sticking

Questions 48–50

For each description of a comminution procedure below, select the process that it best describes.

(A) Trituration
(B) Spatulation
(C) Levigation
(D) Pulverization by intervention
(E) Tumbling

48. Rubbing or grinding a substance in a mortar with a rough inner surface

49. Reducing and subdividing a substance by adding an easily removed solvent

50. Adding a suitable agent to form a paste and then rubbing or grinding the paste in a mortar

Questions 51–54

Match the drug product below with the type of controlled-release dosage form that it represents.

(A) Matrix device
(B) Ion-exchange resin complex
(C) Hydrocolloid system
(D) Osmotic system
(E) Coated granules

51. Biphenamine capsules

52. Thorazine Spansule capsules

53. Valrelease

54. Slow-K

ANSWERS AND EXPLANATIONS

1. The answer is C *[IV A 1 a, 3 d].*
Glucose, urea, and sucrose are nonelectrolytes, whereas sodium chloride (NaCl) is an example of a strong electrolyte. Electrolytes are substances that form ions when dissolved in water and, thus, can conduct an electric current through the solution. Ions are particles that bear electrical charges: cations are positively charged ions, and anions are negatively charged. Strong electrolytes are completely ionized in water at all concentrations; weak electrolytes (e.g., ephedrine) are only partially ionized at most concentrations. Nonelectrolytes do not form ions when in solution and, thus, are nonconductors.

2. The answer is D *[IV A 3 b].*
The pH is a measure of the acidity or hydrogen ion concentration of an aqueous solution. The pH is the logarithm of the reciprocal of the hydrogen ion (H^+) concentration expressed in moles per liter. Because the logarithm of a reciprocal equals the negative logarithm of the number, the pH is the negative logarithm of the H^+ concentration. A pH of 7.0 indicates neutrality; as the pH decreases, the acidity increases. The pH of arterial blood is 7.35 to 7.45; of urine, 4.8 to 7.5; of gastric juice, about 1.4; of cerebrospinal fluid, 7.35 to 7.40. The concept of pH was introduced by Sörensen in the early 1900s. Alkalinity is the negative logarithm of (OH^-) and is inversely related to acidity.

3. The answer is B *[IV A 2 d].*
Osmotic pressure is an example of a colligative property. The osmotic pressure is the magnitude of pressure needed to stop osmosis across a semipermeable membrane between a solution and pure solvent. Colligative properties of a solution depend on the total number of dissociated and undissociated solute particles and are independent of the size of the solute. Other colligative properties of solutes are the reduction in vapor pressure of a solution, elevation of its boiling point, and depression of its freezing point.

4. The answer is C *[IV A 1 b].*
The colligative properties of a solution are related to the total number of solute particles in a solution. Examples of colligative properties are osmotic pressure, lowering of vapor pressure, elevation of the boiling point, and depression of the freezing (or melting) point.

5. The answer is B *[IV A 3 e].*
The Henderson-Hasselbalch equation for a weak acid and its salt is represented as:

$$pH = pK_a + \log \frac{[salt]}{[acid]}$$

where pK_a is the negative log of the dissociation constant of a weak acid, and [salt]/[acid] is the ratio of the molar concentration of salt and acid used to prepare a buffer.

6. The answer is C *[V D 1].*
Although it is true that all of the mechanisms listed in the question can be responsible, the chemical degradation of medicinal compounds is most frequently due to hydrolysis. This is true particularly of esters in liquid formulations, and drugs having ester functional groups are, therefore, formulated in dry form whenever possible. Oxidation, another common mode of degradation, is minimized by including antioxidants, such as ascorbic acid, in drug formulations. Photolysis is reduced by packaging susceptible products in amber or opaque containers. Decarboxylation, the removal of COOH groups, affects carboxylic acid compounds. Racemization neutralizes the effects of an optically active compound by converting half its molecules into the mirror-image configuration, so that the dextro- and levorotatory forms cancel one another out. This form of degradation affects only drugs characterized by optical isomerism.

7. The answer is C *[V E 3 c].*
Testing of a drug formulation to determine its shelf life can be accelerated by applying the Arrhenius equation to data obtained at higher temperatures. The method involves the determination of rate constant (k) values for the degradation of a drug at various elevated temperatures. The log of k is then plotted against the reciprocal of the absolute temperature, and the k value for degradation at room temperature is obtained by extrapolation.

8. The answer is E *[IV A 3].*
The solubility of a weak acid varies as a function of pH. Because pH and pK_a (the dissociation constant) are related, solubility is also related to the degree of ionization. The drug aspirin is a weak acid

and will be completely ionized at pH that is 2 units above its pK_a. Therefore, it will be most soluble at pH 6.0.

9. The answer is B *[VI B 7].*
Aluminum acetate and aluminum subacetate solutions are astringents used as wet dressings for contact dermatitis and as antiperspirants. Strong iodine solution and benzalkonium chloride are topical antibacterial solutions; acetic acid is added to products as an acidifier; and aromatic ammonia spirit is a respiratory stimulant.

10. The answer is A *[IV B 1].*
A suspension is a two-phase system that consists of a finely powdered solid dispersed in a liquid vehicle. The particle size of the suspended solid should be as small as possible to minimize sedimentation; however, the particle size is usually greater than 0.5 μm.

11. The answer is C *[VI E 3].*
Levigation is the process of blending and grinding a substance to separate the particles, reduce their size, and form a paste. It is performed by adding a small amount of suitable levigating agent, such as glycerin, to the solid and then blending the mixture, using a mortar and pestle.

12. The answer is A *[VI D 3].*
Acacia (gum arabic) is the exudate obtained from the stems and branches of various species of Acacia, a woody plant native to Africa. Acacia is a natural emulsifying agent that provides a good stable emulsion of low viscosity. Emulsions consist of droplets of one or more immiscible liquids dispersed in another liquid. Emulsions are inherently unstable: the droplets tend to coalesce into larger and larger drops. The purpose of an emulsifying agent is to keep the droplets dispersed and prevent them from coalescing. Polysorbate 20, polysorbate 80, and sorbitan monopalmitate are also emulsifiers but are synthetic, not natural, substances.

13. The answer is D *[VI E 1 a].*
Ointments are used typically as emollients to soften the skin, as protective barriers, or as vehicles for medication. To serve these functions, a variety of ointment bases are available. Vanishing cream, an emulsion type of ointment base, is an oil-in-water (o/w) emulsion that contains a high percentage of water. Stearic acid is present to create a thin film on the skin when the water evaporates.

14. The answer is B *[VI F 2 a].*
By convention, a rectal suppository for an adult weighs about 2 g; suppositories for infants or children are smaller. Vaginal suppositories typically weigh about 5 g. Rectal suppositories are usually shaped like a rather elongated bullet, being cylindrical and tapered at one end. Vaginal suppositories are usually ovoid.

15. The answer is A *[VI F 4 c].*
In the fusion method of making suppositories, molds made of aluminum, brass, or nickel-copper alloys are used. A mixture of finely powdered drug in melted cocoa butter is poured into a mold that is lubricated very lightly with mineral oil.

16. The answer is B *[VI G; Table 3-8].*
The *United States Pharmacopeia* (USP) definition of a very fine chemical powder is one that will completely pass through a standard #120 sieve (which has 125-μm openings). The USP classification for powdered vegetable and animal drugs differs from that for powdered chemicals. To be classified as very fine, powdered vegetable and animal drugs must pass completely through a #80 sieve (which has 180-μm openings).

17. The answer is C *[VI G 1 c (3)].*
Pulverization by intervention is the milling technique used for drug substances that are gummy and tend to reagglomerate or resist grinding (e.g., camphor, iodine). "Intervention" refers to the addition of a small amount of material that aids milling and that can be removed easily after pulverization is complete. For example, camphor can be reduced readily if a small amount of volatile solvent (e.g., alcohol) is added; the solvent is then allowed to evaporate.

18. The answer is D *[VI G 2 b, c].*
When mixing potent substances with a large amount of diluent, the pharmacist uses geometric dilution. The potent drug and an equal amount of diluent are first mixed in a mortar by trituration. A vol-

ume of diluent equal to the mixture in the mortar is then added, and the mix is again triturated. The procedure is repeated, each time adding diluent equal in volume to the mixture then in the mortar, until all the diluent has been incorporated.

19. The answer is A *[VI G 3 b].*
Hygroscopic and volatile drugs can be protected best by the use of waxed paper, which is waterproof. The packet may be double wrapped with a bond paper to improve the appearance of the completed powder.

20. The answer is A *[VI H 2 c].*
Hard capsules are numbered from 000 (the largest size) to 5 (the smallest size). The approximate capsule capacity ranges from 600 mg to 30 mg; however, the capsule capacity depends on the density of the contents.

21. The answer is A *[VI H 3 a].*
The shells of soft gelatin capsules are plasticized by the addition of a polyhydric alcohol (polyol), such as glycerin or sorbitol. An antifungal preservative can also be added. Both hard and soft gelatin capsules can be filled with a powder or other dry substance; soft gelatin capsules also are useful dosage forms for fluids or semisolids.

22. The answer is C *[VI H 4].*
Different uniformity test, in effect, is a test of potency. To ensure that each tablet or capsule contains the amount of drug substance intended, the *United States Pharmacopeia* (USP) provides two tests: weight variation and content uniformity. The content uniformity test can be used for any dosage unit but is required for coated tablets, for tablets in which the active ingredient comprises less than 50% of the tablet for suspensions in single-unit containers or in soft capsules, and for many solids that contain added substances. The weight variation test can be used for liquid-filled soft capsules, for any dosage-form unit that contains at least 50 mg of a single drug if the drug comprises at least 50% of the bulk, for solids without added substances, and for freeze-dried solutions.

23. The answer is A *[V A 2].*
A number of factors can affect the reaction velocity, or degradation rate, of a pharmaceutical product. Among these are temperature, solvents, and light. The degradation increases two to three times with each 10° increase in temperature. The effect of temperature on reaction rate is given by the Arrhenius equation:

$$k = Ae^{-Ea/RT}$$

where *k* is the reaction rate constant, *A* is the frequency factor, *Ea* is the energy of activation, *R* is the gas constant, and *T* is the absolute temperature.

24. The answer is D *[V B 2 a].*
In zero-order degradation, the concentration of a drug decreases over time; it is the change of concentration with respect to time that is unchanged. In the equation:

$$\frac{-dC}{dt} = k$$

the fact that dC/dt is negative signifies that the concentration is decreasing; however, the *velocity* of concentration change is seen to be constant.

25. The answer is B *[V B 2 b (3)].*
The half-life ($t_{1/2}$) is the time required for the concentration of a drug to decrease by one-half. For a first-order degradation,

$$t_{1/2} = \frac{0.693}{k}$$

Because both k and 0.693 are constants, $t_{1/2}$ is a constant.

26. The answer is D *[VI F 3].*
A satisfactory suppository base should remain firm at room temperature; preferably, it should not melt below 30°C to avoid premature softening during storage and insertion. A satisfactory suppository base should also be inert, nonsensitizing, nonirritating, and compatible with a variety of drugs. Moreover, it

should melt just below body temperature and should dissolve or disintegrate rapidly in the fluid of the body cavity into which it is inserted.

27. The answer is E *[VI F 3 c (1)].*
Cocoa butter is a fat obtained from the seed of *Theobroma cacao.* Chemically, it is a mixture of stearin, palmitin, and other glycerides that are insoluble in water and freely soluble in ether and chloroform. Depending on the fusion temperature, cocoa butter can crystallize into any one of four crystal forms. Cocoa butter is a good base for rectal suppositories but is less than ideal for vaginal or urethral suppositories.

28. The answer is C *[VI I 5].*
To satisfy the *United States Pharmacopeia* (USP) standards, tablets are required to meet a weight variation test (if the active ingredient comprises the bulk of the tablet) or a content uniformity test (if the active ingredient comprises less than 50% of the tablet bulk or if the tablet is coated). Many tablets for oral administration are required to meet a disintegration test, with disintegration times specified in the individual monographs. A dissolution test might be required instead if the active component of the tablet has limited water-solubility. Hardness and friability would affect a tablet's disintegration and dissolution rates, but hardness and friability tests are in-house quality control tests, and are not official USP tests.

29. The answer is D (II, III) *[VI A 1].*
Water for injection USP is water that has been purified by distillation or by reverse osmosis. It is used in preparing parenteral solutions that are subject to final sterilization. For parenteral solutions prepared aseptically and not subsequently sterilized, sterile water for injection USP is used. Sterile water for injection USP is water for injection USP that has been sterilized and suitably packaged; it meets the USP requirements for sterility. Bacteriostatic water for injection USP is sterile water for injection USP that contains one or more antimicrobial agents. It can be used in parenteral solutions if the antimicrobial additives are compatible with the other ingredients in the solution, but it cannot be used in newborn infants. Purified water USP is not used in parenteral preparations.

30. The answer is E (all) *[VI C].*
An ideal suspension would have particles of uniform size, minimal sedimentation, and no interaction between particles. These ideal criteria are rarely realized, although they can be approximated by keeping the particle size as small as possible, the densities of the solid and the dispersion medium as similar as possible, and the dispersion medium as viscous as possible.

31. The answer is D (II, III) *[IV B 2].*
As Stokes' law indicates, the sedimentation rate of a suspension is slowed by reducing its density, reducing the size of the suspended particles, or increasing its viscosity (achieved by incorporating a thickening agent). Sodium benzoate is an antifungal agent and would not reduce the sedimentation rate of a suspension.

32. The answer is C (I, II) *[VI C 3].*
Acacia and methylcellulose are both commonly used as suspending agents. Acacia is a natural product; methylcellulose is a synthetic polymer. By increasing the viscosity of the liquid, these agents enable particles to remain suspended for a longer period of time.

33. The answer is E (all) *[VI D 3].*
Emulsifying agents provide a mechanical barrier to coalescence, reducing the natural tendency of the internal-phase (oil or water) droplets in the emulsion to coalesce. Three mechanisms appear to be involved: some emulsifiers promote stability by forming strong, pliable interfacial films around the droplets. Emulsifying agents also reduce interfacial tension. An electrical charge on the ions in the emulsion can create charge repulsion that causes droplets to repel one another, thereby preventing coalescence.

34. The answer is B (III) *[VI D 3].*
All of the substances listed in the question are emulsifying agents, but only sorbitan esters are nonionic synthetic agents. Tragacanth, like acacia, is a natural emulsifying agent, and sodium lauryl sulfate is an anionic surfactant. Sorbitan esters (known colloquially as spans by virtue of their trade names) are hydrophobic and form water-in-oil (w/o) emulsions. The polysorbates (known colloquially as Tweens) are also nonionic, synthetic sorbitan derivatives, but they are hydrophilic and, therefore, form oil-in-water (o/w) emulsions. Sodium lauryl sulfate, as an alkali soap, is also hydrophilic and, thus, forms o/w emulsions.

35. The answer is C (I, II) *[VI F 2].*
Rectal suppositories are useful for delivering systemic medication under certain circumstances. Absorption of a drug from a rectal suppository involves release of the drug from the suppository vehicle, followed by diffusion of the drug through the rectal mucosa and transport to the circulation by way of the rectal veins. Because the rectal veins bypass the liver, rapid hepatic degradation of certain drugs (first-pass effect) is avoided. The rectal route is also useful when a drug cannot be given orally (e.g., because of vomiting). However, the extent of drug release and absorption is variable; it depends on the properties of the drug, the suppository base, and the environment in the rectum.

36. The answer is E (all) *[VI G 1 c].*
Milling is the process of mechanically reducing the particle size of solids before formulation into a final product. For a lubricant to work effectively, it must coat the surface of the granulation or powder. Hence fine particle size is essential. Decreasing the particle size increases the surface area, and this can enhance the dissolution rate. Possible degradation of thermolabile drugs might occur as a result of heat buildup during milling.

37. The answer is D (II, III) *[VI G 2 a].*
Some solid substances (e.g., aspirin, phenylsalicylate, phenacetin, thymol, camphor) liquefy or form eutectic mixtures when in close and prolonged contact with one another. Such substances are best insulated by the addition of light magnesium oxide or magnesium carbonate; other inert diluents that can be used are kaolin, starch, or bentonite.

38. The answer is B (III) *[VI G 2 b].*
In the mixing of powders, if comminution is especially desired, a porcelain or Wedgwood mortar having a rough inner surface is preferred over the smooth working surface of the glass mortar. A glass mortar cleans more easily after use and, therefore, is preferable for chemicals that may stain a porcelain or Wedgwood mortar and for simple mixing of substances without the need for comminution.

39. The answer is A (I) *[VI G 3 a].*
Powders for oral use can be dispensed by the pharmacist in bulk form or divided into premeasured doses (divided powders). Divided powders are traditionally dispensed in folded paper packets (chartulae) made of parchment, bond paper, glassine, or waxed paper. However, if the powder needs greater protection from humidity or evaporation, the individual doses can be packaged in metal foil or small plastic bags.

40. The answer is C (I, II) *[VI I].*
Tablets for oral ingestion usually contain excipients that are added to the formulation for their special functions. Binders and adhesives are added to promote granulation or compaction. Diluents are fillers added to make up the required tablet bulk; they can also aid in the manufacturing process. Disintegrants aid tablet disintegration in gastrointestinal fluids. Lubricants, antiadherents, and glidants aid in reducing friction or adhesion between particles or between the tablet and the die. For example, lubricants are used in tablet manufacture to reduce friction when the tablet is ejected from the die cavity in which it was formed. Lubricants are usually hydrophobic substances that can affect the dissolution rate of the active ingredient in a tablet.

41. The answer is E (all) *[VI I 2 b (3)].*
Disintegrants are added to tablet formulations to facilitate tablet disintegration in the gastrointestinal fluids. The tablet's disintegration in the body is critical to its dissolution and subsequent absorption and bioavailability. The binder and the compression force used during tablet manufacturing both affect a tablet's hardness, and this also affects tablet disintegration and drug dissolution.

42. The answer is B (III) *[VI H 4 b].*
An enteric-coated tablet has a coating that remains intact in the stomach but dissolves in the intestines to yield the tablet's ingredients there. Enteric coatings include various fats, fatty acids, waxes, and shellacs. Cellulose acetate phthalate remains intact in the stomach because it dissolves only above pH 6. Other enteric-coating materials include povidone (polyvinylpyrrolidone; PVP), polyvinyl acetate phthalate (PVAP), and hydroxypropyl methylcellulose phthalate (HPMCP).

43. The answer is E (all) *[VI J 2 c].*
The delivery of drugs through a transdermal drug delivery system (TDDS) depends on the microporous membranes that act as rate-controlling barriers, the mechanism by which the drug diffuses through these carriers (e.g., reservoir, matrix), and the surface area of the patch.

44–47. The answers are: 44-A, 45-D, 46-B, 47-A *[VI I 4].*
Sticking refers to tablet material adhering to a die wall. Sticking can be caused by excessive moisture or ingredients with low melting temperatures. Mottling is uneven color distribution; it is most often due to poor mixing of the tablet granulation but may also result from a degraded drug that produces a colored metabolite. Capping is the separation of the top or bottom crown of a tablet from the main body of the tablet. Capping implies that compressed powder is not cohesive. Reasons for capping include excessive force of compression, use of insufficient binder, worn tablet tooling equipment, and air entrapment during processing. Picking refers to surface material from a tablet sticking to a punch. Picking can be caused by a granulation that is too damp, by a scratched punch, by static charges on the powder, and particularly by use of a punch tip with engraving or embossing.

48–50. The answers are: 48-A, 49-D, 50-C *[VI G 1 c].*
Comminution is the process of reducing the particle size of a powder to increase the powder's fineness. Several comminution techniques are suitable for small-scale use in a pharmacy. Trituration is used both to comminute and to mix dry powders; if comminution is desired, the substance is rubbed in a mortar with a rough inner surface. Pulverization by intervention is often used for substances that tend to agglomerate or to resist grinding. A small amount of easily removed (e.g., volatile) solvent is added, and after the substance is pulverized, the solvent is allowed to evaporate or is otherwise removed. Levigation is often used to prepare pastes or ointments. The powder is reduced by adding a suitable nonsolvent (levigating agent) to form a paste and then rubbing the paste in a mortar, using a pestle, or on an ointment slab, using a spatula. Spatulation and tumbling are procedures for mixing or blending powders, not for reducing them. Spatulation is blending small amounts of powders together by stirring them with a spatula on a sheet of paper or a pill tile. Tumbling is the process of blending large amounts of powder in a large rotating container.

51–54. The answers are: 51-B, 52-E, 53-C, 54-A *[VI J].*
Controlled-release dosage forms are designed to release a drug slowly for prolonged action in the body. A variety of pharmaceutical mechanisms are employed to provide the controlled release. Ion-exchange resins may be complexed to drugs (e.g., biphenamine capsules) by passing a cationic drug solution through a column containing the resin. The drug is complexed to the resin by replacement of hydrogen atoms. Drug release from the complex depends on the ionic environment within the gastrointestinal tract and on the resin's properties. Coated beads or granules (e.g., Thorazine Spansule capsules) produce blood levels similar to those obtained with multiple dosing. The various coating thicknesses produce a sustained-release effect.

The hydrocolloid system (e.g., Valrelease, a slow-release form of diazepam) includes a unique hydrodynamically balanced drug-delivery system (HBS). Outermost hydrocolloids swell to form a boundary when in contact with gastric fluid, preventing penetration of fluid into the formulation. As outer layers erode, new boundary layers form, allowing a gradual release of the drug.

Matrix devices can employ insoluble plastics, hydrophilic polymers, or fatty compounds, which are mixed with the drug and compressed into a tablet. The primary dose, the portion of the drug to be released immediately, is placed on the tablet as a layer or coat. The remainder of the dose is released slowly from the matrix.

4
Biopharmaceutics and Drug Delivery Systems

Lawrence H. Block
Charles C. Collins

I. INTRODUCTION

A. Biopharmaceutics is the study of the relation of the physical and chemical properties of a drug to its bioavailability, pharmacokinetics, and pharmacodynamic and toxicologic effects.

1. A **drug product** is the finished dosage form (e.g., tablet, capsule, solution) that contains the active drug ingredient in association with nondrug (usually inactive) ingredients (**excipients**) that make up the **vehicle,** or **formulation matrix.**

2. The phrase drug delivery system is often used interchangeably with the terms drug product or dosage form. However, a **drug delivery system** is a more comprehensive concept that includes the drug formulation and the dynamic interactions among the drug, its formulation matrix, its container, and the patient.

3. **Bioavailability** is a measurement of the rate and extent (amount) of systemic absorption of the therapeutically active drug.

B. Pharmacokinetics is the study of the time course of drug movement in the body during absorption, distribution, and elimination (excretion and biotransformation).

C. Pharmacodynamics is the study of the relation of the drug concentration or amount at the site of action (receptor) and its pharmacologic response.

II. DRUG ABSORPTION

A. Transport of drug molecules across cell membranes. Drug absorption requires the drug to be transported across various cell membranes. Drug molecules may enter the bloodstream and be transported to the tissues and organs of the body. Drug molecules may cross additional membranes to enter cells. Drug molecules may also cross an intracellular membrane, such as the nuclear membrane or endoplasmic reticulum, to reach the site of action.

1. **General principles**
   a. A **cell membrane** is a semipermeable structure composed primarily of lipids and proteins.
   b. Drugs may be transported by **passive diffusion, partitioning, carrier-mediated transport, paracellular transport,** or **vesicular transport.**
   c. Usually, **proteins, drugs bound to proteins,** and **macromolecules** do not cross cell membranes easily.
   d. **Nonpolar lipid-soluble drugs** traverse cell membranes more easily than **ionic** or **polar water-soluble drugs.**
   e. **Low–molecular-weight drugs** diffuse across a cell membrane more easily than **high–molecular-weight drugs.**

2. **Passive diffusion and partitioning**
   a. **Within the cytoplasm** or in **interstitial fluid,** most drugs undergo transport by simple **diffusion.**
   b. **Fick's law of diffusion. Simple passive diffusion** involves the transfer of drugs from an area of high concentration (C_1) to an area of lower concentration (C_2) according to Fick's law of diffusion:

$$\frac{dQ}{dt} = \frac{DA}{h}(C_1 - C_2),$$

where dQ/dt is the rate of drug diffusion, D is the diffusion coefficient for the drug, A is the surface area of the plane across which transfer occurs, h is the thickness of the region through which diffusion occurs, and $(C_1 - C_2)$ is the difference between the drug concentration in area 1 and area 2, respectively.

c. Passive drug transport across cell membranes involves the successive **partitioning** of a solute between aqueous and lipid phases as well as **diffusion** within the respective phases. Modifying Fick's law of diffusion to accommodate the partitioning of drug gives the following:

$$\frac{dQ}{dt} = \frac{DAK}{h}(C_1 - C_2),$$

The rate of drug diffusion, dQ/dt, now reflects its direct dependence on K, the oil:water partition coefficient of the drug, as well as on A and $(C_1 - C_2)$.

d. **Ionization of a weak electrolyte** is affected by the pH of the medium in which the drug is dissolved as well as by the pK_a of the drug. The nonionized species is more lipid soluble than the ionized species, and it partitions more readily across cell membranes.

3. **Carrier-mediated transport**
   a. **Active transport** of the drug across a membrane is a carrier-mediated process that has the following characteristics:
      (1) The drug moves against a concentration gradient.
      (2) The process requires energy.
      (3) The carrier may be selective for certain types of drugs that resemble natural substrates, or metabolites that are normally actively transported.
      (4) The carrier system may be saturated at a high drug concentration.
      (5) The process may be competitive (i.e., drugs with similar structures may compete for the same carrier).
   b. **Facilitated diffusion** is also a carrier-mediated transport system. However, facilitated diffusion occurs with a concentration gradient and does not require energy.

4. **Paracellular and convective transport.** Drug transport across tight (narrow) junctions between cells or transendothelial channels of cells is known as **paracellular transport.** It involves the **convective** (bulk) flow of water and accompanying water-soluble drug molecules through the paracellular channels.

5. **Vesicular transport** is the process of engulfing particles or dissolved materials by a cell. Vesicular transport is the only transport mechanism that does not require a drug to be in an aqueous solution to be absorbed. **Pinocytosis** and **phagocytosis** are forms of vesicular transport.
   a. **Pinocytosis** is the engulfment of small solute or fluid volumes.
   b. **Phagocytosis** is the engulfment of larger particles, or macromolecules, generally by macrophages.
   c. **Endocytosis** and **exocytosis** are the movement of macromolecules into and out of the cell, respectively.

B. Routes of drug administration

1. **Parenteral administration**
   a. **Intravenous bolus injection.** The drug is injected directly into the bloodstream, distributes throughout the body, and acts rapidly. Any side effects, including an intense pharmacologic response, anaphylaxis, or overt toxicity, also occur rapidly.
   b. **Intra-arterial injection.** The drug is injected into a specific artery to achieve a high drug concentration in a specific tissue before drug distribution occurs throughout the body. Intra-arterial injection is used for diagnostic agents and occasionally for chemotherapy.
   c. **Intravenous infusion.** The drug is given intravenously at a constant input rate. Constant-rate intravenous infusion maintains a relatively constant plasma drug concentration.
   d. **Intramuscular injection.** The drug is injected deep into a skeletal muscle. The rate of absorption depends on the vascularity of the muscle site, the lipid solubility of the drug, and the formulation matrix.
   e. **Subcutaneous injection.** The drug is injected beneath the skin. Because the subcutaneous region is less vascular than muscle tissues, drug absorption is less rapid. The factors that affect absorption from intramuscular depots also affect subcutaneous absorption.

f. Miscellaneous parenteral routes

(1) Intra-articular injection. The drug is injected into a joint.

(2) Intradermal (intracutaneous) injection. The drug is injected into the dermis (i.e., the vascular region of the skin below the epidermis).

(3) Intrathecal injection. The drug is injected into the spinal fluid.

2. Enteral administration

a. Buccal and sublingual administration. A tablet or lozenge is placed under the tongue (**sublingual**) or in contact with the mucosal (**buccal**) surface of the cheek. This type of administration allows a nonpolar, lipid-soluble drug to be absorbed across the epithelial lining of the mouth. After buccal or sublingual administration, the drug is absorbed directly into the systemic circulation, bypassing the liver and any first-pass effects.

b. Peroral (oral) drug administration. The drug is administered orally, is swallowed, and undergoes absorption from the gastrointestinal tract through the mesenteric circulation to the hepatic portal vein into the liver and then to the systemic circulation. The peroral route is the most common route of administration.

(1) The peroral route is the most convenient and the safest route.

(2) Disadvantages of this route include the following:

(a) The drug may not be absorbed from the gastrointestinal tract consistently or completely.

(b) The drug may be digested by gastrointestinal enzymes or decomposed by the acid pH of the stomach.

(c) The drug may irritate mucosal epithelial cells or complex with the contents of the gastrointestinal tract.

(d) Some drugs may be incompletely absorbed because of first-pass effects or presystemic elimination (e.g., the drug is metabolized by the liver before systemic absorption occurs).

(e) The absorption rate may be erratic because of delayed gastric emptying or changes in intestinal motility.

(3) Most drugs are absorbed from the gastrointestinal tract by **passive diffusion** and **partitioning. Carrier-mediated transport, paracellular transport,** and **vesicular transport** play smaller, but critical, roles.

(4) Drug molecules are absorbed throughout the gastrointestinal tract, but the **duodenal region,** which has a large surface area because of the villi and microvilli, is the primary absorption site. The large blood supply provided by the mesenteric vessels allows the drug to be absorbed more efficiently (see II A 2).

(5) **Altered gastric emptying** affects arrival of the drug in the duodenum for systemic absorption. Factors that affect gastric emptying time include meal content, emotional factors, and drugs that affect gastrointestinal tract motility (e.g., anticholinergics, prokinetic agents).

(6) Normal intestinal motility from **peristalsis** brings the drug in contact with the intestinal epithelial cells. A sufficient period of contact (residence time) is needed to permit drug absorption across the cell membranes from the mucosal to the serosal surface.

(7) Some drugs, such as **cimetidine** and **acetaminophen,** when given in an immediate-release peroral dosage form to fasted subjects, produce a systemic drug concentration time with two peaks. This **double-peak phenomenon** is attributed to variability in stomach emptying, variable intestinal motility, and enterohepatic cycling.

c. Rectal administration. The drug in solution (enema) or suppository form is placed in the rectum. Drug diffusion from the solution or release from the suppository leads to absorption across the mucosal surface of the rectum. Drug absorbed in the lower two-thirds of the rectum enters the systemic circulation directly, bypassing the liver and any first-pass effects.

3. Respiratory tract administration

a. Intranasal administration. The drug contained in a solution or suspension is administered to the nasal mucosa, either as a spray or as drops. The medication may be used for local (e.g., nasal decongestants, intranasal steroids) or systemic effects.

b. Pulmonary inhalation. The drug, as liquid or solid particles, is inhaled perorally (with a nebulizer or a metered-dose aerosol) into the pulmonary tree. In general, **particles larger than 60 μm** are primarily deposited in the **trachea. Particles larger than 20 μm do not reach the bronchioles,** and **particles smaller than 0.6 μm** are not deposited and are

exhaled. Particles between **2 and 6 μm** can reach the **alveolar ducts,** although only particles of **1 to 2 μm are retained in the alveoli.**

4. **Transdermal and topical administration**
   a. **Transdermal** (**percutaneous**) drug absorption is the placement of the drug (in a lotion, ointment, cream, paste, or patch) on the skin surface for systemic absorption. An occlusive dressing or film improves systemic drug absorption from the skin. Small lipid-soluble molecules, such as nitroglycerin, nicotine, scopolamine, clonidine, fentanyl, and steroids (e.g., estradiol-17β, testosterone), are readily absorbed from the skin.
   b. Drugs (e.g., antibacterials, local anesthetic agents) are applied **topically** to the skin for a local effect.

5. Miscellaneous routes of drug administration include **ophthalmic, otic, urethral,** and **vaginal** administration. These routes of administration are generally used for local therapeutic activity. However, some systemic drug absorption may occur.

C. **Local drug activity** versus **systemic drug absorption.** The route of administration, absorption site, and bioavailability of the drug from the dosage form are major factors in the design of a drug product.

1. Drugs intended for **local activity,** such as topical antibiotics, anti-infectives, antifungal agents, and local anesthetics are formulated in dosage forms that minimize systemic absorption. The concentration of these drugs at the application site affects their activity.

2. When **systemic absorption** is desired, the bioavailability of the drug from the dosage form at the absorption site must be considered (e.g., a drug given intravenously is 100% bioavailable because all of the drug is placed directly into the systemic circulation). The amount, or dose, of drug in the dosage form is based on the extent of drug absorption and the desired systemic drug concentration. The type of dosage form (e.g., immediate release, controlled release) affects the rate of drug absorption.

III. BIOPHARMACEUTIC PRINCIPLES

A. Physicochemical properties

1. **Drug dissolution.** For most drugs with limited water solubility, the rate at which the solid drug enters into solution (i.e., the rate of dissolution) is often the rate-limiting step in bioavailability. The **Noyes Whitney** equation describes the diffusion-controlled rate of drug dissolution (dm/dt; i.e., the change in the amount of drug in solution with respect to time):

$$\frac{dm}{dt} = \frac{DA}{\delta}(C_s - C_b),$$

where D is the diffusion coefficient of the solute, A is the surface area of the solid undergoing dissolution, δ is the thickness of the diffusion layer, C_s is the concentration of the solvate at saturation, and C_b is the concentration of the drug in the bulk solution phase.

2. **Drug solubility** in a saturated solution (see Chapter 3 VI) is a static (equilibrium) property. The dissolution rate of a drug is a dynamic property related to the rate of absorption.

3. **Particle size** and **surface area** are inversely related. As solid drug particle size decreases, particle surface area increases.
   a. As described by the Noyes Whitney equation, the dissolution rate is directly proportional to the surface area. An increase in surface area allows for more contact between the solid drug particles and the solvent, resulting in a faster dissolution rate (see III A 1).
   b. With certain **hydrophobic drugs,** excessive particle size reduction does not always increase the dissolution rate. Small particles tend to reaggregate into larger particles to reduce the high surface free energy produced by particle size reduction.
   c. To prevent the formation of aggregates, small drug particles are molecularly dispersed in polyethylene glycol (PEG), polyvinylpyrrolidone (PVP; povidone), dextrose, or other agents. For example, a molecular dispersion of griseofulvin in a water-soluble carrier such as PEG 4000 (e.g., Gris-PEG) enhances dissolution and bioavailability.

4. **Partition coefficient and extent of ionization**

a. The **partition coefficient** of a drug is the ratio of the solubility of the drug, at equilibrium, in a nonaqueous solvent (e.g., *n*-octanol) to that in an aqueous solvent (e.g., water; pH 7.4, buffer solution). Hydrophilic drugs with higher water solubility have a faster dissolution rate than hydrophobic or lipophilic drugs, which have poor water solubility.

b. **Extent of ionization.** Drugs that are weak electrolytes (acids or bases) exist in both an ionized form and a nonionized form. The extent of ionization depends on the pK_a of the weak electrolyte and the pH of the solution. The ionized form is more polar, and therefore more water soluble, than the nonionized form. The **Henderson-Hasselbalch equation** describes the relation between the ionized and nonionized forms of a drug as a function of pH and pK_a. When the pH of the medium equals the pK_a of the drug, 50% of the drug in solution is nonionized and 50% is ionized, as shown in the following equations.

(1) For weak acids:

$$pH = pK_a + \log\left(\frac{[\text{salt}]}{[\text{nonionized acid}]}\right)$$

(2) For weak bases:

$$pH = pK_a + \log\left(\frac{[\text{nonionized base}]}{[\text{salt}]}\right)$$

5. **Salt formation**

a. The choice of salt form for a drug depends on the desired physical, chemical, or pharmacologic properties. Certain salts are designed to provide slower dissolution, slower bioavailability, and longer duration of action. Other salts are selected for greater stability, less local irritation at the absorption site, or less systemic toxicity.

(1) Some soluble salt forms are less stable than the nonionized form. For example, sodium aspirin is less stable than aspirin in the acid form.

(2) A solid dosage form containing buffering agents may be formulated with the free acid form of the drug (e.g., buffered aspirin).

(a) The buffering agent forms an alkaline medium in the gastrointestinal tract, and the drug dissolves in situ.

(b) The dissolved salt form of the drug diffuses into the bulk fluid of the gastrointestinal tract, forms a fine precipitate that redissolves rapidly, and becomes available for absorption.

b. **Effervescent granules** or **tablets** containing the acid drug in addition to sodium bicarbonate, tartaric acid, citric acid, or other ingredients are added to water just before oral administration. The excess sodium bicarbonate forms an alkaline solution in which the drug dissolves. Carbon dioxide is also formed by the decomposition of carbonic acid.

c. For weakly acidic drugs, potassium and sodium salts are more soluble than divalent cation salts (e.g., calcium, magnesium) or trivalent cation salts (e.g., aluminum).

d. For weak bases, common water-soluble salts include the hydrochloride, sulfate, citrate, and gluconate salts. The estolate, napsylate, and stearate salts are less water soluble.

6. **Polymorphism** is the ability of a drug to exist in more than one crystalline form.

a. Different polymorphs have different physical properties, including melting point and dissolution rate.

b. **Amorphous,** or **noncrystalline, forms** of a drug have faster dissolution rates than crystalline forms.

7. **Chirality** is the ability of a drug to exist as **optically active stereoisomers** or **enantiomers.** Individual enantiomers may not have the same pharmacokinetic and pharmacodynamic activity. Because most chiral drugs are used as racemic mixtures, the results of studies with such mixtures may be misleading because the drug is assumed to behave as a single entity. For example, ibuprofen exists as the *R*- and *S*-enantiomers; only the *S*-enantiomer is pharmacologically active. When the racemic mixture of ibuprofen is taken orally, the *R*-enantiomer undergoes presystemic inversion in the gut to the *S*-enantiomer. Because the rate and extent of inversion are site specific and formulation dependent, ibuprofen activity may vary considerably.

8. **Hydrates.** Drugs may exist in a **hydrated,** or **solvated, form** or as an **anhydrous molecule.** Dissolution rates differ for hydrated and anhydrous forms. For example, the anhydrous form of ampicillin dissolves faster and is more rapidly absorbed than the hydrated form.

9. **Complex formation.** A **complex** is a species formed by the reversible or irreversible association of two or more interacting molecules or ions. **Chelates** are complexes that typically involve a ring-like structure formed by the interaction between a partial ring of atoms and a metal. Many biologically important molecules (e.g., hemoglobin, insulin, cyanocobalamin) are chelates. Drugs such as tetracycline form chelates with divalent (e.g., Ca^{++}, Mg^{++}) and trivalent (e.g., Al^{+++}, Bi^{+++}) metal ions. Many drugs adsorb strongly on charcoal or clay (e.g., kaolin, bentonite) particles by forming complexes. Drug complexes with proteins, such as albumin or α_1-acid glycoprotein, often occur.
   a. Complex formation usually alters the physical and chemical characteristics of the drug. For example:
      (1) The chelate of tetracycline with calcium is less water soluble and is poorly absorbed.
      (2) Theophylline complexed with ethylenediamine to form aminophylline is more water soluble and is used for parenteral and rectal administration.
      (3) Cyclodextrins are used to form complexes with many drugs to increase their water solubility.
   b. Large drug complexes, such as drug–protein complexes, do not cross cell membranes easily. These complexes must dissociate to free the drug for absorption at the absorption site, permitting transport across cell membranes or glomerular filtration before the drug is excreted into the urine.

B. Drug product and delivery system formulation

1. **General considerations**
   a. **Design of the appropriate dosage form** or **delivery system** depends on the:
      (1) Physical and chemical properties of the drug
      (2) Dose of the drug
      (3) Route of administration
      (4) Type of drug delivery system desired
      (5) Desired therapeutic effect
      (6) Physiologic release of the drug from the delivery system
      (7) Bioavailability of the drug at the absorption site
      (8) Pharmacokinetics and pharmacodynamics of the drug
   b. **Bioavailability.** The more complicated the formulation of the finished drug product (e.g., controlled-release tablet, enteric-coated tablet, transdermal patch), the greater the potential for a bioavailability problem. For example, the **release** of a drug from a peroral dosage form and its subsequent bioavailability depend on a succession of rate processes (Figure 4-1). These processes may include:
      (1) **Attrition, disintegration,** or **disaggregation** of the drug product
      (2) **Dissolution** of the drug in an aqueous environment
      (3) **Convection** and **diffusion** of the drug molecules to the absorbing surface
      (4) **Absorption** of the drug across cell membranes into the systemic circulation
   c. The **rate-limiting step** in the bioavailability of a drug from a drug product is the slowest step in a series of kinetic processes.
      (1) For most conventional solid drug products (e.g., capsules, tablets), the dissolution rate is the slowest, or rate-limiting, step for bioavailability.
      (2) For a controlled- or sustained-release drug product, the release of the drug from the delivery system is the rate-limiting step.

2. **Solutions** are homogeneous mixtures of one or more solutes dispersed molecularly in a dissolving medium (solvent).
   a. Compared with other oral and peroral drug formulations, a drug dissolved in an aqueous solution is in the most bioavailable and consistent form. Because the drug is already in solution, no dissolution step is necessary before systemic absorption occurs. Peroral drug solutions are often used as the reference preparation for solid peroral formulations.
   b. A drug dissolved in a hydroalcoholic solution (e.g., elixir) also has good bioavailability. Alcohol aids drug solubility. However, when the drug is diluted by gastrointestinal tract fluid and other gut contents (e.g., food), it may form a finely divided precipitate in the lumen of the gastrointestinal tract. Because of the extensive dispersion and large surface area of such finely divided precipitates, redissolution and subsequent absorption occur rapidly.
   c. A viscous drug solution (e.g., syrup) may interfere with dilution and mixing with gastrointestinal tract contents. The solution decreases the gastric emptying rate and the rate of transfer of drug solution to the duodenal region, where absorption is most efficient.

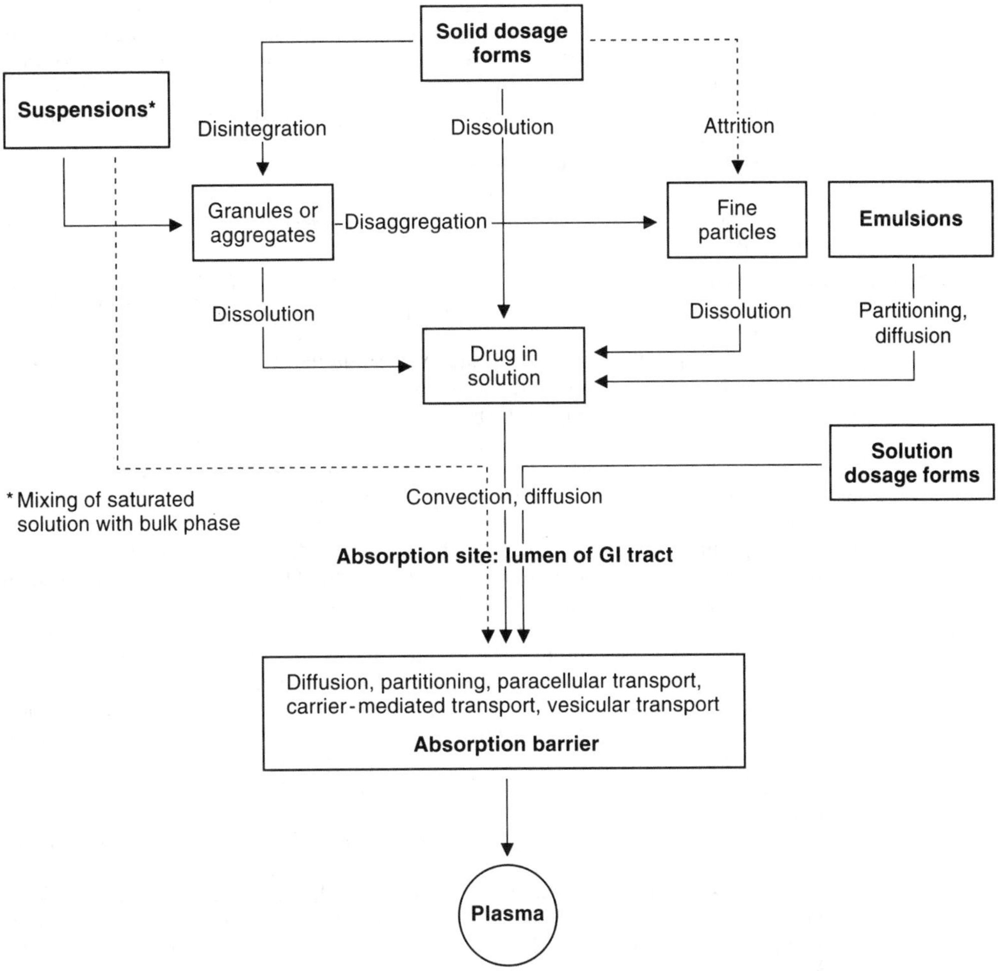

Figure 4-1. Schematic representation of the processes involved in drug release from peroral dosage forms.

3. **Suspensions** are dispersions of finely divided solid particles of a drug in a liquid medium in which the drug is not readily soluble. The liquid medium of a suspension comprises a saturated solution of the drug in equilibrium with the solid drug.
   a. The bioavailability of the drug from suspensions may be similar to that of a solution because the finely divided particles are dispersed and provide a large surface area for rapid dissolution. On the other hand, a slow dissolution rate decreases the absorption rate.
   b. **Suspending agents** are often hydrophilic colloids (e.g., cellulose derivatives, acacia, xanthan gum) added to suspensions to increase viscosity, inhibit agglomeration, and decrease the rate at which particles settle. Highly viscous suspensions may prolong gastric emptying time, slow drug dissolution, and decrease the absorption rate.

4. **Capsules** are solid dosage forms with hard or soft gelatin shells that contain drugs, usually admixed with excipients. **Coating** the capsule shell or the drug particles within the capsule can affect bioavailability.
   a. **Hard gelatin capsules** are usually filled with a powder blend that contains the drug. Typically, the powder blend is simpler and less compacted than the blend in a compressed tablet. After ingestion, the gelatin softens, swells, and begins to dissolve in the gastrointestinal tract. Encapsulated drugs are released rapidly and dispersed easily, and bioavailability is good. Hard gelatin capsules are the preferred dosage form for early clinical trials of new drugs.
   b. **Soft gelatin capsules** may contain a nonaqueous solution, a powder, or a drug suspension. The vehicle may be water miscible (e.g., PEG). The cardiac glycoside digoxin,

dispersed in a water-miscible vehicle (Lanoxicaps), has better bioavailability than a compressed tablet formulation (Lanoxin). However, a soft gelatin capsule that contains the drug dissolved in a **hydrophobic** vehicle (e.g., vegetable oil) may have poorer bioavailability than a compressed tablet formulation of the drug.

c. Aging and **storage conditions** can affect the moisture content of the gelatin component of the capsule shell and the bioavailability of the drug.
   (1) At low moisture levels, the capsule shell becomes brittle and is easily ruptured.
   (2) At high moisture levels, the capsule shell becomes moist, soft, and distorted. Moisture may be transferred to the capsule contents, particularly if the contents are hygroscopic.

5. Compressed tablets are solid dosage forms in which high pressure is used to compress a powder blend or granulation that contains the drug and other ingredients, or excipients, into a solid mass.

a. Excipients, including diluents (fillers), binders, disintegrants, lubricants, glidants, surfactants, dye, and flavoring agents, have the following properties:
   (1) They permit the efficient manufacture of compressed tablets.
   (2) They affect the physical and chemical characteristics of the drug.
   (3) They affect bioavailability. The higher the ratio of excipient to active drug, the greater the likelihood that the excipients affect bioavailability.

b. Examples
   (1) Disintegrants (e.g., starch, croscarmellose, sodium starch glycolate) vary in action, depending on their concentration, the method by which the disintegrant is mixed with the powder formulation or granulation, and the degree of tablet compaction. Although tablet disintegration is usually not a problem because it often occurs more rapidly than drug dissolution, it is necessary for dissolution in immediate-release formulations. Inability to disintegrate may interfere with bioavailability.
   (2) Lubricants are usually hydrophobic, water-insoluble substances such as stearic acid, magnesium stearate, hydrogenated vegetable oil, and talc. They may reduce wetting of the surface of the solid drug particles, slowing the dissolution and bioavailability rates of the drug. Water-soluble lubricants, such as L-leucine, do not interfere with dissolution or bioavailability.
   (3) Glidants (e.g., colloidal silicon dioxide) improve the flow properties of a dry powder blend before it is compressed. Rather than posing a potential problem with bioavailability, glidants may reduce tablet-to-tablet variability and improve product efficacy.
   (4) Surfactants enhance drug dissolution rates and bioavailability by reducing interfacial tension at the boundary between solid drug and liquid and improving the wettability (contact) of solid drug particles by the solvent.

c. Coated compressed tablets have a sugar coat, a film coat, or an enteric coat with the following properties:
   (1) It protects the drug from moisture, light, and air.
   (2) It masks the taste or odor of the drug.
   (3) It improves the appearance of the tablet.
   (4) It may affect the release rate of the drug.

d. In addition, **enteric coatings** minimize contact between the drug and the gastric region by resisting dissolution or attrition and preventing contact between the underlying drug and the gastric contents or gastric mucosa. Some enteric coatings minimize gastric contact because they are insoluble at acidic pHs. Other coatings resist attrition and remain whole long enough for the tablet to leave the gastric area. By resisting dissolution or attrition, enteric coatings may decrease bioavailability. Enteric coatings are used to:
   (1) Minimize irritation of the gastric mucosa by the drug
   (2) Prevent inactivation or degradation of the drug in the stomach
   (3) Delay release of the drug until the tablet reaches the small intestine, where conditions for absorption may be optimal

6. Modified-release dosage forms are drug products that alter the rate or timing of drug release. Because modified-release dosage forms are more complex than conventional immediate-release dosage forms, more stringent quality control and bioavailability tests are required. **Dose dumping,** or the abrupt, uncontrolled release of a large amount of drug, is a problem.

a. Extended-release dosage forms include **controlled-release, sustained-action,** and **long-acting drug delivery systems.** These delivery systems allow at least a twofold reduction in dosing frequency compared with conventional immediate-release formulations.

(1) The extended, slow release of controlled-release drug products produces a relatively flat, sustained plasma drug concentration that avoids toxicity (from high drug concentrations) or lack of efficacy (from low drug concentrations).

(2) Extended-release dosage forms provide an immediate (initial) release of the drug, followed by a slower sustained release.

b. Delayed-release dosage forms release active drug at a time other than immediately after administration at a desired site in the gastrointestinal tract. For example, an enteric-coated drug product does not allow for dissolution in the acid pH environment of the stomach, but rather, in the less acidic pH environment of the small intestine.

7. **Transdermal drug delivery systems, or patches,** are controlled-release devices that contain the drug for systemic absorption after topical application to the skin surface. Transdermal drug delivery systems are available for a number of drugs (nitroglycerin, nicotine, scopolamine, clonidine, fentanyl, 17-β-estradiol, and testosterone). Although the formulation matrices of these delivery systems differ somewhat, they all differ from conventional topical formulations in the following ways:
   - **a.** They have an impermeable **occlusive backing film** that prevents insensible water loss from the skin beneath the patch. This film causes increased hydration and skin temperature under the patch and enhanced permeation of the skin by the drug.
   - **b.** The formulation matrix of the patch maintains the drug concentration gradient within the device after application so that drug delivery to the interface between the patch and skin is sustained. As a result, drug partitioning and diffusion into the skin persist, and systemic absorption is maintained throughout the dosing interval.
   - **c.** Transdermal drug delivery systems are kept in place on the skin surface by an **adhesive layer,** ensuring drug contact with the skin and continued drug delivery.

8. **Targeted (site-specific) drug delivery systems** are drug carrier systems that place the drug at or near the receptor site. Examples include macromolecular drug carriers (protein drug carriers), particulate drug delivery systems (e.g., liposomes, nanoparticles), and monoclonal antibodies. With targeted drug delivery, the drug may be delivered:
   - **a.** To the capillary bed of the active site
   - **b.** To a special type of cell (e.g., tumor cells), but not to normal cells
   - **c.** To a specific organ or tissue by complexing with a carrier that recognizes the target

9. **Inserts, implants, and devices** are used to control drug delivery for localized or systemic drug effects. The drug is impregnated into a biodegradable or nonbiodegradable material and is released slowly. The inserts, implants, and devices are inserted into a variety of cavities (e.g., vagina, buccal cavity, skin). For example, the L-norgestrel implant (Norplant) is inserted beneath the skin of the upper arm. It provides contraceptive protection for nearly 5 years.

STUDY QUESTIONS

Directions: Each of the numbered items or incomplete statements in this section is followed by answers or by completions of the statement. Select the **one** lettered answer or completion that is **best** in each case.

1. Which statement best describes bioavailability?

(A) Relation between the physical and chemical properties of a drug and its systemic absorption
(B) Measurement of the rate and amount of therapeutically active drug that reaches the systemic circulation
(C) Movement of drug into body tissues over time
(D) Dissolution of the drug in the gastrointestinal tract
(E) Amount of drug destroyed by the liver before systemic absorption from the gastrointestinal tract occurs

2. The route of drug administration that gives the most rapid onset of the pharmacologic effect is

(A) intramuscular injection
(B) intravenous injection
(C) intradermal injection
(D) peroral administration
(E) subcutaneous injection

3. The route of drug administration that provides complete (100%) bioavailability is

(A) intramuscular injection
(B) intravenous injection
(C) intradermal injection
(D) peroral administration
(E) subcutaneous injection

4. After peroral administration, drugs generally are absorbed best from the

(A) buccal cavity
(B) stomach
(C) duodenum
(D) ileum
(E) rectum

5. The characteristics of an active transport process include all of the following EXCEPT

(A) active transport moves drug molecules against a concentration gradient
(B) active transport follows Fick's law of diffusion
(C) active transport is a carrier-mediated transport system
(D) active transport requires energy
(E) active transport of drug molecules may be saturated at high drug concentrations

6. The passage of drug molecules from a region of high drug concentration to a region of low drug concentration is known as

(A) active transport
(B) bioavailability
(C) biopharmaceutics
(D) simple diffusion
(E) pinocytosis

7. What equation describes the rate of drug dissolution from a tablet?

(A) Fick's law
(B) Henderson-Hasselbalch equation
(C) Law of mass action
(D) Michaelis-Menten equation
(E) Noyes Whitney equation

8. Which condition usually increases the rate of drug dissolution from a tablet?

(A) Increase in the particle size of the drug
(B) Decrease in the surface area of the drug
(C) Use of the free acid or free base form of the drug
(D) Use of the ionized, or salt, form of the drug
(E) Use of sugar coating around the tablet

9. Dose dumping is a problem in the formulation of

(A) compressed tablets
(B) modified-release drug products
(C) hard gelatin capsules
(D) soft gelatin capsules
(E) suppositories

10. The rate-limiting step in the bioavailability of a lipid-soluble drug formulated as an immediate-release compressed tablet is the rate of

(A) disintegration of the tablet and release of the drug
(B) dissolution of the drug
(C) transport of the drug molecules across the intestinal mucosal cells
(D) blood flow to the gastrointestinal tract
(E) biotransformation, or metabolism, of the drug by the liver before systemic absorption occurs

11. The extent of ionization of a weak electrolyte drug is dependent on the

(A) pH of the media and pK_a of the drug
(B) oil:water partition coefficient of the drug
(C) particle size and surface area of the drug
(D) Noyes Whitney equation for the drug
(E) polymorphic form of the drug

12. The rate of drug bioavailability is most rapid when the drug is formulated as a

(A) controlled-release product
(B) hard gelatin capsule
(C) compressed tablet
(D) solution
(E) suspension

ANSWERS AND EXPLANATIONS

1. The answer is B *[I A 3].*
Bioavailability is the measurement of the rate and extent (amount) of therapeutically active drug that reaches the systemic circulation. The relation of the physical and chemical properties of a drug to its systemic absorption (i.e., bioavailability) is known as its biopharmaceutics. The movement of a drug into body tissues is an aspect of pharmacokinetics, which is the study of drug movement in the body over time. The dissolution of a drug in the gastrointestinal tract is a physicochemical property that affects bioavailability. Significant destruction of a drug by the liver before it is systemically absorbed (known as the first-pass effect because it occurs during the first passage of the drug through the liver) decreases bioavailability.

2. The answer is B *[II B 1 a].*
When the active form of the drug is given intravenously, it enters the systemic circulation directly. The drug is delivered rapidly to all tissues, including the drug receptor sites. For all other routes of drug administration except intra-arterial injection, the drug must be systemically absorbed before it is distributed to the drug receptor sites. For this reason, the onset of pharmacologic effects is slower. If the drug is a prodrug that must be converted to an active drug, oral administration, not intravenous injection, may not provide the most rapid onset of activity if conversion to the active form takes place in the gastrointestinal tract or liver.

3. The answer is B *[II C 2].*
When a drug is given by intravenous injection, the entire dose enters the systemic circulation. With other routes of administration, the drug may be lost before it reaches the systemic circulation. For example, with first-pass effects, a portion of an orally administered drug is eliminated, usually through degradation by liver enzymes, before the drug reaches its receptor sites.

4. The answer is C *[II B 2 b (4)].*
Drugs given orally are well absorbed from the duodenum. The duodenum has a large surface area because of the presence of villi and microvilli. In addition, because the duodenum is well perfused by the mesenteric blood vessels, a concentration gradient is maintained between the lumen of the duodenum and the blood.

5. The answer is B *[II A 2–3].*
Fick's law of diffusion describes passive diffusion of drug molecules moving from a high concentration to a low concentration. This process is not saturable and does not require energy.

6. The answer is D *[II A 2].*
The transport of a drug across a cell membrane by passive diffusion follows Fick's law of diffusion: the drug moves with a concentration gradient (i.e., from an area of high concentration to an area of low concentration). In contrast, drugs that are actively transported move against a concentration gradient.

7. The answer is E *[III A 1].*
The Noyes Whitney equation describes the rate at which a solid drug dissolves. Fick's law is similar to the Noyes Whitney equation in that both equations describe drug movement caused by a concentration gradient. Fick's law generally refers to passive diffusion, or passive transport, of drugs. The law of mass action describes the rate of a chemical reaction, the Michaelis-Menten equation involves enzyme kinetics, and the Henderson-Hasselbalch equation gives the pH of a buffer solution.

8. The answer is D *[III A 1–3].*
The ionized, or salt, form of a drug has a charge and is generally more water soluble and, therefore, dissolves more rapidly than the nonionized (free acid or free base) form of the drug. The dissolution rate is directly proportional to the surface area and inversely proportional to the particle size. An increase in the particle size or a decrease in the surface area slows the dissolution rate.

9. The answer is B *[III B 6].*
A modified-release, or controlled-release, drug product contains two or more conventional doses of the drug. An abrupt release of the drug, known as dose dumping, may cause intoxication.

10. The answer is B *[III B 1 c].*
For lipid-soluble drugs, the rate of dissolution is the slowest (i.e., rate-limiting) step in drug absorption and thus in bioavailability. The disintegration rate of an immediate-release or conventional compressed

tablet is usually more rapid than the rate of drug dissolution. Because the cell membrane is a lipoprotein structure, transport of a lipid-soluble drug across the cell membrane is usually rapid.

11. The answer is A *[III A 4 b].*
The extent of ionization of a weak electrolyte is described by the Henderson-Hasselbalch equation, which relates the pH of the solvent to the pK_a of the drug.

12. The answer is D *[III B 2 a].*
Because a drug in solution is already dissolved, no dissolution is needed before absorption. Consequently, compared with other drug formulations, a drug in solution has a high rate of bioavailability. A drug in aqueous solution has the highest bioavailability rate and is often used as the reference preparation for other formulations. Drugs in hydroalcoholic solution (e.g., elixirs) also have good bioavailability. The rate of drug bioavailability from a hard gelatin capsule, compressed tablet, or suspension may be equal to that of a solution if an optimal formulation is manufactured and the drug is inherently rapidly absorbed.

5
Extemporaneous Prescription Compounding

Loyd V. Allen, Jr.

I. INTRODUCTION

A. Definitions

1. **Extemporaneous compounding** is the preparation, mixing, assembling, packaging, and labeling of a drug product based on a prescription order from a licensed practitioner for the individual patient.

2. **Manufacturing** is the mass production of compounded prescription products for resale to pharmacies and is regulated by the Food and Drug Administration (FDA).

B. Regulation

1. **Current Good Manufacturing Practices** (cGMP) are the standards of practice used in the pharmaceutical industry and are regulated by the FDA. Community pharmacists must comply with state board of pharmacy regulations and guidelines to assure a quality product, which includes using proper materials, weighing equipment, a documented technique, and dispensing and storage instructions.

2. **Legal considerations**
   a. Extemporaneous compounding by the pharmacist or a prescription order from a licensed practitioner, as with the dispensing of any other prescription, is controlled by the state boards of pharmacy.
   b. The legal risk (liability) of compounding is no greater than the risk of filling a prescription for a manufactured product because the pharmacist must assure that the correct drug, dose, and directions are provided. The pharmacist is also responsible for preparing a quality pharmaceutical product, providing proper instructions regarding its storage, and advising the patient of any adverse effects.

II. REQUIREMENTS FOR COMPOUNDING

A. Sources for chemicals and drugs. Pharmacists must obtain small quantities of the appropriate chemicals or drugs from wholesalers or chemical supply houses. These suppliers then may act as consultants to the pharmacists by assuring them of their product's purity and quality.

B. Equipment. The correct equipment is important when compounding. Many state boards of pharmacy have a required minimum list of equipment for compounding prescriptions. Suggested equipment, which varies according to the amount of material needed and the type of compounded prescription (e.g., parenteral), includes:

1. Class A prescription balance and/or electronic balance
2. Hot plate
3. Magnetic stirrers
4. Electric mixer
5. Special containers for packaging (e.g., applicator tip bottles, insufflators).
6. Graduated cylinders from 10 ml to 1000 ml
7. Glass, Wedgwood, and porcelain mortars and pestles of various sizes

8. Funnels of various sizes
9. Spatulas of various sizes, including several plastic spatulas
10. Weighing and filter papers
11. Stirring rods (glass)
12. Ointment/pill tile
13. Capsule filling machine
14. Ointment filling machine
15. Autoclave
16. Laminar flow clean bench
17. Special suppository molds
18. Record-keeping system (compounding log book)
19. Glass beakers from 50 ml to 1000 ml

C. Location of compounding area. Many pharmacies actively involved in compounding have dedicated a separate area in the pharmacy to this process. The ideal location is away from heavy foot traffic and is near a sink where there is enough space to work and store all chemicals and equipment. For compounding of sterile products, a laminar air flow hood (minimal) and a clean room are current practice.

D. Sources of Information

1. Library at a college of pharmacy
2. References
   a. Gennaro AR ed. *Remington: The Science and Practice of Pharmacy.* 19th ed. Easton, Pa: Mack Publishing Co; 1995.
   b. Budavari S ed. *Merck Index.* 12th ed. Whitehouse Station, NJ: Merck & Co; 1996.
   c. *United States Pharmacopeia* (USP) 23; *National Formulary* (NF) 18. United States Pharmacopeial Convention.
   d. Ansel HC, Popovich NG, Allen LV Jr. *Pharmaceutical Dosage Forms and Drug Delivery Systems.* Media, Pa: Williams & Wilkins; 1995.
3. Journals (e.g., *U.S. Pharmacist, Pharmacy Times, Hospital Pharmacy)*
4. Manufacturers' drug product information inserts; compounding specialty suppliers

III. COMPOUNDING OF SOLUTIONS

A. Definition. USP 23 defines **solutions** as liquid preparations that contain one or more chemical substances dissolved (i.e., molecularly dispersed) in a suitable solvent or mixture of mutually miscible solvents. Although the uniformity of the dosage in a solution can be assumed, the stability, pH, solubility of the drug or chemicals, taste (for oral solutions), and packaging need to be considered.

B. Types of solutions

1. **Sterile parenteral and ophthalmic solutions.** These solutions require special consideration for their preparation (see XI).
2. **Nonsterile solutions** include oral, topical, and otic solutions.

C. Preparation of solutions. Solutions are the easiest of the dosage forms to compound extemporaneously, as long as a few general rules are followed.

1. Each drug or chemical is dissolved in the solvent in which it is most soluble. Thus, the solubility characteristics of each drug or chemical must be known.
2. If an alcoholic solution of a poorly water-soluble drug is used, the aqueous solution is added to the alcoholic solution to maintain as high an alcohol concentration as possible.

3. The salt form of the drug, and not the free-acid or base form, which both have poor solubility, is used.

4. Flavoring or sweetening agents are prepared ahead of time.

5. When adding a salt to a syrup, dissolve the salt in a few milliliters of water first; then add the syrup to volume.

6. The proper vehicle (e.g., syrup, elixir aromatic water, purified water) must be selected.

D. Examples

1. **Example 1**
   a. **Medication order**
   Phenobarbital 1 g
   Belladonna Tr 5 ml
   Peppermint water qs 120 ml
   b. **Compounding procedure.** Sodium phenobarbital (equivalent to 1 g of phenobarbital) is dissolved in the aromatic water. This solution is then added slowly in divided portions to the tincture contained in a beaker and is stirred continuously or a magnetic stirrer is used.

2. **Example 2**
   a. **Medication order**
   Potassium chloride 500 mg/10 ml
   Aromatic elixir ad 60 ml
   b. **Compounding procedure.** Potassium chloride (3 g) is dissolved with the smallest amount of purified water possible. A sufficient amount of aromatic elixir is added to bring the final volume up to 60 ml.

3. **Example 3**
   a. **Medication order**
   Salicylic acid 2%
   Lactic acid 6 ml
   Flexible collodion ad 30 ml
   b. **Compounding procedure.** Pharmacists must use caution when preparing this prescription because flexible collodion is extremely flammable. A 1-oz applicator tip bottle is calibrated, using ethanol, which is poured out and allowed to evaporate, resulting in a dry bottle. Salicylic acid (0.6 g) is added directly into the bottle, to which is added the 6 ml of lactic acid. The bottle is agitated or a glass stirring rod is used to dissolve the salicylic acid. Flexible collodion is added up to the calibrated 30-ml mark on the applicator tip bottle.

4. **Example 4**
   a. **Medication order**
   Iodine 2%
   Sodium iodide 2.4%
   Alcohol qs 30 ml
   b. **Compounding procedure.** Iodine (0.6 g) and sodium iodide (0.72 g) are dissolved in the alcohol, and the final solution is placed in an amber bottle. A **rubber or plastic spatula** is used because **iodine is corrosive.**

IV. COMPOUNDING OF SUSPENSIONS

A. Definition. Suspensions are defined by the USP as liquid preparations that consist of solid particles dispersed throughout a liquid phase in which the particles are not soluble.

B. General characteristics

1. Some suspensions should contain an antimicrobial agent as a preservative.

2. Particles settle in all suspensions even when a suspending agent is added; thus, suspensions must be shaken well before use to ensure the distribution of particles for a uniform dose.

3. Tight containers are necessary to ensure the stability of the final product.

4. Principles to keep in mind when compounding include the following:
   a. Insoluble powders should be small and uniform in size to decrease settling.
   b. The suspension should be viscous.
   c. Topical suspensions should have a smooth impalpable texture.
   d. Oral suspensions should have a pleasant odor and taste.

C. **Formation of suspensions.** Suspensions are easy to compound; however, physical stability after compounding the final product is problematic. The following steps may minimize stability problems.

1. The particle size of all powders used in the formulation must be reduced.
2. A thickening agent (suspending agent) may be used to increase viscosity. Common suspending agents include bentonite, Veegum, methylcellulose, and tragacanth.
3. A levigating agent may aid in the initial dispersion of insoluble particles. Common levigating agents include glycerin, propylene glycol, alcohol, syrups, and water.
4. Flavoring agents and preservatives should be selected and added if the product is intended for oral use. Common preservatives include methyl and propylparabens, benzoic acid, and sodium benzoate. Flavoring agents may be any flavored syrup or flavor concentrate (Table 5-1).
5. The source of the active ingredients (e.g., bulk powders versus tablets or capsules) must be considered.

D. **Preparation of suspensions**

1. The insoluble powders are triturated to a fine powder.
2. A small portion of liquid is used as a levigating agent, and the powders are triturated until a smooth paste is formed. The levigating agent is added slowly and mixed deliberately.
3. The vehicle containing the suspending agent is added in divided portions. A high-speed mixer greatly increases the dispersion.
4. The product is brought to the required volume using the vehicle.
5. The final mixture is transferred to a "tight" bottle for dispensing to the patient.
6. All suspensions are dispensed with a "shake well" label.
7. Suspensions are not filtered.
8. The water-soluble ingredients, including flavoring agents, are mixed in the vehicle before mixing with the insoluble ingredients.

Table 5-1. Selected Flavor Applications

Drug Category	Preferred Flavors
Antibiotics	Cherry, maple, pineapple, orange, raspberry, banana-pineapple, banana-vanilla, butterscotch-maple, coconut custard, strawberry, vanilla, lemon custard, cherry custard, fruit-cinnamon
Antihistamines	Apricot, black currant, cherry, cinnamon, custard, grape, honey, lime, loganberry, peach-orange, peach-rum, raspberry, root beer, wild cherry
Barbiturates	Banana-pineapple, banana-vanilla, black currant, cinnamon-peppermint, grenadine-strawberry, lime, orange, peach-orange, root beer
Decongestants and expectorants	Anise, apricot, black current, butterscotch, cherry, coconut custard, custard mint-strawberry, grenadine-peach, strawberry, lemon, coriander, orange-peach, pineapple, raspberry, strawberry, tangerine
Electrolyte solutions	Cherry, grape, lemon-lime, raspberry, wild cherry syrup, black currant, grenadine-strawberry, lime, port wine, sherry wine, root berry, wild strawberry

E. Examples

1. **Example 1**
   a. **Medication order**
      Propranolol HCl 4 mg/ml
      Disp 30 ml
      Sig: 1 ml p.o. t.i.d.
   b. **Calculations.** Propranolol HCl, 4 mg/ml × 30 ml = 120 mg. Propranolol HCl is available as a powder or in immediate-release and extended-release (long-acting) dosage forms. Only the powder or the immediate-release tablets are used for compounding prescriptions; therefore, some combination of propranolol HCl tablets, which yields 120 mg active drug (e.g., 3 × 40 mg tablets), may be used.
   c. **Compounding procedure.** The propranolol tablets are reduced to a fine powder in a mortar. The powder or the comminuted tablets are levigated to a smooth paste, using a 2% methylcellulose solution. To this mixture, about 10 ml of a suitable flavoring agent is added. The mixture is transferred to a calibrated container and brought to the final volume with purified water. A "shake well" label is attached to the prescription container.

2. **Example 2**
   a. **Medication order**
      Zinc oxide 10
      Ppt sulfur 10
      Bentonite 3.6
      Purified water ad 90 ml
      Sig: Apply t.i.d.
   b. **Compounding procedure.** The powders are reduced to a fine uniform mixture in a mortar. The powders are mixed to form a smooth paste using water and transferred to a calibrated bottle. The final volume is attained with purified water. A "shake well" label is attached to the prescription container.

3. **Example 3**
   a. **Medication order**
      Rifampin suspension 20 mg/ml
      Disp 120 ml
      Sig: u.d.
   b. **Calculations.** Rifampin, 20 mg/ml × 120 ml = 2400 mg. Rifampin is available in 150-mg and 300-mg capsules. Hence, 8 capsules containing 300 mg of rifampin in each capsule or 16 capsules containing 150 mg of rifampin per capsule are needed.
   c. **Compounding procedure.** The contents of the appropriate number of rifampin capsules are emptied into a mortar and comminuted with a pestle. This powder is levigated with a small amount of 1% methylcellulose solution. Twenty milliliters of simple syrup are added and mixed. The mixture is brought to the final volume with simple syrup. "Shake well" and "refrigerate" labels are attached to the prescription container.

V. EMULSIONS

A. Definition. Emulsions are **two-phase systems** in which one liquid is dispersed throughout another liquid in the form of small droplets (see Chapter 3 VI D).

B. General characteristics. Emulsions can be used **externally** as lotions and creams or **internally** to mask the taste of medications.

1. The two liquids in an emulsion are immiscible and require the use of an **emulsifying agent.**
2. Emulsions are classified as either **oil-in-water (o/w)** or **water-in-oil (w/o).**
3. Emulsions are **unstable,** and the following steps must be taken to prevent the two phases of an emulsion from separating into two layers after preparation.
   a. The correct **proportions** of oil and water should be used during preparation. The internal phase should represent about 40%–60% of the total volume.
   b. An emulsifying **agent** is needed for emulsion formation.
   c. A **hand homogenizer,** which reduces the size of globules of the internal phase, may be used.

d. **Preservatives** should be added if the preparation is intended to last longer than a few days. Generally, a combination of methylparaben (0.2%) and propylparaben (0.02%) may be used.

e. A **"shake well" label** should be placed on the final product.

f. The product should be **protected** from light and extreme temperature. Both freezing and heat may have an effect on stability.

C. Emulsifying agents

1. **Gums,** such as acacia or tragacanth, are used to form o/w emulsions. These emulsifying agents are for general use, especially for emulsions intended for internal administration (Table 5-2).

a. One gram of acacia powder is used for every 4 ml of fixed oil or 1 g to 2 ml for a volatile oil.

b. If using tragacanth in place of acacia, 0.1 g of tragacanth is used for every 1 g of acacia.

2. **Methylcellulose and carboxymethylcellulose** are used for o/w emulsions. The concentrations of these agents vary, depending on the grade that is used. Methylcellulose is available in several viscosity grades, ranging from 15 to 4000 and designated by a centipoise number, which is a unit of viscosity.

3. **Soaps** can be used to prepare o/w or w/o emulsions for external preparations.

4. **Nonionic emulsifying agents** can be used for o/w and w/o emulsions.

D. Formation and preparation of emulsions. The procedure for preparing an emulsion depends on the desired emulsifying agent in the formulation.

1. A **mortar** and **pestle** are frequently all the equipment that is needed.

a. A mortar with a **rough surface** (e.g., Wedgwood) should be used. This rough surface allows maximal dispersion of globules to produce a fine particle size.

b. A **rapid motion** is essential when triturating an emulsion using a mortar and pestle.

c. The mortar should be able to hold at least three times the **quantity** being made. Trituration seldom requires more than 5 minutes to create the emulsion.

2. **Electric mixers** and hand homogenizers are useful for producing emulsions after the coarse emulsion is formed in the mortar.

3. The **order** of mixing of ingredients in an emulsion depends on the type of emulsion being prepared (i.e., o/w or w/o) as well as the emulsifying agent chosen. Methods used for compounding include the following.

a. **Dry gum** (continental) method is used for forming emulsions using natural emulsifying agents and requires a specific order of mixing.

b. **Wet gum** (English) method is used for forming emulsions using natural emulsifying agents and requires a specific order of mixing.

c. **Bottle method** is used for forming emulsions using natural emulsifying agents and requires a specific order of mixing.

d. **Beaker method** is used to prepare emulsions using synthetic emulsifying agents and produces a satisfactory product regardless of the order of mixing.

4. **Preservatives.** If the emulsion is kept for an extended period of time, refrigeration is usually sufficient. The product should not be frozen. If a preservative is used, it must be soluble in the water phase to be effective.

5. **Flavoring agents.** If the addition of a flavor is needed to mask the taste of the oil phase, the flavor should be added to the external phase before emulsification (Table 5-3).

E. Examples

1. Example 1

a. Medication order

Mineral oil 18 ml
Acacia q.s.
Distilled water q.s. ad 90.0 ml
Sig: 1 tbsp q.d.

b. **Compounding procedure.** With the dry gum method, an initial emulsion (primary emulsion) is formed, using 4 parts (18 ml) of oil, 2 parts (9 ml) of water, and 1 part (4.5 g) of

Table 5-2. Agents Used in Prescription Compounding

Ointments	
Oleaginous or hydrocarbon bases Anhydrous Nonhydrophilic Insoluble in water Not water removable (occlusive) Good vehicles for antibiotics Examples Petrolatum Absorption, or hydrophilic, bases Anhydrous Hydrophilic Insoluble in water Not water removable (occlusive) Examples Hydrophilic petrolatum Lanolin USP (anhydrous)	Hydrous emulsion bases (w/o) Hydrous Hydrophilic Insoluble in water Not water removable (occlusive) Examples Cold cream Hydrous lanolin Emulsion bases (o/w) Hydrous Hydrophilic Insoluble in water Water removable Can absorb 30%–50% of weight Examples Hydrophilic ointment USP Acid mantle cream Water soluble Anhydrous or hydrous Soluble in water Water removable Hydrophilic Example Polyethylene glycol ointment
Suspending Agents	
Acacia 10% Bentonite 6% Carboxymethylcellulose 1%–3% Methylcellulose 1%–7%	Sodium alginate 1%–2% Tragacanth 1%–3% Veegum 6%
Preservatives	
Methylparaben 0.02%–0.2%	Propylparaben 0.01%–0.04%
Emulsifying Agents	
Hydrophilic colloids Acacia Tragacanth Pectin Favor o/w Carboxymethylcellulose Methylcellulose Proteins Gelatin Egg whites Favor o/w Inorganic gels and magmas Milk of magnesia Bentonite Favor o/w	Surfactants, nonionic Concentrations used (1%–30%) Tweens (e.g., polysorbate 80) Spans Soaps Triethanolamine Stearic acid Others Sodium lauryl sulfate Dioctyl sodium sulfosuccinate Cetyl pyridinium chloride

o/w = oil-in-water; w/o = water-in-oil

Table 5-3. Flavor Selection Guide

Taste	Masking Flavor
Salt	Butterscotch, maple
Bitter	Wild cherry, walnut, chocolate mint, licorice
Sweet	Fruit, berry, vanilla
Acid	Citrus

powdered acacia. The mineral oil is triturated with the acacia in a Wedgwood mortar. The 9 ml of water are added all at once and, with rapid trituration, form the primary emulsion, which is triturated for about 5 minutes. The remaining water is incorporated in small amounts with trituration. The emulsion is transferred to a 90-ml prescription bottle, and a "shake well" label is attached to the container.

2. **Example 2**
   a. **Medication order**
      Zinc oxide 8 g
      Calamine 8 g
      Olive oil 30 ml
      Lime water 30 ml
   b. **Compounding procedure.** The olive oil is placed in a suitably sized beaker. Using an electric mixer, the zinc oxide, the calamine, and the lime water are added in that order. This yields a w/o emulsion. This procedure is known as the nascent soap method. The olive oil reacts with the calcium hydroxide solution (lime water) and forms a soap. For this reaction to occur, fresh lime water (calcium hydroxide solution) is required.

3. **Example 3**
   a. **Medication order**
      Mineral oil 50 ml
      Water q.s. 100 ml
      Sig: 2.5 ml p.o. h.s.
   b. **Compounding procedure.** Using a combination of nonionic emulsifying agents, such as Span 40 and Tween 40, the correct hydrophilic–lipophilic balance (HLB) is obtained. Next, the mineral oil is warmed in a water bath to about 60°C, and the Span 40 is dissolved in the heated mineral oil. The water is warmed to about 65°C, and the Tween 40 is dissolved in the heated water. This mixture is added to the mineral oil and dissolved Span 40 and stirred until cooled. An "external use only" label is added to the container.

VI. POWDERED DOSAGE FORMS

A. Definition. Powders are intimate mixtures of dry, finely divided drugs and/or chemicals that may be intended for internal (oral powders) or external (topical powders) use. The major types are powder papers, bulk powders, and insufflations.

B. General characteristics

1. Powder dosage forms are used when **drug stability** or **solubility** is a concern. These dosage forms may also be used when the powders are too bulky to make into capsules and when the patient has difficulty swallowing a capsule.
2. Some **disadvantages** to powders include unpleasant-tasting medications and, occasionally, the rapid deterioration of powders.
3. **Blending** of powders may be accomplished by using trituration in a mortar, stirring with a spatula, and sifting. Geometric dilution should be used if needed. When heavy powders are mixed with lighter ones, the heavier powder should be placed on top of the lighter one and then blended. When mixing two or more powders, each powder should be pulverized separately to about the same particle size before blending together.
   a. The mortar and pestle method is preferred when **pulverization** and a thorough mixing of ingredients are desired (geometric dilution). A Wedgwood mortar is preferable, but glass or porcelain may also be used.
   b. Light powders are mixed best by using the **sifting method.** The sifting is repeated three to four times to ensure thorough mixing of the powders.

C. Preparation of powder dosage forms

1. **Bulk powders,** which may be used internally or topically, include dusting powders, douche powders, laxatives, antacids, and insufflation powders.
2. After a bulk powder has been pulverized and blended, it should be dispensed in an appropriate container.
   a. **Hygroscopic** or **effervescent** salts should always be placed in a tight widemouthed jar.
   b. **Dusting** powders should be placed in a container with a sifter top.
3. **Eutectic mixtures** of powders can cause problems because they may liquefy. One remedy is to add an inert powder, such as magnesium oxide, to separate the eutectic materials.
4. **Powder papers** are also called divided powders.
   a. The entire powder is initially blended. Each dose is then individually weighed.
   b. The dosage should be weighed, then transferred onto a powder paper and folded. This technique requires practice. Hygroscopic, deliquescent, and effervescent powders require the use of glassine paper as an inside lining. Plastic bags or envelopes with snap-and-seal closures offer a convenient alternative to powder papers.
   c. The folded papers are dispensed in a powder box or other suitable container; however, these containers are not child-resistant.

D. Examples

1. **Example 1**
   a. **Medication order**
      Camphor 100 mg
      Menthol 200 mg
      Zinc oxide 800 mg
      Talc 1900 mg
      M foot powder
      Sig: Apply to aa b.i.d.
   b. **Compounding procedure**. The camphor and menthol are triturated together in a glass mortar, where a liquid eutectic is formed. The zinc oxide and talc are blended and mixed with the eutectic, using geometric dilution. This mixing results in a dry powder, which is passed through a wire mesh sieve. The final product is dispensed in a container with a sifter top.
2. **Example 2**
   a. **Medication order**
      Psyllium mucilloid 2 g
      Citric acid 0.3 g
      Sodium bicarbonate 0.25 g
      M. Ft d.t.d. charts v
      Sig: Empty the contents of one chart into a glass of water and take h.s.
   b. **Calculations.** Calculate for one extra powder paper:
      Psyllium mucilloid 2 g × 6 doses = 12 g
      Citric acid 0.3 g × 6 doses = 1.8 g
      Sodium bicarbonate 0.25 g × 6 doses = 1.5 g
      Total weight = 15.3
      15.3 g/6 doses = 2.55 g/dose
   c. **Compounding procedure.** The ingredients are first pulverized and weighed. The citric acid and sodium bicarbonate are mixed together first; the psyllium mucilloid is then added, using geometric dilution. Each dose (2.55 g) of the resultant mixture is weighed and placed into a powder paper. This preparation is an effervescent powder. When dissolved in water, the citric acid and sodium bicarbonate react to form carbonic acid, which yields carbon dioxide, making the solution more palatable.

VII. CAPSULES

A. Definition. Capsules are solid dosage forms in which the drug is enclosed within either a hard or soft soluble container or shell. The shells are usually made from a suitable gelatin. Hard gelatin capsules may be manually filled for extemporaneous compounding.

B. Capsule sizes

1. A list of capsule sizes and the approximate amount of powder that may be contained in the capsule appear on the side of the capsule box (Table 5-4).
2. Capsule sizes for oral administration in humans range from no. 5, the smallest, to no. 000, the largest.
3. No. 0 is usually the largest oral size suitable for patients.
4. Capsules for veterinarians are available in nos. 10, 11, and 12, containing approximately 30, 15, and 7.5 g, respectively.

C. Preparation of hard and soft capsules

1. As with the bulk powders, all ingredients are triturated and blended, using geometric dilution.
2. The correct size capsule must be determined by trying different capsule sizes, weighing them, and then choosing the appropriate size.
3. Before filling capsules with the medication, the body and cap of the capsule are separated. Filling is accomplished by using the "punch" method.
   a. The powder formulation is compressed with a spatula on a pill tile or paper sheet with a uniform depth of approximately half the length of the capsule body.
   b. The empty capsule body is repeatedly pressed into the powder until full.
   c. The capsule is then weighed to ensure an accurate dose. An empty tare capsule of the same size is placed on the pan containing the weights.
   d. For a large number of capsules, capsule-filling machines can be used for small-scale use to save time.
4. The capsule is wiped clean of any powder or oil and dispensed in a suitable prescription vial.

D. Examples

1. **Example 1**
   a. **Medication order**
      Rifampin 100 mg
      dtd #50
      Sig: 1 cap p.o. q.d.
   b. **Calculations.** Calculate for at least one extra capsule.
      51 caps × 100 mg/cap = 5100 mg rifampin
      5100 mg rifampin ÷ 300 mg/cap = 17 caps
   c. **Compounding procedure.** Seventeen rifampin capsules, each containing 300 mg rifampin, are used. The content of each capsule is emptied, and the powder is weighed. The **equivalent** powder equal to 100 mg rifampin is placed in a capsule and sufficient lactose added to fill the capsule. The capsule contents weigh 200 mg. The **equivalent** weight is subtracted to obtain the amount of lactose required per capsule. This is multiplied by 51 capsules. Enough lactose is added to make a total of 10.2 g of powder. The

Table 5-4. Approximate Amount of Powder Contained in Capsules

Capsule Size	Range of Powder Capacity (mg)
No. 5	60–130
No. 4	95–260
No. 3	130–390
No. 2	195–520
No. 1	225–650
No. 0	325–910
No. 00	390–1300
No. 000	650–2000

powders are combined, using geometric dilution, and 50 capsules can be punched out. Each capsule should weigh 10.2 g/51 caps or 200 mg.

2. **Example 2**
   a. **Medication order.** This order is for veterinary use only.
      Castor oil 8 ml
      Disp 12 caps
      Sig: 2 caps p.o. h.s.
   b. **Calculations.** No calculations are necessary.
   c. **Compounding procedure.** A no. 11 veterinary capsule is used. Using a calibrated dropper or a pipette, 8 ml of the oil are carefully added to the inside of each capsule body. Next, the lower inside portion of the cap is moistened, using a glass rod or brush. The cap and body are joined together, using a twisting motion, to form a tight seal. The capsules are placed on a piece of filter paper and checked for signs of leakage. The capsules are dispensed in the appropriate size and type of prescription vial.

VIII. MOLDED TABLETS (TABLET TRITURATES)

A. Definition. Tablet triturates are small, usually cylindrical molded or compressed tablets. They are made of powders created by moistening the powder mixture with alcohol and water. They are used for compounding potent drugs in small doses.

B. Formulation and preparation of tablet triturates

1. Tablet triturates are made in special molds consisting of a pegboard and a corresponding perforated plate.
2. In addition to the mold, a diluent, usually a mixture of lactose and sucrose (80/20), and a moistening agent, usually a mixture of ethyl alcohol and water (60/40), are required.
3. The diluent is triturated with the active ingredients.
4. A paste is then made, using the alcohol and water mixture.
5. This paste is spread into the mold; the tablets are punched out and remain on the pegs until dry.

C. Example

1. **Medication order**
   Atropine sulfate 0.4 mg
   Disp # 500 TT
   Sig. u.d.
2. **Calculations.** For 500 TT: 500 × 0.4 mg = 200 mg atropine sulfate
3. **Compounding procedure.** The mold prepares 70 mg tablets. The 200 mg of atropine sulfate, 6.8 g of sucrose, and 28 g of lactose are weighed and mixed by geometric dilution. The powder is wetted with a mixture of 40% purified water and 60% ethyl alcohol (95%). The paste that is formed is spread onto the tablet triturate mold; the tablets are then punched out of the mold and allowed to dry on the pegs. This procedure is repeated until the required number of tablet triturates has been prepared.

IX. OINTMENTS, CREAMS, PASTES, AND GELS

A. Definitions

1. **Ointments, creams, and pastes** are semisolid dosage forms intended for topical application to the skin or mucous membranes. **Ointments** are characterized as being oleaginous in nature; **creams** are generally o/w or w/o emulsions, and **pastes** are characterized by their high content of solids (about 25%).
2. **Gels** (sometimes called jellies) are semisolid systems consisting of suspensions made up of either small inorganic particles or large organic molecules interpenetrated by a liquid.

B. General characteristics. These dosage forms are semisolid preparations generally applied externally. Semisolid dosage forms may contain active drugs intended to:

1. Act solely on the surface of the skin to produce a local effect (e.g., antifungal agent)
2. Release the medication, which, in turn, penetrates into the skin (e.g., cortisol cream)
3. Release medication for systemic absorption through the skin (e.g., nitroglycerin)

C. Types of ointment bases

1. Hydrophobic bases feel greasy and contain mixtures of fats, oils, and waxes. Hydrophobic bases cannot be washed off using water.
2. Hydrophilic bases are usually emulsion bases. The o/w-type emulsion bases can be easily washed off with water, but the w/o type are slightly more difficult to remove.

D. Preparation of ointments, creams, pastes, and gels

1. Mixing can be done in a mortar or on an ointment slab/tile.
2. Liquids are incorporated by gradually adding them to an absorption-type base and mixing.
3. Insoluble powders are reduced to a fine powder and then added to the base, using geometric dilution.
4. Water-soluble substances are dissolved with water and then incorporated into the base.
5. The final product should be smooth (impalpable) and free of any abrasive particles.

E. Examples

1. **Example 1**
   a. **Medication order**
      Sulfur
      Salicylic acid aa 600 mg
      White petrolatum ad 30 g
      Sig: Apply t.i.d.
   b. **Compounding procedure.** The particle sizes of the sulfur and salicylic acid are reduced separately in a Wedgwood mortar and then blended together. Using a pill tile, the powder mixture is levigated with the base. Using geometric dilution, the base and powders are blended to the final weight. An ointment jar or plastic tube is used for dispensing, and an "external use only" label is placed on the container.

2. **Example 2**
   a. **Medication order**
      Methylparaben 0.25 g
      Propylparaben 0.15 g
      Sodium lauryl sulfate 10 g
      Propylene glycol 120 g
      Stearyl alcohol 250 g
      White petrolatum 250 g
      Purified water 370 g
      Disp 60 g
      Sig: Apply u.d.
   b. **Compounding procedure.** The stearyl alcohol and the white petrolatum are melted on a steam bath and heated to about 75°C. The other ingredients, previously dissolved in purified water at about 78°C, are added. The mixture is stirred until it congeals. An ointment jar is used for dispensing, and an "external use only" label is placed on the jar.

X. SUPPOSITORIES

A. General characteristics

1. Suppositories are **solid bodies** of various weights and shapes, adapted for introduction into the rectal, vaginal, or urethral orifices of the human body. They are used to deliver drugs for their local or systemic effects.

2. Suppositories differ in **size** and **shape** and include:
   a. Rectal
   b. Vaginal
   c. Urethral

B. **Common suppository bases**

1. **Cocoa butter** (theobroma oil), which melts at body temperature, is a fat-soluble mixture of triglycerides that is most often used for rectal suppositories. Witepsol is a synthetic triglyceride. Fatty acid bases include Fattibase®.
2. **Polyethylene glycol** (PEG, Carbowax) derivatives are water-soluble bases suitable for vaginal and rectal suppositories. Polybase® is an example.
3. **Glycerinated gelatin** is a water-miscible base often used in vaginal and rectal suppositories.

C. **Suppository molds**

1. Suppository molds can be made of rubber, plastic, brass, stainless steel, or other suitable material.
2. The formulation and volume of the base depend on the size of the mold used, less the displacement caused by the active ingredient.

D. **Methods of preparing and dispensing suppositories**

1. **Molded suppositories** are prepared by first melting the base and then incorporating the medications uniformly into the base. This mixture is then poured into the suppository mold (fusion method).
2. **Hand-rolled suppositories** require a special technique. With proper technique, it is possible to make a product equal in quality to the molded suppositories.
3. **Containers for the suppositories** are determined by the method and base used in preparation. Hand-rolled and molded suppositories should be dispensed in special boxes that prevent the suppositories from coming in contact with each other.
4. **Storage conditions.** If appropriate, a "refrigerate" label should appear on the container. Regardless of the base or medication used in the formulation, the patient should be instructed to store the suppositories in a cool dry place.

E. **Examples**

1. **Example 1**
   a. **Medication order**
      Naproxen suppository 500 mg
      Disp #12
      Sig: Insert u.d. into rectum
   b. **Calculations.** Each standard adult suppository should weigh 2 g, but depends on the mold used.
      2 g (total weight) − 0.540 g (weight of each 500-mg tablet) naproxen per suppository
      = 1.46 g cocoa butter per suppository × 13 suppositories
      = 18.98 g cocoa butter
   c. **Compounding procedure.** The 13 naproxen 500-mg tablets are triturated to a fine powder, using a Wedgwood mortar. The 18.98 g cocoa butter base is melted in a beaker, using a water bath. The temperature of the water bath should not exceed 36°C. The powder is then added and stirred until mixed. The mixture is poured into an appropriate rectal suppository mold (about 2 g per suppository) and placed into a refrigerator until the suppositories congeal. Any excess is scraped from the top of the mold, and a suppository box is used for dispensing. A "refrigerate" label is placed on the box.
2. **Example 2**
   a. **Medication order**
      Progesterone 50 mg
      Disp #14
      Sig: 1 per vagina once daily on days 14–28 of cycle

b. Calculations. Total weight of each vaginal suppository is 1.9 g.
50 mg progesterone/suppository × 15 = 750 mg progesterone
1.9 g (total weight) − 0.050 g progesterone
= 1.85 g PEG × 15 suppositories
= 27.75 g PEG total

c. Compounding procedure. The PEG is melted to 50°C, and 750 mg progesterone is added. This mixture is poured into a vaginal suppository mold, allowed to cool, cleaned, and dispensed.

XI. PARENTERAL PRODUCTS

A. General requirements. The extemporaneous compounding of sterile products is no longer confined only to the hospital environment; it now is done by community pharmacists engaged in home care practice. Minimum requirements include:

1. Proper equipment and supplies
2. Proper facilities, including a laminar-flow clean bench and a clean room
3. Proper documentation of all products made
4. Quality control, including batch sterility testing
5. Proper storage both at the facility and in transport to the patient's home
6. Proper labeling of the prescription product
7. Knowledge of product's stability and incompatibilities
8. Knowledge of all ancillary equipment involved in production or delivery of the medications

B. Preparation of parenteral products

1. Preparation of sterile products requires special skills and training. Preparing parenteral products or providing this service without proper training should not be attempted.
2. These products must be prepared in a clean room, using aseptic technique (i.e., working under controlled conditions to minimize contamination).
3. Dry powders of parenteral drugs for reconstitution are used for drug products that are unstable as solutions. It is important to know the correct diluents that can be used to yield a solution.
4. Solutions of drugs for parenteral administration may also be further diluted before administration. If further dilution is required, then the pharmacist must know the stability and compatibility of the drug in the diluent.

C. Reconstitution of a dry powder from a vial

1. Work takes place in a laminar-flow clean bench, observing aseptic technique.
2. The manufacturer's instructions should be checked to determine the required volume of diluent.
3. The appropriate needle size and syringe are chosen, keeping in mind that the capacity of the syringe should be slightly larger than the volume required for reconstitution.
4. Using the correct diluent, the surface of the container is cleaned, using an alcohol prep pad, after which the alcohol is permitted to evaporate.
5. The syringe is filled with the diluent to the proper volume.
6. The surface of the vial containing the sterile powder is cleaned, using an alcohol prep pad, after which it is permitted to dry. The diluent is injected into the vial containing the dry powder.
7. The vial is gently shaken or rolled, and the powder is allowed to dissolve.
8. After the powder has dissolved, the vial is inverted and the desired volume is withdrawn.

9. The vehicle is prepared by swabbing the medication port of the bag or bottle with an alcohol prep pad.
10. The solution in the syringe is injected into the vehicle. If a plastic container is used, care must be taken not to puncture the side walls of the container with the tip of the needle.
11. The container should be shaken or kneaded or rotated to assure thorough mixing of the contents.
12. The contents of the container should be checked for particulate matter.
13. A sterile seal or cap is applied over the port of the container.
14. All needles and syringes should be properly discarded.
15. The bag is labeled.

D. Removing the fluid contents from an ampule

1. The ampule is held upright to open it, and the top is tapped to remove any solution trapped in this area.
2. The neck of the ampule is swabbed with an alcohol swab.
3. The ampule is grasped on each side of the neck with the thumb and index finger of each hand and quickly snapped open.
4. A 5- μm filter needle is attached to a syringe of the appropriate size.
5. The ampule is tilted, and the needle is inserted.
6. The needle is positioned near the neck of the ampule, and the solution is withdrawn from the ampule.
7. If the solution is for an intravenous push (bolus injection), the filter needle is removed from the syringe and replaced with a cap.
8. If the solution is for an intravenous infusion, then the filter needle is removed and replaced with a new needle of the appropriate size. The drug is injected into the appropriate vehicle.
9. All materials should be discarded properly, and the final product should be labeled.

E. Removing drug solution from a vial

1. The tab around the rubber closure on the vial is removed, and this surface is swabbed with an alcohol prep pad.
2. An equivalent amount of sterile air is injected into the vial to prevent a negative vacuum from being created and to allow the drug to be removed.
3. Using the appropriate needle size and syringe, the needle is inserted into the rubber closure bevel at a 45° angle.
4. The plunger is pushed down, and air is released into the vial; when the plunger is pulled back, the solution is withdrawn.
5. The solution is then injected into the appropriate vehicle.

STUDY QUESTIONS

Directions: Each of the numbered items or incomplete statements in this section is followed by answers or by completions of the statement. Select the **one** lettered answer or completion that is **best** in each case.

Questions 1–3

The following medication order is given to the pharmacist by the physician:

Olive oil 60.0
Vitamin A 60,000 units
Water 120.0
Sig: 15 ml t.i.d.

1. The final dosage form of this prescription will be

(A) a solution
(B) an elixir
(C) an emulsion
(D) a suspension
(E) a lotion

2. When preparing this prescription, the pharmacist needs to add

(A) Tween 80
(B) acacia
(C) glycerin
(D) alcohol
(E) propylene glycol

3. Which of the following caution labels should the pharmacist affix to the container when dispensing this product?

(A) Do not refrigerate
(B) Shake well
(C) For external use only
(D) No preservatives added

Directions: Each item below contains three suggested answers of which **one or more** is correct. Choose the answer

A if **I only** is correct
B if **III only** is correct
C if **I and II** are correct
D if **II and III** are correct
E if **I, II and III** are correct

4. Correct statements about the prescription below include which of the following?

Morphine 1 mg/ml
Flavored vehicle q.s. ad 120 ml
Sig: 5–20 mg p.o. q 3–4 hours prn pain

I. The amount of morphine needed is 240 mg
II. Powdered morphine alkaloid should be used when compounding this prescription
III. The final dosage form of this prescription is a solution

5. When preparing the following prescription, the pharmacist should:

Podophyllum 5%
Salicylic acid 10%
Acetone 20%
Flexible collodion ad 30 ml
Sig: Apply q h.s.

I. triturate 1.5 g of podophyllum with the 8 ml of acetone
II. add 3 g of salicylic acid to the collodion with trituration
III. affix an "external use only" label to the container

6. Correct statements about the prescription below include which of the following?

Sulfur 6
Purified water
Camphor water aa q.s. ad 60

I. Precipitated sulfur can be used to prepare this prescription
II. The sulfur can be triturated with glycerin before mixing with other ingredients
III. A "shake well" label should be affixed to the bottle

7. Correct statements about the prescription below include which of the following?

Starch 10%
Menthol 1%
Camphor 2%
Calamine q.s. ad 120.0

I. The powders should be blended together in a mortar, using geometric dilution
II. The prescription should be prepared by dissolving the camphor in a sufficient amount of 90% alcohol
III. A eutectic mixture should be avoided

8. When preparing the following prescription, the pharmacist should

Salicylic acid 3 g
Sulfur Ppt 7 g
Lanolin 10 g
White petrolatum 10 g

I. reduce the particle size of the powders, using a mortar and pestle, or using the pill tile with a spatula
II. place on an ointment tile and levigate the ingredients, using geometric dilution
III. package the ointment in an ointment jar or tube

9. An equal volume of air is injected when removing drug solutions from

I. vials
II. ampules
III. syringes

ANSWERS AND EXPLANATIONS

1–3. The answers are: 1-C [*V B 1*], **2-B** [*V B 2, C1*], **3-B** [*V B 3*].
Because olive oil and water are two immiscible liquids, their incorporation requires a two-phase system in which one liquid is dispersed throughout another liquid in the form of small droplets. To accomplish this, an emulsifying agent is necessary. Acacia is the most suitable emulsifying agent when forming an oil-in-water emulsion that is intended for internal use.

Emulsions are physically unstable, and they must be protected against the effects of microbial contamination and physical separation. Shaking before use redistributes the two layers of emulsion. Because light, air, and microorganisms also affect the stability of an emulsion, preservatives can be added.

4. The answer is B (III) [*III A, C 3*].
The concentration of morphine needed for the prescription described in the question is 1 mg/ml, and because 120 ml is the final volume, 120 mg of morphine is needed to compound this prescription. Morphine alkaloid has poor solubility; therefore, one of the salt forms should be used. Because morphine is dissolved in the vehicle, resulting in a liquid preparation, the final dosage form is a solution.

5. The answer is B (III) [*III C 1, 5, D 3*].
Calculating for the amount of each ingredient of the prescription in the question requires 1.5 g of podophyllum, 3 g of salicylic acid, and 6 ml of acetone. The correct procedure would be to triturate the podophyllum with the acetone, then add the triturated salicylic acid to a calibrated bottle containing the podophyllum and acetone. Flexible collodion is then added up to the 30-ml calibration. An "external use only" label should be affixed to the container.

6. The answer is E (all) [*IV B 2, C 5, D 1, 2*].
While precipitated sulfur can be used to prepare the prescription described in the question, it is difficult to triturate; therefore, it must first be levigated with a suitable levigating agent (e.g., glycerin). All suspensions, due to their instability, require shaking before use to redistribute the insoluble ingredients.

7. The answer is A (I) [*VI C 3, D 1*].
The proper procedure for compounding the prescription described in the question is to first form a liquid eutectic. This is done by triturating the menthol and camphor together in a mortar. This eutectic is then blended with the powdered starch and calamine, using geometric dilution.

8. The answer is E (all) [*IX D 1–3, E 1*].
The proper procedure for preparing the prescription given in the question is to reduce the particle size of each powder and mix them together, using geometric dilution. This ensures the proper blending of the powders. Next, this powdered mixture is incorporated, geometrically, with the petrolatum. Then, the lanolin is added geometrically.

9. The answer is A (I) [*XI E 2*].
An equal volume of air must be injected when removing a drug solution from a vial. This is done to prevent the formation of a vacuum within the vial. This problem does not occur with ampules and syringes containing drug solutions; therefore, it is unnecessary to inject any air when removing them.

6
Pharmacokinetics

Leon Shargel

I. PHARMACOKINETICS

A. Introduction

1. **Rates and orders of reactions.** The **rate** of a chemical reaction or process is the velocity with which it occurs. The **order** of a reaction is the way in which the concentration of a drug or reactant in a chemical reaction affects the rate.
   a. **Zero-order reaction.** The drug concentration changes with respect to time at a constant rate, according to the following equation:

$$\frac{dC}{dt} = -k_0$$

   where C is the drug concentration and k_0 is the **zero-order rate constant** expressed in units of concentration per time (e.g., milligrams per milliliters per hour). Integration of this equation yields the linear (straight-line) equation:

$$C = -k_0t + C_0$$

   where k_0 is the slope of the line (see Chapter 3, Figure 3-4) and C_0 is the y intercept, or drug concentration, when time (t) equals zero. The negative sign indicates that the slope is decreasing.
   b. **First-order reaction.** The drug concentration changes with respect to time equal to the product of the rate constant and the concentration of drug remaining, according to the following equation:

$$\frac{dC}{dt} = -kC$$

   where k is the first-order rate constant, expressed in units of reciprocal time, or time-1 (e.g., 1/hr or hr^{-1}).
   (1) Integration of this equation yields the following mathematically equivalent equations:

$$C = C_0e^{-kt}$$
$$\ln C = -kt + \ln C_0$$
$$\log C = -\frac{kt}{2.3} + \log C_0$$

   (2) A graph of the equation in Chapter 3, Figure 3-5, shows the linear relation of the log of the concentration versus time. In Figure 3-5, the slope of the line is equal to $-k/2.3$, and the y intercept is C_0. The values for C are plotted on logarithmic coordinates, and the values for t are shown on linear coordinates.
   (3) The **half-life ($t_{1/2}$)** of a reaction is the time required for the concentration of a drug to decrease by one-half. For a first-order reaction, the half-life is a constant and is related to the first-order rate constant, according to the following equation:

$$t_{1/2} = \frac{0.693}{k}$$

2. **Models and compartments**
   a. A **model** is a mathematic description of a biologic system and is used to express quantitative relations concisely.
   b. A **compartment** is a group of tissues with similar blood flow and drug affinity. A compartment is not a real physiologic or anatomic region.

3. **Drug distribution**
   a. Drugs distribute rapidly to tissues with high blood flow and more slowly to tissues with low blood flow.
   b. Drugs rapidly cross capillary membranes into tissues because of **passive diffusion** and **hydrostatic pressure. Drug permeability** across capillary membranes varies.
      (1) Drugs easily cross the capillaries of the glomerulus of the kidney and the sinusoids of the liver.
      (2) The capillaries of the brain are surrounded by glial cells that create a **blood–brain barrier** that acts as a thick lipid membrane. Polar and ionic hydrophilic drugs cross this barrier slowly.
   c. **Drugs may accumulate in tissues** as a result of their physicochemical characteristics or special affinity of the tissue for the drug.
      (1) Lipid-soluble drugs may accumulate in adipose (fat) tissue because of partitioning of the drug.
      (2) Tetracycline may accumulate in bone because complexes are formed with calcium.
   d. **Plasma protein binding of drugs** affects drug distribution.
      (1) A drug bound to a protein forms a complex that is too large to cross cell membranes.
      (2) **Albumin** is the major plasma protein involved in drug protein binding. **α_1-Glycoprotein,** also found in plasma, is important for the binding of such basic drugs as propranolol.
      (3) Potent drugs, such as phenytoin, that are highly bound (more than 90%) to plasma proteins, may be displaced by other highly bound drugs. The displacement of the bound drug results in more free (nonbound) drug, which rapidly reaches the drug receptors and causes a more intense pharmacologic response.

B. One-compartment model

1. **Intravenous bolus injection.** The entire drug dose enters the body rapidly, and the rate of absorption is neglected in calculations (Figure 6-1). The entire body acts as a single compartment, and the drug rapidly equilibrates with all of the tissues in the body.
   a. **Drug elimination** is a first-order kinetic process, according to the equations in I A 1 b.

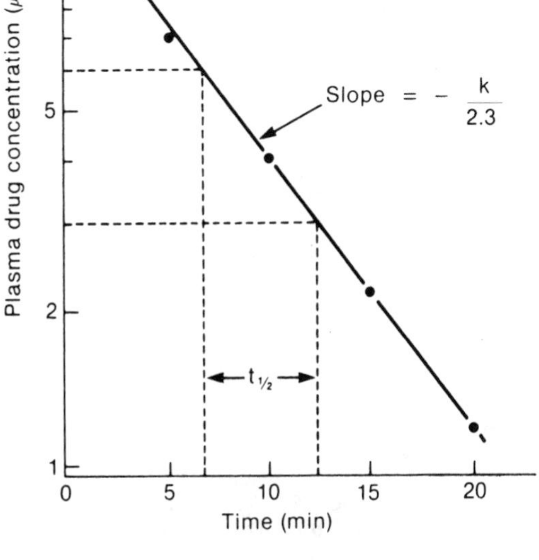

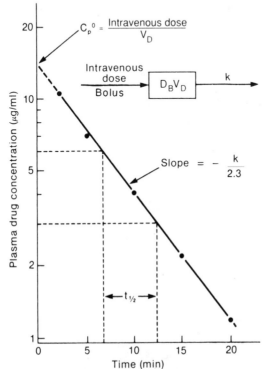

Figure 6-1. Generalized pharmacokinetic model for a drug administered by rapid intravenous bolus injection. C_p0 = extrapolated drug concentration; V_D = apparent volume of distribution; D_B = amount of drug in the body; k = elimination rate constant; $t_{1/2}$ = elimination half-life. (Adapted with permission from Gibaldi M, Perrier D: *Pharmacokinetics,* 2nd ed. New York, Marcel Dekker, 1982, p 4.)

(1) The first-order elimination rate constant (k) is the sum of the rate constants for removal of drug from the body, including the rate constants for renal excretion and metabolism **(biotransformation)** as described by the following equation:

$$k = k_e + k_m$$

where k_e is the rate constant for renal excretion and k_m is the rate constant for metabolism. This equation assumes that all rates are first-order processes.

(2) The **elimination half-life ($t_{1/2}$)** is given by the following equation:

$$t_{1/2} = \frac{0.693}{k}$$

b. Apparent volume of distribution (V_D) is the hypothetical volume of body fluid in which the drug is dissolved. This value is not a true anatomic or physical volume.

(1) V_D is needed to estimate the amount of drug in the body relative to the concentration of drug in the plasma, as shown in the following:

$$V_D \times C_p = D_B$$

where V_D is the apparent volume of distribution, C_p is the plasma drug concentration, and D_B is the amount of drug in the body.

(2) To calculate the V_D after an intravenous bolus injection, the equation is rearranged to give:

$$V_D = \frac{D_B{}^0}{C_p{}^0}$$

where $D_B{}^o$ is the dose (D^o) of drug given by intravenous bolus and $C_p{}^o$ is the extrapolated drug concentration at zero time on the y axis, after the drug equilibrates.

(3) According to the equation, V_D is increased when the drug is distributed more extravascularly into the tissues and $C_p{}^o$ is decreased. When more drug is contained in the vascular space or plasma, $C_p{}^o$ is increased and V_D is decreased.

2. Single oral dose. If the drug is given in a conventional dosage form (e.g., tablet, capsule), the drug is rapidly absorbed by first-order kinetics. Elimination of the drug also follows the principles of first-order kinetics (Figure 6-2).

a. The following equation describes the pharmacokinetics of **first-order absorption and elimination:**

$$C_p = \frac{FD_o k_A}{V_D(k_A - k)} (e^{-kt} - e^{-kt})$$

where k_A is the first-order absorption rate constant and F is the fraction of drug bioavailable. Changes in F, D_o, V_D, k_A, and k affect the plasma drug concentration.

b. The time for maximum, or **peak, drug absorption** is given by the following equation:

$$T_{max} = \frac{2.3 \log (k_A/k)}{k_A - k}$$

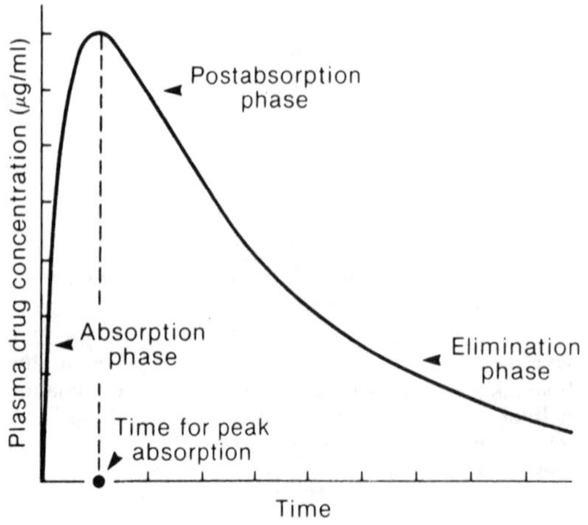

Figure 6-2. Generalized plot for a one-compartment model showing first-order drug absorption and first-order drug elimination. (Adapted with permission from Shargel L, Yu ABC: *Applied Biopharmaceutics and Pharmacokinetics,* 3rd ed. East Norwalk, CT, Appleton & Lange, 1993, p 170.)

T_{max} depends only on the rate constants k_A and k, not on F, D_o, or V_D.

c. After T_{max} is obtained, the peak drug concentration (C_{max}) is calculated, using the equation in I B 2 a and substituting T_{max} for t.

d. The area under the curve (AUC) may be determined by integration of $\int_0^t C_p\,dt$, using the trapezoidal rule, or by the following equation:

$$\int_0^t C_p dt = [AUC]_0^t \int_0^\infty C_p dt = \frac{FD_0}{V_D k'}$$

where changes in F, D_0, k, and V_D affect the AUC. Minor changes in k_A do not affect the AUC.

e. Lag time occurs at the beginning of systemic drug absorption. For some individuals, systemic drug absorption is delayed after oral drug administration because of delayed stomach emptying or other factors.

3. Intravenous infusion. Zero-order absorption and first-order elimination occur (Figure 6-3).

a. A few oral controlled-release drug products release the drug by zero-order kinetics and have **zero-order systemic absorption.**

b. The plasma drug concentration at any time after the start of an intravenous infusion is given by the following equation:

$$C_p = \frac{R}{V_D k}(1 - e^{-kt})$$

where R is the zero-order rate of infusion given in units as milligrams per hour or milligrams per minute.

c. If the intravenous infusion is discontinued, the plasma drug concentration declines by a first-order process. The elimination half-life, or k, may be obtained from the declining plasma drug concentration versus time curve.

d. As the drug is infused, the plasma drug concentration increases to a plateau, or **steady-state concentration.**

(1) Under steady-state conditions, the fraction of drug absorbed equals the fraction of drug eliminated from the body.

(2) The plasma concentration at steady state (C_{ss}) is given by the following equation:

$$C_{ss} = \frac{R}{V_D k}$$

(3) The rate of drug infusion (R) may be calculated from a rearrangement of the equation if the desired C_{ss}, the V_D, and the k are known. These values can often be obtained from the drug literature. To calculate the rate of infusion, the following equation is used:

$$R = C_{ss} V_D k$$

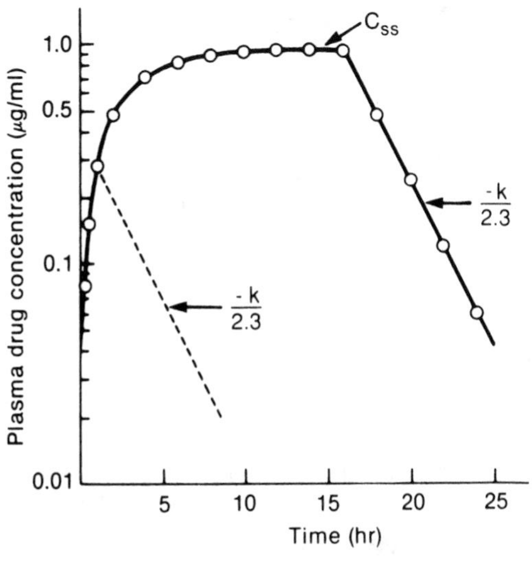

Figure 6-3. Generalized semilogarithmic plot for a drug showing zero-order absorption and first-order elimination. C_{ss} = steady-state concentration; k = elimination rate constant. (Adapted with permission from Gibaldi M, Perrier D: *Pharmacokinetics,* 2nd ed. New York, Marcel Dekker, 1982, p 30.)

where C_{ss} is the desired (target) plasma drug concentration. The product, V_Dk, is also equal to total body clearance, Cl_T.

e. A **loading dose (D_L)** is given as an initial intravenous bolus dose to produce the C_{ss} as rapidly as possible. The intravenous infusion is started at the same time.

(1) The time to reach C_{ss} depends on the elimination half-life of the drug. Reaching 95% or 99% of the C_{ss} without a D_L takes 4.32 or 6.65 half-lives, respectively.

(2) The D_L is the amount of drug that, when dissolved in the apparent V_D, produces the desired C_{ss}. Thus, D_L is calculated by the following equation:

$$D_L = C_{ss}V_D \text{ and } D_L = R/k$$

f. For a drug with a narrow therapeutic window, an intravenous infusion provides a relatively constant plasma drug concentration that does not increase to more than the minimum toxic concentration (MTC) or decrease to less than the minimum effective concentration (MEC).

4. Intermittent intravenous infusions

a. Intermittent intravenous infusions are infusions in which the drug is infused for short periods to prevent accumulation and toxicity.

b. Intermittent intravenous infusions are used for a few drugs, such as the aminoglycosides. For example, gentamicin may be given as a 1-hour infusion every 12 hours. In this case, steady-state drug concentrations are not achieved.

c. The peak drug concentration in the plasma for a drug given by intermittent intravenous infusion may be calculated by the following equation:

$$Cp_n = \frac{R(1 - e^{-kt})\,(1 - e^{-nk\tau})}{Cl\,(1 - e^{-k\tau})}$$

where Cp_n is the peak drug concentration, R is the rate of drug infusion, Cl is total body clearance, T is the dosage interval, and t is the time for the infusion.

5. Multiple doses. Many drugs are given intermittently in a multiple-dose regimen for continuous or prolonged therapeutic activity. This regimen is often used to treat chronic disease.

a. If drug doses are given frequently before the previous dose is completely eliminated, then plasma drug concentrations accumulate and increase to a steady-state level.

b. At **steady state,** plasma drug concentration fluctuates between a maximum (C^{∞}_{max}) and a minimum (C^{∞}_{max}) value (Figure 6-4).

c. When a multiple-dose regimen is calculated, the **superposition principle** assumes that previous drug doses have no effect on subsequent doses. Thus, the predicted plasma drug concentration is the total plasma drug concentration obtained by adding the residual drug concentrations found after each previous dose.

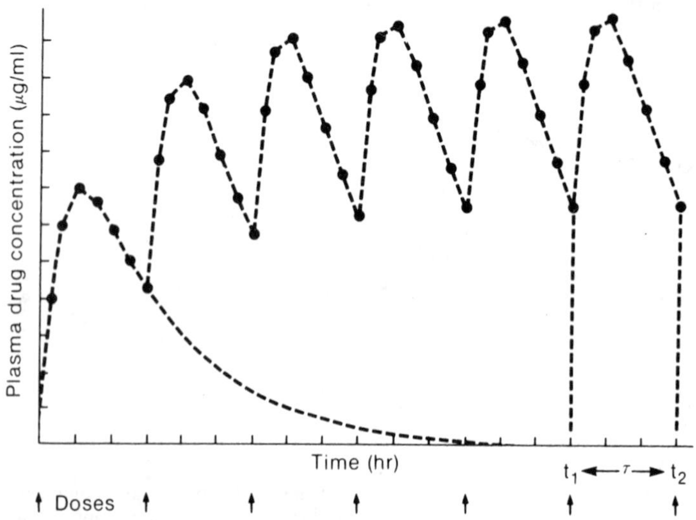

Figure 6-4. Generalized plot showing plasma drug concentration levels after administration of multiple doses and levels of accumulation when equal doses are given at equal time intervals. τ = time interval between doses (t), or the frequency of dosing. (Adapted with permission from Shargel L, Yu ABC: *Applied Biopharmaceutics and Pharmacokinetics,* 3rd ed. East Norwalk, CT, Appleton & Lange, 1993, p 354.)

d. When a multiple-dose regimen is designed, only the **dosing rate** (D_0/τ) can be adjusted easily.

(1) The dosing rate is based on the **size of the dose** (D_0) and the **interval (τ) between doses**, or the **frequency of dosing.**

(2) The dosing rate is given by the following equation:

$$\text{Dosing rate} = D_0/\tau$$

(3) As long as the dosing rate is the same, the expected **average drug concentration at steady state (C^{∞}_{av})** is the same.

(a) For example, if a 600-mg dose is given every 12 hours, the dosing rate is 600 mg/12 hr, or 50 mg/hr.

(b) A dose of 300 mg every 6 hours or 200 mg every 4 hours also gives the same dosing rate (50 mg/hr), with the same expected C^{∞}_{av}.

(c) For a larger dose given over a longer interval (e.g., 600 mg every 12 hours), the C^{∞}_{max} is higher and the C^{∞}_{min} lower compared with a smaller dose given more frequently (e.g., 200 mg every 4 hours).

e. Certain antibiotics are given by **multiple rapid intravenous bolus injections.**

(1) The peak, or **maximum, serum drug concentration** at steady state may be estimated by the following equation:

$$C^{\infty}_{max} = \frac{D_o/V_D}{1 - e^{-k\tau}}$$

(2) The **minimum serum drug concentration** (C^{∞}_{min}) at steady state is the drug concentration after the drug declines one dosage interval. Thus, C^{∞}_{min} is determined by the following equation:

$$C^{\infty}_{min} = C^{\infty}_{max}\, e^{-k\tau}$$

(3) The **average drug concentration** (C^{∞}_{av}) at steady state is estimated with the equation used for multiple oral doses:

$$C^{\infty}_{av} = \frac{FD_o}{kV_D\tau}$$

For intravenous bolus injections, $F = 1$.

f. Orally administered drugs given in **immediate-release dosage forms** (e.g., solutions, conventional tablets, capsules) by multiple oral doses are usually rapidly absorbed and slowly eliminated ($k_A >> k$). C^{∞}_{max} and C^{∞}_{min} for these drugs are approximated by the equations shown in I B 5 e (1) (2).

(1) For more exact calculations of C^{∞}_{min} and C^{∞}_{max} after multiple oral doses, the following equation is used:

$$C^{\infty}_{max} = \frac{FD_o}{V_D}\,\frac{1}{1 - e^{-k\tau}} \quad \text{and}$$

$$C^{\infty}_{min} = \frac{FD_o k_A}{V_D(k_A - k)}\,\frac{1}{1 - e^{-k\tau}}\, e^{-k\tau}$$

(2) The calculation of C^{∞}_{av} is the same as for multiple intravenous bolus injections, using the equation shown in I B 5 e (3).

(3) The term $1/(1 - e^{-k\tau})$ is known as the **accumulation rate.**

(4) The fraction of drug remaining in the body (f) after a dosage interval is given by the following equation:

$$f = e^{-k\tau}$$

(5) An initial loading dose (D_L) is given to obtain a therapeutic steady-state drug level quickly.

(a) For multiple oral doses, D_L is calculated by:

$$D_L = D_M \frac{1}{1 - e^{-k\tau}}$$

where D_M is the maintenance dose.

(b) If D_M is given at a dosage interval equal to the elimination half-life of the drug, then D_L equals twice the maintenance dose.

C. Multicompartment models

1. Drugs that exhibit multicompartment pharmacokinetics distribute into different tissue groups at different rates. Tissues with high blood flow equilibrate with a drug more rapidly than tissues with low blood flow. Drug concentration in various tissues depends on the physical and chemical characteristics of the drug and the nature of the tissue. For example, highly lipid-soluble drugs accumulate slowly in fat (lipid) tissue.

2. **Two-compartment model (intravenous bolus injection)**
   a. After an intravenous bolus injection, the drug distributes and equilibrates rapidly into highly perfused tissues **(central compartment)** and more slowly into peripheral tissues **(tissue compartment)** (Figure 6-5).
   b. The initial rapid decline in plasma drug concentration is known as the **distribution phase.** The slower rate of decline in drug concentration after complete equilibration is achieved is known as the **elimination phase.**
   c. The **plasma drug concentration** at any time is the sum of two first-order processes, as given in the following equation:

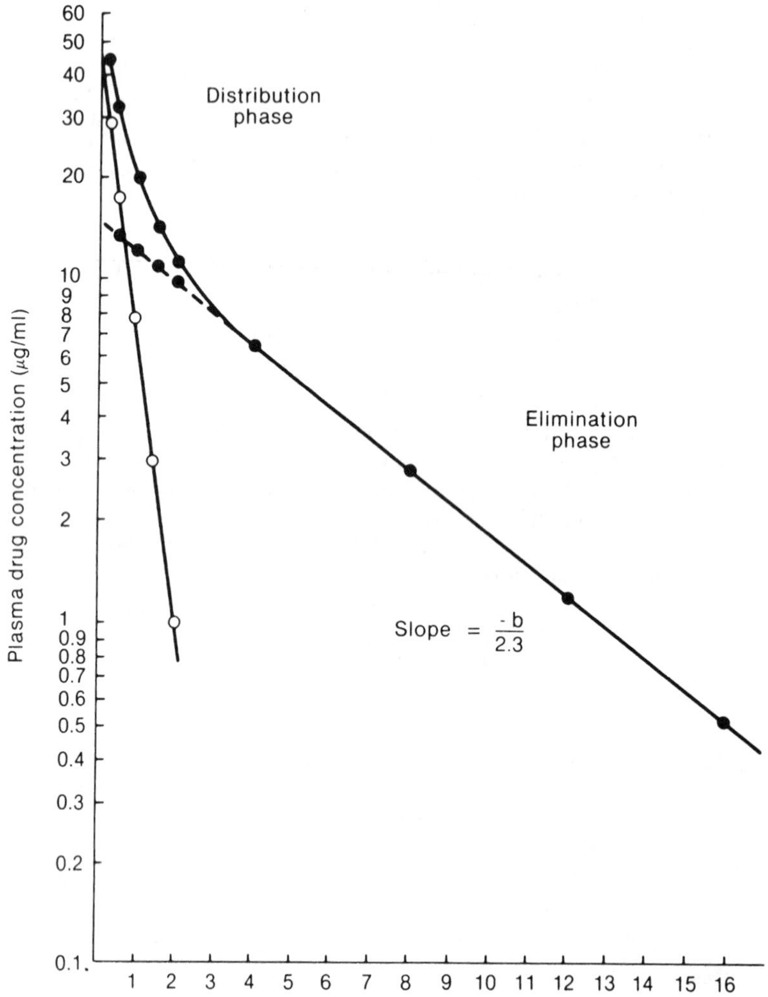

Figure 6-5. Generalized plot showing drug distribution and equilibration for a two-compartment model (intravenous bolus injection). The distribution phase is the initial rapid decline in plasma drug concentration. The elimination phase is the slower rate of decline after complete equilibration of the drug is achieved. (Adapted with permission from Shargel L, Yu ABC: *Applied Biopharmaceutics and Pharmacokinetics,* 3rd ed. East Norwalk, CT, Appleton & Lange, 1993, p 62.)

$$C_p = Ae^{-at} + Be^{-bt}$$

where a and b are hybrid first-order rate constants and A and B are y intercepts.

(1) The **hybrid first-order rate constant b** is obtained from the slope of the elimination phase of the curve (see Figure 6-5) and represents the first-order elimination of drug from the body after the drug equilibrates with all tissues.

(2) The **hybrid first-order rate constant a** is obtained from the slope of the residual line of the distribution phase after the elimination phase is subtracted.

d. The **apparent volume of distribution** depends on the type of pharmacokinetic calculation. Volumes of distribution include the volume of the central compartment (V_p), the volume of distribution at steady state (V_{ss}), and the volume of the tissue compartment (V_t).

3. Two-compartment model (oral drug administration)

a. A drug with a rapid distribution phase may not show two-compartment characteristics after oral administration. As the drug is absorbed, it equilibrates with the tissues so that the elimination half-life of the elimination portion of the curve equals 0.693/b.

b. Two-compartment characteristics are seen if the drug is rapidly absorbed and the distribution phase is slower.

4. Models with additional compartments

a. The addition of each new compartment to the model requires an additional first-order plot.

b. The addition of a third compartment suggests that the drug slowly equilibrates into a deep tissue space. If the drug is given at frequent intervals, the drug begins to accumulate into the third compartment.

c. The terminal linear phase generally represents the elimination of the drug from the body after equilibration occurs. The rate constant from the elimination phase is used to calculate dosage regimens.

d. Adequate pharmacokinetic description of multicompartment models is often difficult and depends on proper plasma sampling and determination of drug concentrations.

D. Nonlinear pharmacokinetics are also known as capacity-limited, dose-dependent, or saturation pharmacokinetics. Nonlinear pharmacokinetics do not follow first-order kinetics as the dose increases (Figure 6-6). Nonlinear pharmacokinetics result from the saturation of an enzyme- or carrier-mediated system.

1. Characteristics of nonlinear pharmacokinetics include:

a. The AUC is not proportional to the dose.

b. The amount of drug excreted in the urine is not proportional to the dose.

c. The elimination half-life may increase at high doses.

d. The ratio of metabolites formed changes with increased dose.

2. Michaelis-Menten kinetics describe the velocity of enzyme reactions. These kinetics are used to describe nonlinear pharmacokinetics.

a. The **Michaelis-Menten equation** describes the rate of change (velocity) of plasma drug concentration after an intravenous bolus injection, as follows:

$$-\frac{dC_p}{dt} = \frac{V_{max}\,C_p}{k_M + C_p}$$

where V_{max} is the maximum velocity of the reaction, C_p is the substrate or plasma drug concentration, and k_M is the rate constant equal to the C_p at 0.5 V_{max}.

b. At low C_p values, where $k_M >> C_p$, this equation reduces to a first-order rate equation because both k_M and V_{max} are constants.

$$-\frac{dC_p}{dt} = \frac{V_{max}\,C_p}{k_M} = k'Cp$$

c. At high C_p values, where $C_p >> k_M$, the Michaelis-Menten equation is a zero-order rate equation, as follows:

$$-\frac{dC_p}{dt} = V_{max}$$

3. Drugs that follow nonlinear pharmacokinetics may show zero-order elimination rates at high drug concentrations, a mix of zero- and first-order elimination rates at intermediate drug concentrations, and first-order elimination rates at low drug concentrations (see Figure 6-6).

E. Clearance is a measurement of drug elimination from the body.

1. **Total body clearance (Cl_T)** is the drug elimination rate divided by the plasma drug concentration. According to the concept of clearance, the body contains an apparent volume of distribution in which the drug is dissolved. A constant portion of this volume is cleared, or removed, from the body per unit time.
   a. The following equations express the measurement of total body clearance:

$$Cl_T = \frac{\text{drug elimination}}{\text{plasma drug concentration}} = \frac{dDe/dt}{C_p},$$

$$Cl_T = V_D k, \text{ and}$$

$$Cl_T = \frac{FD_o}{AUC}$$

   b. For drugs that follow first-order (linear) pharmacokinetics, total body clearance is the sum of the clearances in the body, as shown in the following equation:

$$Cl_T = Cl_R + Cl_{NR}$$

   where Cl_R is renal clearance and Cl_{NR} is nonrenal clearance.
   c. The relation between Cl_T and $t_{1/2}$ is obtained by substituting $0.693/t_{1/2}$ for k in the equation in I E 1 a to obtain the following expression:

$$t_{1/2} = \frac{0.693\ V_D}{Cl_T}$$

   V_D and Cl_T are considered independent variables, and $t_{1/2}$ is considered a dependent variable.
   d. As clearance decreases (e.g., in renal disease), $t_{1/2}$ increases. Changes in V_D also cause proportional changes in $t_{1/2}$.

2. **Renal drug excretion** is the major route of drug elimination for polar drugs, water-soluble drugs, drugs with low molecular weight (mol wt less than 500), or drugs that are biotransformed slowly. The relation between the drug excretion rate and the plasma drug concentration is shown in Figure 6-7. Drugs are excreted through the kidney into the urine by glomerular filtration, tubular reabsorption, and active tubular secretion.
   a. **Glomerular filtration** is a passive process by which small molecules and drugs are filtered through the glomerulus of the nephron.

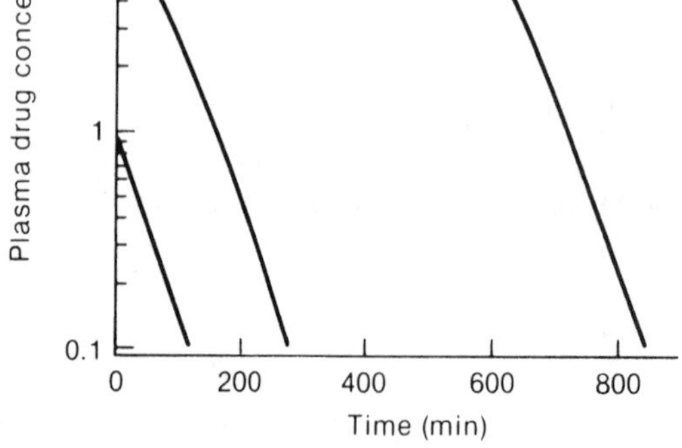

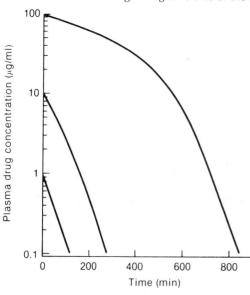

Figure 6-6. Generalized plot showing plasma drug concentration versus time for a drug with Michaelis-Menten (nonlinear) elimination kinetics. For this one-compartment model (intravenous injection), the doses are 1 mg, 10 mg, and 100 mg, and the apparent in vivo rate constant (kM) is 10 mg. The maximum velocity of the reaction (V_{max}) is 0.2 mg/min. (Adapted with permission from Gibaldi M, Perrier D: *Pharmacokinetics,* 2nd ed. New York, Marcel Dekker, 1982, p 271.)

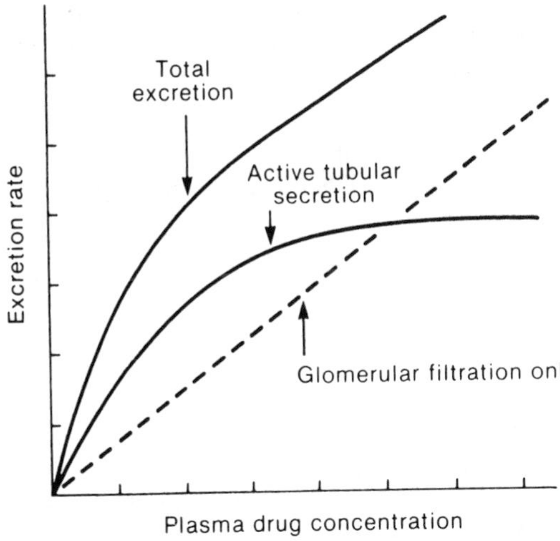

Figure 6-7. Generalized plot showing the excretion rate versus plasma drug concentration for a drug with active tubular secretion and for a drug secreted by glomerular filtration only. (Adapted with permission from Shargel L, Yu ABC: *Applied Biopharmaceutics and Pharmacokinetics,* 3rd ed. East Norwalk, CT, Appleton & Lange, 1993, p 283.)

(1) Drugs bound to plasma proteins are too large to be filtered at the glomerulus.
(2) Drugs such as **creatinine and inulin** are not actively secreted or reabsorbed. They are used to measure the **glomerular filtration rate (GFR).**

b. Tubular reabsorption is a passive process that follows Fick's law of diffusion.

(1) Lipid-soluble drugs are reabsorbed from the lumen of the nephron back into the systemic circulation.
(2) For weak electrolyte drugs, urine pH affects the ratio of nonionized and ionized drug.
  (a) If the drug exists primarily in the nonionized or lipid-soluble form, then it is reabsorbed more easily from the lumen of the nephron.
  (b) If the drug exists primarily in the ionized or water-soluble form, then it is excreted more easily in the urine.
  (c) Depending on the pK_a of the drug, alteration of urine pH alters the ratio of ionized to nonionized drug and affects the rate of drug excretion. For example, alkalinization of the urine by the administration of sodium bicarbonate increases the excretion of salicylates (weak acids).
(3) An increase in urine flow caused by simultaneous administration of a diuretic decreases the time for drug reabsorption. Consequently, more drug is excreted.

c. Active tubular secretion is a carrier-mediated active transport system that requires energy.

(1) Two active tubular secretion pathways exist in the kidney: one system for weak acids and one system for weak bases.
(2) The active tubular secretion system shows competition effects. For example, probenecid (a weak acid) competes for the same system as penicillin, decreasing the rate of penicillin excretion.
(3) The renal clearance of drugs that are actively secreted, such as ***p*-aminohippurate (PAH),** is used to measure **effective renal blood flow (ERBF).**

3. **Renal clearance** is the volume of drug contained in the plasma that is removed by the kidney per unit time. **Units for renal clearance** are expressed in volume per time (e.g., milliliters per minute or liters per hour).

a. Renal clearance may be measured by dividing the rate of drug excretion by the plasma drug concentration, as shown in the following equation:

$$Cl_R = \frac{\text{Rate of drug excretion}}{C_p} = \frac{dD_U/dt}{C_p}$$

b. Measurement of renal clearance may also be expressed by the following equation:

$$Cl_R = k_e V_D$$

where k_e is the first-order renal excretion rate constant and

$$Cl_R = \frac{D_U^\infty}{AUC}$$

where D_U^∞ is the total amount of parent (unchanged) drug excreted in the urine.

c. Renal clearance is measured without regard to the physiologic mechanism of renal drug excretion. The probable mechanism for renal clearance is obtained with a **clearance ratio,** which relates drug clearance to inulin clearance (a measure of GFR).

(1) If the clearance ratio is less than 1.0, the mechanism for drug clearance may result from filtration plus reabsorption.

(2) If the ratio is 1.0, the mechanism may be filtration only.

(3) If the ratio is more than 1.0, the mechanism may be filtration plus active tubular secretion.

4. Hepatic clearance is the volume of drug-containing plasma that is cleared by the liver per unit time.

a. Measurement of hepatic clearance. Hepatic clearance is usually measured indirectly, as the difference between total body clearance and renal clearance, as shown in the following equation:

$$Cl_H = Cl_T - Cl_R$$

where Cl_H is the hepatic clearance. This clearance is equivalent to Cl_{NR}, or nonrenal drug clearance. However, the hepatic clearance can also be calculated as the **product of the liver blood flow (Q)** and the **extraction ratio (ER),** as shown in the following equation:

$$Cl_H = QER$$

(1) The extraction ratio is the fraction of drug that is irreversibly removed by an organ or tissue as the drug-containing plasma perfuses that tissue.

(2) The extraction ratio is obtained by measuring the plasma drug concentration entering the liver and the plasma drug concentration exiting the liver:

$$ER = \frac{C_a - C_v}{C_a}$$

where C_a is the arterial plasma drug concentration entering the liver and C_v is the venous plasma drug concentration exiting the liver.

(3) Values for the ER range from 0 to 1. For example, if the ER is 0.9, then 90% of the incoming drug is removed as the plasma perfuses the liver. If the ER is 0, then no drug is removed by the liver.

b. Blood flow, intrinsic clearance, and **protein binding** affect hepatic clearance.

(1) Blood flow to the liver is approximately 1.5 L/min and may be altered by exercise, food, disease, or drugs.

(a) Blood enters the liver through the hepatic portal vein and hepatic artery and leaves through the hepatic vein.

(b) After oral drug administration, the drug is absorbed from the gastrointestinal tract into the mesenteric vessels and proceeds to the hepatic portal vein, liver, and systemic circulation.

(2) Intrinsic clearance describes the ability of the liver to remove the drug independently of blood flow.

(a) Intrinsic drug clearance primarily occurs because of the inherent ability of the **biotransformation enzymes** (mixed-function oxidases) to metabolize the drug as it enters the liver.

(b) Normally, basal level mixed-function oxidase enzymes biotransform drugs. Levels of these enzymes are increased by various drugs (e.g., phenobarbital) and environmental agents (e.g., tobacco smoke). These enzymes are inhibited by other drugs and environmental agents (e.g., cimetidine, acute lead poisoning).

(3) Protein binding. Drugs that are bound to protein are not easily cleared by the liver or kidney because only the free, or nonplasma protein-bound, drug crosses the cell membrane into the tissue.

(a) The free drug is available to drug-metabolizing enzymes for biotransformation.

(b) A sudden increase in free-drug plasma concentration results in more available drug at pharmacologic receptors, producing a more intense effect in the organs (e.g., kidney, liver) involved in drug removal.

(c) Blood flow (Q), intrinsic clearance (Cl_{int}), and **free-plasma drug concentration (f)** are related to hepatic clearance as shown in the following equation:

$$Cl_H = Q \frac{fCl_{int}}{Q + Cl_{int}}$$

(1) The hepatic clearance of drugs that have high extraction ratios and high Cl_{int} values (e.g., propranolol) is most affected by changes in blood flow and inhibitors of the drug metabolism enzymes.
(2) The hepatic clearance of drugs that have low extraction ratios and low Cl_{int} values (e.g., theophylline) is most affected by changes in Cl_{int} and is affected only slightly by changes in hepatic blood flow.
(3) Only drugs that are highly plasma protein-bound (i.e., more than 95%) and have a low intrinsic clearance (e.g., phenytoin) are affected by a sudden shift in protein binding. This shift causes an increase in free-drug plasma concentration.

c. Biliary drug excretion, an active transport process, is also included in hepatic clearance. Separate active secretion systems exist for weak acids and weak bases.
(1) Drugs that are excreted in bile are usually high–molecular-weight compounds (i.e., mol wt more than 500) or polar drugs, such as reserpine, digoxin, and various glucuronide conjugates.
(2) Drugs may be recycled by the **enterohepatic circulation.**
(a) Some drugs are absorbed from the gastrointestinal tract through the mesenteric and hepatic portal veins, proceeding to the liver. The liver may secrete some of the drug (unchanged or as a glucuronide metabolite) into the bile.
(b) From the bile (stored in the gallbladder), the drug may empty into the gastrointestinal tract through the bile duct.
(c) If the drug is a **glucuronide metabolite,** bacteria in the gastrointestinal tract may hydrolyze the glucuronide moiety, allowing the released drug to be reabsorbed.

d. First-pass effects (presystemic elimination) occur with drugs given orally. A portion of the drug is eliminated before systemic absorption occurs.
(1) First-pass effects generally result from rapid drug biotransformation by liver enzymes. Other mechanisms include metabolism of the drug by gastrointestinal mucosal cells, intestinal flora, or biliary secretion.
(2) First-pass effects are usually observed by measuring the **absolute bioavailability** (F) of the drug. If F is less than 1, then some of the drug was eliminated before systemic absorption occurred.
(3) Drugs that have a **high hepatic extraction ratio,** such as propranolol, show first-pass effects.
(4) If the first-pass effect is high (i.e., more than 90%), then either:
(a) The drug dose could be increased (e.g., propranolol, penicillin).
(b) The drug could be given by an alternate route of administration (e.g., nitroglycerin, insulin).
(c) The dosage form could be modified (e.g., mesalamine).

F. Noncompartment methods. Pharmacokinetic parameters for absorption, distribution, and elimination are estimated with noncompartment methods. These methods usually require comparison of the areas under the curve.

1. Mean residence time

a. Mean residence time (MRT) is the average time for the drug molecules to reside in the body. MRT is also known as the mean transit time or mean sojourn time.

b. The MRT depends on the route of administration and assumes that the drug is eliminated from the central compartment.

c. The MRT is the total residence time for all molecules in the body divided by the total number of molecules in the body, as shown in the following equation:

$$MRT = \frac{\text{Total residence time for all drug molecules in the body}}{\text{Total number of drug molecules}}$$

d. MRT = IV bolus injection
(1) The MRT after a bolus intravenous injection is calculated by the following equation:

$$MRT_{IV} = \frac{AUMC}{AUC_{0-\infty}}$$

where AUMC is the area under the first moment versus time curve from t = 0 to t = infinity and $AUC_{0-\infty}$ is the area under the plasma drug concentration versus time curve from t = 0 to t = infinity. $AUC_{0-\infty}$ is also known as the zero moment curve.

(2) The MRT_{IV} is related to the elimination half-life by the following expression:

$$MRT_{IV} = 1/k$$

(3) During MRT_{IV}, 62.3% of the intravenous bolus dose is eliminated.
(4) The MRT for a drug given by a noninstantaneous input is longer than the MRT_{IV}.

2. **Mean absorption time (MAT)** is the difference between MRT and MRT_{IV} after an extravascular route is used.

$$MAT = MRT_{po} - MRT_{IV}$$

When first-order absorption occurs, MAT = 1/ka.

3. **Steady-state volume of distribution (V_{ss})**
   a. The steady-state volume of distribution is the amount of drug in the body at steady state and the average steady-state drug concentration.
   b. After an intravenous bolus injection, V_{ss} is calculated by the following equation:

$$Vss = \frac{Dose_{IV}\,(AUMC)}{(AUC)^2}$$

II. CLINICAL PHARMACOKINETICS

CLINICAL PHARMACOKINETICS is the application of pharmacokinetic principles for the rational design of an individualized dosage regimen. The two main objectives are **maintenance of an optimum drug concentration at the receptor site** to produce the desired therapeutic response for a specific period and **minimization of any adverse or toxic effects** of the drug.

A. Design factors for an individualized dosage regimen

1. Drug pharmacokinetics in the patient, including absorption, distribution, and elimination profile
2. The patient's normal physiologic condition, including age, weight, sex, and nutritional status
3. Pathophysiologic conditions [e.g., renal disease, congestive heart failure (CHF), liver disease] that may affect drug pharmacokinetics
4. Other factors (e.g., diet) that may affect the predicted therapeutic activity
5. Environmental factors that may affect drug pharmacokinetics (e.g., smoking increases theophylline clearance)
6. The **target concentration** (i.e., plasma or serum drug concentration for optimal therapeutic effect) and **therapeutic window** (i.e., range of plasma drug concentration between MTC and MEC) of the drug
   a. The probability of an adverse response to the drug increases as the plasma drug concentration approaches the MTC.
   b. The probability that the drug lacks efficacy (i.e., does not produce a therapeutic response) increases as the plasma drug concentration approaches the MEC.

B. Responsibilities of the clinical pharmacist.

The appropriate drug must be selected, usually in conjunction with the clinician, and a dosage regimen must be designed for the patient.

1. Dosage regimen
   a. **The target drug concentration** and **dosing rate** must be determined.
      (1) **Dosing rate** (D_o/τ) is the main parameter that the clinical pharmacist may adjust. This rate is based on the target drug concentration, therapeutic window, and estimated clearance of the drug in the patient, as shown in the following equation:

$$\text{Target drug concentration} = \text{dosing rate} \times \frac{1}{\text{clearance}}$$

$$C_{av}^{\infty} = \frac{FD_o}{\tau} \times \frac{1}{Cl_T}$$

where F is the fraction of drug absorbed.

      (2) **Drug dose** should be adjusted to commercially available dosage forms and strengths. For example, if the drug is manufactured in 125-mg, 250-mg, and 500-mg tablets, then the calculated dose is rounded to the nearest strength.

(3) **Dosage interval (τ)** should be set at intervals convenient for the patient. For example, a dose given every 8 hours is more practical than a dose given every 7.3 hours. When the dose and dosage interval are adjusted, the C_{av}^{∞} is the same as long as the dosing rate is maintained. However, the C_{min}^{∞} and C_{max}^{∞} values vary and should be checked.

(4) Many drugs are available as **extended-release drug products.** For some patients, this form is more appropriate than an immediate-release dosage form.

b. **Nomograms** are often used to develop dosage regimens. These are based on average, or population, pharmacokinetic parameters. Although they are easy to use, nomograms may not apply to a specific patient's needs.

2. The **patient's response** to the drug and dosage regimen must be evaluated.

3. **Serum or plasma drug concentrations** must be determined as needed.
   a. **Therapeutic drug monitoring (TDM)** verifies the adequacy of the dosage regimen, using plasma or drug concentrations.
   b. **The number of blood samples** and the **timing of blood sample collection** are important considerations for TDM.
   c. Drug levels in plasma or serum are assayed.
   d. **Pharmacokinetic interpretation** of the serum drug concentration is performed.
   e. The **dosage is readjusted,** if necessary, according to the results obtained by TDM.
   f. Plasma drug concentrations are further monitored.
   g. **Special recommendations** or **patient education** is provided to ensure compliance with the dosage regimen. Patients should understand their drug dosage regimen in relation to meals, other drugs, their daily routines, and sleep habits.

III. PHARMACOKINETICS IN RENAL DISEASE

A. **Overview.** Patients with renal disease pose a special problem because of the role of the kidneys in pharmacokinetics. The kidneys regulate body fluids, electrolyte balance, metabolite waste removal, and drug excretion. **Acute renal failure,** which alters kidney function, may result from a variety of causes, including disease, trauma, and nephrotoxic agents.

1. Renal failure usually causes a **reduced GFR** and a decreased ability of the kidneys to remove metabolite wastes, such as urea and drugs.

2. Renal disease may also **decrease plasma drug–protein binding** because of competition for binding sites by accumulating metabolite wastes, including urea, the active drug, and biotransformation products.

B. Measuring glomerular filtration rate

1. **Criteria for drugs used to measure GFR**
   a. The drug is filtered at the glomerulus.
   b. The drug is not reabsorbed or actively secreted.
   c. The drug is not metabolized.
   d. The drug is not highly bound to plasma proteins.
   e. The drug is nontoxic and does not affect renal function.
   f. The drug is easily measured in plasma and urine.

2. Inulin and creatinine
   a. **Inulin,** a polysaccharide, meets most of these criteria. However, it is exogenous and must be administered in addition to any other drug therapy.
   b. **Creatinine,** an endogenous substance formed from creatinine phosphate during muscle metabolism, is an alternative.
      (1) Creatinine production varies with sex, age, and body weight.
      (2) Creatinine is filtered at the glomerulus and is not reabsorbed.
      (3) A small fraction is actively secreted, and the creatinine clearance value for measurement of GFR may be slightly higher than the inulin clearance value.

3. **Creatinine clearance (Cl_{CR})** is the most common method for obtaining the GFR. Creatinine clearance may be estimated with both urine and serum values or with only the serum creatinine concentration.

a. Measurement with both urine and serum concentrations is more accurate. The value is usually estimated by the following equation:

$$Cl_{CR} = \frac{C_U\,\dot{V}\,100}{C_{CR}\,1440}$$

where CCR is the creatinine serum concentration in milligrams per deciliter of the 12-hour serum value, $\dot{V}$ is the 24-hour urine volume, C_U is the concentration of creatinine in the urine, and Cl_{CR} is the creatinine clearance in milliliters per minute.

b. Creatinine clearance is estimated from the serum creatinine concentration because there is usually an inverse relation between serum creatinine concentration and the GFR.

(1) The **Siersback-Nielsen nomogram** is used to obtain the creatinine clearance using the serum creatinine concentration (milligrams per deciliter) and the patient's body weight and sex (Figure 6-8).

(2) The **Cockcroft and Gault method,** which is also based on body weight, age, and sex, calculates creatinine clearance from serum creatinine, using the following relation.

(a) For male subjects:

$$Cl_{CR} = \frac{(140 - \text{age in years})\ \text{body weight (kg)}}{72\ (C_{CR}\ \text{in mg/dl})} = \text{ml/min}$$

(b) For female subjects, 0.85 of the creatinine clearance obtained for male subjects is used.

(3) These methods assume that renal function is stable; however, renal function may change, depending on the progress of the renal disease, causing changes in the creatinine clearance.

C. Dosage adjustment

1. Dosage adjustment for renal disease is usually based on the following assumptions, which may not be valid for every patient:

a. The desired plasma or serum drug concentration in a patient with renal disease is the same as that for a patient without renal disease. One exception is digoxin. Renal disease may alter normal serum potassium concentrations and change the target digoxin serum concentration. Also, active metabolites may not be excreted.

b. Other pharmacokinetic parameters (e.g., V_D, plasma drug protein binding, nonrenal drug elimination or biotransformation) are not noticeably altered in renal disease.

c. The normal GFR is 100 ml/min or greater. Unless the GFR decreases to significantly below normal, dosage may not be adjusted for a patient with minor renal impairment.

d. Drugs such as gentamicin, which is primarily eliminated by renal excretion, are more significantly affected by diminished renal function than drugs such as theophylline, which is primarily eliminated by biotransformation. Biotransformation is more significantly affected by nonrenal or hepatic clearance.

e. All drug elimination pathways follow first-order pharmacokinetics.

f. When the dosage of a drug is adjusted for a patient with renal disease, therapeutic drug monitoring is important to prevent adverse effects and maintain appropriate drug therapy.

2. In **renally impaired patients,** the dosage is adjusted to estimate the fraction of total body drug clearance remaining.

a. Total body clearance is the sum of renal clearance and nonrenal clearance, as determined by the following equation:

$$Cl_T = Cl_R + Cl_{NR}$$

b. Because V_D is assumed to be constant, then:

$$k = k_R + k_{NR}$$

c. As k_R decreases in renal disease, k (i.e., the overall rate constant for drug elimination) also decreases.

3. The **Guisti and Hayton method** estimates the fraction of k remaining in the patient, using the following equation:

$$\frac{k_U}{k_N} = 1 - f_e\left(1 - \frac{Cl_{CR}{}^{U}}{Cl_{CR}{}^{N}}\right),$$

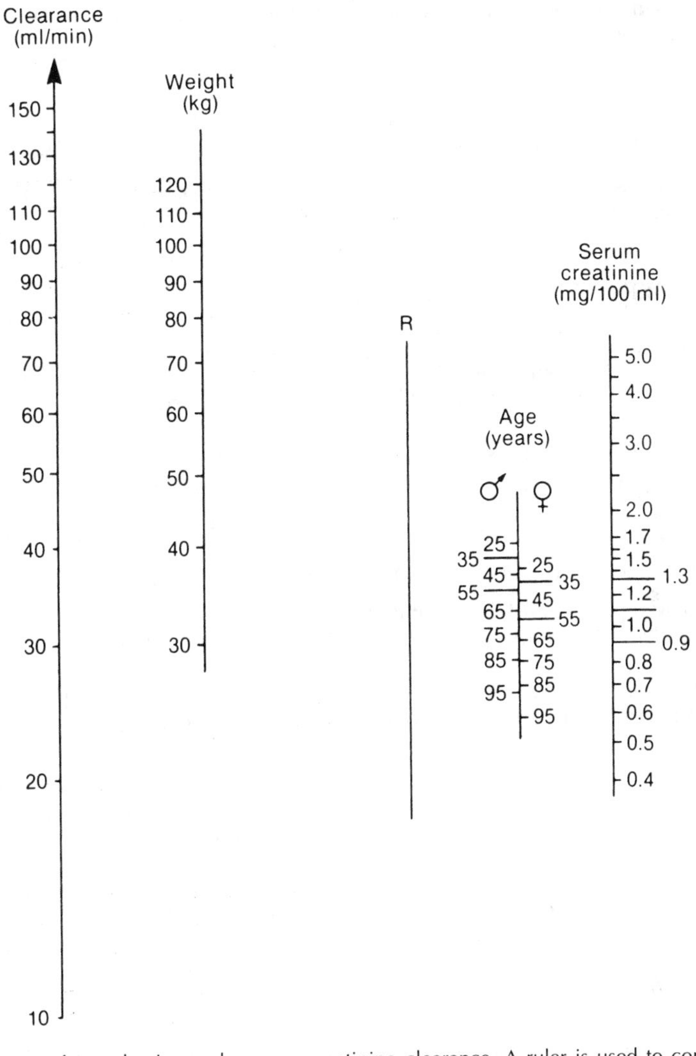

Figure 6-8. Nomogram for evaluating endogenous creatinine clearance. A ruler is used to connect the patient's weight on the second line from the left with the patient's age on the fourth line. The point of intersection on R is noted. The ruler is kept in place, and the right part of the ruler is turned to the serum creatinine value. The left side of the ruler indicates the clearance in milliliters per minute. (Reprinted with permission from Kampmann J, Siersback-Nielsen JM: Rapid evaluation of creatinine clearance. *Acta Med Scand* 196:517–520, 1974.)

where k_U is the first-order elimination rate constant in the renally impaired (uremic) patient; k_N is the patient's normal elimination rate constant; f_e is the fraction of drug excreted unchanged in the urine; Cl_{CR}^{N} is the normal creatinine clearance (GFR), assumed to be 100 ml/min; and Cl_{CR}^{U} is the creatinine clearance in the renally impaired patient, usually estimated from the serum creatinine concentration.

a. The values for k, k_{NR}, and f_e are the standard population pharmacokinetic parameters obtained from the literature.

b. After the value for k_U/k_N is obtained, the dosage regimen is calculated by decreasing the normal dose, prolonging the dosage interval, or both.

(1) To decrease the dose and maintain a constant dosage interval, the following equation is used:

$$D_U^{O} = \frac{k_U}{k_N} \times D_N^{O},$$

where D_U^{0} is the dose in renal disease, D_N^{0} is the normal dose, and k_U/k_N is calculated.

(2) To prolong the interval and maintain a constant dose, the following equation is used:

$$T_U = \frac{k_N}{k_U} \times T_N,$$

where T_U is the dosage interval in renal disease and T_N is the normal dosage interval.

4. Loading dose. Because V_D is assumed to be approximately the same in normal and renally impaired patients, the loading dose (D_L) is usually the same.

IV. PHARMACOKINETICS IN HEPATIC DISEASE

A. Overview. Pharmacokinetic alterations in hepatic disease (e.g., cirrhosis, hepatitis) are more difficult to predict quantitatively than those in renal disease. No reliable measurement of hepatic function is available to estimate hepatic drug clearance.

B. Pharmacokinetic alterations caused by hepatic disease:

1. Decreased hepatic drug clearance

a. Drugs that show significant first-pass effects (e.g., propranolol) have greater bioavailability.

b. The $t_{1/2}$ for drugs that are eliminated by hepatic clearance increases.

2. Decreased plasma protein binding of drugs

a. The liver is the primary organ involved in the synthesis of albumin and other plasma proteins.

b. In hepatic disease, the plasma protein concentration may be quantitatively decreased and proteins that are formed may be qualitatively altered. The result is decreased plasma protein binding.

STUDY QUESTIONS

Directions: Each of the numbered items or incomplete statements in this section is followed by answers or by completions of the statement. Select the **one** lettered answer or completion that is **best** in each case.

1. Creatinine clearance is used as a measurement of

(A) renal excretion rate
(B) glomerular filtration rate (GFR)
(C) active renal secretion
(D) passive renal absorption
(E) drug metabolism rate

Questions 2–5

A new cephalosporin antibiotic was given at a dose of 5 mg/kg by a single intravenous bolus injection to a 58-year-old man who weighed 75 kg. The antibiotic follows the pharmacokinetics of a one-compartment model and has an elimination half-life of 2 hours. The apparent volume of distribution is 0.28 L/kg, and the drug is 35% bound to plasma proteins.

2. What is the initial plasma drug concentration (C_p^0) in this patient?

(A) 0.24 mg/L
(B) 1.80 mg/L
(C) 17.9 mg/L
(D) 56.0 mg/L

3. The predicted plasma drug concentration (C_p) at 8 hours after the dose is

(A) 0.73 mg/L
(B) 1.11 mg/L
(C) 2.64 mg/L
(D) 4.02 mg/L
(E) 15.10 mg/L

4. How much drug remains in the patient's body (D_B) 8 hours after the dose?

(A) 15.3 mg
(B) 23.3 mg
(C) 84.4 mg
(D) 100.0 mg
(E) 112.0 mg

5. How long after the dose is exactly 75% of the drug eliminated from the patient's body?

(A) 2 hours
(B) 4 hours
(C) 6 hours
(D) 8 hours
(E) 10 hours

Questions 6–11

A 35-year-old man who weighs 70 kg and has normal renal function needs an intravenous infusion of the antibiotic carbenicillin. The desired steady-state plasma drug concentration is 15 mg/dl. The physician wants the antibiotic to be infused into the patient for 10 hours. Carbenicillin has an elimination half-life ($t_{1/2}$) of 1 hour and an apparent volume distribution (V_D) of 9 L in this patient.

6. Assuming that no loading dose was given, what rate of intravenous infusion is recommended for this patient?

(A) 93.6 mg/hr
(B) 135.0 mg/hr
(C) 468.0 mg/hr
(D) 936.0 mg/hr
(E) 1350.0 mg/hr

7. Assuming that no loading intravenous dose was given, how long after the initiation of the intravenous infusion would the plasma drug concentration reach 95% of the theoretic steady-state drug concentration?

(A) 1.0 hour
(B) 3.3 hours
(C) 4.3 hours
(D) 6.6 hours
(E) 10.0 hours

8. What is the recommended loading dose?

(A) 93.6 mg
(B) 135.0 mg
(C) 468.0 mg
(D) 936.0 mg
(E) 1350.0 mg

9. To infuse the antibiotic as a solution containing 10 g drug in 500 ml 5% dextrose, how many milliliters per hour of the solution would be infused into the patient?

(A) 10.0 ml/hr
(B) 46.8 ml/hr
(C) 100.0 ml/hr
(D) 936.0 ml/hr
(E) 1141.0 ml/hr

10. What is the total body clearance rate for carbenicillin in this patient?

(A) 100 ml/hr
(B) 936 ml/hr
(C) 4862 ml/hr
(D) 6237 ml/hr
(E) 9000 ml/hr

11. If the patient's renal clearance for carbenicillin is 86 ml/min, what is the hepatic clearance for carbenicillin?

(A) 108 ml/hr
(B) 1077 ml/hr
(C) 3840 ml/hr
(D) 5160 ml/hr
(E) 6844 ml/hr

12. The earliest evidence that a drug is stored in tissue is

(A) an increase in plasma protein binding
(B) a large apparent volume of distribution (V_D)
(C) a decrease in the rate of formation of metabolites by the liver
(D) an increase in the number of side effects produced by the drug
(E) a decrease in the amount of free drug excreted in the urine

13. The intensity of the pharmacologic action of a drug is most dependent on the

(A) concentration of the drug at the receptor site
(B) elimination half-life ($t_{1/2}$) of the drug
(C) onset time of the drug after oral administration
(D) minimum toxic concentration (MTC) of the drug in plasma
(E) minimum effective concentration (MEC) of the drug in the body

14. Drugs that show nonlinear pharmacokinetics have which property?

(A) A constant ratio of drug metabolites is formed as the administered dose increases
(B) The elimination half-life ($t_{1/2}$) increases as the administered dose increases
(C) The area under the plasma drug concentration versus time curve (AUC) increases in direct proportion to an increase in the administered dose
(D) Both low and high doses follow first-order elimination kinetics
(E) The steady-state drug concentration increases in direct proportion to the dosing rate

15. The loading dose (D_L) of a drug is usually based on the

(A) total body clearance (Cl_T) of the drug
(B) percentage of drug bound to plasma proteins
(C) fraction of drug excreted unchanged in the urine
(D) apparent volume of distribution (V_D) and desired drug concentration in plasma
(E) area under the plasma drug concentration versus time curve (AUC)

16. The renal clearance of inulin is used as a measurement of

(A) effective renal blood flow
(B) rate of renal drug excretion
(C) intrinsic enzyme activity
(D) active renal secretion
(E) glomerular filtration rate (GFR)

17. All of the following statements about plasma protein binding of a drug are true EXCEPT

(A) displacement of a drug from plasma protein binding sites results in a transient increased volume of distribution (V_D)
(B) displacement of a drug from plasma protein binding sites makes more free drug available for glomerular filtration
(C) displacement of a potent drug that is normally more than 95% bound may cause toxicity
(D) albumin is the major protein involved in protein binding of drugs
(E) drugs that are highly bound to plasma proteins generally have a greater V_D compared with drugs that are highly bound to tissue proteins

18. The onset time for a drug given orally is the time for the

(A) drug to reach the peak plasma drug concentration
(B) drug to reach the minimum effective concentration (MEC)
(C) drug to reach the minimum toxic concentration (MTC)
(D) drug to begin to be eliminated from the body
(E) drug to begin to be absorbed from the small intestine

19. The initial distribution of a drug into tissue is determined chiefly by the

(A) rate of blood flow to tissue
(B) glomerular filtration rate (GFR)
(C) stomach emptying time
(D) affinity of the drug for tissue
(E) plasma protein binding of the drug

20. Which tissue has the greatest capacity to biotransform drugs?

(A) Brain
(B) Kidney
(C) Liver
(D) Lung
(E) Skin

21. The principle of superposition in designing multiple-dose regimens assumes that

(A) each dose affects the next subsequent dose, causing nonlinear elimination
(B) each dose of drug is eliminated by zero-order elimination
(C) steady-state plasma drug concentrations are reached at approximately 10 half-lives
(D) early doses of drug do not affect subsequent doses
(E) the fraction of drug absorbed is equal to the fraction of drug eliminated

Questions 22–24

A new cardiac glycoside is developed for oral and intravenous administration. The drug has an elimination half-life ($t_{1/2}$) of 24 hours and an apparent volume of distribution (V_D) of 3 L/kg. The effective drug concentration is 1.5 ng/ml. Toxic effects of the drug are observed at drug concentrations greater than 4 ng/ml. The drug is bound to plasma proteins at approximately 25%. The drug is 75% bioavailable after an oral dose.

22. What is the oral maintenance dose, if given once a day, for a 68-year-old man who weighs 65 kg and has congestive heart failure (CHF) and normal renal function?

(A) 0.125 mg
(B) 0.180 mg
(C) 0.203 mg
(D) 0.270 mg
(E) 0.333 mg

23. What is the loading dose (D_L) for this patient?

(A) 0.270 mg
(B) 0.293 mg
(C) 0.450 mg
(D) 0.498 mg
(E) 0.540 mg

24. If the drug is available in tablets of 0.125 mg and 0.250 mg, what is the patient's plasma drug concentration if he has a dosage regimen of 0.125 mg every 12 hours?

(A) 1.39 ng/ml
(B) 1.85 ng/ml
(C) 2.78 ng/ml
(D) 3.18 ng/ml
(E) 6.94 ng/ml

Directions: The question below contains three suggested answers of which **one or more** is correct. Choose the answer

A if **I only** is correct
B if **III only** is correct
C if **I and II** are correct
D if **II and III** are correct
E if **I, II, and III** are correct

25. Which equation is true for a zero-order reaction rate of a drug?

I. $\frac{dA}{dt} = -k$

II. $t_{1/2} = \frac{0.693}{k}$

III. $A = A_o e^{-kt}$

ANSWERS AND EXPLANATIONS

1. The answer is B *[I E 2 a].*
A substance that is used to measure the glomerular filtration rate (GFR) must be filtered, but not reabsorbed or actively secreted. Although inulin clearance gives an accurate measurement of GFR, creatinine clearance is generally used because no exogenous drug must be given. However, creatinine formation depends on muscle mass and muscle metabolism, which may change with age and various disease conditions.

2–5. The answers are: 2-C *[I B 1 b (2)],* **3-B** *[I C 2 c],* **4-B** *[I B 1 b (1)],* **5-B** *[I B 5 f (4)].*
Substituting the data for this patient in the equation for the initial plasma drug concentration (C_p^0) gives:

$$C_p^O = \frac{D_o}{V_D} = \frac{5 \text{ mg/kg}}{0.28 \text{ kg}} = 17.9 \text{ mg/L}$$

To obtain the patient's plasma drug concentration (C_p) 8 hours after the dose, the following calculation is performed:

$$C_p = C_p^O e^{-kt},$$

$$k = \frac{0.693}{t_{1/2}} = \frac{0.693}{2} = 0.347 \text{ hr}^{-1},$$

$$C_p = 17.9 e^{-(0.347)(8)},$$

$$C_p = (17.9)(0.0623) = 1.11 \text{ mg/L}$$

The amount of drug in the patient's body at 8 hours is calculated as follows:

$$D_B = C_pV_D = (1.11)(0.28)(75) = 23.3 \text{ mg}.$$

For any first-order elimination process, 50% of the initial amount of drug is eliminated at the end of the first half-life, and 50% of the remaining drug (i.e., 75% of the original amount) is eliminated at the end of the second half-life. Because the drug in the current case has an elimination half-life ($t_{1/2}$) of 2 hours, 75% of the dose is eliminated in two half-lives, or 4 hours.

6–11. The answers are: 6-D *[I B 3 d (3)],* **7-C** *[I B 3 b],* **8-E** *[I B 5 f (5) (a)],* **9-B** *[I B 3 d (3)],* **10-D** *[I B 3 d (3)],* **11-B** *[I E 4 a].*
The equation for the plasma concentration at steady state (C_{ss}) provides the formula for calculating the rate of an intravenous infusion (R). The equation is:

$$C_{ss} = \frac{R}{kV_D},$$

where k is the first-order elimination rate constant and V_D is the apparent volume of distribution. Rearranging the equation and substituting the data for this patient give the following calculations:

$$R = C_{ss}kV_D = \frac{15 \text{ mg}}{100 \text{ ml}} \times \frac{0.693}{1 \text{ hr}} \times 9000 \text{ ml},$$

$$R = 936 \text{ mg/hr}.$$

The time it takes for an infused drug to reach the C_{ss} depends on the elimination half-life of the drug. The time required to reach 95% of the C_{ss} is equal to 4.3 times the half-life, whereas the time required to reach 99% of the C_{ss} is equal to 6.6 times the half-life. Because the half-life in the current case is 1 hour, the time to reach 95% of the C_{ss} is 4.3 × 1 hour, or 4.3 hours.
The loading dose (D_L) is calculated as follows:

$$D_L = C_{ss} V_D = \frac{15 \text{ mg}}{100 \text{ ml}} \times 9000 \text{ ml} = 1350 \text{ mg}.$$

The answer to question 6 shows that the infusion rate should be 936 mg/hr. Therefore, if a drug solution containing 10 g in 500 ml is used, the required infusion rate is:

$$\frac{936 \text{ mg}}{1 \text{ hr}} \times \frac{500 \text{ ml}}{10{,}000 \text{ mg}} = 46.8 \text{ ml/hr}.$$

The patient's total body clearance (Cl_T) is calculated as follows:

$$Cl_T = kV_D,$$

$$Cl_T = \frac{0.693}{1} \times 9000 \text{ ml} = 6237 \text{ ml/hr.}$$

The hepatic clearance (Cl_H) is the difference between total clearance (Cl_T) and renal clearance (Cl_R):

$$Cl_H = Cl_T - Cl_R$$

$$Cl_H = 6237 - (86 \text{ ml/min} \times 60 \text{ min/hr}) = 1077 \text{ ml/hr.}$$

12. The answer is B *[I B 1 b (1)].*
A large apparent volume of distribution (V_D) is an early sign that a drug is not concentrated in the plasma, but is distributed widely in tissue. An increase in plasma protein binding suggests that the drug is located in the plasma rather than in tissue. A decrease in hepatic metabolism, an increase in side effects, or a decrease in urinary excretion of free drug is caused by a decrease in drug elimination.

13. The answer is A *[I A 3 d (3)].*
As more drug is concentrated at the receptor site, more receptors interact with the drug to produce a pharmacologic effect. The intensity of the response increases until it reaches a maximum. When all of the available receptors are occupied by drug molecules, additional drug does not produce a more intense response.

14. The answer is B *[I D].*
Nonlinear pharmacokinetics is a term used to indicate that first-order elimination of a drug does not occur at all drug concentrations. With some drugs, such as phenytoin, as the plasma drug concentration increases, the elimination pathway for metabolism of the drug becomes saturated and the half-life increases. The area under the plasma drug concentration versus time curve (AUC) of the drug is not proportional to the dose; neither is the rate of metabolite formation. The metabolic rate is related to the effects of the drug.

15. The answer is D *[I B 5 f (5)].*
A loading dose (D_L) of a drug is given to obtain a therapeutic plasma drug level as rapidly as possible. The D_L is calculated on the basis of the apparent volume of distribution (V_D) and the desired plasma level of the drug.

16. The answer is E *[I E 3 c].*
Inulin is neither reabsorbed nor actively secreted. Therefore, it is excreted by glomerular filtration only. The inulin clearance rate is used as a standard measure of the glomerular filtration rate (GFR), a test that is useful both clinically and in the development of new drugs.

17. The answer is E *[I A 3 d].*
Drugs that are highly bound to plasma proteins diffuse poorly into tissue and have a low apparent volume of distribution (V_D).

18. The answer is B *[I B 3 f].*
The onset time is the time from the administration of the drug to the time when absorbed drug reaches the minimum effective concentration (MEC). The MEC is the drug concentration in the plasma that is proportional, but not necessarily equal, to the minimum drug concentration at the receptor site that elicits a pharmacologic response.

19. The answer is A *[I A 3 a].*
The initial distribution of a drug is chiefly determined by blood flow, whereas the affinity of the drug for tissue determines whether the drug concentrates at that site. The glomerular filtration rate (GFR) affects the renal clearance of a drug, not its initial distribution. The gastric emptying time and degree of plasma protein binding affect drug distribution, but are less important than the rate of blood flow to tissue.

20. The answer is C *[I E 4 b (2)].*
The kidney, lung, skin, and intestine all have some capacity to biotransform, or metabolize, drugs, but the brain has little capacity for drug metabolism. The liver has the highest capacity for drug metabolism.

21. The answer is D *[I B 5 c].*
The superposition principle, which underlies the design of multiple-dose regimens, assumes that earlier drug doses do not affect subsequent doses. If the elimination rate constant or total body clearance of the drug changes during multiple dosing, then the superposition principle is no longer valid. Changes in the total body clearance (Cl_T) may be caused by enzyme induction, enzyme inhibition, or saturation of an elimination pathway. Any of these changes would cause nonlinear pharmacokinetics.

22–24. The answers are: 22-D *[I B 5 f (5) (a)],* **23-E** *[I B 5 f (5) (a)],* **24-A** *[I B 1 b (1)].*
The oral maintenance dose (D_o) should maintain the patient's average drug concentration (C_{av}^{∞}) at the effective drug concentration. The bioavailability of the drug (F), the apparent volume of distribution (V_D), the frequency of dosing (τ), and the excretion rate constant (k) must be considered in calculating the dose. The equation used is:

$$C_{av}^{\infty} = \frac{FD_o}{kV_D\tau}$$

For this drug, F = 0.75, k = 0.693/24 hr, V_D = 3 L/kg x 65 kg, τ = 25 hours, and C_{av}^{∞} = 1.5 ng/ml, or 1.5 μg/L. Therefore, by substitution, D_o = 270 μg, or 0.270 mg. When the maintenance dose is given at a dosage frequency equal to the half-life, then the loading dose is equal to twice the maintenance dose, in this case, 540 μg, or 0.540 mg. To determine the plasma drug concentration for a dosage regimen of 0.125 mg every 12 hours, the C_{av}^{∞} formula is used. This time, F = 0.75, D_o = 0.125, k = 0.693/24 hr, V_D = 3 L/kg x 65 kg, and τ = 12 hours. Therefore, C_{av}^{∞} = 1.39 ng/ml. For cardiac glycosides, the peak (C_{max}) and trough (C_{min}) concentrations are calculated, and plasma drug concentrations are monitored after dosing. The loading dose (D_L) may be given in small increments over a specified period, according to the dosage regimen suggested by the manufacturer.

25. The answer is A (I) *[I A 1 a].*
The first equation in the question describes a zero-order reaction (dA/dt) in which the reaction rate increases or decreases at a constant rate (k). A zero-order reaction produces a graph of a straight line with the equation of $A = -kt + Ao$ when A is plotted against time (t). The other equations in the question represent first-order reactions.

7
Bioavailability and Bioequivalence

Leon Shargel

I. INTRODUCTION

A. **Bioavailability** is a measurement of the rate and extent (amount) of therapeutically active drug that is systemically absorbed.

B. **Bioequivalence:** A generic drug product is considered bioequivalent to the brand (Reference) drug product if its rate and extent of systemic absorption (bioavailability) do not show a statistically significant difference when administered at the same dose of the active ingredient, in the same chemical form, in a similar dosage form, by the same route of administration, and under the same experimental conditions.

C. **Generic Drug Product**

1. The generic drug product requires an Abbreviated New Drug Application (ANDA) for Food and Drug Administration (FDA) approval and may be marketed after patent expiration of the Reference drug product.
2. The generic drug product must be a therapeutic equivalent to the Reference drug product but may differ in certain characteristics including shape, scoring configuration, packaging, and excipients (includes colors, flavors, preservatives, expiration date, and minor aspects of labeling).

D. **Pharmaceutical equivalents** are drug products that contain the same therapeutically active drug ingredient (same salt, ester, or chemical form); are of the same dosage form; and are identical in strength and concentration and route of administration.

E. The **Reference drug product** is a currently marketed, brand-named product with a full New Drug Application (NDA) approved by the FDA.

F. **Therapeutic equivalent drug products** are pharmaceutical equivalents that can be expected to have the same therapeutic effect when administered to patients under the same conditions specified in the labeling. Therapeutic equivalent drug products have the following criteria:

1. The products are pharmaceutical equivalents containing the same active drug ingredient in the same dosage form and meet compendia or other applicable standards of strength, quality, purity, and identity.
2. The drug products are bioequivalent.
3. The drug products are adequately labeled.
4. The drug products are manufactured in compliance with current good manufacturing practice regulations.

II. BIOAVAILABILITY

A. **Bioavailability and therapeutic effect. Pharmacologic responses** occur when drugs combine with **receptors** in the body. This drug-receptor interaction is usually reversible. As more drug molecules combine with the receptor, the intensity of the pharmacologic effect increases up to a maximum effect (Figure 7-1). The **time course of the pharmacologic response** depends on the

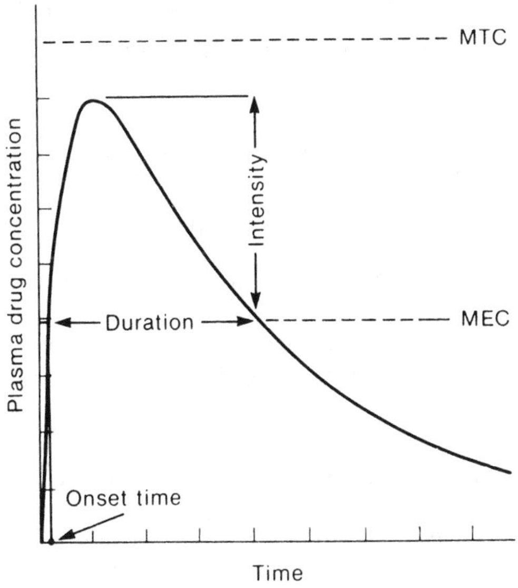

Figure 7-1. Generalized plasma drug concentration versus time curve after oral drug administration. *MEC* = minimum effective concentration; *MTC* = minimum toxic concentration. (Adapted with permission from Shargel L, Yu ABC: *Applied Biopharmaceutics and Pharmacokinetics,* 3rd ed. East Norwalk, CT, Appleton & Lange, 1993, p 34.)

rates of association and dissociation of the drug with the receptor and the drug concentration at the receptor site.

1. **Onset time.** As the drug is systemically absorbed, the drug concentration at the receptor rises to a **minimum effective concentration (MEC)** and a pharmacologic response is initiated. The time from drug administration to the MEC is known as the onset time.
2. **Duration of action.** As long as the drug concentration remains above the MEC, pharmacologic activity is observed. The duration of action is the time for which the drug concentration remains above the MEC.
3. **Therapeutic window.** As the drug concentration increases, other receptors may combine with the drug to exert a toxic or adverse response. This drug concentration is the **minimum toxic concentration (MTC).** The drug concentration range between the MEC and the MTC is the therapeutic window.

B. Measuring bioavailability

1. **Plasma drug concentration versus time curve** measures the bioavailability of a drug from a drug product (Figure 7-2).

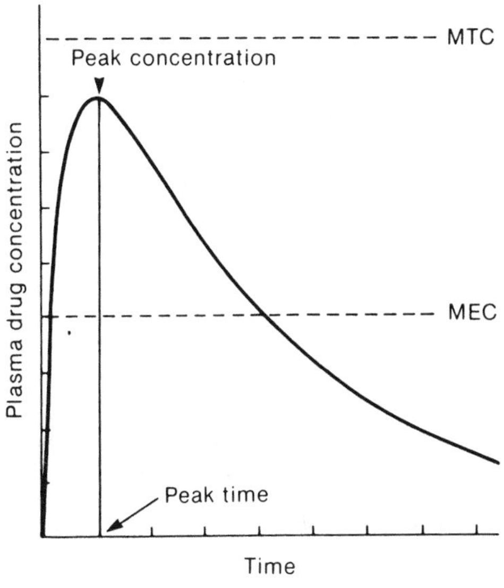

Figure 7-2. Generalized plasma drug concentration versus time curve, showing peak time and peak concentration. *MEC* = minimum effective concentration; *MTC* = minimum toxic concentration. (Adapted with permission from Shargel L, Yu ABC: *Applied Biopharmaceutics and Pharmacokinetics,* 3rd ed. East Norwalk, CT, Appleton & Lange, 1993, p 35.)

a. **Time for peak plasma drug concentration** (T_{max}) relates to the rate constants for systemic drug absorption and elimination. If two oral drug products contain the same amount of active drug but different excipients, the dosage form that yields the faster rate of drug absorption has the shorter T_{max} because the elimination rate constant for the drug from both dosage forms is the same..

b. **Peak plasma drug concentration** (C_{max})—the plasma drug concentration at T_{max}—relates to the intensity of the pharmacologic response. Ideally, C_{max} should be within the therapeutic window.

c. **Area under the plasma drug concentration versus time curve (AUC)** relates to the amount or extent of drug absorption. The amount of systemic drug absorption is directly related to the AUC. The AUC is usually calculated by the **trapezoidal rule** and is expressed in units of concentration multiplied by time (e.g., μg × hr/ml).

2. **Measurement of urinary drug excretion** can determine bioavailability from a drug product. This method is most accurate if the active therapeutic moiety is excreted unchanged in significant quantity in the urine (Figure 7-3).

a. The **cumulative amount** of active drug excreted in the urine (D_U^∞) is directly related to the extent of systemic drug absorption.

b. The **rate of drug excretion** in the urine (dD_U/dt) is directly related to the rate of systemic drug absorption.

c. The **time for the drug to be completely excreted** (t^∞) corresponds to the total time for the drug to be systemically absorbed and completely excreted after administration.

3. **Acute pharmacologic effects,** such as changes in heart rate, blood pressure, electrocardiogram (ECG), or clotting time, can be used to measure bioavailability when no assay for drug concentration is available. Parameters for measuring an acute pharmacologic effect include onset time, duration of action, and intensity of the effect.

4. **Clinical (pharmacodynamic) responses to a drug** can be used to measure bioavailability quantitatively; however, they are less precise than other methods and are highly variable because of individual differences in drug pharmacodynamics and subjective measurements.

5. **The rate of drug dissolution** in vitro for certain drugs correlates with drug bioavailability in vivo. When the dissolution test in vitro is considered statistically adequate to predict

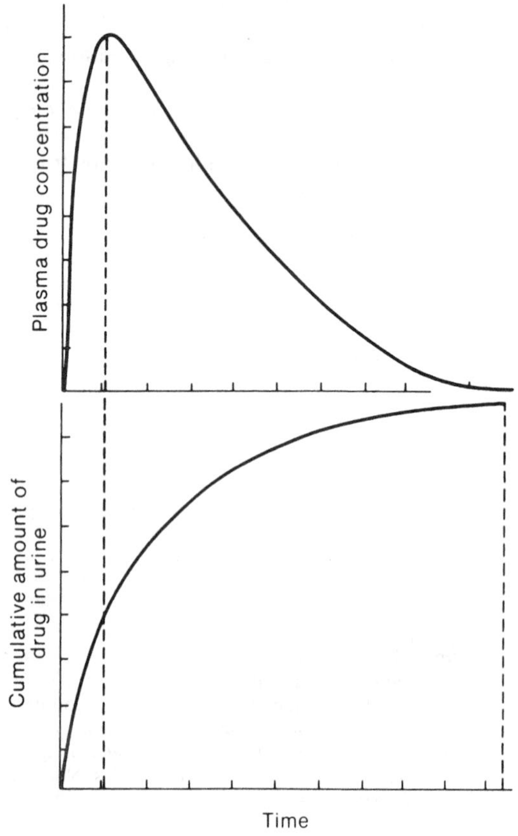

Figure 7-3. These corresponding plots show the relationship of the plasma drug concentration versus time curve to the cumulative amount of drug in the urine versus time curve. (Adapted with permission from Shargel L, Yu ABC: *Applied Biopharmaceutics and Pharmacokinetics,* 3rd ed. East Norwalk, CT, Appleton & Lange, 1993, p 201.)

drug bioavailability, then dissolution may be used in place of an in vivo bioavailability study.

C. Relative and absolute bioavailability

1. **Relative bioavailability**—the systemic availability of the drug from a dosage form as compared to a Reference standard—is calculated as the ratio of the AUC for the dosage form to the AUC for the Reference dosage form. A relative bioavailability of 1 (or 100%) implies that drug bioavailability from both dosage forms is the same but does not indicate the completeness of systemic drug absorption. Determining relative bioavailability is very important in generic drug studies (e.g., bioequivalence studies).
2. **Absolute bioavailability (F)**—the fraction of drug systemically absorbed and the availability of the drug from the dosage form as compared to the availability of the drug after intravenous (IV) administration—is usually calculated as the ratio of the AUC for the dosage form given orally to the AUC obtained after IV drug administration. An F value of 0.80 (or 80%) indicates that only 80% of the drug was systemically available from the dosage form.

III. BIOEQUIVALENCE STUDIES FOR SOLID ORAL DRUG PRODUCTS

A. Design of bioequivalence studies

1. For many drug products, the Division of Bioequivalence, Office of Generic Drugs (FDA), provides guidance for the performance of in vitro dissolution and in vivo bioequivalence studies.
2. **Fasting study:** Bioequivalence studies are usually evaluated by a single-dose, two-period, two-treatment, two-sequence, open-label, randomized **crossover design,** comparing equal doses of the Test and Reference products in fasted, adult, healthy subjects.
   - **a.** Both men and women may be used in the study.
   - **b.** Blood sampling is performed just before (zero time) the dose and at appropriate intervals after the dose to obtain an adequate description of the plasma drug concentration versus time profile.
3. **Food intervention study:** If the bioavailability of the active drug ingredient is known to be affected by food, the generic drug manufacturer must use a single-dose, randomized, three-treatment, three-period, six-sequence, crossover, limited food effects study comparing equal doses of the Test product given under fasting conditions with those of the Test and Reference products given immediately after a standard high-fat content breakfast.
4. **Multiple-dose (steady-state) study:** A multiple dose, steady-state, randomized, two-treatment, two-way, crossover study comparing equal doses of the Test and Reference products in adult, healthy subjects is required for oral-extended (controlled) release drug products in addition to a single-dose fasting study and a food intervention study.
   - **a.** Three consecutive trough concentrations (C_{min}) on three consecutive days should be determined to ascertain that the subjects are at steady-state.
   - **b.** The last morning dose is given to the subject after an overnight fast with continual fasting for at least 2 hours following dose administration. Blood sampling is performed similarly to the single-dose study.
5. **Waiver of an in vivo bioequivalence study**
   - **a.** A comparative in vitro dissolution (drug release) study between the Test and Reference products may be used in lieu of an in vivo bioequivalence study for some immediate-release (conventional) oral drug product.
   - **b.** No bioequivalence study is required for certain drug products such as oral, parenteral, ophthalmic, or other solutions because bioequivalence is self-evident.

B. Pharmacokinetic evaluation of the data

1. **Single-dose studies:** Pharmacokinetic analysis includes calculation for each subject of the AUC to the last quantifiable concentration ($AUC_{0\text{-}t}$) and to infinity ($AUC_{0\text{-}\infty}$), T_{max}, and C_{max}. Additionally, the elimination rate constant, k; the elimination half-life, $t_{1/2}$; and other parameters may be estimated.

2. **Multiple-dose studies:** Pharmacokinetic analysis includes calculation for each subject of the steady-state area-under-the-curve, ($AUC_{0\text{-}T}$), T_{max}, C_{min}, C_{max}, and the percent fluctuation [$100 \times (C_{max} - C_{min})/C_{min}$].

C. **Statistical evaluation of the data**

1. **Single-dose, fasting study:** An analysis of variance (ANOVA) should be performed on the log transformed AUC and C_{max}. There should be no statistical differences between the mean AUC and C_{max} parameters for the Test (generic) and Reference drug products. In addition, the 90% confidence intervals about the ratio of the means for AUC and C_{max} values of the Test drug product should not be less than 0.80 (80%) nor greater than 1.25 (125%) of the Reference product based on log transformed data (Table 7-1).
2. **Single-dose, three-way crossover food/fasting study:** The mean values for the AUC and C_{max} for the Test product when administered with food should be within 20% from the respective mean values of the Reference product when given with food.
3. **Multiple-dose studies:** An ANOVA should be performed on the log transformed AUC and C_{max}. The AUC and C_{max} parameters for the Test (generic) product should be within 80%–25% of the Reference product using the 90% confidence interval.

IV. BIOEQUIVALENCE ISSUES

A. Problems in determining bioequivalence include lack of an adequate study design, inability to accurately measure the drug analytes including metabolites and enantiomers (chiral drugs), and lack of systemic drug absorption (Table 7-2.)

B. Bioequivalence studies for which objective blood drug concentrations cannot be obtained require a clinical study using pharmacodynamic measurements.

1. Pharmacodynamic measurements are more difficult to obtain and tend to be variable, requiring a larger number of subjects compared to the bioequivalence studies for systemically absorbed drugs.

Table 7-1. Bioavailability Comparison of a Generic (Test) and Brand (Reference) Drug Product

Parameter	Units	Test	Reference	Ratio (%) T/R	90% Confidence Limits
$AUC_{0\text{-}t}$	μg hr/mL	1466	1494	98.1	93.0–102.5
$AUC_{0\text{-}\infty}$	μg hr/mL	1592	1606	99.1	94.5–104.1
C_{max}	μg	11.6	12.5	92.8	88.5–98.6
T_{max}	hr	1.87	2.10	89.1	

The results were obtained from a two-way crossover, single dose, fasting study in 24 healthy adult volunteers. Mean values are reported. No statistical differences were observed between AUC and C_{max} values for the Test and Reference products.

Table 7-2. Problem Issues in the Determination of Bioequivalence

Problem Issues	Example
Drugs with highly variable bioavailability	Propranolol
Drugs with active metabolites	Selegilene
Chiral drugs	Ibuprofen
Drugs with nonlinear pharmacokinetics	Phenytoin
Orally administered drugs that are not systemically absorbed	Cholestyramine resin Sulcralfate
Drugs with long elimination half-lives	Probucol
Variable dosage forms	Dyazide, Premarin
Nonoral drug delivery	
Topical drugs	Steroids, antifungals
Transdermal delivery systems	Estrogen patch
Drugs given by inhalation aerosols	Bronchodilators, steroids
Intranasal drugs	Intranasal steroids
Target population used in the bioequivalence studies	Geriatric, pediatric patients

2. A bioequivalence study using pharmacodynamic measurements tries to obtain a pharmacodynamic effect versus time profile for the drug in each subject.
   a. From this profile, the area under the effect versus time profile, peak effect, and time for peak effect are obtained.
   b. Statistical analysis of these parameters is then performed for the Test and Reference products.

V. DRUG PRODUCTION SELECTION

A. Generic substitution

1. **Generic substitution** is the process of dispensing a different brand or unbranded (generic) drug product in place of the prescribed drug product. The substituted product must be a therapeutic equivalent to the prescribed product.
2. The underlying pharmacodynamic principle is that if the generic drug meets all the criteria for a therapeutic equivalent, then the generic drug will produce the same clinical effect as the prescribed product.

B. Therapeutic substitution is the process of dispensing a therapeutic alternative in place of the prescribed drug product. For example, amoxicillin is dispensed for ampicillin.

C. Formulary issues

1. All states have legal requirements that address the issue of drug product selection. States may provide information and guidance in drug product selection through positive or negative formularies.
2. The FDA annually publishes *Approved Drug Products with Therapeutic Equivalence Evaluations* ("The Orange Book"). This publication is also reproduced in the *United States Pharmacopeia*/DI Vol III Approved Drug Products and Legal Requirements, published annually by the USP Convention.
   a. The Orange Book provides therapeutic evaluation codes for drug products (Table 7-3).
      (1) "A" rated drug products are drug products that are considered therapeutic equivalents and may be interchanged.
      (2) "B" rated drug products are not considered therapeutically equivalent to other pharmaceutically equivalent products.
   b. For some drug products, bioequivalence has not been established or no generic product is currently available.

Table 7-3. Therapeutic Equivalence Evaluation Codes

A Codes	Drug products that are considered to be therapeutically equivalent to other pharmaceutically equivalent products
AA	Products in conventional dosage forms not presenting bioequivalence problems
AB	Products meeting bioequivalence requirements
AN	Solutions and powders for aerosolization
AO	Injectable oil solutions
AP	Injectable aqueous solutions
AT	Topical products
B Codes	Drug products that the FDA does not at this time consider to be therapeutically equivalent to other pharmaceutically equivalent products
BC	Extended-release tablets, extended-release capsules, and extended-release injectables
BD	Active ingredients and dosage forms with documented bioequivalence problems
BE	Delayed-release oral dosage forms
BN	Products in aerosol-nebulizer drug delivery systems
BP	Active ingredients and dosage forms with potential bioequivalence problems
BR	Suppositories or enemas for systemic use
BS	Products with drug standard deficiencies
BT	Topical products with bioequivalence issues
BX	Insufficient data

3. Various hospitals, institutions, and health maintenance organizations (HMOs) may have a formulary that provides guidance for drug product substitution.

4. **Prescribability** refers to average bioequivalence in which the comparison of population means of the Test and Reference products falls within acceptable statistical criteria. Prescribability is the current basis for FDA approval of therapeutic equivalent generic drug products.

5. **Switchability** refers to individual bioequivalence, which requires knowledge of individual variability and assures that the generic drug product produces the same response in the individual patient.

STUDY QUESTIONS

Directions: Each of the numbered items or incomplete statements in this section is followed by answers or by completions of the statement. Select the **one** lettered answer or completion that is **best** in each case.

1. The parameters used to describe bioavailability are

(A) C_{max}, AUC_{0-t}, and $AUC_{0-\infty}$
(B) C_{max}, AUC_{0-t}, and $AUC_{0-\infty}$, and T_{max}
(C) C_{max}, AUC_{0-t}, and $AUC_{0-\infty}$, and $t_{1/2}$
(D) C_{max}, and AUC_{0-t}
(E) C_{max}, AUC_{0-t}, and $AUC_{0-\infty}$, T_{max} and $t_{1/2}$

2. To determine the absolute bioavailability of a drug given as an oral extended-release tablet, the bioavailability of the drug must be compared to the drug's bioavailability from

(A) An immediate-release oral tablet containing the same amount of active ingredient.
(B) An oral solution of the drug in the same dose.
(C) A parenteral solution of the drug given by IV bolus or IV infusion.
(D) A Reference (brand) extended-release tablet that is a pharmaceutical equivalent.
(E) An immediate-release hard gelatin capsule containing the same amount of active drug and lactose.

3. A single dose four-way crossover, fasting, comparative bioavailability study was performed in 24 healthy, adult male subjects. Plasma drug concentrations were obtained for each subject and the following results were obtained (Table 7Q-1):

Table 7Q-1

Drug Product	Dose (mg)	C_{max} (μg/ml)	T_{max} (hr)	$AUC_{0-\infty}$ (μg hr/ml)
IV bolus injection	100			1714
Oral solution	200	21.3	1.2	3143
Generic tablet	200	17.0	2.1	2822
Reference tablet	200	16.5	1.9	2715

The *relative bioavailability* of the drug from the generic tablet compared to the Reference tablet is

(A) 82.3%
(B) 69.8%
(C) 91.7%
(D) 96.2%
(E) 103.9%

Directions: Each question below contains three suggested answers of which **one or more** is correct. Choose the answer

A if **I only** is correct
B if **III only** is correct
C if **I and II** are correct
D if **II and III** are correct
E if **I, II, and III** are correct

4. For two drug products, generic (Test) and brand (Reference), to be considered bioequivalent,

I. there should be no statistical difference between the bioavailability of the drug from the Test product compared to the Reference product
II. the ratios of the C_{max} and AUC values for the Test product/Reference product must be within 80%–125% of the Reference product based on 90% confidence intervals
III. there should be no statistical differences between the mean C_{max} and AUC values for the Test product compared to the Reference product

5. For which of the following products is measuring plasma drug concentrations not appropriate to estimate bioequivalence?

I. Metered-dose inhaler containing a bronchodilator
II. Antifungal agent for the treatment of a vaginal infection
III. Enteric-coated tablet containing a nonsteroidal anti-inflammatory agent

ANSWERS AND EXPLANATIONS

1. The answer is B *[II A 2 a]*.
AUC relates to the *extent* of drug absorption. C_{max} and T_{max} relate to the *rate* of drug absorption. The elimination $t_{1/2}$ of the drug is usually independent of the route of drug administration and is not used as a measure of bioavailability.

2. The answer is C *[II A 3 b]*.
After an IV bolus injection or IV infusion all the dose is absorbed into the body. The ratio of the AUC of the drug given orally to the AUC of the drug given by IV injection is used to obtain the absolute bioavailability (F) of the drug.

3. The answer is E *[II A 3 a]*.
The relative bioavailability is determined from the ratio of the AUC of the generic (Test) product to the AUC of the Reference standard. Thus, the relative bioavailability can exceed 100%; whereas, the absolute bioavailability can not exceed 100%.

4. The answer is E *[III C]*.
Although T_{max} is an indication of rate of drug absorption, T_{max} is a discrete measurement and usually too variable to use for statistical comparisons in bioequivalence studies. Statistical comparisons use AUC and C_{max} values from Test and Reference drug products as the basis of bioequivalence.

5. The answer is C *[IV A]*.
Although some systemic absorption may be demonstrated after administering a metered dose inhaler containing a bronchodilator or a vaginal antifungal agent, bioequivalence can only be determined using a clinical response measurement.

8
Organic Chemistry and Biochemistry

Edward F. La Sala
John D. Leary

I. ORGANIC CHEMISTRY

A. Medicinal chemistry is rooted in organic chemistry—the study of organic (carbon-based) compounds. These compounds are classified by **functional group**—a group of atoms that occurs in many molecules and confers on them a characteristic chemical reactivity, regardless of the carbon skeleton. Functional groups are part of the overall structure of the drug and determine such characteristics as water or lipid solubility, reactivity, chemical stability, and in vivo stability, which in turn determine drug properties.

1. Functional groups that impart **hydrophilicity** are likely to increase the drug's water solubility, and functional groups that impart **liposolubility** (lipophilicity) are likely to increase the drug's tendency to cross cellular membranes through passive diffusion.
2. Functional group **reactivity** is most important for reactions occurring under **normal environmental conditions,** primarily air oxidation and hydrolysis. For example, benzene's characteristic reactions occur only with special reagents and under special laboratory conditions. Thus, benzene's shelf life is relatively long, and it requires no special storage conditions.
3. Functional groups affect drug reactivity and, hence, **drug shelf life** and **stability.**
4. Functional groups also affect **in vivo stability** and duration of action—the susceptibility of the drug to biotransformation such as oxidation, reduction, and hydrolysis by metabolic enzymes.

B. Alkanes, which are also called **paraffins** or **saturated hydrocarbons,** have a general formula of $R—CH_2—CH_3$, where R is a radical or molecule fragment.

1. Alkanes are **lipid soluble.**
2. The common reactions of alkanes are **halogenation** and **combustion.**
3. On the shelf, alkanes are **chemically inert** with regard to air, light, heat, acids, and bases.
4. In vivo, alkanes are **stable; terminal carbon** or **side-chain hydroxylation** may occur.

C. Alkenes, also called **olefins** or **unsaturated hydrocarbons,** have a general formula of $R—CH{=}CH_2$.

1. Alkenes are **lipid soluble.**
2. The common reactions of alkenes are the **addition of hydrogen or halogens, hydration** (to form glycols), and **oxidation** (to form peroxides).
3. On the shelf, **volatile alkenes and peroxides may explode** in the presence of oxygen and a spark.
4. In vivo, alkenes are relatively stable. **Hydration, epoxidation, peroxidation, or reduction** may occur.

D. Aromatic hydrocarbons are based on benzene (Figure 8-1). These molecules exhibit multicenter bonding, which confers unique chemical properties.

1. Aromatic hydrocarbons are **lipid soluble.**
2. The common reactions of aromatic hydrocarbons are electrophilic aromatic substitution such as **halogenation, nitration, sulfonation,** and **alkylation.**

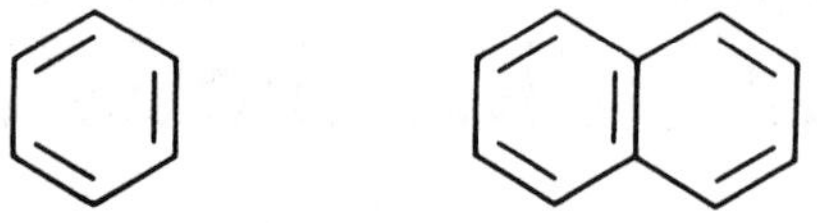

A B

Figure 8-1. Chemical structures of (*A*) benzene and (*B*) naphthalene. Benzene and related compounds, such as naphthalene, are planar molecules in the form of a regular hexagon.

3. On the shelf, aromatic hydrocarbons are **stable.**
4. In vivo, aromatic hydrocarbons undergo **hydroxylation, epoxidation, and diol formation**

E. Alkyl halides, also known as **halogenated hydrocarbons,** have a general formula of R—CH_2—X.

1. Alkyl halides are **lipid soluble.** Their solubility increases with the extent of halogenation.
2. The common reactions of alkyl halides are **nucleophilic substitution** and **dehydrohalogenation.**
3. On the shelf, alkyl halides are **stable.**
4. In vivo, alkyl halides are **not readily metabolized.**

F. Alcohols contain a **hydroxyl group** (—OH) and may be classified as **primary, secondary,** or **tertiary** alcohols with their general formulas shown below (Figure 8-2).

1. Low molecular weight alcohols are **water soluble;** water solubility decreases as hydrocarbon chain length increases. Alcohols are also **lipid soluble.**
2. The common reactions of alcohols are **esterification** and **oxidation.**
   a. Primary alcohols are oxidized to aldehydes and then to acids.
   b. Secondary alcohols are oxidized to ketones.
   c. Tertiary alcohols ordinarily are not oxidized.
3. On the shelf, alcohols are stable.
4. In vivo, alcohols may undergo oxidation, glucuronidation, or sulfation.

G. Phenols are aromatic compounds containing a hydroxyl group (—OH) directly connecting to the aromatic ring. Monophenols have one hydroxyl group, and catechols have two hydroxyl groups next to each other (Figure 8-3).

1. Phenols are **lipid soluble;** phenol itself (carbolic acid) is fairly water soluble. Ring substitutions generally decrease water solubility.
2. The common reactions of phenols are reactions with strong bases to form **phenoxide ion, esterification** with acids, and **oxidation** (to form quinones, usually colored).

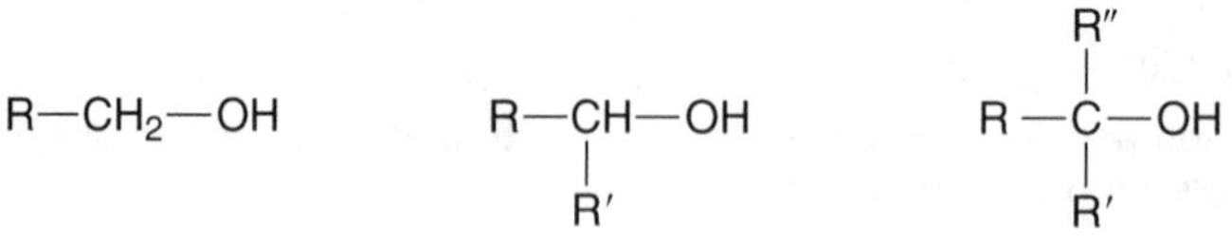

A B C

Figure 8-2. Structures of primary *(A),* secondary *(B),* and tertiary *(C)* alcohols. R, R′ and R″ are either alkyl or aryl groups.

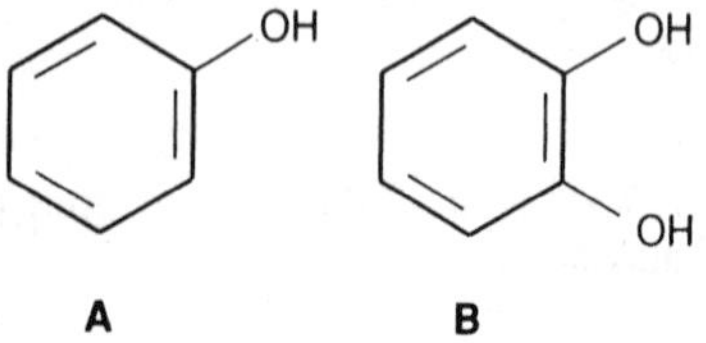

A B

Figure 8-3. Structures of (*A*) monophenol and (*B*) catechol functional groups.

3. On the shelf, phenols are susceptible to **air oxidation** and to **oxidation on contact with ferric ions.**
4. In vivo, phenols undergo **sulfation, glucuronidation, aromatic hydroxylation,** and ***O*-methylation.**

H. Ethers have a general formula of R—O—R, with an oxygen atom bonded to two carbon atoms.

1. **Low molecular weight** ethers are partially **water soluble;** water solubility decreases with an increase in the hydrocarbon portion of the molecule. Ethers are also **lipid soluble.**
2. The common reaction of ethers is **oxidation** (to form peroxides).
3. On the shelf, **peroxides may explode.**
4. In vivo, ethers undergo ***O*-dealkylation.** Stability increases with the size of the alkyl group.

I. Aldehydes have a general formula of R—CHO and contain a carbonyl group (C=O).

1. Aldehydes are **lipid soluble;** low molecular weight aldehydes are also water soluble.
2. The common reactions of aldehydes are **oxidation** and **hemiacetal and acetal formation.**
3. On the shelf, aldehydes **oxidize to acids.**
4. In vivo, aldehydes may also undergo **oxidation** to acids.

J. Ketones have a general formula of R—CO—R and, similar to aldehydes, they contain a carbonyl group (C=O).

1. Ketones are **lipid soluble.** Low molecular weight ketones are also water soluble with solubility decreasing as the hydrocarbon portion of the molecule increases.
2. Ketones are relatively **nonreactive,** although they may exist in equilibrium with their enol forms.
3. On the shelf, ketones are **very stable.**
4. In vivo, ketones may undergo some **oxidation** and **some reduction.**

K. Amines contain an amino group (—NH_2). The amino group can exist in ionized or unionized form. The general formulas of primary, secondary, tertiary, and quaternary amines are shown below (Figure 8-4).

1. Low molecular weight amines are **water soluble;** solubility decreases with increased branching (e.g., primary amines are more water soluble than secondary amines). However, quaternary amines, being ionic, are water soluble, as are most amine salts. Amines are also **lipid soluble.**
2. The common reactions of amines are **oxidation** and, for alkyl amines, **salt formation** with acids. Aromatic amines, which are less basic, have less tendency to react with acids.
3. On the shelf, phenolic amines are **susceptible to air oxidation.**
4. In vivo, amines may undergo **minor glucuronidation, sulfation,** and **methylation.** Primary amines also undergo oxidative deamination. Primary and secondary amines undergo acetylation. Secondary and tertiary amines undergo *N*-dealkylation, and tertiary amines undergo *N*-oxidation.

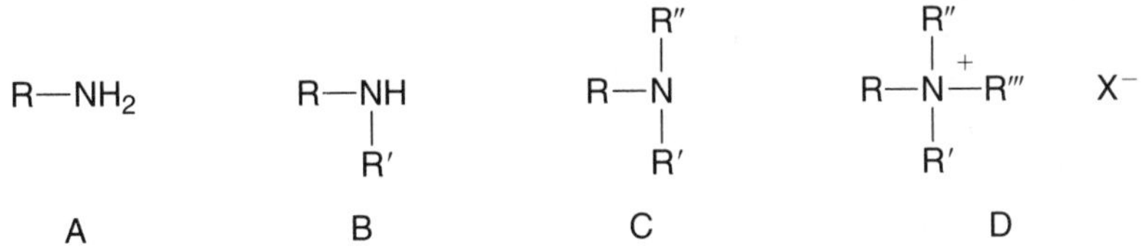

Figure 8-4. Structures of primary (*A*), secondary (*B*), tertiary (*C*), and quaternary (*D*) amines. R, R′, R″, and R‴ are either alkyl or aryl groups.

L. Carboxylic acids have a general formula of R—COOH and contain a carboxyl group (—COOH).

1. Low molecular weight carboxylic acids are **water soluble,** as are sodium and potassium salts. Carboxylic acids are also **lipid soluble.**
2. The common reactions of carboxylic acids are salt formation with bases, esterification, and decarboxylation.
3. On the shelf, carboxylic acids are **very stable.**
4. In vivo, carboxylic acids undergo conjugation (with glucuronic acid, glycine, and glutamine) and β-oxidation.

M. Esters have a general formula of R—COOR.

1. Esters are **lipid soluble;** low molecular weight esters are **slightly water soluble.**
2. The common reaction of esters is **hydrolysis** to form carboxylic acid and alcohol.
3. On the shelf, simple or low molecular weight esters are **susceptible to hydrolysis,** whereas complex, high molecular weight, or water-insoluble esters are **resistant.**
4. In vivo, esters undergo **enzymatic hydrolysis** by esterases.

N. Amides have a general formula of R—$CONH_2$ or R—CONR—R (lactam form).

1. Amides are **lipid soluble;** low molecular weight amides are **fairly water soluble.**
2. Amides have **no common reactions.**
3. On the shelf, amides are **very stable.**
4. In vivo, amides undergo **enzymatic hydrolysis** by amidases, primarily in the liver.

II. BIOCHEMISTRY

A. Introduction. Biochemistry is the study of chemical principles that support life processes. It influences drug metabolism, therapeutic effectiveness, and biotransformation. Biochemically significant molecules include amino acids and proteins, carbohydrates, lipids, pyrimidines, and purines, and biopolymers—enzymes, which are built from amino acids; polysaccharides, which are built from carbohydrates; and nucleic acids, which are built from pyrimidines and purines.

B. Amino acids and proteins

1. Amino acids are the monomeric units of proteins and have the following general formula:

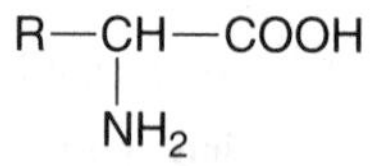

a. Naturally occurring amino acids are mostly L, α-amino acids. Proteins are made up of the 20 different amino acids, which differ in the side chain (R) attached to the α-carbon. The 20 different side chains vary in size, shape, charge, hydrogen bonding capacity, and chemical reactivity. A protein can be hydrolyzed into its component α-amino acids by acids, bases, or enzymes.

b. Amino acids have a **zwitterion structure** (both positive and negative regions of charge), which accounts for their high melting point and low water solubility. Amino acids in solution have the following general formula:

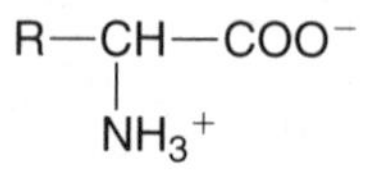

c. **Ionization** of amino acids to the zwitterion form or other forms depends on pH (Figure 8-5).

d. Amino acids are linked to form proteins by the **peptide bond**—a link between the carbonyl carbon and the amino nitrogen (Figure 8-6).

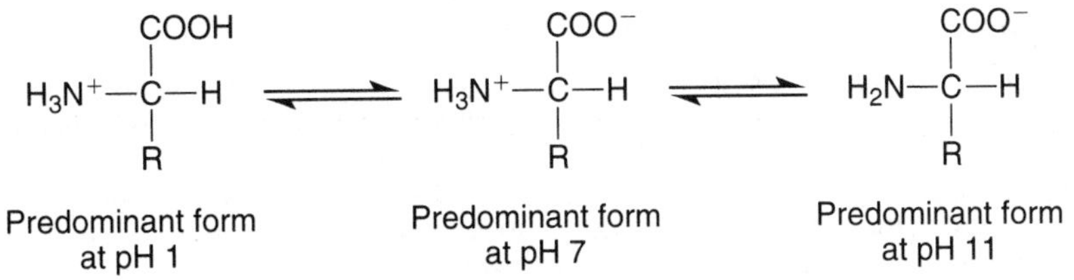

Figure 8-5. Amino acid ionization as solution. The carboxyl and amino groups are either in ionized or unionized form depending on the pH of the solution.

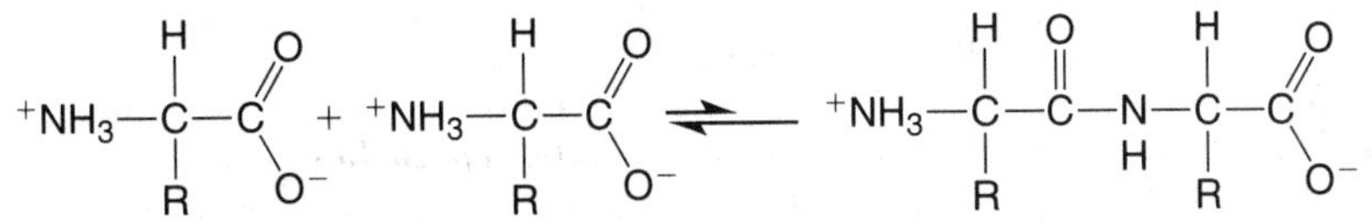

Figure 8-6. Peptide bond formation occurs as a result of the condensation of the carboxyl group of one amino acid with the amino group of another. Water is eliminated during this process.

2. **Proteins,** which result from amino acids linking by means of peptide bonds, have four levels of structure.
   a. **Primary** structure refers to the sequence of amino acids and location of disulfide bond in the protein.
   b. **Secondary** structure refers to the spatial arrangement of sequenced amino acids; for example, α–conformation (helical coil) or β-conformation (pleated sheet).
   c. **Tertiary** structure refers to the three-dimensional structure of a single protein.
   d. **Quaternary** structure refers to the arrangement of individual subunit chains into complex molecules.

C. **Carbohydrates.** These are polyhydroxy aldehydes or ketones. Three major classes of carbohydrates exist.

1. **Monosaccharides** (simple sugars), such as glucose or fructose, consist of a single polyhydroxy aldehyde or ketone unit.
   a. **Aldehydic** monosaccharides are reducing sugars.
   b. Monosaccharides can be linked together by **glycosidic bonds,** which are hydrolyzed by acids but not by bases.

2. **Oligosaccharides,** such as sucrose, maltose, and lactose, consist of short chains of monosaccharides joined covalently.
   a. **Sucrose** cannot be absorbed by the intestine until it is converted by sucrase into its components, glucose and fructose.
   b. **Maltose** is hydrolyzed by maltase into two molecules of glucose.
   c. **Lactose** (or milk sugar) cannot be absorbed by the intestine until it is converted by lactase into its components, galactose and glucose.

3. **Polysaccharides,** such as **cellulose** and **glycogen,** consist of long chains of monosaccharides.

D. **Pyrimidines and purines.** These are bases that, when bonded with ribose, form nucleosides, which when subsequently bonded to phosphoric acid form nucleotides—the structural building blocks of nucleic acids.

1. **Pyrimidine bases** include:
   a. **Cytosine** (C), found in deoxyribonucleic acid (DNA) and ribonucleic acid (RNA)
   b. **Uracil** (U), found in RNA only
   c. **Thymine** (T), found in DNA only

2. **Purine bases** include:
   a. **Adenine** (A), found in DNA and RNA
   b. **Guanine** (G), found in DNA and RNA

3. Pyrimidines and purines exhibit **tautomerism** (a form of stereoisomerism) and can exist in either **keto** (lactam) or **enol** (lactim) forms.

E. Biopolymers

1. **Enzymes**—linked chains of amino acids—are proteins capable of acting as catalysts for biologic reactions. They may be simple or complex and may require cofactors or coenzymes for biologic activity.
   a. An enzyme enhances the rate of a specific chemical reaction by lowering the **activation energy** of the reaction. It does not change the reaction's equilibrium point, and it is not used up or permanently changed by the reaction.
   b. A cofactor may be an **inorganic component** (usually a metal ion) or a **nonprotein organic molecule.** A cofactor may be biologically inactive without an apoenzyme (the protein portion of a complex enzyme). A cofactor firmly bound to the apoenzyme is called a **prosthetic group.** An organic cofactor that is not firmly bound but is actively involved during catalysis is called a **coenzyme.**
   c. A complete, catalytically active enzyme system is referred to as a **holoenzyme.**
   d. Enzymes fall into six major classes.
      (1) **Oxidoreductases** (e.g., dehydrogenases, oxidases, peroxidases) are important in the oxidative metabolism of drugs.
      (2) **Transferases** catalyze the transfer of groups, such as phosphate and amino groups.
      (3) **Hydrolases** (e.g., proteolytic enzymes, amylases, esterases) hydrolyze their substrates.
      (4) **Lyases** (e.g., decarboxylases, deaminases) catalyze the removal of functional groups by means other than hydrolysis.
      (5) **Ligases** (e.g., DNA ligase, which binds nucleotides together during DNA synthesis) catalyze the coupling of two molecules.
      (6) **Isomerases** catalyze various isomerizations, such as the change from D to L forms or the change from cis- to trans-isomers.

2. **Polysaccharides** (also called glycans) are long-chain polymers of carbohydrates and may be linear or branched. They are classified as homopolysaccharides or heteropolysaccharides.
   a. **Homopolysaccharides** (e.g., starch, glycogen, cellulose) contain only one type of monomeric unit.
      (1) **Starch** (a reserve food material of plants) is composed of two glucose polymers—amylose (linear and water soluble) and amylopectin (highly branched and water insoluble). It yields mainly maltose (a glucose disaccharide) after enzymatic hydrolysis with salivary or pancreatic amylase; only glucose after complete hydrolysis by strong acids.
      (2) **Glycogen,** like amylopectin, is a highly branched, compact chain of D-glucose. The main storage polysaccharide of animal cells, it is found mostly in liver and muscle and can be hydrolyzed by salivary or pancreatic amylase into maltose and D-glucose.
      (3) **Cellulose** (a water-insoluble structural polysaccharide found in plant cell walls) is a linear, unbranched chain of D-glucose. It cannot be digested by humans because the human intestinal tract secretes no enzyme capable of hydrolyzing it.
   b. **Heteropolysaccharides** (e.g., heparin, hyaluronic acid) contain two or more types of monomeric unit.
      (1) **Heparin** (an acid mucopolysaccharide) consists of sulfate derivatives of *N*-acetyl-D-glucosamine and D-iduronate. It can be isolated from lung tissue and is used medically to prevent blood clot formation.
      (2) **Hyaluronic acid,** a component of bacterial cell walls as well as of the vitreous humor and synovial fluid, consists of alternating units of *N*-acetyl-D-glucosamine and *N*-acetyl-muramic acid.

3. **Nucleic acids** are linear polymers of nucleotides—pyrimidine and purine bases linked to ribose or deoxyribose sugars (nucleosides) and bound to phosphate groups. The backbone of the nucleic acid consists of alternating phosphate and pentose units with a purine or pyrimidine base attached to each.
   a. Nucleic acids are strong acids, closely associated with **cellular cations** and such basic proteins as **histones** and **protamines.**
   b. The two main types of nucleic acids are **DNA** and **RNA.** RNA exists in three forms.
      (1) **Ribosomal** RNA (rRNA) is found in the ribosomes, but its functions are not fully understood yet.
      (2) **Messenger** RNA (mRNA) serves as the template for protein synthesis and specifies a polypeptide's amino acid sequence.

(3) **Transfer** RNA (tRNA) carries activated amino acids to the ribosomes, where the amino acids are incorporated into the growing polypeptide chain.

c. In both DNA and RNA, the successive nucleotides are joined by **phosphodiester bonds** between the 5′-hydroxy group of one nucleotide's pentose and the 3′-hydroxy group of the next nucleotide's pentose.

d. DNA differs from RNA in that it **lacks a hydroxyl group** at the pentose's C_2' position, and it contains T rather than U.

e. DNA structure consists of two α-helical DNA strands coiled around the same axis to form a double helix. The strands are antiparallel—the 5′, 3′-internucleotide phosphodiester links run in opposite directions.

(1) **Hydrogen bonding** between specific base pairs A—T and cytosine (C)—G holds the two DNA strands together. The strands are complementary (the base sequence of one strand determines the base sequence of the other).

(2) The **hydrophobic bases** are on the inside of the helix; the hydrophilic deoxyribose–phosphate backbone is on the outside.

III. BIOCHEMICAL METABOLISM

A. Overview. Biochemical metabolism is the review of pathways that lead to the synthesis or breakdown of compounds important to the life of an organism.

1. **Control of metabolism.** Metabolism is controlled by substrate concentration, enzymes (constitutive or induced), allosteric (regulatory) enzymes, hormones, and compartmentation.

2. **Catabolism** is the sum of degradation reactions that usually release energy for useful work (e.g., mechanical, osmotic, biosynthetic).

3. **Anabolism** is the sum of biosynthetic (build-up) reactions that consume energy to form new biochemical compounds (metabolites).

4. **Amphibolic pathways** are those that may be used for both catabolic as well as anabolic purposes. **Krebs cycle** breaks down metabolites primarily to release 90% of the total energy of an organism. It also draws off metabolites to form compounds such as amino acids (e.g., aspartic, glutamic, alanine). Hemoglobin has its heme moiety formed from succinyl coenzyme A (succinyl CoA) and glycine followed by a complex set of reactions.

B. Bioenergetics

1. **Substrate level phosphorylation** entails the formation of one unit of A triphosphate (ATP) per unit of metabolite transformed (e.g., succinyl CoA to succinate, phosphoenolpyruvate to pyruvate). These reactions do not need oxygen.

2. **Oxidative phosphorylation** entails the formation of two or three units of ATP per unit of metabolite transformed by oxidoreductase enzymes (e.g., dehydrogenases); these enzymes use flavin A dinucleotide (FAD) formed from the vitamin riboflavin, or nicotinamide A dinucleotide (NAD^+) from the vitamin nicotinamide as cofactors. The reactions are coupled to the electron transport system, and the energy released is used to form ATP in the mitochondria.

C. Carbohydrate metabolism

1. **Catabolism.** This process releases stored energy from carbohydrates.

a. **Glycogenolysis** is the breakdown of glycogen into glucose phosphate in the liver and skeletal muscle, controlled by the hormones glucagon and epinephrine.

b. **Glycolysis** is the breakdown of sugar phosphates (e.g., glucose, fructose, glycerol) into pyruvate (aerobically) or lactate (anaerobically).

2. **Anabolism.** This process consumes energy to build up complex molecules from simpler molecules.

a. **Glycogenesis** is the formation of glycogen in the liver and muscles from glucose consumed in the diet; its synthesis is controlled by the pancreatic hormone insulin.

b. **Gluconeogenesis** is the formation of glucose from noncarbohydrate sources, such as lactate, alanine, pyruvate, and Krebs cycle metabolites; fatty acids cannot form glucose.

D. Krebs cycle. This pathway serves both breakdown and synthetic purposes and occurs in the mitochondrial compartment.

1. **Catabolism.** This pathway converts pyruvate (glycolysis), acetyl CoA (fatty acid degradation), and amino acids to carbon dioxide and water with a release of energy. The cycle is strictly oxygen-dependent (aerobic). Mature red blood cells lack mitochondria; hence, there is no Krebs cycle activity.

2. **Anabolism.** This pathway forms amino acids such as aspartate and glutamate from cycle intermediates; also, the porphyrin ring of heme (e.g., hemoglobin, myoglobin, cytochromes) is formed from a cycle intermediate.

3. **Anaplerotic reactions.** Because metabolites are used to make amino acids or heme (e.g., succinyl CoA), the metabolite must be replaced by intermediates from other sources (e.g., glutamate from the breakdown of protein forms ketoglutarate).

4. **Electron transport.** The electron transport system accepts electrons and hydrogen from the oxidation of Krebs cycle metabolites and couples the energy released to synthesize ATP in the mitochondria.

E. Lipid metabolism

1. **Catabolism. Triglycerides** (triacylglycerols) stored in fat cells (adipocytes) are hydrolyzed by hormone-sensitive lipases into three fatty acids and glycerol.
   a. **Fatty acids** are broken down by beta oxidation to acetyl CoA (two carbon units), which enter the Krebs cycle to complete the oxidation to carbon dioxide and water with release of considerable energy. Too rapid breakdown of fatty acids leads to ketone bodies (ketogenesis) as in diabetes mellitus.
   b. **Glycerol** enters glycolysis and is oxidized to pyruvate and, via the Krebs cycle, to carbon dioxide and water.
   c. **Steroids** may be converted to other compounds such as bile acids, vitamin D, or steroidal hormones (e.g., cortisone, estrogens, androgens); they are not broken down completely.

2. **Anabolism. Biosynthesis** forms fatty acids, steroids, and other terpene-related metabolites.
   a. **Fatty acids** are formed in the cytoplasm, and unsaturation occurs in the mitochondria or endoplasmic reticulum. Humans cannot make linoleic acid; thus, it is important that it be included in the diet (essential fatty acid).
   b. **Terpene compounds** are derived from acetyl CoA via mevalonate and include:
      (1) Cholesterol and other steroids
      (2) Fat-soluble vitamins (i.e., A,D,E,K)
      (3) Bile acids
   c. **Sphingolipids** contain sphingenine formed from palmitoyl CoA and serine. Sphingenine forms a ceramide backbone when joined to fatty acids. The addition of sugars, sialic acid, or choline phosphate forms compounds such as cerebrosides, gangliosides, or sphingomyelin found in nerve tissues and membranes.
   d. **Phosphatidyl compounds,** such as phosphatidyl choline (lecithin), phosphatidyl serine, or ethanolamine, are also important parts of membranes.

F. Nitrogen metabolism. Nitrogen metabolism involves amino acid metabolism and nucleic acid metabolism (see Chapter 9 for a discussion of the nucleic acid role in cell activity).

1. **Catabolism**
   a. **Amino acids.** The amino group is removed by a transaminase enzyme. The carbon skeleton is broken down to acetyl CoA (ketogenic amino acids) or to citric acid cycle intermediates (glycogenic amino acids) and oxidized to carbon dioxide and water for energy. Glycogenic amino acids form glucose as needed via gluconeogenesis; some amino acids are both ketogenic and glycogenic (e.g., tyrosine).
   b. **Purines** are salvaged (90%), and the remaining 10% are degraded in a sequence that includes xanthine oxidase forming uric acid in humans.
   c. **Pyrimidines** are catabolized to β-alanine, ammonia, and carbon dioxide.

2. **Anabolism**
   a. **Amino acids** are formed from the citric acid cycle intermediated (see III D 2); others must be eaten daily in dietary proteins. The latter are called essential amino acids [phenylala-

nine, valine, tryptophan (PVT); threonine, isoleucine, methionine (TIM); histidine, arginine in infants, lysine, leucine (HALL)].

b. **Purines** are formed by complex reactions using carbamoyl phosphate, aspartate, glutamine, glycine, carbon dioxide, and formyl tetrahydrofolate.

c. **Pyrimidines** are formed from aspartate and carbamoyl phosphate in a multistep process.

G. **Nitrogen excretion.** Excess nitrogen must be eliminated because it is toxic. Humans primarily excrete urea but also excrete uric acid.

1. **Urea synthesis.** The **Krebs-Henseleit pathway** is used to form urea principally in the liver. The ammonia is removed from amino acids by amino acid transferases (transaminases) that use pyridoxal phosphate (vitamin B_6) as a coenzyme. **Glutamine** is formed from glutamate (an intermediate) and ammonia; glutamine and carbon dioxide form carbamoyl phosphate, which enters the urea cycle and after several steps forms urea.

2. **Uric acid synthesis.** Although most purines are salvaged, humans excrete the remaining purines as uric acid.

STUDY QUESTIONS

Directions: Each of the numbered items or incomplete statements in this section is followed by answers or by completions of the statement. Select the **one** lettered answer or completion that is **best** in each case.

1. Which of the following classes of organic compounds reacts to form salts with hydrochloric acid?

(A) Tertiary amines
(B) Carboxylic acids
(C) Amides
(D) Ethers
(E) Secondary alcohols

2. Which of the following terms best describes the conversion of

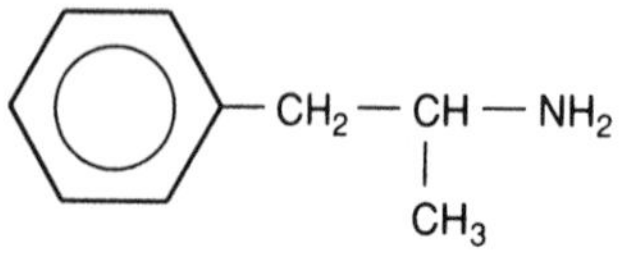

to

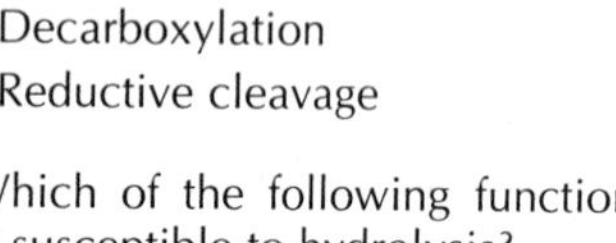

?

(A) *N*-dealkylation
(B) Oxidative deamination
(C) Acetylation
(D) Decarboxylation
(E) Reductive cleavage

3. Which of the following functional groups is most susceptible to hydrolysis?

(A) R—CO—R
(B) R—COOR
(C) R—O—R
(D) $R—NH—CH_3$
(E) R—COOH

4. Monomer units of proteins are known as

(A) monosaccharides
(B) prosthetic groups
(C) amino acids
(D) purines
(E) nucleosides

5. Which of the following formulas represents the zwitterion form of an amino acid?

(A) $H_2N{—}\underset{\displaystyle R}{\underset{|}{CH}}{—}COO^-$

(B) $\overset{+}{H_3N}{—}\underset{\displaystyle R}{\underset{|}{CH}}{—}COOH$

(C) $H_2N{—}\underset{\displaystyle R}{\underset{|}{CH}}{—}COOH$

(D) $\overset{+}{H_3N}{—}\underset{\displaystyle R}{\underset{|}{CH}}{—}COO^-$

(E) $H_2N{—}\underset{\displaystyle R}{\underset{|}{CH}}{—}CONH{—}\underset{\displaystyle R}{\underset{|}{CH}}{—}COOH$

6. Glucose is a carbohydrate that cannot be hydrolyzed into a simpler substance. It is best described as

(A) a sugar
(B) a monosaccharide
(C) a disaccharide
(D) a polysaccharide
(E) an oligosaccharide

7. All of the following carbohydrates are considered to be polysaccharides EXCEPT

(A) heparin
(B) starch
(C) glycogen
(D) maltose
(E) cellulose

8. Which of the following compounds are considered the building blocks of nucleic acids?

(A) Nucleotides
(B) Nucleosides
(C) Monosaccharides
(D) Purines
(E) Amino acids

9. Which of the following terms best describes a cofactor that is firmly bound to an apoenzyme?

(A) Holoenzyme
(B) Prosthetic group
(C) Coenzyme
(D) Transferase
(E) Heteropolysaccharide

10. Enzymes that uncouple peptide linkages are best classified as

(A) hydrolases
(B) ligases
(C) oxidoreductases
(D) transferases
(E) isomerases

11. The sugar that is inherent in the nucleic acids RNA and DNA is

(A) glucose
(B) sucrose
(C) ribose
(D) digitoxose
(E) maltose

Directions: Each item below contains three suggested answers of which **one or more** is correct. Choose the answer

A if **I only** is correct
B if **III only** is correct
C if **I and II** are correct
D if **II and III** are correct
E if **I, II, and III** are correct

12. When certain functional groups are introduced into a benzene nucleus, they tend to decrease the liposolubility of benzene. These groups include

I. an ethyl group
II. a phenolic group
III. a carboxylic acid group

Questions 13–16

The following questions refer to the drug molecule

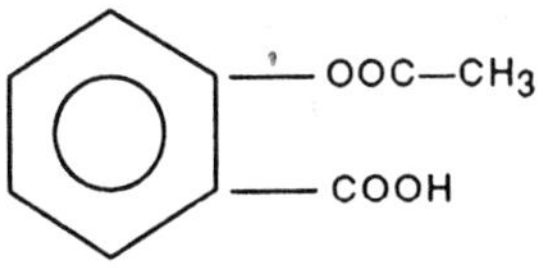

13. The drug molecule is soluble in

I. an aqueous base
II. water
III. an aqueous acid

14. Decomposition of the drug molecule at room temperature most likely would occur by

I. oxidation of the ester
II. reduction of the carboxylic acid
III. hydrolysis of the ester

15. Reactions that would be possible metabolic pathways for the drug molecule include

I. ring hydroxylation
II. enzymatic hydrolysis
III. glucuronide formation

16. Classes of organic compounds that have greater in vitro stability than in vivo stability include

I. carboxylic acids
II. alcohols
III. alkyl halides

ANSWERS AND EXPLANATIONS

1. The answer is A *[I K 2].*
Substances that react with acids to form salts must be bases. Only organic compounds that contain the nitrogen-containing amine group are bases. While amides contain nitrogen, the adjacent carbonyl group decreases the basicity; therefore, they are essentially neutral.

2. The answer is B *[I K 4].*
The reactant depicted contains a primary amine that is lost during the reaction; that is, the molecule is deaminated. The resultant product is a ketone formed from the oxidation of the carbon atom. Thus, this reaction would best be termed oxidative deamination.

3. The answer is B *[I M 2].*
Hydrolysis is a double decomposition reaction in which water is one of the reactants. Esters, particularly simple esters, commonly undergo hydrolysis. Certain types of ethers such as glycosides also undergo hydrolysis, but they usually require strongly alkaline conditions or a catalyst such as an enzyme. Ketones, amines, or carboxylic acids do not undergo hydrolysis.

4. The answer is C *[II B 1].*
Proteins are large molecules with molecular weights ranging from 5000 to more than 1 million daltons. All proteins are composed of chains of amino acids and can be hydrolyzed to yield a mixture of their respective amino acids. There are 20 α- amino acids, which are commonly found in proteins. All the naturally occurring amino acids in proteins are L-enantiomers, with the exception of glycine. All have at least one amino group and one carboxyl group. The amino acids are linked together through the amino group of one amino acid and the carboxyl group of another amino acid with the splitting out of a water molecule to form an amide linkage, which in a protein is referred to as a peptide.

Monosaccharides are simple, nonhydrolyzable sugars. Purines and pyrimidines are organic bases, while a prosthetic group is a cofactor that is firmly bound to an apoenzyme.

5. The answer is D *[II B 1 c, d; Figures 8-5, 8-6].*
A zwitterion is a single species containing both negative and positive charges. It sometimes is referred to as an inner salt. Amino acids have an amino group and a carboxyl group in the same molecule. The amino group, which is basic, attracts the proton from the carboxyl group and becomes positively charged, while the carboxyl group becomes negatively charged when it donates its proton to the amino group. Amino acids exist as zwitterions at near neutral pH such as occurs within a cell or in the bloodstream.

6. The answer is B *[II C 1].*
While glucose is a sugar, it is more specifically a simple sugar that cannot be hydrolyzed into more simple sugars—thus, it is classified as a monosaccharide. Sugars may be simple, such as glucose, or complex, such as sucrose, and are classified as disaccharides or oligosaccharides, respectively. Polysaccharides consist of long chains of monosaccharides such as cellulose and glycogen.

7. The answer is D *[II C 2 b, 3, E 2 a, b].*
Polysaccharides are long-chain polymers of sugars. As the prefix "poly" indicates, there are many sugar units in the molecule. Maltose is composed of two molecules of glucose and is classified as a disaccharide or an oligosaccharide.

8. The answer is A *[II D, E 3].*
Nucleic acids are linear polymers of nucleotides that consist of three different molecules that are covalently linked to form one unit: (1) an organic base of either a purine or a pyrimidine; (2) a 5-carbon sugar (e.g., pentose); and (3) a phosphoric acid group. A nucleoside consists of the organic base and the pentose. A monosaccharide is a simple nonhydrolyzable carbohydrate, which may be considered a building block of polysaccharides. Purines are heterocyclic bases. Adenine and guanine are the two purines found in deoxyribonucleic acid (DNA) and ribonucleic acid (RNA). Amino acids are the building blocks of protein.

9. The answer is B *[II E 1 b].*
Complex, or conjugated, enzymes contain a nonprotein group called a cofactor, which is required for biologic activity. In many cases, the cofactor is quite firmly bound to the protein. In others, the binding

occurs only during the reaction that the enzyme catalyzes. Cofactors that are firmly bound to the protein are known as prosthetic groups, whereas those that are actively bound to the protein only during catalysis are referred to as coenzymes.

A holoenzyme is a complete, catalytically active enzyme system. A transferase is an enzyme that catalyzes the transfer of groups from one substance to another, such as catechol *O*-methyl transferase (COMT). A heteropolysaccharide is a polysaccharide that contains two or more different monomeric units, such as heparin.

10. The answer is A *[II E 1 d (3)].*
A peptide linkage is an amide functional group formed from the loss of a molecule of water from two amino acids. Uncoupling this linkage is the reverse of this reaction, a hydrolysis reaction. A hydrolase is an enzyme that catalyzes hydrolysis reactions. More specific terms for an enzyme that catalyzes the hydrolysis of proteins are amidase or peptidase. A ligase catalyzes the coupling of two molecules. An oxidoreductase catalyzes oxidation reactions. A transferase catalyzes the transfer of groups from one substance to another. An isomerase catalyzes the interconversion of one isomer to another.

11. The answer is C *[E 3].*
Nucleic acids are biopolymers consisting of long chains of nucleotides. Nucleotides contain a pentose monosaccharide as one of their three constituents. RNA contains, as the name suggests, the monosaccharide ribose, whereas DNA contains deoxyribose. The only difference between these two sugars is the absence of oxygen in the 2 position of the ribose ring. Glucose, also known as dextrose, is a hexose. Digitoxose is a deoxyhexose present in the digitalis glycosides. Sucrose and maltose are disaccharides.

12. The answer is D (II, III) *[I A 1, G 1, L 1].*
The overall solubility of the various classes of organic compounds illustrates a tendency for functional groups containing oxygen or nitrogen to demonstrate a degree of water solubility, whereas functional groups containing only carbon and hydrogen have very little water solubility. The phenolic and carboxylic groups both contain oxygen. In addition, they are acidic groups capable of undergoing ionization. Thus, compared to the ethyl group, they are more likely to increase the water solubility of benzene.

13–16. The answers are: 13-A (I) *[I L 1],* **14-B (III)** *[I L 2, 3, M 2, 3],* **15-E (all)** *[I D 4, L 4, M 4],* **16-C (I, II)** *[I A, E, F, L].*
Organic substances generally are nonpolar; thus, they usually are insoluble in water. Since water is a polar solvent, only polar organics are water soluble. The most common type of polar organic compound is a salt. Since the molecule depicted is a carboxylic acid, it reacts with a base to form a water-soluble salt.

The molecule contains both a simple ester and a carboxylic acid. Simple esters are susceptible to hydrolysis from moisture in the air but are not susceptible to oxidation. Carboxylic acids are not reduced easily.

The molecule, acetylsalicylic acid, contains an aromatic hydrocarbon nucleus (which can undergo ring hydroxylation), a simple acetate ester (which can undergo hydrolysis), and a free carboxyl group (which can undergo glucuronide conjugation as well as glycine conjugation).

Molecules that have poor in vitro stability are usually those that are susceptible to air oxidation and hydrolysis, or they may be light sensitive. Alcohols undergo oxidation but not without the presence of oxidizing agents. Also, they do not hydrolyze; thus, they are stable in air and moisture. In the body, there are several common metabolic pathways available for their biotransformation. Acids do not hydrolyze, nor are they susceptible to oxidation; thus, they are stable in the presence of air and moisture. In vivo, acids easily undergo several common metabolic reactions, particularly conjugation reactions. Alkyl halides are not susceptible to either oxidation or hydrolysis and do not undergo common metabolic reactions in the body. Thus, alkyl halides are equally stable in vitro and in vivo.

9
Microbiology

Ralph N. Blomster

I. TAXONOMY AND NOMENCLATURE

A. **Taxonomy** is classification or ordering into groups based on degree of relatedness. Bacteria belong to the **Procaryotae** kingdom and are grouped and named primarily by morphology, biochemical and metabolic differences, and immunologic and genetic relationships. Bacteria are named by the **linnaean** or **binomial** system as a genus and species (e.g., *Homo sapiens* is the genus and species for humans).

B. **Morphology** is classification of bacteria by shape and structure.

1. **Gross morphology** is based on the size, shape, and texture of colonies that are grown in an **axenic, or** pure, culture. Each colony is formed from a **colony-forming unit (CFU)**, which usually consists of a single cell but can have two or more adherent daughter cells.
2. **Microscopic morphology** describes bacteria on the basis of the size, shape, and arrangement of the cell.

C. **Stains.** Because of their small size and relative transparency, bacteria must be stained to be visible. Staining is also used as a classification system. The major types of staining reactions are:

1. **Simple** stain: a single dye (e.g., gentian violet, safranin) that colors the cell to make it visible
2. **Gram** stain: a differential staining procedure that divides cell organisms into either gram positive (blue) or gram negative (red)
3. **Acid-fast** stain: a vigorous procedure that stains cells that have a large amount of lipid material (acid-fast) but not those that have a small amount of lipid material (non–acid-fast)
4. **Spore** stain
5. **Capsule** stain

D. Bacterial cell shape and arrangement

1. **Cocci** are spherical and exist in chains (streptococci), pairs or diplococci *(Streptococcus pneumoniae, Neisseria gonorrhoeae)*, clusters (staphylococci), and packets (sarcinae).
2. **Bacilli** are cylindrical and rod-shaped organisms (pseudomonads, *Escherichia, Bacteroides*).
3. **Coccobacilli** are a combination of small rods or flattened cocci *(Brucella)*.
4. **Spirochetes** are snake shaped *(Treponema pallidum)*.
5. **Fusobacteria** have tapered ends and are slightly curved (i.e., fusiform) *[Fusobacterium mortiferum]*.
6. **Filamentous** organisms are branching *(Haemophilis influenzae)*.
7. **Vibrios** are comma shaped *(Vibrio cholerae)*.
8. **Pleomorphic organisms** exist in varied forms *(Mycobacteria, Corynebacteria)*.

E. **Other parameters** used for classification

1. The **presence** or **absence** of:
   a. **Spores**
   b. **Capsules** or **slime layers**

2. **Motility** and the type of **flagella**
   a. **Monotrichous:** a single flagellum at either pole
   b. **Lophotrichous:** a tuft of flagella at either or both poles
   c. **Amphitrichous:** a flagellum at both poles
   d. **Peritrichous:** flagella distributed evenly over the entire cell

II. STRUCTURE OF THE PROKARYOTIC CELL

A. Overview. Prokaryotic cells (bacteria) are **small** and **simple** in design. They have the following characteristics:

1. **Less complex inside,** but more complex outside, the cytoplasmic membrane than **eukaryotic cells** (true plants, animals, algae, fungi, protozoa, slime molds)
2. Lack a true nucleus, a nuclear membrane, and intracytoplasmic organelles (e.g., plastids, endoplasmic reticulum, vacuoles)
3. Multiply by **binary fission** rather than by mitosis or meiosis
4. **Protein synthesis** is mediated by 70s rather than by 80s ribosomes.
5. Bacterial genetic information is arranged on a single circular strand of DNA, the **nucleoid.**

B. External structures

1. **Capsule and slime layer**
   a. The **capsule** is an expressed, adherent, large polymer surface coat that differs in composition between genera and usually is polysaccharide in nature; however, the surface coat of *Bacilli* can be polypeptide. The capsule has several functions:
      (1) Increases the **virulence** (degree of organism pathogenicity) of a microorganism
      (2) Prevents **phagocytosis** of the organism by macrophages and neutrophiles.
      (3) Aids in **adherence** of the organism to host cells
   b. If the polysaccharide is nonadherent, it is called a **slime layer.**
   c. **Transformation** from smooth to rough colonies on media is indicative of **capsule loss.** Concurrently, there is a loss of virulence. This capsular material is immunogenic and causes the production of **opsonins** (antibodies), which prepare the organism for phagocytosis (**opsonization**).

2. **Flagella** are proteinaceous, helically coiled organs of locomotion that extend outward from the cell wall to the cell surface. Flagella cause bacteria to move toward nutrient chemoattractants and away from repellants.
   a. **Structure**
      (1) Flagella are composed of **flagellin,** a protein that is antigenically distinct from other flagella and cell antigens and is termed **H antigen.**
      (2) **Three parts** comprise flagella:
         (a) **Basal body**
            (i) Attaches the flagella to the cell envelope (cytoplasmic membrane and cell wall)
            (ii) The number of rings that make up the basal body differ in gram-positive (2) and gram-negative (4) organisms.
         (b) **Hook**
         (c) **Filament**
   b. **Periplasmic flagella,** also called **axial filaments,** occur in spirochetes and are embedded into the cell membrane. Because they cause a corkscrew type of motion on contraction, these organisms are not hindered by viscosity of media.

3. **Pili (fimbriae).** Proteinaceous hairs that are shorter than flagella, composed of regularly arranged protein subunits, are called **pilin** or **fimbrilin.** They are more common in gram-negative organisms but can be found in gram-positive organisms. There are two morphological and functional varieties:
   a. **Common** (attachment) pili
      (1) Appear in greater numbers than sex pili
      (2) Have adhesive properties

(3) Are lectins that are responsible for trophism, the ability of the organism to bind to specific receptors on host cells

b. Sex (conjugative or F) pili

(1) Are longer than common pili

(2) Form in groups of less than 10

(3) Are involved in the transport of DNA between donor and recipient cells

C. The cell wall and cytoplasmic membrane

1. The **cell wall** is rigid and provides the general shape of the cell. It has no cholesterol or other sterols (unlike eukaryotic cells) and is composed of a basic **carbohydrate layer** (**peptidoglycan** or **murein layer**). This layer is composed of repeating disaccharide units, with a four amino acid side chain that is covalently linked to amino acids from neighboring disaccharide units, forming a stable cross-linked structure. This complex structure is a polymer of ***N*-acetylglucosamine** and ***N*-acetylmuramic acid.** Most bacteria are designated as either gram positive or gram negative based on fundamental differences in the components of the cell wall.

a. Gram-positive organisms have a thick cell wall with extensive cross linking that is approximately 40 layers thick and forms a sacculus in parallel layers or layered network around the cytoplasmic membrane. Within the cell wall, a variety of elements serve to stabilize the cell wall, maintain its association with the cytoplasmic membrane, and act as antigenic determinants.

(1) **Proteins**

(2) **Polysaccharides**

(3) **Teichoic acid** (glycerol or ribitol phosphodiesters)

(a) **Membrane-associated teichoic acids** (lipoteichoic acid) are covalently linked to glycolipids of the cytoplasmic membrane.

(b) **Wall-associated teichoic acids** are covalently linked to the glycan chain of peptidoglycan.

b. Gram-negative organisms

(1) **Structure.** Gram-negative cell walls are multilayered with a thin peptidoglycan layer that has no teichoic acids. External to this is the **outer membrane,** a complex cell wall layer, linked to the peptidoglycan layer by the **lipoprotein** layer. The outer membrane acts as a hydrophobic diffusion barrier and consists of:

(a) **Phospholipid,** a bilayer similar to the cytoplasmic membrane with protein channels called **porins** for nutrient transport

(b) **Lipopolysaccharide**

(c) **Protein**

(2) Before nutrients enter the cell, they must enter the **periplasmic space,** an area between the cell wall and the cytoplasmic membrane. It contains a gel of several types of molecules (e.g., hydrolytic enzymes, periplasmic-binding proteins) that process molecules before they enter the cytoplasm. It also contains proteins that act as chemoreceptors for chemotaxis, others that act as carriers of nutrient (similar to carriers in the cytoplasmic membrane), and antibiotic inactivating enzymes.

(3) The **lipopolysaccharide (LPS)** component projects from the cell surface and is both toxic and antigenic **(O antigen)**. In the gram-negative organism, the LPS **blocks diffusion** of low–molecular-weight substances into the cell, so antibiotics and chemicals that attack the cell wall (e.g., lysozyme, penicillin) cannot pass through LPS, also known as gram-negative **endotoxin,** is toxic to humans and is composed of three parts:

(a) **Lipid A:** toxic potion that is released into circulation upon lysis of the cell, causing diarrhea, fever, and septic shock

(b) **Core polysaccharide:** similar within genera

(c) **O-specific side chain:** species specific

2. The **cytoplasmic membrane** is a phospholipid bilayer matrix of a fatty acid core (hydrophobic) and glycerol phosphate backbone (hydrophilic). With the presence of proteins embedded in the matrix, these membranes are actively and passively engaged in several **cellular functions.**

a. Transportation of nutrients through:

(1) Passive diffusion

(2) Facilitated diffusion

(3) Active transport (this method is the only one that actively uses energy)
b. The site of **respiration proteins** used for:
(1) **Electron transport** and energy formation
(2) **Enzymes** involved in the assembly of the cell wall components
(3) **Secretion of exotoxins** and other substances for the breakdown of macromolecules

D. Internal structures

1. **Storage granules** have inclusion bodies of metachromatic granules used for food or energy storage (e.g., polyphosphate complexes, carbohydrate).

2. Some gram-positive organisms have an internal membrane structure called a **mesosome,** which develops from the invagination of the cell membrane.

3. **Ribosomes** are cellular units that synthesize protein by the translation of messenger RNA (mRNA)-base sequences into amino-acid protein sequences. These ribosomes, unlike those in eukaryotic cells, are 70s units and are not enclosed in organelles, such as mitochondria and rough endothelial tissue.

4. The **nuclear region** of bacteria is a condensed area containing the bacterial DNA or genome that lacks a nuclear membrane (a nucleoid) and consists of a long, double-stranded, circular DNA molecule.

5. Some organisms contain **plasmids,** circular double-stranded pieces of DNA that are found outside of the bacterial chromosome. These structures are autonomous (not controlled by the bacterial chromosome), contain information for antibiotic resistance, are conjunctive, and carry genetic elements called **transposons.**

III. MICROBIAL PHYSIOLOGY

A. Nutritional types

1. **Autotrophs** use carbon dioxide as the sole or main carbon source.
   a. **Photoautotrophs** use light as an energy source.
   b. **Chemoautotrophs** oxidize organic or inorganic compounds to produce energy.

2. **Heterotrophs** use organic compounds as their main carbon source.
   a. **Photoheterotrophs** use light as an energy source.
   b. **Chemoheterotrophs** oxidize organic and inorganic compounds to produce energy.

3. **Prototrophs** are parent cells that have no special nutritional requirements. They require the same nutrients as the major number of the natural members of the species.

4. **Auxotrophs** are mutated so that they cannot synthesize the same essential nutrients (usually amino acids) as their parent cell.

5. **Subsets**
   a. **Holophytic:** organisms in which nutrients must be in a soluble, diffusible form
   b. **Holozoic:** organisms that need complex nutrients, often solid materials that are ingested and then broken down
   c. **Saprophytic:** organisms whose nutrients are obtained from dead or decaying organic matter
   d. **Parasitic:** organisms whose nutrients are obtained from and at the expense of a living organism

B. Nutritional requirements. Bacteria use a wide variety of nutrients to obtain energy and to construct new cellular components. There are **six macro elements** that are used as the main components of carbohydrates, lipids, proteins, and nucleic acids. These are carbon, oxygen, hydrogen, nitrogen, phosphorus, and sulfur. There are several minor and trace elements as well as cations that play various roles in the microorganisms.

C. Temperature relations

1. **Psychrophile:** an organism that grows well at 0°C, has optimal growth at 15°C or less, and a maximum growth temperature of 20°C

2. **Mesophile:** an organism with optimal growth at 20°C–45°C; minimum growth temperatures between 15°C and 20°C, and maximum approximately 45°C
3. **Thermophile:** an organism that can grow at 55°C or greater, with a minimum growth temperature of approximately 45°C

D. **Oxygen requirements.** How organisms use oxygen can be a major factor in their classification.

1. **Aerobes** have the ability to grow in the presence of atmospheric oxygen.
   a. **Obligate** aerobes are completely dependent on oxygen for growth and serve as terminal electron acceptors in aerobic respiration.
   b. **Facultative** aerobes have the ability to grow with or without oxygen.
2. **Anaerobes** have the ability to grow without oxygen.
   a. **Obligate** anaerobes do not tolerate oxygen at all and die in its presence.
   b. **Facultative** anaerobes do not require oxygen but grow better in its presence.
3. **Microaerophiles** require oxygen levels below normal.

E. **Bacterial growth curve.** Bacterial growth is defined as an increase in cellular constituents. Because bacteria reproduce by **binary fission,** growth can be plotted as a log of the cell number versus time to produce a curve with four distinct phases.

1. **Lag phase** is a transition period when the bacteria produce necessary enzymes so that they can grow in the new environment.
2. **Logarithmic (log) phase** division occurs at constant and maximal rate, and the cells increase in a geometric progression. The generation time, which varies among species, usually is 15–20 minutes but may be hours.
3. **Stationary phase** is when the growth rate tapers off and growth and death rates are nearly equal. A fairly constant population of viable cells results.
4. **Death phase** describes when the concentration of viable cells decreases at a geometric rate because of the accumulation of toxic wastes.

IV. METABOLISM AND ENERGY PRODUCTION

Microorganisms derive energy from nutrients by a series of chemical reactions in which the energy stored in chemical bonds is transferred to newly formed chemical bonds to provide energy storage in a useful form, such as adenosine triphosphate (ATP).

A. ATP generation

1. **Substrate-level phosphorylation** releases energy through direct transfer of high energy phosphate groups from an intermediate metabolic compound to adenosine diphosphate (ADP). No molecular oxygen or other inorganic final electron acceptor is required.
2. **Oxidative phosphorylation** removes electrons from organic compounds and passes these electrons through a series of electron acceptors along an electron transport chain, with molecular oxygen or some other inorganic compound as the final acceptor.

B. **Fermentation** refers to energy-producing oxidative sequences in which organic compounds serve as both electron donors and acceptors. This process occurs in the absence of external electron acceptors.

1. **Glycolysis** is the first step in fermentation and respiration and causes the oxidation of glucose to pyruvic acid with a yield of two moles of ATP. There are different pathways for glycolysis in microorganisms:
   a. The **Embden-Meyerhof (glycolytic) pathway** is the major pathway.
   b. The **Entner-Doudoroff pathway** is an alternate.
   c. The **hexose monophosphate shunt** used with the glycolytic pathway is an alternative.
2. **Secondary fermentation process.** Many bacteria use pyruvate to oxidize **reduced nicotinamide adenine dinucleotide (NADH)** produced in glycolysis to produce a variety of final products.
   a. **Lactic acid fermentation:** the simplest process in which pyruvate produces lactate *(Lactobacillus, Streptococcus)*

b. **Alcohol fermentation:** pyruvate produces ethanol and carbon dioxide *(Saccharomyces)*
c. **Mixed acid fermentation:** a combination of lactic, formic, and acetic acids is produced with ethanol, hydrogen, and carbon dioxide *(Escherichia coli)*
d. **Butanediol fermentation:** pyruvate *(Enterobacter)* produces acetoin, which is reduced to 2,3-butanediol
e. **Butyric acid fermentation:** produces butanol, isopropanol, and acetone *(Clostridium)*
f. **Propionic acid fermentation:** pyruvate is converted to oxaloacetate with the addition of carbon dioxide, then to propionic acid *(Propionibacterium)*

C. **Respiration** refers to energy-producing oxidative sequences in which inorganic compounds act as the last electron acceptor in a series of reactions. This process includes glycolysis, **tricarboxylic acid (TCA) cycle,** and the **electron transport system,** which yields ATP when coupled with oxidative phosphorylation.

1. **Aerobic respiration:** oxygen serves as the final electron acceptor.
   a. Pyruvate is converted to **acetyl coenzyme A** and carbon dioxide and water through the **TCA cycle.**
   b. The **electron transport system** plays a role in the transport of electrons along a series of carriers, found in the cytoplasmic membrane, each with successively higher oxidation potentials. Major components of the electron transport system include:
      (1) Cytochromes
      (2) Flavoproteins
      (3) Ubiquinones

2. **Anaerobic respiration:** an inorganic electron acceptor other than oxygen (e.g., nitrate, sulfate, carbonate) serves as the terminal electron acceptor.

V. GENETICS

A. **Definition and terms.** The study of what genes are, how they carry information, how they are replicated and passed.

1. **Chromosomes** are bodies that have the DNA cells that contain genetic information. Bacteria have only one chromosome: a single, continuous (closed), double-stranded, circular piece of DNA.
   a. **Duplication** occurs by semiconservative replication in which the two strands of the helix separate **(origin)** and at this point **(replication fork)** new strands are synthesized, with the originals serving as templates.
   b. **Structure.** The cell membrane is attached to the chromosome, and as the cell grows it separates the daughter chromosome. Therefore each daughter cell has one original and one new strand.

2. **Genes** are DNA segments that are processed in two steps to produce various proteins. A normal bacterial cell is **haploid** (has one set of chromosomes).

B. **Regulation and expression of genetic information**

1. **DNA** has many **functions.**
   a. It is **duplicated** for transfer to progeny during cell division.
   b. It is **transcribed** into ribonucleic acid that can be translated into a protein.
   c. It contains **control signals** that ultimately control the synthesis of protein.
   d. It can be **mutated** to result in the alteration of specific characteristics that are encoded by genes.
   e. It can be duplicated and transferred to **other specimens** in processes other than cell division (i.e., conjugal transfer).

2. **DNA replication, transcription,** and **translation** affect cellular growth and development.
   a. Bacterial **replication** involves accurate duplication of chromosomal DNA, which enables the formation of two identical daughter cells.
   b. **Transcription** of information from DNA to RNA is the first of two steps needed to produce necessary proteins. One gene can be transcribed into many copies of RNA.
   c. **Translation** is the processing of genetic information to synthesize proteins. RNA polymerase locates the beginning of the gene, and this area undergoes localized unwinding to allow RNA polymerase to **transcribe** RNA (called **mRNA**) from the DNA template.

Before this transcription is completed, a ribosome will attach to the beginning of the message. The 70s bacterial **ribosome** is composed of two subunits, 30s and 50s. The ribosome **translates** the message into protein by reading the **triplet codon** (three nucleotides) as a specific amino acid. This acid is carried to the site by **transfer RNA (tRNA)** and pairs with the codon by an **anticodon.** Amino acids are joined, and the ribosome moves to the next codon. This continues until the complete protein is synthesized.

3. **Regulation.** The products of cellular growth must be produced in correct proportions for the cell to live and function. The two most common mechanisms of metabolic and genetic regulation are as follows:
   a. **Feedback inhibition** of enzyme activity (metabolic regulation) inhibits the synthesis of the cell growth product.
   b. **Repression** of enzyme activity (genetic regulation) inhibits the synthesis of the enzyme.

C. **Other methods of DNA transfer.** Microorganisms can change their genetic constitution by mechanisms other than cell division. Transfer of genetic material from the donor DNA to the recipient DNA is called **recombination**. Most recombinations occur between homologous segments (those that have similar nucleotide sequences). There are three general mechanisms.

1. **Transformation** involves the recipient cell taking up cell-free, fragmented (i.e., naked) DNA and recombining genetic elements.
   a. This process is **primitive** and occurs within only a few genera.
   b. Requirements include competent recipient cells and a **"leaky" bacterial cell wall** so that DNA can be introduced into the cell.
   c. It is generally associated with **recombinant DNA technology** or **cloning,** a technique to amplify a specific gene in preparation for analysis. However, in this process, the bacterial cell walls are made "leaky" by chemical treatment.
      (1) Cloning involves putting a gene into a plasmid DNA **(vector),** resulting in a 50- to 100-fold amplification of the DNA. All vectors share several common characteristics:
         (a) Typically small, well-characterized molecules of DNA
         (b) Contain at least one replicon and can be replicated within the host even when they contain foreign DNA
         (c) Code for a phenotypic trait that can be used to detect the presence of foreign DNA, which often can be used to distinguish parental from recombinant vectors
      (2) **Selectable markers** are used to find cells that contain these vectors.
      (3) **Plasmids** cannot maintain stability unless they are beneficial to the host, so the plasmid should contain a gene essential for cellular survival: either an enzyme required in a metabolic pathway or a gene that resists certain antibiotics (see II D 5).

2. **Conjugation** is an important means of gene transfer, particularly among gram-negative organisms. This process involves two mating types [the donor **(F^+)** and recipient **(F^-)** cells] and the extrachromosomal piece known as the sex or fertility factor **(F factor)**. The F factor (e.g., F plasmid or episome) is not under the control of the chromosome and can replicate autonomously. Plasmid-mediated exchange of genetic information can only occur through the expression of transfer genes. These genes encoded on the plasmid result in the transfer of a single strand of DNA through the pilus into the recipient cell. The F factor has several genes that code for formation and aid in donor attachment of sex pili. During this process, a copy is made, a single strand is transferred, and the recipient becomes F^+. Along with the F plasmids, there can be R plasmids, which encode for resistance to certain antibiotics. When an F plasmid integrates into the cellular chromosome, the bacterial strain is said to be a **high frequency recombination (Hfr)** strain. During the conjugal transfer involving an Hfr strain, the whole bacterial chromosome may be transferred. Antibiotic resistance genes are often parts of **transposons** (see II C 5), which are responsible for additions, deletions, and inversions of large (4–80 kb) sequences. When different transposons "jump" into transferable plasmids, contagious resistance to multiple antibiotics can occur.

3. **Transduction** is the transfer of genetic material by **bacteriophage** (virus that infect bacteria). These viruses can be classified into two different groups:
   a. **Lytic phages** enter the cell, replicate, and package their DNA and then lyse the cell to release mature infective virus particles.
   b. **Lysogenic (temperate) phages** can enter the cell by one of two ways:
      (1) By the lytic pathway

(2) By integrating into the host DNA and remaining dormant
- **(a)** The viral DNA does not replicate but is integrated into the host genome and is known as **prophage.**
- **b)** The prophage suppresses the lytic state by synthesizing a protein known as a repressor, which protects the cell from further infection by a virus.
- **(c)** Some prophages can change the cell's phenotype **(phage** or **lysogenic conversion),** which allows the organism to elaborate materials (exotoxins or virulence factors) that are detrimental to the host if the organism is pathogenic [e.g., *Corynebacterium diphtheriae* (diphtheria), *Streptococcus pyogenes* (scarlet fever), *Clostridium tetani* (tetanus)].

STUDY QUESTIONS

Directions: Each of the numbered items or incomplete statements in this section is followed by answers or by completions of the statement. Select the **one** lettered answer or completion that is **best** in each case.

1. Cell envelopes of both gram-positive and gram-negative bacteria are composed of complex macromolecules. Which of the following statements describes both types of cell envelopes?

(A) They contain significant amounts of teichoic acid
(B) They contain all the common amino acids
(C) Their antigenic specificity is determined by the polysaccharide O antigen
(D) They form a diffusion barrier to large macromolecules

2. Which of the following descriptions best characterizes sex pili? They

(A) enable DNA transport between bacteria during conjugation
(B) play a role in the adhesion of bacteria to their target cells
(C) are numerous on the bacterial cell surface
(D) are found on both gram-positive and gram-negative organisms

3. The mode of gene transfer in which naked DNA is taken up is called

(A) transformation
(B) transduction
(C) conjugation
(D) cell fusion

4. Bacteria that make either a fermentative or respiratory set of enzymes are known as

(A) obligate anaerobes
(B) obligate aerobes
(C) microaerophiles
(D) facultative organisms

5. Which of the following statements describes plasmids? They

(A) are single-stranded DNA molecules
(B) carry optional genes
(C) carry genes essential for growth
(D) are always found in linear form

6. All of the following statements describe the nuclear body EXCEPT it

(A) is referred to as nucleoid
(B) is free of ribosomes
(C) is composed of ribosomes
(D) lacks a nuclear membrane

7. Bacteria that grow at temperatures as high as 55°C are known as

(A) psychrophiles
(B) thermophiles
(C) mesophiles
(D) auxotrophs

8. Which of the following organisms can use only molecular oxygen as the final acceptor?

(A) Obligate anaerobes
(B) Facultative anaerobes
(C) Obligate aerobes
(D) Strict anaerobes

Directions: Each item below contains four suggested answers of which **one or more** is correct. Choose the answer

A if **I, II, and III** are correct
B if **I** and **III** are correct
C if **II** and **IV** are correct
D if **IV** only is correct

9. Gram-negative and gram-positive cell walls share which of the following characteristics?

I. Peptide cross-links between polysaccharides
II. Hydrolysis by lysozyme
III. Rigid polysaccharide framework
IV. A wide variety of complex lipids

10. A declining growth rate occurs during which of the following phases of bacterial cell growth?

I. Lag phase
II. Exponential phase
III. Stationary phase
IV. Death phase

11. The peptidoglycan layer of a bacterial cell contains

I. tetrapeptide chains
II. *N*-acetylmuramic acid
III. teichoic acid
IV. *N*-acetylglucosamine

ANSWERS AND EXPLANATIONS

1. The answer is D *[II C 1].*
The envelope is composed of the cytoplasmic membrane and the cell wall. The membrane is a diffusion barrier for large macromolecules; the cell wall of gram-positive bacteria is a thick layer of peptidoglycan with a large amount of teichoic acids (surface antigens). The gram-negative bacteria have only a small amount of peptidoglycan, no teichoic acid, and an outer membrane composed of lipoprotein and lipopolysaccharide, of which the polysaccharide comprises the O antigen.

2. The answer is A *[II B 3 b].*
Sex pili are found only on gram-negative organisms and in very small numbers (less than 10). They act as fragile transport tubes for DNA exchange. Common pili are adhesions.

3. The answer is A *[V C 1].*
Of the three methods of DNA transfer, only transformation takes up DNA without an intermediary.

4. The answer is D *[III D 1–2].*
Facultative organisms can grow without air and make either a fermentative or a respiratory set of enzymes, depending on the conditions.

5. The answer is B *[II D 5, V C 1].*
The chromosome carries all of the genes essential for growth, whereas plasmids are extrachromosomal, double-stranded, circular pieces of DNA that carry optional genes that add extra properties.

6. The answer is C *[II D 3].*
Ribosomes are found in the cytoplasm, not in the nucleoid (a long, circular, double-stranded DNA without a nuclear membrane).

7. The answer is B *[III C 1–3].*
Thermophiles grow at 55°C and are found in hot springs and compost piles. Mesophiles grow at approximately 37°C, psychrophiles grow at 15°C and lower, and auxotrophs are mutant organisms.

8. The answer is C *[III D 1–2].*
Obligate aerobes require oxygen and lack an alternative fermentative pathway. Obligate anaerobes are strict anaerobes that cannot live in the presence of oxygen. Facultative anaerobes can use oxygen as the final acceptor or to provide an alternate fermentative pathway.

9. The answer is B (I, II) *[II C 1].*
Peptidoglycan is the basic layer of the cell wall in both gram-positive and gram-negative organisms. It provides a rigid framework that is susceptible to the action of lysozyme. Gram-positive cells are deficient in lipids; however, gram-negative cells are rich in complex lipids (e.g., lipopolysaccharide). Both types of cell walls have cross-links between polysaccharides.

10. The answer is D (IV) *[III E 1–4].*
During the lag phase, the cells prepare for growth, so there is no actual growth. Growth is maximal during the exponential phase and levels out during the stationary phase with no net increase in cell number. There is a decline in organism number during the death phase because there are more organisms dying than being produced.

11. The answer is C (II, IV) *[II C 1].*
The cell wall of both gram-positive and gram-negative organisms is composed of repeating disaccharide units. These units contain *N*-acetylglucosamine and *N*-acetylmuramic acid, to which tetrapeptide chains are cross-linked. Only gram-positive organisms have teichoic acid.

10
Immunology

Gail Goodman-Snitkoff
Vincent C. LoPresti

I. THE PHYSIOLOGY OF THE IMMUNE SYSTEM

A. Immunogens, antigens, and haptens

1. **Immunogens** are chemical compounds that cause a specific immune response.
2. **Antigens** are chemical compounds that are recognized and eliminated by a specific immune response.
3. **Immunogen–antigens.** Compounds associated with or secreted by parasitic bacteria, protozoa, fungi, and viruses, and of molecular weight (mol wt) greater than 5000 daltons may act as both immunogens and antigens.
   a. Molecular complexity is as important as molecular weight in determining the status of a compound as an immunogen. Therefore, proteins, glycoproteins, lipoproteins, and nucleoproteins are the most potent immunogen–antigens.
   b. Drugs of sufficient molecular weight (e.g., insulin) can act as immunogen–antigens. The cells of another individual and the cells of one's own body (see III) can act as immunogen–antigens. Immunogen–antigens can be contacted environmentally (e.g., pollens).
4. **Haptens** are low–molecular-weight compounds that act as immunogens after chemically complexing to a larger molecule or cell surface. After they stimulate the immune system in this complex, these compounds act as antigens in the uncomplexed state, with certain exceptions.
   a. Haptens may be present in the environment (e.g., pentadecyl catechol of poison ivy).
   b. Several types of drugs act as haptens (e.g., penicillin).
5. **Tolerogens** are chemical compounds that elicit specific nonresponsiveness. This specific nonresponsiveness may be caused by the ability of the compound to be broken down by the body or by the route of administration of the compound (e.g., oral administration often causes specific nonresponsiveness).
6. In this chapter, the term antigen is used for compounds and cells that are both immunogens and antigens.

B. Cells of the immune system

1. **B lymphocytes and T lymphocytes** are the primary cells of specific immune responses. All B and T lymphocytes are antigen-specific because they have specific antigen receptors as part of their plasma membranes. In this chapter, the terms **B cell** and **T cell** are used instead of B lymphocyte and T lymphocyte.
2. **Antigen receptors of B cells** are antibody molecules.
   a. B cells have thousands of identical antibodies in their membranes that allow them to bind chemically to a small group of chemically related antigens. This group defines the antigen specificity of each B cell. Different B cells have different antigen specificities, but each B cell has only one specificity. B cells recognize specific antigens and divide to form new B cells (**memory B cells**) and **plasma cells (antibody-forming cells),** which secrete free, soluble (humoral) antibody molecules into extracellular fluids.
   b. Virgin B cells have never responded to an antigen since their release into the circulation from bone marrow. Their membrane antibodies are of the immunoglobulin M and D (IgM, IgD) classes (see I D).

c. **Memory B cells** are derived by cell division from another B cell that has responded to an antigen. Their membrane antibodies are of immunoglobulin classes A, E, or G (IgA, IgE, IgG; see I D).

3. **Antigen receptors of T cells** have two membrane proteins (α and β or γ and δ) that define the antigen specificity of each T cell and several other integral membrane proteins known as the **CD3 complex.** Therefore, T cells are **CD3+**. Each T cell has thousands of identical antigen receptors in its membrane. Different T cells of different antigen specificities differ in the conformation of their antigen receptors.
   a. **Major histocompatibility complex (MHC) proteins.** The antigen receptors of T cells do not chemically recognize antigens alone. Rather, they normally recognize **C peptide epitopes** (fragments of antigen) that are chemically combined with MHC proteins on the surface of other body cells (Figure 10-1). MHC proteins are divided into **two major classes:**
      (1) **Class I proteins,** which are present on the surfaces of almost all body cells
      (2) **Class II proteins,** which are present only on the surfaces of special **antigen-presenting cells (APCs).**
   b. **Thymus gland.** T cells do not enter the circulation directly from bone marrow, but first enter the thymus gland to mature. Most T cells die in the thymus. These cells either do not recognize normal self-antigens or produce a response against normal self-antigens.
      (1) T cells that are released from the thymus into the circulation are **virgin T cells.**
      (2) T cells that originate through cell division from the responses of other T cells are **memory T cells.**
   c. **Glycoproteins.** Most T cells can be classified by the presence of a membrane glycoprotein known as **CD4,** the **helper,** or **T_H, group,** or the presence of **CD8,** the **cytotoxic T lymphocyte (CTL) group.** There also may be a group of **suppressor T cells,** or **T_S**. These cells also belong to the CD8 group.
      (1) T_H cells are primarily responsible for regulating the responses of B cells, CTL cells, macrophages, and other cells through secreting compounds known as **lymphokines.** CTL cells directly kill self-cells that are infected by viruses. This process is known as

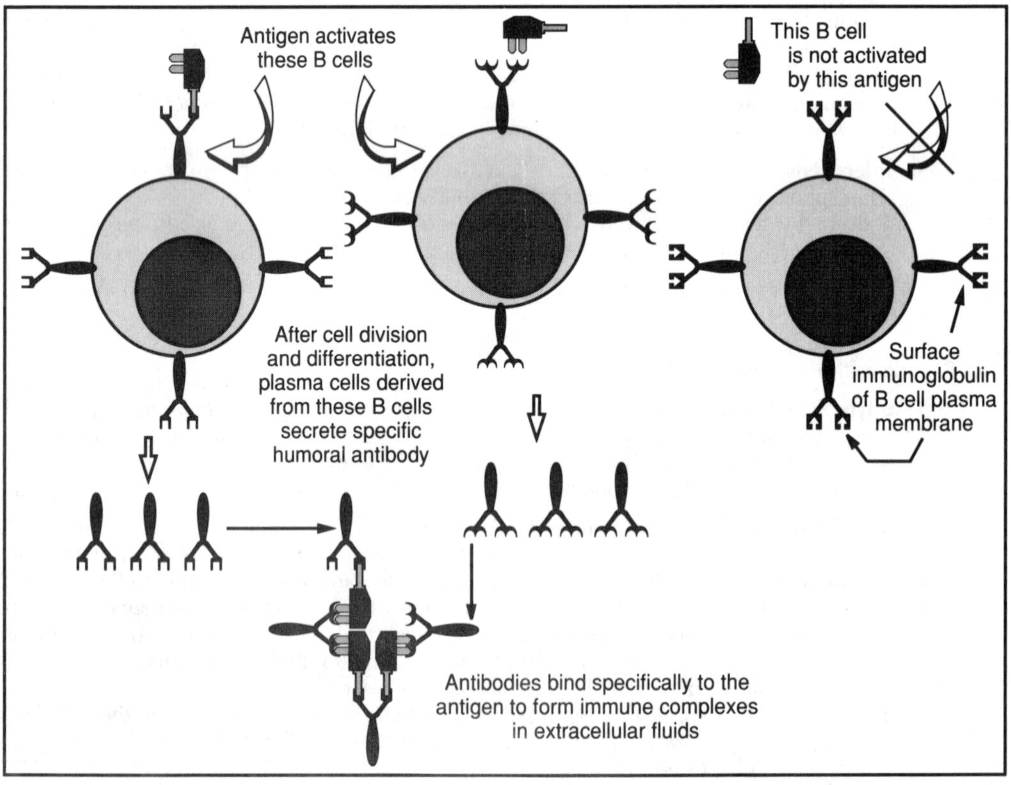

Figure 10-1. B cells: antigen specificity and activation.

cytotoxicity. CTL cells also secrete lymphokines, small proteins that are usually secreted paracrinely.

(2) Lymphokines are part of a larger network of regulatory **cytokines.** This network includes secretions of other cell types in addition to those of lymphocytes. Table 10-1 lists the sources and actions of important cytokines that regulate the immune system and inflammation.

4. **Natural killer (NK) cells** are large, granular lymphocytes without a specific T- or B-cell antigen receptor. Their cytotoxicity appears to be similar to that of CTL cells. NK cells recognize and destroy tumors.

5. **APCs** are essential for most immune responses and define the sites at which these responses originate.
   a. The best understood APCs are the macrophages and **fixed macrophages of the lymph nodes, spleen, and other lymphoid tissue.** These cells include follicular dendritic cells and interdigitating cells. Most immune responses within these organs begin when these cells present epitopes bound to their surface MHC class II molecules to T_H (see Figure 10-1) and secrete cytokines as accessory signals.
   b. Any body cell can act as an APC for a subset of immune responses involving CTL cells. Body cells can present fragments of antigens bound to their surface MHC class I molecules to CTL (CD8) lymphocytes.

Table 10-1. Major Cytokines and Their Actions

Cytokine	Sources of Secretion*	Major Actions
IL-1	Macrophages, antigen-presenting cells, others	T- and B-cell activation, pyrogenic, proinflammatory
TNF-α, TNF-β	Macrophages, T_H cells	Similar to IL-1, but including cytotoxicity
IL-2	T_H cells	T-, B-, and natural killer (NK)-cell activation
IFN-γ	T_H cells	Induction of major histocompatibility complex (MHC), activation of macrophages and NK cells, formation of memory B cells, antiviral
IFN-α, IFN-β	Leukocytes, fibroblasts	Induction of MHC, antiviral and growth inhibition
IL-3	Macrophages, T_H cells	Proliferation of multilineage marrow stem cells
IL-4	T_H cells	B-cell activation and memory B-cell formation, increased mast cell precursors, activation of mast cells
IL-5	T_H cells	Memory B-cell formation, eosinophil production
IL-6	T_H cell, other types	Plasma cell maturation, others similar to IL-1
IL-7	Bone marrow stroma	Lymphocyte maturation
IL-8	T_H cells, macrophages, endothelial cells	Neutrophil activation
IL-9	T_H cells	Proliferation and differentiation of bone marrow cells and thymocytes
IL-10	Macrophages, T_H cells CD8$^+$ T cells, B cells	Increased humoral (antibody), immunity decreased cell-mediated immunity, mast cell growth
IL-11	Bone marrow stroma	Proliferation and differentiation of bone marrow cells and thrombocytes
IL-12	Macrophages, B cells	Promotion of cell-mediated immunity, activation of Tc and NK cells, suppression of humoral immunity
IL-13	T_H cells	IL-4–like effects on B cells, inhibition of production of inflammatory cytokines by monocytes
IL-14	T_H cells	Important for the generation of B memory cells
IL-15	Endothelial cells, epithelial monocytes, muscle cells	IL-2–like effects
GM-CSF	T_H cells, macrophages	Marrow proliferation of myeloid precursors
G-CSF	Fibroblasts, endothelial cells	Proliferation and survival of neutrophil precursors
M-CSF	Fibroblasts, endothelial cells	Survival of monocyte–macrophages

GM-CSF = granulocyte macrophage colony-stimulating factor; IFN = interferon; IL = interleukin; TNF = tumor necrosis factor.

*Not all sources are listed.

c. Both T and B cells continually circulate through the lymph nodes, spleen, and other lymphoid tissue. If their specific antigen is present, an immune response can begin.

6. **Neutrophils, monocyte–macrophages, eosinophils, basophils, platelets,** and **mast cells** assist in eliminating antigens from the body. Their functions may be phagocytic, proinflammatory, cytotoxic, or regulatory.

C. Humoral immunity: primary and memory responses that produce antibodies

1. **Overview.** In most humoral immune responses, antigens are recognized by specific B cells and T_H cells. The T_H cells secrete cytokines, and B and T_H cells divide to increase their cell numbers. Non–antigen-specific B and T_H cells do not respond. Responding B cells produce both memory B cells and plasma cells (Figure 10-2). T_H cells are not involved in some humoral immune responses (e.g., to certain polysaccharide antigens) **[T-independent responses]**. B cells respond alone, producing plasma cells that secrete IgM antibodies, but no memory B cells.

2. **Primary immune response.** The first time a specific antigen is encountered, only **virgin B cells** and T_H cells are present to respond to the antigen. These cells produce plasma cells that secrete IgM antibody and memory cells that produce the other classes of antibody in later immune responses. The primary immune response is detected after 4 days and peaks in 7–11 days. IgM is produced first, followed by IgG.

3. **Memory immune responses.** The second or subsequent encounter with the same antigen or a closely related antigen produces responses by memory B cells and memory T_H cells. These responses are more rapid because more antigen-specific B and T cells are involved. Most antibody produced is IgG, with smaller amounts of IgA and IgE. Significant amounts of antibodies are produced as rapidly as 2–3 days after the entry of antigen, and the absolute amount of antibody (measured in milligrams per deciliter of serum) is greater than in primary immune responses. The duration of memory varies among antigens and probably among individuals. Some, but not all, memory is lifelong.

4. **Major roles of antibodies**

   a. The first function of an antibody is to act as an **antigen receptor** for B cells so that the B cells can recognize and respond to antigens.

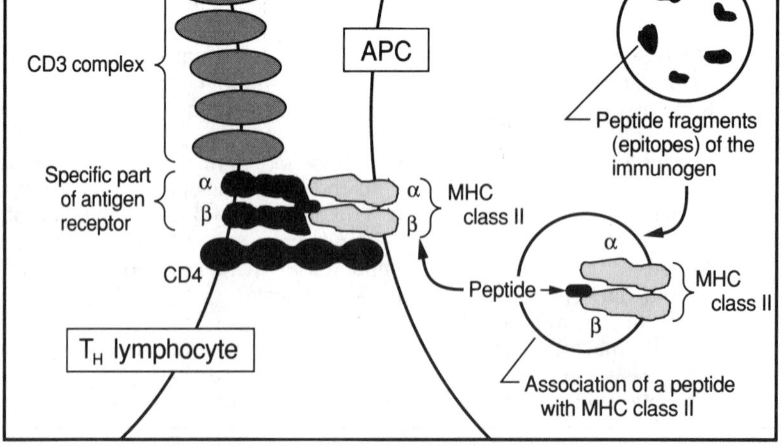

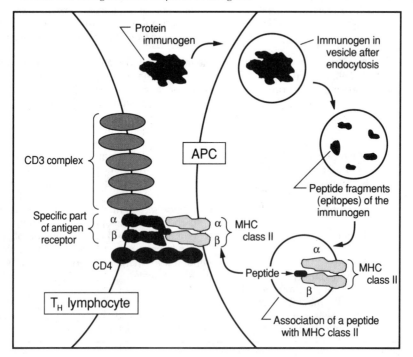

Figure 10-2. Helper T-cell antigen recognition.

b. The second function of an antibody is to aid in the **elimination of antigen.** Elimination occurs through nonspecific functions, such as phagocytosis or complement activation. The mechanism of elimination depends on the class of antibody involved.

c. The third function of an antibody is **neutralization of toxins.** Neutralization occurs when an antibody binds to the toxin and prevents it from reaching the target organ.

D. Immunoglobulins: antigen-binding and class-specific functions. The terms antibody and immunoglobulin are used interchangeably.

1. Structure. The standard immunoglobulin unit has four polypeptide chains: two identical light polypeptide chains and two identical heavy polypeptide chains. The structure is represented as H_2L_2. Each chain can be divided into a **C-terminal constant** region and an **N-terminal variable region** of amino acids (Figure 10-3). The N-terminal variable region formed from the H and L variable domains is responsible for antigen binding by the immunoglobulin. The C-terminal constant regions of the H chain determine the class of the immunoglobulin.

2. Class. There are five general heavy-chain, constant region amino acid sequences. These determine the **five general classes of immunoglobulins: IgM, IgG, IgE, IgA,** and **IgD.** Within some classes, variants of the heavy-chain sequence yield subclasses: IgM1, IgM2, IgG1–4, IgA1, and IgA2. The class of an immunoglobulin defines its nonspecific antigen elimination or inflammatory function. These functions are activated only after immune complexes are formed, not in unbound antibodies.

a. IgM is the first immunoglobulin secreted during primary responses. It plays a minor role in memory responses. It does not leave the blood in significant amounts because of its

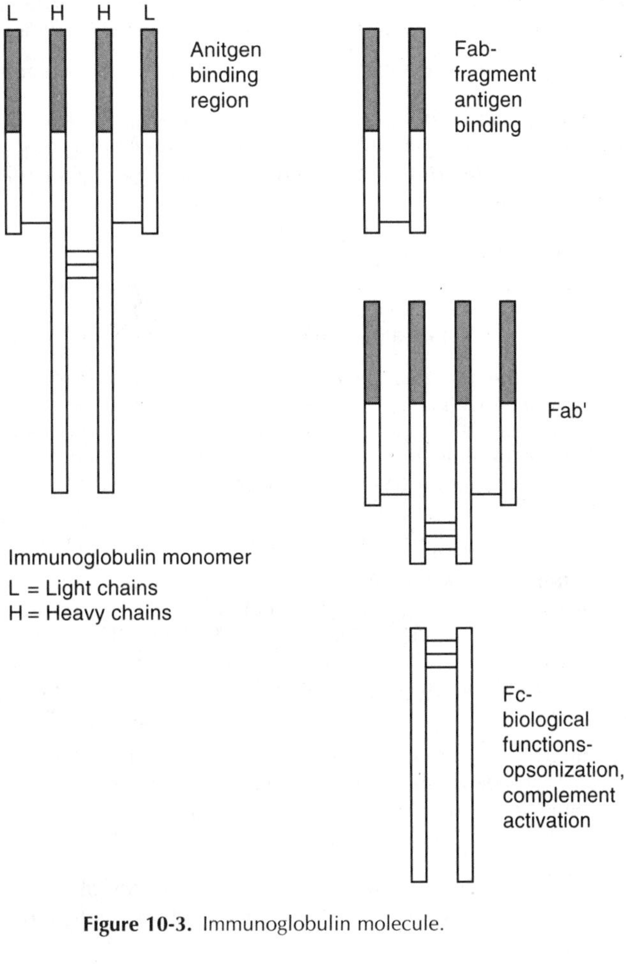

Figure 10-3. Immunoglobulin molecule.

large size (mol wt 900,000 daltons). It accounts for approximately 20% of the adult serum immunoglobulin. IgM **activates the complement system** (see I E 2). Its serum half-life is 9–11 days.

b. **IgG** is the predominant immunoglobulin secreted during memory responses and may also be secreted late during a primary response. It can diffuse from blood into other extracellular fluids, particularly in inflamed microvasculature, and it crosses the placenta to enter the fetal circulation. It accounts for approximately 70% of adult serum immunoglobulin. It **opsonizes antigens** for **phagocytosis** and **activates the complement system.** Its serum half-life is 25–35 days.

c. **IgE** is secreted during memory responses and may also be secreted late during a primary response. It normally accounts for less than 1% of serum immunoglobulin. It **binds to IgE receptors located on the cell surfaces of blood basophils and on connective tissue mast cells** to trigger the secretion of inflammatory mediators from these cells in the presence of specific antigens. Its serum half-life is 2–3 days, but its mast cell-bound half-life is several months.

d. **IgA** is secreted during memory responses and may also be secreted late during a primary response. It accounts for 10% of serum immunoglobulin. It is **secreted across mucosal surfaces into gastrointestinal, respiratory, lacrimal, mammary, and genitourinary secretions, where it protects mucosal colonization** by bacteria and other microorganisms. Its serum half-life is approximately 5 days.

e. **IgD** accounts for less than 1% of serum immunoglobulin and has no known function as a secreted immunoglobulin.

3. **Specificity.** The specificity of each immunoglobulin for antigen binding resides in the two identical antigen-binding sites, each formed by the combination of the variable regions of heavy and light chains. Secreted IgM antibodies have ten identical antigen-binding sites through the combination of five H_2L_2 units with a joining polypeptide chain to form a pentamer. Likewise, IgA typically exists as a dimer with four binding sites.

4. **Quantitation of immunoglobulin: antigen-binding and cross-reactivity.** The immune system forms 10^8 to 10^{11} specificities of immunoglobulin.

   a. Each immunoglobulin specificity can bind to several different, but structurally related, antigens. This ability illustrates the phenomenon of cross-reactivity of a single antibody for multiple antigens. Each immunoglobulin–antigen interaction is quantitated by its **association constant (K_a)**.

   b. Cross-reactivity may also occur through the sharing of some, but not all, antigens by two strains of bacteria, viruses, or other microorganisms.

   c. Because each microorganism has several antigens, each elicits the production of multiple antibody specificities by the immune system. This combination of antibodies is known as a **polyclonal antiserum** and defines the serotype of the immunizing organism.

5. **Fragments of immunoglobulin for clinical use.** Immunoglobulins can be enzymatically cleaved into fragments [e.g., **Fab** and **$F(ab')_2$** (antigen-binding fragments), **Fc** (crystallizable fragment), **Fv** (variable region fragment)]. Fab and $F(ab')_2$ fragments are clinically useful because they retain antigen specificity, but not class-specific (e.g., inflammatory) functions, and are readily excreted renally. Conversely, this characteristic limits their effectiveness.

E. Antigen elimination and acute inflammatory mechanisms of humoral immunity

1. **Opsonization** is the preparation of any extracellular fluid antigen for phagocytosis through the formation of immune complexes. Neutrophils and monocyte–macrophages have a variety of receptors for the constant region of IgG antibodies, which bind immune complexes when the complexes are sufficiently large. This binding triggers phagocytosis of the immune complex and activates the metabolism of the phagocyte, shifting it toward the production of bactericidal oxygen radicals (e.g., superoxide anion, hydrogen peroxide).

2. **Complement** is a group of approximately 20 serum proteins that, when activated, form a proteolytic cascade similar to the clotting and fibrinolytic sequences. Of these, certain proteins inhibit activation. Complement is responsible for increasing the inflammatory response, phagocytosis of antigen, lysis of cells (usually pathogens), and clearance of immune complexes.

   a. In the **classic activation pathway,** immune complexes of IgM or IgG antibodies bind subunits of complement component I (C1) and trigger an initial series of proteolytic cleavages.

b. In the **alternative activation pathway,** the cell walls of certain microorganisms (e.g., gram-negative bacteria) trigger a similar sequence of cleavages that overcome normal inhibitory controls.
c. Certain complement proteins provide opsonization in addition to that provided by IgG in immune complexes.
d. **Pro-inflammatory fragments** of certain complement proteins act both by **direct activity on the microvasculature,** promoting arteriole dilation and increased vascular permeability, and by triggering the release of histamine and other pro-inflammatory mediators from mast cells and basophils.
e. A complex of complement proteins known as the **membrane attack complex (MAC)** can insert into any lipid bilayer membrane, forming a large channel through which ions and water diffuse. Many bacteria, enveloped viruses, and some human or mammalian cells are subject to this osmotic lysis.

3. **Circulating basophils and connective tissue mast cells** are mainly pro-inflammatory cells that rapidly initiate acute inflammation. Triggers of secretion include mechanical and thermal trauma and the immunologic triggers, complement and IgE.
   a. **IgE antibodies,** regardless of antigen specificity, equilibrate between serum and binding noncovalently to high-affinity IgE receptors on mast cell and basophil surfaces. This activity arms the mast cells and basophils, but the triggering of secretion requires that antigen bind to and cross-link antigen-specific IgE molecules already affixed to their receptors.
   b. Mast cells and basophils, when triggered, immediately secrete the contents of their storage granules, including histamine, proteases, and chemotactic proteins for neutrophils and eosinophils. In addition, activation of phospholipase A_2 releases arachidonic acid from membrane phospholipids and results in the synthesis of various leukotrienes, prostaglandins, and thromboxanes. The primary effects of these mediators are:
      (1) Arteriole dilation
      (2) Increased vascular permeability
      (3) Contraction of respiratory and gastrointestinal smooth muscle
      (4) Neutrophil and eosinophil chemotaxis

4. **Antibody-dependent cell-mediated cytotoxicity** is mediated by cells with cytotoxic potential as well as receptors for IgG. These cells, NK cells, macrophages, and some Tc cells bind to and lyse target cells coated with IgG.

5. **Acute inflammation** causes increased ease of movement of crucial components of the blood into the tissues, including phagocytes, particularly neutrophils, IgG antibodies, complement, clotting proteins, and kinins. The adaptive result is the isolation and removal of invading microorganisms and necrotic tissues, followed by tissue repair and regeneration.

F. **Cell-mediated immunity** responses are those in which **antibody is not involved in the elimination of antigen.**

1. **Nonviral intracellular parasites** of monocyte–macrophages, such as *Mycobacteria, Listeria,* and certain protozoa, are primarily eliminated by T-cell–macrophage immunity. $CD4^+$ T cells recognize infected macrophages and secrete lymphokines, particularly interferon- γ (IFN-γ). These lymphokines activate macrophages to produce more bactericidal oxygen radicals (e.g., superoxide anion, hydrogen peroxide). The lymphokines also increase the secretory function of the macrophages and inhibit phagocytosis, enabling the macrophages to kill the parasites in the **extracellular** environment.

2. **Viruses** must be eliminated from both extracellular sites and infected cells.
   a. **Antibodies** opsonize virus particles in blood and tissue fluids for phagocytosis, but antibodies are generally ineffective against infected cells.
   b. **CTL cells** recognize infected cells and directly kill them in an antigen-specific manner, secreting lymphokines, such as tumor necrosis factor-β (TNF-β). Often, the cells are killed before infectious virus particles are assembled. When killed cells release infectious viral particles, they may be opsonized by an antibody. Cell-mediated immunity and humoral immunity must function in concert to provide optimal antiviral defenses.
   c. **NK cells** are believed to kill infected (and tumor) cells in a non–antigen-specific manner.
   d. **IFN-γ,** secreted by CTL, NK, and T_H cells, and **IFN-α** and **IFN-β,** secreted by macrophages and other cells, provide additional antiviral immunity by binding to

receptors on other cells and inducing synthesis of kinases and endonucleases (i.e., antiviral proteins) that inhibit viral and cellular growth. Interferons also upregulate MHC proteins, which make infected cells more visible to CTL cells.

3. **Tumors** are modified host cells and must be eliminated by the immune system, usually by cell-mediated immunity.
   a. **NK cells** are primarily responsible for killing tumor cells. They may act through a nonspecific mechanism or by **antibody-dependent cell-mediated cytotoxicity.**
   b. **CTL cells** recognize tumor cells in an antigen-specific manner and kill them by secreting lymphokines, such as TNF-β.
   c. **Macrophages** also kill tumor cells in a nonspecific manner through the release of TNF-α.

4. **Graft rejection** (see V)

II. HYPERSENSITIVITY REACTIONS

II. HYPERSENSITIVITY REACTIONS describe **exaggerated, inappropriate,** or **prolonged immune responses that cause tissue damage** (Figure 10-4). Four types of hypersensitivity reactions are recognized, primarily on the basis of the mechanisms of pathogenesis. Many etiologies are included within each type. **Allergens** are broadly defined as antigens or haptens that induce hypersensitivity reactions.

A. IgE-mediated type I hypersensitivity reaction

1. A type I hypersensitivity reaction is caused by **inappropriate hypersecretion of IgE** to specific allergens, plus auxiliary factors such as increased mucosal permeability to allergens (e.g., SO_2, NO_x, diesel fumes). The **tendency to hypersecrete IgE is inheritable;** a child's probability of being a hypersecretor is 50% with one hypersecretor parent and 75% with two hypersecretor parents. These individuals are atopic.
   a. IgE is produced locally on nonsystemic exposure to an antigen.
      (1) In normosecretors (1–10 μg/dl), arming of local mast cells occurs (see I B 6).
      (2) In hypersecretors (typically 100 μg–1 mg/dl), IgE spillover occurs, arming basophils and nonlocal mast cells and causing increased occupancy of mast cell and basophil IgE receptors by IgE.
   b. Because there is a lag period for IgE synthesis and cell arming, a type I reaction usually does not occur on the first (or first seasonal) exposure to a specific allergen.

2. **Common allergens**
   a. **Respiratory allergens** include pollens of various plants (e.g., ragweed, grasses, trees), fungi, animal fur, carpet mites, and other shed allergens.
   b. **Gastrointestinal allergens** include dairy products, shellfish, soybeans, and peanuts.
   c. **Skin and mouth allergens** include topically applied drugs (e.g., procaine).
   d. **Intravenous allergens** include insect venoms and drugs that act as cell or plasma protein–bound haptens (e.g., penicillin, cephalosporins, vaccines). These drugs may cause type II or III hypersensitivity reactions in people who do not hypersecrete IgE in response to these drugs.

3. **Activation of mast cell and basophil secretion** by an allergen requires two or more receptor-bound IgE molecules to be cross-linked by a specific allergen. Hapten-sized drugs that provoke this reaction both sensitize the immune system and trigger mast cells bound to a larger molecule (e.g., a protein). Activation leads to an increase in cytoplasmic calcium ion (Ca^{2+}), probably as a result of the second messengers produced by phospholipase C. A transient increase in the cyclic adenosine monophosphate (cAMP) level occurs, followed by an increase in the level of cyclic guanosine monophosphate (cGMP) relative to cAMP. Prolonged increases in cAMP levels inhibit mast cell activation. Immediate secretion of stored inflammatory mediators and activation of phospholipase A_2 follow.

4. **Effects of mediators secreted from mast cells and basophils**
   a. Vasodilation and increased capillary permeability are caused by histamine; the leukotrienes C4, D4, and E4; and prostaglandin D_2 (PGD_2) secreted by mast cells.
   b. Gastrointestinal and respiratory smooth muscle constriction is caused primarily by the leukotrienes C4, D4, and E4; PGD_2; and platelet-activating factor secreted by mast cells and other leukocytes.
   c. Eosinophil and neutrophil infiltration is caused by chemotactic factors secreted by mast cells.

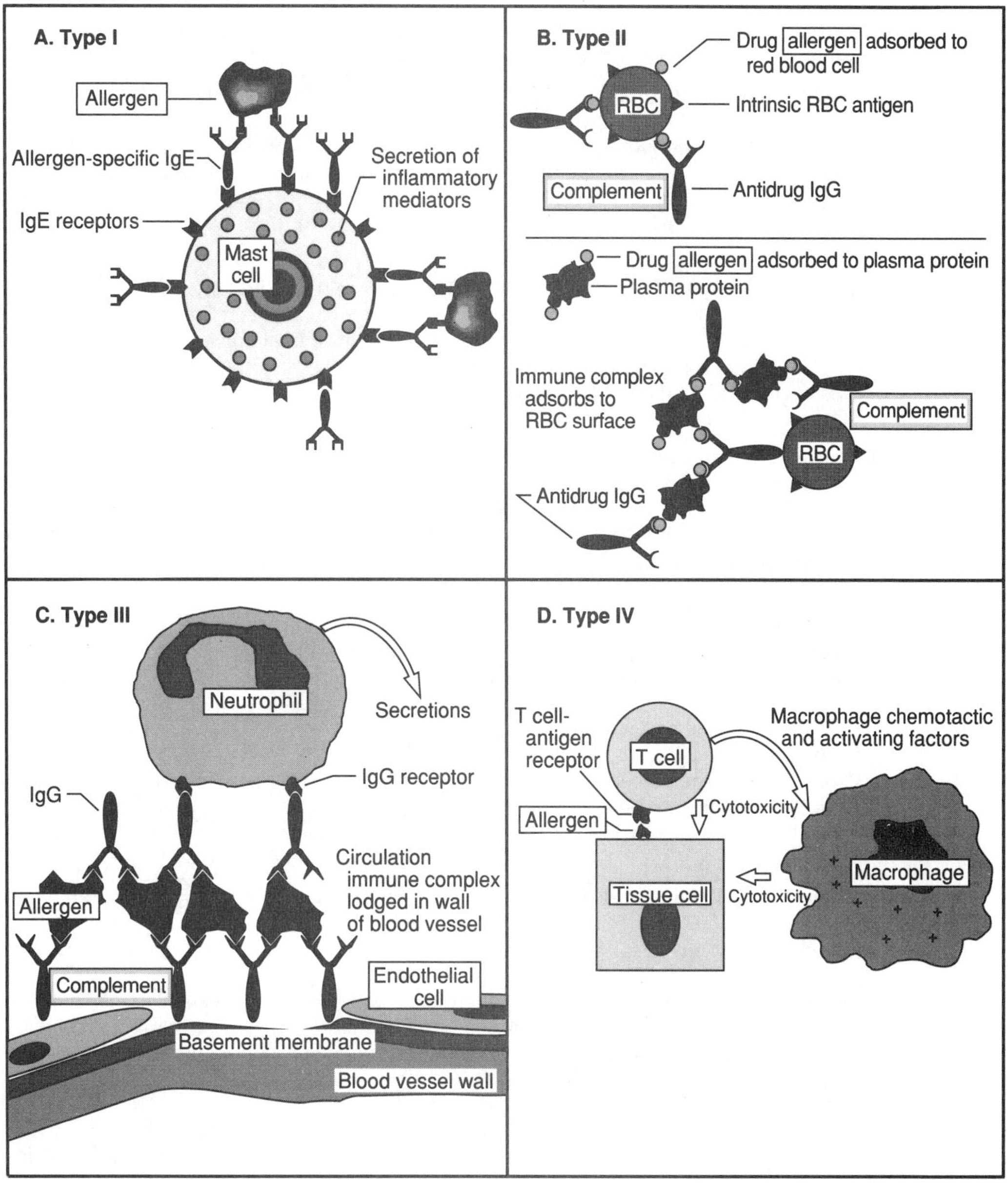

Figure 10-4. The four main types of hypersensitivity reactions.

5. **Local symptoms of pathogenesis** include inflammation of the upper (rhinitis) and lower respiratory tract, gastrointestinal tract, and skin.
   a. Common clinical symptoms include urticaria, pruritus (itching), nasal congestion, bronchoconstriction, mucus and lacrimal hypersecretion, laryngeal edema, vomiting, and diarrhea.
   b. Symptoms may be confined to the portal of allergen entry (e.g., respiratory allergen: respiratory symptoms) or may be more widespread as a result of allergen spillover into the circulation (e.g., food allergen: gastrointestinal, skin, respiratory symptoms).
   c. **Atopic dermatitis** typically includes severe pruritic dermatitis, rhinitis or asthma, food allergies, and changes in the cell-mediated immune system.
   d. The local introduction of allergen sometimes leads to anaphylaxis.

e. Approximately 50% of patients with asthma hypersecrete IgE. This tendency is probably contributory, but ancillary, to the underlying bronchial hyperreactivity present in these patients (see Chapter 48).

6. **Systemic anaphylactic manifestations of pathogenesis.** Intravenous allergen (e.g., bee venom) administered to a sensitized individual causes systemic edema and hypovolemic shock, with cardiac arrhythmia, asphyxiation as a result of bronchoconstriction and mucus hypersecretion, and urticaria. Death usually occurs because of asphyxiation. In some individuals, intravenous drug allergens (e.g., penicillin) cause only mild local symptoms. These differences suggest that there is a continuum of IgE secretion, from normosecretion to hypersecretion.

7. **Time course.** The reaction has two phases. The **early reaction** begins within 1–2 minutes, peaking 1–2 hours after allergen contact, as a result of mediator secretion by mast cells. The **late-phase reaction** begins 3–12 hours after contact with the allergen and lasts for several hours. The late-phase reaction is characterized by increased numbers of eosinophils. Late-phase reactions are initiated by immediate hypersensitivity reactions, but maintained by eosinophil-derived products.

8. **Diagnosis.** In scratch tests, a variety of allergens are injected intradermally to screen for the presence of a wheal and flare (i.e., edema, erythema) response in the skin. **Radioallergosorbent (RAST)** and **radioimmunosorbent (RIST) assays** are radiolabeled tests that detect serum IgE concentrations. The results of these tests do not always agree with each other or with the clinical manifestations.

9. **Prophylaxis**
   a. Identifying and avoiding allergens is the most important measure.
   b. **Hyposensitization** is performed by injecting increasing weekly doses of allergen subcutaneously and later by administering monthly maintenance injections. The best outcome is to elicit decreased allergen-specific IgE synthesis and increased allergen-specific IgG synthesis. IgG binds entering allergen and prevents it from binding to basophil-bound IgE.
   c. Cromolyn sodium (cromoglycate) is a locally administered inhibitor of mast cell activation. Glucocorticoids block the late phase of the response, but have less effect on the early phase.

10. **Therapy**
    a. **Competitive H_1** antagonists of histamine are useful in local forms, but do not completely reverse inflammation because histamine is not the only inflammatory mediator. They have little effect on anaphylaxis. Baths, creams, and corticosteroid ointments are used to treat dermatitis.
    b. **Epinephrine** reverses anaphylaxis through its α- and β-agonist effects. Patients with systemic allergies are given epinephrine self-administration kits. β_2-Agonists (e.g., albuterol) promote bronchodilation, and α_1-agonists (e.g., phenylpropanolamine) decrease nasal congestion.

B. **Non–IgE-mediated type I hypersensitivity reactions.** These reactions are probably of several types, most poorly understood, and sometimes referred to as **anaphylactoid reactions.** The following factors may contribute to and exacerbate non–IgE-mediated type I reactions:

1. Respiratory β_2-receptor unresponsiveness, which leads to a diminished bronchodilatory effect of the sympathetic nervous system

2. Hyperreactivity of mast cells through H_2-receptor unresponsiveness, which decreases negative feedback by histamine on the activation of mast cells

C. **Type II hypersensitivity reactions**

1. **Pathogenesis.** Antibody-mediated cytotoxicity occurs through the production of IgM or IgG, which forms immune complexes that bind to their specific allergens located on cell surfaces.
   a. These allergens may be intrinsic cell surface components or extrinsic compounds adsorbed to the cell surface.
   b. Cytotoxicity may result from activation of complement, phagocytosis of the IgG- or IgM-opsonized cell, or both.

c. A third cytotoxic mechanism, known as antibody-dependent, cell-mediated cytotoxicity, involves the direct killing of antibody-coated cells by macrophages, eosinophils, or NK cells.
d. Type II reactions may become anaphylactic if enough complement is activated. However, they usually do not.

2. **Common allergens.** These subtypes of type II reactions have diverse causes. Only the pathogenic mechanism is common to all of them.
   a. Foreign blood cell surface antigens (allergens) produce **transfusion mismatches** or **Rh disease.**
   b. **Drug allergens** (or drug metabolite allergens) acting as haptens are the **leading cause of hemolytic anemia.**
      (1) These allergens may directly adsorb to blood cell surfaces and be specifically bound by antibodies (e.g., penicillins, cephalosporins, quinidine).
      (2) Alternatively, they may form serum-phase immune complexes, which adsorb nonspecifically to blood cell surfaces as "innocent bystanders" (e.g., rifampin, sulfonamides, chlorpromazine).
   c. **Certain autoimmunities** in which the allergens are self-antigens (e.g., Hashimoto's thyroiditis, myasthenia gravis, autoimmune hemolytic anemia; see III). Autoimmune hemolytic anemia is sometimes associated with the administration of α-methyldopa, which causes autoantibodies against the red blood cell surface.
   d. **Hyperacute rejection** of renal cardiac grafts (see V)

3. **Chemical mediators.** Complement proteins produce cytotoxicity and inflammation and stimulate **macrophages and granulocyte** secretions, which enhance inflammation.

4. **Clinical symptoms** depend on the subtype (see II C 2). Hemolytic anemia and thrombocytopenia are the main symptoms of reactions that involve blood cells. In autoimmune varieties, symptoms depend on the cell type damaged by cytotoxicity. In hyperacute graft rejection, the transplanted tissue does not successfully perfuse because of antibody-mediated cytotoxicity to its vasculature.

5. **Time course**
   a. In the first sensitization to a drug allergen, blood cell lysis and inflammation begin 7–10 days after the initiation of drug therapy. The second exposure to the drug causes symptoms within 3 days.
   b. **Transfusion mismatch.** Hemolysis begins 1–2 hours after transfusion. Peak effects occur after approximately 12 hours.
   c. **Rh disease** does not usually occur in the first RhD^+ pregnancy of an RhD^- mother. In second and subsequent pregnancies, maternal IgG is produced, usually as a result of the mother's sensitization to the RhD antigen by transplacental fetal red blood cells. This sensitization usually occurs near the end of the third trimester. Maternal anti-RhD IgG crosses the placenta, binds to fetal red blood cells, and activates the fetal complement system prenatally, leading to perinatal hemolytic anemia.

6. **Prophylaxis and therapy.** In drug-induced hypersensitivity reactions, withdrawing the drug usually reverses the effect. Preventing recontact is the best prophylaxis. In Rh disease, anti-RhD IgG is administered to the Rh^- mother within 72 hours postpartum for each Rh^+ delivery. The simplest mechanism of action is that this passive immunization (see VI B) binds fetal red blood cells in the maternal circulation and prevents sensitization of the maternal immune system.

D. **Type III hypersensitivity reactions** involve the persistence of immune complexes in the circulation or at local tissue sites when they are not removed after specific antibodies are formed. The subtypes of type III hypersensitivity have diverse causes, and only the pathogenic mechanism is common to all of them.

1. **Pathogenesis.** Immune complexes activate complement, cause inflammation, and induce positive chemotaxis in neutrophils. Persistence of immune complexes may be caused by:
   a. A **high concentration of antigen,** which leads to a disparity in the molar ratio of antigen to antibody. Hyposecretion of antibodies can also produce this type of reaction.
   b. **Chronic formation of immune complexes** in the circulation as a result of **persistence of antigen**

c. Other factors that cause insoluble immune complexes to form and precipitate intravascularly or on basement membranes

2. **Common allergens**
   a. **Self-antigens in most non–organ-specific** (rheumatologic) **autoimmune disorders** (e.g., systemic lupus erythematosus, rheumatoid arthritis)
   b. **Bacterial or protozoan antigens in persistent or chronic infections** and in the initial stages of viremia of certain viral infections [e.g., prodrome of hepatitis B virus (HBV) infection]
   c. **Drugs** (e.g., penicillin, sulfonamides, thiouracil)
   d. **Serum sickness.** Passive immunization with antisera from other species (e.g., horse)
   e. **Fungal and bacterial spores** in the local respiratory form of the reaction

3. **Chemical mediators. Complement proteins** cause inflammation and **stimulate mast cell and basophil secretions,** which enhance inflammation. The increased vascular permeability allows immune complexes to leave the circulation and affix to the basement membrane underlying the endothelial lining of blood vessels. The kidney glomerulus and certain small arteries are particularly susceptible. Complement and mast cell proteins attract neutrophils, which phagocytose immune complexes and release enzymes that damage local tissue and intensify inflammation. Platelets aggregate, and microthrombi may form.

4. **Clinical symptoms** depend on the severity and systemic or local nature of immune complex persistence and deposition.
   a. The first symptoms of systemic reactions are lymphadenopathy, splenomegaly, fever, and rash, which are common in drug- and viremia-induced type III reactions.
   b. More serious symptoms include vasculitis and glomerulonephritis, both of which may become necrotizing. These symptoms often occur with systemic lupus erythematosus (SLE). Arthralgia and arthritis occur in both systemic and local types.
   c. The most common local types are hypersensitivity pneumonitis to inhaled fungi and bacteria to which the patient is occupationally exposed (e.g., moldy hay in **farmer's lung**) and reactions to spores borne in aerosol microdroplets from dirty ultrasonic humidifiers (e.g., **humidifier lung**). The etiology of this disease is not completely understood, but both IgE and IgG are implicated. IgE causes the initial inflammation and trapping of antigen, and IgG is involved in the long-term effects. Symptoms include:
      (1) Nasal congestion and bronchoconstriction
      (2) Joint pain and inflammation of rheumatoid arthritis caused by joint-localized immune complexes involving rheumatoid factor and neutrophil phagocytosis (see Chapter 49).

5. **Time course**
   a. **Systemic.** For patients with no previous exposure, symptoms appear 1–2 weeks, and possibly longer, after exposure. For patients with preexisting antibodies, symptoms appear within several hours to a day after exposure. Severe symptoms, such as glomerulonephritis, usually occur after 2 weeks.
   b. **Local.** In hypersensitivity pneumonitis, symptoms appear 6–8 hours after exposure in patients with preexisting antibodies.

6. **Prophylaxis and therapy.** In drug-induced types, **withdrawing the drug** usually reverses the reaction. Treatment includes antihistamines or corticosteroids. Transient infectious forms resolve spontaneously as complexes are removed by phagocytes.

E. Type IV hypersensitivity reactions

1. **Pathogenesis.** Type IV reactions include prolonged inappropriate and appropriate immune responses. The common factor is the mediation of inflammation and tissue damage by antigen-specific T cells, usually in collaboration with activated macrophages. T cells are of the helper (CD4) category. These cells infiltrate tissues, recruiting and activating macrophages that induce inflammation and disrupt tissue architecture, independent of antibody.
   a. **Reactions to infections** involve a T-cell response against specific intracellular bacterial and protozoan parasites (e.g., *Mycobacteria).* Significant tissue damage occurs when the response is ineffective and prolonged and leads to the formation of granulomas.
   b. **Contact dermatitis** is an inappropriate skin reaction to haptens (e.g., the pentadecyl catechols of poison ivy), which bind to epidermal cell surfaces and elicit a T-cell response.
   c. **Tuberculin reaction** is an appropriate dermal skin inflammation that is caused by intradermal puncture with microorganismal allergens. It indicates a state of either active T-cell

immunity or T-cell memory to the organism. This type IV reaction is a convenient test for the status of a patient's T-cell immunity. The absence of an expected response indicates a state of anergy, or unresponsiveness.

2. Common allergens

a. Infectious allergens. *Mycobacterium tuberculosis, Mycobacterium leprae, Listeria monocytogenes,* trypanosomes, and viruses

b. Contact dermatitis. Pentadecyl catechols from poison ivy, poison oak, chromates, nickel ions (leached from some jewelry clasps), acrylates, hair dyes containing *p*-phenylene diamine, and certain antibiotic ointments (e.g., topical neomycin)

c. Tuberculin. Skin testing with purified protein derivative (PPD) or tuberculin (Mantoux reaction), *Candida,* mumps, and other microorganismal antigens

3. Chemical mediators are important in type IV reactions. Cytokines of activated T cells attract and activate monocyte–macrophages to tissue sites where the pathogen is localized, such as the epidermis (in contact sensitivity), the dermis (in a tuberculin reaction), or the site of a graft. Cytotoxicity occurs as a result of macrophage secretions, such as TNF. Macrophages also secrete inflammatory cytokines.

4. Clinical symptoms depend on the subtype.

a. Granulomas are local aggregations of T cells, monocyte–macrophages, and giant–epithelioid cells that derive from the fusion of activated macrophages. They occur around sites of chronic infectious organisms (e.g., the lungs in tuberculosis).

b. In contact sensitivity, cellular infiltration of the epidermis produces microvesicle formation with spongiosis.

c. Tuberculin tests cause erythema and induration as a result of cellular infiltration of the dermis, but no epidermal spongiosis.

5. Time course

a. Granulomas form at various times after the onset of a chronic immune response, but are generally delayed by 2 weeks.

b. Contact sensitivity may not occur at the first transient exposure, but skin inflammation occurs within 12–24 hours and peaks within 24–48 hours of exposure. Susceptibility and severity vary widely. The same time course applies to tuberculin reactions, often known as **delayed cutaneous hypersensitivity testing.**

6. Prophylaxis and therapy. Treatment depends on the organism involved. Identifying and avoiding the allergen is important in contact sensitivity dermatitis. This condition is treated with topical corticosteroid ointments, which suppress T-cell and macrophage function. Widespread or severe cases may require systemic corticosteroid treatment.

III. AUTOIMMUNITY is a tissue-damaging immune response directed specifically and inappropriately against one or more self-antigens.

A. Etiology. The etiologies of autoreactive immune responses are not generally known and probably involve several deregulations in the network of controls that normally prevent them. Aberration in normal regulation by CD4 T_H and CD8 T_S cells is most often cited; other factors include cross-reactivity with antigens from pathogens and loss of self-tolerance.

B. Epidemiology

1. Familial clustering is evident for many, if not most, reactions, representing a complex inherited predisposition toward autoimmunity. In some cases, this predisposition is associated with specific MHC types (e.g., the strong association of rheumatoid arthritis with MHC class II type DR4).

2. These reactions are more common among women. The female to male incidence ratio is approximately 2 to 1 for myasthenia gravis and 10 to 1 for SLE. Some conditions are more common in men (e.g., Goodpasture's syndrome).

C. Pathogenesis

1. Overview. In a specific autoimmune disorder, the primary pathogenic mechanism may be mediated by antibodies (humoral), with or without a contribution by complement; may be primarily cell-mediated; or may involve both humoral and cell-mediated damage. Alternate exacerbation and remission of pathogenesis is a common feature.

2. **Environmental factors** trigger pathogenesis, but specific factors are known for only a few types. These include associations between *Streptococcus* group A pharyngitis and rheumatic fever, exposure to organic solvents and Goodpasture's syndrome, and ultraviolet radiation and SLE. Environmental factors probably act with genetic predisposition.

3. **Organ-specific or non–organ-specific disorders**
   a. **Organ-specific disorders** (e.g., antithyroid autoimmunity). The immune response is limited to and directed specifically against self-antigens in one organ. Lesions and clinical symptoms are limited primarily to that organ. Cellular damage often arises through antibody- and complement-mediated cytotoxicity (type II pathogenic mechanism) and sometimes through cell-mediated cytotoxicity (type IV pathogenic mechanism).
   b. **Non–organ-specific disorders** (e.g., SLE)
      (1) These disorders are also known as immunologic connective tissue, collagen vascular, or rheumatologic disorders. Autoantibodies are formed against self-antigens common to many or all tissues, particularly those located in the nuclei of cells and containing DNA or RNA (**antinuclear antibodies**). Pathologic changes occur systemically, primarily in connective tissues, and are at least partly caused by the pathogenic mechanisms of type III hypersensitivity reactions (see II D). Symptoms are seen in blood vessels, the kidney glomerulus, skin, joints, and serous membranes. Blood cells and plasma proteins also may be involved.
      (2) Non–organ-specific disorders are sometimes difficult to distinguish from one another because of the similarities in autoantigens and pathogenesis. For example, most patients with SLE have circulating antinuclear antibodies, but these occur in 50%–65% of patients with Sjögren's syndrome and rheumatoid arthritis as well as a small percentage of clinically normal individuals. By contrast, rheumatoid factor (anti-IgG) is seen in 75%–90% of patients with Sjögren's syndrome and rheumatoid arthritis, but also in approximately 35% of patients with SLE. The synovitis of rheumatoid arthritis is often a clinical finding in SLE, and the vasculitis of SLE is found in rheumatoid arthritis (see Chapter 49).

D. Organ-specific autoimmunities

1. **Rheumatic fever** is not technically an autoimmune response because antibodies are produced against group A streptococci and cross-react with cardiac muscle fibers that are damaged by complement. Increased risk is related to a strong immune response to streptococcal M antigen.

2. **Antithyroid autoimmunities** (see Chapter 53). Aspects of several subtypes may occur in the same patient. Increased risk is associated with MHC class II types DR3 and DR5.
   a. **Primary autoimmune myxedema.** Antibodies against the thyroid-stimulating hormone (TSH) receptor on thyroid follicle cells act as antagonists to the stimulation of growth of the follicle cells normally provoked by TSH. The result is thyroid atrophy with hypothyroidism.
   b. **Hashimoto's thyroiditis.** Antibodies against thyroid peroxidase on follicle cells cause cytotoxicity and inflammation through the activation of complement. Antibodies against thyroglobulin (colloid) also may be present. Cell-mediated immunity may cause some cytotoxic damage. The resulting hypothyroidism is treated with synthetic thyroid hormone.
   c. **Graves' disease.** Antibodies act as agonists of TSH, binding to the TSH receptor and stimulating hypersecretion of thyroid hormone [thyroid-stimulating immunoglobulins (TSI)]. The result is hyperthyroidism, which is treated by antithyroid drugs (e.g., propylthiouracil) or thyroid ablation with surgery or radiation.

3. **Myasthenia gravis**
   a. **Pathogenesis.** Antibodies against the nicotinic acetylcholine receptor on skeletal muscle plasma membrane at neuromuscular junctions act as competitive antagonists of **acetylcholine** binding. This activity causes weakness and fatigue in skeletal muscles. In addition to this direct blockage of neuromuscular transmission, down regulation of receptors and complement damage to muscle fibers occur. Many patients have swallowing and respiratory muscle dysfunction that may be caused by penicillamine therapy. Increased risk is associated with MHC class I type B8.
   b. **Therapy.** Anticholinesterase therapy (e.g., neostigmine) increases acetylcholine synaptic concentrations (preservation of endogenous acetylcholine). Immunosuppression with

corticosteroids is used in severe cases; plasmapheresis to remove autoreactive antibodies from the blood is also helpful. Thymectomy helps many patients.

4. **Autoimmune pernicious anemia**
   a. **Pathogenesis.** Antibodies against intrinsic factor are secreted into the stomach lumen, where they inhibit the association of intrinsic factor with vitamin B_{12}. The absorption of vitamin B_{12} is decreased. This condition also can result from antibodies against gastrin receptors on parietal cells of the stomach mucosa that block stimulation of the cells by gastrin and decrease their secretion of intrinsic factor.
   b. **Therapy** is intramuscular injection of cyanocobalamin or oral administration of concentrated intrinsic factor preparations.

5. **Goodpasture's syndrome**
   a. **Pathogenesis.** Antibodies against **glomerular capillary basement membrane (GBM)** activate complement- and neutrophil-mediated damage. This activation leads to glomerulonephritis, with rapid deterioration of renal function. These antibodies cross-react with pulmonary capillary basement membrane, producing pulmonary hemorrhage. Increased risk is associated with MHC class II type DR2.
   b. **Therapy.** Immunosuppressive therapy includes corticosteroids, with plasmapheresis to remove autoreactive antibodies.

6. **Autoimmune hemolytic anemia (red blood cell), thrombocytopenia (platelet), neutropenia (neutrophil), and lymphopenia (lymphocyte)**
   a. **Pathogenesis.** Antibodies against membrane antigens of one or more of the indicated cell types may activate complement and opsonize the cells for rapid splenic phagocytosis. It may also occur as part of the spectrum of autoimmunity in non–organ-specific disorders, particularly SLE. These autoimmune varieties must be distinguished from those precipitated by responses to external antigens (e.g., drugs), but the clinical effects are similar.
   b. **Therapy.** These disorders are acute and self-limiting, but therapy is required when they are chronic. In adults, treatment begins with corticosteroids. Additional options are cyclophosphamide, chlorambucil, and intravenous immune globulin (IVIG).

7. **Insulin-dependent diabetes mellitus (IDDM)** (see Chapter 52)
   Progressive and ultimately complete destruction of pancreatic β-islet cells occurs in diabetes. Although they are predictively useful, antibodies against insulin and surface cytoplasmic antigens of the β-islet cell are present before clinical onset. The main cytotoxic mechanisms appear to be mediated by T cells and macrophages. This view is supported by the beneficial effects of cyclosporine therapy in patients with early-stage IDDM at levels that have little effect on antibody production. Increased risk is associated with MHC class II types DR3 and DR4.

8. **Multiple sclerosis (MS)**
   a. **Pathogenesis.** T cells and macrophages, which are thought to be cytocidal for oligodendrocytes, infiltrate the central nervous system (CNS) and **attack the basic protein of myelin** as an autoantigen. The immunologic component may be secondary to other unknown initiating agents. **CNS demyelination with sclerotic plaques** leads to spasticity. Increased risk is associated with MHC class II type DR2. Guillain Barré syndrome is a related condition that involves peripheral nervous system (PNS) demyelination that, unlike MS, can be acute.
   b. **Therapy.** Spasticity is treated with **baclofen** with variable effectiveness.The peripheral skeletal muscle relaxant **dantrolene** is effective in some patients. **Adrenocorticotropic hormone (ACTH),** rather than corticosteroids, is the favored immunosuppressive therapy. Recombinant IFN-β 1b (Betaseron) is approved by the FDA as a treatment for MS.

E. **Non–organ-specific autoimmunities.** The similarities and differences in this class of disorders are shown by a comparison of Sjögren's syndrome and SLE. Rheumatoid arthritis is discussed in Chapter 49.

1. **Sjögren's syndrome**
   a. **Diagnosis** is usually based on lymphocytic infiltration and the presence of autoantibodies against salivary gland antigens and exocrine glands of the eyes, gastrointestinal and respiratory systems, and vagina. Hypergammaglobulinemia (50%) as a result of hyperactive β-cells, antinuclear antibodies (50%–65%), and rheumatoid factors (anti-IgG; 75%–90%) is present in the indicated percentages of patients.

b. **Pathogenesis.** Primary symptoms include **inhibition of exocrine gland secretion,** with dryness of the eyes, mouth, and gastrointestinal, respiratory, and vaginal mucous membranes; and pain and edema in the salivary glands. Patients with hypergammaglobulinemia often have type III hypersensitivity reactions (e.g., vasculitis with CNS involvement and kidney disease; see II D).

c. **Therapy.** Mild cases are treated with **artificial tears** and frequent drinking of water. For more serious cases (e.g., vasculitis), treatment is similar to that for SLE **(systemic corticosteroids).**

2. **SLE**

a. **Diagnosis** is complicated and depends on the presence of four or more of eleven criteria. The most useful criterion is a high concentration of antinuclear antibodies directed against double-stranded DNA and the Smith (Sm) nuclear antigen, both of which are considered specific for SLE. Other diagnostic criteria include the presence of the lupus erythematosus cell (a neutrophil that has phagocytosed nuclei), a discoid erythematous facial rash, photosensitivity, oral ulcers, arthritis, persistent proteinuria, and anticardiolipin, antierythrocyte, or antileukocyte antibodies.

b. **Pathogenesis** is that of **type III hypersensitivity.** Patients have **hyperactivity of B cells** of unknown origin. This hyperreactivity causes hypergammaglobulinemia, with circulating immune complexes of DNA and other nuclear antigens that precipitate onto vascular basement membranes and activate complement.

(1) Mild arthritis, fever, rash, and fatigue occur.

(2) Progressive necrotizing vasculitis with CNS involvement and glomerulonephritis are the most serious consequences, occurring in approximately 50% of patients.

(3) Hypertension may develop secondary to kidney disease.

(4) Hemolytic anemia and thrombocytopenia are common.

(5) Behavioral changes occur in approximately 25% of patients.

(6) Several drugs (e.g., **procainamide, hydralazine, quinidine, methyldopa, isoniazid, phenytoin, chlorpromazine)** provoke a lupus-like syndrome that usually resolves when the drug is withdrawn. The basis for this syndrome is not understood. No renal disorder occurs in drug-induced SLE.

c. **Therapy.** Mild disease (e.g., low fever, arthritis) is managed with nonsteroidal anti-inflammatory drugs (NSAIDs). Therapy for patients with severe symptoms is usually oral methylprednisolone. Cyclophosphamide may also be used, and plasmapheresis to remove circulating immune complexes may be helpful.

F. **Prospects for more specific immunologic therapies.** Current therapies involve approaches that suppress all immune responses; however, current clinical trials seek to suppress only lymphocytes that are activated; for example:

1. **Feeding autoantigens** to patients to induce immunologic suppression

2. **Vaccination with autoreactive T cells** to induce immunologic suppression

3. Administration of **anti-T_H** monoclonal antibodies (particularly anti-CD4) to eliminate autoreactive T cells

4. Administration of **conjugates of interleukin-2 (IL-2) and toxins** from plants or bacteria to eliminate autoreactive T cells without generalized T-cell suppression

IV. IMMUNODEFICIENCY

IMMUNODEFICIENCY is either primary or secondary. **Primary immunodeficiencies** are either **hereditary** or **congenital,** and at least one element basic to the immune system does not function properly or is absent. **Secondary immunodeficiencies** are the **result of another systemic disorder** or are **iatrogenic in patients given immunosuppressive therapy.** They usually develop in patients who previously showed normal immune function. The expected clinical outcome of an immunodeficiency is governed by the specific portion of the immune system that is affected (e.g., B and T cells, complement).

A. **Primary immunodeficiencies** are, with one exception, rare. Examples are:

1. **X-linked agammaglobulinemia** (hypogammaglobulinemia) is an inherited deficiency in antibody production (humoral immunity) in which T-cell function is relatively normal, but B

cells do not fully mature. Serum immunoglobulin levels are low. Because this disorder is linked to the X-chromosome, it occurs primarily in men.

a. **Pathogenesis** occurs 6–9 months after birth and is representative of situations in which antibody function is deficient, but T-cell function is intact, such as recurrent infections with extracellular pyogenic bacteria (e.g., streptococci, pneumococci, *Haemophilus).* Immunity to fungi and most viruses is generally functional.
b. **Clinical symptoms** include pneumonia, sinusitis, otitis, meningitis, and septicemia.
c. **Therapy** is **passive immunization with intravenous human immune globulin** (IGIV; see VI B 1 c).

2. **Common variable immunodeficiency** is an acquired deficiency of B-cell maturation to plasma cells. It can occur at any age and in either sex. Pathogenesis, symptoms, and treatment are similar to those for X-linked agammaglobulinemia; the pathogenesis and etiology vary significantly.

3. **Selective IgA deficiency** is the most common primary immunodeficiency, affecting approximately 0.5% of the United States population. It appears to be inherited. The low secretory IgA (sIgA) concentration predisposes patients to extracellular bacterial infections of the mucosal surfaces, leading to respiratory, urogenital, and gastrointestinal infections. Some affected individuals are asymptomatic for unknown reasons. Certain autoimmunities may be more prevalent. There is no specific immunologic therapy.

4. **DiGeorge syndrome** results from developmental failure of the thymus and parathyroid glands, accompanied by cardiovascular and other developmental anomalies. Patients have a decrease in total T-cell numbers, but relatively normal immunoglobulin levels.

   a. **Pathogenesis** in severe cases (i.e., little functional thymic tissue) is representative of conditions involving T-cell deficiency, such as recurrent infections of the skin, lung, genitourinary tract, and blood with opportunistic pathogens, particularly viruses (e.g., herpes viruses), fungi (e.g., *Candida),* and protozoa (e.g., *Pneumocystis carinii);* increased incidence of certain cancers; graft-versus-host disease (GVH; see V C) after transfusion of whole blood; and death in infancy or early childhood.
   b. **Therapy** for severe T-cell deficiencies is bone marrow transplantation (see V C).

5. **Nezelof syndrome** is probably inherited and causes lymphopenia and thymic abnormalities, but normal or elevated serum immunoglobulin levels. Gram-negative sepsis may occur in addition to the opportunistic infections associated with T-cell deficiency.

6. **Severe combined immunodeficiency disorders (SCIDs)** are a heterogeneous group of inherited disorders with deficiencies in T cells, B cells (variable), and serum immunoglobulin. Infections with opportunistic organisms occur in the first few months postnatally, and survival for longer than 1 year is rare without successful bone marrow transplantation. One form involves the inherited deficiency of the enzyme adenosine deaminase (ADA). Human trials with gene replacement therapy are underway.

7. **Chronic granulomatous disease (CGD)** is a defect in the ability of phagocytes to kill bacteria. The disease is caused by a genetic defect in the production of oxygen radicals that are important for intra- and extracellular killing of bacteria. The defect can occur in any of the four proteins important for producing oxygen radicals, but the most common defect is X-linked. CGD is characterized by chronic infection with organisms such as *Staphylococcus aureus* and is usually fatal.

8. **Leukocyte adhesion deficiency (LAD)** is associated with a defect in the phagocytic cells. These cells lack intercellular adhesion molecules, the proteins necessary for binding to the endothelial cells of the blood vessels and other cell membranes. This defect leads to an inability to exit the blood and enter the tissues. In addition, the phagocytes have a decreased ability to bind to activated components of complement on a bacterial surface, leading to a decrease in phagocytosis. Patients have severe bacterial infections, especially in the mouth and gastrointestinal tract.

9. **Chédiak-Higashi syndrome** is a deficiency in the fusion of lysosomes with phagocytic vesicles. The cause is unknown, but this syndrome leads to bacterial survival in the phagocyte, with an increase in bacterial infections.

B. **Secondary immunodeficiencies** involve decreased immunologic responsiveness.

1. **Cytotoxic drugs** prevent the division of responding lymphocytes, suppress the production of blood cells in bone marrow, and may directly kill cells. Patients who receive chemotherapy and exhibit a significant loss of neutrophils may be treated with filgrastim, or recombinant G-CSF (Neupogen), to restore the white blood cell count to normal levels. Treatment to increase neutrophil levels in these patients results in decreased morbidity rates as a result of bacterial infection. Corticosteroids broadly suppress immune system cells, including decreased division, cytokine secretion, and chemotaxis, or emigration from the blood into tissues.

2. **Leukemias, lymphomas, and myelomas** are associated with decreased immune responsiveness, at least some of which results from destruction of the architecture of lymphoid organs (e.g., spleen, lymph nodes). Malignancy-related immunodeficiency also occurs in other cancers.

3. **Protein calorie malnutrition** significantly decreases immune competence, particularly in children.

4. **Aging** is associated with decreased immunologic competence.

5. **Acute infections** produce a transient immunodeficiency.

6. **Acquired immune deficiency syndrome (AIDS)** is a secondary immunodeficiency that is usually persistent and is probably an indirect consequence of infection by **human immunodeficiency virus 1 (HIV-1)** and possibly **HIV-2.**
   a. **Pathogenesis.** The viral envelope glycoprotein 120 (gp120) has a strong affinity for CD4 (see I B 3 c), allowing the virus to directly infect T_H cells and certain monocyte–macrophages. Because it is a retrovirus, viral entry and uncoating release the viral RNA genome and the associated reverse transcriptase enzyme, which synthesizes a double-stranded DNA copy of the genome (provirus). The proviral copy is integrated into the genome of the $CD4^+$ cell, and the virus enters a period of latency, during which it is essentially hidden from the immune system.
      (1) During **initial infection,** an acute illness that lasts an average of 3 weeks and resembles mononucleosis occurs in some individuals; others have no symptoms.
      (2) **Seroconversion** (i.e., the appearance of antiviral antibodies) occurs 3 weeks to 6 months after the initial exposure to HIV-1. A period of **asymptomatic infection** typically follows seroconversion.
      (3) Infected T_H cells are killed when **viral genes are reactivated from latency** and viruses bud from the cell. In addition, infected T cells may fuse to form syncytia. This fusion may hasten the spread of virus to uninfected T cells and contribute to cell killing. A **progressive depletion of T_H** cells occurs (normal count, 800–1000/mm^3). However, even before an obvious loss of $CD4^+$ T cells occurs, there is evidence of a defect in $CD4^+$ T-cell function. The functional defect is a failure of these cells to respond to antigens to which they were previously sensitized (e.g., tetanus toxoid). The defect in responsiveness may be a function of the $CD4^+$ T cells, the APCs, or both.
      (4) Monocyte–macrophages may produce new virus without being killed and may spread the virus to uninfected T cells and other cell types. $CD4^-$ cell lines that are susceptible to HIV infection include neurons, liver, and fibroblasts. In direct cell-to-cell transfer of the virus, minimal exposure to the extracellular immune system (e.g., antibody) may occur.
      (5) **APCs** are also affected by the infection. There is a loss of follicular dendritic cells and interdigitating cells in the lymphoid tissue. This loss leads to decreased antigen presentation to the $CD4^+$ T cells. In addition, the cytokines produced by the APCs may produce $CD4^+$ T cells that increase B-cell activation, but do not produce the appropriate cytokines for T-cell proliferation. This activity changes the T_H-cell ratios.
   b. **Clinical symptoms**
      (1) **Persistent generalized lymphadenopathy** (extrainguinal) is an indicator of impending progression to full disease. Unexplained fever, night sweats, diarrhea, and other symptoms known as **AIDS-related complex (ARC)** may occur.
      (2) Progression to full-blown AIDS may occur 8 years or longer after the initial infection. Depletion of the T_H-cell level to less than 200/mm^3 and oral candidiasis suggest imminent disease. Because CD8 T cells are not significantly affected, the ratio of circulating CD4 to CD8 cells is inverted. In addition, the number of virgin T_H cells relative

to memory T_H cells increases. T_H cells are lost, and memory T_H cells are lost in relatively larger numbers. There is also a shift in the type of T_H cell help being generated.

(3) A diagnosis of AIDS involves the occurrence of **opportunistic infections** or **neoplasms as a result of the progressive immunodeficiency** caused by severe depletion of T_H-cell (CD4) function. Also included in this diagnosis are the HIV wasting syndrome and encephalopathy.

(a) Opportunistic infections are the major consequence of AIDS, particularly by *P. carinii* (as many as 80% of patients), *Candida albicans, Mycobacterium avium-intracellulare,* herpes simplex virus (HSV), cytomegalovirus (CMV), and others. Tuberculosis occurs as a reactivation of a latent infection in carriers. Cumulatively, **these opportunistic infections are the primary cause of death.**

(b) **Kaposi's sarcoma,** an otherwise rare cancer, occurs in fewer than one-half of patients with AIDS. Non-Hodgkin's lymphoma is also more common than in the general population.

(4) **HIV-associated dementia complex (HADC)** affects more than one-half of patients with AIDS. In HADC, macrophages infiltrate the brain and are the most productively infected cell in comparison with neurons or glia. Some patients show demyelination.

(5) Other immune system abnormalities include polyclonal B-cell activation and hypergammaglobulinemia with a concomitant decreased ability to mount humoral immune responses to specific antigens. Chemotaxis, cytokine secretion, and cytotoxic ability of monocyte–macrophages are all diminished. These problems are consequences of impaired T-cell regulation.

c. Therapy

(1) Current therapies include antibiotics; azidothymidine (AZT), a viral reverse transcriptase inhibitor; dideoxyinosine; and IFN-α (see VII D 1) for the treatment of Kaposi's sarcoma. Many other drugs and immunomodulators are being tested.

(2) An effective active vaccine is necessary to limit the spread of HIV infection. Because of viral antigenic variation, cell-to-cell transmission, and the uncertain role of antibodies in protection, the process of vaccine development is difficult. A live, attenuated vaccine (see VI C 2) is considered too great a risk. Trials of subunit vaccines are imminent.

V. GRAFT REJECTION

A. Overview. Individual differences in the molecular structures of cells and tissues occur, except in identical twins, because of the genetic variation inherent in humans. Because of these molecular differences, transplanted tissues or organs (i.e., grafts) are likely to be antigenically different from the recipient and therefore may stimulate an immune response.

1. Although MHC class I and II glycoproteins play an essential role in all T-cell immune responses (see I B 3 a), these molecules are particularly antigenic and variant in structure among different humans (polymorphic).

2. Each person's set of MHC glycoproteins is called his **human leukocyte antigen (HLA),** or **histocompatibility, type.** Class I glycoproteins are known as HLA-A, -B, and -C antigens. Class II glycoproteins are known as HLA-DR, -DP, and -DQ antigens. Each person receives one set of genes (a haplotype) encoding these protein antigens from each parent.

3. Identical twins have the same histocompatibility type. In others, the probability is approximately 25% (0.25) that two siblings with the same parents are HLA-identical, or matched, and approximately 50% that they are one-half HLA-matched, or haploidentical. Parents and children are almost always haploidentical. Some transplanted tissues are rejected because of HLA incompatibility. In other cases, the reason for rejection is unknown. HLA matching is not always a factor in rejection.

B. Common solid-organ transplants are kidney, heart, liver, heart–lung, and pancreas. Organs are obtained from cadavers or living donors. The probability of an exact HLA match in a cadaver graft is approximately 1 in 10 million.

1. HLA matching

a. The primary problem with organ donation is rejection of the transplanted organ by the host's immune response, a host-versus-graft response. Donation of an organ by an HLA-matched sibling is the best way to avoid this problem.

b. Although HLA-DR and HLA-B matching decreases the rejection reaction in renal and cardiac grafts, rejection occurs in HLA-matched situations. HLA matching is not important in liver transplantation.

2. **Types of rejection of organ grafts**
   a. **Hyperacute rejection** is mediated by preexisting antibody in the recipient, usually against ABO mismatches. Complement is activated, clotting occurs, and the vasculature of the transplanted organ is occluded. Rejection occurs within 2 days after transplantation. An ABO-mismatched graft is rarely attempted. Rejection is essentially untreatable.
   b. **Acute rejection** is most likely a T-cell–macrophage–mediated attack on the graft based on HLA and other tissue antigen mismatches. T cells and monocyte–macrophages infiltrate the graft and, in 10 to 14 days, cause cellular necrosis and inflammation perivascularly. The entire graft begins to necrose if untreated.
   c. **Chronic rejection** occurs several months to several years after transplantation. It causes fibrosis and occlusion of small arteries and arterioles in the kidneys and atherosclerosis in the heart. It may be controlled by immunologic injury, through antibody or cells, and includes the release of inflammatory cytokines by macrophages. Despite the high success rate of MHC-matched, pharmacologically treated grafts in the first year after transplantation (85%–90% kidney grafts), the rejection rate after 5 years is nearly 50%. This form of rejection is resistant to therapy.

C. **Bone marrow transplantation** is sometimes attempted in patients with immunodeficiency diseases, aplastic anemias, some leukemias, and certain genetic diseases. The graft contains a high proportion of donor lymphocytes that respond to the host HLA and other antigens. This response causes GVH disease.

1. Graft T-cell recognition of the host is important in GVH disease, as shown by the decreased incidence of GVH disease after procedures that purge T cells from the donor marrow.

2. **Clinical symptoms** of GVH disease are seen in the skin (e.g., rash, desquamation), gastrointestinal tract (e.g., pain, vomiting, intestinal bleeding), and liver (e.g., necrosis indicated by increased serum bilirubin levels). Death commonly occurs.

3. HLA matching is important in bone marrow transplantation, but the failure rate, even of matched grafts, as a result of GVH disease is high.

4. Because the recipient of the marrow (host) is immunosuppressed by drugs or radiation, the host-versus-graft response is less important.

D. **Prophylaxis and treatment of graft rejection**

1. **Immunosuppression of the graft recipient**
   a. **Corticosteroids** (e.g., methylprednisolone, prednisone) are administered just before transplantation and rapidly tapered because of their side effects. Corticosteroids are used in combination with azathioprine, cyclosporine, or **antilymphocyte globulins/antithymocyte globulins (ALG/ATG).**
   b. **Azathioprine** is given before transplantation. Maintenance doses are given afterward.
   c. **Methotrexate** is used primarily for bone marrow transplantation in combination with ALG/ATG. It is administered either a few days before or at the time of transplantation.

2. **Specific suppression of T cells**
   a. **Cyclosporine** binds to an intracellular protein known as cyclophilin and blocks the transcription of cytokine genes in a T cell that has recognized antigens. In this way, it inhibits T-cell secretion of IL-2 and IFN-γ and prevents complete T-cell activation. It is administered prophylactically because it is more effective if it is present when rejection begins. Cyclosporine is commonly combined with other agents. The major side effect is nephrotoxicity.
   b. **Tacrolimus (FK-506)** is an immunosuppressive agent that inhibits T_H-cell function in the same way as cyclosporine. Both drugs function through the same pathway and are not used together.
   c. **Rampamycin** inhibits T_H-cell response to IL-2 and prevents T_H-cell activation. It works through a different pathway than either cyclosporine or tacrolimus and is especially effective in combination with the other drugs.

d. **ALG** and **ATG** are antisera derived from animals. They contain a variety of antibody specificities against T-cell antigens. They are used both prophylactically and therapeutically in bone marrow and organ transplantation.

e. **Muromonab-CD3** (OKT3) is a mouse monoclonal antibody specific for the CD3 antigen, which is present on all peripheral T cells. OKT3 is used therapeutically to halt and reverse acute rejection as soon as it is diagnosed.

(1) Its main action is the opsonization of T cells for enhanced phagocytosis. It is administered daily for 10–14 days. Only one course is typically used because it causes an immune response against the foreign mouse antibody.

(2) Acute side effects are common, probably because of nonspecific T-cell activation that causes the release of cytokines. Side effects include high fever, chills, blood pressure changes, vomiting, diarrhea, and respiratory distress. OKT3 is contraindicated in patients who have fluid overload because it may cause fatal pulmonary edema.

(3) OKT3 may also be used in vitro to purge donor bone marrow of T cells to reduce the risk of GVH disease.

3. **Investigational agents** that are being tested to prevent or reverse graft rejection include anti-T-cell immunotoxins (see VII C 1); conjugates of IL-2 and a toxin; and other monoclonals that prevent T cells from adhering to foreign graft cells. These agents are administered to the graft recipient. In addition, monoclonal antibodies are used to mask HLA antigens on the graft tissue before it is transplanted into the recipient.

VI. VACCINATION

A. Overview

1. **Passive vaccination** is the intramuscular or intravenous injection of antibody preparations to enhance a patient's immune competence. Protection depends on the serum half-life of the injected antibody and is limited to several weeks to several months for each administration (human sera).

2. **Active vaccination** is the intramuscular, subcutaneous, or oral introduction of one or more antigens designed to stimulate the immune system to produce a specific immune response. This response generates antibody, activated T cells, and specific memory. Protection through memory varies with the vaccine, but immunity is long-lasting.

B. Passive vaccination (Table 10-2)

1. **Preparations.** Doses of intramuscular preparations are sometimes given in units per kilogram and sometimes in milliliters per kilogram. The dose varies with the vaccine and patient population. Intravenous preparations are commonly used in high doses.

a. **Standard human serum immune globulin for intramuscular vaccination (IGIM)** is a polyclonal antiserum prepared from pooled plasma of donors. It contains 165 mg/ml human immunoglobulin, predominantly the four subclasses of IgG. Side effects are rare, minimal, and usually confined to minor inflammation and pain at the site of injection. This preparation is unsuitable for intravenous injection because antibody aggregates form and may activate complement and platelets.

b. **Special IGIMs** are individual sera prepared from plasma lots of subjects actively immunized against or recovering from specific diseases. Each serum is enriched for antibodies of the desired specificity [e.g., tetanus immune globulin (TIG) contains more antibodies against tetanus toxin than would be found in IGIM].

c. **IVIGs** are prepared from pooled human serum and modified to minimize antibody aggregation. Chills, nausea, and abdominal pain occur in approximately 10% of patients. Side effects are diminished by reducing the rate of intravenous infusion. Premedication with corticosteroids is recommended, and intravenous epinephrine is used if anaphylaxis occurs.

d. **Animal antisera.** Equine (horse) antisera are used in certain situations (see Table 10-2). Mouse monoclonal antibody (muromonab-CD3) is used in acute renal rejection (see V D 2 e). The half-lives of animal antibodies are shorter in humans.

2. **Rationales for passive vaccination**

a. **Prophylaxis of infectious disease.** Antibodies are given prophylactically to prevent clinical symptoms of a viral or bacterial infectious process, particularly in a patient without

Table 10-2. Passive Vaccines

Illness	Vaccine	Rationale
Intramuscular		
Hepatitis B (HBV)	Hepatitis B immune globulin (HBIG)	Prophylaxis
Hepatitis A (HAV)	Immune globulin IM (IGIM)	Prophylaxis
Non-A, non-B hepatitis	IGIM	Prophylaxis, therapy
Measles	IGIM	Prophylaxis, therapy
Rabies	Rabies immune globulin (RIG)	Prophylaxis
Rubella	IGIM	Fetal prophylaxis in exposed mother
Varicella	Varicella zoster immune globulin (VZIG)	Prophylaxis and therapy in immunocompromised individual
Tetanus	Tetanus immune globulin (TIG)	Prophylaxis
Hypogammaglobulinemia	IGIM	Therapy for antibody deficiency
Rh disease	Rh_o (D) immune globulin (RhoGAM)	Prophylaxis during pregnancy and after delivery of Rh^+ fetus by Rh^- mother
Diphtheria	Diphtheria antitoxin (equine)	Prophylaxis, therapy
Botulism	Botulism antiserum (equine)	Prophylaxis, therapy
Snakebite	Polyvalent antivenin (equine)	Prophylaxis, therapy
Black widow bite	Black widow antivenin (equine)	Prophylaxis, therapy
Intravenous*		
Hypogammaglobulinemia	Intravenous immune globulin (IVIG)	Therapy for antibody deficiency
Idiopathic thrombocytopenic purpura (ITP)	IVIG	Therapy
Chronic lymphocytic leukemia	IVIG	Therapy for antibody deficiency
Cytomegalovirus (CMV) infection	CMV IVIG	Therapy in renal transplant patients
Acute renal rejection	Muromonab-CD3 (murine)	Reversal of acute rejection

*Food and Drug Administration (FDA)–approved uses; many others currently in trials.

previous exposure and therefore without memory. The vaccine protects the recipient during the incubation period for infection. For example:

(1) *Clostridium tetani* infection has an incubation period of approximately 5 days before significant quantities of tetanus toxin are produced. A primary immune response of 7–10 days is too slow. Passive vaccination with TIG binds the toxin and prevents disease.

(2) **Hepatitis B immune globulin (HBIG)** is administered to exposed individuals as soon as possible after exposure to prevent viral infection.

b. Prophylaxis or therapy prevents or attenuates the effects of infection in special populations. Examples are the use of **varicella zoster immune globulin (VZIG)** in immunocompromised patients and the use of IGIM in pregnant women who are exposed to rubella and have not been actively vaccinated.

c. Treatment of antibody deficiency. Persons who are deficient in antibody production, either because of primary immunodeficiency (see IV) or as a result of chronic lymphocytic leukemia, receive IVIG or IGIM every 2–4 weeks to maintain humoral immunity. IVIG is preferred.

d. Other situations. IVIG is used for idiopathic (autoimmune) thrombocytopenia purpura. Intramuscular Rh_o(D) immune globulin (RhoGAM) is used prophylactically for Rh disease (see II C 5 c). Muromonab-CD3 (see V D 2 e) is used for acute renal graft rejection.

C. Active vaccination (Table 10-3) is used for prophylaxis.

1. Overview

a. Contents. Active vaccines contain one or more antigens or whole pathogenic organisms, but may also contain preservatives, low doses of antibiotics, and other compounds that result from vaccine preparation in cells of nonhuman origin. The valence of a vaccine indicates the number of strains of organism included (e.g., trivalent polio vaccine includes three strains of poliovirus).

b. **Administration.** Active vaccines are administered subcutaneously, intramuscularly, or intradermally. Some are introduced adsorbed to aluminum hydroxide or aluminum phosphate adjuvants. An adjuvant increases the antigenicity of the vaccine. A few vaccines are administered orally or intranasally.

c. **Seroconversion.** For most active vaccines, the success of the series of vaccinations is indicated by seroconversion of the patient. Seroconversion indicates that a person who previously did not have specific serum antibodies (i.e., seronegative) now has these antibodies (i.e., seropositive). Seroconversion does not indicate established immunity for certain vaccines [e.g., bacillus Calmette-Guérin (BCG) vaccine for tuberculosis].

d. **A schedule of active vaccination** is recommended for infants and children (see Table 10-3). The first vaccination is given after the infant is 6 weeks old because responses are normally inadequate in newborns and because maternal antibodies remain in the newborn circulation. Some vaccines are intended for use primarily in noninfant populations.

e. Most vaccines require **a series of vaccinations;** others are effective with a single vaccination. For those that require a series, intervals between vaccinations greater than those recommended do not generally diminish protection. The duration of memory varies with each vaccine, and **booster vaccinations** are often necessary.

f. **Side effects** include inflammation at the site of vaccination, malaise, mild fever, chills, headache, myalgia, and arthralgia. More severe side effects include febrile illness, somnolence, seizures, or anaphylactic hypersensitivity to vaccine antigens or accessory components (e.g., antibiotic, chicken protein). Severe reactions contraindicate continuation of a series. A person with severe febrile illness should not be actively vaccinated until the illness resolves.

2. **Types of active vaccines**

a. **Live, attenuated vaccines** consist of whole organisms (usually viruses). These organisms multiply after vaccination, but are attenuated to reduce their pathogenicity.

(1) A small dose produces a strong immune response because the antigen concentration increases when the organism multiplies. Some vaccines elicit lifelong immunity in two doses [e.g., measles, mumps, rubella vaccine (MMR)]. Because of their relative genetic instability, viruses can revert to virulence and cause the disease against which the patient is vaccinated [e.g., oral polio vaccine (OPV)].

(2) Live, attenuated viral vaccines are not recommended for pregnant women or those intending to become pregnant within 3 months of vaccination. Live, attenuated viral or bacterial vaccines are not given to immunocompromised individuals.

b. **Killed, inactivated vaccines** may contain whole killed cells (e.g., phenol-killed *Bordetella pertussis)* or any antigenic fraction isolated from the organism. They are usually given adsorbed to adjuvant.

(1) Isolated antigens may require inactivation before they are used in a vaccine [e.g., formaldehyde-modified toxin of *Clostridium tetani,* known as **tetanus toxoid (Td)** after modification]. Inactivation eliminates pathogenicity, but preserves some antigenicity.

(2) Because no live organisms are present, reversion to pathogenicity is not a problem. However, doses of cells or antigens must be higher than in live, attenuated vaccines, and hypersensitivity reactions to vaccine components are more common. Minimum effective doses are usually measured in numbers of cells or micrograms of antigen.

(3) Vaccines in which the antigenic fragment is a polysaccharide (e.g., *Haemophilus b*) are usually poor at eliciting immune responses and memory, probably because they do not evoke T-cell activation. These vaccines have been improved by conjugating the polysaccharide to another antigenic compound (e.g., Td). These are known as **conjugate vaccines.**

c. **Subunit vaccines.** Proteins and glycoproteins of an organism are produced by recombinant DNA technology in bacteria, yeast, or mammalian cells, and are used as the antigens for vaccination. One vaccine containing recombinant HBV surface antigen (rHBsAg) is approved by the United States Food and Drug Administration (FDA).

d. **Experimental vaccines** include other subunit vaccines; peptides produced by chemical, cell-free synthesis; recombinant DNA viruses containing genes for the antigens of multiple organisms; and anti-idiotype antibodies used for active vaccination.

Table 10-3. Commonly Administered Food and Drug Administration (FDA)–Approved Active Vaccines

Vaccine	Target Population*	Number of Vaccinations	Schedule	Notes
Live, attenuated viral				
Oral polio (OPV; trivalent)	Infants, children, health and day care workers	4	2, 4, 15–18 months; one at school entry	Approximately 1 in 2.6 million risk of vaccine-induced paralysis
Measles, mumps, rubella (MMR)	Infants, children	2	15 months (<12 months if high risk); one at school entry	Generally affords lifelong immunity
Rubella	Adolescent girls not previously vaccinated	1	Postpuberty	Protects future fetus from congenital rubella injury
Bacterial				
BCG tuberculosis	Persons exposed to sputum-positive tuberculosis patients	Varies	Depends on success of initial vaccination	Unpredictable effectiveness; induces cell-mediated immunity
Killed, inactivated viral				
Influenza (tri- or polyvalent)	Geriatric patients, health care workers, those at risk for complications of flu	1/year	Annually for maximal protection	Variant strains may appear each year; vaccine must be updated annually
Hepatitis B (HBV)	Homosexual men, prostitutes, health care workers, newborn of carrier mothers, preadolescents	1 with boosters	Booster every 5 years for those with continuing risk	HBsAg from plasma of chronic carriers; routine infant vaccination now approved
Inactivated polio (IPV; trivalent)	Immunodeficient children and families; as booster in health and day care workers	4	2, 4, 15–18 months; one at school entry	No sIgA; thus, reduced protection; no paralysis risk
Rabies (HDCV)	Animal care workers	4 or 5^+ with boosters	7 days apart; boosters as required to maintain immunoglobulin (Ig)	Two doses to exposed, already immune individual
Bacterial				
Diphtheria, tetanus, pertussis (DTP)	Infants, children	4 with boosters	2, 4, 15–18 months; one at school entry	Tetanus toxoid (Td) booster every 10 years or on exposure through a wound

Tetanus and diphtheria toxoids (Td)	Children 7 years or older, adults with no vaccination	3 with boosters	Second dose in 4–8 weeks; third dose 6 months later	Td booster every 10 years or on exposure through a wound
Haemophilus b (Hib)	Infants, children, HIV-infected adults	Depends on formulation	Depends on formulation	Polysaccharide capsule is poor antigen; conjugate vaccines enhance potency
Pneumococcus (polyvalent)	At-risk adults or children 2 years or older (e.g., immunocompromised patients, geriatric patients)	1 or 1/year	As necessary in at-risk patients; not given during active infection; 1/year in geriatric patients	Poor response to polysaccharide antigen in children younger than 2 years old
Subunit				
Recombinant HBV	See hepatitis B	See hepatitis B	See hepatitis B	Generally interchangeable with plasma-derived vaccine

BCG = bacille Calmette-Guérin; *HBsAg* = hepatitis B surface antigen; *HDCV* = human diploid cell vaccines; *HIV* = human immunodeficiency virus; *sIgA* = secretory immunoglobulin A.

*Entire target population is not listed in all cases.

†Five doses to already exposed individuals.

3. **Specific vaccines** in common use and recommended administration schedules are listed in Table 10-3.

D. **Simultaneous administration of active and passive vaccines.** Sometimes active and passive vaccines against a pathogenic organism are administered simultaneously to maximize postexposure prophylaxis. The immune globulin offers immediate protection, and the active vaccine stimulates an immune response. These vaccines are given at separate sites to prevent antibody (passive) and antigen (active) from reacting and inactivating one another.

1. Infants with **HBV** who are born to mothers who have the hepatitis B surface antigen (HBsAg) are significantly protected from becoming chronic carriers by this combined prophylaxis.

2. **Rabies.** Postexposure prophylaxis typically includes the combined use of active and passive vaccines because of the lethal nature of the unchecked infection. The exception is patients with a previous active vaccination who have sufficient existing serum antibody concentration.

3. **Tetanus.** Combined prophylaxis is sometimes used, depending on the type of wound and the patient's history of active vaccination. Recommended guidelines are as follows:
   a. **A tetanus-prone wound** is one that produces anaerobic conditions (e.g., deep puncture) or one in which exposure to *Clostridium* or its spores is probable (e.g., contaminated with animal feces). If the patient's history of active vaccination is uncertain or includes fewer than three doses, both TIG and Td are administered. The patient returns to complete the toxoid series.
      (1) If the wound is tetanus-prone but the patient received a full series of active vaccination, no treatment is necessary if the last Td dose was received within the last 5 years.
      (2) If the last dose was received more than 5 years ago, Td, but not TIG, is given to boost memory immunity and antibody production.
   b. For a **clean, minor wound,** if the patient's history of active vaccination is uncertain or includes fewer than three doses, Td is administered.
      (1) If the patient received a full series of active vaccinations, no treatment is necessary if the last Td dose was received within 10 years.
      (2) If the last dose was received more than 10 years ago, Td, but not TIG, is given to boost memory immunity and antibody production.

VII. PROSPECTS FOR IMMUNOMODULATION

A. **Fab antidigoxin antibody** preparations obtained from sheep are approved for the reversal of toxicity associated with toxic digoxin serum levels. The antibody binds digoxin and prevents it from binding to its normal receptor site. The Fab–digoxin complex is excreted renally.

B. **Monoclonal antibodies** are generally produced through the in vitro fusion of a cancerous plasma cell (myeloma) with an activated mouse B cell. The resulting **hybridoma** secretes murine (mouse) antibodies of a single defined specificity and has the immortality characteristic of the myeloma. Techniques for the production of human monoclonal antibodies and a variety of hybrid mouse–human monoclonal antibodies are not as well refined as the hybridoma technology.

1. **Monoclonal antibodies** [e.g., whole antibodies or Fab or $F(ab')_2$ fragments] are routinely used for in vitro diagnostic tests (e.g., blood group and tissue typing for HLA); screening for cancer-related antigens [e.g., carcinoembryonic antigen (CEA)]; urine testing for drugs and metabolites; and testing for HIV infection. In these and many other diagnostic applications, monoclonal antibodies are often conjugated to enzymes, radioisotopes, or fluorescent dyes.

2. **Muromonab-CD3** is used to treat acute graft rejection. Several other monoclonal antibodies are being tested (see V D 2 e).

3. In clinical trials, **monoclonal antibodies against T cells** show improvement in certain autoimmune disorders.

4. **Monoclonal antibodies against neoplastic cells** show limited success, but are useful in treating certain leukemias and lymphomas.

C. **Monoclonal antibodies are conjugated to enzymes, drugs, prodrugs, radioisotopes, or plant and bacterial toxins** to provide specific delivery of the conjugated agent to one or more focused in vivo sites of action. Several problems are associated with the use of these agents.

1. **Immunotoxins** are usually produced by the conjugation of a monoclonal antibody to a biologic polypeptide toxin (e.g., diphtheria toxin) that is modified to reduce nonspecific toxicity.
2. Although they are being tested for graft rejection and autoimmunity, immunotoxins are primarily used as antineoplastic agents. Clinical trials show moderate success in treating leukemia and lymphoma, with lower success rates against tumors such as breast carcinoma.
3. **Monoclonal antibodies conjugated to radioisotopes** (e.g., ^{90}Y) cause remissions in patients with Hodgkin's disease and acute T-cell leukemia.
4. **Monoclonal antibodies conjugated to enzymes** that activate a prodrug to the active drug at a specific tissue site (e.g., neoplastic cell surface) are in the early stages of human trials.

D. **Immunostimulation** has been attempted with a variety of compounds, ranging from cytokines (see Table 10-1) to bacterial products.

1. IFN-α has many subtypes. Two are currently FDA-approved. Because it inhibits cell growth, it is used to treat hairy cell leukemia, Kaposi's sarcoma in patients with AIDS, and genital warts. At low doses, interferons stimulate immune cellular function (e.g., T cells, NK cells, macrophages), but at high doses, they are immunosuppressive. The use of IFN-α against other cancers produces variable results.
2. IFN-γ provides greater immunostimulation in the intact immune system, but its effects depend on dose and timing. The combined use of IFN-α and IFN-γ yields better results. The most common side effects of interferon therapy are influenza-like symptoms. IFN-γ is approved for use as a macrophage-activating factor in chronic granulomatous disease.
3. Several protocols using **IL-2** show promising results, with apparently complete remissions in some patients with melanoma. With this technique, known as adoptive immunotherapy, a patient's peripheral blood lymphocytes, or tumor-infiltrating lymphocytes, are removed. They are cultured with IL-2 and reinfused with additional IL-2. These IL-2–responsive cells are likely T cells and NK cells. Severe capillary leak syndrome, with some patients dying, is a problematic side effect.
4. **Hormones of the thymus** that induce T-cell maturation and other functions are used to increase certain cell-mediated immune functions, with variable results.
5. Sulfur-containing compounds, such as **levamisole** (a phenylimidothiazole anthelmintic) and diethyldithiocarbamate **(Imuthiol),** have immunostimulatory activity. Their effect is greater on cell-mediated immunity than on humoral immunity. Levamisole is approved as an oral agent for use in colon cancer in combination with fluorouracil.
6. **Inosine pranobex** is licensed for use in many countries as an immunostimulant. It induces T-cell differentiation and augments cell-mediated immune functions, with minimal toxicity.
7. As a component of mycobacterial cell walls, **muramyl dipeptide (MDP)** stimulates macrophage activation and may be used as an adjuvant, given with antigen (see I), or given alone as an immunostimulant.

STUDY QUESTIONS

Directions: Each of the numbered items or incomplete statements in this section is followed by answers or by completions of the statement. Select the **one** lettered answer or completion that is **best** in each case.

1. A man has symptoms of a viral infection of about 4 days' duration. To confirm the diagnosis, the physician draws a blood sample and requests the antibody titer (level) for the suspected agent. The first blood sample shows a low titer of antibody. A week later, another blood sample is drawn, and the titer against the virus is much higher. This situation is an example of

(A) an inflammatory response to the viral infection
(B) a primary immune response to the viral infection
(C) a secondary immune response to the viral infection
(D) a cellular response to the viral infection

2. Which class of antibody has the longest serum half-life and opsonizes antigens for phagocytosis through two different pathways?

(A) Immunoglobulin G (IgG)
(B) Immunoglobulin M (IgM)
(C) Immunoglobulin A (IgA)
(D) Immunoglobulin E (IgE)

3. Urticaria that appears rapidly after the ingestion of food usually indicates which type of hypersensitivity reaction?

(A) Type I
(B) Type II
(C) Type III
(D) Type IV

4. In which autoimmune disorder is the mechanism of pathogenesis classified as type II hypersensitivity?

(A) Systemic lupus erythematosus (SLE)
(B) Insulin-dependent diabetes mellitus (IDDM)
(C) Graves' disease
(D) Hashimoto's thyroiditis

5. A patient receives long-term, high-dose therapy with a sulfonamide. After approximately 3 weeks of therapy, the patient has a low-grade fever, rash, and muscle and joint pain. Which type of hypersensitivity accounts for these symptoms?

(A) Type I
(B) Type II
(C) Type III
(D) Type IV

6. In which type IV hypersensitivity reaction is the tissue-damaging disorder considered an inappropriate response by the immune system?

(A) Poison ivy dermatitis
(B) Chronic tuberculosis
(C) Acute graft rejection
(D) Tuberculin test

7. Which agent is commonly used to treat multiple sclerosis (MS)?

(A) Neostigmine
(B) Cyanocobalamin
(C) Adrenocorticotropic hormone (ACTH)
(D) Propylthiouracil

8. The therapeutic role of muromonab-CD3 in acute renal graft rejection is probably based on

(A) activation of T-cell function and secretion of cytokines
(B) destruction of T cells by complement
(C) opsonization of T cells for phagocytosis
(D) selective inhibition of T_H-cell function

9. Which is a current clinical application of intravenous human immune globulin (IVIG)?

(A) Prophylaxis after hepatitis B virus (HBV) exposure
(B) Treatment of humoral immunodeficiency
(C) Prophylactic infant immunization for polio
(D) Prophylaxis for Rh disease by infant immunization

10. Which cytokine is approved for the treatment of certain forms of cancer?

(A) Interleukin-2 (IL-2)
(B) Interferon-α (IFN-α)
(C) Interferon-γ (IFN-γ)
(D) Imuthiol

Questions 11 and 12

A 6-year-old child has a deep puncture wound. The parent is unsure of the child's history of vaccination.

11. If no other information is available, what should the physician recommend?

(A) No vaccination
(B) Tetanus immune globulin (TIG)
(C) Tetanus toxoid (Td)
(D) Both TIG and Td at separate sites

12. If the child received a full series of diphtheria, pertussis, tetanus (DPT) vaccinations, the last at entry into school, what should the physician recommend?

(A) No vaccination
(B) Tetanus immune globulin (TIG)
(C) Tetanus toxoid (Td)
(D) Both TIG and Td at separate sites

13. Persistent infections by opportunistic pathogens, such as *Candida albicans* and *Pneumocystis carinii,* could indicate all of the following EXCEPT

(A) inherited T-cell immunodeficiency
(B) humoral immunodeficiency
(C) AIDS
(D) combined immunodeficiency

14. Which statement about human immunodeficiency virus (HIV) infection is NOT correct?

(A) Individuals who become infected with human immunodeficiency virus-1 (HIV-1) always show overt symptoms shortly after infection
(B) Seroconversion to positive status for anti-HIV-1 antibodies is the primary criterion for diagnosis of a viral carrier
(C) The incubation period for the pathogenesis of acquired immune deficiency syndrome (AIDS) is believed to be 8 years or longer after the initial infection with HIV
(D) $CD4^+$ T cells and macrophages may be able to spread HIV to uninfected $CD4^+$ cells without releasing any extracellular virus particles

Directions: Each question below contains three suggested answers of which **one or more** is correct. Choose the answer

A if **I only** is correct
B if **III only** is correct
C if **I and II** are correct
D if **II and III** are correct
E if **I, II, and III** are correct

15. Which statement about the currently approved sheep Fab fragment used to counteract digoxin overdose is true?

I. It is obtained by the immunization of sheep with a digoxin–protein conjugate and subsequent proteolytic cleavage of the collected antibody
II. It specifically binds digoxin, preventing its activity
III. It has a serum half-life of approximately 3 weeks

16. $CD4^+$ T cells specifically recognize antigens in which form?

I. Bound to major histocompatibility (MHC) class I molecules on the surface of any body cell
II. In free, soluble form in extracellular fluids
III. Bound to MHC class II molecules on the surface of special antigen-presenting cells (APCs)

17. Which is a normal outcome of the activation of the complement system by either the classic or alternative pathway?

I. Acute inflammation
II. Opsonization of immune complexes
III. Cytolytic action

18. In antiviral immunity, what directly recognizes and kills viral-infected cells?

I. Cytotoxic T cells (CTLs)
II. Antiviral antibodies
III. Interferons

19. A patient is treated with penicillin and produces antibodies against the drug. They are still mostly present. An emergency situation requires administration of an intravenous dose of penicillin. If the patient has a type I penicillin hypersensitivity reaction, which pathologic consequence would be expected, and within what time course of clinical onset?

I. Hemolytic anemia, with an onset of 1–2 hours after the intravenous dose
II. Anaphylaxis, with an onset of a few minutes after the intravenous dose
III. Cutaneous urticaria and pruritus, with an onset of a few minutes after the intravenous dose

20. Which situation occurs in all type IV hypersensitivity reactions?

I. Infiltration of the affected tissue by mononuclear cells
II. A delay of 12 hours or longer in the onset of clinical symptoms after allergen contact
III. Significant beneficial effect of the administration of H_1-antagonists

21. Which immunologic finding is NOT unique to systemic lupus erythematosus (SLE)?

I. Hypergammaglobulinemia
II. The presence of circulating antinuclear antibodies
III. The presence of circulating rheumatoid factors

22. An organ donor who is human leukocyte antigen (HLA)-matched with the recipient of a graft is sought. Which individual is at least somewhat likely to provide a total HLA match?

I. A sibling of the graft recipient
II. A parent of the graft recipient
III. A cadaver

23. Graft-versus-host (GVH) disease is associated primarily with which type of transplantation?

I. Kidney
II. Heart
III. Bone marrow

24. The prophylactic use of cyclosporine in graft rejection is probably based on its ability to

I. inhibit synthesis of antibodies, thereby preventing hyperacute rejection
II. inhibit activation of T cells, thereby preventing acute rejection
III. block transcription of the interleukin-2 (IL-2) gene and synthesis or secretion of IL-2

25. Which is a valid comparison of live, attenuated and killed, inactivated active vaccines?

I. Replication of the organisms in a live, attenuated vaccine increases the stimulation of the immune system, and a lower dose is often required
II. Attenuated vaccines often require multiple doses
III. A killed, inactivated vaccine probably produces lifelong immunity in one or two doses

26. Which active vaccine is recommended for health care workers, but is not routinely given to infants?

I. Measles, mumps, rubella (MMR) vaccine
II. Influenza polyvalent
III. Tetanus toxoid (Td)

27. Which statement about inactivated polio vaccine (IPV) versus oral polio vaccine (OPV) is true?

I. IPV is administered to immunocompromised children and families; otherwise, OPV is used
II. OPV provides superior protection because it is introduced through the normal route of entry for poliovirus infection
III. The risks of severe side effects are greater for OPV than for IPV

ANSWERS AND EXPLANATIONS

1. The answer is B *[1 C 2, 3].*
A primary immune response to an infection is characterized by the initial production of IgM, beginning about 4 days after antigen is encountered. A switch to a different immunoglobulin isotype (i.e., IgG, IgE, or IgA) occurs before the peak of antibody production is reached. The peak primary immune response occurs 10–14 days after the antigen is encountered, and the serum contains both IgM and IgG.

2. The answer is A *[I D 2 b, E].*
Immunoglobulin G (IgG) has a serum half-life of 25–35 days, longer than that of any other class, although mast cell–bound immunoglobulin E (IgE) has the longest half-life. In general, immune complexes containing IgG are opsonized for phagocytosis through binding to the IgG receptors on neutrophils and macrophages, and additionally through the activation of complement. Immunoglobulin M (IgM) also opsonizes, but only through the activation of complement.

3. The answer is A *[II A 5 a, b].*
Food allergies are usually type I reactions. In a patient with preexisting hypersecreted immunoglobulin E (IgE) specific to a food allergen and bound to mast cells, the allergic response usually occurs shortly after ingestion. Mast cell secretions lead to vomiting. Systemic spillover of allergen into the circulation may lead to milder effects in other tissues (e.g., urticaria).

4. The answer is D *[II C 2 c; III D 2 b].*
Antithyroid peroxidase antibodies produce complement-mediated cytotoxicity to thyroid follicle cells (a type II pathogenic mechanism). In systemic lupus erythematosus (SLE), persistent circulating immune complexes are responsible for much of the pathogenesis (type III); in Graves' disease, an antibody acting as a thyroid-stimulating hormone (TSH) agonist hyperstimulates the thyroid; in insulin-dependent diabetes mellitus (IDDM), T-cell cytotoxicity to beta islet cells is probably responsible for the major pathogenesis (type IV).

5. The answer is C *[II D 2 c, 4 a, b, 5 a].*
One of the most common causes of type III hypersensitivity is the response to drugs. This type of reaction is often seen after long-term, high-dose therapy. The treatment of choice is to discontinue treatment and substitute an unrelated drug.

6. The answer is A *[II E 1].*
Poison ivy contains a hapten, pentadecyl catechol, which is not known to be toxic. Therefore, its capacity to elicit an immune response is inappropriate because it serves no useful function. In chronic tuberculosis, the immune response is attempting, although unsuccessfully, to eliminate the mycobacterial pathogen. Acute graft rejection is also appropriate, but unfortunate, because it is a response against foreign tissue. A tuberculin test is an appropriate manifestation of the existence of active immunity or memory to *Mycobacterium.*

7. The answer is C *[III D 8 b].*
Adrenocorticotropic hormone (ACTH) is the immunosuppressive agent of choice in multiple sclerosis (MS). Neostigmine is used as an anticholinergic agent in myasthenia gravis. Cyanocobalamin is administered in autoimmune pernicious anemia to replace nonabsorbed vitamin B_{12}. Propylthiouracil is used as an antithyroid in Graves' disease.

8. The answer is C *[V D 2 e].*
Muromonab-CD3 is a mouse anti-CD3 monoclonal antibody that binds to all T cells because CD3 is a constant part of the antigen receptor of each T cell. The binding of muromonab-CD3 opsonizes the T cells for phagocytosis. Therefore, the total number of T cells is reduced. Mouse antibodies are inefficient at activating human complement. Some T-cell activation with cytokine secretion occurs, but it is an undesirable side effect of muromonab-CD3 administration.

9. The answer is B *[VI B 1 c; Table 10-2].*
Intravenous human immune globulins (IVIGs) are used to replace antibody in immunodeficient individuals. Hepatitis B immune globulin (HBIG) is administered intramuscularly. Anti-Rh antibody is also administered intramuscularly to the mother immediately postpartum (sometimes during pregnancy), but not to the infant. Prophylactic infant immunization for polio is provided through active, not passive, vaccination.

10. The answer is B *[VII D].*
Interferon-α (IFN-α) is approved for use in patients with hairy cell leukemia and patients with acquired immune deficiency syndrome (AIDS) and Kaposi's sarcoma. Some of its beneficial effects probably derive from its ability to inhibit growth. The other cytokines are in various stages of clinical trials as antineoplastic therapies, although interferon-γ (IFN-γ) is approved for use in patients with chronic granulomatous disease. Imuthiol is not a cytokine, but a synthetic drug.

11 and 12. The answers are: 11-D, 12-A *[VI D 3 a; Table 10-3].*
A patient with an uncertain history of vaccination and a tetanus-prone wound requires both active and passive vaccination. The tetanus immune globulin (TIG) provides immediate protection if the individual does not have memory. The tetanus toxoid (Td) begins the series that leads to the establishment of memory. A tetanus-prone wound in an individual with a full series of active vaccinations requires no treatment if the last vaccination in the series was administered less than 5 years earlier. These recommendations are general guidelines.

13. The answer is B *[IV A, B 6].*
Opportunistic infections by fungi, viruses, and parasites other than extracellular pyogenic bacteria suggest a deficiency of T-cell function. Inherited T-cell immunodeficiency and acquired immune deficiency syndrome (AIDS) are inherited and acquired T-cell deficiencies, respectively. Combined immunodeficiency includes both humoral and T-cell deficiency. Only humoral immunodeficiency is a primarily humoral deficiency in which the expected signs are recurrent infections by extracellular pyogenic bacteria.

14. The answer is A *[IV B 6 a (1)].*
It is not known what percentage of individuals shows overt symptoms after initial infection. Those who do, however, generally show mononucleosis-like symptoms for approximately 3 weeks. Some individuals display no overt symptoms.

15. The answer is C (I, II) *[I A 4, D 2, 5; VII A].*
Digoxin is a hapten, a molecule that is too small to stimulate responses (be an immunogen) in its free form, but can be recognized by antibodies. To obtain sheep antidigoxin antibodies, the sheep is immunized with digoxin that has been coupled to a larger molecule, in this case, a protein. The antibodies obtained from the sheep are cleaved with proteolytic enzymes to yield the Fab fragment. This fragment is specific to and can bind digoxin, blocking its biologic activity. Animal antibodies have a shorter serum half-life when injected into humans, and all Fab fragments, even human, have a short half-life compared with complete antibody molecules. Only complete human immunoglobulin G (IgG) has a half-life of approximately 1 month.

16. The answer is B (III) *[I B 3, 5].*
$CD4^+$, or helper, T cells have receptors that recognize fragments (epitopes) of immunizing antigens (immunogens) only when the fragments are bound to an MHC class II molecule on the surface of antigen-presenting cells (APCs). As a result, T cells cannot be activated inappropriately by soluble antigens. $CD8^+$ T cells recognize fragments bound to MHC class I molecules.

17. The answer is E (all) *[I E 2].*
When complement is activated, different proteins of the complement sequence have functions that lead to all three actions. Acute inflammation allows greater movement of plasma proteins and phagocytes from blood to tissue. Opsonization of immune complexes enhances their phagocytosis. Cytolysis of microorganisms often results in their killing.

18. The answer is A (I) *[I F 2].*
Antiviral antibodies are probably most important in extracellular immunity to viruses, binding virus particles for opsonization and preventing additional infection of cells. Interferons are secreted from viral-infected and other cells (e.g., macrophages, T cells) and, after binding to receptors, induce the appearance of antiviral proteins in other cells. Cytotoxic T cells (CTLs) recognize viral-infected cells and cause direct cytotoxicity.

19. The answer is D (II, III) *[II A 2 d, 6, 7, C 1 b, 5].*
If the patient produced antibodies that are still present and the hypersensitivity reaction is type I, these antibodies are hypersecreted immunoglobulin E (IgE), mostly bound to mast cell and basophil IgE re-

ceptors. Their half-life is several months. Intravenous introduction of penicillin causes rapid activation of and secretion by blood basophils. Symptoms of type I hypersensitivity occur within minutes. These symptoms may be severe (anaphylaxis) or less severe (cutaneous, gastrointestinal, or respiratory), depending on the individual. Hemolytic anemia is an expected result of a type II hypersensitivity reaction to penicillin, based on the presence of immunoglobulin M (IgM) or immunoglobulin G (IgG) antibodies in the serum. The onset is delayed by a few hours in a patient with preexisting antibodies.

20. The answer is C (I, II) *[II E 3–6].*
Type IV hypersensitivity reactions are delayed after the introduction of allergen because allergen-specific T cells become activated and attract other cells, such as macrophages, to the site of allergen introduction (e.g., the epidermis of the skin in contact sensitivity, the lungs in tuberculosis). These sites are infiltrated by mononuclear cells. Inflammation is primarily caused by tissue disruption and necrosis as well as by secretion of cytokines by the infiltrating cells. Although histamine secretion can also occur from local mast cells, H_1 antagonists of histamine usually do not have significant effects because T-cell and macrophage activation, migration, and secretion are not greatly affected by these drugs.

21. The answer is E (all) *[III C 3 b, E 1, 2].*
All three findings are common to more than one non–organ-specific autoimmune disorder, but occur in different percentages of patients with specific disorders. For example, antinuclear antibodies are probably present in all patients with systemic lupus erythematosus (SLE), but are found in only a fraction of patients with rheumatoid arthritis and Sjögren's syndrome. Rheumatoid factors are more common in rheumatoid arthritis than in SLE or Sjögren's syndrome, and hypergammaglobulinemia is more prevalent in SLE than in Sjögren's syndrome.

22. The answer is A (I) *[V A 3, B].*
Parents and children are rarely human leukocyte antigen (HLA)-matched, but are usually half-matched. An HLA match from a cadaver-derived organ is unlikely. The probability that two siblings are HLA-matched is 25%; the probability that they are half-matched is 50%.

23. The answer is B (III) *[V B 2, C 1].*
In bone marrow transplantation, marrow containing competent lymphocytes is transplanted to a generally immunosuppressed host. The greatest problem is an immune response by the graft against human leukocyte antigens (HLA) and other tissue antigens of the host. In renal and cardiac transplantation, the greatest problem is rejection of the foreign organ by the immune system of the host [host-versus-graft (HVG) disease].

24. The answer is D (II, III) *[V B 2, D 2 a].*
Cell-mediated immune mechanisms are thought to be more important in acute graft rejection, and the inhibition of T-cell activation appears to be the key element in immunosuppression. Responding T cells require signaling from interleukin-2 (IL-2) to reach full activation and progress to cell division. IL-2 is produced by activated T cells and can act autocrinely. Cyclosporine blocks transcription of the IL-2 gene during T-cell activation, inhibits the synthesis of IL-2, and prevents full T-cell activation and division. Its effects are limited to activated T cells. Because it has no direct effect on antibody synthesis, it is not useful in the hyperacute rejection phenomena that are based on antibody-mediated mechanisms. Hyperacute rejection is essentially untreatable because it depends on the presence of antibodies in the graft recipient.

25. The answer is A (I) *[VI C 2 a, b].*
Live, attenuated vaccines introduce organisms that are competent to replicate. This replication stimulates the immune response. For this and probably other reasons, a live, attenuated vaccine (but not a killed, inactivated vaccine) probably provides lifelong immunity in one or two doses.

26. The answer is D (II, III) *[VI C 1 d; Table 10-3].*
The measles, mumps, rubella (MMR) vaccine is administered to infants within or shortly after the first year. A second dose is recommended at school entry. Influenza active vaccine is targeted toward specific adult populations. Health care workers are included in this target population, as are infants and children at risk; however, the vaccine is not routinely administered to infants. Tetanus toxoid (Td) is not routinely administered to infants, who instead receive diphtheria, tetanus, pertussis (DTP). Td is used primarily for initial vaccinations in adults who were not previously vaccinated and for 10-year booster vaccinations in all individuals, including health care workers.

27. The answer is E (all) *[VI C 2; Table 10-3].*
Because oral polio vaccine (OPV) is a live, attenuated vaccine, it is not used in immunocompromised individuals who would have difficulty clearing the replicating virus. In general, live, attenuated vaccines are not given to immunocompromised individuals. Because individuals who are vaccinated with OPV become transient carriers of the attenuated virus, family members of these individuals are not vaccinated, except with inactivated polio vaccine (IPV). OPV is the vaccine of choice for others and is given orally, the normal route of viral entry. This route of administration induces secretory immunoglobulin A (sIgA) in addition to immunoglobulin G (IgG), providing increased protection. The risk of reversion to virulence (vaccine-induced polio) is small for OPV and probably nonexistent for IPV.

11 Biotechnological Products

Andrew B. C. Yu
Godwin W. Fong

I. INTRODUCTION.

Advances in biotechnology have resulted in formerly unstable products becoming available for therapeutic use. Some life-threatening diseases are being treated with biotechnological products.

A. Biotechnological products

1. **Interferon** is an example of a successful drug genetically engineered to inhibit certain types of cancer cells and some viruses.
2. Cellular hormones known as **interleukins, lymphotoxins,** and the **tumor necrosis factor** are used to treat cancer and immune deficiency diseases.
3. **Monoclonal antibodies (MAB)** can deliver toxins specifically to cancer cells and destroy these cells. MAB are also used with radioisotopes to diagnose and visualize cancer cells.

B. Modified biotechnological products

1. In animal studies synthetic analogue of **thyrotropin-releasing hormone** has proved effective in preventing paralysis after spinal-cord injuries.
2. In the future, **superoxide dismutase** might be used to prevent damage to tissues deprived of oxygen.
3. New drugs are developed for emphysema, congestive heart failure, ulcers, atherosclerosis, and an increasing number of new medical conditions. Biotechnological products approved for human use are listed in Table 11-1.

II. BASIC TERMINOLOGY

A. Antigen is a substance that stimulates the production of antibodies in the body.

B. Antibody is an immunoglobulin produced by the body in response to stimulation from an antigen.

C. Antisense DNA refers to a complementary strand of DNA specifically synthesized to attach to the sense DNA, thereby preventing genetic transcription. The sense DNA that carries the information impacting the disease process is usually elucidated before an antisense drug is designed.

D. Colony-stimulating factor (CSF) refers to a class of glycoprotein hormones that regulate the differentiation and formation of blood cells from precursor cells.

E. Cytokine refers to a group of special proteins (nonantibody) released by cells to trigger action in other cells.

F. Deoxyribonucleic acid (DNA) is the molecule that contains the genetic instruction of a cell. DNA consists of deoxyribose, phosphate, and repeating bases as building blocks. The four bases are adenine, guanine, thymine, and cytosine.

G. DNA ligase is an enzyme that seals single-stranded nicks between nucleotides in double-stranded DNA. This enzyme enables DNA fragments from different sources to be joined.

Table 11-1. Approved Recombinant and Other Biotechnological Products

Drug	**Indication**	**Company (Year introduced)**
Human insulin (Humulin, Novolin)	Diabetes	Eli Lilly/Genentech (1982); Novo Nordisk
Somatrem for injection (Protropin)	hGH deficiency in children	Genentech (1985)
Interferon-α-2a (Roferon-A)	Hairy cell leukemia	Hoffmann-La Roche (1986)
Interferon-α-2b (Intron A)	Hairy cell leukemia	Schering-Plough/Biogen (1986)
Hepatitis B vaccine, MSD (Recombivax HB)	Hepatitis B prevention	Merck; Chiron (1986)
Muromonab-CD3 (Orthoclone OKT3)	Reversal of acute kidney transplant rejection	Ortho Biotech (1986)
Somatropin for injection (Humatrope)	hGH deficiency in children	Eli Lilly (1987)
Alteplase (TPA) (Activase)	Acute myocardial infarction	Genentech (1987)
	Acute pulmonary embolism	(1990)
Interferon-α-2a (Roferon-A)	AIDS-related Kaposi's sarcoma	Hoffmann-La Roche (1988)
Interferon-α-2b (Intron A)	AIDS-related Kaposi's sarcoma	Schering-Plough/Biogen
	Genital warts	(1988)
	Hepatitis C	(1991)
Interferon-α-n3 (Alferon N injection)	Genital warts	Interferon Sciences (1989)
Hepatitis B vaccine (Engerix-B)	Hepatitis B prevention	SmithKline Beecham; Biogen (1989)
Erythropoietin (Epogen)	Anemia associated with chronic renal failure	Amgen; Johnson & Johnson; Kirin (1989)
Erythropoietin (Procrit)	Anemia associated with AIDS	Amgen; Ortho Biotech (1990)
Erythropoietin (Procrit)	Anemia associated with chronic renal failure	Ortho Biotech (1990)
Erythropoietin (Procrit)	Chemotherapy-associated anemia in nonyloid malignancy patients	Amgen; Ortho Biotech (1993)
Erythropoietin (Procrit)	Anemia associated with cancer and chemotherapy	Ortho Biotech (1993)
PEG-adenosine	ADA-deficient SCID	Enzon; Eastman Kodak (1990)
Interferon-γ-1b (Actimmune)	Management of chronic granulomatous disease	Genentech (1990)
Alteplase (TPA) (Activase)	Acute pulmonary embolism	Genentech (1990)
CMV immune globulin (CytoGam)	CMV prevention in kidney transplant	Medimmune (1990)
Filgrastim; G-CSF (Neupogen)	Chemotherapy-induced neutropenia	Amgen (1991)
β-glucocerebrosidase (Ceredase)	Type I-Gaucher's disease*	Genzyme (1991)
Glucocerebrosidase (Cerezyme)	Type I-Gaucher's disease*	Genzyme (1994)

*__Gaucher's disease__ is an autosomal dominant or recessive disorder due to excess of glucocerebroside in the reticuloendothelial cells due to lack of a metabolic enzyme, cerebrosidase. Proliferation of abnormal cells lead to **splenomegaly, hepatomegaly,** skeletal lesions, and other symptoms.

Table 11-1. *Continued*

Drug	Indication	Company (Year introduced)
Didanosine, ddI (Videx)[a]	HIV/AIDS	Bristol-Myers Squibb (1991)
Sargramostim (GM-CSF) (Prokine)	Autologous bone marrow transplantation	Hoechst-Roussel; Immunex (1991)
Sargramostim (GM-CSF) (Leukine)	Neutrophil recovery following bone marrow transplantation	Immunex; Hoechst-Roussel (1991)
Antihemophilic factor (Mononine)	Hemophilia B	Armour (1992)
Antihemophilic factor (Recombinate)	Hemophilia A	Genetics Institute; Baxter Healthcare (1992)
Aidesleukin (Interleukin-2) (Proleukin)	Renal cell carcinoma	Chiron (1992)
Indium-111 labeled antibody (OncoScint CR103)	Detection, staging, and follow-up of colorectal cancer	Cytogen; Knoll (1992)
Indium-111 labeled antibody (OncoScint OV103)	Detection, staging, and follow-up of ovarian cancer	(1992)
Zalcitabine, ddC (Hivid)[b]	HIV/AIDS	Hoffmann La-Roche (1992)
Interferon-β (Betaseron)	Relapsing/remitting multiple sclerosis	Chiron; Berlex (1993)
DNase (Pulmozyme)	Cystic fibrosis	Genentech (1993)
Factor VIII (Kogenate)	Hemophilia A	Genentech; Miles (1993)
Filgrastim (G-CSF) (Neupogen)	Bone marrow transplant	Amgen (1994)
PEG-L-asparaginase (Oncaspar)	Refractory childhood acute lymphoblastic leukemia	Enzon (1994)
Human growth hormone (Nutropin)	Short stature caused by human growth hormone deficiency	Genentech (1994)
Abciximab, (ReoPro)	Anti-platelet prevention of blood clots	Centocor (1994)
Lamivudine, 3 TC (Epivir)	HIV/AIDS	Glaxo Wellcome; Biochem Pharma (1995)
Saquinavir (Invirase)[+] Protease Inhibitor**	HIV/AIDS	Hoffman La-Roche (1995)
Riluzole (Rilutek)	ALS (amyotrophic lateral sclerosis)	Rhone-Poulenc Rorer (1995)
Ritonavir (Norvir)[+] Protease Inhibitor**	HIV/AIDS	Abbott Laboratories (1996)
Indinavir (Crixivan)[+] Protease Inhibitor**	HIV/AIDS	Merck (1996)

[a]Based on ACTG 175 study results. Videx is recommended by the Antiviral Drugs Advisory Committee (on 2/28/96) as first-line therapy in HIV infection in asymptomatic patients. This will make Videx the first nucleoside analog to compete with Retrovir (AZT) as the first-line monotherapy. Clinical data showed that ddI monotherapy is better than AZT monotherapy. Note: ddI uses a buffer system to slow rapid degradation by acid in the stomach. BMS is developing an oral caplet and an enteric-coated product to address the gastrointestinal side effects issue.

[b]Based on ACTG 175 study results, Hivid/AZT combination is recommended by the Antiviral Drugs Advisory Committee (on 2/28/96) as first-line therapy in HIV infection in antiretroviral naive patients.

[+]The NDAs for Invirase and Norvir were approved by FDA under accelerated approval in only 97 and 72 days, respectively, a record-breaking speed by FDA for a life-threatening disease.

****Protease inhibitors** are a new class of potent anti-HIV therapeutic agents. Indinovir (Crixivan, Merck) is considered to be the most potent of the three (3) protease inhibitors available on the U.S. market.

H. DNA polymerase is an enzyme that catalyzes the synthesis of DNA by using a single strand of DNA as the template and nucleotides as the substrates.

I. Enzyme is a protein that catalyzes a substrate during its conversion to a product.

J. Gene is a segment of DNA that codes for a specific polypeptide.

K. Genome refers to the genetic information content.

L. Hormone is an endogenous substance secreted by one type of cell and acting on another type of cell.

M. Hybridoma is a hybrid cell produced by the fusion of a myeloma cell and a specific antibody-producing B lymphocyte. A single hybridoma will produce only a single antibody.

N. Interferon is any of a class of glycoproteins produced by animal cells in response to viral infection.

O. Interleukin (IL) is a group of proteins synthesized by macrophages and T lymphocytes in response to antigen and other stimulation.

P. Lymphokine is any of a class of soluble proteins produced by some white blood cells that stimulate other white blood cells as part of the immune response.

Q. Plasmid is a circular piece of duplex DNA that is not part of the chromosome and can replicate independently. Plasmids are used as vectors for the transfer of DNA in the process of recombinant DNA technology.

R. Ribonucleic acid (RNA) is a macromolecule involved in executing information during protein synthesis. The three types of RNA are ribosomal RNA (rRNA), transfer RNA (tRNA), and messenger RNA (mRNA). RNA is also the genetic material of some viruses.

S. Recombinant DNA (rDNA) is a hybrid DNA that is formed by the joining of pieces of DNA from different sources. The process is also known as gene splicing.

T. Restriction endonuclease is an enzyme that cleaves DNA at sequence-specific sites.

U. Tumor necrosis factor (TNF) is a lymphokine produced by macrophages that can be activated to kill tumor cells.

III. PROTEINS AND PEPTIDES.

III. PROTEINS AND PEPTIDES. Proteins and peptides (macromolecules that consist of amino acids) play an essential role in all aspects of cellular functions. Many endogenous substances synthesized in the body are essential proteins, and many enzymes that catalyze vital reactions in the body are proteins.

A. Examples of these proteins include:

1. **Hemoglobin:** a large protein involved in oxygen transport
2. **Globulins:** special proteins in the plasma involved in immunogenic response and antibody formation
3. **Albumin:** a plasma protein that binds to many drugs and is used as a carrier for new drugs; **albumin human 5%** [USP]: used to reverse hypovolemia in shock, burn, and chronic hypoalbuminemia patients
4. **Insulin** and the digestive enzymes

B. Glycoproteins. Many special proteins acquire biological activity because of their covalent linking with a polymer of sugar or **carbohydrate.** The covalently linked protein–carbohydrate molecule is referred to as **glycoprotein.** Glycoproteins form natural structural membranes in human and animal cells, including bacteria.

Table 11-2. Immunoglobulin Applications

Gammaglobulinemia
Hepatitis A prophylaxis
Measles and rubella prophylaxis
Multiple myeloma with specific antibody deficiency
Prophylaxis-infants/children with HIV exposure
Chronic inflammatory demyelinating neuropathy
Acquired hemophilia
Orphan drug: treatment of juvenile rheumatoid arthritis
Orphan drug: polymyositis, acute myocarditis
Immune thrombocytopenic purpura

1. ***N*-acetylglucosamine (NAG)** forms the cell membrane in bacteria, an example of a carbohydrate chain linked to a protein via a chain of amino acids. Bacterial resistance to penicillin is linked to the integrity of the **NAG** in the cell membrane.

2. The extent and site of **glycosylation** of the protein molecule may affect the physicochemical properties, stability, and specificity of surface receptors in a cell. Glycoproteins in the surface of red blood cells are involved in recognizing the specific blood type of a person.

3. The **charge** in a site of the glycoprotein molecule might play a role in receptor orientation and interaction and can be modified by **sialic acid, sulfate,** and **phosphate groups.** Change in glycosylation is a powerful tool in engineering preferred configuration and stability in designing recombinant glycoprotein for therapeutic use. The protein molecule presents potential sites for ***N*-glycosylation** and ***O*-glycosylation.**

4. **Examples** of carbohydrates that contribute to activities include terminal sialic acids of glycoproteins by various viruses and bacteria, recognition of polylactosamines on **erythrocytes** by autoimmune antibodies, and recognition of sialylated, fucosylated lactosaminoglycans on leukocytes by E-selectin of endothelial cells.

C. **Immunoglobulin (IgG)** is an important class of globulin protein involved in immunity and allergic response. IgG is used therapeutically to modulate and replace antibodies in various immunodeficiencies (Table 11-2). Intramuscular and intravenous preparations are available from various manufacturers as shown in Table 11-3. Most of these products have limited shelf-life and must be stored at 2°C–8°C.

D. **Recombinant human granulocyte colony-stimulating factor (rHuG-CSF)**

1. **Definition.** CSFs are **glycoproteins** and include **macrophages, eosinophils, neutrophils, basophils,** and **platelets** (see II D).

2. **Uses. Natural** and **modified** CSFs are produced to treat a variety of congenital disorders and several forms of cancer.

3. **Structure**

   a. **Lenograstim,** a rHuG-CSF derived from Chinese hamster ovary cells, is glycosylated at the same site as natural HuG-CSF (threonine:133 amino acids) and consists of 174 amino acids.

Table 11-3. Immunoglobulin Products

Gamimune-N
Gammagard
Polygram
Gammar
Iveegam
Sandoglobulin
Polygam
Venoglobulin

b. **Filgrastim,** an *Escherichia coli*-derived rHuG-CSF, is not glycosylated and differs from natural HuG-CSF in structure. Colony-forming assays have indicated that lenograstim is approximately three times as potent as filgrastim, whereas cell proliferation assays have shown these agents as similarly potent.

4. **Functions.** As with natural HuG-CSF and filgrastim, lenograstim selectively promotes the proliferation, differentiation, and maturation of blood-cell precursors. Dose-related increases in blood neutrophil counts are observed after lenograstim administration.
   a. Both natural and recombinant HuG-CSF products stimulate the release of mature **neutrophils** from hematopoietic tissue, prolong cell survival, and enhance cell phagocytic and cytotoxic activity.
   b. Other actions of rHuG-CSF include **synergism** with:
      (1) **Interleukin-3** to induce megakaryocyte formation
      (2) **Granulocyte-macrophage** colony-stimulating factor (GM-CSF)
   c. Lenograstim reduces the:
      (1) Duration of **neutropenia**
      (2) Severity of **infection** in patients receiving **cytotoxic chemotherapy** for **nonmyeloid malignancy**

IV. DNA

A. **Definition.** DNA is the genetic material in all organisms except some viruses, which have genetic material in the form of RNA (see II F).

B. **Structure**

1. Most organisms have **double-stranded** DNA. α However, some viruses contain **single-stranded** DNA and replicate by entering a host cell and making a complementary copy of themselves, temporarily forming a double strand.

2. All DNA molecules consist of many covalently linked subunits called **nucleotides,** which consist of deoxyribose, phosphate, and one of the nitrogen-containing bases (e.g., adenine, guanine, thymine, cytosine).

C. **Function.** DNA **encodes information** to produce all proteins needed by the organism. The DNA sequence can be modified or recombined with new strands. This recombinant technology can be applied to correct genetic defects in living organisms.

V. ANTISENSE DRUGS

A. **Overview.** Many diseases occur as a result of genetic defects or errors in the gene involved in producing essential enzymes or proteins in the body. Genetic information resides in **chromosomes,** which house helical strands known as DNA within the nucleus (see II F).

B. **Definition.** The process of targeting DNA or RNA using the following technique is called **antisense** drug (see II C).

1. **Strategies** to alter or block the **transcriptional process** in DNA can moderate many disease processes.

2. By changing the DNA sequence so that the **complementary strand** is transcribed instead of the normal "sense" gene, the DNA would be unable to make a copy of normal RNA, which participates in protein synthesis.

3. The aberrant copies of RNA may "pair up" **(hybridize)** with other RNAs that complement it and block protein synthesis.

4. Many **oligonucleotides** have been designed to target viral disease and cancer cells in the body. To further stabilize the drug, **phosphodiesters** are substituted for **phosphothioates.** Antisense drugs against CMV, HIV, and other viruses and cancers are now in various phases of clinical trial.

C. Developments. When the **nucleotide** base sequence of a gene that controls a specific body function is known, the antisense DNA strands can be synthesized. These strands can be introduced into cells where they attach themselves to the complementary sense DNA strands, depressing the transcription of these genes. This has been done successfully in cell culture for the cancer-causing gene that produces human **larynx squamous carcinoma.**

D. Human Genome Initiative. This research group was created several years ago to study all human genes. This national effort is now yielding information on many diseases, including congenital defects, cancer, AIDS, and other immune system disorders.

VI. GENE THERAPY. The first example of human gene therapy started in 1990 when an FDA-approved PEG-ADA (made by Enzon Inc., Piscataway, NJ) for **adenosine deaminase (ADA)** deficiency, a rare genetic disorder that weakens the immune system. Two girls were reinfused with genetically altered white blood cells (drawn from their bodies) with the gene corrected. The altered cells lived and functioned normally, allowing the two girls to live a relatively normal life.

VII. MISCELLANEOUS BIOTECHNOLOGIC PRODUCTS

A. Alteplase (Activase, Genentech) is a **thrombolytic** agent formerly known as **tissue-type plasminogen activator (tPA).**

1. **Intravenous (IV)** alteplase is **effective** in:
   a. Producing recanalization of occluded coronary arteries following acute **myocardial infarction** (recommended dosage is 100 mg in divided doses)
   b. Treating acute massive **pulmonary embolism** (recommended dose is 100 mg infused intravenously over 2 hours)
2. **Adverse effects** include:
   a. Bleeding complications
   b. Reperfusion arrhythmias
   c. Reinfarction
   d. **Systemic fibrinolysis**, which is less than that seen with streptokinase

B. Antithrombin III (heparin cofactor, human antithrombin III) has been designated an orphan drug product for use as replacement therapy in congenital deficiency states for prevention or treatment of thromboembolic episodes. The **amount** of IV antithrombin (AT) III concentrate given is based on the AT III levels.

1. Between 80% and 120% of normal AT III levels is the desired goal in patients with congenital or acquired AT III deficiency.
2. A daily dose of AT III should maintain serum levels above 80% of normal; levels should be monitored twice daily until stabilization, then daily, that is, immediately prior to the next dose.

C. Interleukin-3 (IL-3) is a **hematopoietic growth factor** used in the treatment of patients with bone marrow failure.

1. **Functions.** Recombinant human IL-3 alone has improved:
   a. **Neutrophil** and **platelet counts** in patients with chemotherapy-related bone marrow failure and myelodysplastic syndromes
   b. Hematopoiesis slightly in aplastic anemia
   c. Responses with the sequential combined use of recombinant human IL-3 and other hematopoietic growth factors, such as GM-CSF
2. Recombinant human IL-3 may be given subcutaneously (SQ) or IV. IV doses can be 30–1000 $\mu g/m^2$/day infused over 4 hours.

D. Aldesleukin, a lymphokine, is a human recombinant IL-2 product used for treating **metastatic renal cell carcinoma.**

1. **Dosage.** The starting dosage is 0.037 mg/kg every 8 hours by a 15-minute IV infusion.

2. **Function.** Aldesleukin is absorbed erratically after intramuscular (IM) or SC injection. It follows two compartment pharmacokinetics, with an α–half-life of 13 minutes and a β–half-life of 85 minutes, and is eliminated renally.

3. **Side effects.** The principal side effects are hypotension and flu-like symptoms. Most adverse effects are dose related.

E. **Abciximab (c7E3 Fab)** is a chimeric monoclonal antibody antigen-binding fragment (Fab) specific to platelet glycoprotein IIb–IIIa receptors.

1. **Use.** In recent tests, this drug was extremely effective in **reducing fatalities** (more than 50%) in subjects with **unstable angina** after receiving **angioplasty** treatment.

2. **Dosage.** The recommended dosage of abciximab (ReoPro) is an IV bolus of 0.25 mg/kg administered 10–60 minutes before the start of percutaneous transluminal coronary angioplasty (PTCA). This is followed by a continuous infusion of 10 μg/min for 12 hours. Platelet aggregation is almost completely inhibited 2 hours after initiation of abciximab therapy.

3. **Side effects.** The major complication of abciximab infusion is dose-related bleeding.

F. **Campath-1** consists of monoclonal antibodies that target human lymphocytes and monocytes.

1. **Uses**
   a. This product is used for **immunosuppression** in organ transplants.
   b. Campath-1 has been used experimentally to treat refractory **autoimmune disorders**, including rheumatoid arthritis and vasculitis.
   c. Campath-1 antibodies are used for the **prevention** of graft-versus-host disease and the **treatment** of lymphoid malignancy immunosuppressants in organ transplants.

2. **Dosage.** The IV dosage is 25 mg once or twice daily.

G. **Edobacomab** is an **immune globulin** directed against gram-negative bacterial endotoxins. The drug is being investigated for the treatment of gram-negative sepsis and septic shock.

1. **Dosage.** For **septic shock,** single IV doses of 2–15 mg/kg every 24 hours are used. The distribution volume of edobacomab ranges from 4 L to 8 L, and the elimination half-life is approximately 10–18 hours.

2. **Side effects.** The main side effects are hypersensitivity and adverse reactions related to antibody production.

H. **Muromonab-CD3** is an immunosuppressive agent that is effective in reversing **acute renal allograft rejection.**

1. **Dosage.** The usual IV dosage is 5 mg/day for 10–14 days following initial signs and symptoms of rejection. The volume of distribution is approximately 6.5 L, and the half-life is 18 hours.

2. **Side effects.** The main side effects include a flu-like symptom complex, which appears to be associated with the release of cytokines. Symptoms may be self-limited or severe and life-threatening.

I. **Nebacumab** is an **immune globulin** directed against gram-negative bacterial endotoxins. The drug is being investigated for the treatment of **gram-negative sepsis** and **septic shock.** Signs and symptoms of septic shock usually resolve during the first 7 days after treatment with nebacumab. Its half-life is 15.9 hours, and the volume of distribution is 48.5 ml/kg.

J. **Satumomab pendetide** is a **monoclonal antibody conjugate** produced from the murine monoclonal antibody, B72.3. It requires radiolabelling to form indium (In^{111}) chloride satumomab pendetide. It is used as a **diagnostic imaging** agent in the staging of patients with known **colorectal** and **ovarian carcinoma.** The metabolic fate of this agent is unclear. The antibody conjugate is cleared slowly with a terminal half-life of approximately 56 hours, and approximately 10% of an administered dose appears in the urine.

K. **Zolimomab aritox** (Orthozyme-CD5 Plus, Xoma/Ortho Biotech) is an **immunoconjugate** of monoclonal anti-CD5 murine IgG and the ricin A-chain toxin.

1. **Uses**
   a. The product's main use is to treat steroid-resistant graft-versus-host disease after **allogeneic bone marrow transplants** for hematopoietic neoplasms, such as acute myelogenous leukemia.
   b. Potential uses of the drug include treatment of **rheumatoid arthritis** and **Type I diabetes mellitus.**

2. **Dosage.** After therapeutic doses of zolimomab aritox, peak serum levels are 1–5 μg/ml. The serum half-life is 1.5–4 hours. The dose varies depending on indications.

L. **Betaseron (Berlex Laboratories).** Interferon (IF)-β is a **glycoprotein** with antiviral, antiproliferative, and immunomodulatory activity. Many of its effects are similar to those of IF-α. IF-β has been administered intravenously, intramuscularly, subcutaneously, intrathecally, topically, and intralesionally for a variety of indications. A new competing product, Avonex (Biogen, Inc.), was approved recently by the FDA for multiple sclerosis treatment.

1. **Uses**
   a. This drug is used for multiple sclerosis, AIDS, malignant melanoma, herpesvirus, and papillomavirus infections.
   b. IF-β is recommended for reducing exacerbations in patients with relapsing–remitting multiple sclerosis.

2. **Dosage.** For patients with relapsing–remitting multiple sclerosis, 8 million units SC every other day is recommended.

3. **Serum levels.** Biological activity of IF-β is evident in the absence of detectable serum levels; serum concentrations are not consistently detectable after SC or IM administration. IF-β can cross the disrupted blood–brain barrier. The compound does not appear in urine following systemic administration.

4. **Side effects.** Adverse effects include flu-like symptoms, bone marrow suppression, neurotoxic effects with high doses, anorexia, other gastrointestinal symptoms, and elevations of liver enzymes and serum creatinine.

STUDY QUESTIONS

Directions: Each of the numbered items or incomplete statements in this section is followed by answers or by completions of the statement. Select the **one** lettered answer or completion that is **best** in each case.

1. Which of the following cells definitely contains double-stranded DNA?

(A) Human cells
(B) Bacteria cells
(C) HIV viral cells

2. Which enyzme is used for HIV to form DNA in the host cell?

(A) Restriction endonuclease
(B) DNA-directed polymerase
(C) Reverse transcriptase
(D) Restriction endonuclease and DNA-directed polymerase

3. γ-Immunoglobulin is considered to be which of the following structures?

(A) DNA
(B) RNA
(C) Protein
(D) None of the above

4. Glycoprotein is considered to be a protein linked to which of the following?

(A) Carbohydrate
(B) Hormone
(C) Lipid
(D) None of the above

5. An enzyme that will cleave DNA at a specific site is called

(A) restriction endonuclease
(B) restriction ribonuclease
(C) trypsin
(D) none of the above

6. Which of the following is an example of a cytokine?

(A) Interleukin
(B) Insulin
(C) Gonadotropin
(D) Thyroxine
(E) None of the above

7. Which of the following storage conditions is most common for most biotechnology products after reconstitution?

(A) Room temperature
(B) Cool temperature
(C) Warm temperature
(D) No excessive heat

8. A drug that is used to prevent embolisms in the lung and during myocardial infarction is called

(A) tissue-type plasminogen activator (tPA)
(B) human γ-globulin
(C) granulocyte-macrophage colony-stimulating factor (GM-CSF)
(D) erythropoietin
(E) none of the above

9. The bases found in DNA are

(A) cytosine, thymine
(B) adenine, thymine
(C) guanine, thymine
(D) thymine, cytosine, adenine, and guanine

ANSWERS AND EXPLANATIONS

1. The answer is A *[IV].*
Human cells contain double-stranded DNA, whereas lower organisms (e.g., bacteria and viruses) do not.

2. The answer is C *[IV].*
Reverse transcriptase is the enzyme that a virus uses to assemble its DNA from RNA. Unlike higher animals, viral particles have genetic material in the RNA and need a host cell for reproduction.

3. The answer is C *[III C].*
Gamma globulin is a subclass of immunoglobulin protein involved in immunity and allergic response.

4. The answer is A *[III B].*
Glycoprotein consists of a carbohydrate linked to a protein.

5. The answer is A *[II T].*
Restriction endonuclease is an enzyme that specifically cleaves DNA molecules. Ribonuclease will cleave RNA only, and trypsin is a digestive enzyme found in the gastrointestinal tract.

6. The answer is A *[II O].*
Interleukin is a "messenger" substance synthesized by the cell (cytokine) to communicate and trigger cellular response.

7. The answer is B *[II C].*
Most biological compounds are heat labile and must be stored at low temperature.

8. The answer is A *[VII A].*
Alteplase is a thrombolytic agent formerly known as tissue plasminogen activator (tPA).

9. The answer is D *[IV B 2].*
All DNA molecules consist of nucleotides, which consist of deoxyribose, phosphate, and one of the nitrogen-containing bases, such as adenine, guanine, thymine, or cytosine.

12 Medicinal Chemistry and Drug Metabolism

Marc W. Harrold

I. DRUG SOURCES AND MAJOR CLASSES

A. Natural products are drugs obtained from plant and animal sources.

1. **Alkaloids** are nitrogen-containing compounds obtained primarily from plants through extraction and purification, which possess pharmacologic activity. The majority of alkaloids are basic compounds (e.g., **morphine,** from the opium poppy; **atropine,** from the belladonna plant); however, some are neutral amides (e.g., **colchicine,** from the autumn crocus). Alkaloids end in the suffix "-ine."

2. **Peptides and polypeptides** are polymers of amino acids, are obtained from either human or animal sources, and are smaller than **proteins.** The amino acid length distinctions between these three classifications are vague and often vary from one source to another. Naturally occurring peptides have little to no oral activity and short half-lives (e.g., **somatostatin,** a 14 amino acid peptide; **glucagon,** a 29 amino acid polypeptide).

3. **Steroids** are chemical derivatives of cyclopentanoperhydrophenanthrecene and can be obtained from either human or animal sources (e.g., **estradiol, testosterone, hydrocortisone**).

4. **Hormones** are chemical substances that are formed in one organ or part of the body and carried in the blood to another organ or part. They are principally proteins or steroids and can be obtained either synthetically, through recombinant DNA technology (e.g., **insulin**), or from animal sources (e.g., **thyroid hormones** and **conjugated estrogens**).

5. **Glycosides** are organic substances consisting of a sugar moiety bound to a non-sugar (aglycone) moiety by means of a glycosidic bond (i.e., a bond between the anomeric carbon of the sugar and a hydroxy group on the aglycone). They can be of either plant (e.g., **digitoxin**) or microbial (e.g., **streptomycin, doxorubicin**) origin.

6. **Vitamins** are organic substances that are present in foods and are essential to normal metabolism.
   a. **Water-soluble vitamins** include thiamine (B_1), riboflavin (B_2), niacin (B_3), pyridoxine (B_6), cyanocobalamine (B_{12}), ascorbic acid (C), folic acid, pantothenic acid, and biotin (H).
   b. **Lipid-soluble vitamins** include retinol (A), ergocalciferol (D), α-tocopherol (E), and phytonadione (K).

7. **Polysaccharides** are polymers of sugars that can be obtained from either human or animal sources (e.g., **heparin**).

8. **Antibiotics** are chemical substances produced by microorganisms that either suppress or kill other microorganisms (e.g., **penicillin, tetracycline, doxorubicin**).

B. Synthetic products are drugs synthesized from organic compounds.

1. Synthetic products can have **chemical structures closely resembling those of active natural products** (e.g., **hydroxymorphone,** which resembles morphine; **ampicillin,** which resembles penicillin).

2. Synthetic products also can be **completely new products,** obtained by screening synthesized materials for drug activity (e.g., **barbiturates, antibacterial sulfonamides, thiazide diuretics, phenothiazine antipsychotics, benzodiazepine anxiolytics**).

C. Major chemical and pharmacologic classes of drugs (Table 12-1, Figures 12-1, 12-2, 12-3)

Table 12-1. Major Chemical and Pharmacologic Classes of Drugs

Classification		Acid–Base Character	Example (See Figures 12-1–12-3 for structures)
A.	**Polyhalogenated ethers and hydrocarbons** General anesthetics	Nonelectrolytes	Isoflurane
B.	**Barbiturates** Sedative/hypnotics; anticonvulsants	Acidic	Phenobarbital
C.	**Benzodiazepines** Antianxiety agents; sedative/hypnotics	Basic	Diazepam
D.	**Hydantoins** Anticonvulsants	Acidic	Phenytoin
E.	**Succinimides** Anticonvulsants	Acidic or nonelectrolyte	Methsuximide
F.	**Phenothiazines** Antipsychotics; antihistamines; antiemetics	Basic	Chlorpromazine
G.	**Thioxanthenes** Antipsychotics	Basic	Thiothixene
H.	**Butyrophenones** Antipsychotics	Basic	Haloperidol
I.	**Tricyclic antidepressants** Antidepressant agents	Basic	Imipramine
J.	**Methyl xanthines** CNS stimulants; bronchodilators	Basic (weak)	Theophylline
K.	**Opioids** Narcotic analgesics; antitussives	Basic	Codeine
L.	**4-Phenylpiperidines** Narcotic analgesics	Basic	Meperidine
M.	**Phenylpropylamines** Narcotic analgesics	Basic	Methadone
N.	**Direct-acting cholinergics** GI smooth muscle stimulant; cataract therapy	Quaternary ammonium salt	Bethanechol
O.	**Aminoalkyl esters** Anticholinergic agents	Basic or quaternary salt	Dicyclomine
P.	**Aminoalkyl ethers** Anticholinergic agents; antihistamines (H_1 antagonists)	Basic	Benztropine
Q.	**Aminoalcohols** Anticholinergic agents	Basic or quarternary salt	Biperiden
R.	**Ethylenediamines** Antihistamines (H_1 antagonists)	Basic	Tripelennamine
S.	**Alkylamines (propylamines)** Antihistamines (H_1 antagonists)	Basic	Chlorpheniramine
T.	**Piperazines** Antihistamines (H_1 antagonists); antivertigo; antiemetics	Basic	Cyclizine
U.	**Phenylethylamines** Sympathomimetics (α- and β-adrenergic agonists)	Basic	Isoproterenol
V.	**Aryloxypropylamines** β-adrenergic blockers	Basic	Propranolol

(Continued on next page)

Table 12-1. Continued

Classification		Acid–Base Character	Example (See Figures 12-1–12-3 for structures)
W.	**Prostaglandins** Eicosanoids	Acidic	PGE_2
X.	**Salicylates** Non-steroidal anti-inflammatory agents (NSAIDs)	Acidic	Aspirin
Y.	**Fenamates** NSAIDs	Acidic	Mefenamic acid
Z.	**Pyrazolidinediones** NSAIDs	Acidic	Phenylbutazone
AA.	**Arylacetic acids (includes indoleacetic acids, pyrrolacetic acids, and propionic acids)** NSAIDs	Acidic	Tolmetin
BB.	**Coumarins** Oral anticoagulants	Acidic	Warfarin
CC.	**Indandiones** Oral anticoagulants	Acidic	Anisindione
DD.	**Benzothiadiazides (thiazides)** Diuretics	Acidic	Chlorthiazide
EE.	**Organic nitrates** Antianginal agents	Nonelectrolytes	Isosorbide dinitrate
FF.	**Dihydropyridines** Antihypertensives; Antianginal agents; Antiarrhythmics	Basic (weak)	Nifedipine
GG.	**Angiotensin-converting enzyme inhibitors** Antihypertensive agents	Amphoteric	Enalapril
HH.	**HMG CoA reductase inhibitors** Cholesterol lowering agents	Acidic	Pravastatin
II.	**Fibrates** Cholesterol and triglyceride lowering agents	Acidic	Gemfibrozil
JJ.	**Steroids** Estrogens; progestins; androgens; adrenocorticoids	Nonelectrolytes	Dexamethasone
KK.	**Sulfonylureas** Oral hypoglycemics	Acidic	Tolbutamide
LL.	**H_2Receptor antagonists** Antiulcer agents	Basic	Cimetidine
MM.	**β-Chloroethylamines (nitrogen mustards)** Antineoplastic agents	Basic	Mechlorethamine
NN.	**Nitrosoureas** Antineoplastic agents	Nonelectrolytes	Carmustine
OO.	**Folate antimetabolites** Antineoplastic agents; antibacterial agents; antifungals	Amphoteric	Methotrexate
PP.	**Purine antimetabolites** Antineoplastic agents; antiviral agents	Basic	6-Mercaptopurine
QQ.	**Pyrimidine antimetabolites** Antineoplastic agents; antiviral agents	Basic	Cytarabine

Table 12-1. Continued

Classification	Acid–Base Character	Example (See Figures 12-1–12-3 for structures)
RR. **Sulfonilamides** Antibacterial agents	Acidic	Sulfamethoxazole
SS. **Penicillins** Antibacterial agents	Acidic	Ampicillin
TT. **Cephalosporins** Antibacterial agents	Acidic	Cefoxitin
UU. **Tetracyclines** Antibacterial agents	Amphoteric	Tetracycline
VV. **Aminoglycosides** Antibacterial agents	Basic	Gentimycin
WW. **Macrolides** Antibacterial agents	Basic	Erythromycin
XX. **4-Quinolones** Antibacterial agents	Amphoteric	Enoxacin
YY. **Imidazoles** Antifungal agents	Basic	Oxiconazole
ZZ. **Polyenes** Antifungal agents	Amphoteric	Amphotericin B

Table 12-1 is not an inclusive list of all drugs or classifications. It is organized according to chemical structure and includes only those classifications that contain multiple compounds with a similar structure. In some instances (e.g., **direct acting cholinergic agonists and H_2 antagonists**), drugs are chemically similar, but are usually denoted only by pharmacological classifications. The acid–base character of each class is a general notation and there are some specific singular agents that fall outside of these general notations (i.e., **ampicillin** is amphoteric, whereas the **penicillins,** in general, are acidic molecules).

II. DRUG ACTION AND PHYSICOCHEMICAL PROPERTIES

A. Drug action results from the interaction of drug molecules with either normal or abnormal physiological processes. Drugs normally interact with receptors, which can be either proteins, enzymes, cell lipids, or pieces of DNA or RNA.

1. Systemically active drugs must **enter** and **be transported by body fluids.**
   - **a.** The drug must **pass various membrane barriers, escape excessive distribution** into sites of loss, and **penetrate to the active site.**
   - **b.** At the active site, the drug molecules must orient themselves and interact with the receptors to **alter function.**
   - **c.** The drug must be removed from the active site and **metabolized** to a form that is easily **excreted** by the body.
2. Drug absorption, metabolism, utilization, and excretion all depend on the **drug's physicochemical properties** and the **host's physiologic** and **biochemical properties.** A drug's physicochemical properties can be altered via the synthesis of chemical analogs, whereas the host's properties usually cannot be altered.

B. Two of the most important **physicochemical properties** of a drug molecule are its polarity and its acid–base nature.

1. **Drug polarity** is a relative measure of a drug's lipid and water solubility and is usually expressed in terms of a **partition coefficient.**
   - **a.** The partition coefficient (P) of a drug is defined as the ratio of the solubility of the compound in an organic solvent to the solubility of the same compound in an aqueous

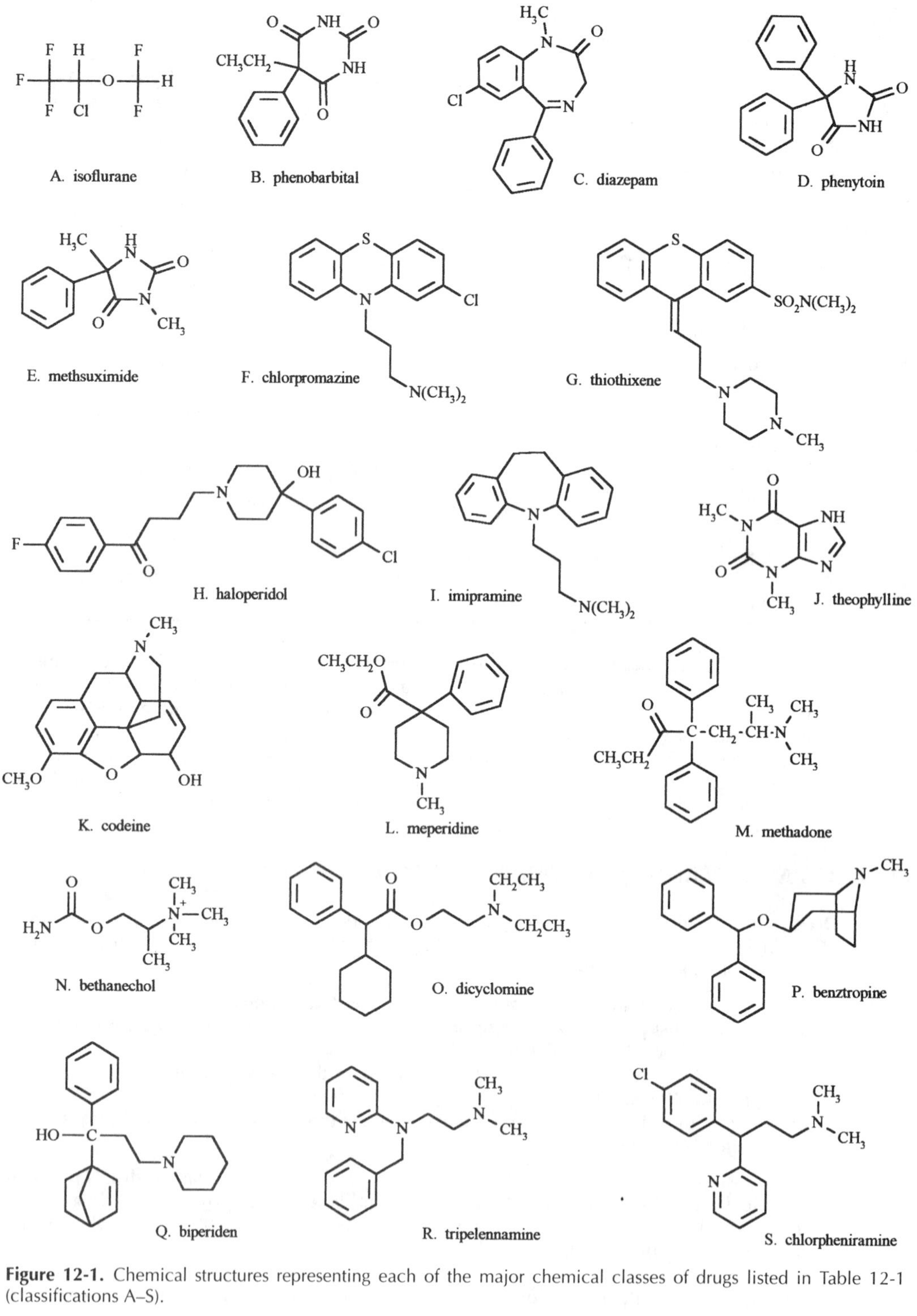

Figure 12-1. Chemical structures representing each of the major chemical classes of drugs listed in Table 12-1 (classifications A–S).

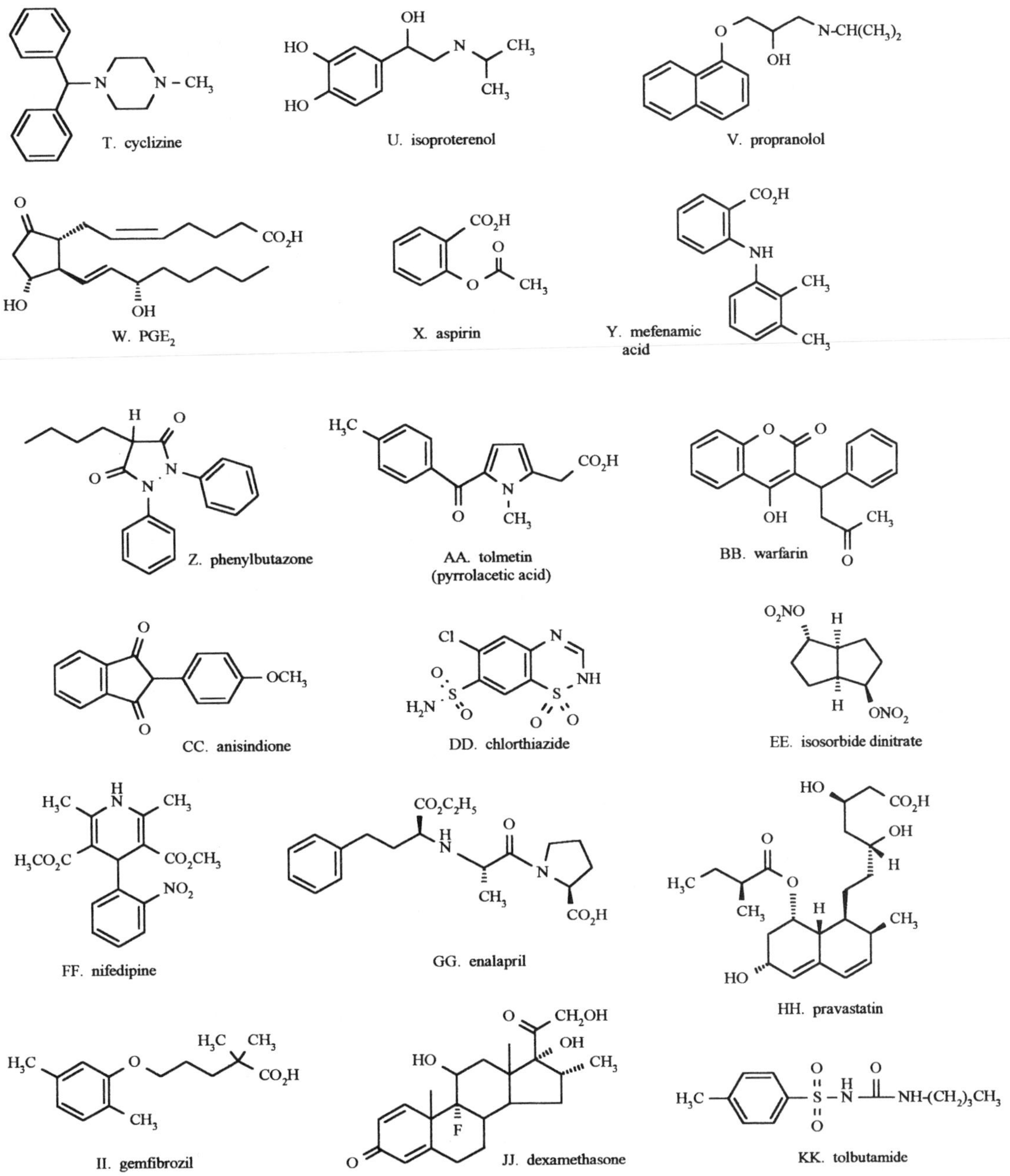

Figure 12-2. Chemical structures representing each of the major chemical classes of drugs listed in Table 12-1 (classifications T–KK).

environment (i.e., **P = [Drug]**$_{lipid}$**/[Drug]**$_{aqueous}$). The partition coefficient is often expressed as a log value.

b. Water solubility (or **hydrophilicity**) depends primarily on two factors: ionic character and hydrogen-bonding capabilities. The presence of oxygen and nitrogen containing functional groups usually enhances water solubility. Water solubility is required for:

(1) Dissolution in the gastrointestinal (GI) tract

(2) Preparation of parenteral solutions (as opposed to suspensions)

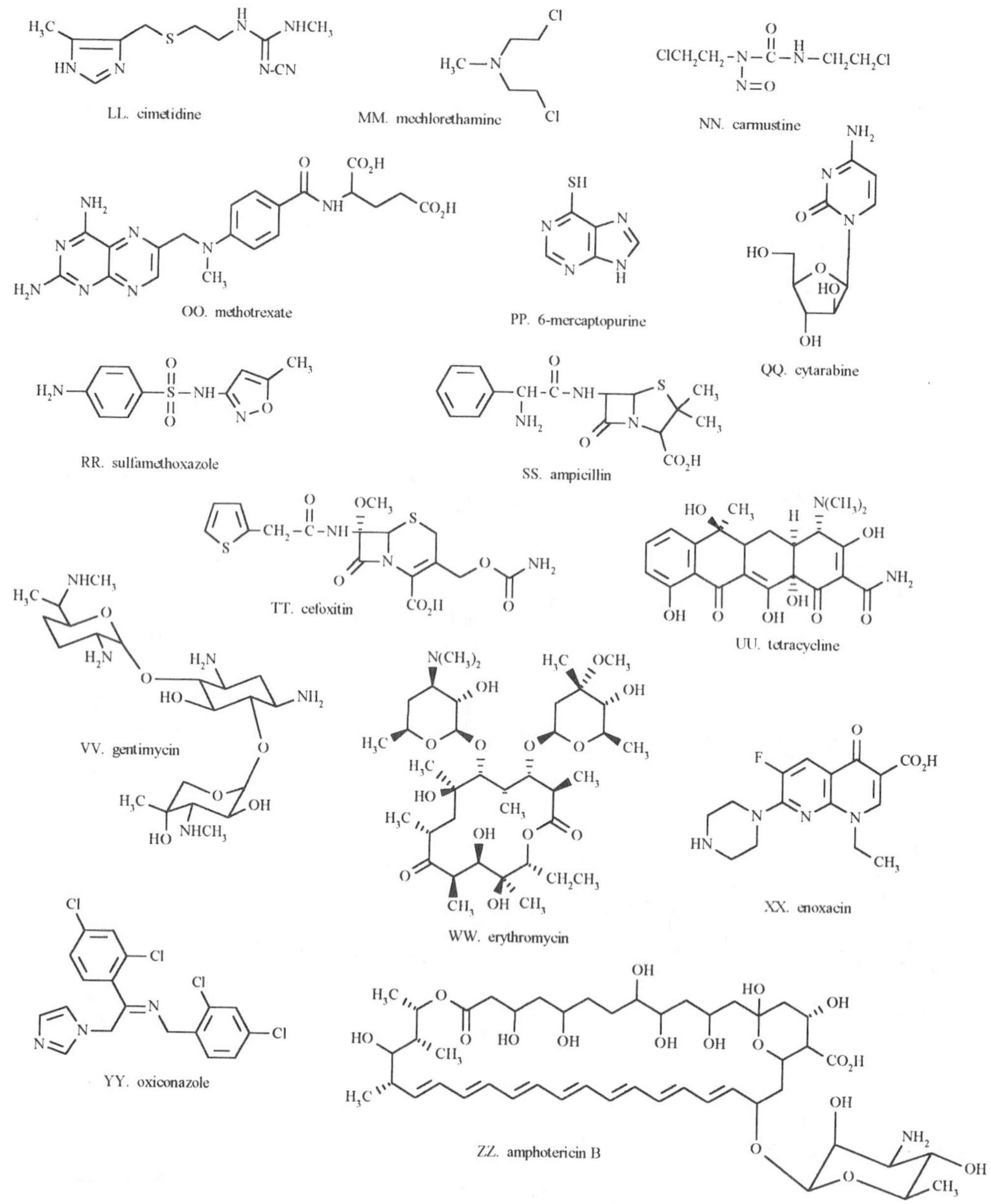

Figure 12-3. Chemical structures representing each of the major chemical classes of drugs listed in Table 12-1 (classifications LL–ZZ).

(3) Preparation of ophthalmic solutions

(4) Adequate urine concentrations (pertains primarily to antibiotics)

c. **Lipid solubility (or lipophilicity)** is enhanced by nonionizable hydrocarbon chains and ring systems. Lipid solubility is required for:

(1) Penetration through the lipid bilayer in the GI tract

(2) Penetration through the blood brain barrier

(3) Preparation of intramuscular (IM) depot injectable formulations

2. **Ionization of acids** and **bases** plays a role with substances that dissociate into ions.

a. The **ionization constant (K_a)** indicates the relative strength of the acid or base. An acid with a K_a of 1×10^{-3} is stronger (more ionized) than one with a K_a of 1×10^{-5}, whereas a base with a K_a of 1×10^{-7} is weaker (less ionized) than one with a K_a of 1×10^{-9}.

b. The **negative log** of the **ionization constant (pK_a)** also indicates the relative strength of the acid or base. An acid with a pK_a of 5 ($K_a = 1 \times 10^{-5}$) is weaker (less ionized) than one with a pK_a of 3 ($K_a = 1 \times 10^{-3}$), whereas a base with a pK_a of 9 (K_a of 1×10^{-9}) is stronger (more ionized) than one with a pK_a of 7 (K_a of 1×10^{-7}).

c. **Strong acids** [e.g., **hydrochloric acid** (HCl), sulfuric acid (H_2SO_4), nitric acid (HNO_3), hydrobromic acid (HBr), iodic acid (HIO_3), perchloric acid ($HClO_4$)] are completely ionized. Almost all other acids, including organic acids, are weak. **Organic acids** contain one or more of these functional groups:

(1) Carboxyl group (—COOH)
(2) Phenolic group (Ar—OH)
(3) Sulfonic acid group ($—SO_2H$)
(4) Sulfonamide group ($—SO_2NH—R$)
(5) Imide group (—CO—NH—CO—)
(6) β-Carbonyl group (—CO—CHR—CO—)

d. **Strong bases** [e.g., sodium **hydroxide** (NaOH), potassium hydroxide (KOH), magnesium hydroxide [$Mg(OH)_2$], calcium hydroxide [$Ca(OH)_2$], barium hydroxide [$Ba(OH)_2$], and quaternary ammonium hydroxides] are also completely ionized. Almost all other bases, including organic bases, are weak.

(1) **Organic bases** contain a primary, secondary, or tertiary aliphatic or alicyclic amino group ($—NH_2$, —NHR, or $—NR_2$).

(2) Most aromatic or unsaturated heterocyclic nitrogens are so weakly basic that they do not readily form salts with acids. Saturated heterocyclic nitrogens, in contrast, are similar to aliphatic amines.

e. **Weak acids.** Ionization of a weak acid (e.g., acetic acid, which has a pK_a of 4.76) takes place as follows:

$$CH_3COOH \rightleftharpoons CH_3COO^- + H^+$$

(1) When a weak acid (such as acetic acid) is placed in an **acid medium,** the equilibrium shifts to the left, suppressing ionization. This decrease in ionization conforms to **Le Chatelier's principle,** which states that when a stress is placed on an equilibrium reaction, the reaction will move in the direction that tends to relieve the stress.

(2) When a weak acid is placed in an **alkaline medium,** ionization increases. The H^+ ions from the acid and the OH^- ions from the alkaline medium combine to form water, shifting the equilibrium to the right.

(3) **Weakly acidic drugs** are less ionized in acid media than in alkaline media. When the pK_a of an acidic drug is greater than the pH of the medium in which it exists, it will be more than 50% in its nonionized (molecular) form and, thus, more likely to cross lipid cellular membranes.

f. **Weak bases.** Ionization of a weak base is the opposite of that for a weak acid.

(1) Weak bases are less ionized in a **basic (alkaline) medium** and more ionized in an **acid medium.**

(2) **Weakly basic** drugs are less ionized in alkaline media than in acid media. When the pK_a of a basic drug is less than the pH of the medium in which it exists, it will be more than 50% in its nonionized (molecular) form and, thus, more likely to cross lipid cellular membranes.

g. **Percent ionization** can be approximated by using the **rule of nines.** If the $|pH - pK_a| = 1$, then a 90 to 10 ratio (note that there is one nine in the ratio) exists. If the $|pH - pK_a| = 2$, the ratio becomes 99 to 1 (two nines in the ratio), and if the $|pH - pK_a| = 3$, the ratio is 99.9 to 0.1 (three nines in the ratio). The predominant form, ionized or unionized, in these ratios can easily be determined [see II B 2 e (3), f (2)].

3. A **salt** is the combination of an acid and a base.

a. With a few minor exceptions (mercuric and cadmium halides and lead acetate), **all salts are strong electrolytes.**

b. Because the vast majority of drugs are organic molecules, drug salts can be divided into two classes based upon the chemical nature of the substance forming the salt.

(1) **Inorganic salts** are made by combining drug molecules with inorganic acids and bases, such as hydrochloric acid, sulfuric acid, potassium hydroxide, and sodium hydroxide. The salt form of the drug has increased water solubility in comparison with the parent molecule. Inorganic salts are generally used to increase the aqueous dissolution of a compound.

(2) **Organic salts** are made by combining two drug molecules, one acidic and one basic. The salt formed by this combination has increased lipid solubility and generally is used to make depot injections (e.g., procaine penicillin).

c. **Amphoteric compounds** contain both acidic and basic functional groups and are capable of forming **internal salts,** or zwitterions, which often have dissolution problems.

d. **Dissolution of salts** can alter the pH of an aqueous medium.

(1) Salts of **strong acids** (i.e., HCl, H_2SO_4) and **basic drugs** (i.e., cimetidine) dissociate in an aqueous medium to yield an **acidic solution.**

(2) Salts of **strong bases** (i.e., NaOH, KOH) and **acidic drugs** (i.e., phenobarbital) dissociate in an aqueous medium to yield a **basic solution.**

(3) Salts of **weak acids** and **weak bases** dissociate in an aqueous medium to yield an **acidic, basic,** or **neutral solution,** depending on the respective ionization constants involved.

(4) Salts of **strong acids** and **strong bases** (i.e., NaCl) do not significantly alter the pH of an aqueous medium.

4. A **neutralization reaction** might occur when an acidic solution of an organic salt (a solution of a salt of a strong acid and a weak base) is mixed with a basic solution (a solution of a salt of a weak acid and a strong base). The nonionized organic acid or the nonionized organic base is likely to **precipitate** in this case. This reaction is the basis for many **drug incompatibilities,** particularly when intravenous solutions are mixed. Neutralization reactions can be avoided by knowing how to predict the approximate pH of the aqueous solutions of common drug salts.

a. Generally, a drug's **salt form** can be recognized when the generic or trade name consists of two separate words, indicating a **cation** and an **anion.**

b. Drugs with **nitrate, sulfate,** or **hydrochloride notations** (e.g., pilocarpine nitrate, morphine sulfate, meperidine hydrochloride) are salts of **strong acids.** Thus, their cation portions (e.g., pilocarpine, morphine, meperidine) must be **bases.**

c. Drugs with **sodium** or **potassium cations** (e.g., warfarin sodium, potassium penicillin G) are salts of **strong bases.**

d. Drugs whose cation name ends with the suffix **"-onium"** or **"-inium"** and whose anion is a chloride, bromide, iodide, nitrate, or sulfate (e.g., benzalkonium chloride, cetylpyridinium chloride), are known as quaternary ammonium salts and form **neutral aqueous solutions.**

III. STRUCTURAL FEATURES AND PHARMACOLOGIC ACTIVITY.

Drugs can be classified as structurally nonspecific and structurally specific.

A. Structurally nonspecific drugs are those for which the drug's interaction with the cell membrane depends more on the drug molecule's physical characteristics than on its chemical structure. Usually, the interaction is based on the **cell membrane's lipid nature** and the **drug's lipid attraction.** Most **general anesthetics,** as well as some **hypnotics** and some **bactericidal agents,** act through this mechanism.

B. Structurally specific drugs are those for which pharmacologic activity is determined by the drug's ability to bind to a **specific endogenous receptor.**

1. **Receptor site theory** describes the pharmacologic activity of such drugs.

a. The **lock-and-key theory** postulates a completely complementary relationship between the drug molecule and a specific area on the surface of the receptor molecule (i.e., the **active,** or **catalytic, site**). This theory does not account for conformational changes in either drug or receptor molecules and is an oversimplification of a complex process.

b. The **induced fit theory** also postulates a complementary relationship between the drug molecule and its active site; however, it provides for **mutual conformational changes** between the drug and its receptor. Conformational changes in the receptor molecule are then translated into biologic responses. This theory explains many more phenomena (e.g., **allosteric inhibitors**) than the lock-and-key model.

c. The **occupational theory of response** further postulates that, for a structurally specific drug, the intensity of the pharmacologic effect is directly proportional to the number of receptors occupied by the drug.

2. **Receptor site binding.** The **ability to bind to a specific receptor,** while not independent of the drug's physical characteristics, is primarily determined by the drug's **chemical structure.**
   a. In such an interaction, the drug's **chemical reactivity** plays an important role, reflected in its **bonding ability** and in the **exactness of its fit** to the receptor.
   b. **Drug interaction** with a specific receptor is analogous to the fitting together of jigsaw puzzle pieces. Only drugs of similar shape (i.e., similar chemical structure) can bind to a specific receptor and initiate a biologic response.
   c. Often, only a **critical portion of the drug molecule** (rather than the whole molecule) is involved in receptor-site binding.
      (1) The functional group making up this critical portion is known as a **pharmacophore.**
      (2) Drugs with **similar critical regions** but differences in other parts may have similar qualitative (although not necessarily quantitative) pharmacologic activity.
   d. In general, the **better a drug fits** the receptor site, the **higher the affinity** between the drug and the receptor and the **greater** the observed biologic response. A drug that binds to a receptor and elicits a biological response is called an **agonist.**
   e. Some drugs, lacking the specific pharmacophore for a receptor, can nonetheless bind to that receptor. Such a drug will have little or no pharmacologic effect and also might prevent a molecule having the specific pharmacophore from binding, blocking the expected biologic response. A drug that blocks a natural agonist and prevents it from binding to its receptor is called an **antagonist.**

3. The **stereochemistry** of both the receptor site surface and the drug molecule helps determine the nature and efficiency of the drug-receptor interaction. Stereoisomers can be divided into three main groups: **optical isomers, geometric isomers,** and **conformational isomers.**
   a. **Optical isomers** contain at least one asymmetric, or **chiral,** carbon atom (i.e., a carbon atom which is covalently bonded to four different substituents). Each asymmetric carbon atom can exist in one of two non-superimposable isomeric forms (Figure 12-4).
      (1) **Enantiomers** are optical isomers that are mirror images of one another. Enantiomers have identical physical and chemical properties except that one rotates the plane of polarized light in a clockwise direction (**dextrorotatory,** designated D or +) and the other in a counterclockwise direction (**levorotatory,** designated L or −).
      (2) An equal mixture of D and L enantiomers is called a **racemic mixture** and is optically inactive.
      (3) Enantiomers can have large differences in potency, receptor fit, biologic activity, transport and metabolism. These differences result when the drug molecule has an asymmetric interaction with a receptor, a transport protein, or a metabolizing enzyme. For example, **levorphanol** has narcotic, analgesic, and antitussive properties, whereas its mirror image, **dextror-phanol,** has only antitussive activity.
      (4) **Diastereomers** are stereoisomers, which are neither mirror images nor superimposable. A drug must have at least two chiral centers in order to exist in diastereomers. Unlike enantiomers, in which all stereochemical centers are opposite, diastereomers have some stereochemical centers that are identical and some that are opposite. Diastereomers possess different physicochemical properties and, thus, differ in properties, such as solubility, volatility, and melting points.
      (5) **Epimers** are a special type of diastereomers because all epimers are also diastereomers; however, the opposite is not true. Epimers are compounds that are structurally identical in all respects except for the stereochemistry about one chiral center. The process of **epimerization** (in which the stereochemistry of one chiral center is inverted) is important in drug degradation and inactivation (Figure 12-5).
   b. **Geometric isomers (*cis—trans* isomers)** occur as a result of restricted rotation about a chemical bond, owing to double bonds or rigid ring systems in the molecule.

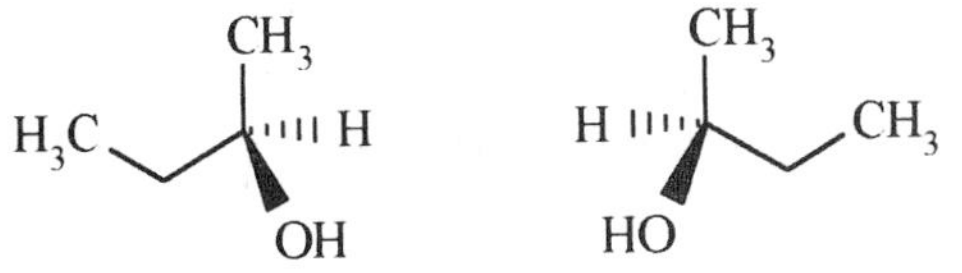

Figure 12-4. The two enantiomers of 2-hydroxybutane. The chiral, or asymmetric, carbon is bonded to four different groups: a methyl group, an ethyl group, a hydroxy group, and a hydrogen. The structures shown are mirror images that cannot be superimposed.

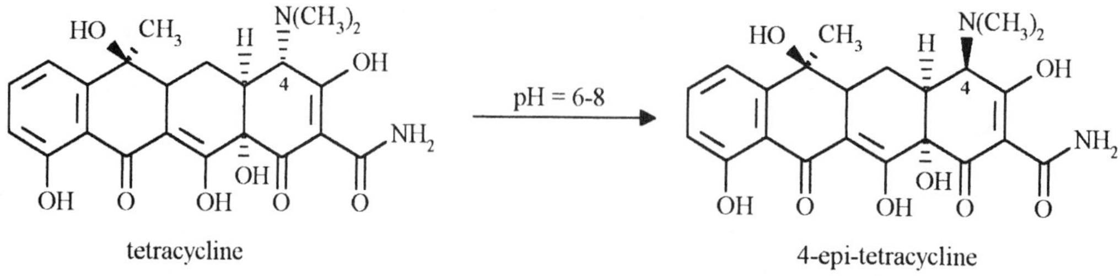

Figure 12-5. Epimerization of tetracycline to 4-epi-tetracycline. The stereochemistry of the 4-dimethylamino group is inverted; however, the stereochemistry of all other chiral centers remains unchanged.

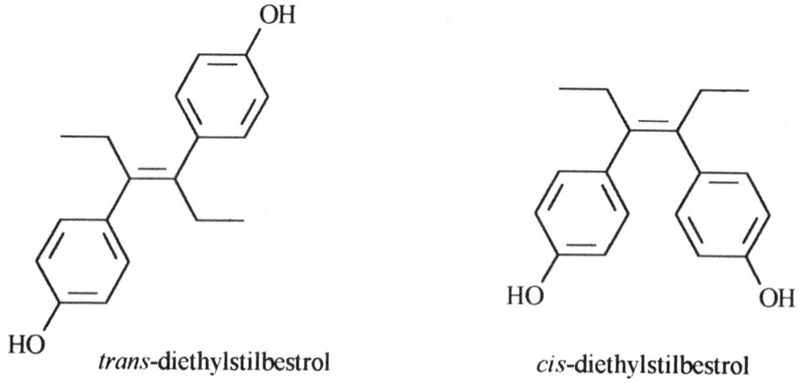

Figure 12-6. The presence of the double bond in diethylstilbestrol allows for the formation of *cis* and *trans* geometric isomers. Only the *trans* isomer has estrogenic activity.

(1) ***Cis—trans* isomers** are not mirror images and have different physicochemical properties and pharmacologic activity.

(2) Because the functional groups of these isomers are separated by different distances, they generally do not fit the same receptor equally well. If these functional groups are pharmacophores, the isomers will **differ in biologic activity.** For example, *cis*-diethylstilbestrol has only 7% of the estrogenic activity of *trans*-diethylstilbestrol (Figure 12-6).

c. **Conformational isomers,** also known as **rotamers** or **conformers,** are non-superimposable orientations of a molecule which result from the rotation of atoms about single bonds. Almost every drug can exist in more than one conformation, and this ability allows many drugs to bind to multiple receptors and receptor subtypes. For example, the *trans* conformation of acetylcholine binds to the muscarinic receptor, whereas the *gauche* conformation binds to the nicotinic receptor (Figure 12-7).

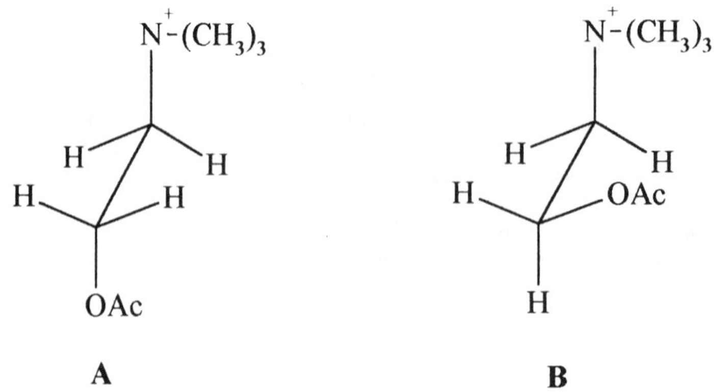

Figure 12-7. The *trans* **(A)** and *gauche* **(B)** conformations of acetylcholine occur as the result of rotation about the carbon-carbon single bond.

d. Bioisosteres are molecules containing groups that are spatially and electronically equivalent and, thus, interchangeable without significantly altering the molecules' physicochemical properties. **Isosteric replacement** of functional groups can increase potency, decrease side effects, separate biologic activities, and increase the duration of action by altering metabolism. Additionally, **isosteric analogs** may act antagonistically to the parent molecule.

(1) **Procainamide,** an amide, has a longer duration of action than **procaine,** an ester, because of the isosteric replacement of the ester oxygen with a nitrogen atom (Figure 12-8).

(2) **Alloxanthine** is an inhibitor of xanthine oxidase. It is also an isostere of **xanthine,** the normal substrate for the enzyme (see Figure 12-8).

IV. MECHANISMS OF DRUG ACTION

A. Interaction with receptors (see III B 1–2)

1. **Agonists** interact with specific cellular constituents, known as receptors, and elicit an observable biologic response. Agonists have both **affinity** for the receptor and **intrinsic activity.**

2. **Partial agonists** interact with the same receptors as full agonists but are unable to elicit the same maximum response. Partial agonists have lower intrinsic activity than full agonists; however, their affinity for the receptor can be greater than, less than, or equal to that of full agonists.

3. **Antagonists** inhibit the actions of agonists.

   a. **Pharmacologic antagonists** bind to the same receptor as the agonist, either at the same site or at an allosteric site. They have affinity for the receptor but lack intrinsic activity. Pharmacologic antagonists can be subdivided into reversible, irreversible, competitive, and noncompetitive categories similar to enzyme inhibitors (see IV B 2).

   b. **Chemical antagonists** react with one another, resulting in the inactivation of both compounds.

      (1) The anticoagulant **heparin,** an acidic polysaccharide, is chemically antagonized by **protamine,** a basic protein, via an acid–base interaction.

      (2) **Chelating agents** can be used as **antidotes for metal poisoning. Ethylenediaminetetraacetic acid** (EDTA) chelates calcium and lead; **penicillamine** chelates copper; and **dimercaprol** chelates mercury, gold, antimony, and arsenic.

   c. **Functional (or physical) antagonists** produce antagonistic physiologic actions through binding at separate receptors. The adrenergic and cholinergic nervous systems frequently produce this type of antagonism. **Acetylcholine** constricts the pupil by acting on recep-

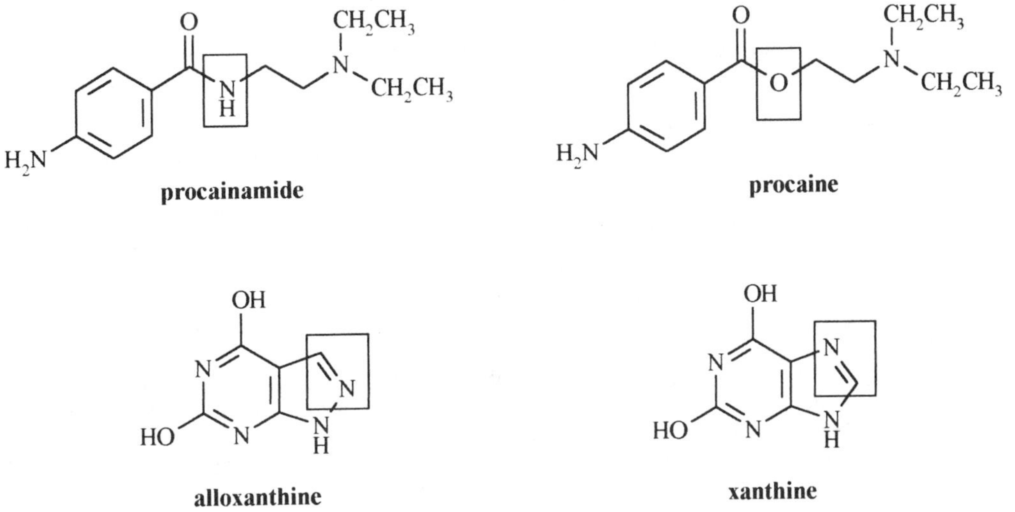

Figure 12-8. Bioisosteric pairs procainamide/procaine and alloxanthine/xanthine. The isosteric replacements are highlighted.

tors that control the circular muscles of the eye, whereas **norepinephrine** dilates the pupil by acting on receptors that control ocular dilator muscles.

B. Interaction with enzymes

1. **Activation,** or **increased enzyme activity,** can result from induction of enzyme protein synthesis by such drugs as barbiturates, phenytoin and other antiepileptics, rifampin, antihistamines, griseofulvin, and oral contraceptives.
   a. **Allosteric binding.** A drug can enhance enzyme activity by allosteric binding, which triggers a conformational change in the enzyme system and, thus, alters its affinity for substrate binding.
   b. **Coenzymes** play a role in optimizing enzyme activity. Coenzymes include **vitamins** (particularly the **vitamin B complex**) and **cofactors** [mainly metallic ions such as sodium (Na^+), potassium (K^+), magnesium (Mg^{2+}), calcium (Ca^{2+}), zinc (Zn^{2+}), and iron (Fe^{2+})]. Coenzymes activate enzymes by complexation and stereochemical interaction.
2. **Inhibition,** or **decreased enzyme activity,** can result from drugs that interact with the apoenzyme, the coenzyme, or even the whole enzyme complex. The drug might modify or destroy the apoenzyme's protein conformation, react with the coenzyme (thus reducing the enzyme system's capacity to function), or bind with the enzyme complex (rendering it unable to bind with its substrate).
   a. **Reversible inhibition** results from a **noncovalent interaction** between the enzyme and the drug. The drug is free to associate and dissociate with the enzyme, and an equilibrium exists between bound and free drug.
   b. **Irreversible inhibition** results from a stable, **covalent interaction** between the enzyme and the drug. Once bound to the enzyme, the drug is not able to dissociate.
   c. **Competitive inhibition** occurs when there is **mutually exclusive binding** of the substrate and the inhibitor. While it is possible for competitive inhibitors to bind to allosteric sites, these inhibitors are usually structurally similar to the natural substrates and compete with the substrates for common binding sites. Competitive inhibition can be overcome by increasing the concentration of the substrate.
   d. **Noncompetitive inhibition** occurs when a drug binds to an **allosteric site** on the enzyme. This binding induces a conformational change in the enzyme that inhibits enzyme action, even if a substrate is bound to the enzyme. Increasing substrate concentration does not overcome this type of inhibition.

C. Interaction with DNA/RNA formation and function

1. **Inhibition of nucleotide biosynthesis** occurs when folate, purine, and pyrimidine **antimetabolites** interfere with the biosynthesis of purine and pyrimidine building blocks.
   a. **Folic acid analogs** (e.g., methotrexate, trimetrexate) inhibit purine and thymidylate synthesis by inhibiting dihydrofolate reductase.
   b. **Purine analogs** (e.g., 6-mercaptopurine, thioguanine) act as antagonists in the synthesis of purine bases. These analogs do not act as active inhibitors until they are converted to their respective nucleotides.
   c. **Pyrimidine analogs** (e.g., 5-fluorouracil) inhibit the synthesis of thymidylic acid by inhibiting thymidine synthetase. As with purine analogs, pyrimidine analogs are not active until they are converted to their respective nucleotides.
2. **Inhibition of DNA or RNA biosynthesis** occurs when drugs interfere with nucleic acid synthesis. These drugs are used primarily as antineoplastic agents for cancer chemotherapy.
   a. Drugs that interfere with DNA replication and function include intercalating agents (e.g., the **anthracyclines, dactinomycin**), alkylating agents (e.g., **nitrogen mustards, nitrosoureas**), and antimetabolites.
   b. Drugs that can damage and destroy DNA include compounds that produce free radicals (e.g., **bleomycin,** the **anthracyclines**) and compounds that inhibit topoisomerases (e.g., **epipodophyllotoxins, mitoxantrone**).
   c. Drugs that interfere with microtubule assembly in the metaphase of **cell mitosis** include the **vinca alkaloids** and **paclitaxel.**

D. Inhibition of protein synthesis

1. **Tetracyclines** interfere with protein synthesis by inhibiting transfer RNA (tRNA) binding to the ribosome and blocking the release of completed peptides from the ribosome.
2. **Chloramphenicol** and **erythromycin** (which compete for the same binding site) bind to the ribosome and inhibit peptidyl transferase, blocking formation of the peptide bond and interrupting formation of the peptide chain.
3. **Aminoglycosides** decrease the fidelity of transcription by binding to the ribosome, which permits formation of an abnormal initiation complex and prohibits addition of amino acids to the peptide chain. Additionally, aminoglycosides cause misreading of the messenger RNA (mRNA) template, so that incorrect amino acids are incorporated into the growing polypeptide chain.

E. Interaction with cell membranes

1. **Digitalis glycosides** inhibit the cell membrane's sodium-potassium pump, inhibiting the influx of K^+ and the outflow of Na^+.
2. **Quinidine** affects the membrane potential of myocardial membranes by prolonging both the polarized and depolarized states.
3. **Local anesthetics** block impulse conduction in nerve cell membranes by interfering with membrane permeability to Na^+ and K^+.
4. **Polyene antifungal drugs** (e.g., amphotericin B, nystatin) affect cell membrane permeability, causing leakage of cellular constituents.
5. **Certain antibiotics** (e.g., polymyxin B, colistin) affect cell membrane permeability through an unknown mechanism.
6. **Acetylcholine** increases membrane permeability to cations.
7. **Omeprazole** and **lansoprazole** inhibit the H^+/K^+ pump (located in parietal cell membranes), thus decreasing the efflux of protons into the stomach.

F. Nonspecific action

1. Structurally nonspecific drugs form a monomolecular layer over entire areas of certain cells. Because they involve such large surfaces, these drugs are usually given in relatively large doses.
2. Drugs that act by nonspecific action include the **volatile general anesthetic gases** (e.g., ether, nitrous oxide), some **depressants** (e.g., ethanol, chloral hydrate), and many antiseptic compounds (e.g., phenol, rubbing alcohol).

V. INTRODUCTION TO DRUG METABOLISM. Drug metabolism (also called **biotransformation**) refers to the biochemical changes that drugs and other foreign chemicals **(xenobiotics)** undergo in the body, leading to the formation of different metabolites with different effects. Xenobiotics can undergo a variety of biotransformation pathways, resulting in the production of a mixture of intermediate metabolites and excreted products, including unchanged parent drug. Rarely is only one metabolite produced from a single drug.

A. Inactive metabolites. Some metabolites are inactive (i.e., their pharmacologically active parent compounds become inactivated or detoxicated).

1. The hydrolysis of **procaine** to *p*-aminobenzoic acid and diethylethanolamine results in loss of anesthetic activity.
2. The oxidation of **6-mercaptopurine** to 6-mercapturic acid results in loss of anticancer activity.

B. Metabolites that retain similar activity. Certain metabolites retain the pharmacologic activity of their parent compounds to a greater or lesser degree.

1. **Imipramine** is demethylated to the essentially equiactive antidepressant, **desipramine.**
2. **Acetohexamide** is reduced to the more active hypoglycemic, **l-hydroxyhexamide.**
3. **Codeine** is demethylated to the more active analgesic, **morphine.**

C. Metabolites with altered activity. Some metabolites develop activity different from that of their parent drugs.

1. The antidepressant **iproniazid** is dealkylated to the antitubercular, **isoniazid.**

2. The vitamin **retinoic acid** (vitamin A) is isomerized to the anti-acne agent, **isoretinoic acid.**

D. Bioactivated metabolites. Some pharmacologically inactive parent compounds are converted to active species within the body. These parent compounds are known as **prodrugs.**

1. The prodrug **enalapril** is hydrolyzed to **enalaprilat,** a potent antihypertensive.

2. The prodrug **sulindac,** a sulfoxide, is reduced to the active sulfide.

3. The antiparkinsonian **levodopa** is decarboxylated in the neuron to active **dopamine.**

VI. BIOTRANSFORMATION PATHWAYS

A. Phase I reactions are those in which polar functional groups are introduced into the molecule or unmasked by oxidation, reduction, or hydrolysis.

1. **Oxidation** is the most common phase I biotransformation.
   a. The majority of oxidations occur in the **liver;** however, extrahepatic tissues, such as the **intestinal mucosa, lungs,** and **kidney,** can also serve as metabolic sites.
   b. The vast majority of oxidations are catalyzed by a group of mixed-function oxidases known as **cytochrome P_{450}.** These oxidases are bound to the smooth endoplastic reticulum of the liver and require both NADPH and a porphyrin prosthetic group. Unlike most enzymes, cytochrome P_{450} uses a variety of oxidative biotransformations to metabolize a diverse group of substrates.
   c. The variety of substrates undergoing cytochrome P_{450} oxidation is attributed to the presence of **multiple isoforms** of the enzyme. At least 20 different isoforms of the enzyme have been identified.
   d. Additional oxidations (e.g., ethanol to acetaldehyde) are catalyzed by nonmicrosomal oxidases located in cytosol and mitochondria of extrahepatic tissues.
   e. Cytochrome P_{450} and nonmicrosomal oxidases catalyze aromatic, aliphatic, olefinic, benzylic, allylic, and α-hydroxylations; *N*-, *O*-, and *S*-dealkylations, oxidative deamination: *N*-and *S*-oxidations; desulfuration; dehalogenation; and oxidations of alcohols and aldehydes (Table 12-2).
   f. The **increased polarity** of the oxidized products (metabolites) enhances their water solubility and reduces their tubular reabsorption to some extent, thus favoring their excretion in the urine. These metabolites are somewhat **more polar** than their parent compounds and very commonly undergo further biotransformation by phase II pathways (see VI B)

2. **Reduction** is less commonly encountered than oxidation; however, the overall goal is the same: to create polar functional groups that can be eliminated in the urine. There is evidence suggesting that the cytochrome P_{450} system might be involved in some reductions. Additionally, bacteria resident in the GI tract are known to be involved in azo and nitro reductions. Reactions catalyzed by reductases are shown in Table 12-3.

3. **Enzymatic hydrolysis,** the addition of water across a bond, also results in more polar metabolites (Table 12-3).
   a. **Esterase enzymes,** usually present in plasma and various tissues, are nonspecific and catalyze de-esterification, hydrolyzing relatively nonpolar esters into two polar, more water-soluble compounds: an alcohol and an acid. Esterases are responsible for converting many prodrugs into their active forms.
   b. **Amidase enzymes** hydrolyze amides into amines and acids (deamidation). Deamidation occurs primarily in the liver.
   c. **Ester drugs** susceptible to plasma esterases (e.g., procaine) are usually shorter acting than structurally similar **amide drugs** (e.g., procainamide), which are not significantly hydrolyzed until they reach the liver.

B. Phase II reactions are those in which the functional groups of the original drug (or metabolite formed in a phase I reaction) are masked by a **conjugation reaction.** Most phase II conjugates are very polar, resulting in rapid drug elimination from the body.

Table 12-2. Phase I Metabolism: Oxidative Pathways

Type of Reaction (Examples)		Reaction Pathway
1. Aromatic hydroxylation (phenytoin, phenylbutazone)	1.	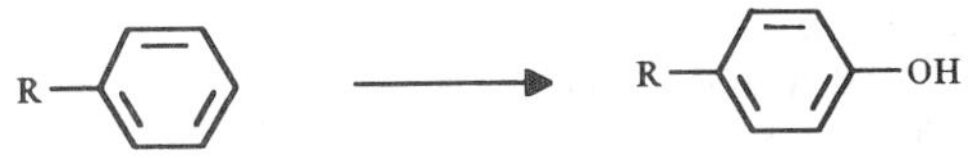
2. Aliphatic hydroxylation (pentobarbital, meprobamate)	2.	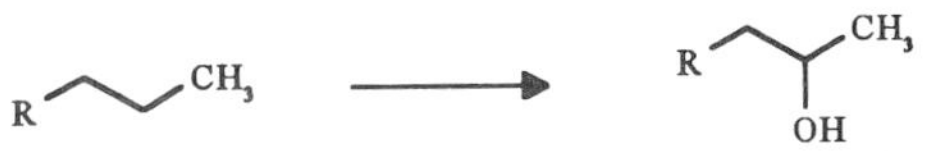
3. Olefinic hydroxylation (carbamazepine, cyproheptadine)	3.	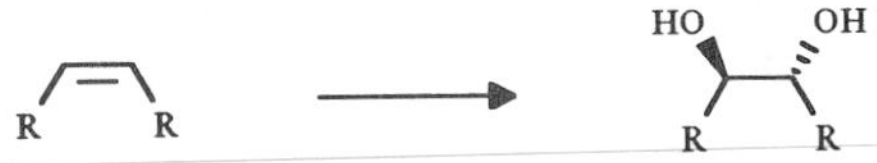
4. Benzylic hydroxylation (tolbutamide, imipramine)	4.	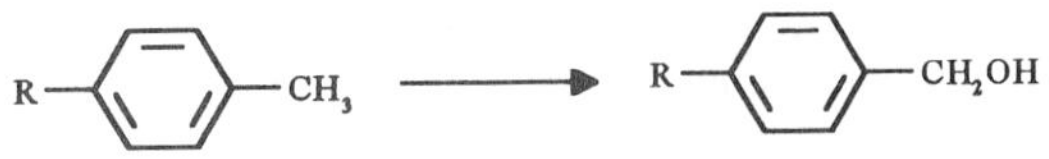
5. Allylic hydroxylation (pentazocine, hexobarbital)	5.	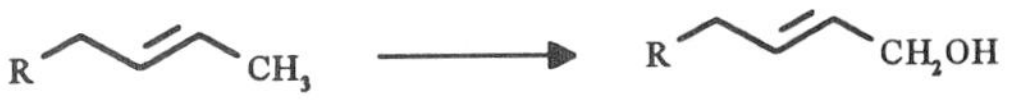
6. Hydroxylation α to a carbonyl (diazepam, ketamine)	6.	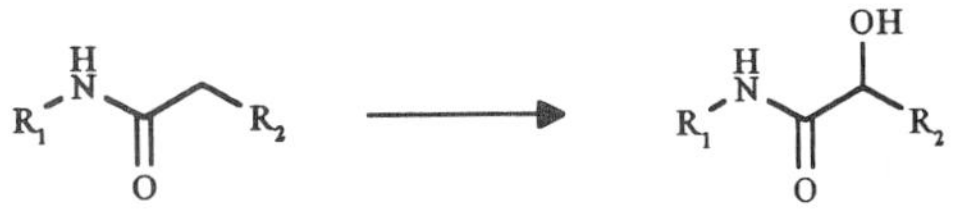
7. Oxidative deamination (amphetamine, dopamine)	7.	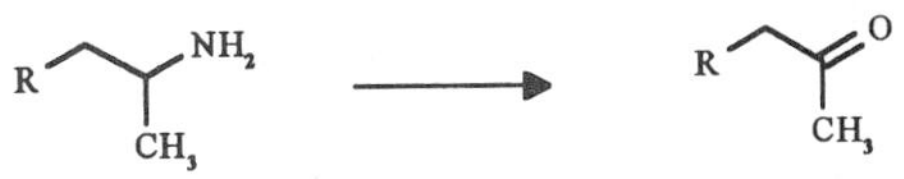
8. *N*-Dealkylation (morphine, ephedrine)	8.	$R-NH-CH_3 \longrightarrow R-NH_2$
9. *N*-Oxidation (acetaminophen, guanethidine)	9.	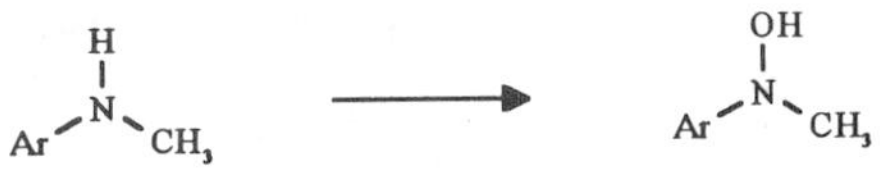
10. *O*-Dealkylation (codeine, papaverine)	10.	$R-O-CH_3 \longrightarrow R-OH$
11. *S*-Dealkylation (6-methylmercaptopurine)	11.	$R-S-CH_3 \longrightarrow R-SH$
12. *S*-Oxidation (chlorpromazine, mesoridazine)	12.	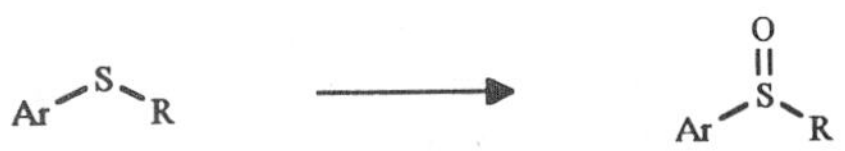
13. Desulfuration (thiopental)	13.	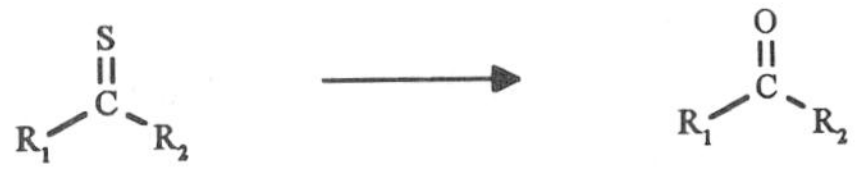
14. Dehalogenation (halothane, chloramphenicol)	14.	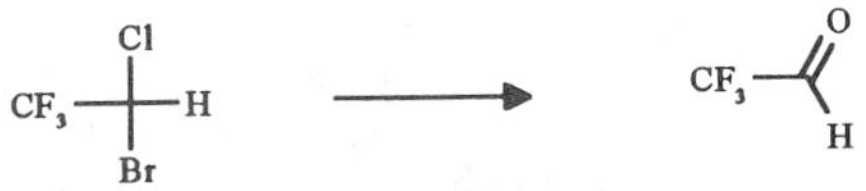
15. Oxidation of alcohols (ethanol, estradiol)	15.	$R-CH_2OH \longrightarrow R-CHO$
16. Oxidation of aldehydes (acetaldehyde, PGE_2)	16.	$R-CHO \longrightarrow R-CO_2H$

Table 12-3. Phase I Metabolism: Reductive and Hydrolytic Pathways

Type of Reaction (Examples)		Reaction Pathway
Reduction		
1. Carbonyl reduction (acetohexamide)	1.	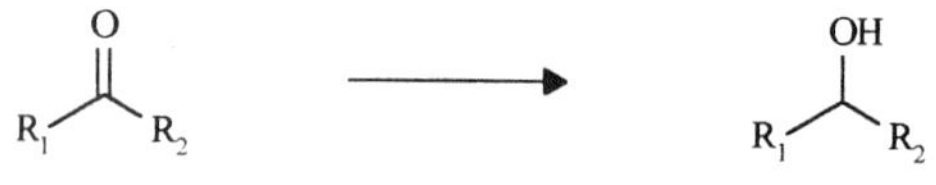
2. Azoreduction (sulfasalazine, olsalazine)	2.	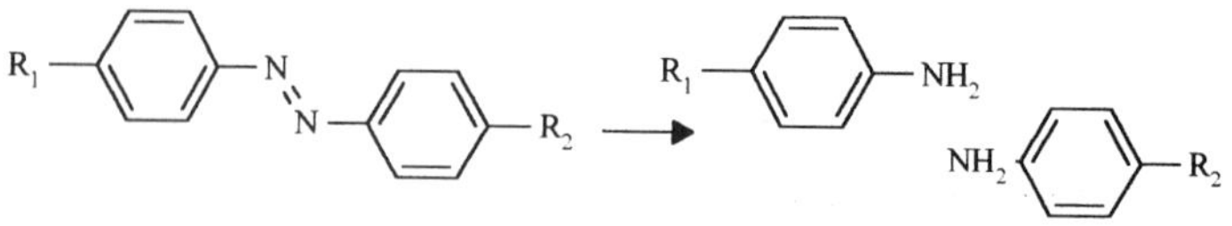
3. Nitroreduction (chloramphenicol, clonazepam)	3.	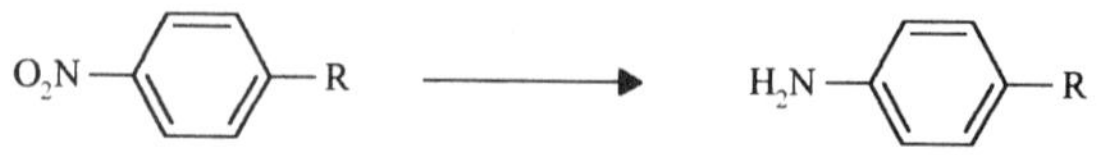
Hydrolysis		
4. Ester hydrolysis (procaine, meperidine)	4.	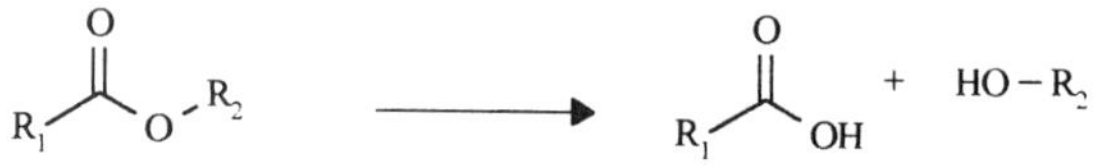
5. Amide hydrolysis (lidocaine, indomethacin)	5.	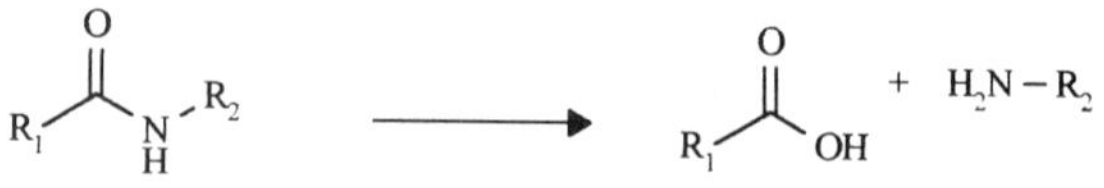

1. **Conjugation reactions** combine the **parent drug** (or its metabolites) with certain **natural endogenous constituents,** such as glucuronic acid, glycine, glutamine, sulfate, glutathione, the two-carbon acetyl fragment, or the one-carbon methyl fragment. These reactions generally require both a **high-energy molecule** and an **enzyme.**
   a. The **high-energy molecule** consists of a **coenzyme** bound to the endogenous substrate, the parent drug, or the drug's phase I metabolite.
   b. The **enzymes** (called **transferases**) that catalyze conjugation reactions are found mainly in the liver and, to a lesser extent, in the intestines and other tissues.
   c. Most conjugates are **highly polar** and **unable to cross cell membranes,** making them almost always **pharmacologically inactive** and of little or no toxicity. Exceptions to this are acetylated and methylated conjugates. These conjugates do not possess increased polarity; however, they are usually pharmacologically inactive.
2. There are **six conjugation pathways** (Table 12-4).
   a. **Glucuronidation** is the **most common** conjugation pathway because of a readily available supply of glucuronic acid as well as a large variety of functional groups, which can enzymatically react with this sugar derivative.
      (1) The high-energy form of glucuronic acid, **uridine diphosphate glucuronic acid,** reacts with a variety of functional groups under the influence of glucuronyl transferase.
      (2) Drugs that possess **hydroxyl** or **carboxyl** functional groups readily undergo glucuronidation to form ethers and esters, respectively. In addition, *N*-, *S*-, and *C*-glucuronides are also possible.
      (3) As shown in Table 12-4, the addition of glucuronic acid to a drug molecule adds three hydroxyl groups and one carboxyl group. This addition greatly increases the **hydrophilicity** of the drug molecule. As a result, it is unlikely to penetrate cell membranes and elicit pharmacologic activity. It is also poorly reabsorbed by the renal tubules and, thus, readily excreted.
      (4) Glucuronides with **high molecular weight** (more than 500) are often excreted into the bile and, eventually, into the intestines. The intestinal enzyme β-glucuronidase can then hydrolyze the conjugate, releasing the unaltered drug (or its primary metabolite) for reabsorption by the intestine.

Table 12-4. Phase II Metabolism: Conjugation Pathways

Type of Conjugate	Reaction Pathway R = Drug Molecule; X = Functional Group
1. Glucuronide (X = OH, NR_2, CO_2H, SH, acidic carbon atoms)	1. 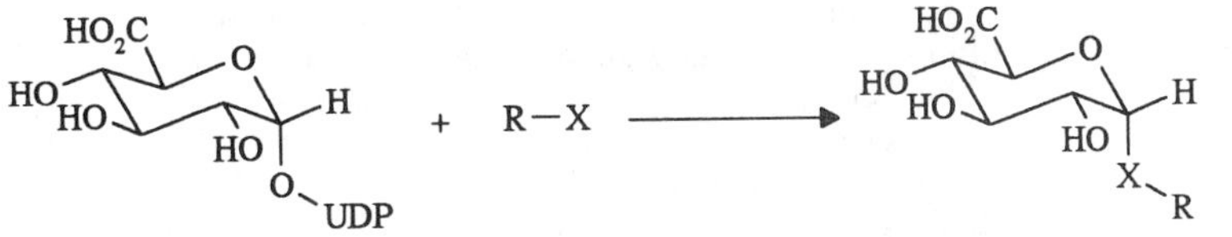
2. Sulfate (X = OH, arylamines, NH-OH)	2. 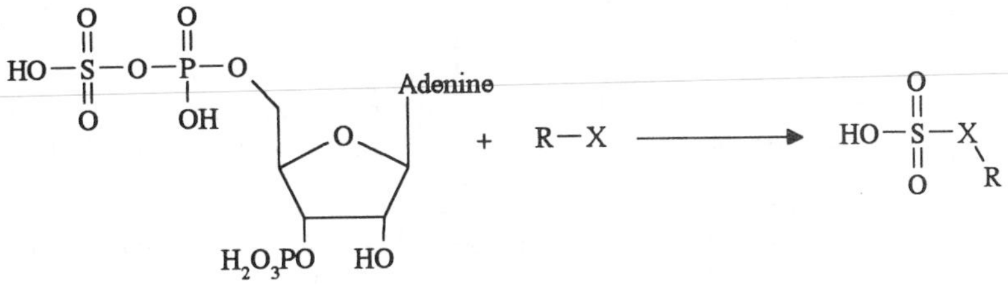
3. Amino acid (Occurs only with acid functional groups)	3. 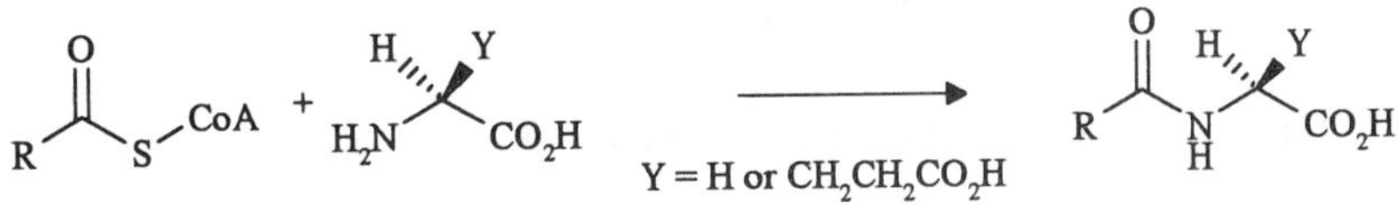
4. Glutathione (X = electrophilic center such as halide, epoxide, or Michael acceptor)	4. 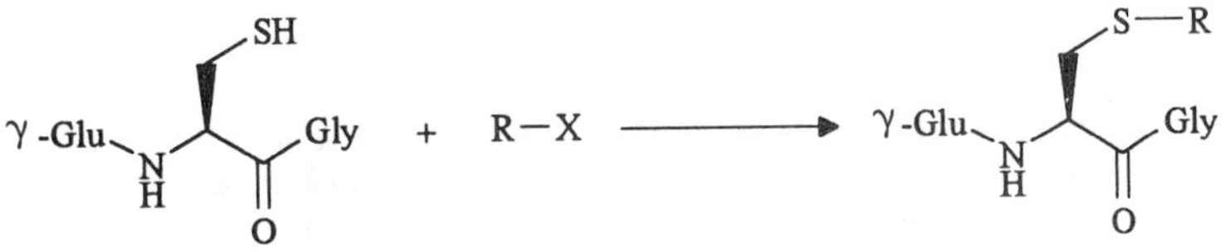
5. Methyl (X = OH, NH_2, SH)	5. 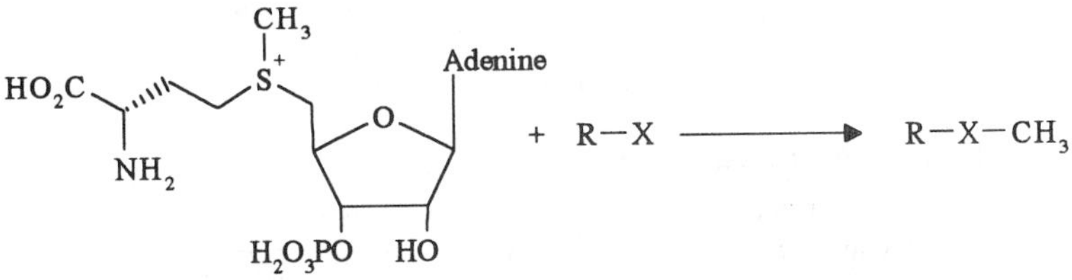
6. Acetylation (X = NH_2, $NHNH_2$, SO_2NH_2, $CO\text{-}NH_2$)	6. 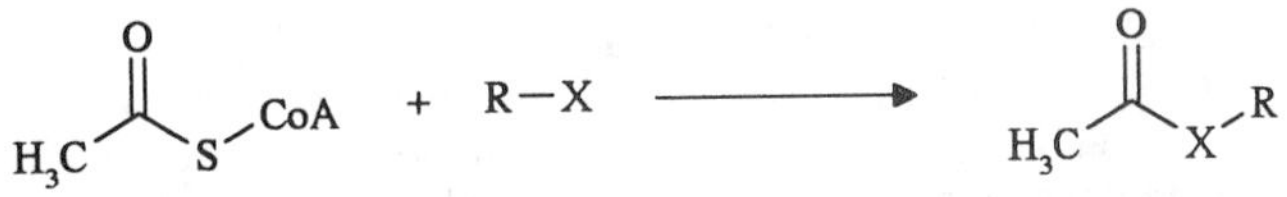

b. **Sulfate conjugation** is much less common than glucuronide conjugation because there is not an available pool of endogenous sulfate. Additionally, there are fewer functional groups capable of forming sulfate conjugates. The high-energy form of sulfate, **3′-phosphoadenosine-5′-phosphosulfate (PAPS),** reacts with phenols, alcohols, arylamines, and *N*-hydroxyl compounds under the influence of **sulfotransferase** to form highly polar metabolites.

c. **Amino acid conjugation** involves the reaction of either glycine or glutamine with aliphatic or aromatic acids to form amides. A drug molecule is first converted to an acyl coenzyme A intermediate. An *N*-acyltransferase enzyme then catalyzes the conjugation of the activated drug molecule with the amino acid.

d. Glutathione conjugation is extremely important in preventing toxicity from a variety of harmful electrophilic agents. Glutathione, a tripeptide containing a nucleophilic sulfhydryl group, is present in almost all mammalian tissues. Under the influence of **glutathione *S*-transferase,** glutathione can react with halides, epoxides, and other electrophilic compounds to form harmless inactive products. When glutathione has reacted with an electrophile, it undergoes a series of reactions to produce a mercapturic acid derivative, which is eliminated.

e. Methylation of oxygen-, nitrogen-, and sulfur-containing functional groups results in metabolites that are usually less polar than the unaltered drugs. Methylation can inactivate certain compounds (e.g., catechol *O*-methyl transferase methylates, a number of catecholamine neurotransmitters), but it plays a **minor role** in the elimination of drugs. Its **major role** is in the biosynthesis of endogenous compounds (e.g., epinephrine). The high-energy form required for **methyltransferase** enzymes is ***S*-adenosylmethionine (SAM).**

f. Acetylation can occur with primary amines, hydrazides, sulfonamides, and, occasionally, amides. It leads to the formation of *N*-acetylated products. These products are usually less polar than the unaltered drug and can retain pharmacologic activity.

(1) *N*-acetylated metabolites can accumulate in tissue or in the kidneys, as in the case of certain **antibacterial sulfonamides.** Crystalluria and subsequent tissue damage may result.

(2) The high-energy molecule for acetylation is **acetyl-CoA.** The reaction is **catalyzed by *N*-acetyltransferase.**

VII. FACTORS INFLUENCING DRUG METABOLISM

A. Chemical structure specifically influences a drug's metabolic pathway. The presence or absence of certain functional groups will determine the necessity, route, and extent of metabolism.

B. Species differences

1. **Qualitative differences** are in the actual metabolic pathway. Such a variation can result from a genetic deficiency of a particular enzyme or a difference in a particular endogenous substrate. In general, qualitative differences occur primarily with **phase II reactions.**

2. **Quantitative differences** are differences in the extent to which the same type of metabolic reaction occurs. Such a variation can result from a difference in the enzyme level, the presence of species specific isozymes, a difference in the amount of endogenous inhibitor or inducer, or a difference in the extent of competing reactions. In general, quantitative differences occur primarily with **phase I reactions.**

C. Physiologic or disease state

1. Because the liver is the major organ involved in biotransformation, **pathologic factors** that **alter liver function** can affect a drug's hepatic clearance.

2. **Congestive heart failure** decreases hepatic blood flow by reducing cardiac output, which alters the extent of drug metabolism.

3. An **alteration in albumin production** (the plasma's major drug-binding protein) can alter the fraction of bound to unbound drug. Thus, a decrease in plasma albumin can increase the fraction of unbound (free) drug, which then becomes available to exert a more intense pharmacologic effect. The reverse is true when plasma albumin increases.

D. Genetic variations

1. The **acetylation rate** depends on the amount of *N*-acetyltransferase present, which is determined by genetic factors. The general population can be divided into **fast acetylators** and **slow acetylators.** For example, fast acetylators are more prone to **hepatotoxicity** from the antitubercular agent isoniazid than slow acetylators, whereas slow acetylators are more prone to isoniazid's other toxic effects.

2. The discovery of isoforms and families of cytochrome P_{450} enzymes has shown that genetic variations exist in isoforms that oxidize **debrisoquine.** Individuals who are poor metabolizers of this compound **(PM phenotype)** also exhibit impaired metabolism of over 20 other therapeutic agents, including β-blockers, antiarrhythmics, opioids, and antidepressants. Approximately 5%–10% of whites, 2% of Asians, and 1% of Arabs express the PM phenotype and are at risk for adverse drug reactions

E. Drug dosage

1. An **increase** in drug dosage results in increased drug concentrations and can saturate certain metabolic enzymes. As drug concentration exceeds 50% saturation for a particular enzyme, drug elimination via this path no longer follows solely first-order kinetics, but rather is a mix of zero- and first-order kinetics. At 100% saturation, metabolism via this enzyme follows zero-order kinetics.

2. **When the metabolic pathway is saturated** (either because of an exceedingly high drug level or because the supply of an endogenous conjugated agent is exhausted), an alternative pathway may be pursued. For example, at normal doses, 98% of a dose of acetaminophen undergoes conjugation with either glucuronic acid or sulfate; however, at toxic doses, conjugation pathways become saturated and acetaminophen undergoes extensive *N*-hydroxylation, which can lead to hepatotoxicity.

F. Nutritional status

1. The levels of some **conjugating agents** (or endogenous substrates), such as sulfate, glutathione, and (rarely) glucuronic acid, are sensitive to body nutrient levels. For example, a **low-protein diet** can lead to a deficiency of certain amino acids, such as glycine. Low-protein diets also decrease oxidative drug metabolism capacity.

2. Diets **deficient in essential fatty acids** (particularly linoleic acid) reduce the metabolism of ethyl-morphine and hexobarbital by decreasing synthesis of certain drug-metabolizing enzymes.

3. A **deficiency of certain dietary minerals** also affects drug metabolism. Calcium, magnesium, and zinc deficiencies decrease drug-metabolizing capacity, whereas iron deficiency appears to increase it. A copper deficiency leads to variable effects.

4. **Deficiencies of vitamins** (particularly vitamins A, C, E, and the B group) affect drug-metabolizing capacity. For example, a vitamin C deficiency can result in a decrease in oxidative pathways, whereas a vitamin E deficiency can retard dealkylation and hydroxylation.

G. Age

1. Metabolizing enzyme systems are not fully developed at birth, thus **infants** and **young children** need to receive smaller doses of drugs than adults to avoid toxic side effects. This is particularly true of drugs which require glucuronide conjugation.

2. In **older children,** some drugs may be less active than in adults, particularly if the dosage is based on weight. The liver develops faster than the increase in general body weight and, thus, represents a greater fraction of total body weight.

3. In the **elderly,** metabolizing enzyme systems decline. The lowered level of enzyme activity slows the rate of drug elimination, causing higher plasma drug levels per dose than in young adults.

H. Gender. Metabolic differences between the sexes have been observed for a number of compounds, suggesting that androgen, estrogen, and/or adrenocorticoid activity might affect the activity of certain cytochrome P_{450} enzyme isozymes.

1. Metabolism of diazepam, prednisolone, caffeine, and acetaminophen is **slightly faster in women.**

2. Oxidative metabolism of propranolol, chlordiazepoxide, lidocaine, and some steroids occurs **faster in men** than in women.

Table 12-5. Examples of Drugs That Undergo First-Pass Metabolism

Acetaminophen	Fluorouracil	Oxprenolol
Albuterol	Imipramine	Pentazocine
Alprenolol	Isoproterenol	Progesterone
Aspirin	Lidocaine	Propoxyphene
Cortisone	Meperidine	Propranolol
Cyclosporin	Methyltestosterone	Salbutamol
Desipramine	Metoprolol	Terbutaline
Dihydropyridines	Nortriptyline	Testosterone
Estradiol	Organic Nitrates	Verapamil

I. Circadian rhythms. The **nocturnal plasma levels** of drugs, such as theophylline and diazepam, are lower than the **diurnal plasma levels.**

J. Drug administration route

1. **Oral administration.** The drug is absorbed from the GI tract and transported to the liver through the hepatic portal vein before entering the systemic circulation. Thus, the drug is subject to hepatic metabolism before it reaches its site of action. This is an effect known as the **first-pass effect,** or **presystemic elimination** (Table 12-5).
   a. The first-pass effect can cause **significant clinical problems.** Because drugs are metabolized in the liver from their active forms to inactive forms, this effect must be counteracted to achieve the desired plasma or tissue drug level.
   b. A common approach is to **increase the oral dose,** offsetting the loss of drug activity from the first-pass effect.
2. **Intravenous administration** bypasses the first-pass effect because the drug is delivered directly to the bloodstream without being metabolized in the liver. Thus, intravenous doses of drugs undergoing considerable first-pass effects are much smaller than oral doses.
3. **Sublingual administration** and **rectal administration** also bypass first-pass effects, although rectal administration can produce variable effects.

K. Enzyme induction or inhibition can pose significant problems for the patient on a multiple-drug regimen, in which drug interactions are likely.

1. **Sequential** or **concurrent administration** of many structurally diverse drugs and environmental chemicals can increase the metabolism of some drugs, a phenomenon known as **enzyme induction.**

Table 12-6. Examples of Drug Interactions Involving Enzyme Induction

Activity of	Decreased by
Carbamazepine	Phenobarbital
Digitoxin	Phenobarbital, Rifampin
Oral Anticoagulants	Phenobarbital, Rifampin
Oral Contraceptives	Carbamazepine, Phenobarbital, Rifampin
Oral Hypoglycemics	Rifampin
Theophylline	Phenobarbital, Rifampin

Table 12-7. Examples of Drug Interactions Involving Enzyme Inhibition

Activity of	Increased by
Diazepam	Cimetidine
Ethanol	Disulfiram
Oral Anticoagulants	Chloramphenicol, Cimetidine, Disulfiram, Metronidazole
Phenytoin	Chloramphenicol, Cimetidine, Disulfiram, Isoniazid
Theophylline	Cimetidine

a. Drugs such as phenobarbital, carbamazepine, and rifampin appear to act as enzyme inducers by increasing the synthesis or decreasing the degradation of drug-metabolizing enzymes (Table 12-6).
b. Environmental chemicals, such as the **polycyclic aromatic hydrocarbons** and the **chlorinated insecticides,** also act as enzyme inducers. Cigarette smokers, for example, have lower plasma levels of drugs such as theophylline than do nonsmokers. The polycyclic aromatic hydrocarbon components of cigarette smoke appear to induce the *N*-demethylation pathway.

2. **Enzyme inhibition.** Some drugs and xenobiotics can **decrease the metabolism** of other drugs. This is a phenomenon known as enzyme inhibition. Inhibition can occur by the destruction of drug-metabolizing enzymes, inhibition of enzyme synthesis, or complexation and inactivation of the drug-metabolizing enzymes (Table 12-7).

3. **Opposite effects** on drug activity occur when prodrugs are involved because these are inactive when administered and must be metabolized to their active forms.

4. **Tolerance** that develops with certain drugs, such as barbiturates, is related to enzyme induction. Induction results in **increased metabolism** and **decreased activity** compared to the effects of initial doses.

VIII. EXTRAHEPATIC METABOLISM

A. **Definition.** Extrahepatic metabolism refers to drug biotransformation that takes place in **tissues other than the liver.** The most common sites include the **portals of entry** (e.g., GI mucosa, nasal passages, and lungs) and the **portals of excretion** (e.g., kidneys). However, metabolism can occur throughout the body.

B. **Metabolism sites**

1. **Plasma** contains **esterases,** which are responsible primarily for hydrolysis of esters. **Simple esters** (e.g., procaine, succinylcholine) are rapidly hydrolyzed in the blood. Additionally, plasma esterases can activate a variety of ester prodrugs.

2. Metabolizing enzymes in the **intestinal mucosa** are especially important for drugs undergoing microsomal oxidation, glucuronide conjugation, and sulfate conjugation.
   a. As a lipid-soluble drug passes through the intestinal mucosa during drug absorption, it can be metabolized into polar or inactive metabolites before entering the blood. The result is **comparable to a first-pass effect.**
   b. The intestinal mucosa's drug-metabolizing capacity compares to that of the liver. However, it shows much greater individual variation because of its greater exposure to the environment.

3. **Intestinal bacterial flora** secrete a number of enzymes capable of metabolizing drugs and other xenobiotics.
   a. Any factor that **modifies the intestinal flora** may also **modify drug activity.** Age, diet, disease state, and exposure to environmental chemicals or drugs may all be important.
      (1) Certain **diseases,** particularly **intestinal disease,** affect intestinal flora. Ulcerative colitis, for example, promotes bacterial growth. Diarrhea reduces the number of bacteria.
      (2) Certain **environmental chemicals** and **drugs** also act on intestinal flora. Antibiotics, for example, decrease the number of bacteria.
   b. Bacterial flora **secrete** β-glucuronidase, which hydrolyzes the polar glucuronide conjugates of bile and allows the free, nonpolar bile acids to be reabsorbed. This **enterohepatic circulation** partially maintains the pool of bile acids. This same principle applies to certain glucuronide conjugates of drugs.
   c. Certain bacterial flora **convert** vitamin precursors to their **active forms,** as with vitamin K.
   d. Bacterial flora can also **convert** certain substances to their **toxic forms,** as with the conversion of the artificial sweetener cyclamate to cyclohexylamine, a suspected carcinogen.
   e. Intestinal bacteria produce **azoreductase,** which reduces the prodrug sulfasalazine to the active anti-inflammatory aminosalicylic acid and the active antibacterial sulfapyridine. Sulfasalazine is one of the few agents effective in the treatment of ulcerative colitis.

4. The **acidic environment** of the **stomach** produces nonenzymatic degradation of a number of drug molecules, including penicillin G, carbenicillin, erythromycin, and tetracycline. Additionally, gastric acid assists in the degradation of proteins and peptides (e.g., insulin).

5. The **nasal mucosa** provides a high level of cytochrome P_{450} activity, which can significantly alter the amount of drug that reaches the systemic circulation. Nasal decongestants, anesthetics, nicotine, cocaine, and other compounds have been shown to undergo nasal metabolism.

6. The **lung** is responsible for first-pass metabolism of drugs administered intravenously, intramuscularly, transdermally, or subcutaneously.
   a. The **total amount** of **metabolizing enzymes** present in the lungs is less than that in the liver; however, the specific activities of the enzymes are comparable to those in the liver.
   b. The lungs provide **second-pass metabolism** for drugs leaving the liver.

C. Placental and fetal metabolism

1. **Placenta.** In general, if a drug or other xenobiotic is lipid soluble enough to be absorbed into the circulation when administered to a pregnant woman, it will likely also pass through the placenta.
   a. The placenta is not a physical or metabolic barrier to xenobiotics. Very little xenobiotic-metabolizing enzyme activity has been demonstrated in the placenta.
   b. Drugs present in their **active form** in the maternal circulation likely pass **unchanged** into the fetal circulation.
   c. An exception to this lack of enzyme activity in the placenta is the presence of a small amount of **aryl aromatic hydroxylase,** which is **inducible in pregnant women who smoke cigarettes.** A potential consequence is an increase in the production of penultimate carcinogens from the action of this enzyme on the polycyclic aromatic hydrocarbons present in cigarette smoke and other environmental sources.

2. **Fetus.** In terms of fetal metabolism, there are varying degrees of drug-metabolizing activity dependent upon a number of factors including fetal age.
   a. A **major deficiency** is that of **glucuronic acid conjugating activity** both in the **fetus** and the **neonate.**
   b. Two consequences of this are the **gray baby syndrome,** resulting from decreased chloramphenicol glucuronidation, and **neonatal hyperbilirubinemia,** resulting from a decrease in bilirubin glucuronide formation.

IX. STRATEGIES TO MANAGE DRUG METABOLISM.

A variety of methods have been used to circumvent the rapid metabolism of certain drugs. These methods seek to improve drug therapy by decreasing the overall extent of metabolism and increasing the duration of action. In some instances, these methods have provided increased site specificity.

A. Pharmaceutical strategies

Pharmaceutical strategies involve the use of different **dosage forms** to either avoid or compensate for rapid metabolism.

1. **Sublingual tablets** are useful for delivering drugs directly into the systemic circulation and bypassing hepatic first-pass metabolism. **Nitroglycerin,** a rapidly acting antianginal agent, is essentially ineffective when administered orally due to an extremely high first-pass effect but is very effective in treating acute attacks of angina if given sublingually.

2. **Transdermal patches** and **ointment formulations** provide a continuous supply of drug over an extended period of time and are useful for rapidly metabolized compounds such as nitroglycerin. These delivery systems, while not suited to treat acute anginal symptoms, are effective in providing prophylactic concentrations of nitroglycerin.

3. **Intramuscular depot injections** also provide a continuous supply of drug over an extended period of time. Highly lipid soluble esters of **estradiol** and **testosterone** (e.g., estradiol benzoate, testosterone enanthate) are slowly absorbed from their administration site. Hydrolysis of these prodrugs (see X) produces a steady supply of these rapidly metabolized hormones.

4. **Enteric-coated formulations** can protect acid sensitive drugs as they pass through the acidic environment of the stomach. **Methenamine, erythromycin,** and **omeprazole** are examples of acid-sensitive agents that are available as enteric-coated preparations.

5. **Nasal administration** allows for the delivery of peptides, such as **calcitonin salmon,** which have very low (if any) oral bioavailability. Characteristics of the lung make it ideal for the administration of peptides. Aerosolized drugs only need to penetrate a thin epithelial layer to reach abundant capillary beds. Additionally, the lungs contain protease inhibitors, which allow for greater stability of the peptides.

B. **Pharmacologic strategies** involve the concurrent use of **enzyme inhibitors** to decrease drug metabolism. In some instances, the concurrent use of an additional agent does not prevent metabolism but rather prevents the toxicity caused by metabolites of the therapeutic agent.

1. **Levodopa (L-dopa),** the amino acid precursor of dopamine, is used in the treatment of parkinsonism. Unlike dopamine, L-dopa can penetrate the blood–brain barrier and reach the central nervous system (CNS). When in the brain, it is decarboxylated to dopamine. To assure that adequate concentrations of L-dopa reach the CNS, peripheral metabolism of the drug must be blocked. The concurrent administration of **carbidopa,** a DOPA decarboxylase inhibitor that cannot penetrate the blood–brain barrier, prevents peripheral formation of dopamine and allows site-specific delivery of dopamine to the CNS.

2. **β-Lactam antibiotics.** The antibacterial activity of a number of β-lactam antibiotics is reduced by microorganisms capable of secreting the enzyme, β-lactamase. This enzyme hydrolyzes the β-lactam ring and inactivates the antibiotic. To counter this resistance mechanism, a β-lactamase inhibitor, such as **clavulanic acid,** is used in conjunction with a penicillin, such as **amoxicillin,** to successfully treat infections caused by β-lactamase producing bacteria.

3. **Ifosfamide** is an alkylating agent which must undergo in vivo metabolism to produce an active nitrogen mustard. In the process of this metabolic activation, significant concentrations of **acrolein** are produced. These acrolein molecules react with nucleophiles on renal proteins and produce hemorrhagic cystitis. To prevent this toxicity, ifosfamide is always coadministered with **mesna,** a sulfhydryl-containing compound that reacts with and neutralizes any acrolein that is present in the kidney.

C. **Chemical strategies** involve the addition, deletion, or isosteric modification of key functional groups. These molecular modifications hinder or completely eliminate metabolic transformations (Figure 12-9).

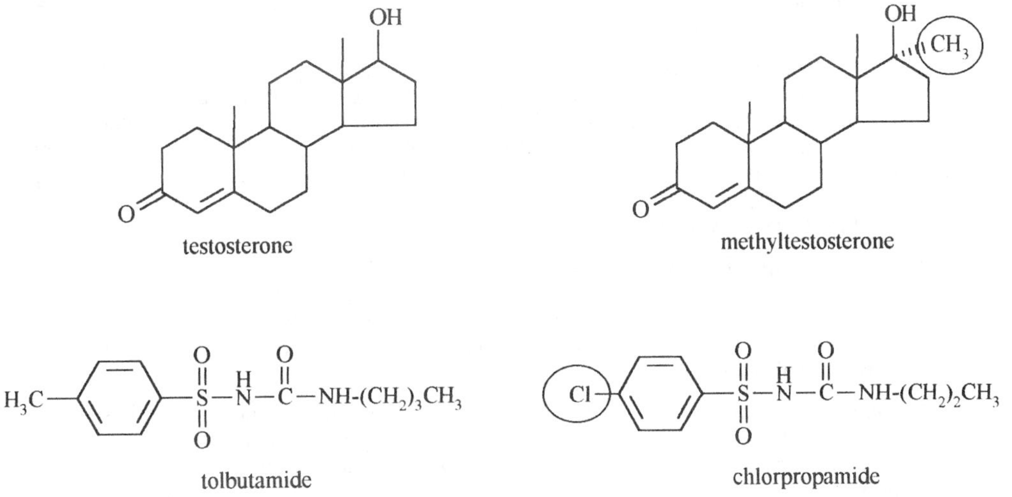

Figure 12-9. Selected examples of chemical modification that eliminate metabolic transformations. Methylation of testosterone blocks the rapid oxidation of the 17-hydroxyl group and allows oral activity, whereas replacement of the metabolically labile *para*-methyl group on tolbutamide with a chloro group allows for a much longer duration of action.

1. **Testosterone** is not orally active due to rapid oxidation of its 17-hydroxyl group to a ketone. Addition of a 17α-methyl group converts the labile secondary alcohol to a stable tertiary alcohol. The resulting compound, **methyltestosterone,** is only half as potent as testosterone; however, it is not subject to rapid first-pass metabolism and can be used orally. A similar strategy has been used to make orally active estradiol analogs.

2. **Tolbutamide** is an oral hypoglycemic with a short duration of action. This sulfonylurea rapidly undergoes oxidation of its *para*-methyl group. A structurally similar compound, **chlorpropamide,** has a non-metabolizable *para*-chloro group and, as a result, has a much longer duration of action.

3. **Isoproterenol** is a potent β-adrenergic agonist used for the relief of bronchospasm associated with bronchial asthma. Because it is a catechol (i.e., 3,4-dihydroxy substituted benzene ring), isoproterenol is subject to rapid metabolism by catechol *O*-methyl transferase (COMT) and, thus, has poor oral activity. Alteration of the 3,4-dihydroxy substitution to a 3,5-dihydroxy substitution produces **metaproterenol,** a bronchodilator that is not susceptible to COMT, is orally active, and has a longer duration of action than isoproterenol.

4. **Octreotide** is a synthetic octapeptide used to suppress or inhibit severe diarrhea associated with certain tumors. Octreotide mimics the actions of **somatostatin,** a naturally occurring, 14 amino acid peptide. Somatostatin undergoes rapid proteolysis, has a half-life of 1–3 minutes, and must be administered as a continuous intravenous infusion. Octreotide contains the amino acids essential for clinical efficacy but replaces two of the amino acids with their *D*-enantiomers. These unnatural *D*-amino acids are more resistant to hydrolysis. As a result, octreotide has an increased half-life and can be administered as a subcutaneous injection.

X. PRODRUGS.

These drugs are molecules that are either inactive or very weakly active and require in vivo biotransformation to produce the physiologically active drug. The phase I metabolic processes discussed previously are used to activate prodrugs. A variety of **advantages** can be gained by using a prodrug instead of the active form of the drug.

A. An **increase in water solubility** is useful for the preparation of ophthalmic and parenteral formulations. **Sodium succinate esters** and **sodium phosphate esters** have been used to make a number of water-soluble steroid prodrugs.

B. An **increase in lipid solubility** is useful for a variety of reasons.

1. **Increased duration of action.** Lipid-soluble esters of estradiol, such as benzoate, valerate, and cypionate, are used to prolong estrogenic activity. IM injections of these esters in oil result in a deposit of drug that is slowly hydrolyzed, thereby releasing free stradiol over a prolonged period of time (see IX A 3).

2. **Increased oral absorption** is obtained by converting carboxylic acid groups to esters. These esters can then be rapidly converted to the active acids by plasma esterases. **Enalaprilat** is a potent angiotensin-converting enzyme (ACE) inhibitor that is used for parenteral administration, but, due to its high polarity, it is orally inactive. Its monomethyl ester, **enalapril,** is considerably more lipophilic and, thus, provides good oral absorption. This strategy has been successfully used for a variety of other compounds, including additional ACE inhibitors, fibric acid derivatives, ampicillin, and several cephalosporins.

3. **Increased topical absorption** of steroids is obtained by masking hydroxyl groups as esters or acetonides. These prodrugs are much less polar than the parent compounds and allow increased dermal permeability for the treatment of inflammatory, allergic, and pruritic skin conditions. Examples include **triamcinolone acetonide, diflorasone diacetate,** and **betamethasone valerate.**

4. **Increased palatability.** Antibiotics such as **sulfisoxazole** have a bitter taste and are not suitable for administration to young children who cannot yet swallow tablets or capsules. Esterification to produce **sulfisoxazole acetyl** decreases the water solubility of the antibiotic and, thus, decreases its interaction with bitter taste receptors on the tongue. This compound is marketed as a flavored suspension. Similar strategies have been used to mask the bitter taste of **chloramphenicol** and other antibiotics

C. A decrease in GI irritation. Nonsteroidal anti-inflammatory agents (NSAIDs) produce gastric irritation and ulceration via two mechanisms: a direct irritant effect of the acidic molecule and inhibition of gastroprotective prostaglandin production. The prodrugs **sulindac** and **nabumetone** produce less GI irritation because the gastric and intestinal mucosa are not exposed to high concentrations of active drug during oral administration. Additionally, nabumetone is a ketone, not an acid, and lacks any direct irritant effects.

D. Site specificity is useful for increasing the concentration of drug at the active site and for decreasing side effects.

1. **Methyldopa** is a prodrug which is structurally similar to L-dopa. As a result, methyldopa is transported into the CNS and metabolized to the active compound, **α-methyldopamine,** via the same path used for the synthesis of dopamine. This allows a significant amount of α-methyldopamine to reach the CNS and bind to central α_2 adrenergic receptors.

2. **Omeprazole** is used to treat gastric ulcers and other hypersecretory disorders. After oral absorption, it is selectively activated at the acidic pH levels (pH less than 1) seen in gastric parietal cells. This allows the active form of the drug to be produced in close proximity to the enzyme H^+/K^+-ATPase (proton pump) resulting in irreversible inhibition of the enzyme and a decrease in gastric acid secretion. Activation in the stomach prior to absorption can be prevented by the use of enteric coated formulations (see IX A 4).

3. **Formaldehyde** is an effective urinary tract antiseptic; however, oral administration results in significant toxicity. To avoid this problem, the prodrug **methenamine** is administered instead. Methenamine is stable and nontoxic at normal physiologic pH, but is selectively hydrolyzed to formaldehyde and ammonium ions in the acidic urine (pH less than 5.5). As with omeprazole, activation before absorption can be prevented by the use of enteric-coated formulations (see IX A 4).

4. **Olsalazine** is a highly polar dimer of 5-aminosalicylic acid that is poorly absorbed after oral administration. On reaching the large intestine, colonic bacteria cleave the azo bond and liberate the active anti-inflammatory agent. Olsalazine and a related compound, **sulfasalazine,** are useful in treating inflammatory bowel disease.

5. **Diethylstilbestrol** is a synthetic estrogen that can produce undesirable, feminizing side effects when used in the treatment of prostate cancer. These side effects can be avoided by the use of the ester prodrug, **diethylstilbestrol diphosphate.** This prodrug is inactive until dephosphorylated by acid phosphatase, an enzyme that is highly active in prostate tumor cells. This allows for a localized release of active compound and a decrease in systemic side effects.

E. Increased shelf life of both solids and parenteral admixtures can be obtained by the use of prodrugs.

1. **Cefamandole** is a second-generation cephalosporin that is unstable in solid dosage forms. Esterification of the α-hydroxyl group with formic acid produces **cefamandole nafate,** a stable prodrug that is hydrolyzed by plasma esterases to produce the parent antibiotic.

2. **Cyclophosphamide** is a prodrug that requires in vivo oxidation, followed by nonenzymatic decomposition, to produce the active phosphoramide mustard. As a result, aqueous solutions of cyclophosphamide are much more stable than those of other nitrogen mustards (i.e., mechlorethamine). **Mechlorethamine** is highly reactive, does not require in vivo activation, and can rapidly decompose in aqueous environments before administration.

STUDY QUESTIONS

Directions: Each of the numbered items or incomplete statements in this section is followed by answers or by completions of the statement. Select the **one** lettered answer or completion that is **best** in each case.

1. Which of the following acids has the highest degree of ionization in an aqueous solution?

(A) Aspirin $pK_a = 3.5$
(B) Indomethacin $pK_a = 4.5$
(C) Warfarin $pK_a = 5.1$
(D) Ibuprofen $pK_a = 5.2$
(E) Phenobarbital $pK_a = 7.4$

2. Which of the following salts will most likely yield an aqueous solution with a pH below 7?

(A) Sodium salicylate
(B) Potassium chloride
(C) Magnesium sulfate
(D) Potassium penicillin
(E) Atropine sulfate

3. Which of the following salts forms an aqueous solution that is alkaline to litmus?

(A) Sodium chloride
(B) Benzalkonium chloride
(C) Meperidine hydrochloride
(D) Cefazolin sodium
(E) Chlordiazepoxide hydrochloride

4. All of the following medicinal agents are classified as natural products EXCEPT

(A) atropine
(B) diazepam
(C) digitoxin
(D) penicillin
(E) morphine

5. All of the following statements about a structurally specific agonist are true EXCEPT

(A) activity is determined more by its chemical structure than by its physical properties
(B) the entire molecule is involved in binding to a specific endogenous receptor
(C) the drug cannot act unless it is first bound to a receptor
(D) a minor structural change in a pharmacophore can produce a loss in activity
(E) the higher the affinity between the drug and its receptor, the greater the biologic response

6. The dextro (D) form of β-methacholine (structure shown) is approximately 500 times more active than the levo (L) enantiomer. The observed difference in pharmacologic activity between the two isomers is most likely due to differences in

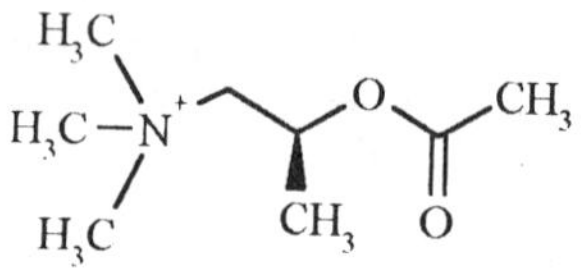

(A) receptor selectivity
(B) dissolution
(C) distribution
(D) interatomic distance between pharmacophore groups
(E) solubility

7. The compound shown below can be classified as a

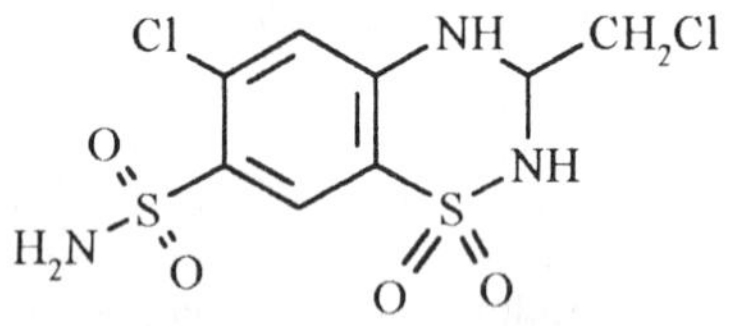

(A) penicillin
(B) thiazide
(C) coumarin
(D) phenothiazine
(E) hydantoin

8. Which of the following statements concerning the structure shown below is NOT correct? The compound

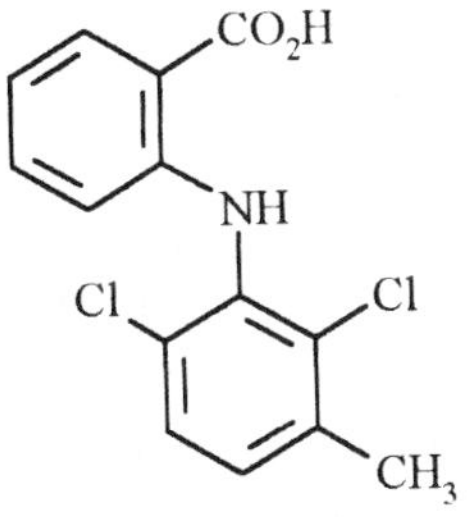

(A) is an acid
(B) can be used to treat arthritis
(C) is a fenamate
(D) increases prostaglandin production
(E) is an NSAID

9. All of the following classes of drugs are used to treat hypertension EXCEPT

(A) aryloxypropylamines
(B) thiazides
(C) fibrates
(D) dihydropyridines
(E) angiotensin-converting enzyme inhibitors

10. Flurazepam has pK_a of 8.2. What percentage of flurazepam will be ionized at a urine pH of 5.2?

(A) 0.1%
(B) 1%
(C) 50%
(D) 99%
(E) 99.9%

11. Which of the following statements concerning drug metabolism is true?

(A) Generally, a single metabolite is excreted for each drug administered
(B) Often a drug may undergo a phase II reaction followed by a phase I reaction
(C) Drug-metabolizing enzymes are found only in the liver
(D) All metabolites are less active pharmacologically than their parent drugs
(E) Phase I metabolites more likely are able to cross cellular membranes than phase II metabolites

12. Which of the following metabolites would be the least likely urinary excretion product of orally administered aspirin (see structure below)?

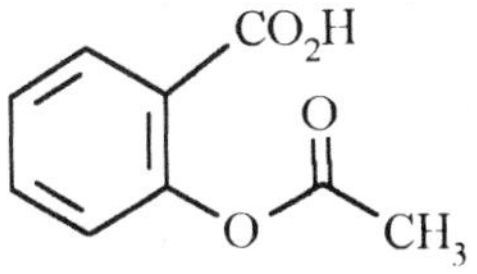

(A) Glycine conjugate
(B) Ester glucuronide
(C) Unchanged drug
(D) Ether glucuronide
(E) Hydroxylated metabolite

13. Sulfasalazine (see structure below) is a prodrug that is activated in the intestine by bacterial enzymes. The enzyme most likely responsible is

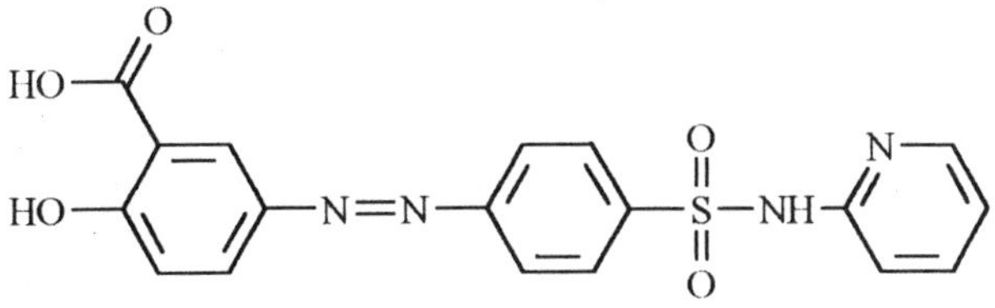

(A) azoreductase
(B) pseudocholinesterase
(C) *N*-acetyltransferase
(D) β-glucuronidase
(E) methyltransferase

14. Chloramphenicol (see structure below) is considered to be toxic in infants (gray baby syndrome). This is due to tissue accumulation of unchanged chloramphenicol, resulting from an immature metabolic pathway. Which of the following enzymes would most likely be deficient?

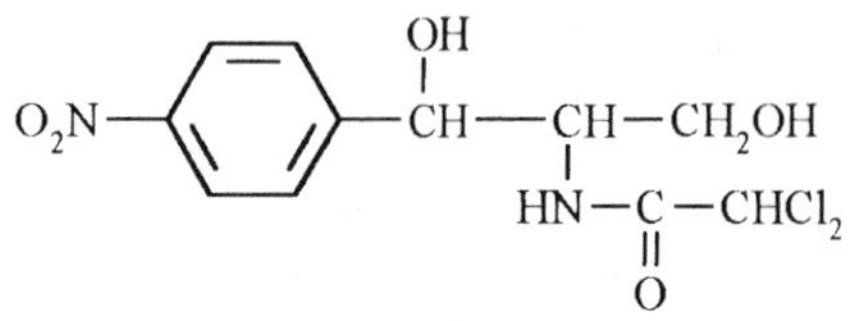

(A) Pseudocholinesterase
(B) Glucuronyl transferase
(C) *N*-acetyltransferase
(D) Azoreductase
(E) Methyltransferase

15. Which of the following therapeutic advantages cannot be obtained by the use of prodrugs? Increased

(A) oral absorption
(B) water solubility
(C) duration of action
(D) potency
(E) palatability

Directions: Each question below contains three suggested answers, of which **one or more** is correct. Choose the answer

A if **I only** is correct
B if **III only** is correct
C if **I and II** are correct
D if **II and III** are correct
E if **I, II, and III** are correct

16. Drugs that act systemically must

I. undergo biotransformation into an active form after reaching their active site
II. be in a form capable of passage through various membrane barriers
III. be in or be converted to a form that is readily excreted from the body

17. Examples of strong electrolytes (i.e., completely dissociated in an aqueous solution) include

I. acetic acid
II. pentobarbital sodium
III. diphenhydramine hydrochloride

18. Precipitation may occur when mixing aqueous solutions of meperidine hydrochloride with which of the following solutions?

I. Sodium bicarbonate injection
II. Atropine sulfate injection
III. Sodium chloride injection

19. Drugs classified as antimetabolites include

I. 5-fluorouracil
II. sulfisoxazole
III. digoxin

20. The excretion of a weakly acidic drug generally is more rapid in alkaline urine than in acidic urine. This process occurs because

I. a weak acid in alkaline media will exist primarily in its ionized form, which cannot be reabsorbed easily
II. a weak acid in alkaline media will exist in its lipophilic form, which cannot be reabsorbed easily
III. all drugs are excreted more rapidly in an alkaline urine

Questions 21–24

All of the following questions refer to the drug meperidine (see structure below).

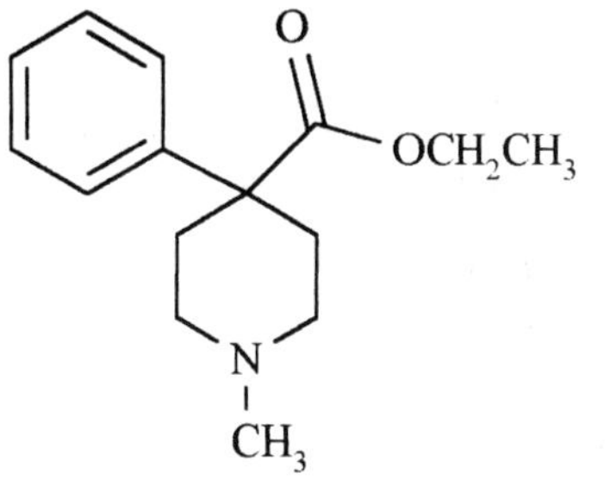

21. Functional groups present in the molecule shown include

I. an ester
II. a tertiary amine
III. a carboxylic acid

22. Meperidine is classified as a

I. weak acid
II. salt
III. weak base

23. Assuming that meperidine is absorbed after oral administration and that a large percentage of the dose is excreted unchanged, the effect of alkalinization of the urine will increase its

I. duration of action
II. rate of excretion
III. ionization in the glomerular filtrate

24. The appropriate chemical classification for meperidine is

I. phenylpropylamines
II. piperazines
III. 4-phenylpiperidines

25. Terms that may be used to describe the following metabolic reaction include

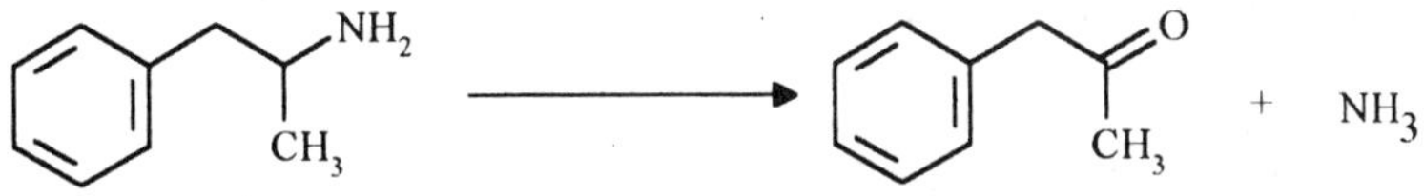

I. *N*-dealkylation
II. oxidative deamination
III. phase I metabolism

26. Which of the following reactions can be classified as phase II metabolism?

I. 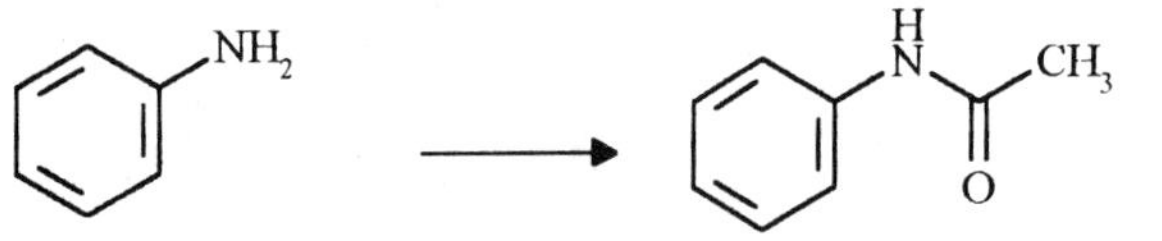

II. 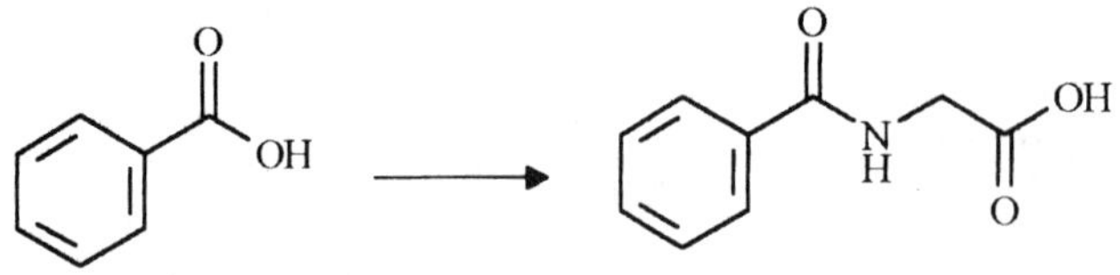

III. 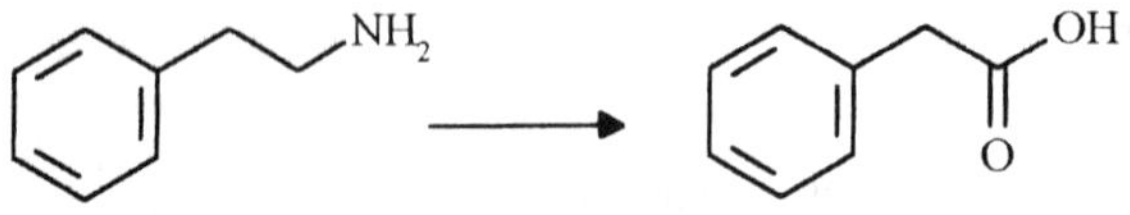

27. Conditions that tend to increase the action of an orally administered drug that undergoes phase II metabolism include

I. enterohepatic circulation
II. enzyme saturation
III. first-pass effect

28. Metabolic reactions likely to be affected by a protein-deficient diet include

I. glycine conjugation
II. hydrolysis
III. glucuronidation

Directions: The group of items in this section consists of lettered options followed by a set of numbered items. For each item, select the **one lettered** option that is most closely associated with it. Each lettered option may be selected once, more than once, or not at all.

Questions 29–33

For each pair of molecules, select the term that best fits the relationship.

(A) Geometric isomers
(B) Enantiomers
(C) Diastereomers
(D) Bioisosteres
(E) Conformational isomers

29. 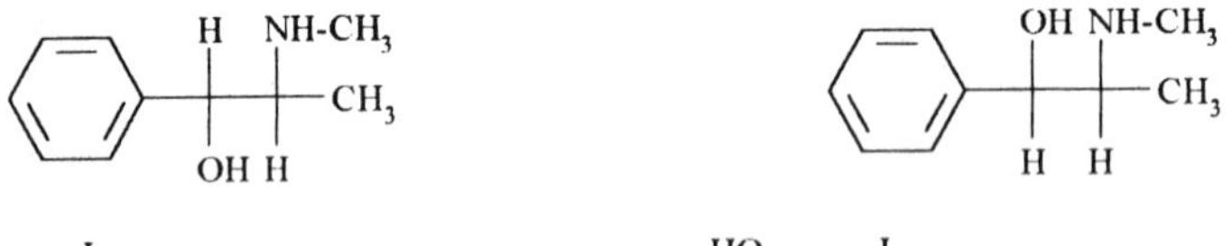

30. 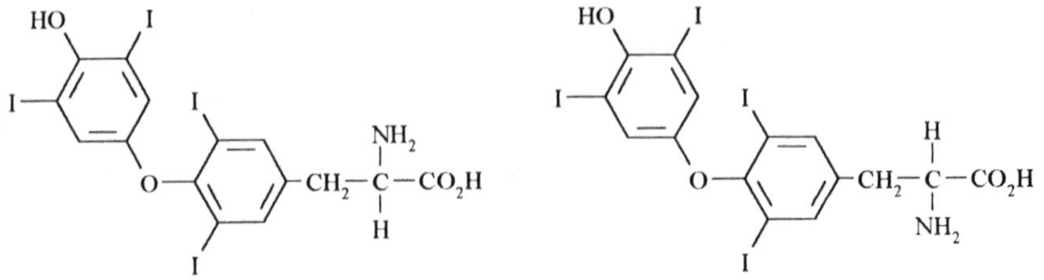

31. 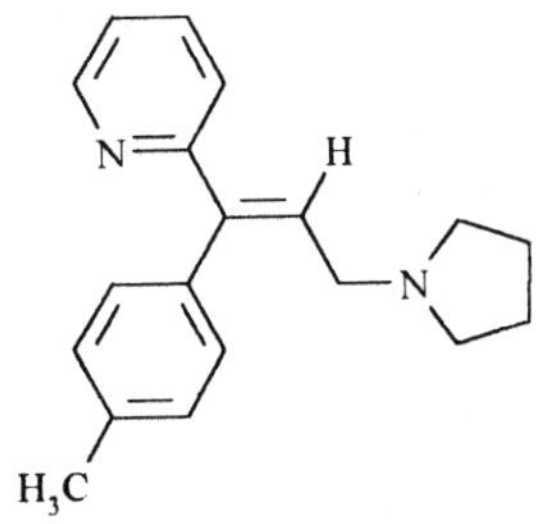 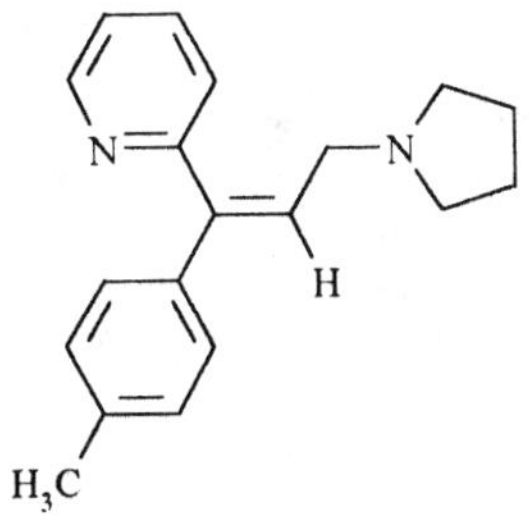

32. 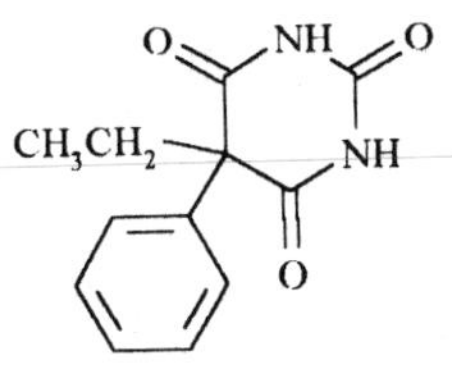 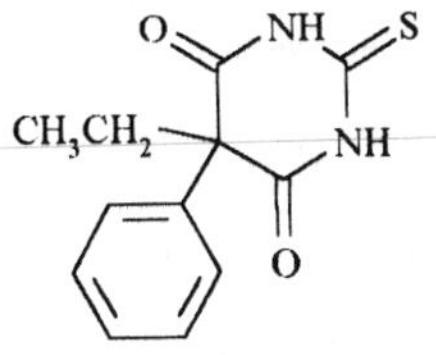

33. 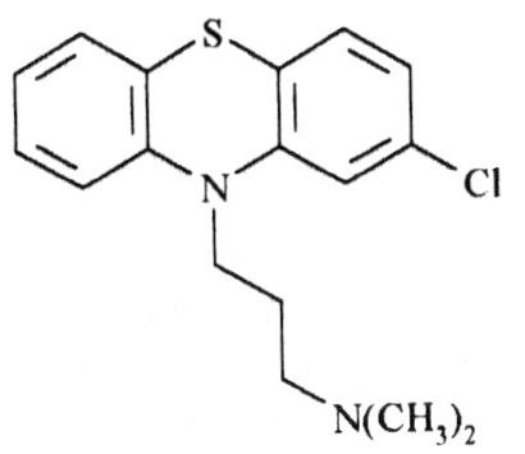 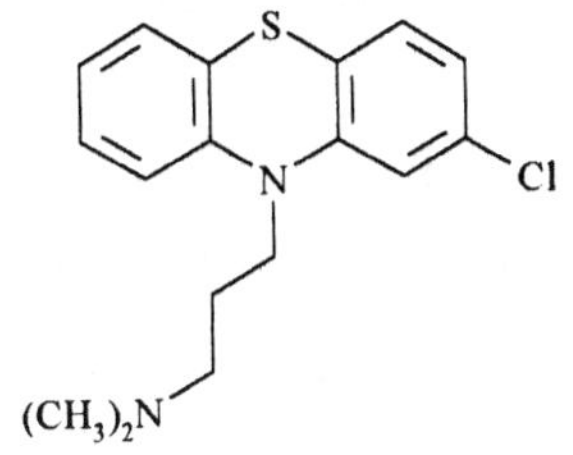

Questions 34–37

For each drug, select its most likely metabolic pathway.

34. Benzoic Acid

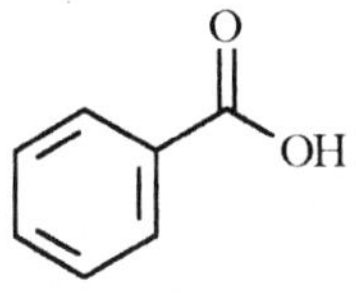

35. Procaine

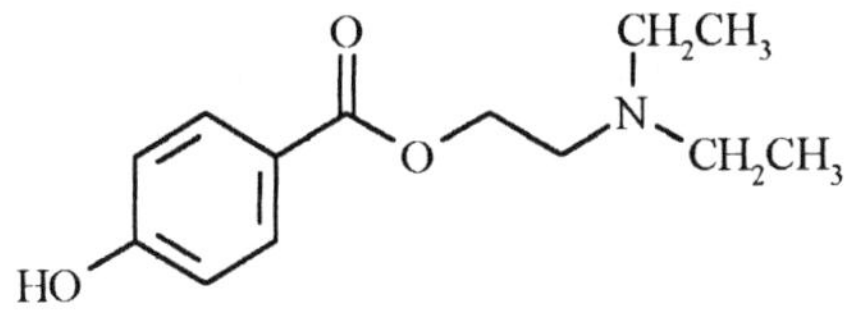

36. Acetaminophen

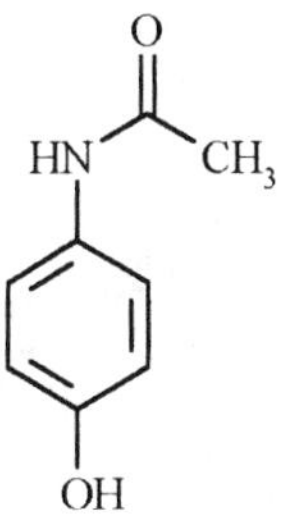

37. Amphetamine

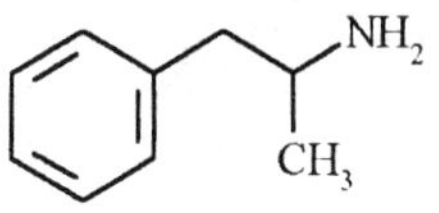

(A) Ether glucuronidation
(B) Ester glucuronidation
(C) Nitroreduction
(D) Oxidative deamination
(E) Ester hydrolysis

ANSWERS AND EXPLANATIONS

1. The answer is A *[II B 2 b].*
The pK_a (the negative log of the acid ionization constant) is indicative of the relative strength of an acidic drug. The lower the pK_a of an acidic drug, the stronger it is as an acid. A strong acid is defined as one that is completely ionized or dissociated in an aqueous solution; therefore, the stronger the acid, the greater the ionization.

2. The answer is E *[II B 3 d].*
The solution must contain an acidic substance to have a pH below 7. Atropine sulfate is a salt of a weak base and a strong acid; therefore, its aqueous solution is acidic. Sodium salicylate and potassium penicillin are both salts of strong bases and weak acids; therefore, their aqueous solutions are alkaline. Magnesium sulfate and potassium chloride are salts of strong bases and strong acids; therefore, their aqueous solutions are neutral.

3. The answer is D *[II B 3 d].*
Only an aqueous solution of cefazolin sodium, which is a salt of a strong base and a weak acid, may be alkaline. Meperidine hydrochloride and chlordiazepoxide hydrochloride are salts of weak bases and strong acids, and their solutions are acidic. Sodium chloride is a salt of a strong acid and a strong base, whereas benzalkonium chloride is a quaternary ammonium salt. Aqueous solutions of these types of salts are neutral.

4. The answer is B *[I A, B].*
Diazepam is a benzodiazepine anxiolytic, which, while it is a heterocyclic nitrogen-containing molecule, is not an alkaloid and is prepared synthetically. Natural products refer to those substances biosynthesized in plants or animals. Natural products include alkaloids, such as atropine and morphine; peptides, such as glucagon; steroids, such as estradiol; hormones, such as insulin; glycosides, such as digitoxin; vitamins, such as riboflavin; polysaccharides, such as heparin; and antibiotics, such as penicillin.

5. The answer is B *[III B].*
The binding of a drug to its receptor usually involves only specific functional groups. These groups comprise what is known as the pharmacophore of the drug molecule. Although the entire drug molecule is present at the receptor site, only a portion of it, the pharmacophore, is required for a biological response.

6. The answer is A *[III B 3 a; Figure 12-4].*
The term enantiomer and the D and L indicate that the β-methacholine has a chiral center and exhibits optical isomerism. Because the optical isomers have different orientations in space, one orientation will give a better fit than the other and will most likely have greater biologic activity than the other. Dissolution, distribution, interatomic distances, and solubility are all related to the physical and chemical properties of the two compounds, which are identical because the compounds are enantiomers.

7. The answer is B *[Table 12-1; Figures 12-1 to 12-3].*
Key structural features of a thiazide, a benzothiadiazine ring with an electron withdrawing chloride atom and a sulfonyl group on the benzene ring, identify this compound as a thiazide.

8. The answer is D *[Table 12-1, Figure 12-2].*
The carboxylic acid identifies this compound as an acid. Other structural features identify it as a fenamate. Fenamates are NSAIDs (non-steroidal anti-inflammatory drugs), which can be used for inflammatory disorders (e.g., arthritis, bursitis). The mechanism of action of NSAIDs is inhibition of cyclooxygenase, which results in a decrease in the production of prostaglandins.

9. The answer is C *[Table 12-1].*
Fibrates decrease cholesterol and triglyceride levels. All of the other chemical classes can be used to treat hypertension. Aryloxypropylamines are β-blockers, thiazides are diuretics, dihydropyridines are calcium channel blockers, and ACE inhibitors decrease the synthesis of angiotensin II, a potent vasoconstrictor.

10. The answer is E *[II B 2 f–g; Table 12-1].*
Flurazepam (take note of the suffix which helps classify the compound) is a benzodiazepine and thus a basic compound. Because the pH is less than the pK_a, flurazepam is in an acidic environment and, therefore, exists primarily in the ionized form. The percent ionized can be easily calculated by using

the rule of nines. The lpH − pKal is 3, so the ratio is 99.9%:0.01% in favor of the ionized form.

11. The answer is E *[V; VI A 1, B].*
Phase I metabolites are often somewhat more polar than their parents. With the exception of acetylated and methylated metabolites, phase II metabolites are always much more polar than their parents. Thus, phase I metabolites are more likely to retain some liposolubility and are more likely to cross cellular membranes.

It is unusual for a single metabolite to be excreted for a given drug. Most drugs yield a mixture of metabolites. Because of the high polarity and subsequent high excretion of phase II metabolites, they are not likely to undergo further metabolism. Phase I metabolites, on the other hand, are less polar and are very likely to undergo further phase II metabolic reactions.

Whereas the major site of metabolism is the liver, there are many extrahepatic sites that secrete drug-metabolizing enzymes. Although many metabolites are less pharmacologically active than their parents, there are many drugs whose metabolites have equal or greater pharmacologic activity and sometimes greater toxicity as well. Prodrugs (i.e., drugs inactive in the form administered) always form at least one active metabolite.

12. The answer is C *[VI A 1 e, 3 a, B 2 a (2), c; Tables 12-2, 12-3, and 12-4].*
Because of the types of functional groups present, aspirin may undergo a number of different metabolic reactions. These include hydroxylation of the aromatic nucleus, conjugation of the carboxyl group with glycine, conjugation of the carboxyl group with glucuronic acid with the formation of an ester glucuronide, hydrolysis of the acetate ester, and conjugation of the phenol group (resulting from hydrolysis of the acetate ester) with glucuronic acid to form an ether glucuronide.

Because the acetate ester is a simple ester, aspirin is susceptible to hydrolysis in the acid media of the stomach before absorption takes place. In addition, any acetylated molecules that are absorbed are subjected to hydrolysis and are catalyzed by the many esterases present in the circulation. Any acetylated molecules not hydrolyzed in the circulation are subject to hydrolysis in the liver. All of these processes occur before the drug reaches the glomerular filtrate; therefore, excretion of the unchanged acetylated drug is highly unlikely.

13. The answer is A *[VI A 2; Table 12-3].*
Sulfasalazine has both anti-inflammatory and antibacterial activity when converted to aminosalicylic acid and sulfapyridine in the body. This reaction occurs by reductive cleavage of the "azo" linkage contained in the sulfasalazine molecule and is catalyzed in the intestine by bacterial azoreductase. This is a form of site-specific delivery because the intact drug is not absorbed from the stomach or upper intestine and reaches the colon, where it is metabolized. Sulfasalazine is one of a few drugs that is effective for the treatment of ulcerative colitis.

14. The answer is B *[VI B 2 a (2); VII G 1; Tables 12-2, 12-3, and 12-4].*
The chloramphenicol molecule contains an aromatic nucleus, which would be subject to hydroxylation, a nitro group that is subject to reduction, an amide group that is subject to liver hydrolysis, and alcohol groups that are subject to glucuronidation. Of all the enzyme systems responsible for these reactions, the system responsible for glucuronidation is developed poorly in premature infants and infants up to approximately 6–8 weeks of age.

15. The answer is D *[X A, B 1–4].*
By definition, prodrugs are inactive or very weakly active molecules that require in vivo activation to the parent molecule. Thus, conversion of a drug molecule to a prodrug does not increase potency because the original molecule, with whatever potency it contains, is produced after administration. A variety of advantages, including increased water solubility, duration of action, oral absorption, and palatability, can be obtained through the use of prodrugs, but none of these advantages results in an increase in potency of the parent molecule.

16. The answer is D (II, III) *[II A 1, 2].*
Generally, drugs must be lipophilic to pass through lipoprotein membranes and hydrophilic to be excreted by the kidney. Drugs do not have to be converted into an active form at their active site, although most drugs must be in their active form when they reach their active site. Many drugs are active in the form in which they are administered. Some drugs, usually referred to as prodrugs, are biotransformed into their active form after administration. Theoretically, drugs that reach their active site and then are metabolically activated should be more specific in their action and have fewer side effects. Currently, research efforts are underway to develop site-specific delivery systems and processes.

17. The answer is D (II, III) *[II B 2 c, 3 a, 4 a].*
Almost all salts (with very few exceptions) are strong electrolytes, and the terminology pentobarbital sodium and diphenhydramine hydrochloride indicate that both compounds are salts. Acetic acid is a weak acid; therefore, it is a weak electrolyte.

18. The answer is A (I) *[II B 3, 4].*
When meperidine hydrochloride solution is mixed with the alkaline solution of sodium bicarbonate, a neutralization reaction occurs with the possible precipitation of the water-insoluble free base meperidine. A neutralization reaction occurs when acidic solutions are mixed with basic solutions, or conversely. No reaction, in terms of acid–base, occurs when solutions are mixed with other acidic or neutral solutions or when basic solutions are mixed with other basic or neutral solutions. There should be no reaction, then, when the meperidine hydrochloride solution, which is acidic, is mixed with the acidic solution of atropine sulfate or the neutral solution of sodium chloride.

19. The answer is C (I, II) *[III B 3 d; IV C 1; IV E 1].*
Both sulfisoxazole and 5-fluorouracil compete with and antagonize isosteric normal biologic molecules and, therefore, are antimetabolites. Digoxin is a drug that is thought to inhibit $Na^{+}-K^{+}$—ATPase or to affect intracellular influx or use of calcium ion (Ca^{2+}). Because digoxin is steroidal, it is not isosteric with either an enzyme, which is a protein, or an ion; therefore, it is not classified as an antimetabolite.

20. The answer is A (I) *[II B 1, 2 e].*
A weakly acidic drug will be more ionized in an alkaline urine; therefore, it will be more polar and, thus, more soluble in the aqueous urine. It would also be less liposoluble, less likely to undergo tubular reabsorption, and thus be more likely to be excreted.

21–24. The answers are: 21-C (I, II), 22-B (III), 23-A (I), 24-B (III) *[II B 2, 3; Figure 12-1].*
The molecule contains a basic nitrogen, which is bonded to three carbon atoms (e.g., a tertiary amine), and an ethyl carboxylate, which is an ester group. An ester is the product of the reaction of an alcohol with a carboxylic acid that forms an alkyl carboxylate. There is no free carboxylic acid present. However, if this molecule is subjected to hydrolysis, it forms a carboxylic acid and ethyl alcohol.

Because meperidine contains a tertiary amine, it is classified as a base; because it is an organic base, it is considered weak. The nitrogen is not protonated. It is not ionic and, therefore, is not a salt.

Alkalinization of the urine decreases the ionization of meperidine, making it more liposoluble and, thus, more likely to undergo reabsorption in the kidney tubule. This results in a decreased rate of excretion and an increased duration of action. The six-member, nonaromatic ring is a piperidine ring which is substituted at the 4-position (nitrogen is position 1) with a phenyl ring. The compound does not contain either a piperazine ring or a propyl group.

25. The answer is D (II, III) *[VI A; Table 12-2].*
The reaction shown in the question involves the conversion of one functional group to another (amine to carbonyl); thus, it is classified as a phase I reaction. The introduction of oxygen into the molecule indicates oxidation, and the loss of the amino group signifies deamination; thus, the reaction also can be classified as oxidative deamination. *N*-Dealkylation implies the removal of an alkyl group from a nitrogen. The nitrogen in the parent molecule does not have an alkyl group attached to it.

26. The answer is C (I, II) *[VI A, B; Table 12-4].*
Phase II metabolic reactions involve masking an existing functional group with a natural endogenous constituent. The formulas shown in choices I and II represent this type of reaction, with choice I being an acetylation reaction and choice II, a glycine conjugation reaction. Choice III represents a change in an existing functional group and, thus, represents a phase I reaction. It is an oxidative deamination reaction.

27. The answer is C (I, II) *[VI B 2 a (4), VII E 1, 2; VIII B 3 b].*
Enterohepatic circulation refers to the process by which glucuronides, which are secreted into the intestine with the bile, are hydrolyzed by intestinal bacterial β-glucuronidase. The hydrolyzed free drug, which is no longer polar, becomes available for intestinal reabsorption into the system and subsequent penetration to its active site.

If an enzyme system becomes saturated, then the active drug cannot be inactivated by that pathway. If the drug cannot undergo an alternative pathway, the increased plasma levels of an unchanged active drug can result in increased activity or toxicity.

The first-pass effect results in metabolism of a drug by the liver before the drug reaches its site of action, resulting in an overall decrease in its activity. Drugs that undergo first-pass metabolism generally are effective in much smaller intravenous rather than oral doses.

28. The answer is A (I) *[VII F 1].*
Phase II metabolic reactions require natural endogenous substrates, which normally are supplied in the diet. A deficiency of these substances results in decreasing the biotransformation of drugs that use these pathways. Glycine conjugation is a phase II reaction. Glycine is an amino acid that requires dietary protein. A diet deficient in protein, therefore, could lead to a deficiency of glycine and, thus, a decrease in glycine conjugation. Glucuronidation is also a phase II reaction that requires endogenous glucuronic acid, but this substance is supplied by dietary carbohydrates. Hydroxylation is a phase I metabolic reaction and does not require dietary protein.

29–33. The answers are: 29-C, 30-B, 31-A, 32-D, 33-E *[III B 3 a–d].*
The first pair of molecules are isomers that have two asymmetric carbon atoms. They are not superimposable and are not mirror images; therefore, they are known as diastereomers.

The second pair of molecules are isomers that have one asymmetric carbon atom. They are nonsuperimposable mirror images; therefore, they are enantiomers.

The third pair of molecules have different spatial arrangements; however, these molecules do not have an asymmetric center. The presence of the double bond, which restricts the rotation of the groups on each carbon atom involved in the double bond, characterizes this type of isomerism as geometric.

The fourth pair of molecules are neither isomers nor the same compound because one contains three oxygens, whereas the other contains two oxygens and a sulfur. Because oxygen and sulfur are in the same periodic family, they are isosteric and are known as bioisosteres.

The final pair of structures are actually two views of the same compound. Rotation about the side chain single bonds connecting the ring nitrogen to the tertiary nitrogen produces these two different conformations. Thus, these are conformational isomers.

34–37. The answers are: 34-B *[VI B 2 a (2)],* **35-E,** *[VI A 3 a],* **36-A** *[VI B 2 a (2)],* **37-D** *[VI A 1 e].*
A common metabolic pathway of carboxylic acids is conjugation with the endogenous substrate, glucuronic acid, with the net equation involving the splitting out of a molecule of water by combining the hydrogen of the carboxyl group with the anomer OH of glucuronic acid. This is essentially a reaction of an acid and an alcohol, which results in the formation of an ester linkage. Carboxylic acids also undergo glycine or glutamine conjugation, which results in the formation of an amide linkage. Theoretically, it is also possible for benzoic acid to undergo ring hydroxylation, which is a common phase I pathway for aromatic nuclei.

Procaine is an ester-type local anesthetic. It is a simple ester and, therefore, very susceptible to hydrolysis in the body, due to the wide distribution of esterase enzymes and body water. This susceptibility to hydrolysis is the major reason why local anesthetics of this type have short durations of action when compared to other types of local anesthetics.

One of the principal functional groups in acetaminophen is the phenol, which commonly undergoes glucuronidation. The net result of the reaction is the splitting out of a molecule of water from the loss of the hydrogen atom of the phenol and the hydroxyl group of glucuronic acid, forming an ether linkage. Phenols also commonly undergo sulfate conjugation reactions and occasionally undergo *O*-methylation reactions. They can also undergo ring hydroxylation, due to the aromatic nucleus.

The principal functional group in amphetamine is a primary amine. Amines have a very low in vivo stability. Primary amines commonly undergo phase I oxidative deamination and phase II acetylation reactions.

13
Pharmacodynamics

Nelson S. Yee
Leon Shargel

I. INTRODUCTION. Pharmacodynamics is a branch of pharmacology that focuses on the study of the biochemical and physiological effects of drugs and the mechanisms by which they produce such effects. Analysis of drug action provides the basis for rational design of therapeutic agents and also provides insight into the regulation of cellular functions.

II. EFFECTS OF DRUGS

A. Perturbation of normal physiological processes. The actions of drugs are the consequences of the dynamic interactions between drug molecules and cellular components. Such interactions lead to alteration in the functions of these components, called **receptors**. The resulting biochemical and physiological changes form the basis of the cellular response to the drug. Drugs act by modulating the ongoing processes inside the cells.

B. Agonists and Antagonists

1. Potentially, any macromolecular component may act as a **drug receptor**.
2. Certain drug receptors normally serve as receptors for endogenous ligands and, thus, are **physiological receptors.** For example, adrenergic receptors are physiological receptors for catecholamines.
3. Drugs whose responses resemble the effects of the endogenous molecules are receptor **agonists**. For example, bethanechol directly stimulates cholinergic receptors, and it is thus an agonist.
4. **Pharmacologic antagonists** are drugs that lack **intrinsic activity** and produce effects by **competitively** or **noncompetitively** inhibiting the action of the endogenous molecules at the receptor.
   a. **Competitive antagonists** produce effects by competitively inhibiting the action of the endogenous molecules at the receptor. For example, propranolol competes with catecholamines for binding with adrenergic β-receptors.
   b. **Noncompetitive antagonists** produce effects by noncompetitive inhibition of the action of the endogenous molecules at the receptor. For example, **monamine oxidase (MAO)** inhibitors such as tranycylpromine (Parnate) initially interact with MAO in a reversible manner but then form covalent adducts that irreversibly inhibit MAO.
5. **Partial antagonists** inhibit the endogenous ligand from binding the receptor but possess some intrinsic activity. Nalorphine is a partial antagonist for the opiate receptor.
6. **Physiological antagonism** occurs when the drugs act independently at different receptor sites, often yielding opposing actions. For example, epinephrine and acetylcholine act on the sympathetic and parasympathetic autonomic nervous system respectively, and their effects are antagonistic to each other.
7. **Neutralizing antagonism** occurs when two drugs bind with each other to form an inactive compound. For example, digoxin-binding antibody used in digoxin overdose acts by sequestering the drug, resulting in the formation of an inactive complex.

III. MECHANISMS OF DRUG ACTION

A. Cell surface receptors

1. Receptors can be **proteins, glycoproteins,** or **nucleic acids.** Receptors can be located at the cell surface, within the cytoplasm, or inside the nucleus.
2. The binding of drugs to receptors is highly specific and can involve a variety of interactions, including hydrophobic interactions, van der Waals forces with ionic, hydrogen, and covalent bonds. The type of interaction and the binding affinity can influence the duration and reversibility of the drug action.
3. The interaction and binding affinity are related to the chemical structure of both the drug and ligand. Chemical modification of the structure of the drug molecule can change the pharmacologic and pharmacokinetic properties of drugs.
4. Through structure–activity relationship studies, synthetic drug analogs can be developed to achieve a high selectivity of drug action, a desirable ratio of therapeutic to toxic effect with better tolerated side effect profile.

B. Signal transduction by cell-surface receptors

1. Cell surface receptors are composed of extracellular domains that bind the ligands (drugs or physiological molecules).
2. The ligand binding serves as a triggering signal that can be propagated in the target cell through intracellular regulatory molecules, known as **second messengers** or **effectors.** For example, isoproterenol binds with the β-adrenergic receptor, which is functionally coupled to adenylate cyclase via the stimulatory G protein G_s. As a result, adenylate cyclase is activated and the cyclic adenosine monophosphate (cAMP) level increases.
3. Ligand binding of receptors often leads to interaction of the receptors with the cytoplasmic effectors, which in turn become activated. Integration of the multiple signal transducing events along the receptor–effector system might change the cellular phenotype or gene expression, leading to new protein synthesis.

C. Signaling mediated by intracellular receptors. Thyroid hormone, steroid hormones, vitamin D, and the retinoids act through binding cytoplasmic receptors, which translocate into the nucleus. These receptors are soluble, DNA-binding proteins that regulate the transcription of specific genes.

D. Target cell desensitization and hypersensitization

1. Cells have the ability to **respond** to endogenous regulatory molecules or exogenously added drugs over a wide range of concentrations. However, protective mechanisms are available for maintaining homeostatic control to prevent overstimulation or understimulation of the target cells.
2. Cell **regulation** can occur at different levels along the signal transduction pathway. Regulation can involve changes in the level of the receptors or alterations in the downstream effector molecules.
3. The expression of receptors is normally under homeostatic control through receptor internalization, recycling, and *de novo* synthesis.
4. **Down-regulation and desensitization**
   a. **Down-regulation** of receptors is caused by continuous prolonged exposure of receptors to drugs that disrupt the homeostatic equilibrium and result in altered levels of the receptors. This disruption involves endocytosis of ligand-bound receptors, resulting in sequestration of receptors from the cell surface and possibly accelerated degradation of the receptors, or inactivation of the receptors.
   b. **Desensitization** is the result of down-regulation. The target cells become desensitized and the effect of subsequent exposure to the same concentration of the drug is reduced. Therefore, an increased concentration of the drug is required to produce an effect of the same magnitude as the initial exposure with a smaller drug concentration.
   c. Repeated doses of bronchodilator such as albuterol inhaler for the treatment of asthma can lead to down-regulation of β-adrenergic receptors in the bronchial cells. The patient develops tolerance and requires increased dosage of the drug to achieve relief of the initial extent. In this case, the target cells become desensitized only to ligands that bind to those receptors; this is called **homologous desensitization.**

5. **Heterologous desensitization.** Some forms of desensitization involve alteration of components in the signaling pathway, such as a G protein. When cultured fibroblasts are exposed to prostaglandin (PGE_1), which normally activates adenylate cyclase through a G_s protein, the cells lose responsiveness not only to PGE_1 but also to other ligands binding to other receptors that act through the G_s-adenylate cyclase pathway.
6. **Hyperreactivity** or **supersensitivity** to receptor agonists is expected when target cells are subject to long-term exposure to receptor antagonists followed by abrupt cessation of administration of the drug. This can involve receptor up-regulation through synthesis of new receptors.

E. **Pharmacologic effects not mediated by receptors.** The effects of some drugs do not involve binding with specific receptors because of interaction with molecules or ions, which are not typically defined as receptors.

1. **Colligative** drug effects are characterized by a lack of requirement for highly specific chemical structure.
   a. Volatile general **anesthetic** agents with diverse structures are lipophilic and interact with the lipid bilayer of cell membranes, resulting in depressed excitability.
   b. **Cathartics,** such as magnesium sulfate and sorbitol, act by increasing the osmolarity of intestinal fluids and, thus, changing the distribution of water.
2. Methotrexate, cytarabine, and 5-fluorouracil are examples of **antimetabolites.** Antimetabolites are structural analogs of endogenous molecules and are incorporated into cellular components that interfere with the normal cellular functions.
3. Certain drugs interact with specific ions normally found in body fluids. For example, **antacids** such as aluminum hydroxide, calcium carbonate and magnesium hydroxide act by neutralizing gastric acid.

IV. RELATIONSHIP BETWEEN DRUG CONCENTRATION AND EFFECT

A. **Dose-response relationship.** In general, the larger the drug dose, the higher the drug concentration at its site of action and the greater the effect of the drug, up to a maximum effect. Higher drug concentrations (or doses) will not produce an effect greater than the maximum effect.

B. A **quantal dose-response curve** describes the relationship between the number of patients exhibiting a defined response (e.g., a 50% increase in peak flow) produced by a specified dose of a drug (e.g., minimum doses of albuterol for 50% increase in peak flow). This relationship often follows a gaussian (bell-shaped) distribution (Figures 13-1 and 13-2).

C. A **graded dose-response curve** describes the relationship between the magnitude of the effect of a drug (e.g., reduction of blood pressure by nifedipine) in an individual and the doses of the drug (Figure 13-3).

1. Generally, as the dose of a drug increases, the effect produced will reach a maximum level.
2. Graded dose-response curves for different drugs allow comparison of their efficacies and potencies.

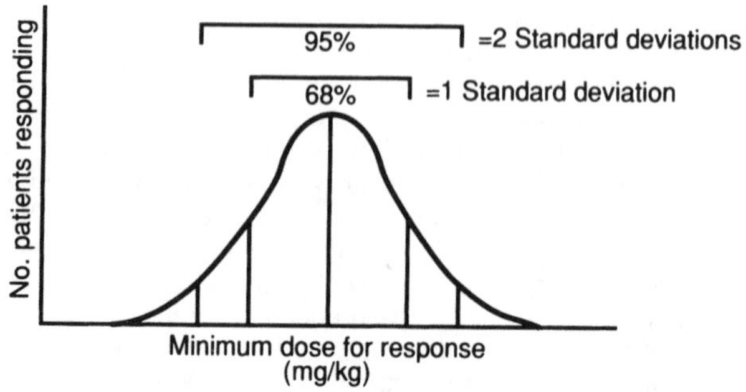

Figure 13-1. Frequency distribution curve, plotting the number of patients showing a quantal response to a drug against the minimum dose needed to produce the response.

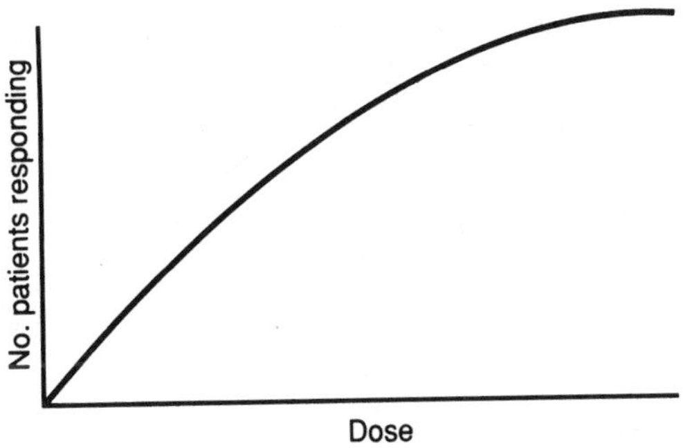

Figure 13-2. Quantal dose-response curve, cumulating the data used in plotting Figure 13-1.

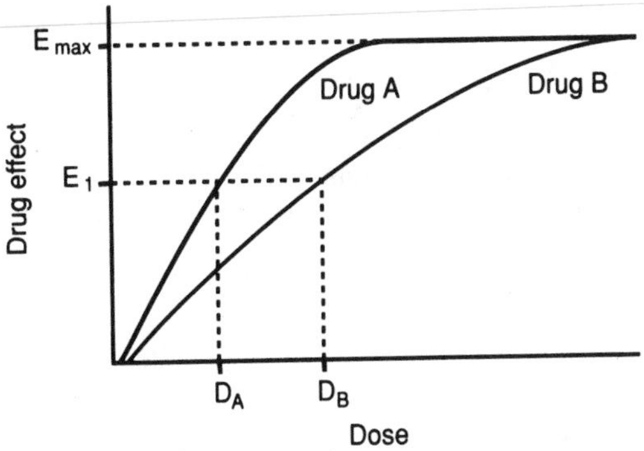

Figure 13-3. Graded dose-response curves for two drugs, A and B. E_{max} = maximum effect; D_A and D_B = amount (dose) of drug A and drug B, respectively, needed to produce the drug effect, E_1.

a. **Efficacy** of a drug is measured by its maximum effect.
b. **Potency** of a drug is a relative measure that compares the different doses (molar doses) of different drugs needed to produce the same effect. From a clinical viewpoint, potency is considered in drug selection (e.g., triazolam is preferred for the treatment of insomnia instead of diazepam).
c. In **selecting** drugs in clinical situations, a drug with greater efficacy might be needed to achieve the therapeutic outcome (e.g., hydromorphone is preferred to acetaminophen for controlling bone pain in a patient with metastatic breast cancer).

D. A **log dose-response curve** describes the relationship between the drug effect and the log of the dose. This curve facilitates comparison of potency and efficacy among different drugs with the same mechanism of action (and thus they have the same slopes) [Figure 13-4].

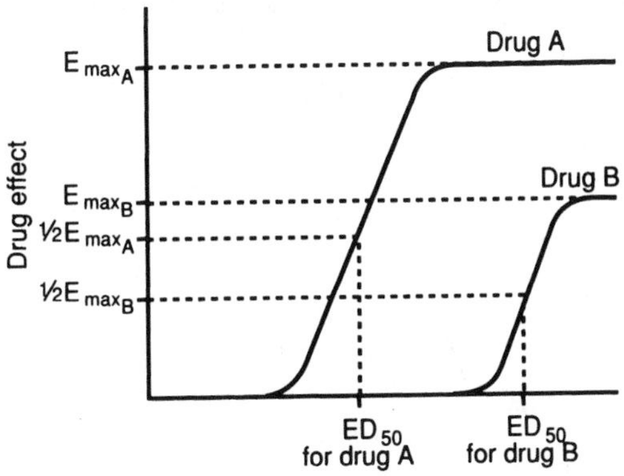

Figure 13-4. Log dose-response curves for two drugs, A and B. E_{max} = maximum effect; ED_{50} = smallest dose showing an effect that is 50% of the E_{max}.

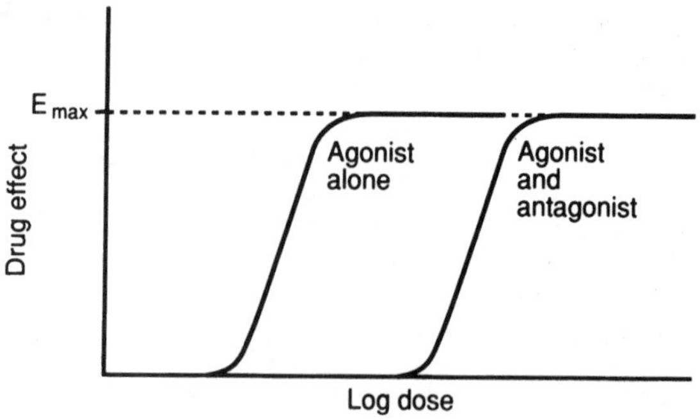

Figure 13-5. Shift in the log dose-response curve that occurs when an agonist is administered in the presence of a competitive antagonist.

1. The **efficacy** of a drug is determined by the **height** of its log dose-response curve (**E_{max}**); the higher the curve, the greater the E_{max} and efficacy.
2. The **potency** of two drugs can be compared by determining their **ED_{50}**. The ED_{50} is the **dose** of each drug producing 50% of the corresponding maximum effect (50% of E_{max}). The smaller the ED_{50}, the greater the potency.
3. A **competitive antagonist** shifts the log-dose response curve to the **right** and the shift is **parallel.** A greater concentration of the agonist is required to produce the same response than when the competitive antagonist is absent. Even in the presence of the antagonist, the **same E_{max}** can be achieved if enough agonist is added (Figure 13-5).
4. A **noncompetitive antagonist** binds to the same receptor or binds to another site that prevents the agonist from producing a response. The shift of the log dose-response curve is to the **right** and **nonparallel**, resulting in a **lower E_{max}**. The action of the antagonist cannot be overcome even if more agonist is present (Figure 13-6).

V. ENHANCEMENT OF DRUG EFFECTS

A. Addition occurs when two different drugs with the same effect are given together, resulting in a drug effect that is equal in magnitude to the sum of the individual effects of the two drugs. For example, trimethoprim and sulfamethoxazole inhibit different steps in the synthesis of folic acid, resulting in suppressing bacterial growth.

B. Synergism occurs when two drugs with the same effect are given together, producing a drug effect that is greater in magnitude than the sum of the individual effects of the two drugs. For example, penicillin and gentamycin are synergistic in their anti-pseudomonal activities.

C. Potentiation occurs when one drug, lacking an effect of its own, increases the effect of another drug that is active. For example, carbidopa is an inactive analog of dopa. When carbidopa

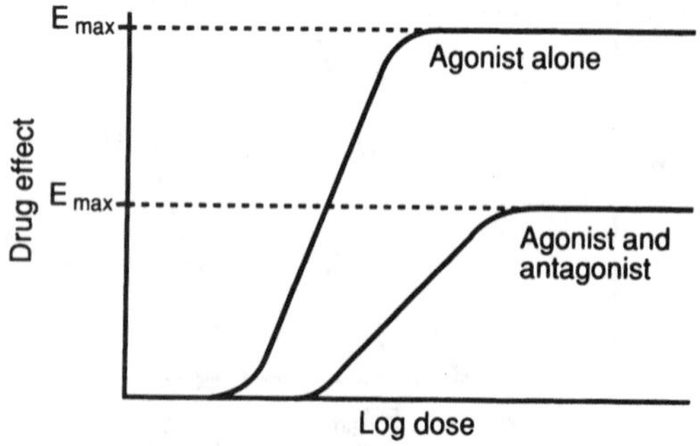

Figure 13-6. Shift in the log dose-response curve and lowering of the maximum effect (E_{max}) that occur when an agonist is given in the presence of a noncompetitive antagonist.

blocks the degradation of dopa and is given with dopa, it prolongs the half-life of dopa and the duration of the anti-Parkinsonian effect.

VI. SELECTIVITY OF DRUG ACTION

A. The **therapeutic index** and the **margin of safety** are the relationship (ratio) between the dose of a drug required to produce undesired effects (toxic or lethal) and the dose required to produce the desired effects (therapeutic).

1. The **therapeutic index** of a drug is a relative measure of the safety and effectiveness in laboratory studies.
2. The **therapeutic index** is the ratio of the minimum dose that is toxic for 50% of the population (**TD_{50}** or **median toxic dose**) to the minimum dose that is effective for 50% of the population (**ED_{50}** or **median effective dose**).

B. In general, the greater the TD_{50} or the smaller the ED_{50}, the greater the therapeutic index, and thus the safer the drug when used at the effective dosage.

C. The **margin of safety** is a more practical term to describe the relative safety and effectiveness of a drug. The margin of safety is the ratio of the minimum toxic dose for 0.1% of the population (**$TD_{0.1}$** or **minimal toxic dose**) to the minimum effective dose for 99.9% of the population (**$ED_{99.9}$** or **minimal effective dose**).

STUDY QUESTIONS

Directions: Each of the numbered items or incomplete statements in this section is followed by answers or by completions of the statement. Select the **one** lettered answer or completion that is **best** in each case.

1. A 40-year-old man complains of dysuria and urinary urgency and is diagnosed to have uncomplicated gonococcal urethritis. He is given procaine penicillin G intramuscularly. In addition, probenecid is given to prolong the duration of action of penicillin. This type of combined drug effect is known as

(A) synergism
(B) competitive antagonism
(C) addition
(D) potentiation
(E) noncompetitive antagonism

2. A 65-year-old woman with intractable pain secondary to bony metastasis of breast cancer had been receiving escalating doses of morphine sulfate intravenously. At 10 a.m., she was found to be unresponsive, her respiratory rate was 4 per minute, and her pupils were pin-pointed. Naloxone, a competitive antagonist of the opiate receptor, was given intravenously and then repeated once. She gradually became conscious and began to complain of pain unrelieved by morphine given at the previous dose. This is most likely because

(A) naloxone directly aggravates the pain due to the bony metastasis.
(B) naloxone reduces the E_{max} for morphine.
(C) naloxone reduces the ED_{50} for morphine.
(D) naloxone increases the E_{max} for morphine.
(E) naloxone increases the ED_{50} for morphine.

3. Which of the following statements regarding signal transduction is true?

(A) Thyroxine-bound receptors act on DNA and regulate specific transcription of genes
(B) Cyclic adenosine monophosphate can act as second messenger
(C) The level of drug receptors at the cell surface increases with chronic stimulation by receptor agonists
(D) Binding of ligand to cell-surface receptors can lead to synthesis of proteins
(E) Antacids act by interacting with small ions normally found in the gastrointestinal tract

4. A pharmacist is consulted regarding selecting a drug that is relatively safe and effective for treating the patient. He searches the literature and obtains the following data that may help guide his decision. The $TD_{0.1}$ and $ED_{99.9}$ for drug A are 20 mg and 0.4 mg respectively, whereas the $TD_{0.1}$ and $ED_{99.9}$ for drug B are 15 mg and 0.2 mg respectively. Which of the following statements is true?

(A) Drug A has a higher $TD_{0.1}$ and, thus, should be the drug of choice
(B) Both drugs have the same margin of safety, so more information is needed
(C) Drug B has a higher margin of safety and thus is preferred to drug A
(D) Drug A is preferred because it has a greater margin of safety than drug B
(E) The information obtained is irrelevant

5. Which of the following statements concerning a drug receptor is true?

(A) It mediates the nonspecific action of volatile anesthetics
(B) Its expression is induced only by exogenously added drugs
(C) It can bind endogenous ligand to produce physiological activity
(D) It mediates the cathartic activity of magnesium citrate
(E) Down-regulation of receptor level can lead to sensitization of the target cell to the receptor agonist

6. Which of the following statements concerning morphine and hydromorphone is true?

(A) Hydromorphone is a more effective analgesic because it has a smaller ED_{50} than morphine
(B) Morphine and hydromorphone are equally potent because they have the same E_{max}
(C) Morphine has a greater ED_{50} and is thus a less effective analgesic than hydromorphone
(D) Hydromorphone is a more potent analgesic because it has a greater E_{max} than morphine
(E) Hydromorphone has a smaller ED_{50} and is thus a more potent analgesic than morphine

7. A 72-year-old man with hypertension has been taking high-dose propranolol for 20 years. He left home for a week and forgot to bring his medication with him. One day he was found collapsed on the floor and then brought to the emergency room. His blood pressure was 300/180, heart rate 180 beats per minute, and retinal hemorrhage was observed. Which of the following best explains this situation?

(A) The β-adrenergic receptors in the cardiac muscles underwent spontaneous mutation and became hyperactive
(B) Reduction in the chronic antagonism of the β-adrenergic receptor led to down-regulation of the β-adrenergic receptor
(C) The propranolol that he had previously ingested remained in his body and acted as a receptor agonist
(D) Long-term administration of propranolol results in desensitization of cardiac muscles to endogenous β-adrenergic stimulation
(E) Reduction in the chronic level of receptor blockade results in supersensitivity to stimulation with endogenous catecholamines

ANSWERS AND EXPLANATIONS

1. The answer is D *[V C]*.
Probenecid alone is inactive against gonococci. However, it can compete with penicillin for urinary excretion. Thus, probenecid can reduce the elimination rate of penicillin whose duration of action becomes prolonged. Therefore, probenecid potentiates the activity of penicillin when the two are given together.

2. The answer is E *[IV D 3]*.
Naloxone is a competitive antagonist of opiate receptor. If one compares the log dose-response curve seen with both morphine and naloxone to that seen with morphine alone, the morphine-naloxone curve would be shifted to the right of the morphine curve. As a result, the ED_{50} for morphine is increased. This means that a larger than previous dose of morphine is required for achieving the same analgesic effect.

3. The answer is C *[III D 4]*.
The level of drug receptors at the cell surface usually decreases when the target cells are chronically stimulated by receptor agonists. Down-regulation of receptors is a protective mechanism that can prevent the target cells from being over-stimulated.

4. The answer is C *[VI C]*.
The margin of safety of the two drugs can be helpful in guiding selection of a drug. Margin of safety is the ratio of $TD_{0.1}$ to $ED_{99.9}$. Thus, the margin of safety for drug A is 20 mg / 0.4 mg, that is 50; whereas the margin of safety for drug B is 15 mg / 0.2 mg, that is 75. Because drug B has a greater margin of safety than drug A, drug B is relatively safe at the dosage given to produce the desired effect.

5. The answer is C *[II B 2, III D 4, III E 1 a, b]*.
A drug receptor, such as muscarinic cholinergic receptor that can bind atropine, normally binds endogenous acetylcholine to produce the physiological responses controlled by the parasympathetic autonomic nervous system. Volatile anesthetics act colligatively as solutes in the lipid bilayer of the cell membrane. Drug receptors are endogenously expressed, but their level can be modulated by exogenously added drugs. The cathartic activity of magnesium citrate is a consequence of increase in the osmolarity of the gastrointestinal fluids. Down-regulation of receptor level can lead to desensitization, not sensitization, of the target cell to the receptor agonist.

6. The answer is E *[IV D 1,2]*.

The efficacy of a drug is determined by its E_{max}, whereas its potency is measured by the ED_{50}. Hydromorphone has a smaller ED_{50} and, thus, is a more potent analgesic than morphine. Hydromorphone and morphine are both agonists for opiate receptors, and they have the same analgesic efficacy (that is, they have the E_{max}) if sufficient amounts of both drugs are used.

7. The answer is E *[III D 6]*.
Chronic level of blocking the β-adrenergic receptors by propranolol results in up-regulation of the receptor level. When the patient ceased taking the drug, the cardiac muscles became supersensitive to stimulation with endogenous catecholamines. This resulted in the hypertensive crisis that caused cerebral hemorrhage and loss of consciousness.

14 Drugs Affecting the Autonomic Nervous System and the Neuromuscular Junction

David C. Kosegarten
Edward F. LaSala

I. INTRODUCTION. Drugs affecting the **autonomic nervous system** and the **neuromuscular junction** mimic or modify the actions of neurohumoral transmitters. These drugs fall into five major categories: cholinergic agonists, cholinergic antagonists, adrenergic agonists, adrenergic antagonists, and neuromuscular blocking agents. Table 14-1 defines basic pharmacologic concepts.

Table 14-1. Basic Pharmacologic Concepts

Concept	Definition
Receptor	A specific cellular site that interacts with an endogenous substance or a drug molecule and mediates that compound's action. Receptors are located in or on the cell membranes or within the cell itself. They are affected by micromolar to nanomolar concentrations, demonstrate relative stereospecificity, and can be selectively blocked by antagonists.
Affinity	The ability of a chemical compound to combine with a specific receptor.
Efficacy	The ability of a compound to produce a physiologic/pharmacologic response. Also referred to as intrinsic activity.
Agonist	A compound that has both affinity for a receptor and efficacy upon occupation of that receptor. A drug that has affinity but little or low efficacy is considered a partial agonist (or partial antagonist).
Antagonist	A compound that has affinity for a receptor but lacks efficacy.
Pharmacologic antagonism	The process that occurs when an antagonist combines with a receptor, preventing or limiting an agonist's ability to produce a physiologic/pharmacologic effect through that receptor.
Physiologic antagonism	The process that occurs when separate compounds act independently on two different receptors or physiologic systems to produce opposing effects. For example, a drug that mimics the activity of the parasympathetic system may be antagonized by a drug that mimics the activity of the sympathetic system.
Potency	The ability of a compound to produce an effect relative to its concentration. The more potent a drug is, the less concentration (dose) required to produce a maximal effect.
Potentiation	The process that occurs when administration of a second drug increases the effectiveness of a first drug that is minimally effective or ineffective when given alone.
Additivity	The process that occurs when co-administration of two drugs causes a therapeutic effect equal to the sum of effects obtained by administration of either drug individually.
Synergism	The process that occurs when co-administration of two drugs causes a therapeutic effect that is greater than the sum of effects obtained by administration of either drug individually.
Therapeutic index (margin of safety)	The relationship between the dosage that produces an undesirable effect (death) and the dosage that produces a desirable (therapeutic) effect. Therapeutic index is defined as the ratio of median lethal dose to median effective dose. The greater the ratio of these dosages, the safer the drug and the higher its therapeutic index.
Tolerance	The phenomenon of decreased responsiveness to a drug following chronic administration.

(Continued on next page)

Table 14-1. Continued

Concept	Definition
Tachyphylaxis	The rapid development of tolerance.
Anaphylaxis	An acute systemic reaction (commonly characterized by urticaria, respiratory distress, and vascular collapse) that occurs in a previously sensitized individual after exposure to the sensitizing antigen.
Anaphylactoid reaction	A dose-dependent, idiosyncratic reaction, clinically similar to anaphylaxis, that can occur after the first administration of certain drugs.

II. CHOLINERGIC AGONISTS

A. Chemistry

1. **Acetylcholine,** the natural endogenous mediator and the most potent cholinergic agonist, is an ester of acetic acid and choline, a quaternary amino alcohol (Figure 14-1). A hygroscopic simple ester, it is unstable and quickly hydrolyzed both in vitro and in vivo. Thus, it is extremely short-acting and usually is not a satisfactory therapeutic agent.

$$CH_3\overset{\overset{\displaystyle C}{\|}}{C}OCH_2CH_2\overset{+}{N}(CH_3)_3 \ Cl^-$$

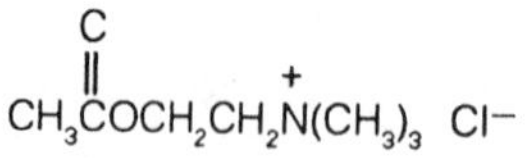

Figure 14-1. The structural formula of acetylcholine.

2. **Therapeutically useful cholinergic agonists** may be direct-acting or indirect-acting.
   a. **Direct-acting agonists** may be produced by replacing the acetyl group of acetylcholine with a carbamoyl group or by substituting a methyl group of the β-carbon. These actions decrease the drug's hydrolysis rate, providing such stable, useful agonists as methacholine chloride (Provocholine) and bethanechol chloride (Urecholine) (Figure 14-2).
   b. **Indirect-acting agonists** (e.g., acetylcholinesterase inhibitors) are divided into two major classes.
      (1) **Reversible (short-acting) agents** are principally carbamic esters, such as physostigmine (Eserine) and neostigmine (Prostigmin) (Figure 14-3).
      (2) **Irreversible (long-acting) agents** are principally organophosphate esters, such as isoflurophate and echothiophate (Phospholine) (Figure 14-4).

B. Pharmacology

1. **Cholinergic responses** are mediated by both muscarinic and nicotinic receptors.
   a. **Muscarinic receptors** are present at parasympathetic postganglionic neuroeffector cell sites (Table 14-2).

$$CH_3\overset{\overset{\displaystyle O}{\|}}{C}OCH_2\underset{\underset{\displaystyle CH_3}{|}}{C}H\overset{+}{N}(CH_3)_3 \ Cl^-$$

A

$$NH_2\overset{\overset{\displaystyle O}{\|}}{C}OCH_2\underset{\underset{\displaystyle CH_3}{|}}{C}H\overset{+}{N}(CH_3)_3 \ Cl^-$$

B

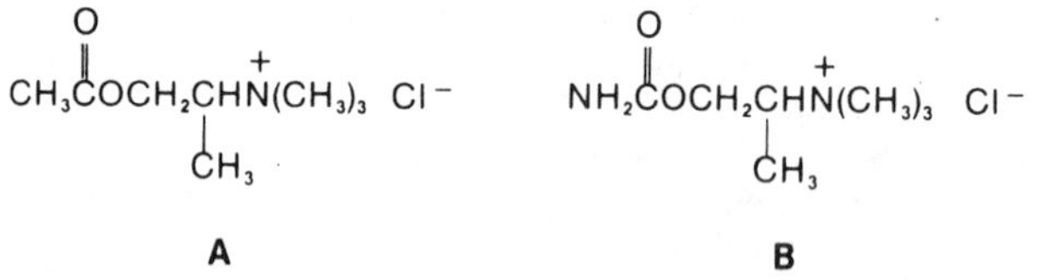

Figure 14-2. Clinically useful direct-acting cholinergic agonists include *(A)* methacholine chloride (Provocholine) and *(B)* bethanechol chloride (Urecholine).

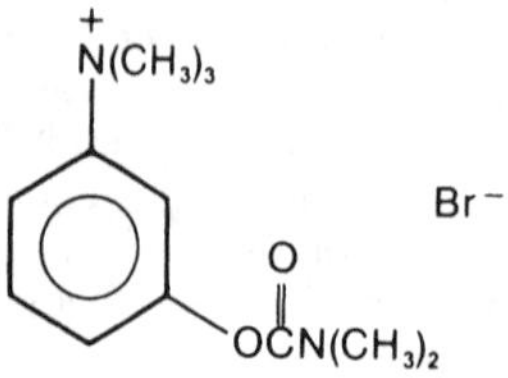

Figure 14-3. The structural formula of neostigmine bromide (Prostigmin), a reversible acetylcholinesterase inhibitor.

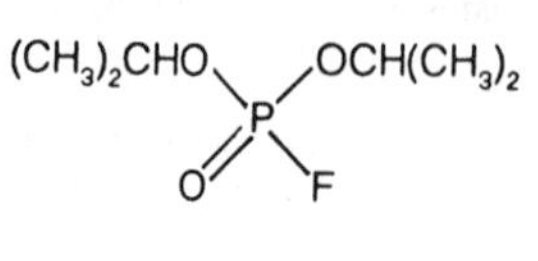

Figure 14-4. The structural formula of isoflurophate (Floropryl), an irreversible acetylcholinesterase inhibitor.

Table 14-2. Muscarinic Receptor-Mediated Responses to Cholinergic Agonists

Organ	Response
Heart	Decreases conduction velocity Decreases contraction force Decreases contraction rate
Eye	Contracts the iris sphincter muscle and the ciliary muscle, producing miosis
Lung	Contracts tracheal and bronchial muscles
Intestine	Increases peristalsis Increases secretions Relaxes sphincter
Urinary bladder	Relaxes trigone and sphincter muscles Contracts detrusor muscle

b. **Nicotinic receptors** are present at the ganglia of both the parasympathetic and sympathetic nervous systems and also at the neuromuscular junctions of the somatic nervous system (see VI A 1).

2. **Cholinergic agonists act by mimicking the activity of endogenous acetylcholine** at muscarinic and nicotinic receptor sites.
   a. **Direct-acting agonists** interact directly with these receptors.
   b. **Indirect-acting agonists** inhibit or block the activity of cholinesterase enzymes (e.g., acetylcholinesterase, pseudocholinesterase), which metabolize endogenous acetylcholine to inactive metabolites. Thus, these agonists allow endogenous acetylcholine to accumulate at cholinergic receptors, producing cholinergic stimulation. Organophosphate cholinesterase inhibitors (e.g., certain agricultural insecticides and so-called nerve gases) bind to the enzyme to form a long-lasting enzyme inhibitor complex and may be extremely toxic.

C. Therapeutic indications

1. **Direct-acting agonists** are indicated to:
   a. Initiate micturition in acute nonobstructive urinary retention (e.g., bethanechol)
   b. Produce miosis in the treatment of glaucoma (e.g., pilocarpine)

2. **Indirect-acting agonists** are indicated to:
   a. Produce miosis in the treatment of glaucoma (e.g., physostigmine, isoflurophate, echothiophate)
   b. Treat myasthenia gravis (e.g., ambenonium, neostigmine, pyridostigmine)
   c. Aid in the differential diagnosis of myasthenia gravis and cholinergic crisis (e.g., edrophonium)
   d. Counteract intoxication or adverse effects from compounds with anticholinergic activity (e.g., physostigmine)

D. Adverse effects

1. **Topical adverse effects** include congested conjunctivae, myopic accommodation, and transient lenticular opacity.

2. **Systemic adverse effects** include headache, syncope, nausea, vomiting, bradycardia, hypotension, bronchospasm, abdominal cramps, diarrhea, epigastric distress, salivation, sweating, lacrimation, flushing, and tremors.

III. CHOLINERGIC ANTAGONISTS

A. Chemistry

1. **Atropine,** an alkaloid obtained from the belladonna plant, is the prototypical cholinergic antagonist (anticholinergic agent). A portion of the atropine molecule is structurally similar to

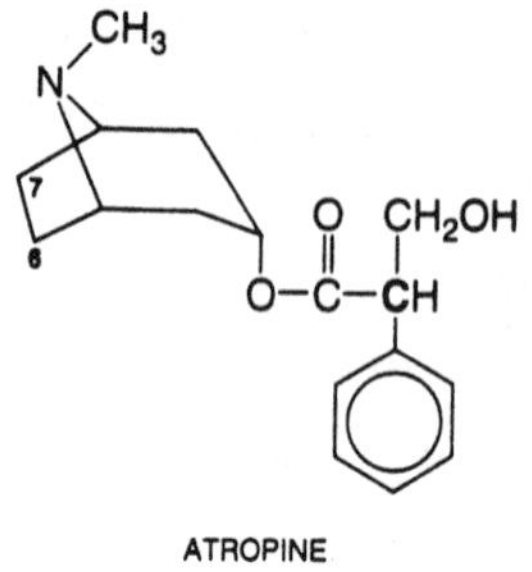

Figure 14-5. Structural formula of atropine, a cholinergic antagonist.

acetylcholine (Figure 14-5), permitting the molecule to bind to postganglionic receptors. However, the molecule has no intrinsic activity, and its bulky shape prevents acetylcholine from binding to the receptor.

2. **Synthetic anticholinergic agents** [e.g., dicyclomine (Bentyl), glycopyrrolate (Robinul), propantheline] are also available. These agents, like atropine, are bulky analogues of acetylcholine (Figure 14-6).

B. Pharmacology

1. Cholinergic antagonists **competitively inhibit** the activity of endogenous acetylcholine.
2. Antagonists that inhibit muscarinic receptor-mediated responses are called **antimuscarinic agents;** those that inhibit nicotinic receptor-mediated responses at the ganglia are called **ganglionic blocking agents,** whereas those that inhibit nicotinic receptor-mediated responses at the neuromuscular junction are called **neuromuscular blockers** (see III C).

C. Therapeutic indications

1. **Antimuscarinic agents** are indicated to:
   a. Reduce glandular and bronchiolar secretions before anesthesia (e.g., atropine, glycopyrrolate)
   b. Induce sedation (e.g., scopolamine)
   c. Alleviate motion sickness (e.g., scopolamine)
   d. Reduce vagal stimulation of the myocardium (e.g., atropine)
   e. Produce ophthalmic mydriasis and cycloplegia (e.g., homatropine)
   f. Reduce gastrointestinal (GI) smooth muscle spasms (e.g., propantheline)
   g. Treat bronchospasm associated with chronic obstructive pulmonary disease (e.g., ipratropium)
   h. Control Parkinson's disease and some neuroleptic-induced extrapyramidal disorders (e.g., benztropine, trihexyphenidyl)
   I. Treat intoxication by cholinergic agonists or by the rapid form of mushroom poisoning (e.g., atropine)
2. **Ganglionic blocking agents** are indicated to treat hypertensive crisis (e.g., trimethaphan, mecamylamine).

D. Adverse effects

1. **Topical adverse effects** include hyperopic accommodation and increased intraocular pressure.

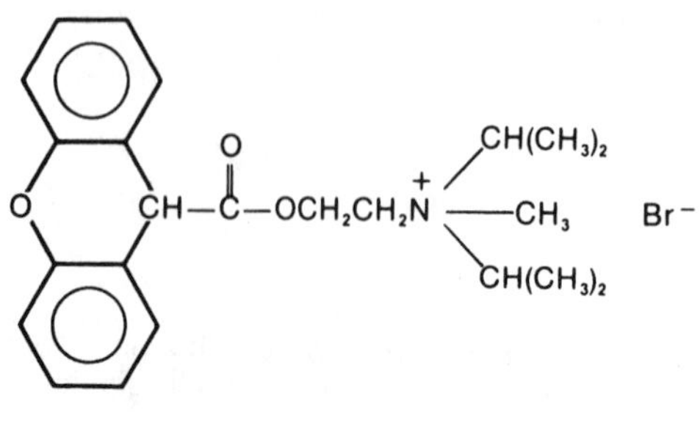

Figure 14-6. Structural formula of propantheline bromide (Pro-Banthine), a synthetic cholinergic antagonist.

2. **Systemic adverse effects** include headache, nervousness, drowsiness, dizziness, palpitations, tachycardia, dry mouth, mydriasis, blurred vision, nausea, vomiting, constipation, urinary retention, and fever.

IV. ADRENERGIC AGONISTS

A. Chemistry

1. **Direct-acting adrenergic agonists** include norepinephrine and epinephrine (naturally occurring catecholamines) as well as their derivatives. Catecholamines are biosynthesized from tyrosine, an amino acid (Figure 14-7). Examples of direct-acting adrenergic agonists include naphazoline, terbutaline, and dobutamine, which is also an indirect-acting agonist (Figure 14-8).
   a. The ethyl amine chain common to these agonists is essential to their activity.
   b. N-substituents alter drug activity. Small substituents (e.g., hydrogen, a methyl group) produce α-receptor activity, as with norepinephrine; larger substituents (e.g., an isopropyl group) produce β-receptor activity, as with isoproterenol.
   c. Removal of the **para (4) hydroxyl group** leaves only α-receptor activity, as with phenylephrine.
   d. The **meta (3) hydroxyl group** is essential for direct α- and β-activity. However, drugs in which the meta hydroxyl is replaced by a sulfonamide or a hydroxymethyl group retain activity.

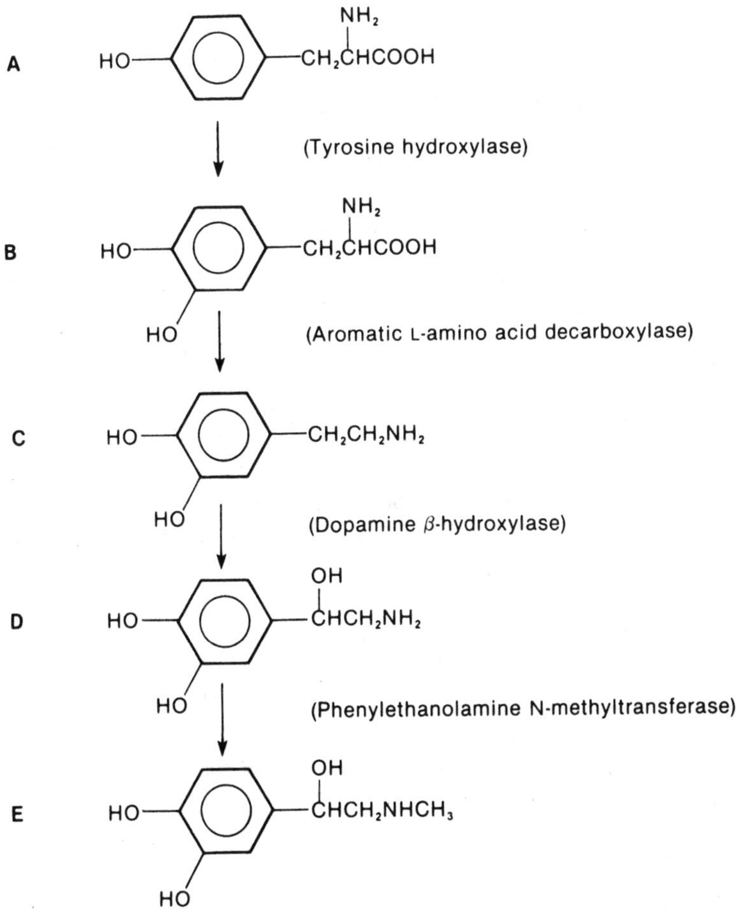

Figure 14-7. Synthesis of catecholamines from the amino acid tyrosine. In the presence of tyrosine hydroxylase, *(A)* tyrosine is converted to *(B)* dihydroxyphenylalanine (dopa). Further substitutions permit the synthesis of *(C)* dopamine, *(D)* norepinephrine, and *(E)* epinephrine.

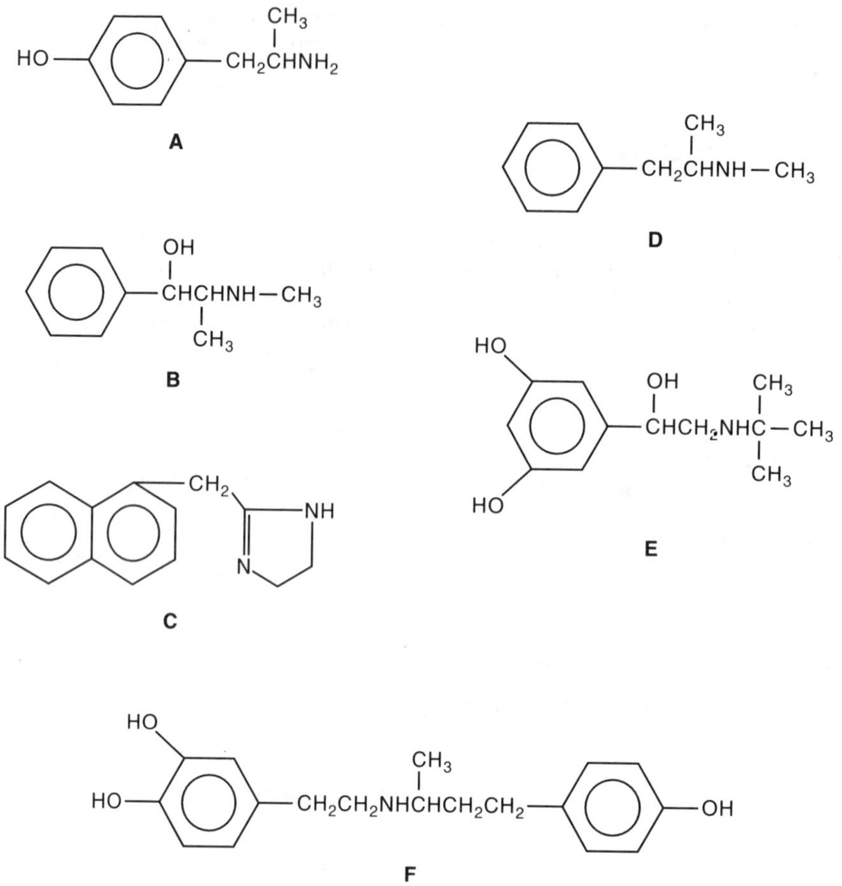

Figure 14-8. Structural formula of representative sympathomimetic amines. *(A)* Hydroxyamphetamine (Paredrine); *(B)* ephedrine or pseudoephedrine (Sudafed); *(C)* naphazoline (Privine); *(D)* methamphetamine (Methedrine); *(E)* terbutaline (Brethine); *(F)* dobutamine (Dobutrex).

e. The catecholamines are inactivated by methylation of the meta hydroxyl group (catalyzed by catechol O-methyltransferase) and by oxidative deamination [catalyzed by monoamine oxidase (MAO)].

2. Indirect-acting agonists (sympathomimetic amines) are compounds that are chemically related to the catecholamines and have similar effects. These are primarily synthetic compounds; examples include hydroxyamphetamine, ephedrine, methamphetamine, and dobutamine (see Figure 14-8).

a. Sympathomimetic amines may have one, two, or no hydroxyl groups. The fewer hydroxyl groups, the less intestinal destruction and the greater the drug's lipophilic character; thus, the greater the absorption and the duration of activity after oral administration.

b. The benzene ring of these drugs may be replaced by cyclohexyl, naphthalene, or other rings or by aliphatic chains.

c. Alkyl substitution at the α-carbon (adjacent to the amino group) retards destruction of phenol and phenyl compounds and increases lipophilic character, contributing to prolonged activity.

d. N-substituents with bulky groups increase β-receptor activity, as with direct-acting agents.

B. Pharmacology

1. Adrenergic peripheral responses are mediated by both α- and β-receptors (Table 14-3).

a. α-Receptors fall into two groups.

Table 14-3. Adrenergic Receptor-Mediated Responses to Adrenergic Agonists

Organ/Tissue	Receptor Type	Response
Heart	β_1	Increases conduction velocity
	β_1	Increases contraction force
	β_1	Increases contraction rate
Arterioles	α_1	Constricts cerebral arterioles
	α_1	Constricts cutaneous arterioles
	α_1	Constricts visceral arterioles
	β_2	Dilates skeletal muscle arterioles
Eye	α_1	Contracts iris sphincter muscle, producing mydriasis
Lung	β_2	Relaxes tracheal and bronchial muscles
Intestine	α, β	Decreases peristalsis
	α_1	Contracts sphincter
Urinary bladder	α_1	Contracts trigone and sphincter muscles
	β_1	Relaxes detrusor muscle
Uterus	α_1	Excites uterine contractions
	β_2	Inhibits uterine contractions
Adipose tissue	β_1	Mobilizes fatty acids

(1) **Postjunctional α_1-adrenergic receptors** are found in the radial smooth muscle of the iris; in the arteries, arterioles, and veins; in the splenic capsule; and in the GI tract. Drugs that are **α_1-selective agonists** include phenylephrine and methoxamine.

(2) **Prejunctional α_2-adrenergic receptors** mediate the inhibition of release of adrenergic neurotransmitter. Drugs that are **α_2-selective agonists** include α-methylnorepinephrine and clonidine.

b. **β-Receptors** also fall into two groups.

(1) **Postjunctional β_1-adrenergic receptors** are found in the myocardium, the intestinal smooth muscle, and adipose tissue. Drugs that are **β_1-selective agonists** include dobutamine.

(2) **Postjunctional β_2-adrenergic receptors** are found in bronchiolar and vascular smooth muscle. Drugs that are **β_2-selective agonists** include terbutaline.

2. **Direct-acting adrenergic agonists** (e.g., phenylephrine, clonidine, dobutamine, terbutaline) produce their effects primarily by direct stimulation of adrenergic receptors. They may be receptor-selective, as with the drugs listed above, or they may be nonselective. For example, the adrenergic neurotransmitter norepinephrine affects α_1-, α_2-, and β_1-receptors, whereas the adrenal medullary hormone epinephrine affects α_1-, α_2-, β_1-, and β_2-receptors. Isoproterenol affects both β_1- and β_2-receptors.

3. **Indirect-acting adrenergic agonists** work through other routes. For example, tyramine acts by releasing norepinephrine from storage sites in adrenergic neurons.

4. Certain agonists (e.g., ephedrine, dopamine, metaraminol, mephentermine) produce their effects through both direct and indirect mechanisms.

C. Therapeutic indications

1. **Epinephrine** (an α- and β-adrenergic agonist) is indicated to treat bronchospasm and hypersensitivity reactions and is the agent of choice for anaphylactic reactions. It is also used to prolong the activity of local anesthetic solutions and to restore cardiac activity in cardiac arrest. Epinephrine is also used topically in the treatment of glaucoma, presumably decreasing intraocular pressure through enhanced outflow of aqueous humor and vasoconstriction-induced decreases in production of aqueous humor.

2. **Phenylephrine** (an α_1-selective agonist) is used to provide pressor activity, to prolong the activity of local anesthetic solutions, and to relieve paroxysmal atrial tachycardia.

3. **Clonidine and related α_2**-selective agonists (methyldopa, guanfacine, guanabenz) are used as antihypertensives, via inhibition of central sympathetic outflow. Apraclonidine is used topically to decrease intraocular pressure during surgery.

4. **Isoproterenol** (a β-adrenergic agonist) is used as a bronchodilator and as a cardiac stimulant in shock and cardiac arrest.

5. **Dobutamine** (a β_1-selective agonist) is used to improve myocardial function in congestive heart failure in emergency situations.

6. Terbutaline and other β_2-selective agonists (metaproterenol, albuterol, pirbuterol, bitolterol, salmeterol) are used as bronchodilators both locally and systemically.

7. The β_2-selective agonist ritodrine is used exclusively to relax uterine smooth muscle in the treatment of premature labor.

D. Adverse effects. Adrenergic agonists may cause cardiac dysrhythmias, cerebral hemorrhage, pulmonary hypertension and edema, anxiety, headache, and rebound nasal congestion.

V. ADRENERGIC ANTAGONISTS

A. Chemistry

1. **α-Adrenergic antagonists** (α-blockers) have varied structures and bear little resemblance to the adrenergic agonists. Antagonists include the ergot alkaloids (e.g., ergotamine), the dibenzamines (e.g., phenoxybenzamine), the benzolines (e.g., tolazoline), and the quinazolines (e.g., prazosin) [Figure 14-9].

2. **β-Adrenergic antagonists** (β-blockers) are structurally similar to β-agonists (Figure 14-10).
   a. The **catechol ring system** can be replaced by a variety of other ring systems, ranging from the prototypical naphthalene (propranolol) to phenylether (oxprenolol), amides (atenolol), indoles (pindolol), and others.
   b. The **side chain** may be either the unchanged isopropyl-aminoethanol or an aryloxyaminopropranol. Side-chain hydroxyl groups are essential for activity.
   c. The **N-substituents** must be bulky; an isopropyl group is the minimum effective size.

B. Pharmacology

1. Adrenergic antagonists inhibit or block adrenergic receptor-mediated responses.

2. **α-Adrenergic antagonists** may be α_1-selective (e.g., prazosin) or nonselective (e.g., phenoxybenzamine, which forms a covalent irreversible bond with α-receptors).

3. β-Adrenergic antagonists may be β_1-selective (e.g., metoprolol) or nonselective (e.g., propranolol). However, β_1-selective agents may loose their selectivity at higher doses and block β_2-receptors as well.

C. Therapeutic indications

1. **Prazosin** and related α_1-selective antagonists (doxazosin, terazosin, and trimazosin) are used to produce vasodilation and are important antihypertensive agents.

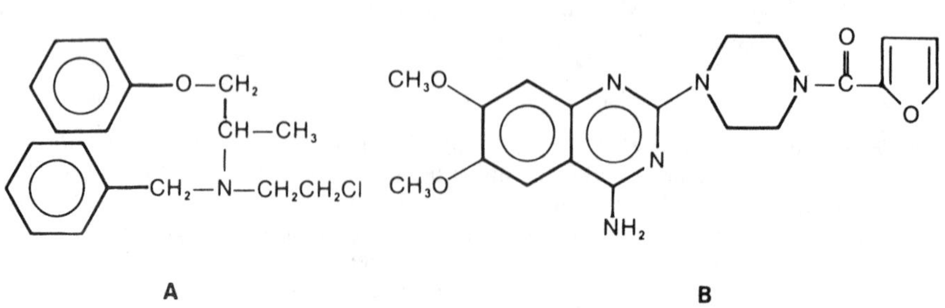

Figure 14-9. The structural formulas of *(A)* phenoxybenzamine (Dibenzyline) and *(B)* prazosin (Minipress), representative α-blockers.

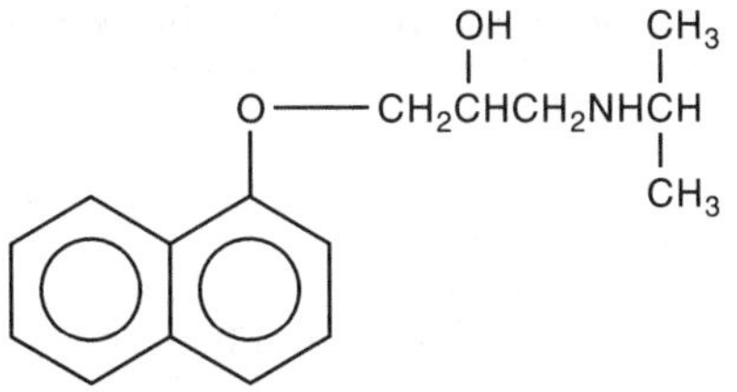

A

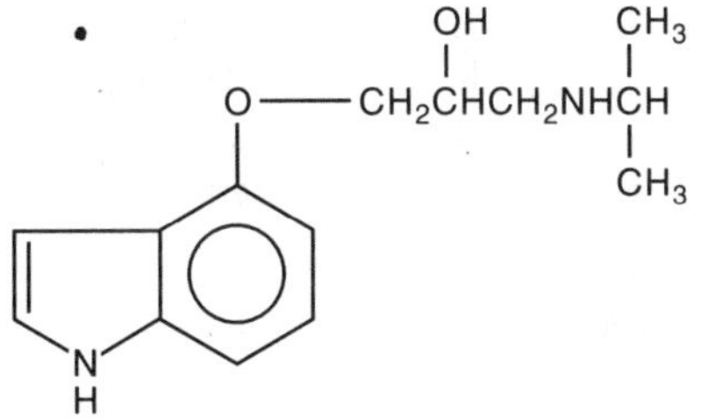

B

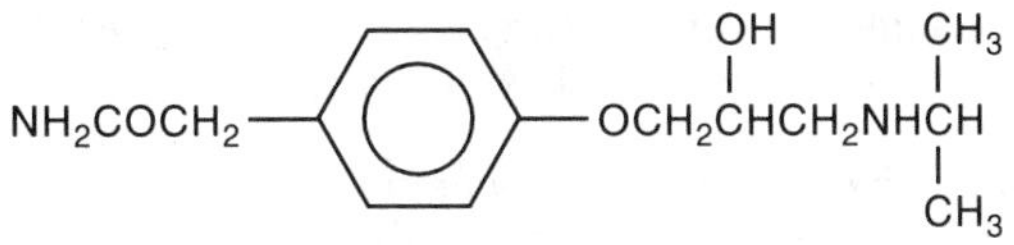

C

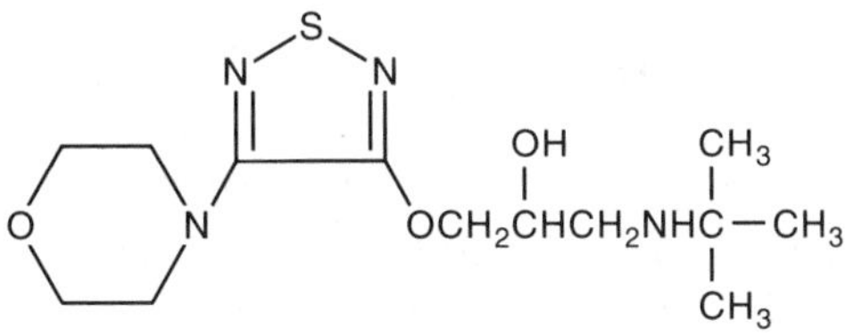

D

Figure 14-10. The structural formulas of *(A)* propranolol (Inderal); *(B)* pindolol (Visken); *(C)* atenolol (Tenormin); and *(D)* timolol (Blocadren), representative β-blockers.

2. **Phenoxybenzamine** and **phentolamine** (nonselective α-blockers) can be used to relieve vasospasm in Raynaud's syndrome and for acute hypertensive emergencies resulting from MAO inhibitors, sympathomimetics, or pheochromocytoma. Tolazoline, a similar agent, is used to treat persistent neonatal pulmonary hypertension.

3. **Labetalol,** an agent that possesses both selective α_1- and nonselective β-blocking activity, is used in the treatment of hypertension.

4. **Propranolol** (a nonselective β-antagonist) is used for the prophylaxis of angina pectoris, supraventricular and ventricular dysrhythmias, and migraine headache. It is also used as an antihypertensive, a negative inotropic agent in hypertrophic obstructive cardiomyopathies, and a negative chronotropic agent in anxiety and hyperthyroidism.

5. β_1-Selective antagonists (metoprolol, betaxolol, atenolol, acebutolol, esmolol, and bisoprolol) may be used in the treatment of hypertension, arrhythmias, and angina.

6. Both β_1-Selective (betaxolol) and nonselective blockers (timolol, metipranolol, and levobunolol) may by used topically in the treatment of glaucoma, via decreased production of aqueous humor.

D. Adverse effects

1. **Prazosin** can cause sudden syncope with the first dose, orthostatic hypotension, dizziness, headache, drowsiness, palpitations, fluid retention, and priapism.
2. **Phenoxybenzamine** can cause orthostatic hypotension, tachycardia, inhibition of ejaculation, miosis, and nasal congestion.
3. **Propranolol** can cause bradycardia and congestive heart failure, increased airway resistance, increased serum triglycerides, decreased high-density lipoprotein cholesterol, blood dyscrasias, psoriasis, depression, hallucinations, organic brain syndrome, and transient hearing loss. Sudden withdrawal can be cardiotoxic.
4. **Metoprolol** has adverse effects similar to those of propranolol, except that it is less likely to increase airway resistance because of its β_1-selectivity.

VI. NEUROMUSCULAR BLOCKING AGENTS

A. Chemistry

1. **Neuromuscular blocking agents** can be competitive (as with the prototypical curare alkaloids) or depolarizing (as with succinylcholine). They act by blocking the effects of acetylcholine at the skeletal neuromuscular junction.
2. The competitive **nondepolarizing agents** are alkaloids of **curare** (the arrow poison of South American Indians) as well as several synthetic analogues. They are primarily bulky, rigid molecules.
   a. The **principal active alkaloid** is tubocurarine chloride (Figure 14-11). A closely related trimethylate derivative is metocurine iodide (Metubine). Their most important structural feature is the presence of a tertiary-quaternary amine in which the distance between the two cations is rigidly fixed at about 14 Å, twice the length of the critical moiety of acetylcholine.
   b. A number of **potent synthetic analogues** have been developed. These include the **structurally similar** pancuronium bromide (Pavulon), vecuronium bromide (Norcuron), pipecuronium bromide (Arduan), doxacurium chloride (Nuromax), and the **structurally dissimilar** gallamine triethiodide (Flaxedil) and atracurium besylate (Tracrium). All of these agents possess at least one quaternized nitrogen.
3. The noncompetitive **depolarizing agents** include decamethonium bromide and succinylcholine chloride (Figure 14-12).
   a. Unlike the large, bulky competitive agents, noncompetitive agents are slender aliphatic molecules. However, they do contain two quaternary nitrogens.
   b. **Succinylcholine** has a short duration of action compared with the other neuromuscular blocking agents. This results from its simple ester functional group, which is rapidly hy-

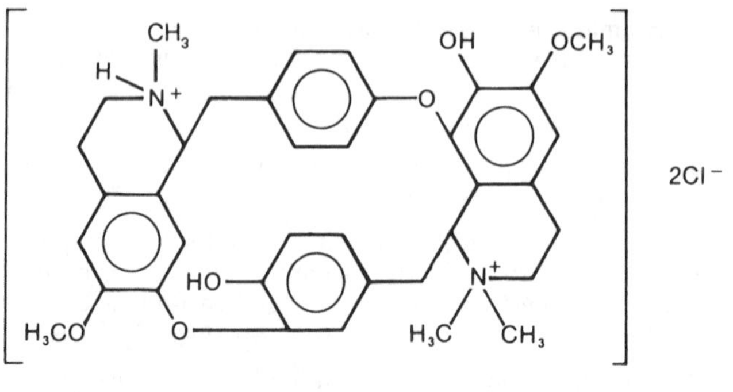

Figure 14-11. Structural formula of tubocurarine chloride (Tubarine), a competitive nondepolarizing agent.

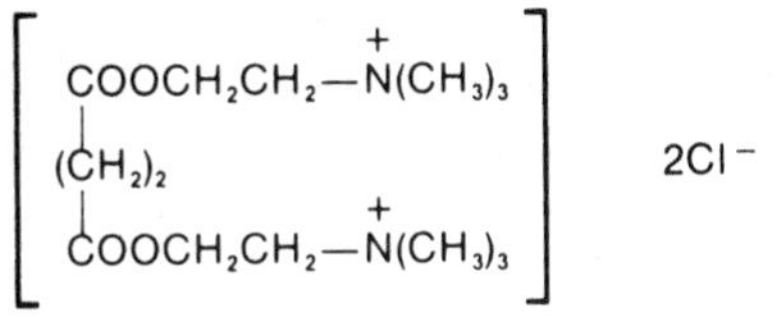

$$\left[\begin{array}{l} \text{COOCH}_2\text{CH}_2-\overset{+}{\text{N}}\text{(CH}_3)_3 \\ (\text{CH}_2)_2 \\ \text{COOCH}_2\text{CH}_2-\overset{+}{\text{N}}\text{(CH}_3)_3 \end{array}\right] \quad 2\text{Cl}^-$$

Figure 14-12. Structural formula of succinylcholine chloride (Anectine), a noncompetitive depolarizing agent.

drolyzed by plasma and liver pseudocholinesterases. Its action may be prolonged, however, in patients with a genetic pseudocholinesterase deficiency.

B. Pharmacology

1. The **competitive nondepolarizing agents** compete with acetylcholine for nicotinic receptors at the neuromuscular junction. These agents decrease the end-plate potential so that the depolarization threshold is not reached.

2. The **noncompetitive depolarizing agents** desensitize the nicotinic receptors at the neuromuscular junction. These agents react with the nicotinic receptors, decreasing receptor sensitivity in a manner similar to that of excess released acetylcholine. They depolarize the excitable membrane for a prolonged period (2–3 minutes); the membrane then becomes unresponsive (desensitized).

C. Therapeutic indications. Neuromuscular blocking agents, which cause only skeletal muscle paralysis (the patient remains conscious and capable of feeling), are used to:

1. Promote skeletal muscle relaxation and facilitate endotracheal intubation, as an adjunct to surgical anesthesia

2. Limit trauma associated with skeletal muscle contraction during electroconvulsive shock therapy

D. Adverse effects

1. Competitive nondepolarizing agents can cause respiratory paralysis, histamine release, bronchospasm, and hypotension (e.g., tubocurarine) or respiratory paralysis, tachycardia, and hypertension (e.g., gallamine, pancuronium).

2. Noncompetitive depolarizing agents (e.g., succinylcholine, decamethonium) can cause respiratory paralysis, muscle fasciculation with pain, extraocular muscle contraction with increased intraocular pressure, and increased intragastric pressure. In addition, succinylcholine may cause muscarinic responses such as bradycardia, increased glandular secretions, and cardiac arrest. In combination with halothane, succinylcholine may cause malignant hyperthermia in genetically predisposed individuals.

STUDY QUESTIONS

Directions: Each of the numbered items or incomplete statements in this section is followed by answers or by completions of the statement. Select the **one** lettered answer or completion that is **best** in each case.

1. Which of the following drugs would most likely be used in the treatment of bronchospasm that is associated with chronic obstructive pulmonary disease?

(A) Edrophonium
(B) Ipratropium
(C) Ambenonium
(D) Propantheline
(E) Homatropine

2. All of the following adverse effects are manifestations of cholinergic agonists EXCEPT

(A) bradycardia
(B) bronchoconstriction
(C) xerostomia
(D) lacrimation
(E) myopic accommodation

3. Which of the following drugs is considered to be the agent of choice for anaphylactic reactions?

(A) Clonidine
(B) Isoproterenol
(C) Epinephrine
(D) Phenylephrine
(E) Terbutaline

4. Which of the following neuromuscular blocking agents can cause muscarinic responses such as bradycardia and increased glandular secretions?

(A) Tubocurarine
(B) Succinylcholine
(C) Pancuronium
(D) Decamethonium
(E) Gallamine

5. Which of the following agents would not appropriate in the treatment of glaucoma?

A. Atropine
B. Pilocarpine
C. Physostigmine
D. Timolol
E. Epinephrine

6. Adverse reactions to atropine include all of the following EXCEPT

A. photophobia
B. dry mouth
C. sedation
D. diarrhea
E. tachycardia

Directions: Each item below contains three suggested answers of which **one or more** is correct. Choose the answer

A if **I only** is correct
B if **III only** is correct
C if **I and II** are correct
D if **II and III** are correct
E if **I, II, and III** are correct

7. True statements concerning therapeutic indications of cholinesterase inhibitors include

I. they can be used as miotic agents in the treatment of glaucoma
II. they can be used to increase skeletal muscle tone in the treatment of myasthenia gravis
III. they decrease GI and urinary bladder smooth muscle tone

8. Antimuscarinic agents are used in the treatment of Parkinson's disease and in the control of some neuroleptic-induced extrapyramidal disorders. These agents include

I. ipratropium
II. benztropine
III. trihexyphenidyl

9. Certain drugs are sometimes incorporated into local anesthetic solutions to prolong their activity and reduce their systemic toxicity. These drugs include

I. dobutamine
II. phenylephrine
III. epinephrine

Directions: Each group of items in this section consists of lettered options followed by a set of numbered items. For each item, select the **one** lettered option that is most closely associated with it. Each lettered option may be selected once, more than once, or not at all.

Case study: B.J. is a 58-year-old white man who has a history of essential hypertension, bronchial asthma, and has recently been diagnosed with prostatic hypertrophy. His medication history includes the following drugs (used to answer the questions below)

A. Propranolol, for hypertension
B. Ipratropium, for asthma
C. Metaproterenol, for asthma
D. Proscar, for prostatic hypertrophy
E. Prazosin, for hypertension

10. Which of these agents could worsen the urinary retention Mr. J. is experiencing as a result of his prostate problems?

11. Which agent could worsen or cause an acute asthma attack?

12. Which agent acts selectively at β_2-receptors?

Case study: M.D. is a 55-year-old black woman. She has a history of moderate hypertension, glaucoma, and mild osteoarthritis. Her medication history includes

A. Metoprolol, for hypertension
B. Pilocarpine gel, for glaucoma
C. Epinephrine drops, for glaucoma
D. Isoflurophate, for glaucoma
E. Timolol, for glaucoma

13. Which of her glaucoma medicines acts via an indirect mechanism?

14. Which two (2) agents could have an additive effect to produce excessive bradycardia?

15. Which two (2) glaucoma agents could lessen the effects of each other?

ANSWERS AND EXPLANATIONS

1. The answer is B *[II C 2 b, c; III C 1 e–g].*
Ipratropium is a newly approved antimuscarinic agent used to treat bronchospasm. Propantheline and homatropine are antimuscarinic agents used as a gastrointestinal (GI) antispasmodic and as a mydriatic, respectively. Edrophonium and ambenonium are indirect-acting cholinergic agonists and, as such, would be expected to induce bronchospasm.

2. The answer is C *[II D].*
Xerostomia, or dry mouth, results from reduced salivary secretions and, therefore, is not a manifestation of cholinergic agonist activity. All of the other effects listed in the question are extensions of therapeutic effects of cholinergic agonists to the point of being adverse effects.

3. The answer is C *[IV C 1].*
Of the adrenergic agonists listed in the question, only epinephrine, because of its broad, nonselective α- and β-activity, is an agent of choice for anaphylactic reactions. Epinephrine improves circulatory and respiratory function and counteracts the vascular effects of histamine-related anaphylaxis.

4. The answer is B *[VI D 2].*
Neuromuscular blocking agents interact with nicotinic receptors at the skeletal neuromuscular junction. Succinylcholine is also capable of eliciting autonomic muscarinic responses, such as bradycardia, increased glandular secretions, and cardiac arrest.

5. The answer is A *[II B–D].*
Both direct (pilocarpine) and indirect acting (physostigmine) cholinergics may be used in glaucoma to increase cholinergic activity and facilitate outflow of aqueous humor. Similarly, both β-agonists (epinephrine) and antagonists (timolol) may be used respectively to increase outflow and decrease production of aqueous humor. Atropine is contraindicated in glaucoma because its anticholinergic effects can block the outflow of aqueous humor and consequently increase intraocular pressure.

6. The answer is D *[III D].*
Classic signs and symptoms of muscarinic blockade as with atropine include mydriasis, which may make the patient light sensitive (photophobia), dry mouth and constipation by decreasing secretory activity and motility in the gastrointestinal (GI) tract, and tachycardia by inhibiting the normal inhibitory cholinergic control of the cardiac system. Diarrhea is one of the common signs of cholinergic agonists (SLUD—salivation, lacrimation or tearing, urination, and diarrhea).

7. The answer is C (I, II) *[II C 2].*
Cholinesterase inhibitors are indirect-acting cholinergic agonists useful in treating myasthenia gravis and glaucoma. Their effects on gastrointestinal (GI) and urinary bladder smooth muscle would be to increase smooth muscle tone, not decrease it.

8. The answer is D (II, III) *[III C 1 g, h].*
All three compounds listed in the question are antimuscarinic agents; however, only benztropine and trihexyphenidyl are used to control Parkinsonism and some neuroleptic-induced extrapyramidal disorders. Ipratropium is a newly approved agent for the treatment of bronchospasm.

9. The answer is D (II, III) *[IV B 1 b, C 1, 2].*
Dobutamine is a β_1-selective adrenergic agonist. It would be inappropriate to use dobutamine to decrease blood flow at the site of local anesthetic administration. Epinephrine is a nonselective α- and β-agonist, and phenylephrine is an α_1-selective agonist; both of these drugs can be used to limit the systemic absorption of local anesthetics and prolong their activity.

10. The answer is B *[II C 1].*
This anticholinergic, if absorbed systemically, could cause classic anticholinergic effects, which include urinary retention.

11. The answer is A *[V C 4].*
Because this is a nonselective β-blocker, there could be some inhibition of β_2-receptors in the bronchial tree, causing bronchoconstriction and possible complication of his asthma.

12. The answer is C *[IV C 6].*
Propranolol is a nonselective β-blocker and prazosin is a selective α_1-blocker. Neither Ipratropium nor Proscar work through the adrenergic system. Metaproterenol is a selective β_2-agonist.

13. The answer is D *[II A 2, C 2].*
Pilocarpine acts directly at the muscarinic receptor whereas epinephrine and timolol both act directly at β-receptors. Isoflurophate inhibits the metabolism of acetylcholine, indirectly increasing levels of the endogenous neurotransmitter.

14. The answers are A and E *[V B 3, D 4].*
Metoprolol, a β_1-selective agent, can cause bradycardia alone. The addition of topical timolol, while limiting systemic absorption, could have an additive β-blocking effect to decrease heart rate (negative chronotropy).

15. The answers are B and D *[II C 1, 2].*
Pilocarpine and isoflurophate could limit the effects of each other because ultimately both act via cholinergic receptors. Pilocarpine acts directly on the receptor while isoflurophate indirectly increases acetylcholine levels. Pilocarpine and acetylcholine could compete for each other at the receptor site, effectively decreasing the effects of both. Epinephrine and timolol are β-agonists and antagonists, respectively. Although both agents are effective in treating glaucoma alone, the use of both concomitantly could result in a pharmacologic antagonism, effectively decreasing the effects of both.

15 Drugs Affecting the Central Nervous System

David C. Kosegarten
Edward F. LaSala
Scott F. Long

I. INTRODUCTION. Drugs affecting the central nervous system (CNS) provide anesthesia, treat psychiatric disorders, relieve anxiety, provide sleep or sedation, prevent epileptic seizures, suppress movement disorders, and relieve pain. These drugs include general and local anesthetics, antidepressants and antipsychotics, anxiolytics, sedative–hypnotics, antiepileptics, antiparkinsonian agents, and opioid analgesics and antagonists.

II. GENERAL ANESTHETICS

A. Chemistry

1. **Inhalation anesthetics** are drugs inhaled as gases or vapors. These diverse drugs are relatively simple lipophilic molecules. They range from the inorganic agent nitrous oxide (N_2O) to the rarely used **flammable** ethers (e.g., ethyl ether) and hydrocarbons (e.g., cyclopropane), to the frequently used **nonflammable** halogenated hydrocarbons (halothane) and ethers (methoxyflurane, isoflurane, desflurane, sevoflurane).

2. **Nonvolatile anesthetics** are also lipophilic molecules. These range from water-soluble salts to aqueous propylene glycol solutions and emulsions.
   a. The **water-soluble salts** include the ultra–short-acting barbiturates (thiopental, methohexital, thiamylal), cyclohexamines (ketamine), benzodiazepines (midazolam), butyrophenones (droperidol), and opioids (fentanyl).
   b. The **aqueous propylene glycol solution** includes the imidazole, etomidate, which is compatible with many preanesthetics.
   c. The dialkylphenol, propofol, is administered as an **emulsion,** which should not be mixed with other therapeutic agents before administration (Figure 15-1).

B. Pharmacology

1. **General anesthetics** depress the CNS, producing a reversible loss of consciousness and loss of all forms of sensation.

2. **Inhalational anesthetics** are absorbed and primarily excreted through the lungs. Frequently, these drugs are supplemented with analgesics, a skeletal muscle relaxant, and antimuscarinic agents.
   a. **Analgesics** permit a reduction in the required concentration of inhalational anesthetic.
   b. **Skeletal muscle relaxants** cause adequate muscle relaxation during surgery.
   c. **Antimuscarinic agents** decrease bronchiolar secretions.

3. **Nonvolatile anesthetics** are usually administered intravenously (e.g., thiobarbiturates, benzodiazepines).

C. Therapeutic indications

1. **Inhalation anesthetics** are indicated to provide general surgical anesthesia.

2. **Nonvolatile anesthetics** are indicated to induce drowsiness and provide relaxation before the induction of inhalational general anesthesia (e.g., thiopental, diazepam, midazolam).

D. Adverse effects. General anesthetics depress respiration, circulation, and the CNS. They can also decrease hepatic and kidney function (e.g., methoxyflurane) and cause cardiac dysrhythmias as a result of increased myocardial sensitivity to catecholamines (e.g., halothane).

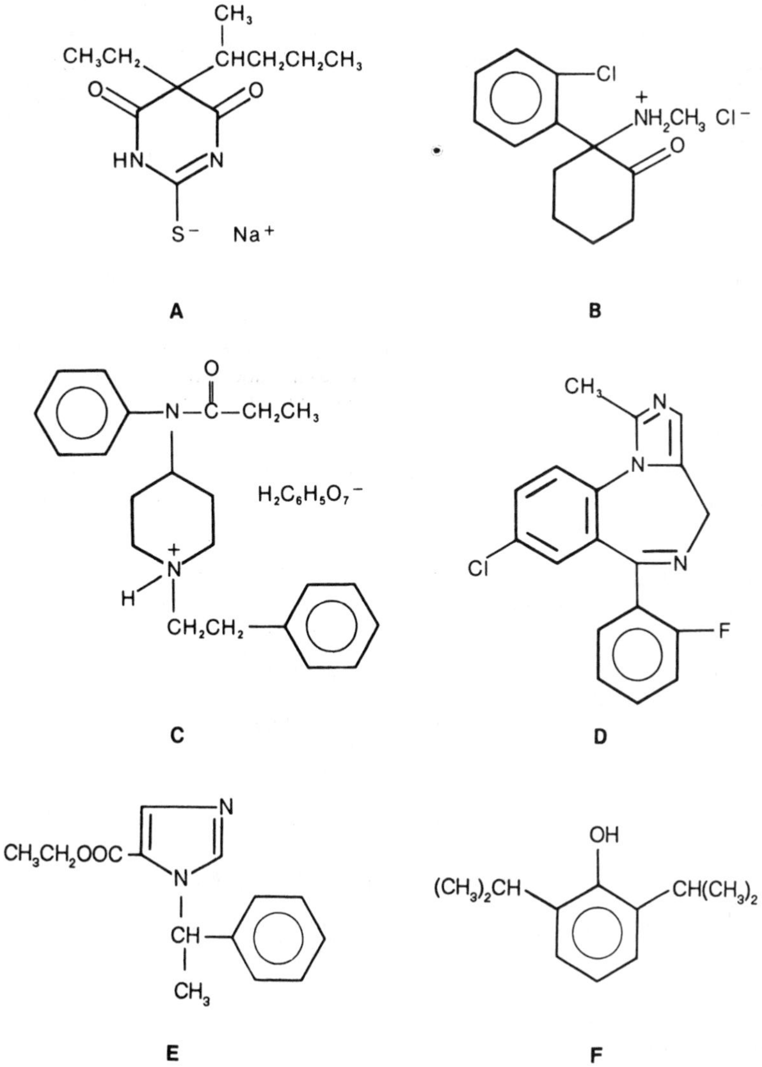

Figure 15-1. Structural formulas of nonvolatile general anesthetics: (*A*) thiopental sodium (Pentothal), (*B*) ketamine hydrochloride (Ketaject), (*C*) fentanyl citrate (Sublimaze), (*D*) midazolam (Versed), (*E*) etomidate (Amidate), and (*F*) propofol (Diprivan).

III. LOCAL ANESTHETICS

A. Chemistry. Most local anesthetics are structurally similar to the alkaloid cocaine (Figure 15-2). These drugs consist of a hydrophilic amino group linked through an ester or amide connecting group to a lipophilic aromatic moiety. A few phenols and aromatic alcohols also have local anesthetic activity.

1. Ester-type agents are generally short acting and are hydrolyzed by plasma esterases. These agents include cocaine, procaine, chloroprocaine, proparacaine, tetracaine, benzocaine, and butamben.

2. Amide-type agents are generally longer acting and are metabolized in the liver. Examples of the amide-type local anesthetics include lidocaine, dibucaine, prilocaine, mepivacaine, bupivacaine, and etidocaine.

3. The drug's pK_a (see Chapter 12) influences its state. At tissue pH, the drug can exist either as a lipophilic, uncharged, secondary or tertiary amine that crosses connective tissue and

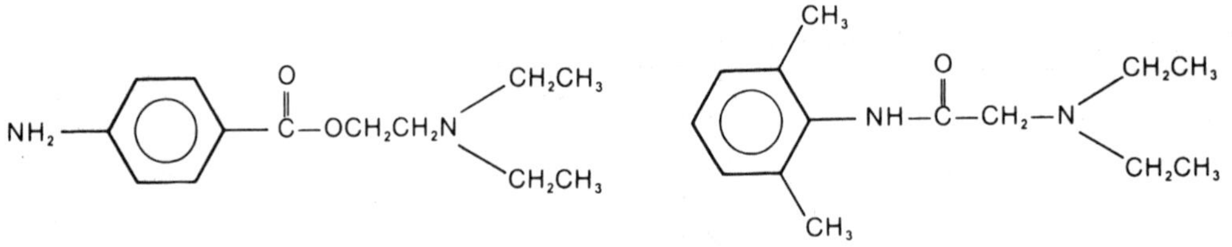

Figure 15-2. Structural formulas of local anesthetics structurally similar to cocaine: (*A*) procaine (Novocaine) and (*B*) lidocaine (Xylocaine).

enters nerve cells or as a charged ammonium cation that appears to block the generation of action potentials by means of a membrane receptor complex.

B. Pharmacology

1. Local anesthetics **reversibly block nerve impulse conduction** and **produce reversible loss of sensation** at their administration site. They do not produce a loss of consciousness.
   a. Small, nonmyelinated nerve fibers, which conduct pain and temperature sensations, are affected first.
   b. Local anesthetics appear to become incorporated within the nerve membrane or to bind to specific membrane sodium ion (Na^+) channels, restricting Na^+ permeability in response to partial depolarization.
2. Local anesthetic solutions frequently contain the vasoconstrictor **epinephrine,** which reduces vascular blood flow at the administration site. This reduces systemic absorption, prolongs the duration of action, and reduces systemic toxicity.

C. Therapeutic indications.
Local anesthetics are indicated to:

1. Produce regional nerve block for the relief of pain when injected close to the innervating nerve
2. Provide anesthesia for minor operations when infiltrated around the tissue site
3. Provide anesthesia for surgery of the lower limbs and pelvis and for obstetric surgery when injected into the epidural space or the subarachnoid space of the spinal cord
4. Provide anesthesia of the skin and mucous membranes when applied locally. This includes two miscellaneous local anesthetics: **dyclonine,** used primarily in throat lozenges and sprays, and **pramoxine,** used primarily in antihemorrhoidal preparations.

D. Adverse effects

1. Ester-type local anesthetics can cause hypersensitivity reactions in susceptible individuals.
2. Systemic absorption of toxic concentrations of local anesthetics can cause seizures; CNS, respiratory, and myocardial depression; and circulatory collapse.

IV. ANTIPSYCHOTICS.
The classic antipsychotics are phenothiazines, thioxanthenes, and butyrophenones. Additional chemical classes having antipsychotic activity include the dihydroindolones (molindone), dibenzoxazepines (loxapine), dibenzodiazepines (clozapine), diphenylbutylpiperidines (pimozide), and benzisoxazoles (risperidone).

A. Chemistry

1. **Phenothiazines** (e.g., chlorpromazine, triflupromazine, thioridazine, prochlorperazine, trifluoperazine, fluphenazine) must have a **nitrogen-containing side-chain substituent** on the ring nitrogen for antipsychotic activity (Table 15-1). The ring and side-chain nitrogens must be separated by a three-carbon chain; phenothiazines, in which the ring and side-chain nitrogens are separated by a two-carbon chain, have antihistaminic or sedative activity only.
   a. The side chains are either dimethylaminopropyl, piperazine, or piperidine derivatives. Piperazine side chains confer the greatest potency.

Table 15-1. Antipsychotic Phenothiazines

General Phenothiazine Structure*

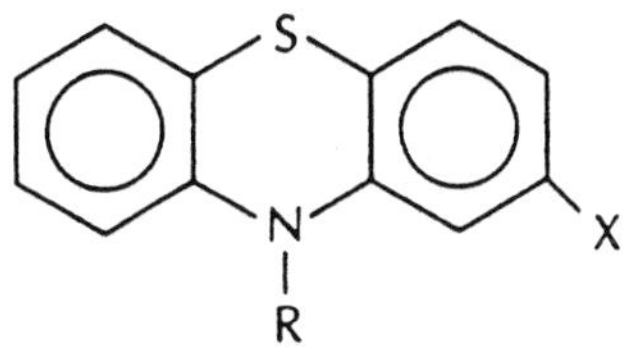

Drug	**X-Substituent**	**R-Substituent**
Chlorpromazine (Thorazine)	–Cl	$-(CH_2)_3-N(CH_3)_2$
Triflupromazine (Vesprin)	$-CF_3$	$-(CH_2)_3-N(CH_3)_2$
Thioridazine (Mellaril)	$-SCH_3$	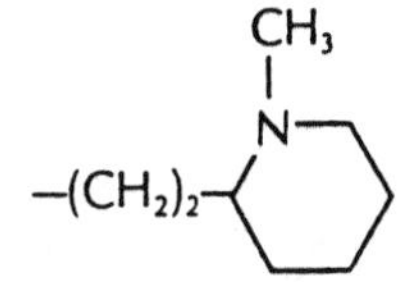
Prochlorperazine (Compazine)	–Cl	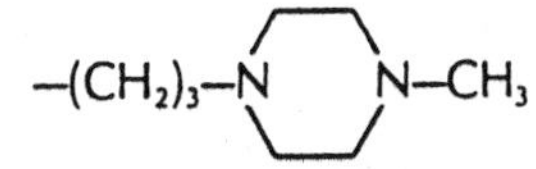
Trifluoperazine (Stelazine)	$-CF_3$	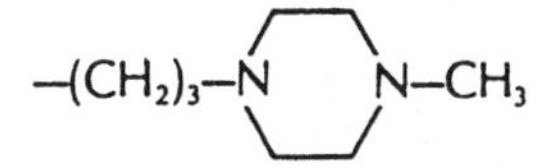
Fluphenazine (Prolixin)	$-CF_3$	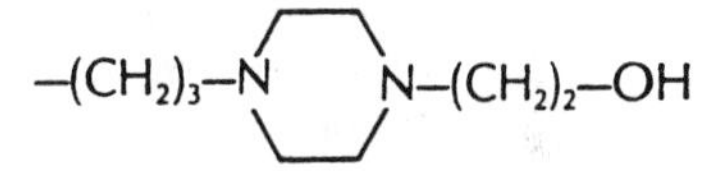

*Antipsychotic phenothiazines have the general structure illustrated in the table. Substituents at positions marked X and R result in different drugs.

b. The ring substituent in position 2 must be electron attractive for optimum activity. A trifluromethyl substituent confers the greatest activity.
c. Fluphenazine and long-chain alcohols form stable, **highly liposoluble esters** (e.g., enanthate, decanoate), which possess markedly prolonged activity.

2. **Thioxanthenes** (e.g., chlorprothixene, thiothixene) lack the ring nitrogen of phenothiazines and have a side chain attached by a double bond (Figure 15-3).

3. **Butyrophenones** (e.g., haloperidol) are chemically unrelated to phenothiazines but have similar activity (Figure 15-4).

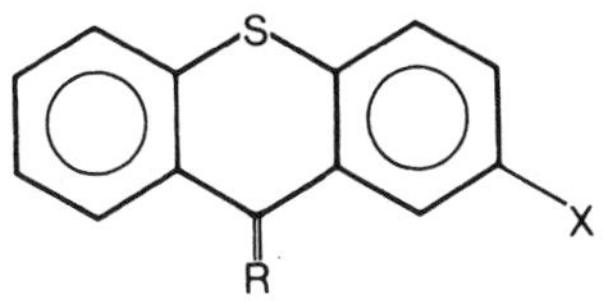

Figure 15-3. Thioxanthenes, similar to phenothiazines, have substituents at *X* and *R* positions that alter drug activity. Chlorprothixene (Taractan) has a $-Cl$ substituent at *X* and $CH-(CH_2)_2-N(CH_3)_2$ at *R*. Thiothixene (Navane) has a $-SO_2\ N(CH_3)_2$ substituent at *X* and the group:

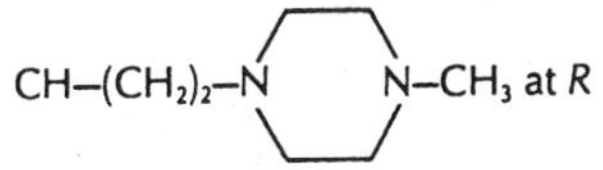

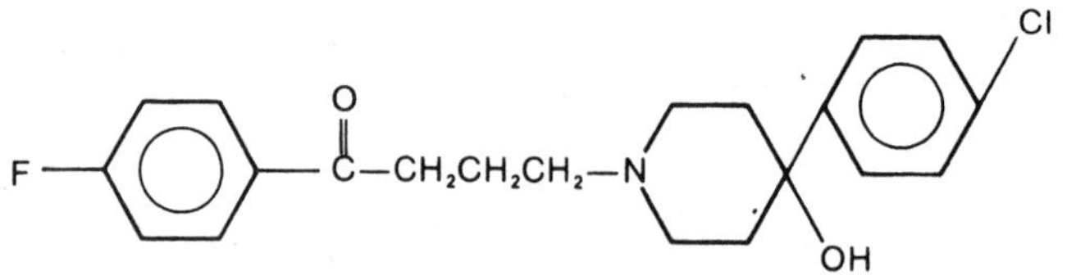

Figure 15-4. Structural formula of haloperidol (Haldol), a butyrophenone antipsychotic.

4. Newer, miscellaneous chemical classes also differ in their structure from the phenothiazines but also possesses antipsychotic activity.

5. **Lithium** is an elemental compound that, as the carbonate salt, is used in the treatment of specific psychotic disorders (manic depression).

B. Pharmacology

1. These agents have similar **pharmacologic effects.** Their antipsychotic effects (i.e., improvement of mood and behavior) and their neuroleptic effects (i.e., emotional quieting, development of extrapyramidal symptoms) appear to result from their ability to antagonize central dopamine-mediated synaptic neurotransmission.

2. Other effects vary among the classes of antipsychotics. These include antiemetic activity and blockade of muscarinic, α_1-adrenergic, and H_1-histaminergic receptors.

C. Therapeutic indications.

C. Therapeutic indications. Antipsychotics are indicated primarily for the treatment of psychosis associated with schizophrenia (clozapine), paranoia, the manic phase of manic-depressive illness (lithium), and Tourette's syndrome (pimozide).

D. Adverse effects

1. **Centrally mediated adverse effects** include:
   a. Drowsiness
   b. Extrapyramidal symptoms, such as akathisia, acute dystonia, akinesia, and tardive dyskinesia
   c. Alteration of temperature-regulating mechanisms, including poikilothermy
   d. Increased appetite and weight gain
   e. Alterations in hypothalamic and endocrine function, such as increased release of corticotropin, gonadotropins, prolactin, growth hormone, and melanocyte-stimulating hormone

2. **Peripheral adverse effects** include:
   a. Postural hypotension and reflex tachycardia
   b. Hepatotoxicity and jaundice
   c. Failure of ejaculation
   d. Bone marrow depression
   e. Photosensitivity
   f. Xerostomia and blurred vision
   g. Fine hand tremors, increased urination, and thirst occur with lithium therapy, however these side effects will diminish with continued therapy.

V. ANTIDEPRESSANTS

V. ANTIDEPRESSANTS are classified into three structurally unrelated groups: the monoamine oxidase (MAO) inhibitors, tricyclic antidepressants, and atypical antidepressants.

A. Chemistry

1. **MAO inhibitors** may be weakly potent **hydralazines** [e.g., phenelzine isocarboxazid (Marplan)] or extremely potent **phenylcyclopropylamines** (i.e., ring-closed amphetamine derivatives, such as tranylcypromine) [Figure 15-5].

2. **Tricyclic** antidepressants, which are used commonly, are secondary or tertiary amine derivatives of molecules that have a fused three-ring system.
   a. The principal tricyclic antidepressants are derivatives of dibenzazepine (imipramine, desipramine, clomipramine, trimipramine) and dibenzocycloheptadiene (amitriptyline, nortriptyline, protriptyline) [Figures 15-6 and 15-7].

A B

Figure 15-5. Structural formulas of (*A*) phenelzine (Nardil), a hydralazine derivative monoamine oxidase (MAO) inhibitor, and (*B*) tranylcypromine (Parnate), a cyclopropylamine derivative MAO inhibitor.

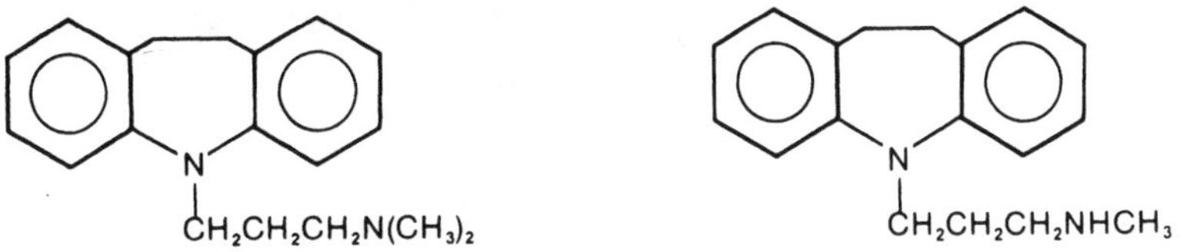

A B

Figure 15-6. Structural formulas of tricyclic antidepressants derived from dibenzazepine: (*A*) imipramine (Tofranil) and (*B*) desipramine (Norpramin).

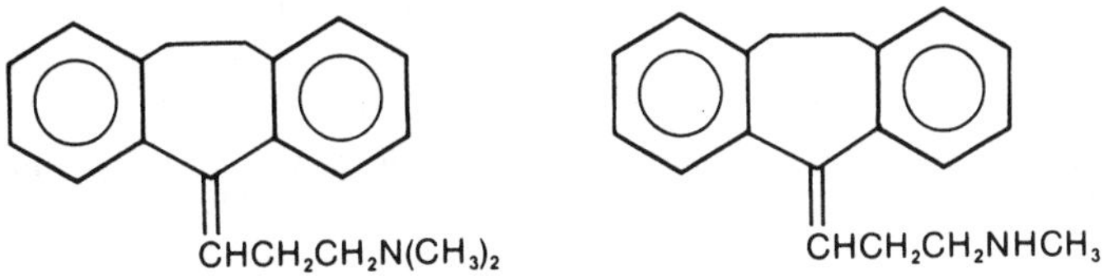

A B

Figure 15-7. Structural formulas of tricyclic antidepressants derived from dibenzocycloheptadiene: (*A*) amitriptyline (Elavil), (*B*) nortriptyline (Aventyl).

b. Other closely related tricyclic antidepressants include doxepin, a dibenzoxepine and amoxapine, a dibenzoxazepine.
c. A closely related **tetracyclic** agent is maprotiline (Ludiomil).

3. **Atypical** antidepressants have varied structures. They range from the complex heterocycles trazodone and nefazodone, to the chemically unrelated serotonin-uptake inhibitors (fluoxetine, fluvoxamine, paroxetine, sertraline, and venlafaxine) and the aminopropiophenone bupropion (Figure 15-8).

B. Pharmacology

1. **MAO inhibitors** appear to produce their antidepressant effects by blocking the intraneuronal oxidative deamination of brain biogenic amines (i.e., norepinephrine, serotonin). This increases the availability of biogenic amines at central aminergic receptors. Other biochemical events (e.g., the down-regulation of central β-adrenergic and serotoninergic receptors) that result from chronic inhibition of MAO and re-uptake blockade can also explain the therapeutic action of antidepressants. This explanation is suggested by the latency period of MAO inhibitors, which take 2–4 weeks to become effective.

2. **Tricyclic** antidepressants appear to act principally by reducing CNS neuronal re-uptake of biogenic amines (i.e., norepinephrine, serotonin). This prolongs the availability of biogenic amines at central aminergic receptors.

3. **Atypical** antidepressants have varying effects on re-uptake of biogenic amines. Trazodone and fluoxetine selectively inhibit serotonin re-uptake.

C. Therapeutic indications

1. **MAO inhibitors** are indicated to treat depression, phobic anxiety, and narcolepsy that has not responded to other treatments. However, their use is limited by their adverse effects (see V D).

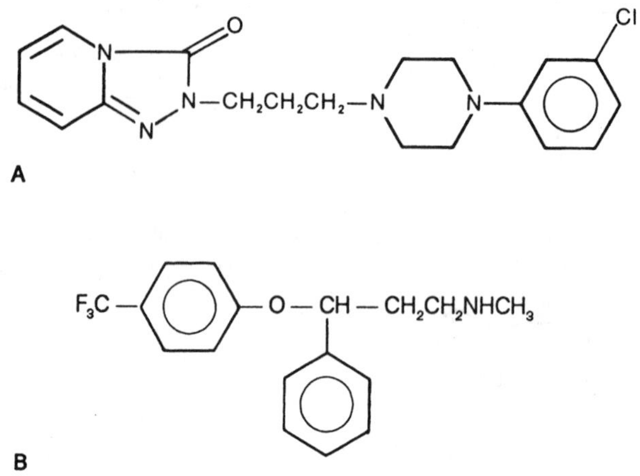

Figure 15-8. Structural formulas of (*A*) trazodone (Desyrel) and (*B*) fluoxetine (Prozac), atypical antidepressants.

2. Tricyclic and atypical antidepressants are the agents of choice for endogenous depression. Additionally, imipramine in use to treat enuresis; clomipramine, fluoxetine, and fluvoxamine are used in obsessive-compulsive disorder; and doxepin, for anxiety.

D. Adverse effects

1. **MAO inhibitors** interact with sympathomimetic drugs and with foods that have a high tyramine concentration, such as cheese, wine, and sausage. Hypertensive crisis can result. In addition, MAO inhibitors can cause a wide range of adverse effects, including:
   a. CNS effects, such as CNS stimulation, tremors, agitation, overactivity, hyperreflexia, mania, and insomnia followed by weakness, fatigue, and drowsiness
   b. Cardiovascular effects, such as postural hypotension
   c. Gastrointestinal (GI) effects, such as nausea, abdominal pain, and constipation
   d. Antimuscarinic effects, such as dry mouth, urinary retention, and constipation

2. **Tricyclic** antidepressants can cause adverse effects including:
   a. CNS effects, such as drowsiness, dizziness, weakness, fatigue, and confusion
   b. Cardiovascular effects, such as orthostatic hypotension, tachycardia, and interference with atrioventricular conduction
   c. Antimuscarinic effects, such as dry mouth, urinary retention, and constipation
   d. GI effects, such as nausea, vomiting, diarrhea, and anorexia
   e. Bone marrow depression
   f. Mania (in patients with manic-depressive illness)

3. **Atypical antidepressants** can cause adverse effects including:
   a. CNS effects, such as dizziness, nightmares, confusion, drowsiness, fatigue, headache, insomnia, impaired memory, akathisia, numbness, and tonic–clonic seizures
   b. Cardiovascular effects, such as hypertension, hypotension, tachycardia, chest pain, and syncope
   c. GI effects, such as nausea, vomiting, diarrhea, and constipation
   d. Blurred vision and tinnitus
   e. Antimuscarinic effects, such as urinary retention, dry mouth, and constipation
   f. Bone marrow depression
   g. Sexual dysfunction and menstrual irregularities

VI. ANXIOLYTICS fall into four major classes: the highly effective benzodiazepines and azaspirodecanediones and the less effective propanediol carbamates and diphenylmethanes.

A. Chemistry

1. **Benzodiazepines** (e.g., chlordiazepoxide, diazepam, halazepam, clorazepate, prazepam, oxazepam, lorazepam, alprazolam) have varying durations of action, which can be correlated with their structures in some cases (Table 15-2).

a. Agents with a 3-hydroxyl group are easily metabolized by phase II glucuronidation and are short acting (see R_3-substituent column in Table 15-2).

b. Agents lacking a 3-hydroxyl group must undergo considerable phase I metabolism, including 3-hydroxylation. These agents are long acting. Most long-acting agents form the intermediate metabolite desmethyldiazepam, which has a very long half-life. Thus, these agents can have a cumulative action.

c. Triazolobenzodiazepines (e.g., alprazolam) undergo a different pattern of metabolism and are intermediate in activity.

Table 15-2. Benzodiazepine Anxiolytics

General Benzodiazepine Structure*

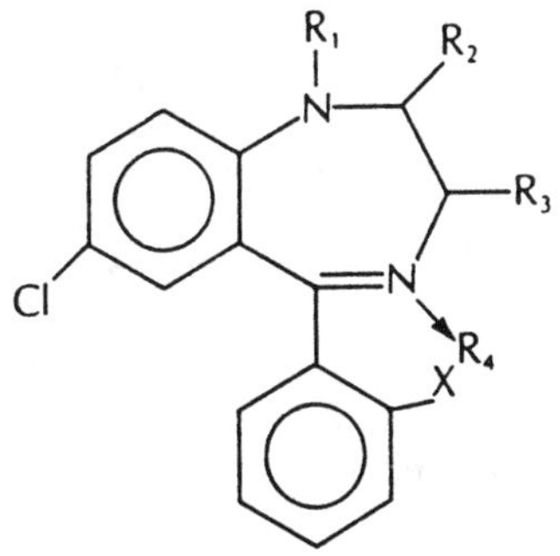

Drug	R_1-Substituent	R_2-Substituent	R_3-Substituent	R_4-Substituent	X-Substituent
Chlordiazepoxide (Librium)	=	$-NHCH_3$	. . .	O	. . .
Diazepam (Valium)	$-CH_3$	=O	. . .	. . .	. . .
Halazepam (Paxipam)	$-CH_2CF_3$	=O	. . .	. . .	. . .
Clorazepate dipotassium (Tranxene)	–H	–OH; –OK	–COOK	. . .	. . .
Prazepam (Centrax)	$-CH_2-CH\langle^{CH_2}_{CH_2}$	=O	. . .	. . .	. . .
Oxazepam (Serax)	–H	=O	–OH	. . .	. . .
Lorazepam (Ativan)	–H	=O	–OH	. . .	–Cl
Alprazolam (Xanax)	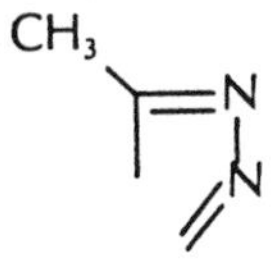		. . .	. . .	. . .

*Benzodiazepine anxiolytics have the general structure illustrated in the table. Substituents at the position marked R_1, R_2, R_3, R_4, and X result in different drugs.

d. Agents lacking an amino side chain are not basic enough to form water-soluble salts with acids. For example, intravenous solutions of diazepam contain propylene glycol as a solvent. Precipitation can occur if these solutions are mixed with aqueous solutions.

2. **Azaspirodecanediones** (e.g., buspirone) have anxiolytic activity resembling that of the benzodiazepines. However, these agents lack other CNS depressant activity (Figure 15-9).

3. **Propanediol carbamates** (e.g., meprobamate) **and diphenylmethanes** (e.g., hydroxyzine) are used much less commonly than the benzodiazepines for the treatment of anxiety (Figure 15-10).

B. Pharmacology

1. **Benzodiazepines** appear to produce their calming effects by depressing the limbic system and reticular formation through potentiation of the inhibitor neurotransmitter γ-aminobutyric acid (GABA).
   a. Anxiolytic activity correlates with the drug's binding affinity to a macromolecular GABA-chloride ionophore receptor complex.
   b. It possesses no hypnotic or anticonvulsant properties and does not appear to add to the depressant effects of alcohol or other CNS depressant drugs.
   c. Benzodiazepines increase the depressant effects of alcohol and other CNS depressant drugs.

2. **Azaspirodecanediones.** Buspirone has an unknown mechanism of action.
   a. **Buspirone** binds to central dopamine and serotonin receptors rather than to GABA chloride ionophore receptor complexes.
   b. It possesses no hypnotic or anticonvulsant properties and does not appear to add to the depressant effects of alcohol or other CNS depressant drugs.

C. Therapeutic indications

1. Benzodiazepines and the azaspirodecanedione buspirone are indicated to treat anxiety.

2. Benzodiazepines are also indicated for use as a preanesthetic medication (see II A 2, C 2), as sedative–hypnotics (see VII), anticonvulsants (see VIII), and during acute alcohol withdrawal.

D. Adverse effects

1. Adverse effects associated with **benzodiazepines** include:

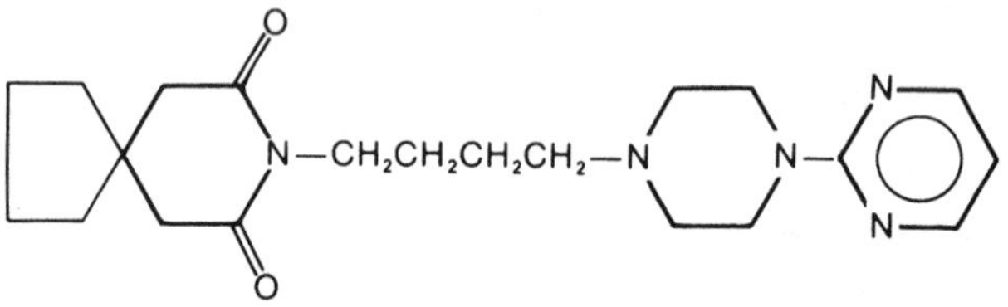

Figure 15-9. Structural formulas of buspirone (Buspar), the prototypical azaspirodecanedione anxiolytic.

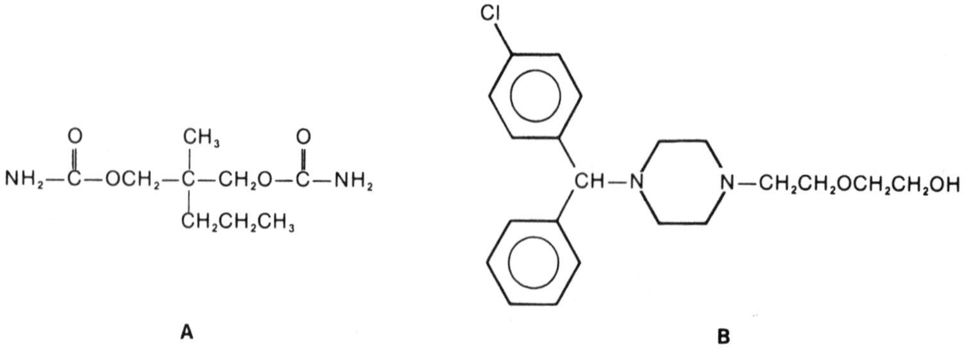

Figure 15-10. Structural formulas of (*A*) meprobamate (Miltown, Equanil), a propanediol carbamate anxiolytic, and (*B*) hydroxyzine (Atarax, Vistaril), a diphenylmethane anxiolytic.

- **a.** CNS effects, such as CNS depression, drowsiness, sedation, ataxia, confusion, and dysarthria
- **b.** GI effects, such as nausea, vomiting, and diarrhea
- **c.** Psychiatric effects (rare), such as paradoxical excitement, insomnia, paranoia, and rage reactions
- **d.** Abuse potential and possibly dependence

2. Adverse effects of **buspirone** are limited to restlessness, dizziness, headache, nausea, diarrhea, and paresthesias. However, tardive dyskinesia is possible with long-term therapy.

VII. SEDATIVE–HYPNOTICS.

Sedatives are principally long-acting or intermediate-acting barbiturates (e.g., phenobarbital, amobarbital), whereas **hypnotics** can be the widely used benzodiazepines (e.g., flurazepam, alprazolam), short-acting barbiturates (e.g., pentobarbital, secobarbital), piperidinediones (e.g., glutethimide), or aldehydes (e.g., chloral hydrate).

A. Chemistry

1. Barbiturates are 5,5-disubstituted derivatives of barbituric acid, a saturated triketopyramidine (Table 15-3).

- **a.** Two side chains in position 5 are essential for sedative-hypnotic activity.
- **b.** Long-acting agents have a phenyl and an ethyl group in position 5.
- **c.** Branched side chains, unsaturated side chains, or side chains longer than an ethyl group increase lipophilicity and metabolism rate. Increased lipophilicity leads to a shorter onset of action, a shorter duration of action, and increased potency.

Table 15-3. Barbiturate Sedative–Hypnotics

General Barbiturate Structure*

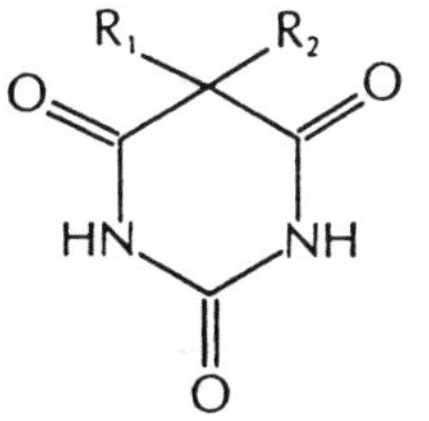

Drug	R_1-Substituent	R_2-Substituent	Duration of Action
Phenobarbital (Luminal)	$-CH_2CH_3$	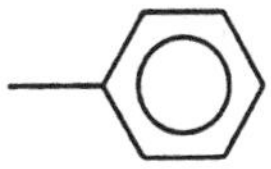	Long
Amobarbital (Amytal)	$-CH_2CH_3$	$-CH_2CH_2CH(CH_3)_2$	Intermediate
Butabarbital (Butisol)	$-CH_2CH_3$	$-CH(CH_3)CH_2CH_3$	Intermediate
Pentobarbital (Nembutal)	$-CH_2CH_3$	$-CH(CH_3)CH_2CH_2CH_3$	Short
Secobarbital (Seconal)	$-CH_2CH{=}CH_2$	$-CH(CH_3)CH_2CH_2CH_3$	Short

*Barbiturate sedative–hypnotics have the general structure illustrated in the table. Substituents at R_1 and R_2 positions result in different drugs with different durations of action.

d. Replacement of the position 2 oxygen with sulfur produces an extremely lipophilic molecule that distributes rapidly into lipid tissues outside the brain.

(1) These ultra–short-acting barbiturates are not useful as sedative–hypnotics but do act as effective induction anesthetics (see II A 2). The action of these drugs is terminated very quickly.

(2) The prototype ultra–short-acting barbiturate is thiopental (Pentothal), the 2-thio isostere of pentobarbital.

e. The barbiturates and many of their metabolites are weak acids, and changes in urinary pH greatly influence their excretion. This is particularly true with overdoses, when a relatively large amount of unchanged drug appears in the glomerular filtrate.

f. Phenobarbital is one of the most powerful and versatile agents that can induce certain enzyme systems (e.g., the Cytochrome P_{450} metabolic system). This increases the potential for drug interactions and includes interaction with any drug metabolized by this system. Other barbiturates have less enzyme-inducing effect, except when they are used continuously in higher-than-normal doses.

2. Benzodiazepine sedative–hypnotics (e.g., flurazepam, quazepam, triazolam, estazolam, temazepam) have varying durations of action, depending on their structures, as is true for the benzodiazepine anxiolytics (Table 15-4) [see VI A 1 and Table 15-2].

Table 15-4. Benzodiazepine Sedative–Hypnotics

General Benzodiazepine Structure*

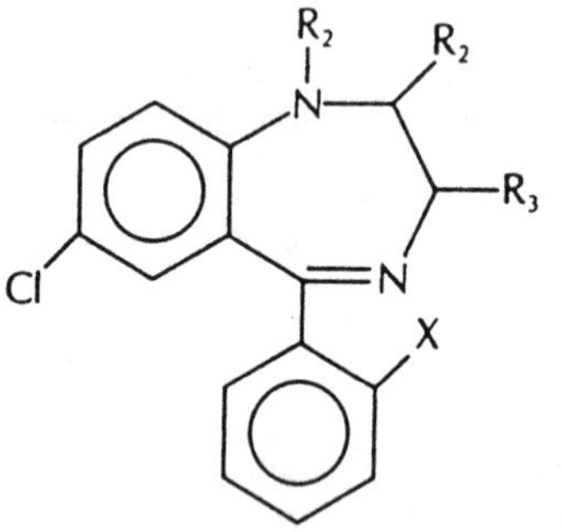

Drug	R_1-Substituent	R_2-Substituent	R_3-Substituent	X-Substituent	Duration of Action
Flurazepam (Dalmane)	$CH_2CH_2N(C_2H_5)_2$	=O	–H	–F	Long
Quazepam (Doral)	$–CH_2CF_3$	=S	–H	–F	Intermediate to long
Triazolam (Halcion)	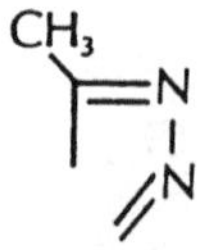		–H	–Cl	Intermediate
Estazolam (ProSom)	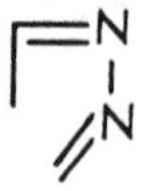		–H	–H	Intermediate
Temazepam (Restoril)	$–CH_3$	=O	–OH	–H	Short

*Benzodiazepine sedative–hypnotics have the general structure illustrated in the table. Substituents at the positions marked R_1, R_2, R_3, and X result in different drugs with different durations of action.

3. **Piperidinediones** (e.g., glutethimide) and **aldehydes** (e.g., chloral hydrate) are used less commonly than the benzodiazepines as sedative–hypnotics (Figure 15-11).

B. Pharmacology

1. **Barbiturates** are less selective than benzodiazepines and produce generalized CNS depression.
   a. The mechanism of action is unclear. However, barbiturate binding sites have been identified on a macromolecular GABA-chloride ionophore receptor complex, and barbiturates appear to mimic or enhance GABA's inhibitory actions.
   b. Barbiturates have a wide range of dose-dependent pharmacologic actions related to CNS depression, including sedation, hypnosis, and anesthesia. They also act as potent respiratory depressants and inducers of hepatic microsomal drug-metabolizing enzyme activity.

2. **Benzodiazepine sedative–hypnotics** act in the same way as benzodiazepine anxiolytics (see VI B 1). Unlike barbiturates, they do not significantly induce hepatic microsomal drug-metabolizing enzyme activity.

3. **Piperidinediones, aldehydes,** and other nonbarbiturate sedative–hypnotics have similar pharmacologic actions related to CNS depression.
   a. Chloral hydrate is a drug of choice to induce sleep in pediatric or geriatric patients.
   b. Chloral hydrate's activity is mediated by the formation of the active metabolite trichloroethanol. Chloral hydrate induces hepatic microsomal drug-metabolizing enzyme activity.

C. Therapeutic indications

1. **Barbiturates** are no longer considered appropriate as sedative–hypnotics in view of the availability of the safer benzodiazepines.
   a. Long-acting barbiturates are widely used as antiepileptics (see VIII).
   b. Ultra–short-acting barbiturates are used for the induction of general anesthesia and as general anesthetics for short surgical procedures (see II, A, 2, C 2).

2. **Benzodiazepines** are indicated to produce drowsiness and promote sleep. They are also indicated for use as a preanesthetic medication (see II A 2, C 2), anticonvulsants (see VIII), anxiolytics (see VI), and during acute alcohol withdrawal.

3. Chloral hydrate is indicated for use as a pediatric or geriatric hypnotic, and also as a preanesthetic agent for minor surgical and dental procedures

D. Adverse effects

1. **Barbiturates** can cause a variety of adverse effects, including:
   a. CNS effects, such as drowsiness, confusion, nystagmus, dysarthria, depressed sympathetic ganglionic transmission, hyperalgesia, impaired judgment, impaired fine motor skills, paradoxic excitement (in geriatric patients), and potentiation of other CNS depressant drugs
   b. Respiratory and cardiovascular effects, such as respiratory depression, bradycardia, and orthostatic hypotension
   c. GI effects, such as nausea, vomiting, constipation, diarrhea, and epigastric distress

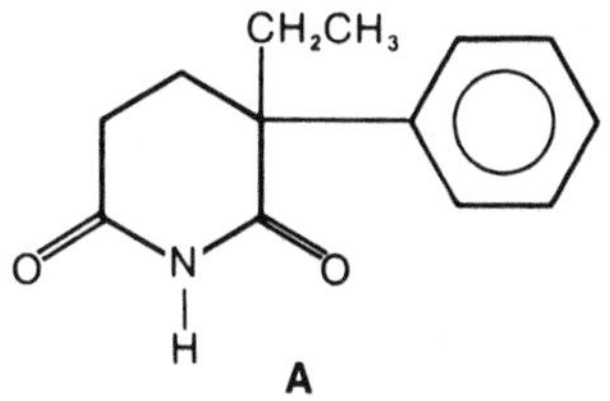

A

$Cl_3C{-}CH(OH)_2$

B

Figure 15-11. Structural formulas of (*A*) glutethimide (Doriden), a piperidinedione sedative-hypnotic, and (*B*) chloral hydrate (Noctec), an aldehyde sedative–hypnotic.

d. Exfoliative dermatitis and Stevens-Johnson syndrome
e. Headache, fever, hepatotoxicity, and megaloblastic anemia (with the chronic use of phenobarbital)

2. **Benzodiazepine sedative–hypnotics** have the same adverse effects as benzodiazepine anxiolytics (see VI D 1). In addition, they have abuse potential and can cause dependence.

3. **Chloral hydrate** has the following adverse effects:
   a. GI effects, such as GI irritation and upset, nausea, and vomiting
   b. CNS effects, such as CNS depression, disorientation, incoherence, drowsiness, ataxia, headache, and potentiation of other CNS depressants (particularly alcohol)
   c. Leukopenia

VIII. ANTIEPILEPTICS

A. Chemistry. Antiepileptics (anticonvulsants) vary widely in structure (Figure 15-12).

1. **Older agents,** which are still widely used, include derivatives of the long-acting barbiturates (e.g., phenobarbital, primidone), hydantoins (e.g., phenytoin), succinimides (e.g., ethosuximide), oxazolidinediones (e.g., trimethadione), and dialkylacetates (valproic acid).

2. Newer agents, which are more structurally diverse, include the iminostilbenes (carbamazepine), benzodiazepines (diazepam, clonazepam, clorazepate), GABA-analogue gabapentin, phenyltriazine derivative lamotrigine, and dicarbamate felbamate.

B. Pharmacology

1. Antiepileptics prevent or reduce excessive discharge and reduce the spread of excitation from CNS seizure foci.

2. The mechanisms of action of antiepileptics appear to be alteration of Na^+ neuronal concentrations by promotion of Na^+ efflux (e.g., hydantoins) and restoration or enhancement of GABA-ergic inhibitory neuronal function (e.g., barbiturates, benzodiazepines, valproic acid).

C. Therapeutic indications. These agents are generally categorized by the type of seizure against which they are effective.

1. Drugs that are indicated for the treatment of tonic–clonic (grand mal) seizures include phenobarbital, phenytoin, primidone, and carbamazepine.

2. Drugs that are indicated for the treatment of absence (petit mal) seizures include phenobarbital, ethosuximide, trimethadione, clonazepam, and valproic acid.

3. Clonazepam is indicated for the treatment of myoclonic seizures.

4. Agents that are effective against partial seizures include clorazepate, felbamate, gabapentin, and lamotrigine.

5. Phenytoin, phenobarbital, primidone, and carbamazepine are effective against psychomotor seizures.

6. Intravenous diazepam, phenytoin, and phenobarbital are indicated for the treatment of status epilepticus.

D. Adverse effects

1. **Barbiturates** (see VII D 1) and **benzodiazepines** (see VI D 1) analeptics have the same adverse effects as those compounds used as sedative–hypnotics. Intravenous use of these agents could cause cardiovascular collapse and respiratory depression.

2. All analeptics have the ability to cause these general side effects:
   a. GI irritation, nausea, and vomiting
   b. CNS sedation, diplopia, nystagmus, ataxia, dizziness, and confusion
   c. Blood dyscrasias, including aplastic anemia and bleeding disorders
   d. Allergic-type reactions, including Stevens-Johnson syndrome
   e. Various organ-systems toxicities, including renal and liver failure, pancreatitis, and cardiotoxicity

3. The hydantoins (phenytoin) can also cause specific **arrhythmias** and **gingival hyperplasia.**

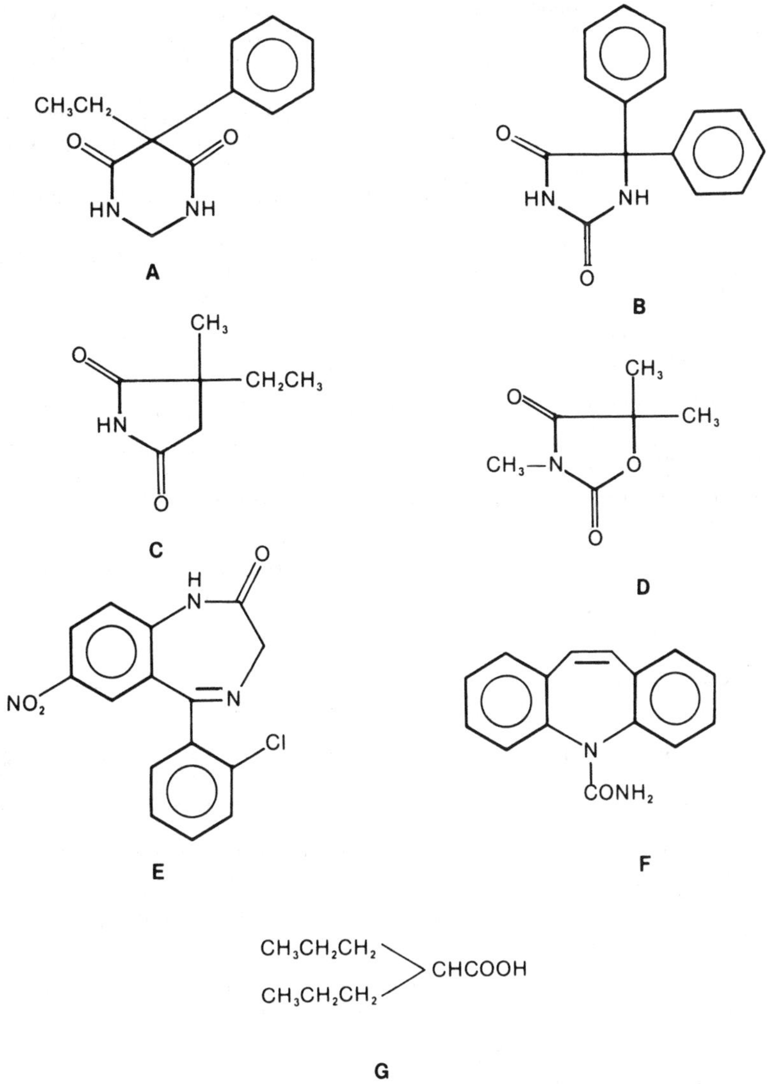

Figure 15-12. Structural formulas of the antiepileptic agents: (*A*) primidone (Mysoline), (*B*) phenytoin (Dilantin), (*C*) ethosuximide (Zarontin), (*D*) trimethadione (Tridione), (*E*) clonazepam (Klonopin), (*F*) carbamazepine (Tegretol), and (*G*) valproic acid (Depakene).

4. Analeptics as a class also have the potential to cause various **birth defects** including cleft palate (carbamazepine, phenytoin) and neural tube defects (valproic acid). These effects present a unique problem in treating pregnant women with convulsive disorders. Discontinuation of analeptic therapy can result in a seizure state that could harm the fetus. However, continued therapy can increase the risk of birth defects and place the mother at risk during delivery, due to bleeding disorders. Compounding the situation, pregnancy can either increase or decrease seizure incidence of the mother. Risk benefit evaluation of therapy should be made on individual cases based upon the patient's history.

IX. ANTIPARKINSONIAN AGENTS

A. Chemistry. The principal antiparkinsonian agents are either **anticholinergic** or **dopaminergic.**

1. **Anticholinergics** are structurally related to **atropine** (e.g., benzatropine, trihexyphenidyl) or **antihistamines** (e.g., ethopropazine). Other anticholinergics include procyclidine (Kemadrin) and biperiden (Akineton).

2. The prototypical **dopaminergic** is the **catecholamine,** levodopa (Figure 15-13). Newer dopaminergics are **ergot alkaloid derivatives** known as **ergolines** (e.g., bromocriptine (Parlodel), pergolide (Permax). There are two agents available that increase the therapeutic efficacy of levodopa.
   a. **Carbidopa,** a levodopa analogue, is a **decarboxylase inhibitor** that diminishes the decarboxylation and subsequent inactivation of levodopa in **peripheral tissues.** A combination of levodopa and carbidopa (Sinemet) is available (see Chapter 12).
   b. **Selegiline,** an **alkylpropynylphenethylamine** is a **selective MAO-B inhibitor** that inhibits the intracerebral degradation of dopamine.

B. Pharmacology. Antiparkinsonian agents act by restoring the striatal balance of dopaminergic and cholinergic neurotransmitters, which is disturbed in parkinsonism.

1. **Levodopa,** which can cross the blood–brain barrier, is the immediate precursor of the striatal inhibitory neurotransmitter dopamine and is converted to dopamine in the body.
2. **Amantadine,** an antiviral agent, appears to stimulate the release of dopamine from intact striatal dopaminergic terminals.
3. **Bromocriptine,** a dopaminergic receptor agonist, mimics the activity of striatal dopamine.
4. **Selegiline,** an inhibitor of the central MAO-B isoenzyme, blocks the central catabolism of dopamine, increasing its availability in the basal ganglia.
5. **Anticholinergics,** such as trihexyphenidyl and benztropine, block the excitatory cholinergic striatal system.
6. **Antihistamines,** such as diphenhydramine, possess anticholinergic properties.

C. Therapeutic indications

1. **Levodopa** is indicated to treat idiopathic, postencephalitic, or arteriosclerotic parkinsonism.
2. **Amantadine** is indicated to treat idiopathic, postencephalitic, or arteriosclerotic parkinsonism, as well as extrapyramidal symptoms induced by antipsychotic drugs (with the exception of tardive dyskinesia).
3. **Bromocriptine** is indicated to treat idiopathic or postencephalitic parkinsonism.
4. **Selegiline, anticholinergics,** and **antihistamines** are indicated for use as adjunctive therapy for all types of parkinsonism, including drug-induced extrapyramidal symptoms (with the exception of tardive dyskinesia).

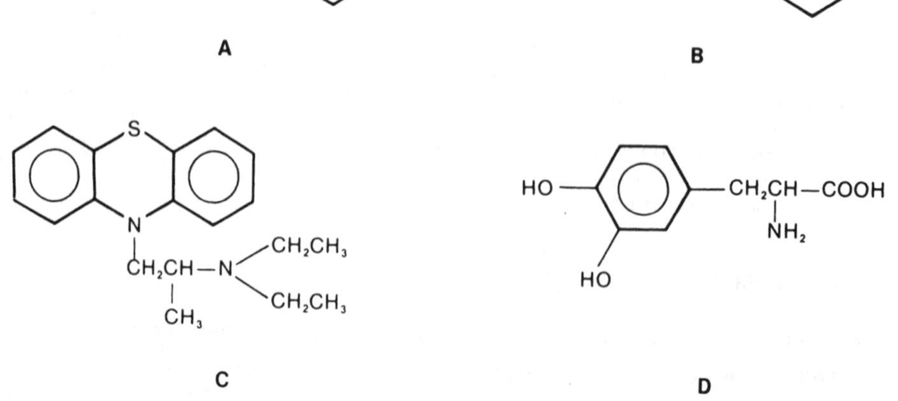

Figure 15-13. Structural formulas of antiparkinsonian agents: (*A*) benztropine (Cogentin), (*B*) trihexyphenidyl (Artane), (*C*) ethopropazine (Parsidol), and (*D*) levodopa (Larodopa).

D. Adverse effects

1. **Levodopa** is associated with these adverse effects:
   a. GI effects, such as GI upset, nausea, vomiting, anorexia, and excessive salivation
   b. Cardiovascular effects, such as orthostatic hypotension, tachycardia, and dysrhythmias
   c. CNS effects, such as headache, dizziness, and insomnia
   d. Abnormal involuntary movements, such as dyskinesia and choreiform or dystonic movements
   e. Psychiatric effects, such as delusions, hallucinations, confusion, psychoses, and depression

2. **Amantadine** is associated with these adverse effects:
   a. CNS effects, such as drowsiness, insomnia, dizziness, slurred speech, and nightmares
   b. Urinary retention and ankle edema
   c. Livedo reticularis (mottling of skin on the extremities)
   d. Psychiatric effects, such as hallucinations and confusion

3. **Bromocriptine** is associated with these adverse effects:
   a. Nausea
   b. Hypotension
   c. Psychiatric effects, such as confusion and hallucinations
   d. Livedo reticularis
   e. Abnormal involuntary movements, such as dyskinesia and choreiform or dystonic movements

4. **Selegiline** is associated with adverse effects that are similar to those of bromocriptine, including dyskinesias and hallucinations.

5. Anticholinergic antiparkinsonian agents have the same adverse effects as other cholinergic antagonists (see Chapter 14).

6. Antihistaminic antiparkinsonian agents have the same adverse effects as other antihistamines (see Chapter 16).

X. OPIOID ANALGESICS consist of natural opiate alkaloids and their synthetic derivatives.

A. Chemistry. The opiate alkaloids are derived from opium, which is considered the oldest drug on record. **Opium** (the dried exudate of the poppy seed capsule) contains about 25 different alkaloids. Of these, morphine is the most important, both quantitatively and pharmacologically (Figure 15-14).

1. The **morphine molecule** can be altered in a variety of ways; related compounds also can be synthesized from other starting materials.

2. Morphine's **phenolic hydroxyl group** is extremely important; however, analgesic activity appears to depend on a *p*-phenyl-*N*-alkylpiperidine moiety, in which the piperidine ring is in the chair form and is perpendicular to the aromatic ring. The alkyl group is usually methyl. Morphine's amphoteric character (phenolic hydroxyl and tertiary amine) contributes to its erratic absorption when administered orally.

3. The **piperidine moiety** of morphine is common to most opioid analgesics, including the morphine analogues (e.g., codeine, heroin, hydromorphone, oxycodone) and the piperidines (meperidine, diphenoxylate). The methadones (e.g., methadone, propoxyphene) appear to assume a pseudopiperidine ring configuration in the body (Figure 15-15).

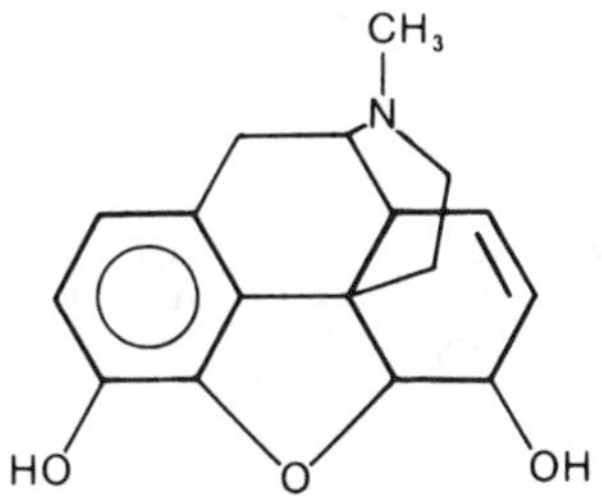

Figure 15-14. Structural formula of morphine.

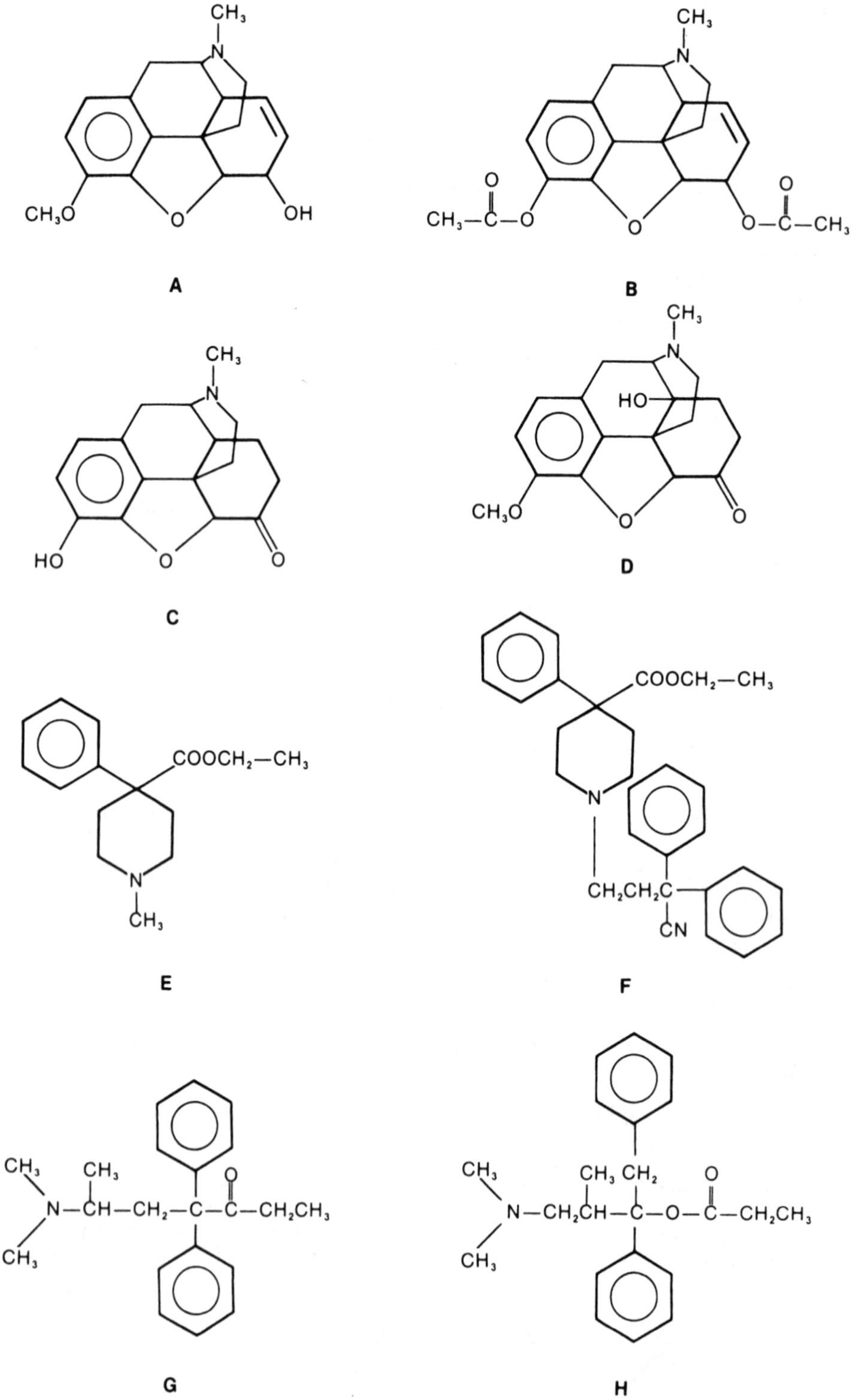

Figure 15-15. Structural formulas of selected opioid agonists, including (*A*) codeine, (*B*) heroin, (*C*) hydromorphone (Dilaudid), and (*D*) oxycodone (Percodan), morphine analogues; (*E*) meperidine (Demerol) and (*F*) diphenoxylate (Lomotil), piperidine analgesics; and (*G*) methadone (Dolophine) and (*H*) propoxyphene (Darvon), methadone analgesics.

4. **Newer agents,** chemically unrelated to the natural, semisynthetic, and synthetic opium derivatives, include **tramadol.**

B. Pharmacology

1. Opioid analgesics mimic endogenous enkephalins and endorphins at CNS opiate receptors, raising the pain threshold and increasing pain tolerance.
2. Opioid analgesics also cause chemoreceptor trigger zone stimulation and decrease α_1-adrenergic receptor responsiveness.
3. Tramadol acts specifically at the μ opioid receptors and also inhibits reuptake of norepinephrine and serotonin.

C. Therapeutic indications. Opioid analgesics are indicated to relieve moderate-to-severe pain, such as the pain associated with myocardial infarction. They are used also as preanesthetic medications, analgesic adjuncts during anesthesia, antitussives, and antidiarrheals.

D. Adverse effects. Opioid analgesics are associated with these adverse effects:

1. CNS effects, including CNS depression, miosis, dizziness, sedation, confusion, disorientation, and coma
2. GI effects, including nausea, vomiting, constipation, biliary spasm, and increased biliary tract pressure
3. Cardiovascular effects, such as orthostatic hypotension, peripheral circulatory collapse, dysrhythmias, and cardiac arrest
4. Respiratory depression
5. Bronchoconstriction
6. Psychiatric effects, such as euphoria, dysphoria, and hallucinations
7. Abuse potential and dependence
8. Precipitation of withdrawal symptoms in opioid-dependent patients (when opioid agonist–antagonists, such as pentazocine or nalbuphine, are used as analgesics)
9. Classic opioid analgesics can also prompt the release of histamine, causing intense pruritus, vasodilation, and bronchoconstriction, that can be confused with a true allergic reaction.
10. Tramadol appears to have significantly less respiratory depressant effects that the classic opioids. It also does not appear to cause the release of histamine. It has less cardiovascular effects with the exception of orthostatic hypotension, which is produced. Tramadol does possess the typical μ-mediated side effects of constipation, nausea, vomiting, and sedation.

XI. OPIOID ANTAGONISTS

A. Chemistry. Replacement of the *N*-methyl group of morphine or a morphine derivative (see X A) with an allyl or cycloalkyl group results in drugs that are pure opioid antagonists (e.g., naloxone, naltrexone, nalmefene) or mixed opioid agonists-antagonists (e.g., pentazocine, butorphanol, buprenorphine, nalbuphine) [Figure 15-16].

B. Pharmacology

1. The pure opioid antagonist naloxone reverses or prevents the effects of opioids but has no opioid-receptor agonist activity.
2. The mixed opioid agonist–antagonist pentazocine has both opioid agonistic actions (e.g., analgesia, sedation, respiratory depression) and weak opioid antagonistic activity.

C. Therapeutic indications

1. Pure opioid antagonists are used as antidotes to reverse the adverse effects of opioid agonists or opioid agonist–antagonists (e.g., respiratory depression, cardiovascular depression, sedation). Naltrexone is the only orally active compound that possesses pure antagonistic activity. It is also used in the treatment of opioid addiction.

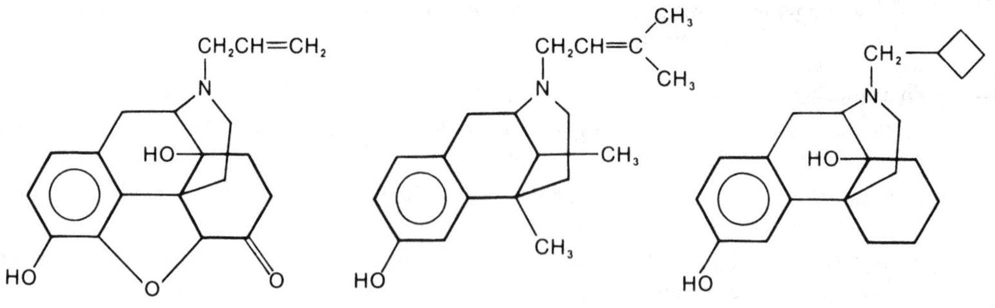

A B C

Figure 15-16. Structural formulas of opioid antagonists: (*A*) naloxone (Narcan), (*B*) pentazocine (Talwin), and (*C*) butorphanol (Stadol).

2. The mixed agonist–antagonists are used as analgesics.

D. Adverse effects

1. Pure opioid antagonists can precipitate withdrawal syndrome in opioid-dependent patients. Pure antagonists, given in the absence of opioid agonists or agonists–antagonists, produce no clinically significant effects.

2. In the absence of opioids, mixed agonist–antagonists produce opioid-like effects, such as respiratory depression (see X D).

STUDY QUESTIONS

Directions: Each of the numbered items or incomplete statements in this section is followed by answers or by completions of the statement. Select the **one** lettered answer or completion that is **best** in each case.

1. Which of the following drugs is a volatile substance that is administered by inhalation?

(A) Thiopental
(B) Halothane
(C) Alprazolam
(D) Buspirone
(E) Phenytoin

2. The structure of prochlorperazine is shown below. Which of the following medications, because of its chemical relationship to prochlorperazine, would most likely cause similar side effects?

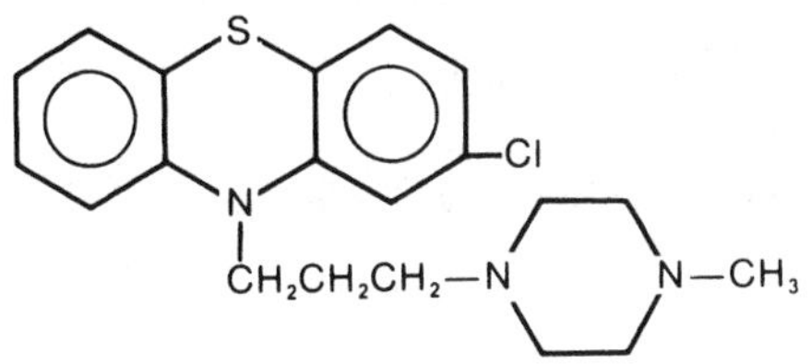

(A) Fluphenazine
(B) Thioridazine
(C) Alprazolam
(D) Buspirone
(E) Pentobarbital

3. The brief duration of action of an ultra–short-acting barbiturate is due to a

(A) slow rate of metabolism in the liver
(B) low lipid solubility, resulting in a minimal concentration in the brain
(C) high degree of binding to plasma proteins
(D) rapid rate of redistribution from the brain due to its high liposolubility
(E) slow rate of excretion by the kidneys

4. Which of the following mechanisms of action most likely contributes to the treatment of parkinsonism?

(A) The direct-acting dopaminergic agonist amantadine mimics the activity of striatal dopamine
(B) The antimuscarinic activity of diphenhydramine contributes to the restoration of striatal dopaminergic-cholinergic neurotransmitter balance
(C) Striatal H_1-receptors are blocked by the antihistaminic trihexyphenidyl
(D) The ergoline bromocriptine stimulates the release of striatal dopamine from intact terminals
(E) The ability of dopamine to cross the blood-brain barrier allows it to restore striatal dopaminergic-cholinergic neurotransmitter balance

5. All of the following adverse effects are associated with the use of levodopa EXCEPT

(A) sialorrhea
(B) orthostatic hypotension
(C) delusions, confusion, and depression
(D) dyskinesia and dystonia
(E) livedo reticularis

6. The activity of which of the following drugs is dependent upon a *p*-phenyl-*N*-alkylpiperidine moiety?

(A) Phenobarbital
(B) Chlorpromazine
(C) Diazepam
(D) Imipramine
(E) Meperidine

7. Opioids are used as all of the following agents EXCEPT

(A) antitussives
(B) analgesics
(C) anti-inflammatories
(D) antidiarrheals
(E) preanesthetic medications

8. Which of the following agents would not be an alternative to phenobarbital in the treatment of partial seizures?

(A) Trimethadione
(B) Gabapentin
(C) Felbamate
(D) Lamotrigine
(E) None of the above

Directions: Each question below contains three suggested answers of which **one or more** is correct. Choose the answer

A if **I only** is correct
B if **III only** is correct
C if **I and II** are correct
D if **II and III** are correct
E if **I, II, and III** are correct

9. Improper administration of local anesthetics can cause toxic plasma concentrations that may result in

I. seizures and central nervous system (CNS) depression
II. respiratory and myocardial depression
III. circulatory collapse

10. In addition to their anxiolytic properties, benzodiazepines are indicated for use

I. as preanesthetic medications
II. as anticonvulsants
III. during acute withdrawal from alcohol

Directions: Each group of items in this section consists of lettered options followed by a set of numbered items. For each item, select the **one** lettered option that is most closely associated with it. Each lettered option may be selected once, more than once, or not at all.

Questions 11–13

For each statement below, choose the drug that it most closely describes.

(A) Tranylcypromine
(B) Imipramine
(C) Buspirone
(D) Trazodone
(E) Phenelzine

11. An anxiolytic drug that does not possess either hypnotic or anticonvulsant properties

12. A prototype tricyclic antidepressant with antimuscarinic properties that make it useful in the treatment of enuresis

13. An antidepressant that inhibits serotonin reuptake and may cause adverse effects such as impaired memory, akathisia, and menstrual irregularities

Questions 14–16

For each of the following structures, select the most appropriate pharmacologic category.

(A) General anesthetic
(B) Local anesthetic
(C) Antidepressant
(D) Anxiolytic
(E) Opioid antagonist

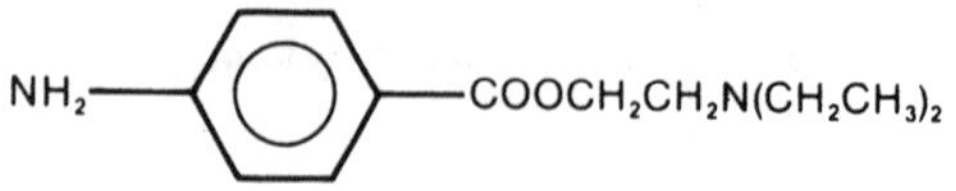

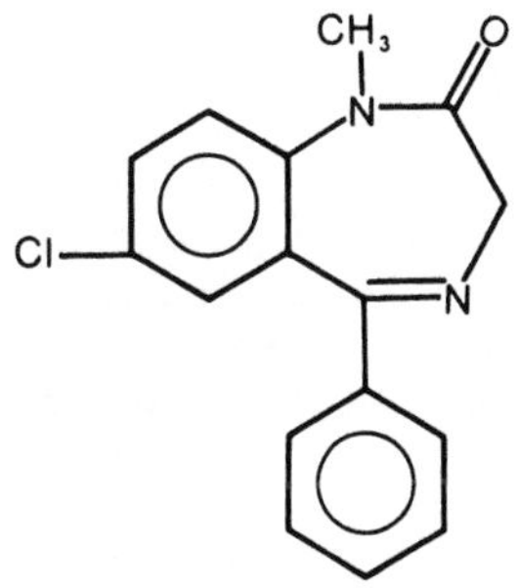

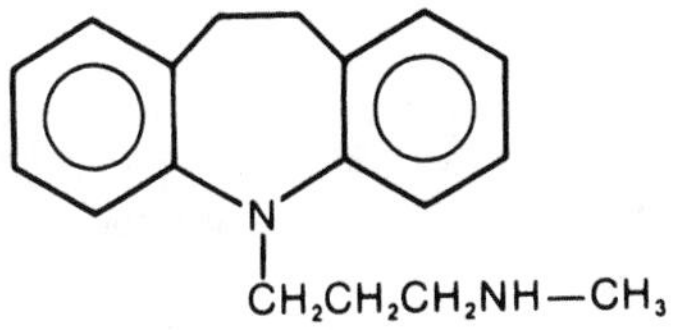

Questions 17–19

A 38-year-old man has a history of affective disorders including schizophrenia, depression, obsessive-compulsive disorder, and situational anxiety. His past medications include thiothixene, chlorpromazine, amitriptyline, and diazepam. His current medication profile includes the following drugs (used to answer the questions below).

A. Clozapine
B. Fluoxetine
C. Buspirone
D. Risperidone

17. Which agent is most likely being used to treat his schizophrenic psychosis?

18. Which agent is most likely being used to treat OCD?

19. Which agent would NOT be likely to cause tardive dyskinesia with chronic use?

ANSWERS AND EXPLANATIONS

1. The answer is B *[II A 1].*
The general anesthetics are divided into two major classes of drugs: those that are gases or volatile liquids, which are administered by inhalation, and those that are nonvolatile salts, which are administered as intravenous solutions. Halothane is a halogenated hydrocarbon, which belongs to the former class. It has the advantage over older volatile anesthetics (e.g., ethyl ether, cyclopropane) of being nonflammable. Thiopental sodium, alprazolam, buspirone, and phenytoin are all nonvolatile substances that are administered orally or parenterally. Thiopental is a general anesthetic and is sometimes referred to as a basal anesthetic because it does not produce significant third-stage surgical anesthesia. Alprazolam and buspirone are anxiolytics, whereas phenytoin is an anticonvulsant.

2. The answer is A *[IV A 1; Table 15-1].*
Fluphenazine, like prochlorperazine, is a piperazinyl phenothiazine antipsychotic and would be likely to cause similar side effects. Whereas thioridazine is also a phenothiazine antipsychotic, it is a piperidyl derivative rather than a piperazinyl derivative. Alprazolam, phenytoin, and pentobarbital are not phenothiazines; therefore, structurally, they are not similar to prochlorperazine.

3. The answer is D *[VII A 1 c, d; Figure 15-1].*
Ultra–short-acting barbiturates are characterized by having branched or unsaturated 5,5-side chains and by having a sulfur atom in place of oxygen in the 2 position of the barbituric acid molecule. These modifications of barbituric acid result in an extremely liposoluble molecule that is very soluble in lipid tissues. After administration, an ultra–short-acting barbiturate readily crosses the blood–brain barrier but then is quickly redistributed into extracerebral tissue, resulting in a rapid loss of activity. Whereas these agents do remain in the body for a long time and seem to have slow rates of metabolism and excretion, their long retention time is due more to their slow rate of leaching out of lipid tissue.

4. The answer is B *[IX B].*
The H_1 antagonist diphenhydramine possesses antimuscarinic activity, which allows it to be of use in the restoration of striatal dopaminergic–cholinergic neurotransmitter balance. Amantadine appears to stimulate the release of striatal dopamine; it does not mimic the action of dopamine. Trihexyphenidyl is an antimuscarinic agent, not antihistaminic; it blocks cholinergic, not H_1, receptors. Bromocriptine is a dopaminergic agonist and mimics the activity of striatal dopamine. The neurotransmitter dopamine is not able to cross the blood–brain barrier and is, therefore, not effective as an antiparkinsonian drug.

5. The answer is E *[IX D 1].*
Livedo reticularis is a circulatory disorder characterized by large, bluish areas on the extremities. It is an adverse effect associated with the use of amantadine and bromocriptine but not with the use of levodopa.

6. The answer is E *[X A 2, 3; Figure 15-15, E].*
The *p*-phenyl-*N*-alkylpiperidine moiety is common to the structurally specific opioid analgesics. Meperidine is an opioid analgesic and is an *N*-methyl-*p*-phenylpiperidine derivative. Its chemical name is ethyl 1-methyl-4-phenylpiperidine-4-carboxylate. Phenobarbital is a barbiturate sedative. Chlorpromazine is a phenothiazine antipsychotic. Diazepam is a benzodiazepine anxiolytic. Imipramine is a tricyclic dibenzazepine antidepressant.

7. The answer is C *[X C].*
Unlike the salicylates, opioids do not possess anti-inflammatory activity. Opioids do suppress the cough reflex and are preeminent analgesics. Opioids cause constipation and are, thus, effective antidiarrheal agents. When used as preanesthetic medication, opioids permit a reduction in the amount of general anesthetic required for surgical anesthesia.

8. The answer is A *[VIII A 1, C 2].*
Whereas many analeptics are useful in controlling more than one seizure type, trimethadione is effective primarily against absence seizures. Additionally, its side effect profile is more extensive than the newer agents (lamotrigine, gabapentin, felbamate) that are effective in treating partial seizures.

9. The answer is E (all) *[III D 2].*
Careful administration of a local anesthetic by a knowledgeable practitioner is essential to prevent sys-

temic absorption and consequent toxicity. This is especially important when the patient has cardiovascular disease, poorly controlled diabetes, thyrotoxicosis, or peripheral vascular disease.

10. The answer is E (all) *[VII C 2].*
Benzodiazepines can serve as induction agents for general anesthesia; they also have anxiolytic properties. In addition, intravenous diazepam is used to treat status epilepticus, whereas clonazepam is used orally for myoclonic and absence (petit mal) seizures. Benzodiazepines also diminish alcohol withdrawal symptoms.

11–13. The answers are: 11-C *[VI B 2],* **12-B** *[V C 2],* **13-D** *[V B 3, D 3].*
Buspirone's mechanism of anxiolytic action is unknown. Unlike the benzodiazepines, buspirone lacks hypnotic and anticonvulsant properties. The tricyclic antidepressant imipramine is useful in the treatment of enuresis because the compound blocks muscarinic receptors mediating micturition. Trazodone is categorized as an atypical antidepressant that selectively blocks serotonin re-uptake.

14–16. The answers are: 14-B *[III A; Figure 15-2],* **15-D** *[VI A; Table 15-2],* **16-C** *[V A 2; Figure 15-6].*
The structure shown in question 14 is that of procaine, which is a diethylaminoethyl *p*-aminobenzoate ester. It contains a hydrophilic amino group in the alcohol portion of the molecule and a lipophilic aromatic acid connected by the ester linkage. The procaine molecule is typical of ester-type local anesthetics.

The structure in question 15 is that of diazepam, which has a benzo-1,4-diazepine as its base nucleus. The widely used benzo-1,4-diazepine derivatives have significant anxiolytic, hypnotic, and anticonvulsant activities.

The structure in question 16 is that of desipramine, which has a dibenzazepine as its base nucleus. Dibenzazepine derivatives that have a methyl- or dimethylaminopropyl group attached to the ring nitrogen have significant antidepressant activity. Similarly substituted dibenzocycloheptadienes also have antidepressant activity. Together these two chemical classes make up the majority of the tricyclic antidepressants.

17. The answer is A *[IV C].*
Clozapine, while therapeutically defined as a general antipsychotic, is used almost exclusively in the treatment of schizophrenia.

18. The answer is B *[V A 3, C 2].*
Fluoxetine is most likely being used in this patient in an attempt to treat his depression and obsessive-compulsive disorder with the same drug. Clinical trials have shown fluoxetine to improve both situations. The use of a single agent for both conditions will minimize the risk of drug–drug interactions, as well as reduce the chances for adverse effects.

19. The answer is B *[IV D 1, V D 3, VI B 2, D 2].*
Fluoxetine is the only agent that does not interfere directly with the dopaminergic system. Clozapine and risperidone are classical antipsychotics, a class that is closely associated with the development of tardive dyskinesia with long-term therapy. Buspirone, an anxiolytic, also acts through the dopaminergic system and can cause this side effect with chronic therapy.

16
Autacoids and Their Antagonists, Non-narcotic Analgesic–Antipyretics, and Nonsteroidal Anti-inflammatory Drugs

David C. Kosegarten
Edward F. LaSala
Scott F. Long

I. INTRODUCTION

A. **Autacoids,** also called autopharmacologic agents or local hormones, have widely differing structures and pharmacologic actions. The two most important autacoids are **histamine** and the **prostaglandins.** Their antagonists also have important pharmacologic roles.

B. **Non-narcotic analgesic–antipyretics** have dissimilar structures but share certain therapeutic actions, including relief of pain, fever, and sometimes inflammation. They appear to work by inhibiting synthesis of prostaglandins and related autacoids.

C. **Nonsteroidal anti-inflammatory drugs (NSAIDs)** differ in structure and activity from the non-narcotic analgesic–antipyretics, but they all have anti-inflammatory properties and appear to inhibit prostaglandin synthesis.

II. AUTACOIDS AND THEIR ANTAGONISTS

A. Histamine and antihistaminics

1. **Chemistry**
   a. **Histamine** (Figure 16-1) is a bioamine derived principally from dietary histidine, which is decarboxylated by L-histidine decarboxylase.
   b. **Antihistaminics** (histamine antagonists) can be classified as **H_1-receptor antagonists** or **H_2-receptor antagonists.**
      (1) **H_1-receptor antagonists,** the classic antihistaminic agents, are chemically classified as **ethylenediamines** (e.g., tripelennamine), **alkylamines** (e.g., chlorpheniramine), **ethanolamines** (e.g., diphenhydramine), **piperazines** (e.g., cyclizine), **phenothiazines** (e.g., promethazine), and **piperidines** (e.g. cyproheptadine). Less sedating, second-generation antihistaminics currently available include astemizole, loratadine, and terfenadine (Figure 16-2).
      (2) **H_2-receptor antagonists** are heterocyclic congeners of histamine. These include cimetidine, ranitidine, famotidine, and nizatidine (Figure 16-3).
      (3) **Alternatives** to the H_2-receptor antagonists include omeprazole and lansoprazole, **specific inhibitors of H^+,K^+-ATPase,** the ultimate mediator of gastric acid secretion. Structurally, these agents are substituted benzimidazoles linked to a pyridine ring by a sulfinyl bridge that is required for H^+,K^+-ATPase inhibition.
2. **Pharmacology**
   a. **Histamine** has powerful pharmacologic actions, mediated by two specific receptor types (Table 16-1).

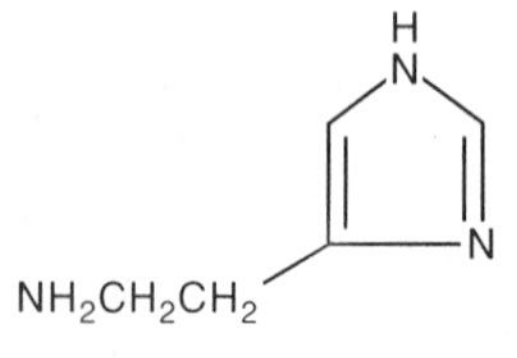

Figure 16-1. Structural formula of histamine, an autacoid.

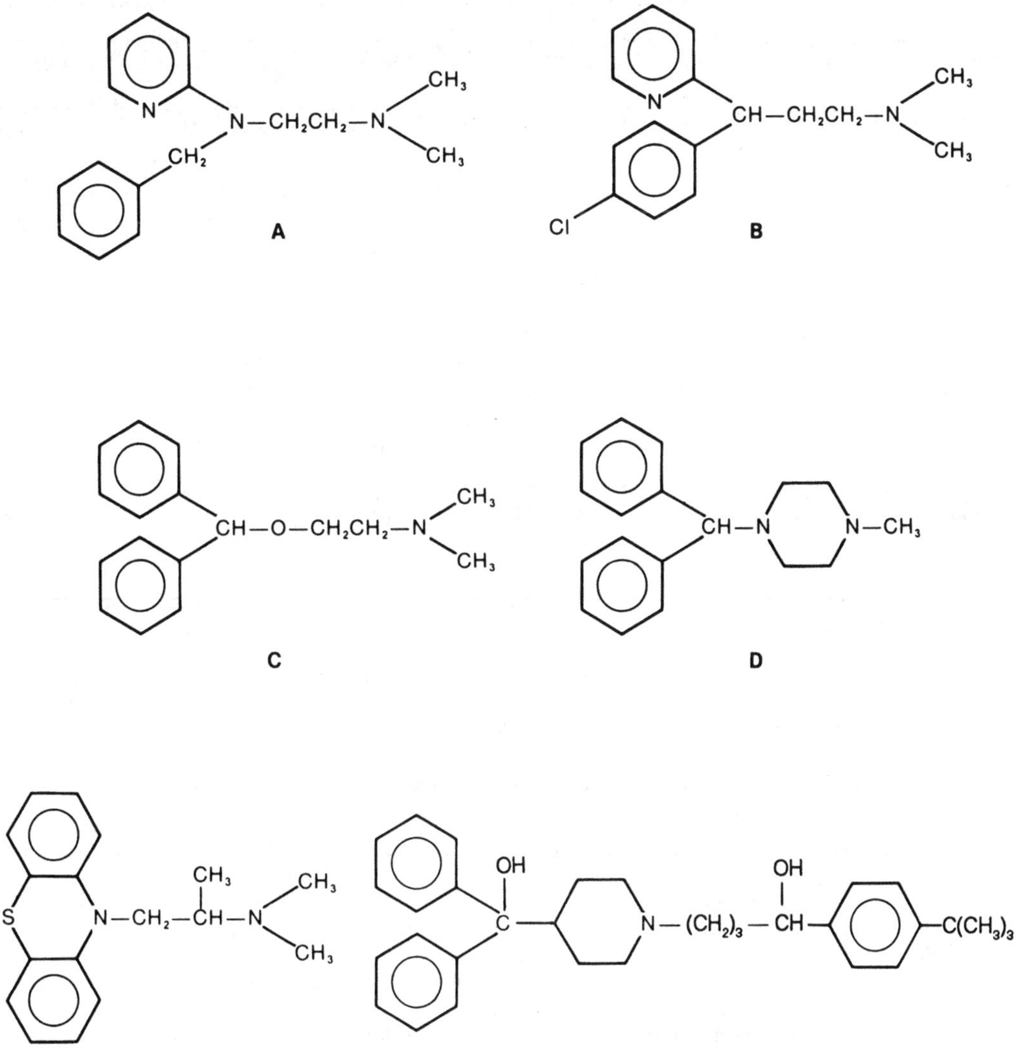

Figure 16-2. Structural formulas of (*A*) tripelennamine (Pyribenzamine), (*B*) chlorpheniramine (Chlor-Trimeton), (*C*) diphenhydramine (Benadryl), (*D*) cyclizine (Marezine), (*E*) promethazine (Phenergan), (*F*) terfenadine (Seldane), H_1-receptor antagonists.

(1) **H_1-receptors mediate** typical allergic and anaphylactic responses to histamine, such as bronchoconstriction, vasodilation, increased capillary permeability, and spasmodic contractions of gastrointestinal (GI) smooth muscle.

(2) **H_2-receptors mediate** other responses to histamine, such as increased secretion of gastric acid, pepsin, and Castle's factor (also known as intrinsic factor).

b. H_1-receptor antagonists competitively block H_1-receptors, thus limiting the histamine's effects on bronchial smooth muscle, capillaries, and GI smooth muscle. These antago-

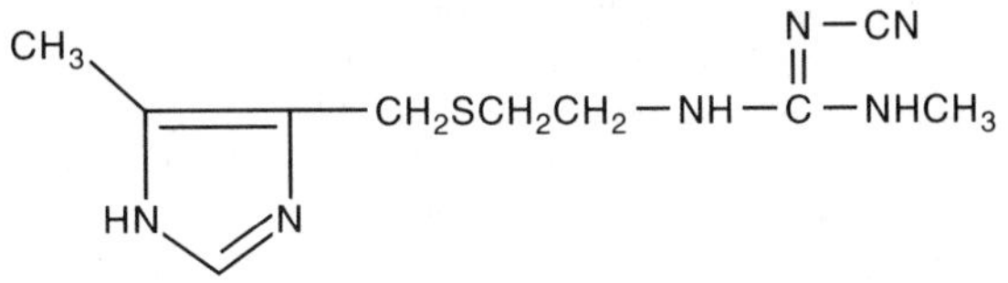

Figure 16-3. Structural formula of cimetidine, and H_2-receptor antagonist.

Table 16-1. Selected Actions of Endogenous Histamine

Site	Action	Receptor Type
Cardiovascular		
Vascular	Arterial contraction	H_1
	Arteriolar relaxation	H_1 and H_2
	Venule contraction	H_1
	Venule relaxation	H_2
	Endothelial cells, release of EDRF	H_1
	Endothelial cells, contraction	H_1
Heart	Increased heart rate	H_2
	Increased force of contraction	H_2
	Slowed atrioventricular conduction	H_1
Respiratory		
	Bronchiolar smooth muscle contraction	H_1
Gastrointestinal		
Gastric mucosa	Increased secretion of acid and pepsin	H_2
Gastrointestinal smooth muscle	Contraction	H_1
Various		
Cutaneous nerve endings	Pain and itch	H_1

EDRF = Endothelium-derived relaxing factor.

nists also prevent histamine-induced pain and itching of the skin and mucous membranes.

c. **H_2-receptor antagonists** competitively block H_2-receptors, thus limiting the effects of histamine on gastric secretions.

d. A new **antisecretory agent, omeprazole,** inhibits the proton pump H^+,K^+-ATPase.

3. **Therapeutic indications**

a. **Exogenous histamine** can be used as a **diagnostic agent** for testing gastric function. However, other stimulants of gastric secretion are more suitable and safer.

b. **H_1-receptor antagonists** are used to provide symptomatic relief of **allergic symptoms,** such as seasonal rhinitis and conjunctivitis. Their antihistaminic effects also make them useful for symptomatic relief of urticaria.

c. **H_2-receptor antagonists** are used to treat **gastric hypersecretory** conditions, such as duodenal ulcer and Zollinger-Ellison syndrome.

d. The **proton pump inhibitor,** omeprazole, is used to treat **duodenal ulcers.**

4. **Adverse effects**

a. **Histamine** may cause numerous adverse effects related to its basic pharmacology (see II A 2 a).

b. **H_1-receptor antagonists** are associated with the following **adverse effects:**

(1) Central nervous system (CNS) effects, such as CNS depression, sedation, fatigue, tinnitus, hallucinations, and ataxia

(2) GI effects, such as nausea and vomiting

(3) Antimuscarinic effects, such as dry mouth, urinary retention, and constipation

(4) Teratogenic effects (possible with piperazine compounds)

c. **Peripheral H_1-receptor antagonists,** terfenadine and astemizole, are devoid of significant sedative and antimuscarinic effects. However, elevated plasma levels of both astemizole and terfenadine have been associated with electrocardiographic QT prolongation, cardiac arrest, torsades de pointes, and other ventricular arrhythmias. Moreover, concomitant use of terfenadine with the antifungal ketoconazole or the macrolide antibiotics, erythromycin and troleandomycin, is contraindicated because such a combination results in significantly elevated terfenadine plasma levels.

d. **H_2-receptor antagonists** are associated with these adverse effects:

(1) CNS effects, such as confusion and dizziness

(2) Hepatic and renal dysfunction

(3) Inhibition of the hepatic microsomal drug-metabolizing enzyme system (with cimetidine)

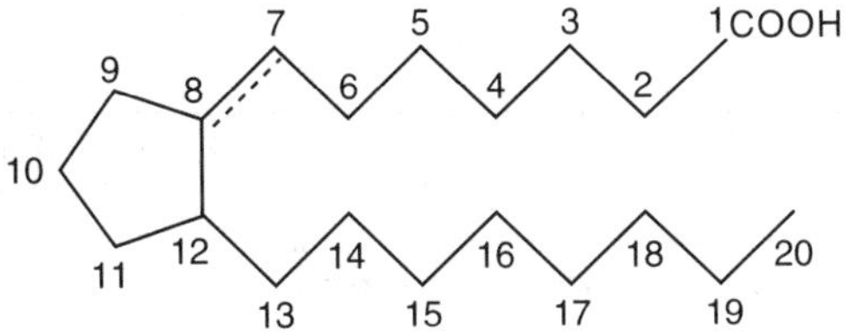

Figure 16-4. Structural formula of prostanoic acid from which the prostaglandins are derived.

(4) Androgenic effects (with high doses of cimetidine), such as impotence and gynecomastia in men and galactorrhea in women

e. The **H^+,K^+-ATPase inhibitors** have been reported to cause diarrhea, GI pain, and headache as their most frequent adverse effects. Additionally, they may interfere with the metabolism of diazepam, warfarin, phenytoin, and theophylline.

B. Prostaglandins

1. Chemistry

a. Prostaglandins are **derivatives** of prostanoic acid, a 20-carbon fatty acid containing a 5-carbon ring (Figure 16-4). In the body, prostaglandins are principally synthesized from arachidonic acid, a component of membrane phospholipids.

b. **Classification** of prostaglandins as prostaglandin A (PGA), prostaglandin B (PGB), prostaglandin E (PGE), and so forth relates to the presence or absence of keto or hydroxyl groups at positions 9 and 11 (see Figure 16-4). Subscripts relate to the number and position of double bonds in the aliphatic chains (Figure 16-5).

2. Pharmacology

a. **Endogenous** prostaglandins appear to affect every body function. They are released in response to many chemical, bacterial, mechanical, and other insults, and they appear to contribute to the signs and symptoms of the inflammatory process, including pain and edema.

b. **Physiologic responses** to prostaglandins include vasodilatation in most vascular beds, although vasoconstriction can occur in isolated areas. PGEs inhibit platelet aggregation, relax bronchial and GI smooth muscle, contract uterine smooth muscle, and (along with PGI) inhibit gastric acid secretion. Alternatively, PGDs and PGFs contract bronchial and GI smooth muscle. Prostaglandins also increase renal blood flow, promote diuresis, natriuresis, and kaliuresis, but paradoxically increase renin secretion. They also possess diverse endocrine and metabolic effects.

3. Therapeutic indications

a. **PGE_1 analogues**

(1) **Alprostadil (Prostin VR Pediatric)** is used for temporary maintenance of a patent ductus arteriosus in awaiting corrective surgery for congenital heart defects.

(2) **Alprostadil (Caverject)** is used in treating impotence due to erectile dysfunction.

(3) **Misoprostol (Cytotec)** is used for the prevention of NSAID-induced GI ulcers (see Figure 16-5).

b. **PGE_2 analogues and derivatives, dinoprostone (Prostin E_2, Prepidil, Cervidil) and carboprost (Hemabate),** are used for their abortifacient effects and to induce cervical "ripening" in pregnancy.

4. **Adverse effects** associated with PGE include:

a. CNS effects, such as CNS irritability, fever, seizures, and headache

b. Cardiovascular effects, such as hypotension, dysrhythmias, vasodilation, and flushing and cardiac arrest

c. Respiratory effects, such as respiratory depression and distress

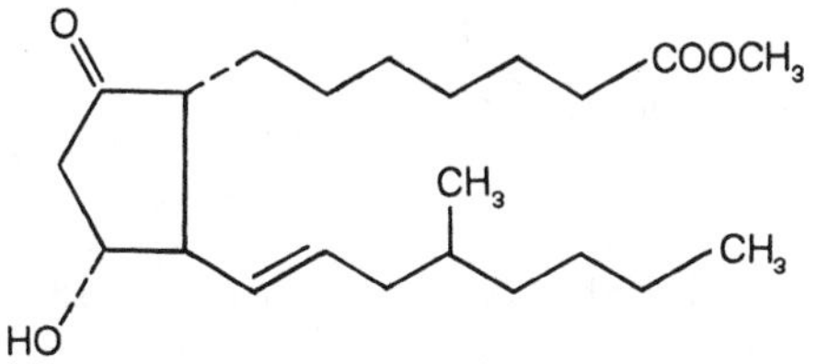

Figure 16-5. Structural formula of misoprostol (Cytotec), a derivative of prostaglandin E_1 (PGE_1).

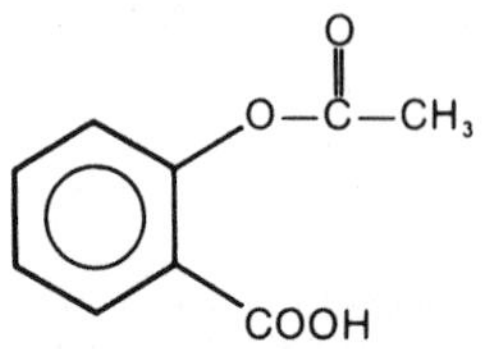

Figure 16-6. Structural formula of aspirin, the prototypical salicylate analgesic-antipyretic.

d. Hematologic effects, such as anemia, thrombocytopenia, and disseminated intravascular coagulation (DIC)
e. Diarrhea
f. Decreased renal function
g. Spotty bleeding and menstrual irregularities, abortion, and penile pain

III. NON-NARCOTIC ANALGESIC–ANTIPYRETICS AND NSAIDS

A. Salicylates

1. Chemistry

a. Salicylates are **derivatives of salicylic acid,** which is found as the glycoside salicin in willow bark. The prototypical drug is **aspirin,** the acetyl ester of salicylic acid (Figure 16-6). A simple ester, aspirin hydrolyzes easily, is unstable in aqueous media and is affected by moisture.

b. More stable salicylates include **diflunisal** and the topical agent **methyl salicylate** (wintergreen oil) [Figure 16-7].

c. Most salicylates are **weak acids.** Their excretion is influenced by changes in urinary pH.

2. Pharmacology

a. Salicylates **inhibit** the enzyme cyclooxygenase and, thus, inhibit local prostaglandin synthesis (see II B 2 a). As a result, they are analgesic for low-intensity integumental pain, antipyretic, and anti-inflammatory.

b. Salicylates also **block** platelet cyclooxygenase and subsequent formation of thromboxane A_2. As a result, they inhibit platelet aggregation and eventual thrombus formation.

3. Therapeutic indications

a. Salicylates are indicated for use as:

(1) Analgesics, for relief of skeletal muscle pain, headache, neuralgias, myalgias, and spasmodic dysmenorrhea

(2) Anti-inflammatory agents, for relief of rheumatoid arthritis symptoms and acute rheumatic fever

(3) Antipyretic agents, for relief of fever. (Children with varicella or influenza-type viral infections should not be given salicylates because of the observed association between salicylate use in these situations and Reye's syndrome.)

b. Aspirin is also indicated for **prophylaxis of myocardial infarction.**

c. Methyl salicylate (wintergreen oil) is used topically as a **counter irritant.**

4. Adverse effects

a. Salicylates are associated with the following effects:

(1) GI effects, such as nausea, vomiting, and GI irritation, discomfort, ulceration, and hemorrhage

(2) Increased depth of respirations

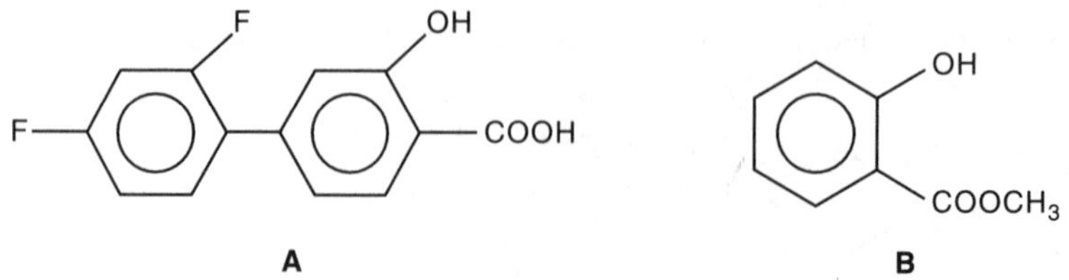

Figure 16-7. Structural formulas of (*A*) diflunisal (Dolobid) and (*B*) methyl salicylate (wintergreen oil), salicylate derivatives.

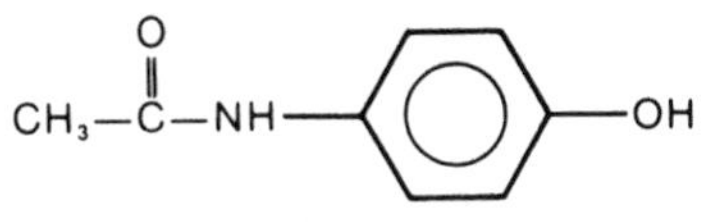

Figure 16-8. Structural formula of acetaminophen, the prototypical *p*-aminophenol derivative.

(3) Antagonism of vitamin K with associated hypoprothrombinemia
(4) Uncoupling of oxidative phosphorylation, hyperglycemia, glycosuria, and reduced lipogenesis
(5) Delayed onset of labor
(6) Salicylism (salicylate toxicity, usually marked by tinnitus, nausea, and vomiting)

b. Low daily doses of salicylates (2 g) decrease renal urate excretion and increase serum uric acid levels. **High daily doses** (5 g) have the opposite effect.

c. Ingestion of one teaspoon of the topical agent **methyl salicylate** (wintergreen oil) can cause **fatal intoxication.**

B. *p*-Aminophenol derivatives

1. Chemistry. The prototypical *p*-aminophenol derivative is **acetaminophen,** an active metabolite of phenacetin and acetanilid (Figure 16-8).

2. Pharmacology

a. *p*-Aminophenol derivatives inhibit central prostaglandin synthesis (see II B 2 a). They are analgesic for low-intensity pain and are antipyretic.

b. Because they are less effective than salicylates in blocking peripheral prostaglandin synthesis, they have no anti-inflammatory activity and do not affect platelet function.

3. Therapeutic indications

a. Acetaminophen and **phenacetin** are indicated for use as **analgesics** and **antipyretics,** particularly in the patient unable to tolerate salicylates.

b. Acetaminophen may be safely used as an **alternative antipyretic** in the child with varicella or an influenza-type viral infection (see III A 3 a [3]).

4. Adverse effects

a. When given in therapeutic doses, adverse effects are limited to:
(1) Skin rash
(2) Hemolytic anemia (with long-term phenacetin use)
(3) Methemoglobinemia
(4) Renal dysfunction and tubular necrosis

b. Acute acetaminophen overdose causes severe hepatotoxicity with necrosis and liver failure.

C. Pyrazolone derivatives

1. Chemistry. The most important pyrazolone derivatives are **phenylbutazone,** its metabolite **oxyphenbutazone,** and the uricosuric agent **sulfinpyrazone** (Anturane). Phenylbutazone is the prototypical agent (Figure 16-9).

2. Pharmacology

a. Phenylbutazone and **oxyphenbutazone** inhibit prostaglandin synthesis (see II B 2 a) and stabilize lysosomal membranes. As a result, they have analgesic, antipyretic, and anti-inflammatory effects.

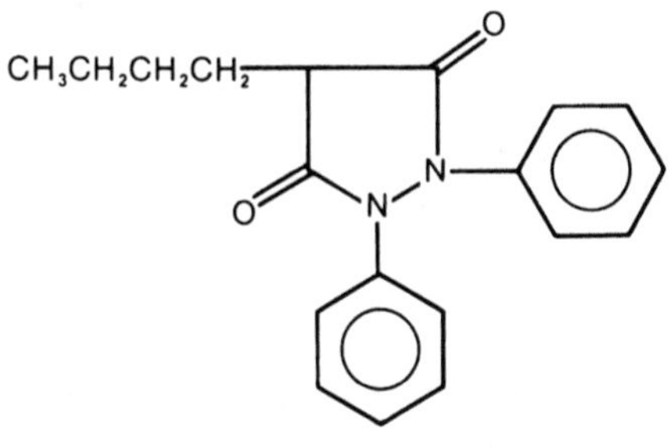

Figure 16-9. Structural formula of phenylbutazone (Butazolidin), a pyrazolone derivative.

b. **Sulfinpyrazone** inhibits proximal tubular absorption of urate and has a uricosuric effect. However, it is devoid of analgesic, antipyretic, or anti-inflammatory effects.

3. **Therapeutic indications**

a. **Phenylbutazone** and **oxyphenbutazone** are used for short-term treatment of acute rheumatoid arthritic conditions and acute gout. However, they should be given only after other therapeutic measures have failed.

b. **Sulfinpyrazone** is used to control hyperuricemia in the treatment of intermittent and chronic gout.

4. **Adverse effects**

a. The adverse effects of **phenylbutazone** and **oxyphenbutazone** often limit their use and include:

(1) GI effects, such as discomfort, nausea, vomiting, dyspepsia, and peptic ulceration

(2) Blood dyscrasias, such as agranulocytosis, aplastic anemia, hemolytic anemia, thrombocytopenia, and petechiae

(3) Cardiovascular effects, such as congestive heart failure with edema and dyspnea

(4) Renal effects, such as nephrotic lithiasis, renal necrosis, impaired renal function, and renal failure

(5) CNS effects, such as drowsiness, agitation, confusion, headache, lethargy, numbness, weakness, tinnitus, and hearing loss

(6) Hyperglycemia

(7) Skin rash

b. **Sulfinpyrazone** is associated with these adverse effects:

(1) GI effects, such as discomfort and upset

(2) Blood dyscrasias, as with phenylbutazone and oxyphenbutazone

(3) Renal failure

D. Agents used for the treatment of gout

1. **Chemistry**

a. Acute attacks of gout result from an inflammatory response to joint depositions of sodium urate crystals. Therapeutic agents counter this response by reducing plasma uric acid concentrations or inhibiting the inflammatory response.

b. Agents used for the treatment of gout have widely varying structures and include the pyrazolone derivative, sulfinpyrazone (see III C 2 b, 3 b, 4 b) the alkaloid colchicine, isopurines such as allopurinol, and benzoic acid derivatives, such as probenecid (Figure 16-10).

2. **Pharmacology**

a. Although **colchicine's** exact mechanism of action is unknown, it appears to reduce the inflammatory response to deposited urate crystals by inhibiting leukocyte migration and phagocytosis. It also interferes with kinin formation and reduces leukocyte lactic acid production.

b. **Allopurinol** reduces serum urate levels by blocking uric acid production. It competitively inhibits the enzyme xanthine oxidase, which converts xanthine and hypoxanthine to uric acid.

c. **Probenecid,** a uricosuric agent, inhibits the proximal tubular reabsorption of uric acid, increasing uric acid excretion, thus reducing plasma uric acid concentrations.

3. **Therapeutic indications**

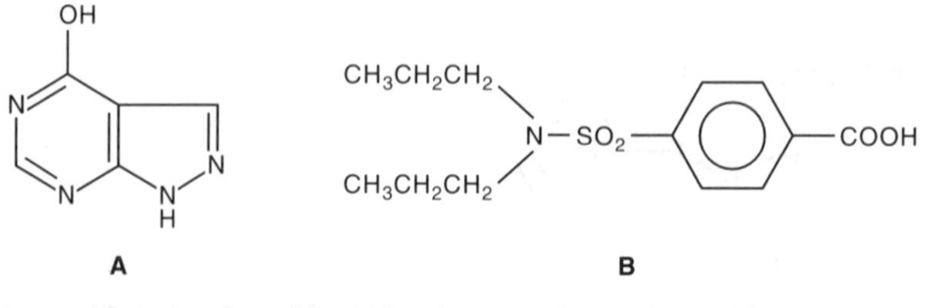

Figure 16-10. Structural formulas of (*A*) allopurinol (Zyloprim) and (*B*) probenecid (Benemid), agents used in the treatment of gout.

a. **Colchicine** is used principally for the treatment of acute gout attacks.
b. **Allopurinol,** which reduces uric acid synthesis and facilitates the dissolution of tophi (chalky urate deposits), is used to prevent the development or progression of chronic tophaceous gout.
c. **Probenecid** is used to treat chronic tophaceous gout. It is also used in smaller doses to prolong the effectiveness of penicillin-type antibiotics by inhibiting their tubular secretion.

4. Adverse effects

a. Chronic use of **colchicine** is associated with these adverse effects:
   (1) Agranulocytosis, aplastic anemia, myopathy, hair loss, and peripheral neuritis
   (2) Nausea, vomiting, abdominal pain, and diarrhea (indications of impending toxicity)
b. **Allopurinol** is associated with these adverse effects:
   (1) GI effects, such as GI distress, nausea, vomiting, and diarrhea
   (2) Skin rash, Stevens-Johnson syndrome, and hepatotoxicity
   (3) Precipitation of an acute gout attack (with initial allopurinol therapy due to initial mobilization of stored urate).
c. **Probenecid** is associated with these adverse effects:
   (1) Headaches, nausea, vomiting, urinary frequency, sore gums, and dermatitis
   (2) Dizziness, anemia, hemolytic anemia, and renal lithiasis

E. NSAIDs

1. Chemistry. The NSAIDs consist of many structurally diverse acids. These include **propionic** acid derivatives (fenoprofen, flurbiprofen, ibuprofen, ketoprofen, naproxen, and oxaprozin), **acetic acid** derivatives (diclofenac, etodolac, indomethacin, ketorolac, nabumetone, sulindac, and tolmetin), **fenamates** or **anthranilic** acid derivatives (meclofenamate and mefenamic acid), and the **oxicams** (piroxicam) [Figure 16-11].

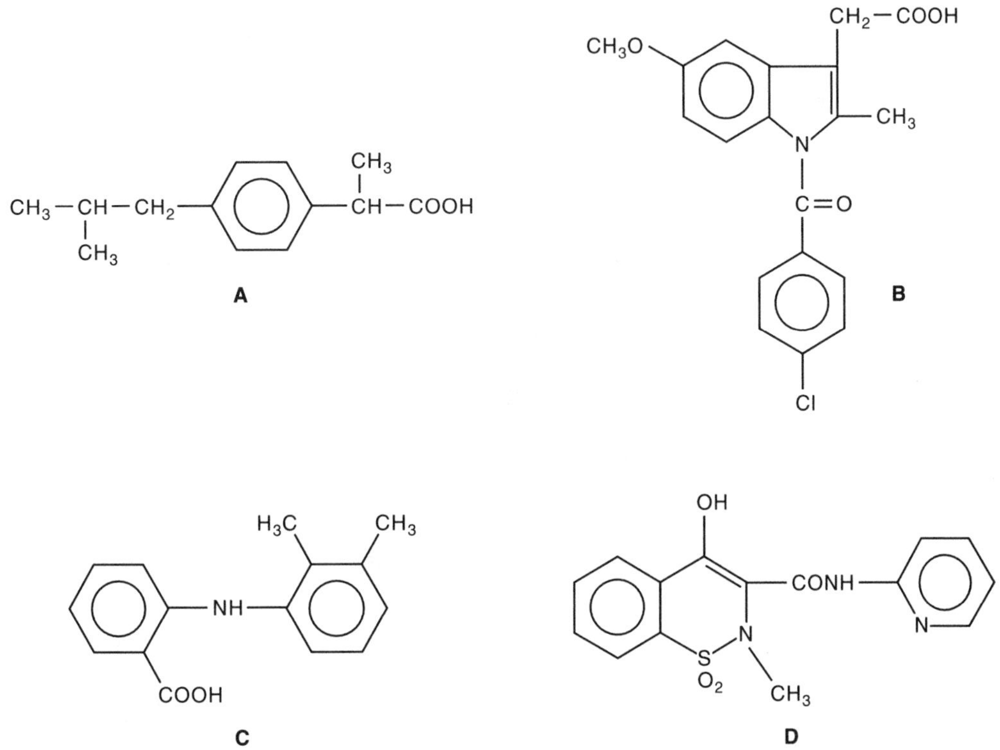

Figure 16-11. Structural formulas of (*A*) ibuprofen, (*B*) indomethacin, (*C*) mefenamic acid, and (*D*) piroxicam, representative nonsteroidal anti-inflammatory drugs (NSAIDs).

2. Pharmacology

a. NSAIDs have anti-inflammatory effects, resulting from their ability to inhibit the cyclooxygenase enzyme system and, thus, reduce local prostaglandin synthesis (see II B 2 a).

b. NSAIDs also have analgesic and antipyretic effects.

3. Therapeutic indications. NSAIDs, like aspirin, are agents of choice for the treatment of rheumatoid arthritis, osteoarthritis, and ankylosing spondylitis.

4. Adverse effects. NSAIDs are associated with these adverse effects:

a. GI effects, such as GI distress and irritation, erosion of gastric mucosa, nausea, vomiting, and dyspepsia

b. CNS effects, such as CNS depression, drowsiness, headache, dizziness, visual disturbances, ototoxicity, and confusion

c. Hematologic effects, such as thrombocytopenia, altered platelet function, and prolonged bleeding time

d. Skin rash

e. Nephrotoxicity

STUDY QUESTIONS

Directions: Each of the numbered items or incomplete statements in this section is followed by answers or by completions of the statement. Select the **one** lettered answer or completion that is **best** in each case.

1. All of the following are therapeutic indications for salicylates EXCEPT

(A) rheumatoid arthritis
(B) fever in children with influenza or varicella
(C) fever in adults with influenza
(D) spasmodic dysmenorrhea
(E) prophylaxis against myocardial infarction

2. All of the following statements describing acetaminophen are true EXCEPT

(A) it has anti-inflammatory activity similar to or greater than that of salicylates
(B) it acts as an analgesic and antipyretic
(C) it may cause skin rash
(D) it may be used in children with varicella or influenza-type viral infections
(E) acute overdose is characterized by severe hepatotoxicity

3. All of the following are therapeutic indications for prostaglandins EXCEPT

(A) impotence
(B) miscarriage with retained fetus
(C) premature labor
(D) delayed labor

Directions: Each question below contains three suggested answers of which **one or more** is correct. Choose the answer

A if **I only** is correct
B if **III only** is correct
C if **I and II** are correct
D if **II and III** are correct
E if **I, II, and III** are correct

4. Correct statements regarding agents used in the treatment of gout include

I. allopurinol inhibits proximal tubular reabsorption of uric acid and may cause renal lithiasis and urinary frequency
II. probenecid blocks the conversion of xanthine and hypoxanthine to uric acid
III. impending colchicine toxicity is heralded by abdominal pain, nausea, vomiting, and diarrhea

5. Pharmacologic properties of histamine include

I. constriction of capillaries
II. elevated blood pressure
III. increased gastric secretions

6. True statements concerning cimetidine and ranitidine include

I. they are useful in the treatment of duodenal ulcers
II. they may cause dizziness, mental confusion, and hepatic dysfunction
III. they are useful in the treatment of allergic reactions

7. The antihistaminic drug famotidine is classified as

I. classic antihistamine
II. H_1-receptor antagonist
III. H_2-receptor antagonist

Directions: The group of items in this section consists of lettered options followed by a set of numbered items. For each item, select the **one** lettered option that is most closely associated with it. Each lettered option may be selected once, more than once, or not at all.

Questions 8–12

For each characteristic given below, select the drug that most appropriately corresponds to it.

(A) Acetaminophen
(B) Indomethacin
(C) Aspirin
(D) Diphenhydramine
(E) Ibuprofen

8. Hydrolyzed in the bloodstream

9. An active metabolite of another drug

10. Classified as a salicylate

11. Excretion somewhat increased in an acidified urine

12. Classified as an arylacetic acid

Questions 13–15

A 32-year-old woman has recently discovered she is pregnant. Use the following medications, which she is currently taking, to answer the questions.

(A) Piroxicam, for arthritis
(B) Misoprostol, for prevention of ulcers
(C) Cyclizine, for car sickness
(D) Cimetidine, for gastric ulcers

13. Which of these agents could induce a miscarriage in this patient?

14. Which agent should be discontinued during this patient's pregnancy due to the increase risk to the fetus?

15. Which agent could increase the risk of galactorrhea, postpartum?

ANSWERS AND EXPLANATIONS

1. The answer is B *[III A 3].*
The association of Reye's syndrome with the use of salicylates in febrile children with varicella or influenza-type viral infections warrants that a nonsalicylate antipyretic be used if needed in such circumstances.

2. The answer is A *[III B 2 b, 3, 4].*
Acetaminophen has a limited peripheral effect on prostaglandin synthesis and, therefore, lacks anti-inflammatory capability. Acetaminophen is a nonsalicylate alternative antipyretic that may be used in children with varicella or influenza-type viral infections. Adverse effects include skin rash or other allergic reactions, and acute overdose is accompanied by severe liver damage.

3. The answer is C *[II B 3].*
Prostaglandins are indicated for erectile dysfunction and stimulate uterine contraction. Therefore, use of prostaglandins are contraindicated in premature labor because they would increase uterine contractions and hasten delivery.

4. The answer is B (III) *[III D 2, 4].*
Gastrointestinal upset, with adverse effects such as nausea, vomiting, and diarrhea, is associated with the early stages of colchicine toxicity. Probenecid inhibits the proximal tubular reabsorption of uric acid, whereas allopurinol inhibits the formation of uric acid from xanthine and hypoxanthine. Probenecid, not allopurinol, can cause renal lithiasis and urinary frequency.

5. The answer is B (III) *[II A 2 a].*
While gastric secretions are stimulated by histamine, the autacoid causes increased capillary permeability, capillary dilation, vasodilation, and hypotension.

6. The answer is C (I, II) *[II A 3, 4 d].*
Cimetidine and ranitidine are examples of H_2-receptor antagonists. They restrict H_2-mediated gastric secretions. They are ineffective in the treatment of allergic reactions because they are not H_1-receptor antagonists. Adverse effects that limit their duration of use include altered hepatic and renal function, as well as dizziness and confusion.

7. The answer is B (III) *[II A 1 b].*
The generic name famotidine more closely resembles those of the widely used H_2-receptor antagonists, cimetidine and ranitidine. All three have the common suffix, -tidine. The generic names of most of the H_1-receptor antagonists end in the suffix, -amine, such as diphenhydramine and chlorpheniramine. The H_1-receptor antagonists, which are much older drugs, are now often called the classic antihistamines.

8–12. The answers are: 8-C *[III A 1 a],* **9-A** *[III B 1; Figure 16-8],* **10-C** *[III A 1 a; Figure 16-6],* **11-D** *[II A 1 b; Figure 16-2],* **12-E** *[III E 1; Figure 16-11].*
Esters, particularly simple esters, readily undergo in vivo hydrolysis both with and without the aid of catalytic enzymes. Amides also undergo hydrolysis but require the aid of catalytic enzymes. There are many specific and nonspecific esterases circulating in the bloodstream but few, if any, amidases. Aspirin (acetylsalicylic acid) is the phenolic acetyl ester of *p*-hydroxybenzoic acid (i.e., salicylic acid) and, thus, is classified as a salicylate. Aspirin is readily hydrolyzed in the bloodstream and is the only drug listed that contains an ester linkage.

Acetaminophen is a metabolite of phenacetin. Phenacetin (*N*-acetyl-*p*-ethoxyaniline) undergoes oxidative O-dealkylation in the body, forming *N*-acetyl-*p*-aminophenol (acetaminophen).

In order for its excretion to be increased in an acidic urine, a drug must be a weak base. Aspirin, indomethacin, and ibuprofen are all weak acids, as are the other nonsteroidal anti-inflammatory agents (NSAIDs). Acetaminophen is a neutral molecule. Diphenhydramine, as the generic name implies, has an amino group present in its molecule. As can be seen in its structure (see Figure 16-2C), it contains a tertiary amine. Amines are weak bases; thus, diphenhydramine would be more ionized in acidic media and less likely to undergo tubular reabsorption from the glomerular filtrate. It would, therefore, be more easily excreted in acidic urine.

The NSAIDs are all acids, which contributes to their ability to penetrate synovial fluids. The NSAIDs are often classified as arylacetic acids or heteroarylacetic acids. Ibuprofen does not contain any hetero atoms and, thus, is classified as an arylacetic acid. Indomethacin, an indene derivative, contains a nitrogen in the pyrrole ring and, thus, is a heteroarylacetic acid. Aspirin, although an acid, is a salicylic acid derivative. Diphenhydramine is a base, and acetaminophen is neutral.

13–15. The answers are 13-B *[II B 3 a],* **14-C** *[II A 1 b],* **15-D** *[II A 4 d].*
Misoprostol is normally contraindicated during pregnancy because of its ability to stimulate uterine contractions. Cyclizine, a piperazine anti-histaminic, may cause teratogenicity and could result in birth defects. Cimetidine, through its endocrine effects, may cause galactorrhea. Postpartum, when lactation is greatest, this effect could be augmented.

17 Drugs Affecting the Cardiovascular System

David C. Kosegarten
Edward F. La Sala
J. Edward Moreton

I. INTRODUCTION.

Numerous categories of drugs affect the cardiovascular (CV) system. Certain drugs can be used to treat heart failure (e.g., cardiac glycosides), relieve angina pectoris (e.g., antianginal agents), and control dysrhythmias (e.g., antiarrhythmic agents). Others can reduce hypertension (e.g., antihypertensives, including a variety of diuretics, β-blocking agents, arteriolar smooth muscle dilators), treat the hyperlipidemias (e.g., antihyperlipidemic agents), reduce clotting and treat such conditions as venous thrombosis and pulmonary embolism (e.g., anticoagulants), and treat anemias (e.g., antianemic agents).

II. CARDIAC GLYCOSIDES AND POSITIVE INOTROPES

A. Chemistry

1. Almost all the cardiac glycosides (also called **cardiotonics**) are naturally occurring steroidal glycosides obtained from plant sources. **Digitoxin** is obtained from *Digitalis purpurea,* **digoxin** from *Digitalis lanata,* and **ouabain** from *Strophanthus gratus.*
2. The cardiac glycosides are closely related structurally, consisting of one or more sugars (i.e., **glycone portion**) and a steroidal nucleus (i.e., **aglycone or genin portion**) bonded through an **ether (glycosidic) linkage.** These agents also have an **unsaturated lactone substituent (cyclic ester)** on the genin portion. The prototypical agent is **digitoxin** (Figure 17-1).
   a. **Digoxin** (Lanoxin) has an additional hydroxyl group at position 12 (see Figure 17-1).
   b. **Ouabain** has a rhamnose glycone portion and additional hydroxyl groups at positions 1, 5, 11, and 19 (see Figure 17-1).
3. Removing the glycone portion causes decreased activity and increased toxicity from changes in polarity that cause erratic absorption from the gastrointestinal (GI) tract.
4. The **duration of action** of a cardiac glycoside is **indirectly proportional to the number of hydroxyl groups,** which increase polarity. Increased polarity results in decreased protein binding, liver biotransformation, and tubular reabsorption.
   a. **Digitoxin** has a long duration of action and may accumulate.
   b. **Ouabain,** in contrast, has an extremely short duration of action and is effective only when given intravenously.
5. **Amrinone and milrinone** are bipyridine derivatives with positive inotropic action (Figure 17-2).

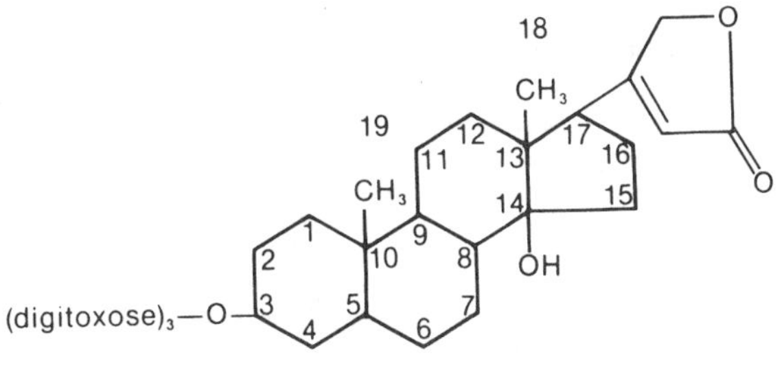

Figure 17-1. Structural formula of digitoxin (Crystodigin), the prototypical cardiac glycoside.

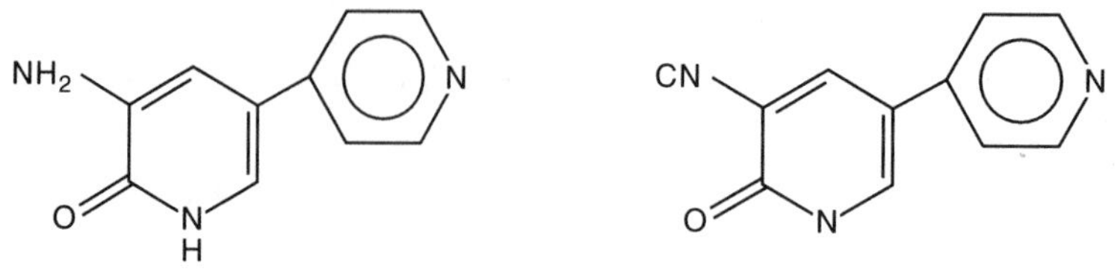

A **B**

Figure 17-2. Structural formulas of bipyridine derivatives *(A)* amrinone (Inocor) and *(B)* milrinone (Primacor).

B. Pharmacology. Cardiac glycosides increase myocardial contractility and efficiency, improve systemic circulation, improve renal perfusion, and reduce edema. The electrophysiologic effects of cardiac glycosides are summarized in Table 17-1.

1. When given in therapeutic doses, cardiac glycosides produce positive inotropic effects by inhibiting membrane bound Na^+/K^+ activated ATPase. These effects of cardiac glycosides increase the rate of tension development, the contractility, and the rate of relaxation of cardiac muscle. The effects include:
   a. Increase in intracellular sodium concentration
   b. Reduction in calcium transport from the cell by the sodium-calcium exchanger
   c. Facilitation of calcium entry via voltage-gated membrane channels
   d. Increased release of calcium from sarcoplasmic reticulum
2. Therapeutic doses of cardiac glycosides also cause:
   a. A negative chronotropic effect from increased vagal tone of the sinoatrial (SA) node
   b. Diminished central nervous system (CNS) sympathetic outflow from increased carotid sinus baroreceptor sensitivity
   c. Systemic arteriolar and venous constriction, which increases venous return and, thus, increases cardiac output
3. Amrinone and milrinone produce positive inotropic effects via selective inhibition of cyclic guanosine monophosphate (cGMP)-inhibited, Type III cyclic adenosine monophosphate (cAMP) phosphodiesterase (PDE) isozyme found in cardiac and smooth muscle. Inhibition of PDE Type III produces:
   a. Vasodilation and fall in vascular resistance
   b. Increased force of cardiac contraction
   c. Increased velocity of cardiac relaxation

C. Therapeutic indications

1. Congestive heart failure
2. Atrial fibrillation
3. Atrial flutter

Table 17-1. Effects of Cardiac Glycosides on the Heart

	Atria	AV Node	Ventricles
Direct effects	Contractility ↑ ERP ↑ Conduction velocity ↓	ERP ↑ Conduction velocity ↓	Contractility ↑ ERP ↓ Automaticity ↑
Indirect effects	ERP ↓ Conduction velocity ↑	ERP ↑ Conduction velocity ↓	No effect
Effects on electrocardiogram	P changes	P-R interval ↑	Q-T ↓; T and ST depressed
Adverse effects	Extrasystole Tachycardia	AV depression or block	Fibrillation Extrasystole Tachycardia

AV = atrioventricular; ERP = effective refractory period. Arrows indicate changes: ↑ = increased; ↓ = decreased.
Reprinted with permission from Jacob LS: *Pharmacology,* 3rd ed. Malvern, PA, Harwal, 1992, p 96.

4. Paroxysmal atrial tachycardia
5. Amrinone and milrinone are indicated for short-term treatment of congestive heart failure.

D. Adverse effects

1. **Early adverse effects** of cardiac glycosides represent the early stages of toxicity, including:
   a. GI effects, such as anorexia, nausea, vomiting, and diarrhea
   b. CNS effects, such as headache, visual disturbances (green or yellow vision), confusion, delirium, neuralgias, and muscle weakness
2. **Later adverse effects** represent intoxication and include such serious cardiac disturbances as premature ventricular contractions, paroxysmal and nonparoxysmal atrial tachycardia, atrioventricular (AV) dissociation or block, ventricular tachycardia, and ventricular fibrillation.

III. Drugs for Treatment of Myocardial Ischemia

A. Chemistry

1. **Antianginal agents** include **nitrites** (i.e., organic esters of nitrous acid), such as amyl nitrite; **nitrates** (i.e., organic esters of nitric acid), such as nitroglycerin and isosorbide; **β-blockers,** such as propranolol; and **calcium antagonists,** such as verapamil and nifedipine (Figure 17-3).
   a. **Amyl nitrite** is a very volatile and flammable liquid, administered by inhalation. It requires special precautions (especially restriction of smoking) during administration.
   b. **Nitroglycerin** is also a very volatile and flammable liquid and requires great care during storage. It must be dispensed from its original glass containers and protected from body heat.
      (1) When given intravenously, nitroglycerin requires the use of special plastic administration sets to avoid absorption and loss of potency.

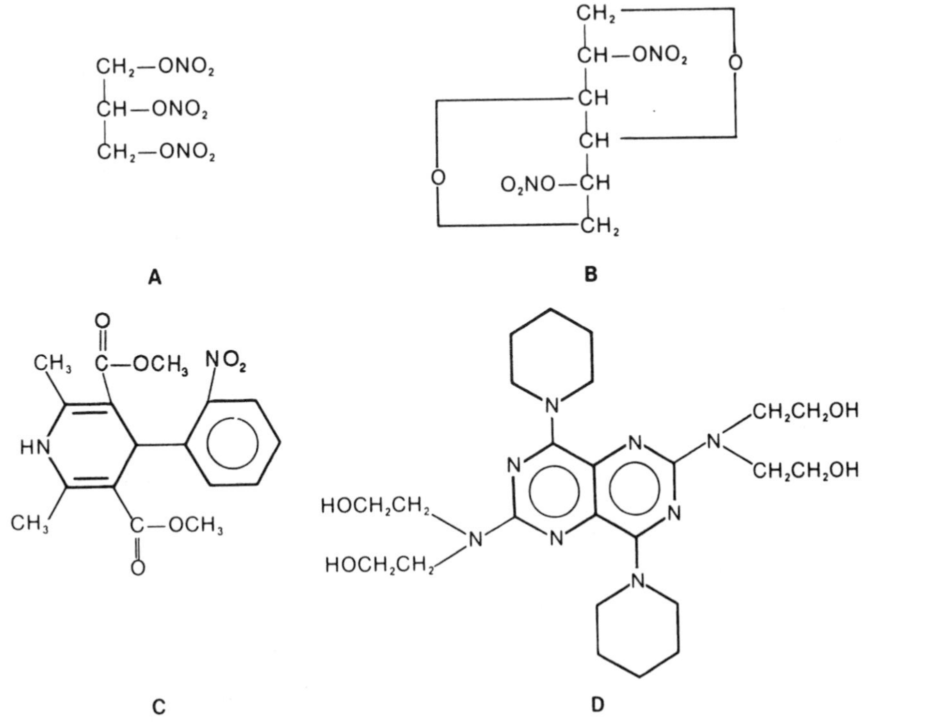

Figure 17-3. Structural formulas of *(A)* nitroglycerin (Nitrostat), *(B)* isosorbide dinitrate (Isordil), *(C)* nifedipine (Procardial), and *(D)* dipyridamole (Persantine), antianginal agents.

(2) **Nitroglycerin** is metabolically unstable and undergoes extensive first-pass metabolism.

2. **Peripheral vasodilators** include the dipiperidino-dipyrimidine dipyridamole (see Figure 17-3).

B. Pharmacology

1. **Nitrites and nitrates** are fast-acting antianginal agents that directly relax vascular smooth muscle by formation of the free radical nitric oxide (NO), which is identical to endothelium-derived relaxing factor (EDRF). NO activates guanylyl cyclase to increase synthesis of cGMP within smooth muscle, resulting in dephosphorylation of light chain myosin and muscle relaxation. This causes peripheral pooling of the blood, diminished venous return (reduced preload), decreased systemic vascular resistance, and decreased arterial pressure (reduced afterload). These vascular effects:
   a. Reduce myocardial oxygen demand
   b. Cause redistribution of coronary blood flow along the collateral coronary arteries, improving perfusion of the ischemic myocardium

2. **β-Adrenergic blockers** decrease sympathetic-mediated myocardial stimulation (see Chapter 14 V A 2, C 3). The resulting negative inotropic and negative chronotropic effects reduce myocardial oxygen requirements.

3. **Calcium antagonists** (also known as **calcium channel blockers**) block calcium entry through the membranous calcium ion (Ca^{2+}) channels of coronary and peripheral vascular smooth muscle.
   a. Peripheral arterioles dilate and total peripheral resistance decreases, reducing afterload and reducing myocardial oxygen requirements.
   b. Calcium antagonists also increase oxygen delivery to the myocardium by dilating coronary arteries and arterioles.

4. **Dipyridamole** relaxes smooth muscles, decreasing coronary vascular resistance and increasing coronary blood flow.

C. Therapeutic Indications

1. **Nitrites and nitrates** are used to relieve acute anginal attacks, as prophylaxis during anticipation of an acute anginal attack, and for long-term management of recurrent angina pectoris.

2. **β-Adrenergic blockers** are used for adjunctive prophylaxis of chronic stable angina pectoris in combination with nitrites or nitrates.

3. **Calcium antagonists** are used to treat chronic stable angina pectoris and variant (Prinzmetal's) angina.

4. **Dipyridamole** is used primarily for prophylaxis of angina pectoris, although its beneficial effects are not well understood.

D. Adverse Effects

1. **Nitrites and nitrates** are associated with:
   a. CNS effects, such as headache, apprehension, dizziness, and weakness
   b. CV effects, such as hypotension, tachycardia, palpitations, and syncope
   c. Skin effects, such as rash and dermatitis
   d. Methemoglobinemia

2. **β-Adrenergic blockers** are associated with:
   a. Worsening of congestive heart failure
   b. Bradycardia and hypotension
   c. Reduced kidney blood flow and glomerular filtration

3. **Calcium antagonists** generally produce only mild adverse effects.
   a. When given in conjunction with β-adrenergic blockers, their CV effects may be enhanced, resulting in bradycardia, hypotension, peripheral edema, congestive heart failure, AV block, and asystole.

b. **Verapamil** may also cause sleeplessness, muscle fatigue, nystagmus, and emotional depression. During the first week of therapy, verapamil increases serum digitalis levels and may cause digitalis toxicity.

4. **Dipyridamole** is associated with:
   a. GI effects, such as nausea, vomiting, and diarrhea
   b. CNS effects, such as headache and dizziness
   c. CV effects, such as hypotension (with excessive doses)

IV. ANTIARRHYTHMIC AGENTS

A. **Chemistry.** Antiarrhythmic agents have widely diverse chemical structures. They include representatives of these groups:

1. **Cinchona alkaloids** (e.g., quinidine, an optical isomer of quinine)
2. **Amides** (e.g., procainamide [Pronestyl], flecainide [Tambocor]; disopyramide [Norpace])
3. **Xylyl derivatives** (e.g., lidocaine [Xylocaine], mexiletine [Mexitil])
4. **Quaternary ammonium salts** (e.g., bretylium [Bretylol])
5. **Diiodobenzyloxyethylamines** (e.g., amiodarone [Cordarone])
6. **β-Blockers** (e.g., nadolol [Corgard], propranolol [inderal], esmolol [Brevibloc], acebutolol [Sectral])
7. **Calcium antagonists** (e.g., diltiazem [Cardizem], verapamil [Calan])
8. **Hydantoins** (e.g., phenytoin [Dilantin])

B. **Pharmacology.** Antiarrhythmic agents are classified according to their ability to alter the action potential of cardiac cells (Tables 17-2 and 17-3).

1. **Class 1A compounds** (e.g., quinidine, procainamide, disopyramide) produce state dependent sodium channel blockade to slow the rate of rise of phase 0 (the phase of rapid depolarization and reversal of transmembrane voltage) and prolong repolarization and effective refractory period.
2. **Class IB compounds** (e.g., lidocaine, tocainide, mexiletine, phenytoin) have a minimal effect on the rate of rise of phase 0 and shorten repolarization.
3. **Class IC compounds** (e.g., encainide, flecainide, propafenone) have a marked effect in slowing the rate of rise of phase 0 and in slowing conduction. They have little effect on repolarization. Encainide was withdrawn from the market but is available on a limited basis.

Table 17-2. Major Effects of Antiarrhythmic Drugs on Electrocardiogram

Drug	QRS	Q-T	P-R*
Quinidine Procainamide Amiodarone	↑	↑	→↑
Disopyramide	↑	↑	→
Lidocaine Phenytoin Tocainide Mexiletine	→	↓	→↑↓
Propranolol	→	↓	→↑

Arrows indicate changes: ↑ = increased; ↓ = decreased; → = no change.

*P-R intervals: All antiarrhythmic drugs have a variable response, usually with little observable effect. However, lidocaine hardly ever affects the P-R interval, whereas phenytoin and propranolol usually increase the P-R interval.

Reprinted with permission from Jacob LS: *Pharmacology,* 3rd ed. Malvern, PA, Harwal, 1992, p 102.

Table 17-3. Effects of Antiarrhythmic Drugs on Electrophysiologic Properties of the Heart

Drug Class	Automaticity		Effective Refractory Period		Membrane Responsiveness
	SA Node	Purkinje Fibers	AV Node	Purkinje Fibers	Purkinje Fibers
IA	→↑	↓→	↑→↓	↑↓	↓
IB	→	↓	→↓	↓	→↓
IC	→	↓	↑	↓	↓
II	↓	↓	↑	↓→↑	↓
III	↑↓	↑↓	↓→↑	↑	→
IV	↓	→↓	↑	→	→

4. **Class II compounds** (e.g., propranolol, nadolol, esmolol, acebutolol) are β-adrenergic antagonists that competitively block catecholamine-induced stimulation of cardiac β-receptors and depress depolarization of phase 4.
5. **Class III compounds** (e.g., bretylium, amiodarone, sotalol) prolong repolarization.
6. **Class IV compounds** (e.g., verapamil) are calcium antagonists that block the slow inward current carried by calcium during phase 2 (i.e., long-sustained depolarization or the plateau of the action potential) and increase the effective refractory period; and depress phase 4 depolarization.
7. **Digoxin and adenosine.** Digitalis glycosides (Digoxin) elicit a vagotonic response that increases AV nodal refractoriness. Adenosine acts at G-protein coupled adenosine receptors to increase AV nodal refractoriness.

C. Therapeutic indications. Antiarrhythmic agents are used to reduce abnormalities of impulse generation (ectopic pacemaker automaticity) and to modify the disturbances of impulse conduction within cardiac tissue. (For indications for specific agents, see Table 17-4.)

D. Adverse Effects

1. **Class IA compounds** are associated with CV effects, such as myocardial depression, AV block, ventricular dysrhythmias, asystole, and hypotension; and GI effects, such as GI upset, nausea, vomiting, and diarrhea. In addition:
   a. **Quinidine** can cause cinchonism, with tinnitus, confusion, photophobia, headache, and psychosis.

Table 17-4. Use of Antiarrhythmic Drugs in Common Cardiac Arrhythmias

Arrhythmia	Treatment of Choice	Alternatives
I. Supraventricular		
Atrial fibrillation or flutter	Digitalis to control ventricular rate, direct current (DC) shock for conversion	Quinidine to suppress recurrences after DC shock
Paroxysmal atrial or nodal tachycardia	Vagotonic maneuver; digitalis	Verapamil (quinidine, procainamide, disopyramide, and β-adrenergic antagonists may all be useful, especially prophylactically)
II. Ventricular		
Ventricular premature depolarization	Lidocaine	Procainamide, quinidine, or disopyramide for prolonged suppression
Ventricular tachycardia	DC shock	Lidocaine, procainamide, or mexiletine
III. Digitalis-induced	Lidocaine or phenytoin	Procainamide is somewhat useful; β-adrenergic antagonists are useful but have a high incidence of adverse effects

Reprinted with permission from Jacob LS: *Pharmacology,* 3rd ed. Malvern, PA, Harwal, 1992, p 102.

b. **Procainamide** can cause systemic lupus erythematosus-like syndrome.
c. **Disopyramide** can cause congestive heart failure and antimuscarinic effects.

2. **Class IB compounds** are associated with CNS effects, including CNS depression, drowsiness, disorientation, and paresthesias; CV effects, including hypotension and circulatory collapse; and hepatitis. In addition:
   a. **Lidocaine** can cause seizures and respiratory arrest.
   b. **Tocainide** can cause pneumonitis and blood dyscrasias.
   c. **Mexiletine** can cause hepatic injury and blood dyscrasias.
   d. **Phenytoin** can cause nystagmus, decreased mental function, and blood dyscrasias.

3. **Class IC compounds** are associated with:
   a. CV effects, including worsening of arrhythmias in patients with ventricular arrhythmias, particularly patients with a history of myocardial infarction (MI). They can worsen sinus node dysfunction and aggravate heart failure.
   b. Visual disturbances, such as blurred or double vision

4. **Class II compounds** are associated with:
   a. CV effects, such as hypotension, AV block, and asystole
   b. Respiratory effects, such as bronchospasm

5. **Class III compounds** are associated with:
   a. CV effects, such as hypotension and initially increased dysrhythmias
   b. GI effects, such as nausea and vomiting

6. **Class IV compound verapamil** is associated with CV adverse effects, such as hypotension, bradycardia, AV block, congestive heart failure, and asystole.

7. **Cardiac glycosides** (see II D). **Adenosine** causes asystole lasting less than 5 seconds and is the therapeutic objective.

V. Antihypertensive Agents

A. **Chemistry.** Antihypertensive agents vary so widely in chemical structure that they are usually classified by mechanism of action rather than chemical class (Table 17-5).

B. **Pharmacology.** Antihypertensive agents lower blood pressure by reducing total peripheral resistance or cardiac output through a variety of mechanisms (see Table 17-5).

1. **Diuretics** (thiazides) create a negative sodium balance, reduce blood volume, and decrease vascular smooth muscle responsiveness to vasoconstrictors (see Chapter 17 IV).

2. **Vasodilators** such as diazoxide and minoxidil are potassium channel activators that produce membrane hyperpolarization, while hydralazine may stimulate formation of EDRF (NO) to decrease arterial resistance. Sodium nitroprusside releases NO to relax both arterioles and veins.

3. **Peripheral sympatholytics** interfere with adrenergic function by blocking postganglionic adrenergic receptors (e.g., propranolol, prazosin), limiting the release of neurotransmitters from adrenergic neurons (e.g., guanethidine), or depleting intraneuronal catecholamine storage sites (e.g., reserpine).

4. **Central α_2-sympathomimetics** (e.g., clonidine, methyldopa) appear to mediate their effects by stimulating presynaptic α_2-inhibitory receptors, resulting in a negative sympathetic outflow and lowered peripheral resistance.

5. **Calcium channel blockers** (e.g., amlodipine, diltiazem felodipine, isradipine, nicardipine, nifedipine, verapamil) lower vascular resistance and blood pressure via blockade of voltage-gated calcium channels. Arterioles are more sensitive than veins.

6. **Angiotensin-converting enzyme (ACE) inhibitors** (e.g., captopril) block the conversion of inactive angiotensin I to the potent vasoconstrictor angiotensin II. The reduced angiotensin II level also lowers aldosterone levels, which limits sodium retention.

7. **Angiotensin II receptor antagonists** (e.g., losartan) are nonpeptide antagonists of the AT_1 angiotensin II receptor subtype located in vasculature, myocardium, brain, kidney, and adrenal

Table 17-5. Classification of Antihypertensive Agents by Their Mechanism of Action

Mechanism of Action	Drug
Diuretic	Hydrochlorothiazide (Hydrodiuril)
Vasodilators	
Arteriolar	Diazoxide (Hyperstat IV) Hydralazine (Apresoline) Minoxidil (Loniten)
Arteriolar and venous	Nitroprusside (Nipride)
Peripheral sympatholytics	Atenolol (Tenormin) Guanadrel (Hylorel) Guanethidine (Ismelin) Labetalol (Trandate) Metoprolol (Lopressor) Nadolol (Corgard) Pindolol (Visken) Prazosin (Minipress) Propranolol (Inderal) Reserpine (Serpasil)
Central α_2-sympathomimetics	Clonidine (Catapres) Guanabenz (Wytensin) Guanfacine (Tenex) Methyldopa (Aldomet)
Calcium channel blockers	Amlodipine (Norvasc) Diltiazem (Cardizem) Felodipine (Plendil) Isradipine (DynaCirc) Nicardipine (Cardene) Nifedipine (Procardia) Verapamil (Calan)
Angiotensin II receptor antagonist	Losartan (Cozaar)
Angiotensin-converting enzyme inhibitors	Benazepril (Lotensin) Captopril (Capoten) Enalapril (Vasotec) Fosinopril (Monopril) Lisinopril (Prinivil) Moexipril (Univasc) Quinapril (Accupril) Ramipril (Altace)

glomerulosa. They produce vasodilation, cause loss of salt and water to decrease plasma volume, and decrease myogenic activity.

C. Therapeutic Indications

1. Antihypertensive agents are used separately or in combination to **treat high blood pressure.**
2. These agents may also be administered parenterally to **treat hypertensive emergencies,** such as malignant hypertension, eclampsia, or the severe hypertension associated with excess catecholamines. Parenteral therapy may include some combination of these agents:
   a. **Arteriolar and venous vasodilator,** such as nitroprusside
   b. **Arteriolar vasodilator,** such as diazoxide or hydralazine
   c. **α-Adrenergic blocking agent** and **β-adrenergic blocking agent,** such as labelalol
   d. **β-Blocking agent,** such as propranolol
   e. **Ganglionic blocking agent,** such as trimethaphan

D. Adverse Effects

1. **Diuretics (thiazides)** can cause:
   - a. Fluid and electrolyte imbalances, such as hypokalemia, hypercalcemia, hyperuricemia, hypomagnesemia, hyponatremia, and hyperglycemia
   - b. Increased serum low-density lipoprotein cholesterol and triglyceride levels
   - c. Other effects (see Chapter 18 IV D)

2. **Vasodilators** are associated with:
   - a. GI effects, such as GI upset
   - b. CNS effects, such as headache and dizziness
   - c. CV effects, such as tachycardia, fluid retention, and aggravation of angina
   - d. Other effects, such as nasal congestion, hepatitis, glomerulonephritis, and systemic lupus erythematosus-like syndrome

3. **Peripheral sympatholytics** are associated with a variety of adverse effects, depending on the specific agent.
   - a. **β-Blockers** (e.g., propranolol) are associated with:
     - (1) CV effects, such as bradycardia, congestive heart failure, and Raynaud's phenomenon
     - (2) GI effects, such as GI upset
     - (3) Blood dyscrasias
     - (4) CNS effects, such as depression, hallucinations, organic brain syndrome, and transient hearing loss
     - (5) Other effects, such as increased airway resistance, increased serum triglyceride levels, decreased high-density lipoprotein cholesterol levels, and psoriasis
     - (6) Cardiac arrhythmias if withdrawal is abrupt
   - b. **Prazosin** is associated with:
     - (1) CV effects, such as sudden syncope with the first dose, palpitations, and fluid retention
     - (2) CNS effects, such as headache, drowsiness, weakness, dizziness, and vertigo
     - (3) Antimuscarinic effects and priapism
   - c. **Guanethidine** is associated with:
     - (1) CV effects, such as bradycardia, orthostatic hypotension, and sodium and water retention
     - (2) Diarrhea
     - (3) Aggravation of bronchial asthma
   - d. **Reserpine** is associated with:
     - (1) CNS effects, such as nightmares, depression, and drowsiness
     - (2) CV effects, such as bradycardia
     - (3) GI effects, such as GI upset and activation of peptic ulcer
     - (4) Nasal stuffiness

4. **Central** α_2-sympathomimetics also have adverse effects that vary with the specific agent.
   - a. **Clonidine** is associated with:
     - (1) CNS effects, such as sedation and drowsiness
     - (2) Dry mouth and severe rebound hypertension
     - (3) Insomnia, headache, and cardiac dysrhythmias (with sudden withdrawal)
   - b. **Methyldopa** is associated with:
     - (1) CV effects, such as orthostatic hypotension and bradycardia
     - (2) CNS effects, such as sedation and fever
     - (3) GI effects, such as colitis
     - (4) Other effects, such as hepatitis, cirrhosis, Coombs-positive hemolytic anemia, and systemic lupus erythematosus-like syndrome

5. **Calcium channel blockers** are associated with CV effects, resulting in hypotension, dizziness, headache, and flushing. When given with β-adrenergic blockers their effects may be enhanced resulting in bradycardia, hypotension, peripheral edema, congestive heart failure, AV block, and asystole.

6. **ACE inhibitors** are associated with:
   - a. CV effects, such as hypotension
   - b. Hematologic effects, such as neutropenia and agranulocytosis

c. Other effects, such as anorexia, polyuria, oliguria, acute renal failure, and cholestatic jaundice

7. **Angiotensin II receptor antagonists** are associated with adverse effects similar to ACE inhibitors except that cough and angioedema, which are independent of angiotensin antagonism, may occur less frequently.

VI. Antihyperlipidemic Agents

A. Chemistry. Antihyperlipidemic agents vary in chemical structure and are usually classified by their site of action—locally in the intestine (nonabsorbable agents) or systemically (absorbable agents).

1. **Nonabsorbable agents** are **bile acid sequestrants.** These agents are hydrophilic, water-insoluble resins that bind to bile acids in the intestine. Examples include **cholestyramine chloride,** a basic anion-exchange resin consisting of trimethylbenzylammonium groups in a large copolymer of styrene and divinylbenzene, and **colestipol hydrochloride,** a copolymer of diethylpentamine and epichlorohydrin (Figure 17-4).

2. **Absorbable agents** include **nicotinic acid** (but not the structurally similar nicotinamide), the aryloxyisobutyric acid derivatives **clofibrate** (a prodrug ester) and **gemfibrozil,** the sulfur-containing bis-phenol **probucol,** the 3-hydroxy-3-methylglutaryl-coenzyme A (HMG-CoA) reductase inhibitor **lovastatin,** and the fatty fish oils containing large amounts of **eicosapentaenoic acid (EPA)** and **docosahexaenoic acid (DHA)** [Figure 17-5].

B. Pharmacology. Antihyperlipidemic agents **increase catabolism** or **reduce lipoprotein production** (e.g., lovastatin, clofibrate, gemfibrozil) or **increase the efficiency of lipoprotein removal** (e.g., cholestyramine, colestipol).

C. Therapeutic indications. These agents are used (in conjunction with appropriate diet and exercise) to reduce plasma lipoprotein levels.

D. Adverse effects

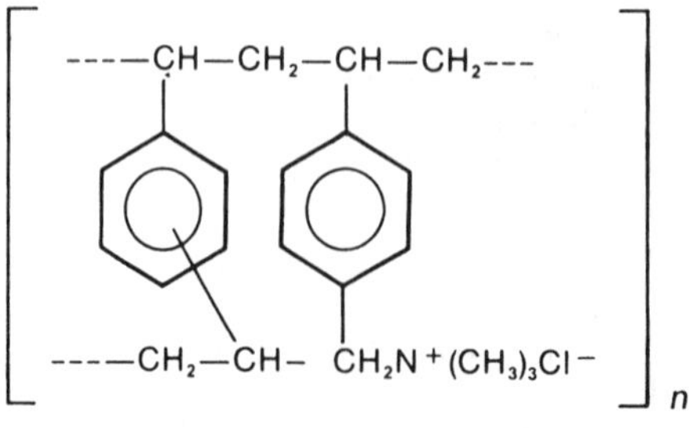

A

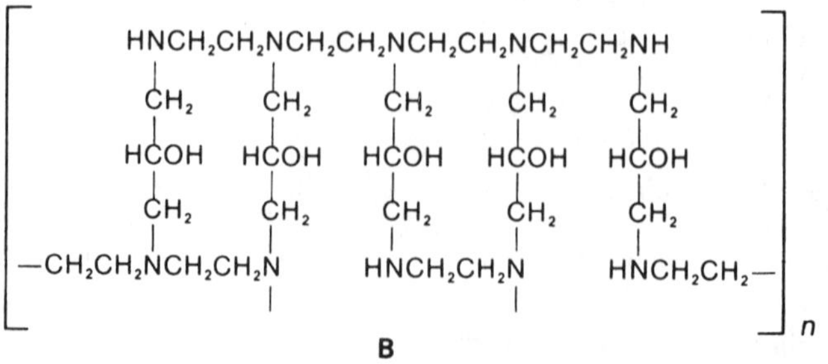

B

Figure 17-4. Structural formulas of *(A)* cholestyramine chloride (Questran) and *(B)* colestipol hydrochloride (Colestid), nonabsorbable antihyperlipidemic agents.

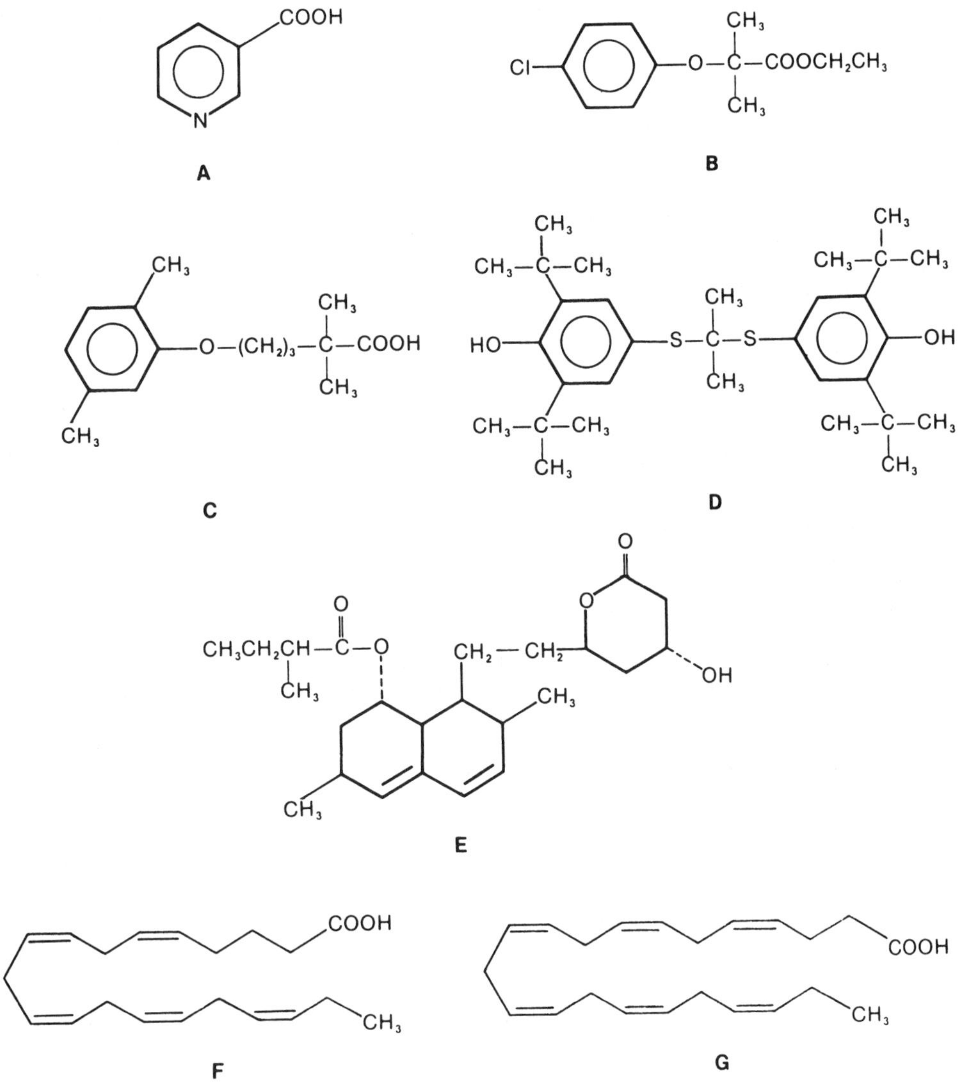

Figure 17-5. Structural formulas of *(A)* nicotinic acid (niacin), *(B)* clofibrate (Atromid-S), *(C)* gemfibrozil (Lopid), *(D)* probucol (Lorelco), *(E)* lovastatin (Mevacor), *(F)* eicosapentaenoic acid (found in Promega, Proto-Chol, and others), and *(G)* docosahexaenoic acid (found in Promega, Proto-Chol, and others). These agents are absorbable antihyperlipidemics.

1. **Nonabsorbable agents** (e.g., cholestyramine, colestipol) are associated with GI distress, including abdominal bloating, nausea, dyspepsia, steatorrhea, and constipation or diarrhea.
2. **Absorbable agents** (e.g., lovastatin, clofibrate, gemfibrozil) are associated with GI distress, skin rash, and leukopenia.
   a. **Lovastatin** and other statins (simvastatin, pravastatin, fluvastatin) may increase blood transaminase and creatinine phosphokinase activity associated with myopathy, especially when combined with fibrates or cyclosporins
   b. **Clofibrate** may cause nausea, vomiting, dysphagia, weight gain, alopecia, and breast tenderness.
   c. **Gemfibrozil** may also cause skeletal muscle pain, blurred vision, and anemia.
   d. **Nicotinic acid** produces flushing associated with pruritus to which tolerance develops in 1–2 weeks and which may be alleviated by one aspirin per day. High doses of nicotinic acid (2 g/day) may produce hepatic damage.
   e. **Probucol** may be associated with prolonged QT interval, syncope, ventricular arrhythmia, and sudden death and should not be given to patients with a history of myocardial

infarct or to patients taking Class I or Class II antiarrhythmic drugs, tricyclic antidepressants, or phenothiazines.

VII. ANTICOAGULANT, ANTIPLATELET, AND THROMBOLYTIC AGENTS

A. Anticoagulants

1. **Chemistry.** The major anticoagulant agents are **heparin** and the **oral anticoagulants.**
   a. **Heparin** is a large, highly acidic mucopolysaccharide composed of sulfated D-glucosamine and D-glucuronic acid molecules (Figure 17-6). **Low molecular weight heparin (LMWH) fragments** (1–10 kDa) **enoxaparin** and **dalteparin** are produced through controlled depolymerization of heparin but they are not interchangeable with heparin in their actions and use.
      (1) Because they are highly acidic, heparin and LMWH fragments exist as anions at physiologic pH and are very poorly absorbed from the GI tract. Thus, they are usually administered parenterally as the sodium salt.
      (2) The action of heparin and LMWH fragments are quickly terminated by **protamine sulfate,** a highly basic protein that combines chemically with them in approximately equal amounts (mg:mg).
   b. **Oral anticoagulants** consist of the highly effective **coumarin derivatives** and the relatively unimportant **indanedione derivatives.**
      (1) The **coumarin derivatives** (e.g., **warfarin, dicumarol**) are water insoluble, weakly acidic 4-hydroxycoumarin lactones (Figure 17-7).
         (a) These agents are **chemically related to vitamin K,** and their mechanism of action is directly related to their antagonism of the reductase responsible for reducing vitamin K epoxide to the reduced hydroquinone.
         (b) These agents are also highly protein bound and extensively metabolized in the liver. These characteristics, in addition to their relatively narrow therapeutic index, make them very susceptible to significant drug interactions.
      (2) **Phenindione** represents a typical **indanedione derivative** (Figure 17-8).
2. **Pharmacology**
   a. Heparin catalyzes the inhibition of thrombin by antithrombin III (heparin cofactor) preventing the conversion of fibrinogen to fibrin. LMWH fragments are unable to catalyze inhibition of thrombin, but catalyze inhibition by antithrombin III of factor Xa, which is responsible for conversion of prothrombin to thrombin. Heparin prolongs blood clotting time both in vivo and in vitro while LMWH fragments have minimal *in vitro* effect.
   b. **Oral anticoagulants interfere with the vitamin K–dependent hepatic synthesis of the active clotting factors** II (prothrombin), VII, IX, and X and the anticoagulant proteins C and S. These agents prolong blood clotting time in vivo only.
3. **Therapeutic indications**
   a. **Heparin** is indicated:

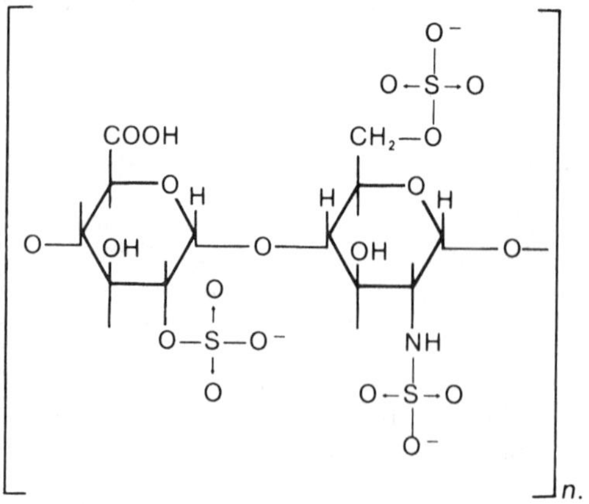

Figure 17-6. Structural formula of heparin, a mucopolysaccharide anticoagulant agent.

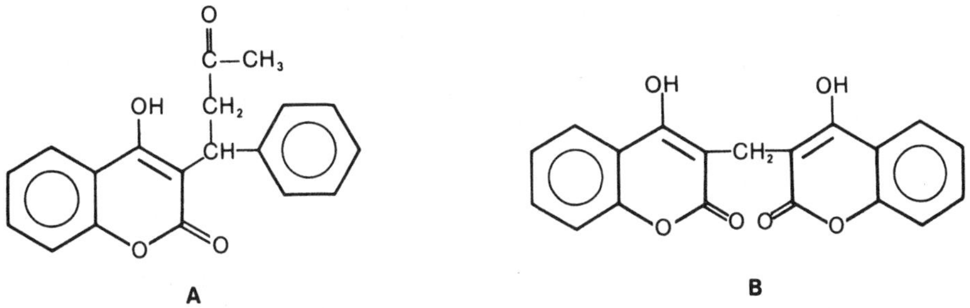

Figure 17-7. Structural formulas of *(A)* warfarin (Coumadin) and *(B)* dicumarol, coumarin-derivative oral anticoagulants.

(1) For the prophylaxis and treatment of venous thrombosis, pulmonary embolism, peripheral arterial embolism, and atrial fibrillation with embolization
(2) To prevent clotting during arterial surgery and cardiac surgery
(3) To diagnose and treat disseminated intravascular coagulation (DIC)
(4) To prevent postoperative venous thrombosis and pulmonary embolism (in low-dose form)
(5) To prevent cerebral thrombosis during an evolving stroke
(6) As adjunct therapy to prevent coronary occlusion with acute MI

b. Warfarin sodium, an oral anticoagulant, is indicated:
(1) For the prophylaxis and treatment of venous thrombosis, pulmonary embolism, and atrial fibrillation with embolization
(2) As adjunct therapy to prevent coronary occlusion with acute MI

4. Adverse effects

a. Heparin
(1) Heparin is associated with:
(a) Hematologic effects, such as hemorrhage, local irritation, thrombocytopenia, hematoma, ulceration, erythema, and pain
(b) Other effects, such as hypersensitivity reactions, fever, chills, and urticaria
(2) Severe adverse effects may be treated by administering protamine sulfate, the specific antidote for heparin.

b. LMWH fragments. LMWH fragments are absorbed more uniformly than heparin, have a longer biological half-life, and may be associated with a lower incidence of side effects than heparin.

c. Warfarin
(1) The oral anticoagulant warfarin sodium is associated with these adverse effects:
(a) Hemorrhage
(b) Anorexia, urticaria, purpura, and alopecia
(2) Severe adverse effects may be treated by administering vitamin K (phytonadione), the specific antidote for warfarin sodium.

B. Antiplatelet agents

1. Chemistry. Antiplatelet drugs include aspirin, a salicylate; ticlopidine, a thienopyridine; dipyridamole, a dipiperidino dinitro pyrimidine; and the Fab fragments of human monoclonal antibody to the GPIIb/IIa receptor.

2. Pharmacology

a. Aspirin in low doses inhibits platelet cyclo-oxygenase production of thromboxane A_2, preventing platelet aggregation. Cyclo-oxygenase is permanently inhibited for the life the platelet (7–10 days).

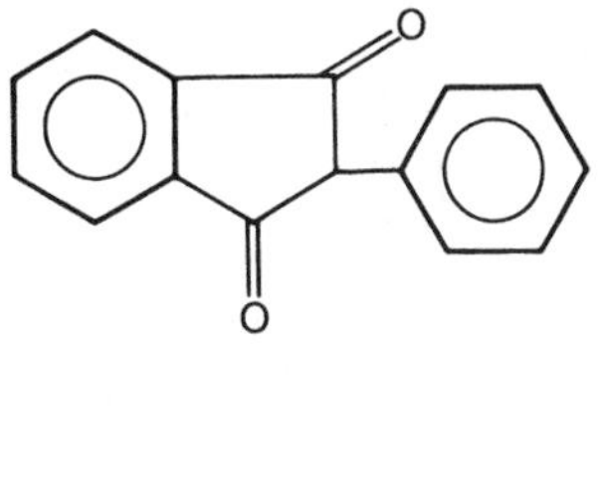

Figure 17-8. Structural formula of phenindione (Hedulin), an indanedione-derivative oral anticoagulant.

b. **Ticlopidine** or an active metabolite inhibits platelet-platelet interaction perhaps via inhibition of expression of or an induced conformational change in the GPIIb/IIa receptor.
c. **Fab fragments** (e.g., Abciximab) are monoclonal antibodies against the GPIIb/IIa receptor that permanently inhibit platelet-platelet interaction.
d. **Dipyridamole** may inhibit platelet aggregation via inhibition of:
(1) Red blood cell adenosine, which acts on A_2 receptors of platelets
(2) Phosphodiesterase to increase intracellular concentrations of cAMP
(3) Thromboxane A_2 formation

3. **Therapeutic indications**
a. **Aspirin** is indicated for reduction of mortality in post-MI, prophylactic treatment of MI to prevent reinfarction, and prophylaxis following transient ischemic attacks and minor stroke.
b. **Ticlopidine** is approved to reduce the risk of thrombotic stroke in patients with demonstrated risk but who cannot tolerate aspirin.
c. **Abciximab** is indicated for use with aspirin and heparin in patients undergoing percutaneous transluminal coronary angioplasty or atherectomy.
d. **Dipyridamole** is indicated for prophylaxis against thromboembolism after cardiac valve replacement.

4. **Adverse effects**
a. **Aspirin** in doses used for treatment of thrombotic disease is associated with epigastric pain, heartburn, nausea, rash, nasal polyps, gout, and anaphylactic reactions in sensitive individuals.
b. **Ticlopidine** is associated with a high incidence of adverse reactions including diarrhea, rash, nausea, vomiting, GI pain, and neutropenia.
c. **Abciximab** is associated with major and minor bleeding events, thrombocytopenia, human antichimeric antibody formation, cardiac arrhythmias, AV block, bradycardia, diarrhea, abnormal thinking, and dizziness.
d. **Dipyridamole** is associated with nausea, epigastric pain, dizziness, headache, and rash.

C. Thrombolytic agents

1. **Chemistry**
a. **Tissue plasminogen activator** (t-PA) is a 527 amino acid serine protease derived from recombinant DNA technology.
b. **Streptokinase** is a nonenzymatic 47-kDa protein derived from cultures of Group C β hemolytic streptococci.
c. **Anistreplase** (anisoylated plasminogen streptokinase activator complex, APSAC) is a complex of human lys-plasminogen and streptokinase with a anisoyl group blocking the catalytic site.
d. **Urokinase** is a two-chain serine protease obtained from cultured human kidney cells.

2. **Pharmacology.** Thrombolytic agents facilitate the conversion of plasminogen to plasmin that subsequently hydrolyzes fibrin to dissolve clots.
a. **t-PA** (Alteplase) is referred to as clot selective because conversion of plasminogen to plasmin by t-PA is enhanced several hundred-fold in the presence of fibrin.
b. **Streptokinase,** which has no enzymatic activity, forms a 1 to 1 complex with plasminogen resulting in a conformational change that exposes the catalytic site of plasminogen. The stable activated complex subsequently cleaves free plasminogen to form plasmin.
c. **Anistreplase** is a prodrug activated in vivo by deacylation of the anisole moiety from the active site of the plasminogen-streptokinase complex. The activated complex converts plasminogen to plasmin in the blood stream or thrombus.
d. **Urokinase,** in contrast to streptokinase, is enzymatic and directly converts plasminogen to plasmin.

3. **Therapeutic indications**
a. **t-PA** is indicated for treatment of acute MI and acute massive pulmonary embolism.
b. **Streptokinase** is indicated for acute MI, deep vein thrombosis, arterial thrombosis, and arterial emboli except those originating from the left side of the heart.
c. **Anistreplase** is indicated for treatment of acute MI and lysis of coronary arterial thrombi.
d. **Urokinase** is indicated for treatment of coronary artery thrombosis and pulmonary emboli.

4. **Adverse effects**
   a. **t-PA** is associated with:
      (1) Internal bleeding of the GI and genitourinary tract, retroperitoneal bleeding, and intracranial bleeding
      (2) Superficial bleeding at catheter insertion sites, arterial punctures, and surgical sites
      (3) Other adverse effects including hypersensitivity reactions, nausea, vomiting, hypotension, and fever
   b. **Streptokinase** may be associated with:
      (1) Internal and superficial bleeding as above
      (2) Allergic reactions including bronchospasm, angioneurotic edema, urticaria, headache, and delayed hypersensitivity reactions
   c. **Anistreplase** may be associated with:
      (1) Internal and superficial bleeding as above
      (2) Cardiac arrhythmias and hypotension
      (3) Allergic type reactions such as bronchospasm, angioneurotic edema, urticaria, delayed purpuric rash
   d. **Urokinase** may be associated with:
      (1) Internal and superficial bleeding as above
      (2) Allergic reactions leading to bronchospasm, and skin rash

VIII. ANTIANEMIC AGENTS

A. **Chemistry.** The major antianemic agents are iron preparations, cyanocobalamin (vitamin B_{12}), and folic acid.

1. **Most iron preparations consist of ferrous salts,** which are better absorbed from the GI tract than ferric salts or elemental iron.
   a. Typical oral preparations include **ferrous sulfate** (e.g., Feosol), **ferrous gluconate** (e.g., Fergon), and **ferrous fumarate** (e.g., Feostat).
   b. When parenteral administration is indicated, **iron dextran** (e.g., Imferon) may be used. This preparation consists of a complex of ferric hydroxide and low molecular weight dextrans, forming a colloidal solution.

2. **Cyanocobalamin** (vitamin B_{12}) is a nucleotide-like macromolecule with a modified porphyrin unit (a corrin ring) containing a trivalent cobalt atom. A cyanide ion is also coordinated to the cobalt atom, as is a benzimidazole group. The benzimidazole group is bonded to an α-ribosyl phosphate.

3. **Folic acid** consists of three major components: a pteridine nucleus bonded to the nitrogen of p-aminobenzoic acid, which is bonded through an amide linkage to glutamic acid (Figure 17-9).

B. **Pharmacology**

1. **Iron preparations** (ferrous salts) are readily absorbed from the GI tract and stored in the bone marrow, liver, and spleen as **ferritin** and **hemosiderin.** They are subsequently incorporated as needed into hemoglobin, where the iron reversibly binds molecular oxygen. A lack of body iron causes iron deficiency anemia with hypochromic, microcytic red blood cells, which transport oxygen poorly.

2. **Cyanocobalamin** is readily absorbed from the GI tract in the presence of intrinsic factor (Castle's factor), a glycoprotein produced by gastric parietal cells, which is necessary for GI absorption of cyanocobalamin.

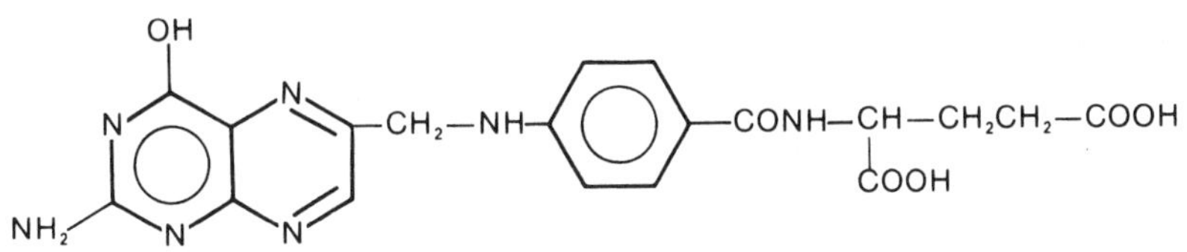

Figure 17-9. Structural formula of folic acid, an antianemic agent.

a. Cyanocobalamin is transported to tissue by transcobalamin II. It is essential for cell growth, for maintaining normal nerve cell myelin, and for the metabolic functions of folate.

b. Lack of dietary cyanocobalamin (or lack of intrinsic factor) causes a vitamin B_{12} deficiency and megaloblastic anemia with hyperchromic, macrocytic, immature red blood cells. Demyelination of nerve cells also occurs, causing irreversible CNS damage.

3. **Folic acid** is readily absorbed from the GI tract, transported to tissue, and stored intracellularly. It is a precursor of several coenzymes (derivatives of tetrahydrofolic acid) that are involved in single carbon atom transfers. A lack of dietary folic acid causes folic acid deficiency and megaloblastic anemia with hyperchromic, macrocytic, immature red blood cells. However, folic acid deficiency causes no neurologic impairment.

C. Therapeutic indications

1. **Iron preparations** (ferrous salts) are used to treat iron deficiency anemia.
2. **Cyanocobalamin** is used to treat megaloblastic anemia resulting from vitamin B_{12} deficiency.
3. **Folic acid** is used to treat megaloblastic anemia resulting from folic acid deficiency.

D. Adverse effects

1. **Iron preparations** are associated with GI effects, such as GI distress, nausea, heartburn, diarrhea, and constipation.
2. **Cyanocobalamin** has only rare adverse effects.
3. **Folic acid** is associated only with rare allergic reactions after parenteral administration.

STUDY QUESTIONS

Directions: Each of the numbered items or incomplete statements in this section is followed by answers or by completions of the statement. Select the **one** lettered answer or completion that is **best** in each case.

1. Calcium channel blockers have all of the following characteristics EXCEPT

(A) they block the slow inward current carried by calcium during phase 2 of the cardiac action potential
(B) they dilate peripheral arterioles and reduce total peripheral resistance
(C) they constrict coronary arteries and arterioles and decrease oxygen delivery to the myocardium
(D) they are useful in treating stable angina pectoris and Prinzmetal's angina
(E) their adverse effects include aggravation of congestive heart failure

2. The termination of heparin activity by protamine sulfate is due to

(A) a chelating action
(B) the inhibition of gastrointestinal absorption of heparin
(C) the displacement of heparin—plasma protein binding
(D) an acid-base interaction
(E) the prothrombin-like activity of protamine

3. Which of the following cardiovascular agents is classified chemically as a glycoside?

(A) Nifedipine
(B) Digoxin
(C) Flecainide
(D) Cholestyramine
(E) Warfarin

4. Cardiac glycosides may be useful in treating all of the following conditions EXCEPT

(A) atrial flutter
(B) paroxysmal atrial tachycardia
(C) congestive heart failure
(D) ventricular tachycardia
(E) atrial fibrillation

5. Ingestion of which of the following vitamins should be avoided by a patient taking the oral anticoagulant?

(A) Vitamin A
(B) Vitamin B
(C) Vitamin D
(D) Vitamin E
(E) Vitamin K

Directions: Each item below contains three suggested answers of which **one or more** is correct. Choose the answer

A if **I only** is correct
B if **III only** is correct
C if **I and II** are correct
D if **II and III** are correct
E if **I, II, and III** are correct

6. In the oral treatment of iron deficiency anemias, iron is preferably administered as

I. ferrous iron
II. ferric salts
III. elemental iron

7. Parenterally administered antihypertensive agents used in treating hypertensive emergencies include the

I. centrally acting antiadrenergic clonidine
II. arteriolar and venous vasodilator nitroprusside
III. ganglionic-blocking agent trimethaphan

8. Certain factors contribute to the longer duration of action of digitoxin when compared with that of digoxin. These include

I. greater protein binding
II. reduced polarity
III. greater tubular reabsorption

9. Correct statements concerning the properties of oral anticoagulants include

I. oral anticoagulants interfere with vitamin K-dependent synthesis of active clotting factors II, VII, IX, and X
II. adverse effects associated with oral anticoagulants are hemorrhage, urticaria, purpura, and alopecia
III. oral anticoagulants prolong the clotting time of blood both in vivo and in vitro

Directions: The group of items in this section consists of lettered options followed by a set of numbered items. For each item, select the **one** lettered option that is most closely associated with it. Each lettered option may be selected once, more than once, or not at all.

Questions 10–12

For each group of adverse effects, select the class of drug that most closely relates to it.

(A) Cardiac glycosides
(B) Calcium channel blockers
(C) Angiotensin-converting enzyme (ACE) inhibitors
(D) β-Adrenergic blockers
(E) Nitrites and nitrates

10. Bradycardia, hypotension, increased airway resistance, and congestive heart failure

11. Visual disturbances (yellow or green vision), confusion, anorexia, vomiting, atrioventricular block, and ventricular tachycardia

12. Hypotension, acute renal failure, cholestatic jaundice, and agranulocytosis

ANSWERS AND EXPLANATIONS

1. The answer is C *[III B 3, C 3, D 3].*
Calcium channel blockers are used in the treatment of angina because they dilate coronary arteries and arterioles, thus decreasing coronary vascular resistance and increasing coronary blood flow.

2. The answer is D *[VII A 1, 4; Figure 17-6].*
Heparin is a highly acidic mucopolysaccharide, whereas protamine is a highly basic protein. When administered subsequently to heparin, protamine chemically combines with it (presumably by an acid-base interaction) and inactivates its anticoagulant effect. Hence, it is an effective antidote for heparin. Caution must be employed when using protamine because an excess of protamine can cause an anticoagulant effect itself.

3. The answer is B *[II A 1].*
Most glycosides are natural products obtained from plant material. Although there are very few medicinal agents that are glycosides, the group known as the cardiac glycosides are extremely important and are widely used for treating congestive heart failure. Digoxin is a cardiac glycoside obtained from *Digitalis lanata.* Other cardiac glycosides include digitoxin, which is obtained from *Digitalis purpurea,* and ouabain, which is obtained from *Strophanthus gratus.*

4. The answer is D *[II C; Table 17-4].*
Ventricular tachycardia is produced by toxic cardiac glycoside dosage and would not be a therapeutic indication for the agents. Cardiac glycosides increase systolic contraction velocity and increase the refractory period of the atrioventricular (AV) node. They also have a positive inotropic effect.

5. The answer is E *[VII A 2 b, 4 c].*
The oral anticoagulants, such as warfarin, act by inhibiting the liver biosynthesis of prothrombin, which is the precursor of the enzyme thrombin that catalyzes the conversion of soluble fibrinogen to the insoluble polymer fibrin, which results in clot formation. One of the principal factors in the biosynthesis of prothrombin is vitamin K, with which warfarin competes to inhibit this process. Since this is a reversible competition, vitamin K acts as an antagonist to the oral anticoagulants.

6. The answer is A (I) *[VIII A 1].*
Absorption of orally administered iron is significantly more complete with ferrous iron than with either ferric salts or elemental iron, presumably because of its better solubility characteristics. Iron preparations (ferrous salts) are more readily absorbed from the gastrointestinal tract and are stored in the bone marrow, liver, and spleen as ferritin and hemosiderin.

7. The answer is D (II, III) *[V B 4, C 2 a, e].*
Clonidine is not recognized as a drug of choice for hypertensive emergencies, possibly because of its central mechanism of action and the latent period required for its effect, compared with other peripheral agents.

8. The answer is E (all) *[II A; Figure 17-1].*
Structurally, digitoxin has only one alcohol group on its steroidal nucleus, whereas digoxin has two. This slight difference in structure has a significant effect on the polarity of the molecule. Owing to its greater liposolubility, digitoxin is more likely to undergo tubular reabsorption, to undergo enterohepatic cycling, to penetrate into the liver microsomes and undergo metabolism, and to be protein-bound, all of which contribute to its longer duration of action and potential cumulative effects.

9. The answer is C (I, II) *[VII A 2 b, 4 c (1)].*
Oral anticoagulants are only effective in vivo since they block hepatic synthesis of vitamin K–dependent coagulation factors (factors II, VII, IX, and X). This also explains the latency period associated with initiation of oral anticoagulant therapy.

10–12. The answers are: 10-D *[III D 2],* **11-A** *[II D],* **12-C** *[V D 6].*
Nonselective β-adrenergic blockers (e.g., propranolol) produce adverse effects associated with their mechanism of action on the autonomic nervous system. Thus, bronchospasm, lowering of blood pressure, and reduced heart rate result from blockade of autonomic β-adrenergic receptors. Visual disturbances (yellow or green vision) are peculiar to cardiac glycoside overdose. Atrioventricular (AV) dissociation and ventricular tachycardia are obviously more significant adverse effects. Angiotensin-converting enzyme inhibitors reportedly may cause blood dyscrasias in addition to cholestatic jaundice and acute renal failure.

18
Diuretics

David C. Kosegarten
Edward F. LaSala
J. Edward Moreton

I. INTRODUCTION. Diuretics increase the rate of urine formation, increasing urine volume and water and solute excretion. Diuretics fall into five major categories: osmotic diuretics, carbonic anhydrase inhibitors, benzothiadiazide diuretics, loop diuretics, and potassium-sparing diuretics.

II. OSMOTIC DIURETICS

A. Chemistry. Osmotic diuretics (e.g., mannitol, urea) are highly polar, water-soluble agents with a low renal threshold (Figure 18-1).

B. Pharmacology

1. Osmotic diuretics are relatively inert chemicals that are freely filtered at the glomerulus and poorly reabsorbed from the renal tubule. By increasing the osmolarity of the glomerular filtrate, they **limit tubular reabsorption of water** and, thus, **promote diuresis.**

2. Because these agents increase water, sodium, chloride, and bicarbonate excretion, they cause an **increase in urinary pH.**

C. Therapeutic indications. Osmotic diuretics are used to:

1. Help prevent and treat oliguria and anuria

2. Reduce cerebral edema and decrease intracranial pressure

3. Reduce intraocular pressure

D. Adverse effects. Osmotic diuretics are associated with:

1. Headache and blurred vision

2. Increased blood volume (aggravates congestive heart failure)

III. CARBONIC ANHYDRASE INHIBITORS

A. Chemistry. Carbonic anhydrase inhibitors are aromatic or heterocyclic sulfonamides with a prominent thiadiazole nucleus. **Acetazolamide** is the prototypical agent (Figure 18-2).

B. Pharmacology

1. Carbonic anhydrase inhibitors **noncompetitively inhibit the enzyme carbonic anhydrase.** This prevents the enzyme from providing the tubular hydrogen ions needed for exchange with sodium in the proximal tubule, resulting in sodium bicarbonate diuresis.

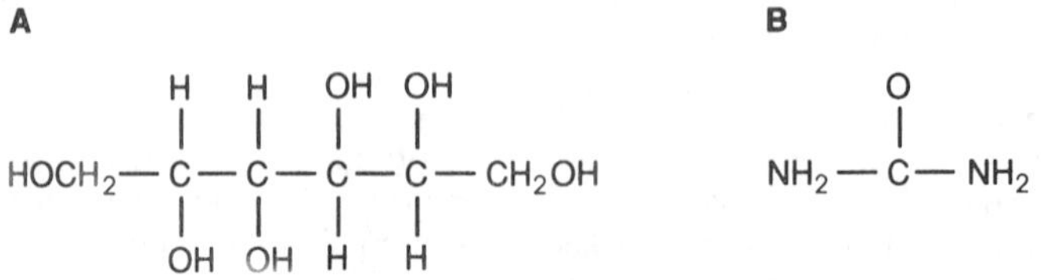

Figure 18-1. Structural formulas of (*A*) mannitol (Osmitrol) and (*B*) urea (Ureaphil), osmotic diuretics.

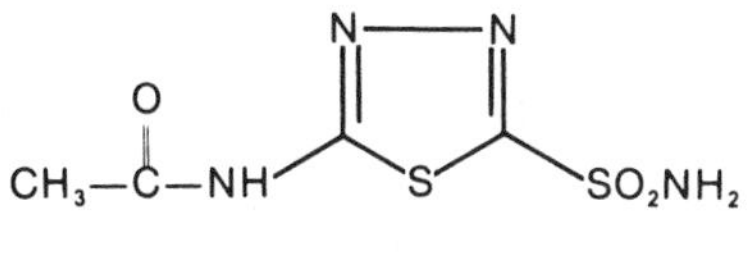

Figure 18-2. Structural formula of acetazoamide (Diamox), the prototypical carbonic anhydrase inhibitor.

2. Because these agents increase water, sodium, potassium, and bicarbonate excretion, they cause an **alkaline urinary pH.**

C. Therapeutic indications. Carbonic anhydrase inhibitors are used to:

1. Reduce edema (as adjunct diuretic therapy)
2. Reduce intraocular pressure (retard aqueous humor formation)
3. Alkalinize the urine, enhancing excretion of acidic drugs and their metabolites
4. Treat motor disorders as petit mal epilepsy, paroxysmal chorea and dystonia, periodic ataxia, and some cases of essential tremor

D. Adverse effects. Carbonic anhydrase inhibitors are associated with:

1. Central nervous system (CNS) effects, such as CNS depression, drowsiness, sedation, fatigue, disorientation, and paresthesia
2. Gastrointestinal (GI) effects, such as GI upset, nausea, vomiting, and constipation
3. Hematologic effects, such as bone marrow depression, thrombocytopenia, hemolytic anemia, leukopenia, and agranulocytosis
4. Hyperchloremic metabolic acidosis
5. Sulfonamide-type hypersensitivity reactions

IV. BENZOTHIADIAZIDE DIURETICS

A. Chemistry

1. The commonly used benzothiadiazide diuretics **(thiazides)** are primarily closely related **benzothiadiazides with variable substituents.** The prototypical agent is chlorothiazide (Figure 18-3, see Figure 18-3*A*).
2. Optimal diuretic activity depends on certain **structural features.**
   - **a.** The benzene ring must have a sulfonamide group (preferably unsubstituted) in position 7 and a **halogen** (usually a chloro group) or a **trifluoromethyl group** in position 6 (see Figure 18-3).
   - **b. Saturation of the 3,4-double bond** increases potency, as with hydrochlorothiazide (see Figure 18-3*B*).
   - **c. Lipophilic substituents** at position 3 or **methyl groups** at position 2 enhance potency and prolong activity, as with cyclothiazide and bendroflumethiazide (see Figure 18-3*C*).
   - **d. Replacement of the sulfonyl group** in position 1 by a **carbonyl group** results in prolonged activity, as with quinethazone (see Figure 18-3*D*).
3. A few **sulfamoylbenzamides** (e.g., indapamide, chlorthalidone) have activity similar to that of the benzothiadiazides (Figure 18-4).
4. **Benzothiadiazines without the sulfonamide group** (e.g., diazoxide) exhibit antihypertensive activity but lack diuretic activity (Figure 18-5).

B. Pharmacology

1. Benzothiadiazides **directly inhibit sodium and chloride reabsorption** on the luminal membrane of the early segment of the distal convoluted tubule.
2. These agents increase water, sodium, chloride, potassium, and bicarbonate excretion and decrease calcium excretion and uric acid secretion. They may cause an **alkaline urinary pH** by inhibiting carbonic anhydrase.

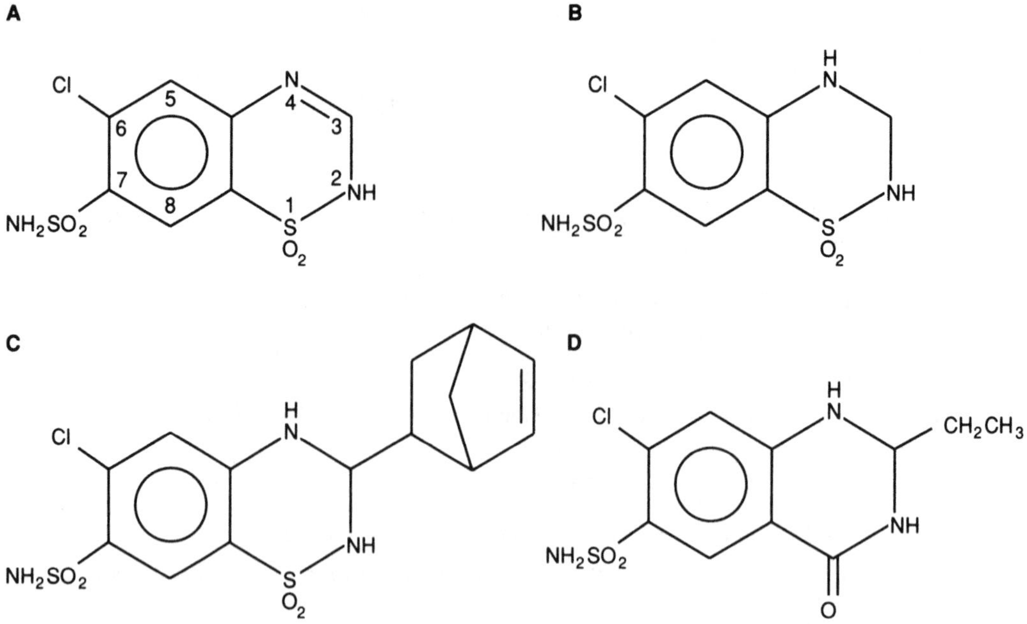

Figure 18-3. Structural formulas of (*A*) chlorothiazide (Diuril), the prototypical benzothiadiazide diuretic, and (*B*) hydrochlorothiazide (Hydrodiuril) as well as (*C*) cyclothiazide (Anhydron) and (*D*) quinethazone (Hydromox), related compounds with substituents that prolong activity and enhace potency.

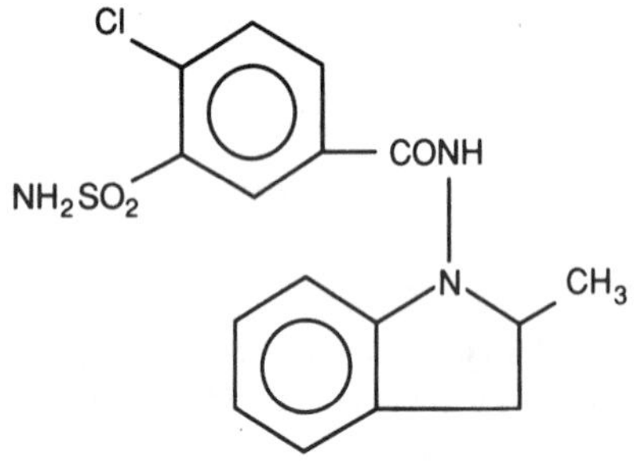

Figure 18-4. Structural formula of indapamide (Lozol), a sulfamoybenzamide with pharmacologic activity similar to that of the benzothiadiazide diuretics.

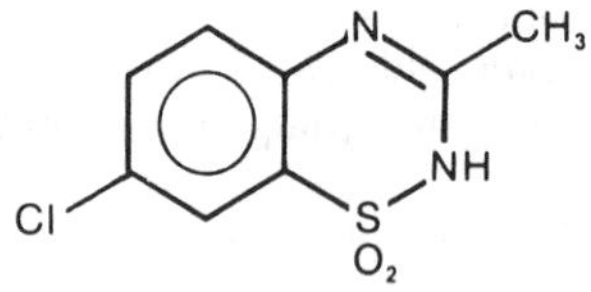

Figure 18-5. Structural formula of diazoxide (Hyperstat), a benzothiadiazine lacking a sulfonamide group and diuretic action.

C. Therapeutic indications. Benzothiadiazides are used to:

1. Treat chronic edema
2. Treat hypertension
3. Treat congestive heart failure (as adjunctive edema therapy)

D. Adverse effects. Benzothiadiazides are associated with:

1. CNS effects, such as headache, dizziness, paresthesias, drowsiness, and restlessness
2. GI effects, such as GI irritation, nausea, vomiting, abdominal bloating, and constipation
3. Cardiovascular effects, such as orthostatic hypotension, palpitations, hemoconcentration, and venous thrombosis
4. Hematologic effects, such as blood dyscrasias, leukopenia, thrombocytopenia, agranulocytosis, aplastic anemia, hemolytic anemia, and rash

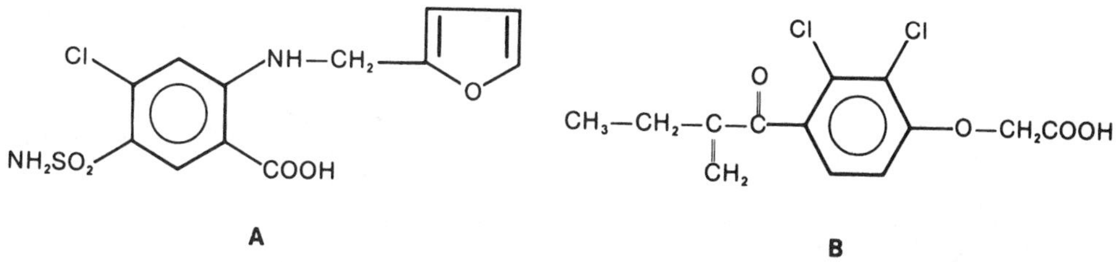

Figure 18-6. Structural formulas of (*A*) furosemide (Lasix) and (*B*) ethacrynic acid (Edecrin), loop diuretics.

5. Fluid and electrolyte imbalances, such as hypokalemia and hypercalcemia, and hyperuricemia
6. Muscular cramps
7. Hyperuricemia and acute gout attacks
8. Hypercholesterolemia and hypertriglyceridemia
9. Sulfonamide-type hypersensitivity reaction

V. LOOP DIURETICS

A. Chemistry. Loop diuretics are anthranilic acid derivatives with a sulfonamide substituent (e.g., furosemide and bumetanide) or aryloxyacetic acids without a sulfonamide substituent (e.g., Fig. 18-6 ethacrynic acid) [Figure 18-6].

B. Pharmacology

1. These agents act principally at the thick ascending limb of the loop of Henle, where they **inhibit the cotransport of sodium and chloride from the luminal filtrate.**
2. Loop diuretics increase excretion of water, sodium, potassium, calcium, and chloride; decrease uric acid secretion; and cause **no change in urinary pH.**

C. Therapeutic indications. Loop diuretics are used to:

1. Treat edema from congestive heart failure, hepatic cirrhosis, and renal disease
2. Treat pulmonary edema and ascites

D. Adverse effects. Loop diuretics are associated with:

1. Fluid and electrolyte imbalances, such as hypokalemia, azotemia, dehydration, hyperuricemia, and hypercalciuria
2. CNS effects, such as headache, vertigo, blurred vision, tinnitus, and (rarely) irreversible hearing loss
3. Hematologic effects, such as thrombocytopenia and agranulocytosis
4. Cardiovascular effects, such as orthostatic hypotension
5. GI effects, such as nausea, vomiting, and diarrhea
6. Leg cramps
7. Hypercholesterolemia and hypertriglyceridemia
8. Sulfonamide-type hypersensitivity reaction

VI. POTASSIUM-SPARING DIURETICS

A. Chemistry. The potassium-sparing diuretics are pteridine or pyrazine derivatives (e.g., triamterene, amiloride) or steroid analogue antagonists of aldosterone (e.g., spironolactone) [Figure 18-7].

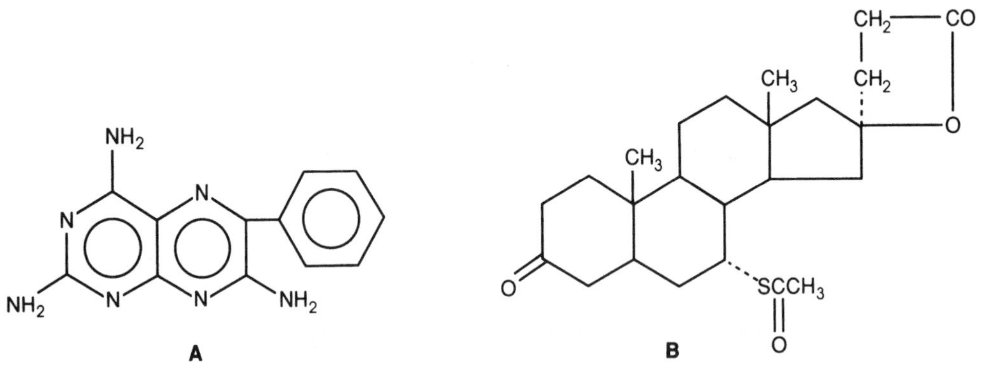

Figure 18-7. Structural fromulas of (*A*) triamterene (Dyrenium) and (*B*) spironolactone (Aldactone), potassium-sparing diuretics.

B. Pharmacology

1. **Spironolactone** acts as a **competitive inhibitor of aldosterone** at mineralocorticoid receptors in the late distal tubule and collecting duct. It interferes with aldosterone-mediated sodium-potassium exchange, decreasing potassium secretion.

2. **Triamterene and amiloride,** which are not aldosterone antagonists, act directly on the late distal tubule and collecting duct. They disrupt sodium exchange with potassium and hydrogen by blocking sodium channels and decreasing the driving force for secretion of potassium and hydrogen.

3. The potassium-sparing diuretics increase bicarbonate excretion and cause an **alkaline urinary pH.**

C. Therapeutic indications.

Potassium-sparing diuretics are used:

1. As adjunctive therapy, to treat edema from congestive heart failure, hepatic cirrhosis, nephrotic syndrome, and hyperaldosteronism (primary and secondary)
2. As adjunctive therapy (with thiazides and loop diuretics), to treat hypertension
3. To treat or prevent hypokalemia

D. Adverse effects

1. **Spironolactone** is associated with:
   a. Hyperkalemia
   b. GI effects, such as GI upset, GI bleeding, gastritis, nausea, abdominal cramps, and diarrhea
   c. Endocrine effects, such as gynecomastia, menstrual irregularities, and hirsutism
   d. CNS effects, such as mental confusion and lethargy

2. **Triamterene** and **amiloride** are associated with:
   a. Hyperkalemia
   b. GI effects, such as GI upset, GI bleeding, nausea, and vomiting
   c. CNS effects, such as headache and dizziness
   d. Increased uric acid levels in patients with gouty arthritis (with triamterene)
   e. Methemoglobinemia in patients with alcoholic cirrhosis (with triamterene, which inhibits dihydrofolate reductase)

STUDY QUESTIONS

Directions: Each of the numbered items or incomplete statements in this section is followed by answers or by completions of the statement. Select the **one** lettered answer or completion that is **best** in each case.

1. The structure shown below is characteristic of which of the following agents?

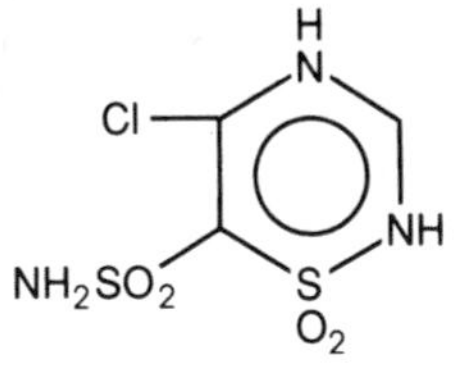

(A) Osmotic diuretics
(B) Carbonic anhydrase inhibitors
(C) Thiazides
(D) Loop diuretics
(E) Potassium-sparing diuretics

2. Which of the following diuretics is most similar in chemical structure to the antihypertensive agent diazoxide?

(A) Furosemide
(B) Spironolactone
(C) Mannitol
(D) Acetazolamide
(E) Chlorothiazide

Directions: The group of items in this section consists of lettered options followed by a set of numbered items. For each item, select the **one** lettered option that is most closely associated with it. Each lettered option may be selected once, more than once, or not at all.

Questions 3–5

For each statement listed below, select the drug that it most closely characterizes.

(A) Furosemide
(B) Hydrochlorothiazide
(C) Spironolactone
(D) Mannitol
(E) Acetazolamide

3. It interferes with distal tubular aldosterone-mediated sodium-potassium exchange, renders the urine alkaline, and may cause hyperkalemia, gynecomastia, and menstrual irregularities

4. Freely filtered, this drug limits tubular reabsorption of water and is useful in reducing cerebral edema and intracranial pressure

5. The principal site of action of this drug is on the thick ascending limb of Henle's loop; it is useful in treating pulmonary edema and ascites

ANSWERS AND EXPLANATIONS

1. The answer is C *[IV A; Figure 18-3].*
The structure can be recognized as a benzothiadiazine, which is known also as a thiazide. It represents the structure of hydrochlorothiazide, a sulfonamide diuretic. Other sulfonamide diuretics include the carbonic anhydrase inhibitors, such as acetazolamide, and the loop diuretics, such as furosemide. Neither of these subclasses contains drugs with a benzothiadiazine nucleus.

2. The answer is E *[IVA; Figures 18-3, 18-5].*
Diazoxide is a benzothiadiazine derivative; therefore, it would be most similar to chlorothiazide, which is also a benzothiadiazine. While both the thiazides and the diazoxides have antihypertensive activity, only the thiazides have significant diuretic activity. One of the structural requirements of the thiazide diuretics is an electron-withdrawing group, such as a halogen, ortho to the sulfonamide group on the benzene nucleus. The diazoxide molecule lacks such a group.

3–5. The answers are: 3-C *[VI B 1, D 1],* **4-D** *[II B 1, C 2],* **5-A** *[V B 1, C 1].*
Spironolactone interferes with aldosterone-mediated sodium-potassium exchange, reducing the amount of potassium excreted and is often used with other diuretics that promote the excretion of potassium, such as the benzothiadiazides. Mannitol increases the osmolarity of the glomerular filtrate since it is reabsorbed poorly. By increasing the osmolarity of the glomerular filtrate, mannitol limits tubular reabsorption of water, thus promoting diuresis. In this way, it reduces cerebral edema and decreases intracranial pressure. Furosemide is a diuretic of choice for treating acute congestive heart failure because it promotes a significant rapid excretion of water and sodium.

19
Hormones and Related Drugs

Marc W. Harrold
Pui-Kai Li

I. INTRODUCTION. Hormones are substances secreted by specific tissues and transported to other specific tissues, where they exert their effects. They can be classified pharmacologically as drugs. Hormones can be obtained from natural substances (animal preparations), or they may be synthetic or semisynthetic compounds resembling the natural products. They are often used for replacement therapy (e.g., exogenous insulin for treatment of diabetes mellitus). However, they can also be used for a variety of other therapeutic and diagnostic purposes. Certain drugs (e.g., thyroid hormone inhibitors, oral antidiabetic agents), while not hormones themselves, influence the synthesis or secretion of hormones. Therapeutically useful hormones and related drugs include the pituitary hormones, the gonadal hormones, the adrenocorticosteroids, the thyroid hormones and inhibitors, and the antidiabetic agents.

II. PITUITARY HORMONES

A. Chemistry. Pituitary hormones are divided into two groups by their site of secretion.

1. **Posterior pituitary hormones.** The two posterior pituitary hormones, **oxytocin** (Pitocin) and **vasopressin** (Pitressin), are closely related octapeptides. They differ from each other in only two of their eight amino acids but have different biologic actions.

2. **Anterior pituitary hormones**
   a. **Protein molecules** are anterior pituitary hormones that are used therapeutically.
      (1) **Corticotropin** (Acthar), known as **adrenocorticotropic hormone (ACTH),** is a single-chain polypeptide containing 39 amino acids. It has a molecular weight (mol wt) of 4600.
      (2) **Thyrotropin** (Thytropar), known as **thyroid-stimulating hormone (TSH),** is a glycoprotein with a mol wt of 28,000.
      (3) **Thyrotropin-releasing hormone (TRH)** [Relefact], known as protirelin, is a tripeptide with a mol wt of 363.
      (4) **Growth hormone** (Asellacrin), known as somatotropin, consists of 191 amino acids and has a mol wt of 21,500.
   b. **Pituitary gonadotropins** are anterior pituitary hormones that are not available for therapeutic use. These include **follicle-stimulating hormone (FSH), luteinizing hormone (LH),** and **prolactin [luteotropic hormone (LTH)].** However, several related nonpituitary gonadotropins have FSH-like or LH-like actions and are used therapeutically. These include:
      (1) **Menotropins** (Pergonal), known as hMG (human menopausal gonadotropin), are high in FSH-like and LH-activity and are obtained from the urine of postmenopausal women.
      (2) **Urofollitropin** (Metrodin) is high in FSH-like activity and is obtained from the urine of postmenopausal women.
      (3) **Human chorionic gonadotropin (hCG)** [Follutein] has LH-like activity and is obtained from the urine of pregnant women.

B. Pharmacology. The therapeutically important pituitary hormones include the **anterior pituitary agents** (corticotropin), **growth hormone** (somatotropin), and **menotropins** (gonadotropin), and the **posterior pituitary agents** (vasopressin and oxytocin).

1. **Corticotropin** is secreted from the anterior pituitary, stimulating the adrenal cortex to produce and secrete adrenocorticosteroids (see IV).

2. **Growth hormone** stimulates protein, carbohydrate, and lipid metabolism to promote increased cell, organ, connective tissue, and skeletal growth, causing a rapid increase in the overall rate of linear growth.

3. **Menotropins** produce ovarian follicular growth and induce ovulation by means of FSH-like and LH-like actions.

4. **Vasopressin** has vasopressor and antidiuretic hormone (ADH) activity. It acts primarily on the distal renal tubular epithelium, where it promotes the reabsorption of water.

5. **Oxytocin** stimulates uterine contraction and plays an important role in the induction of labor.

C. Therapeutic indications

1. **Corticotropin** is used primarily for the diagnosis and differentiation of primary and secondary adrenal insufficiency.

2. **Growth hormone** is used for the long-term treatment of children whose growth failure is the result of lack of endogenous growth hormone secretion.

3. **Menotropins** are used to induce ovulation and pregnancy in anovulatory infertile women whose anovulation is not the result of primary ovarian failure. In men, menotropins are used to induce spermatogenesis.

4. **Vasopressin** is used to treat neurogenic diabetes insipidus and to treat postoperative abdominal distention.

5. **Oxytocin** is used to promote delivery by initiating and improving uterine contractions and to control postpartum bleeding or hemorrhage.

D. Adverse effects

1. **Corticotropin** is only rarely associated with adverse effects, which represent hypersensitivity reactions or corticosteroid excess.

2. **Growth hormone** is associated with adverse effects primarily related to the development of antibodies to growth hormone. The antibodies are nonbinding in most cases and do not interfere with continued growth hormone treatment.

3. **Menotropins** are associated with:
   a. **Hypersensitivity,** arterial thromboembolism, febrile reactions, ovarian enlargement hyperstimulation syndrome, hemoperitoneum, and (rarely) birth defects in women
   b. **Gynecomastia** in men

4. **Vasopressin** is associated with:
   a. Gastrointestinal (GI) effects, such as abdominal cramps, flatulence, nausea, and vomiting
   b. Central nervous system (CNS) effects, such as tremor, sweating, vertigo, and headache
   c. Other effects, such as urticaria, bronchoconstriction, and anaphylaxis

5. **Oxytocin** is associated with:
   a. Sever water intoxication with convulsions and coma after slow (24-hour) infusion
   b. Uterine hypertonicity, with spasm, tetanic contraction, or uterine rupture
   c. Postpartum hemorrhage
   d. Nausea, vomiting, and anaphylaxis
   e. Fetal effects, such as bradycardia, neonatal jaundice, cardiac dysrhythmias, and premature ventricular contractions

III. GONADAL HORMONES.

Most natural and synthetic gonadal hormones are derivatives of cyclopentanoperhydrophenanthrene (Figure 19-1). All hormones having this fused reduced 17-carbon-atom ring system are classified as steroids.

A. Estrogen

1. **Natural and semisynthetic estrogens.** The basic nucleus of the natural estrogens has a methyl group designated as C-18 on position C-13 of cyclopentanoperhydrophenanthrene. This basic nucleus is known as **estrane.**

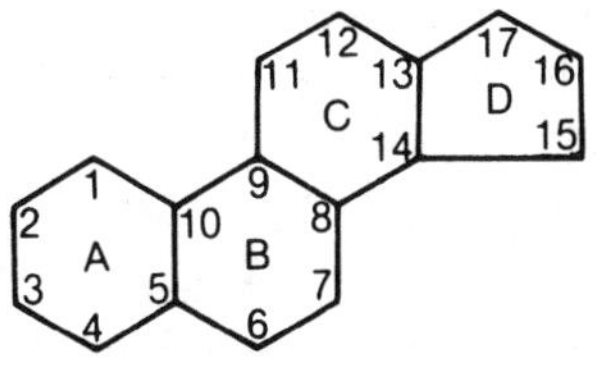

Figure 19-1. Structural formula of cyclopentanoperhydrophenanthrene, from which the gonadal hormones are derived. The letters *A* through *D* indicate the rings, which may be modified during subsequent conversions; the numbers 1 through 17 refer to carbon atom positions on the rings.

a. Unlike other steroid hormones, all estrogens have an aromatic A ring (see Figure 19-1).

b. Estradiol (Estrace), the principal estrogenic hormone, exists in the body in equilibrium with estrone, which is converted to estriol prior to excretion (Figure 19-2).

c. Several estradiol esters, such as estradiol cypionate and estradiol valerate (Figure 19-3), are prepared as intramuscular injections in oil, to prolong their action. These estradiol esters are slowly hydrolyzed in muscle tissues before absorption and, thus, are considered to be prodrugs.

d. Several 17α-substituted estradiols increase resistance to first-pass metabolism and enhance oral effectiveness. Two of these estradiol derivatives, ethinyl estradiol and its 3-methyl ether mestranol, are used principally as the estrogenic components of serial-type oral contraceptives (Figure 19-4). Another, quinestrol (Estrovis), is used principally for estrogen replacement therapy.

2. **Nonsteroidal synthetic estrogens** (e.g., diethylstilbestrol, dienestrol, chlorotrianisene) are nonsteroidal stilbene derivatives that appear to assume an estradiol-like conformation in vivo (Figure 19-5).

3. **Estrogen antagonists** (antiestrogens). The antiestrogens clomiphene and tamoxifen citrate are stilbene derivatives that are structurally related to chlorotrianisene (Figure 19-6). However, these agents have different in vivo binding sites and activities.

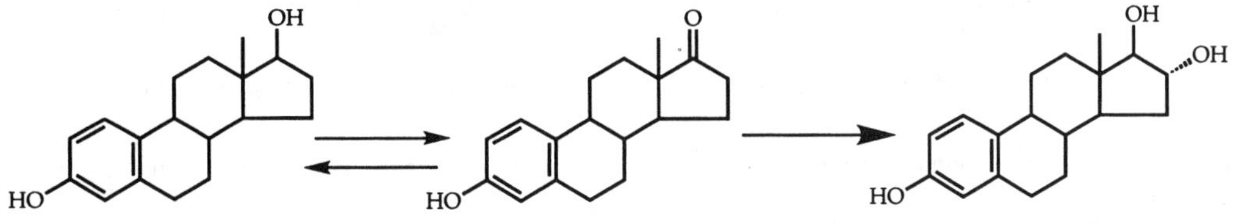

A B C

Figure 19-2. Structural formulas of (*A*) estradiol, which exists in the body in equilibrium with (*B*) estrone, which in turn is converted to (*C*) estriol before excretion.

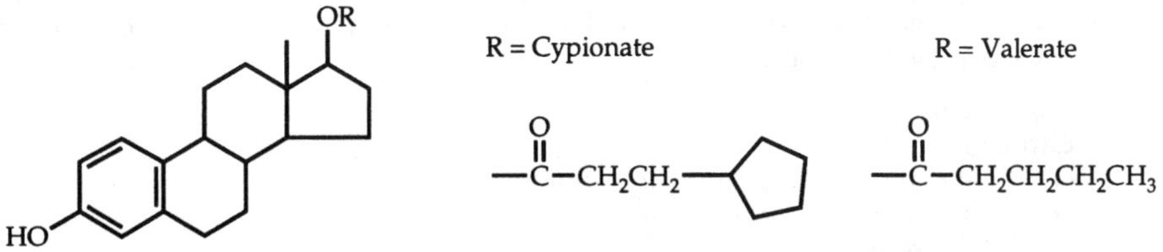

Figure 19-3. Structural formulas of estradiol cypionate and valerate.

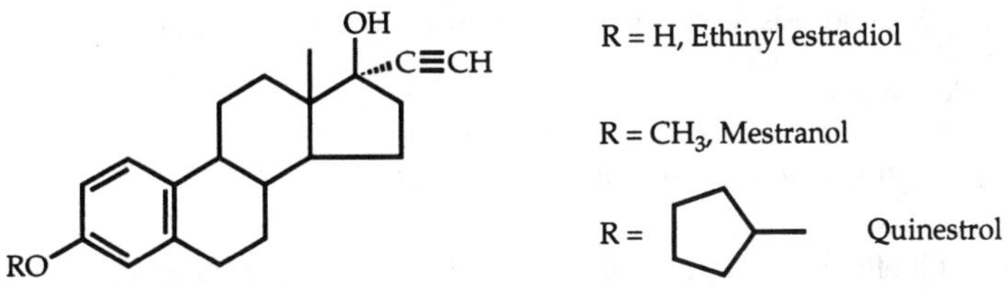

Figure 19-4. Structural formulas of ethinyl estradiol, mestranol and quinestrol.

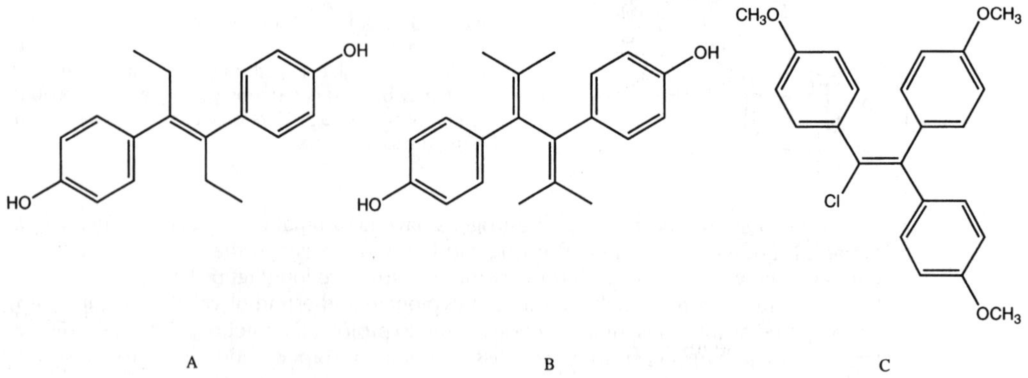

Figure 19-5. Structural formulas of (*A*) diethylstilbestrol (DES), (*B*) dienestrol and (*C*) chlorotrianisene (Tace), synthetic estrogens derived from stilbene.

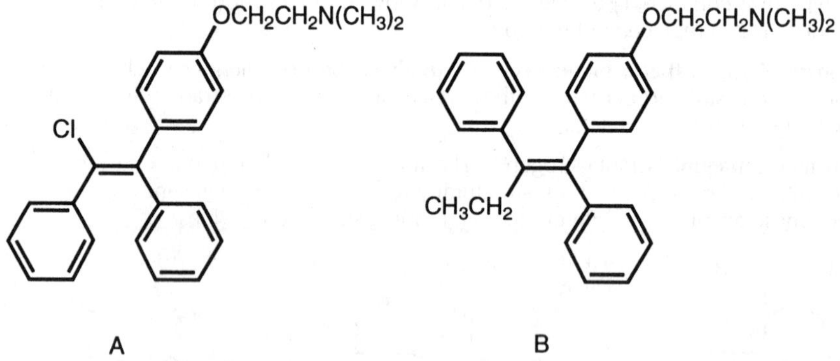

Figure 19-6. Structural formulas of antiestrogens (*A*) clomiphene and (*B*) tamoxifen. They are structurally similar to chlorotrianisene.

4. **Pharmacology** (estrogen). The specificity of estrogen actions is due to the presence of estrogen receptors in estrogen-responsive tissues (e.g., vagina, uterus, mammary glands, anterior pituitary, hypothalamus). The receptors are located in the nucleus. When the estrogen has bound to the estrogen receptor, the receptor undergoes a conformational change that activates the estrogen-receptor complex, increases its affinity for DNA, and alters the production of messenger RNA (mRNA). This ultimately leads to either an increase or decrease in enzyme or protein synthesis.

5. **Therapeutic uses**
   a. **Estrogens**
      (1) Oral contraceptives (in combination with progestins)
      (2) Treatment of menopausal symptoms
         (a) Vasomotor disorder
         (b) Urogenital atrophy
         (c) Psychological disorder
      (3) Acne
      (4) Osteoporosis, both senile and postmenopausal osteoporosis
      (5) Prostate cancer
   b. **Antiestrogen**
      (1) Tamoxifen is used to treat estrogen-dependent breast cancer.
      (2) Clomiphene is used to induce ovulation in women who have ovulation failure.

6. **Adverse effects** of estrogens
      (1) GI effects, such as GI distress, nausea, vomiting, anorexia, and diarrhea
      (2) Cardiovascular effects, such as hypertension and an increased incidence of thromboembolic diseases, stroke, and myocardial infarction

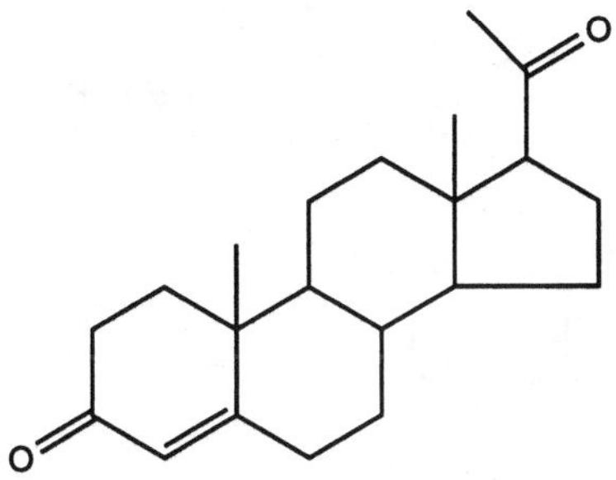

Figure 19-7. Structural formula of progesterone, which is a derivative of pregnane.

(3) Fluid and electrolyte disturbances, such as increased fluid retention and increased triglyceride level
(4) An increased incidence of endometrial cancer and hepatic adenomas (associated with long-term use)

B. Progestins

1. The **naturally occurring** progestin progesterone is C-21 steroid. Its basic nucleus is known as pregnane (Figure 19-7).
2. **Synthetic progestins,** which are also steroids, consist of two types.
   a. The 17α-hydroxyprogesterone derivatives (e.g., medroxyprogesterone acetate, megestrol acetate) typically introduce a methyl group at position C-6 progesterone and an acetoxyl group at position C-17. These substitutions increase lipid solubility and decrease firstpass metabolism, enhancing oral activity and the progestin effect (Figure 19-8).
   b. The 17α-ethinylandrogens are structurally classified as androgens but contain progestational activities.
      (1) The 17α-ethinylandrogens are more liposoluble than progesterone and undergo less first-pass metabolism.
      (2) These agents have potent oral activity and are extensively used as oral contraceptive. Other 17α-ethinylandrogens include the positional isomer of norethindrone, norethynodrel, its 18-methyl homologue norgestrel, and its 3, 17-diacetate analogue ethynodiol diacetate (Figure 19-9).
3. **Pharmacology.** The mechanism of action of progestins is similar to estrogen. Progestins bind to progesterone receptor located in the nucleus of progestin responsive tissues. The formation of progestin receptor complex results in the increase in the synthesis of mRNA and specific enzyme or protein synthesis.
4. **Therapeutic uses**
   a. Oral contraceptives (alone or in combination with estrogens)

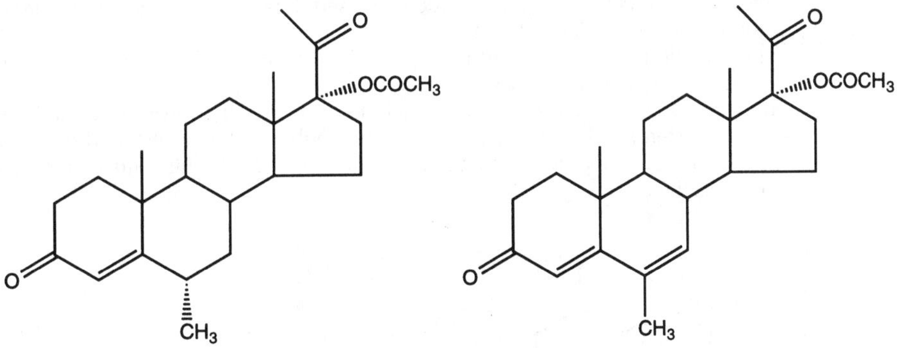

A B

Figure 19-8. Structural formulas of (*A*) medroxyprogesterone acetate (Provera) and (*B*) megestrol acetate (Megace), synthetic progestins.

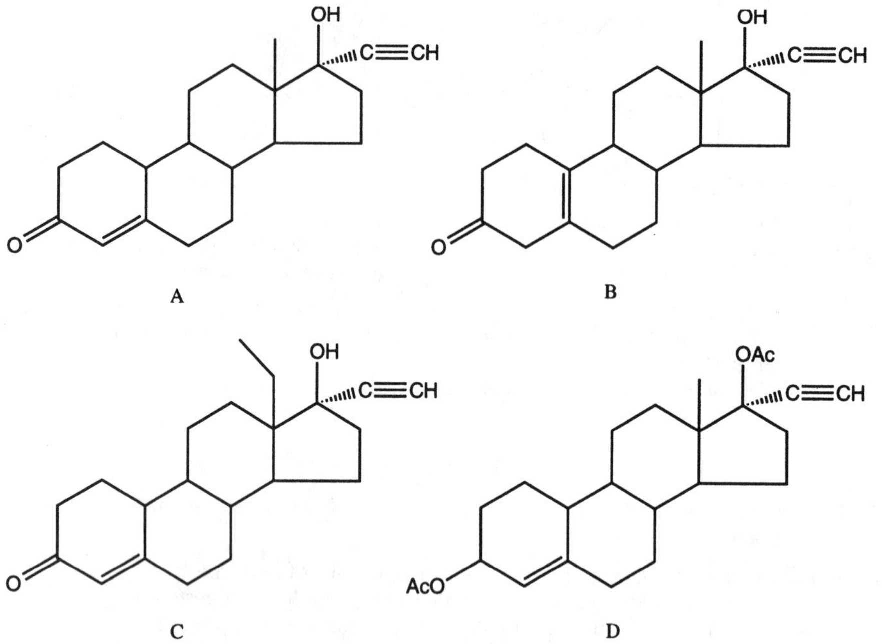

Figure 19-9. Structural formulas of (*A*) Norethindrone, (*B*) Norethynodrel, (*C*) Norgestrel and (*D*) Ethynodiol Diacetate

b. Menstrual disorder (dysfunctional uterine bleeding, dysmenorrhea)
c. Endometriosis

5. **Adverse effects**
   a. Gynecologic effects, such as irregular menses, breakthrough bleeding, and amenorrhea
   b. Weight gain and edema
   c. Exacerbation of breast carcinoma

C. Androgens and anabolic steroids

1. The primary natural androgen is **testosterone,** a C-19 steroid (Figure 19-10). Testosterone has two physiologic effects, androgenic and anabolic effects.
   a. Compounds used for **androgenic effects**
      (1) Esters of testosterone, such as testosterone 17-enanthate (Delatestryl), resemble estradiol esters in that they provide increased duration of action when administered intramuscularly (Figure 19-11).
      (2) Introduction of a methyl group at position C-17 results in potent, orally active androgens, such as fluoxymesterone (see Figure 19-11).
   b. Compounds used for **anabolic effects** include drugs resulting from structural modifications of testosterone. These drugs have a much-enhanced anabolic–androgenic activity ratio (e.g., oxandrolone, dromostanolone) [Figure 19-12]. Agents with 17-methyl groups are orally active.

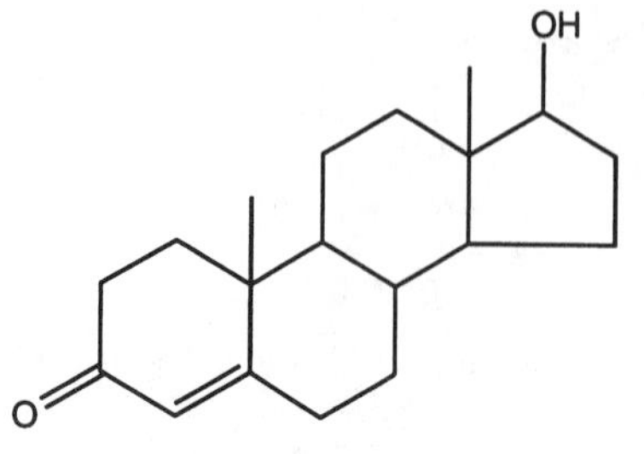

Figure 19-10. Structural formula of testosterone.

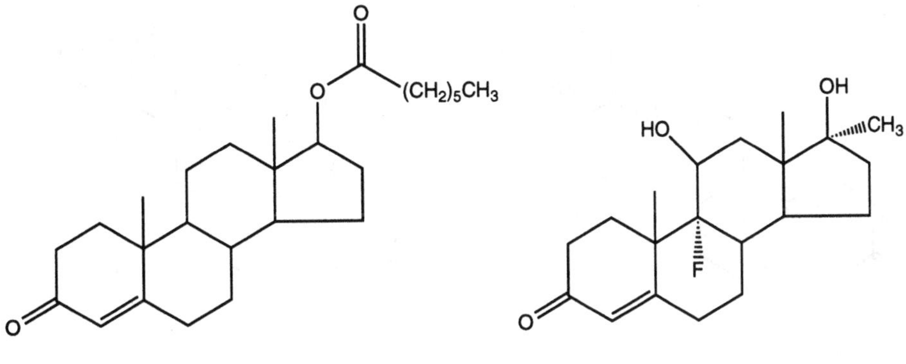

B

A

Figure 19-11. Structural formula of (*A*) testosterone enanthate and (*B*) fluoxymesterone.

2. **Pharmacology** (androgen). The mechanism of action of androgen is similar to estrogen. However, the molecule that binds to an androgen receptor is not testosterone. Testosterone is converted to dihydrotestosterone in the cytoplasm of androgen responsive tissue by the enzyme 5α-reductase. Dihydrotestosterone binds to an androgen receptor in the nucleus. The formation of androgen receptor complex results in the increase in the synthesis of mRNA and specific enzyme or protein synthesis.

3. **Therapeutic uses**
   (1) Androgen-replacement therapy
   (2) Breast cancer and endometriosis
   (3) Female hypopituitarism, in combination with estrogen therapy
   (4) Anabolic therapy, use in patients with negative nitrogen balance
   (5) Anemia

4. **Adverse effects**
   (1) Fluid retention
   (2) Increase LDL and decrease HDL cholesterol levels
   (3) Psychological changes
   (4) Liver disorders
   (5) Development of masculine features in female
   (6) Decreased fertility in male

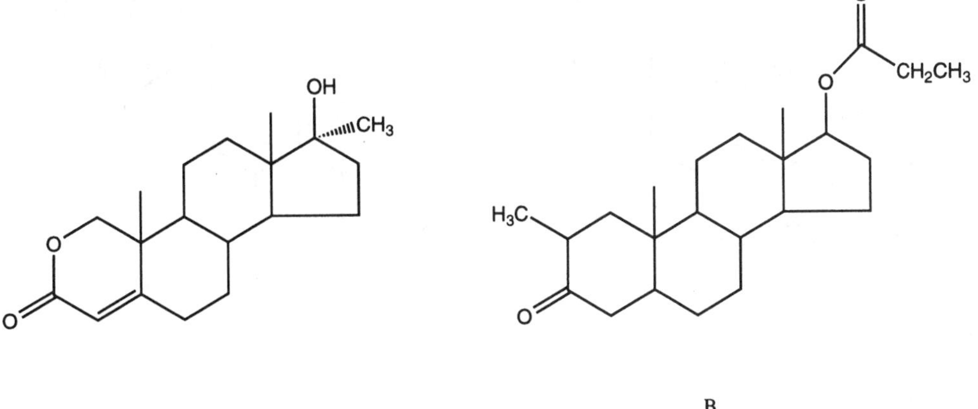

A

B

Figure 19-12. Structural formulas of (*A*) oxandrolone and (*B*) dromostanolone.

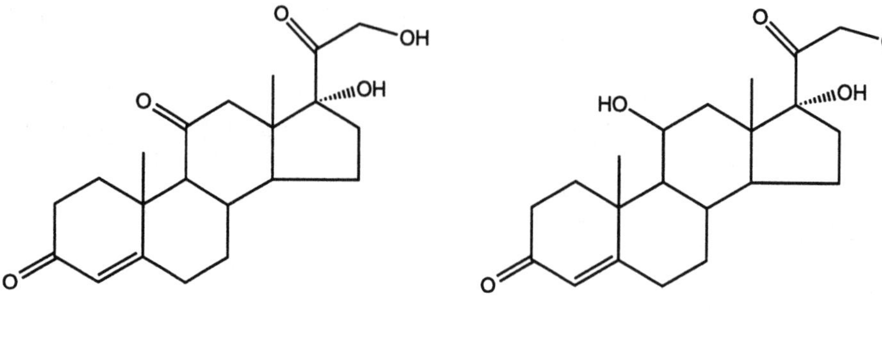

A B

Figure 19-13. Structural formulas of (*A*) cortisone and (*B*) hydrocortisone.

IV. ADRENOCORTICOSTEROID

A. Chemistry. The adrenal cortex synthesizes adrenocorticosteroids. Adrenocorticoids are divided into two classes. The first class is **mineralocorticoids,** possessing sodium-retaining and potassium-excreting effects, and the second class is **glucocorticoids,** possessing anti-inflammatory, protein-catabolic, and immunosuppressant effects. However, most naturally occurring adrenocorticosteroids have some degree of both mineralocorticoid and glucocorticoid activity. All adrenocorticosteroids are derived from the C-21 pregnane steroidal nucleus.

1. **Cortisone** and **hydrocortisone,** which are formed in the middle (fascicular) layer of the adrenal cortex (Figure 19-13), are the prototypical glucocorticoids.
   a. The 17 β-ketol side chain ($-COCH_2OH$), the 4-ene, and the 3-ketone structures are found in all clinically useful adrenocorticosteroids (see Figure 19-13).
   b. Many natural, semisynthetic, and synthetic glucocorticoids are available. **Modifications** of the prototypes cortisone and hydrocortisone represent attempts to increase glucocorticoid activity while decreasing mineralocorticoid activity.
      (1) The oxygen atom at position C-11 is essential for glucocorticoid activity.
      (2) A double bond between positions C-1 and C-2 increases glucocorticoid activity without increasing mineralocorticoid activity as with prednisolone (Figure 19-14).
      (3) Fluorination at position C-9 greatly increases both mineralocorticoid and glucocorticoid activity, as with fludrocortisone; whereas fluorination at position C-6 increases glucocorticoid activity with less effect on mineralocorticoid activity, as with fluprednisolone (see Figure 19-14).

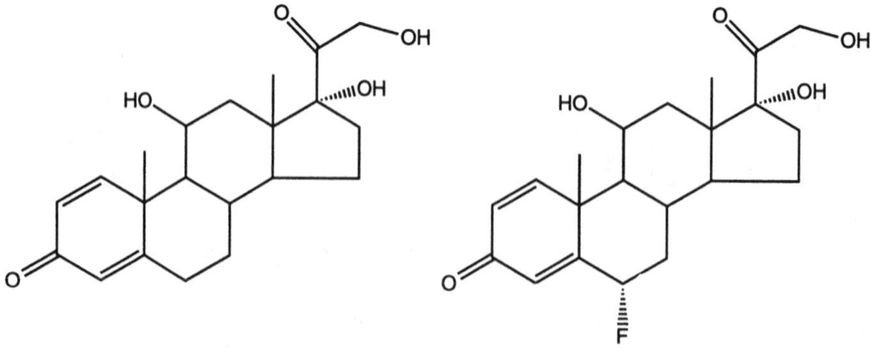

A B

Figure 19-14. Structural formulas of (*A*) prednisolone, and (*B*) fluprednisolone.

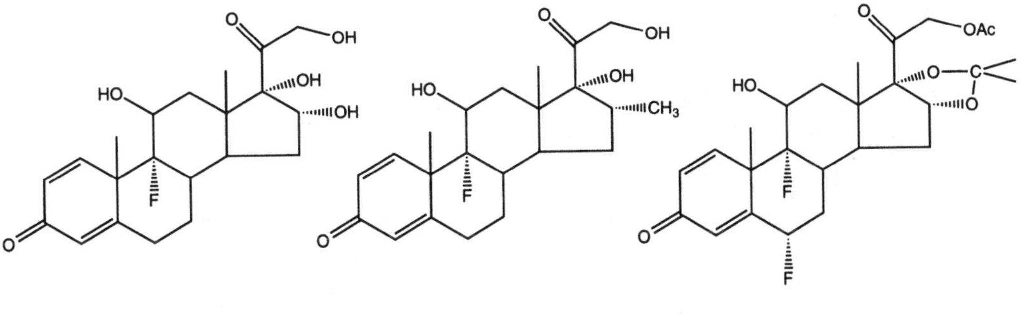

A B C

Figure 19-15. Structural formulas of (*A*) triamcinolone, (*B*) dexamethasone and (*C*) fluocinonide.

(4) A hydroxyl group at position C-17 and a hydroxyl group (as with triamcinolone) or a methyl group (as with dexamethasone) at position C-16 enhance glucocorticoid activity and abolish mineralocorticoid activity (Figure 19-15).

(5) An acetate ester or a 16α-, 17α-isopropylidenedioxy group (also known as an acetonide group) at position C-21 enhances topical absorption, as with fluocinonide (see Figure 19-15).

2. **Aldosterone,** which is formed in the outer (glomerular) layer of the adrenal cortex, is the prototypical mineralocorticoid. The two clinically useful mineralocorticoids are **desoxycorticosterone acetate** and **fludrocortisone acetate** (Figure 19-16).

B. Pharmacology

1. Therapeutically useful adrenocorticosteroids mimic the activity of the natural glucocorticoids and have metabolic, anti-inflammatory, and immunosuppressive activity.

2. Adrenocorticosteroid require cytoplasmic receptors for transportation to the nuclei of target tissue cells, where they stimulate production of messenger and ribosomal RNA. Adrenocorticosteroid also act in the feedback regulation of pituitary corticotropin.

C. Therapeutic indications.

Adrenocorticosteroids are used:

1. As replacement therapy, to treat acute and chronic adrenal insufficiency
2. As the therapy of last resort, to treat severe, disabling arthritis
3. To treat severe allergic reactions

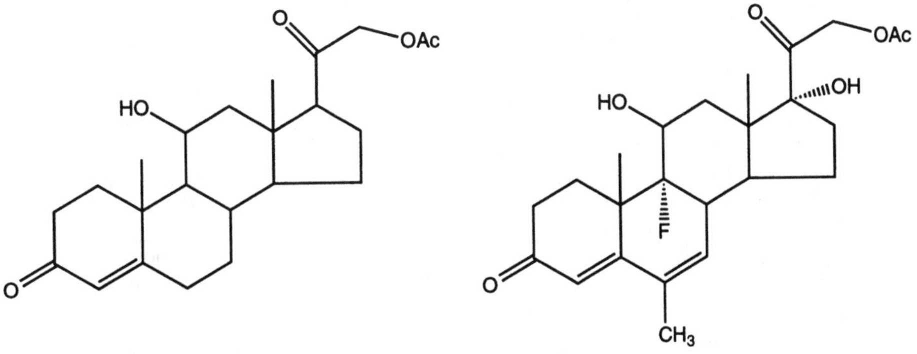

A B

Figure 19-16. Structural formulas of (*A*) desoxycorticosterone acetate and (*B*) fludrocortisone acetate, the clinically useful mineralocorticoids.

4. To treat chronic ulcerative colitis
5. To treat rheumatic carditis
6. To treat renal diseases, including nephrotic syndrome
7. To treat collagen vascular diseases
8. To treat cerebral edema
9. As topical agents, to treat skin disorders and inflammatory ocular disorders

D. **Adverse effects.** Adrenocorticosteroids are associated with:

1. Suppression of pituitary-adrenal integrity
2. GI effects, such as peptic ulcer, GI hemorrhage, ulcerative esophagitis, and acute pancreatitis
3. CNS effects, such as headache, vertigo, increased intraocular and intracranial pressures, muscle weakness, and psychological disturbances (euphoria or dysphoria, depression, suicidal tendencies)
4. Cardiovascular effects, such as edema and hypertension
5. Other effects, including weight gain, osteoporosis, hyperglycemia, flushed face and neck, acne, hirsutism, cushingoid "moon face" and "buffalo hump," and increased susceptibility to infection

V. THYROID HORMONES AND INHIBITORS

A. Chemistry

1. **Synthesis of thyroid hormones** is a four-step process beginning with the concentration of iodide in the thyroid gland. The enzyme iodoperoxidase then catalyzes steps two and three: iodination of tyrosine residues located on thyroglobulin, a 650,000 mol wt glycoprotein located within the thyroid gland; and coupling of the iodinated tyrosine precursors. Finally, proteolysis of thyroglobulin produces the two naturally occurring thyroid hormones, **thyroxine (levothyroxine, T_4)** and **triiodothyronine (liothyronine, T_3)** in a ratio of 4 to 1.
   a. Levothyroxine is less potent than liothyronine but possess a longer duration of action (6–7 days versus 1–2 days).
   b. Peripheral deiodination by **5′-deiodinase** converts T_4 to T_3.
   c. **Regulation** of thyroid hormone production involves a hypothalamic-pituitary-thyroid feedback system. **TRH** is secreted by the hypothalamus and stimulates the release of **TSH (thyrotropin)** from the anterior pituitary. Thyrotropin stimulates the thyroid gland to produce T_4 and T_3. These hormones then regulate their own synthesis by binding to specific sites in the anterior pituitary and inhibiting the release of TSH.
2. **Available thyroid preparations**
   a. The **sodium salts** of T_3 and T_4 are used therapeutically (Figure 19-17). Due to peripheral conversion, the administration of levothyroxine sodium alone will produce the natural 4 to 1 ratio of T_4 to T_3.
   b. **Liotrix** (Euthroid, Thyrolar) is a 4 to 1 mixture of levothyroxine sodium to liothyronine sodium which is equivalent to, but offers no advantages over, levothyroxine only.
   c. **Thyroid USP** is made from dried, defatted thyroid glands of domestic animals and is standardized based on iodine content.
   d. **Thyroglobulin** (Proloid) is a partially purified extract of frozen porcine or bovine thyroid gland. It contains both T_3 and T_4 and conforms to USP iodine content requirements.
3. **Inhibitors** of thyroid function directly or indirectly interfere with the synthesis of thyroid hormones. These agents include ionic inhibitors, potassium or sodium iodide, radioactive iodine (e.g., $Na^{131}I$), and the thiourylenes (e.g., propylthiouracil, methimazole) [Figure 19-18].

B. Pharmacology

1. **Thyroid hormone preparations** mimic the activity of endogenous and thyroid hormones. These hormones regulate growth and development, have calorigenic and metabolic activ-

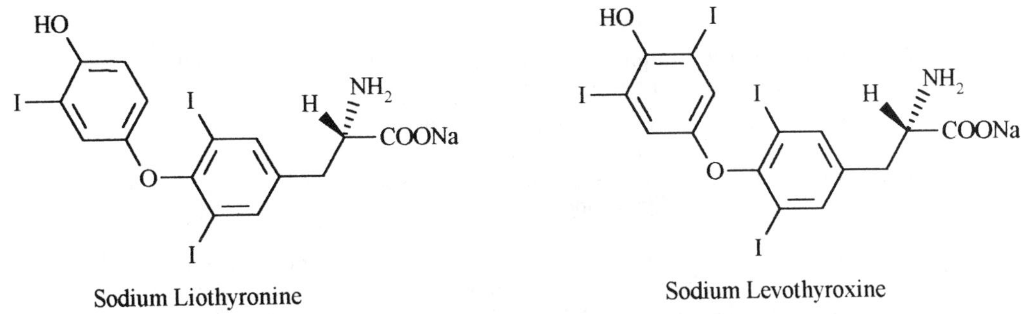

Figure 19-17. Sodium salt forms of the naturally occurring thyroid hormones, liothyronine (T_3) and levothyroxine (T_4).

ity, and (through sensitization of β-adrenergic receptors) have positive inotropic and chronotropic effects on the myocardium.

2. **Thyroid inhibitors** act via several different mechanisms.
   a. **Ionic inhibitors,** such as thiocyanate (SCN) and perchlorate (ClO_4^-), are inorganic, monovalent anions that interfere with the concentration of iodide ion by the thyroid gland.
   b. **Iodides in high concentrations** (e.g., Lugol's solution) have profound effects in all aspects of thyroid synthesis, release, and metabolism. Iodides limit their own transport, inhibit the synthesis of both iodotyrosine and iodothreonine, and most importantly, inhibit the release of thyroid hormones.
   c. **Radioactive iodine (^{131}I)** is administered as a sodium salt, is rapidly trapped by the thyroid gland, and is incorporated into both tyrosine precursors and mature thyroid hormones. Radioactive β-particle decay produces localized destruction of thyroid cells and the desired therapeutic effect.
   d. **Thiourylenes** inhibit the enzyme iodoperoxidase, thereby inhibiting two crucial steps in thyroid synthesis: the incorporation of iodine into tyrosine precursor molecules and the coupling of iodinated tyrosines to form T_4 and T_3.

C. Therapeutic indications

1. The major indications for **thyroid hormone preparations** are hypothyroidism (i.e., myxedema), myxedema coma, cretinism, and simple goiter. Other indications include endemic goiter and thyrotropin-dependent carcinoma.

2. **Thyroid Inhibitors** are used to treat hyperthyroidism. The two most common types of hyperthyroidism are **Grave's disease** and **toxic adenoma.** Less common causes are toxic multinodular goiter, thyroiditis and single hyperfunctioning thyroid nodules.
   a. **Ionic inhibitors** are rarely used therapeutically; however, the metabolism of some foods (e.g., cabbage) and drugs (e.g., sodium nitroprusside) can produce significant amounts of thiocyanate.
   b. **High concentrations of iodide** (Lugol's solution) are used before thyroid surgery to make the thyroid gland firmer and reduce its size.
   c. ^{131}I is useful particularly in treating hyperthyroidism in older patients and in patients with heart disease.
   d. **Thiourylenes** (e.g., propylthiouracil, methimazole) are used to control mild cases of hyperthyroidism, in conjunction with ^{131}I, and to prepare patients before thyroid surgery. They are less effective in producing permanent remission of Grave's disease.

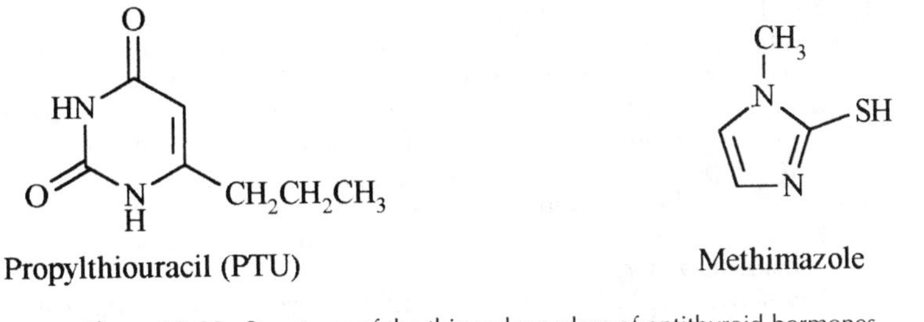

Figure 19-18. Structures of the thiourylene class of antithyroid hormones.

D. Adverse effects

1. **Thyroid hormone preparations** are only **rarely associated** with adverse effects. Overdosage can cause palpitations, nervousness, insomnia, and weight loss.

2. **Thyroid inhibitors** are associated with adverse effects that depend on the agent used.
   a. **Iodides** are associated with these adverse effects:
      (1) Iodism, including increased salivation, brassy taste, sore teeth and gums, swollen eyelids, inflamed larynx and pharynx, frontal headache, skin lesions, and skin eruptions
      (2) Hypersensitivity reactions with fever, arthralgia, eosinophilia, and angioedema
      (3) Large doses of iodides given over long periods can cause goiter and hypothyroidism which can be corrected by the administration of thyroid hormone.
   b. ^{131}I is associated with:
      (1) Delayed hypothyroidism (relatively high incidence)
      (2) Possible effects on the future offspring of young adults
   c. **Thiourylenes** are associated with:
      (1) Dermatologic effects, such as urticarial papular rash and dermatitis
      (2) Hematologic effects, such as agranulocytosis, thrombocytopenia and granulocytopenia
      (3) GI effects, such as nausea, vomiting, and GI distress
      (4) Pain, stiffness in the joints, headache, and paresthesias
      (5) Other effects such as drug fever, hepatitis, nephritis, and systemic lupus erythematosus-like syndrome are rare.

VI. ANTIDIABETIC AGENTS

A. Chemistry. Antidiabetic agents include insulin preparations and oral hypoglycemic agents.

1. **Insulin** is an endocrine hormone secreted by the β-cells of the pancreas. It is composed of **two polypeptide chains:** an A chain of 21 amino acids and a B chain of 30 amino acids. Two disulfide bonds connect the A and B chains and a third disulfide bond is found within the A chain.
   a. **Source.** Insulin is available as bovine insulin (differs from human insulin by three amino acids), porcine insulin (differs from human insulin only in the terminal amino acid), and human insulin.
      (1) **Single-species** insulins contain only bovine or only porcine insulin.
      (2) **Mixed** insulins contain both bovine and porcine insulin.
      (3) **Human** insulins are prepared either by enzymatic conversion of the terminal amino acid of porcine insulin (Novolin) or by means of recombinant DNA technology (Humulin).
      (4) Purified insulins (or single-peak insulins) are preparations containing less than 10 parts per million (ppm) of the insulin precursor proinsulin.
   b. **Duration of action.** Insulins are classified by their duration of action as well as by their source and purity.
      (1) **Short-acting** insulins include crystalline zinc insulins and semilente insulin.
         (a) **Crystalline zinc** insulin (also called regular insulin or CZI) is a soluble insulin prepared at neutral pH. It is the only type of insulin that can be mixed with all other insulins and also the only type forming a clear solution, which can be given intravenously.
         (b) **Semilente** insulin is a finely divided, amorphous preparation also called prompt insulin zinc suspension. The lente insulins [see VI A 1 b (2) (b), (3) (b)] contain no modifying protein and are prepared with an acetate buffer. Lente insulins can be mixed with each other but cannot be mixed with either isophane insulin (NPH) or protamine zinc insulin (PZI). Semilente insulin has a duration of action comparable to that of CZI.
      (2) **Long-acting** insulins include PZI and ultralente insulin.
         (a) PZI consists of insulin complexed with zinc and an excess of protamine in a phosphate buffer.
         (b) Ultralente insulin is a large, crystalline form, also known as extended insulin zinc suspension. Its duration of action is comparable to that of PZI.

(3) **Intermediate-acting** insulins include NPH and lente insulin.
(a) NPH is similar to PZI but contains less protamine.
(b) Lente insulin, also known as insulin zinc suspension, is a mixture of 70% ultralente crystals and 30% semilente powder. Its duration of action is comparable to that of NPH.

2. **Oral hypoglycemic agents** can be classified as either sulfonylureas, biguanides, or α-glucosidase inhibitors.
   a. **Sulfonylureas,** shown in Table 19-1, are acidic compounds and include both first and second generation agents. Second generation agents (**glyburide, glipizide,** and **glimepride**) have larger groups attached to the aromatic ring (i.e., larger R_1 substituents), are more lipid soluble, and are more potent as compared to first generation agents (**tolbutamide, chlorpropamide, tolazamide,** and **acetohexamide**).
   b. **Biguanides** are basic compounds and include **metformin** and **phenformin** (Figure 19-19). Of these two agents, only metformin is available in the United States. Phenformin was withdrawn from the market in 1977 because of a high incidence of fatal lactic acidosis.
   c. **Acarbose,** a basic tetrasaccharide derived from α1-4 linked sugar units, is currently the only available **α-glucosidase inhibitor** (see Figure 19-19).

B. Pharmacology

1. Insulin **preparations** mimic the activity of endogenous insulin, which is required for the proper utilization of glucose in normal metabolism. Insulin interacts with a specific cell-surface receptor to facilitate the transport of glucose and amino acids.

2. **Oral hypoglycemic agents** act through a variety of mechanisms.
   a. **Sulfonylureas** block ATP-sensitive potassium channels which stimulates the release of insulin from pancreatic β-cells. Additionally, sulfonylureas can enhance the peripheral response to a given amount of insulin by increasing the number or affinity of cell-surface insulin receptors. The clinical significance of this extrahepatic effect has been questioned.
   b. **Biguanides** do not stimulate the release of insulin, do not cause hypoglycemia, and thus are best described as antihyperglycemic agents. The reduction in glucose levels seen with these agents is thought to be caused by an increase in insulin action in peripheral tissues as well as an inhibition of gluconeogenesis.
   c. **α-Glucosidase inhibitors** inhibit the digestion of carbohydrates in the small intestine and therefore decrease the postprandial rise in glucose levels.

C. Therapeutic indication

1. Insulin preparations are used to treat diabetes mellitus that cannot be controlled by diet alone.

2. Oral hypoglycemic agents are used as an adjunct to diet in treating non–insulin-dependent diabetes mellitus (NIDDM) that cannot be controlled by diet alone. Each class of compounds can be used either as monotherapy or in combination with one another.

D. Adverse effects

1. Insulin preparations are associated with these adverse effects:
   a. **Hypoglycemia,** with sweating, tachycardia, and hunger; possibly progressing to insulin shock with hypoglycemic convulsions
   b. **Hypersensitivity** reactions
   c. **Local irritation** at the injection site

2. **Oral hypoglycemic agents** produce a variety of adverse effects which depend upon both the class and mechanism of the compounds
   a. **Sulfonylureas** are associated with the following adverse effects:
      (1) Hypoglycemia, particularly in patients with renal or hepatic insufficiency who are taking longer-acting agents (e.g., chlorpropamide).
      (2) GI effects, such as nausea, vomiting, diarrhea, and constipation
      (3) Hypersensitivity reactions, such as skin rash and photosensitivity. Cross sensitivity is seen among classes of compounds that also contain the benzene sulfonamide functional group (e.g., **sulfanilamide antibacterials, thiazides, loop diuretics,** and **carbonic anhydrase inhibitors**).

Table 19-1. Oral Hypoglycemic Agents: The Sulfonylureas

General Sulfonylurea Structure

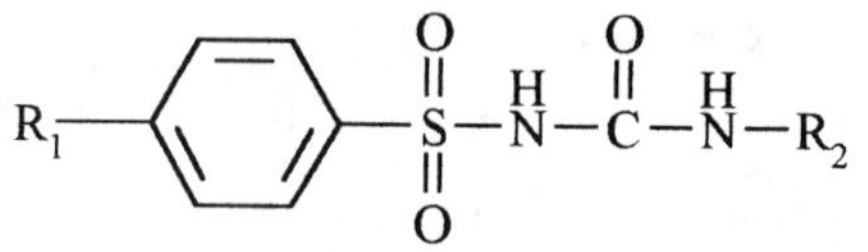

Drug	**R_1 Substituent**	**R_2 Substituent**
First-generation agents		
Tolbutamide (Orinase)	CH_3	$CH_2CH_2CH_2CH_3$
Chlorpropamide (Diabinese)	Cl	$CH_2CH_2CH_3$
Tolazamide (Tolinase)	CH_3	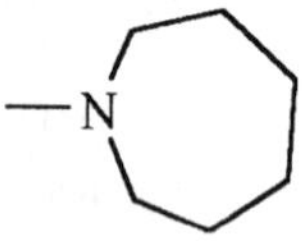
Acetohexamide (Dymelor)	$H_3C-C(=O)$	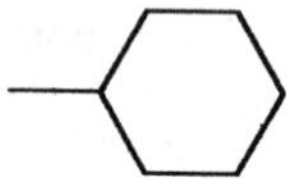
Second-generation agents		
Glyburide (DiaBeta, Micronase)	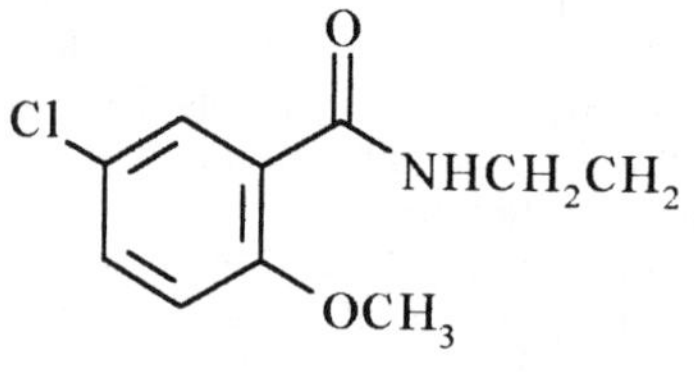	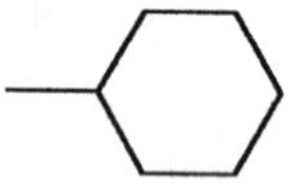
Glipizide (Glucotrol)	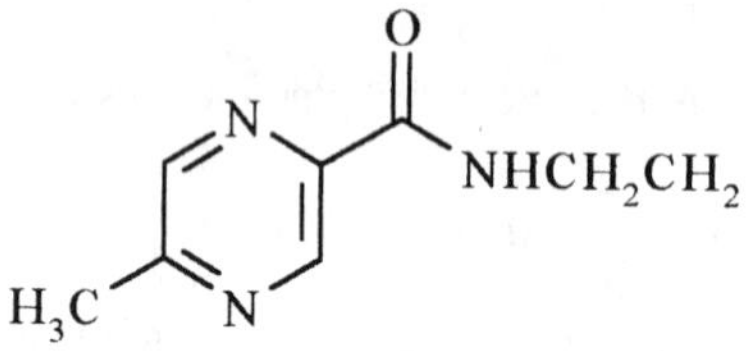	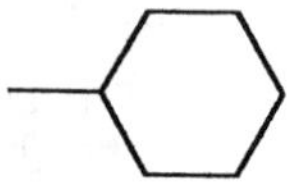
Glimipride (Amaryl)	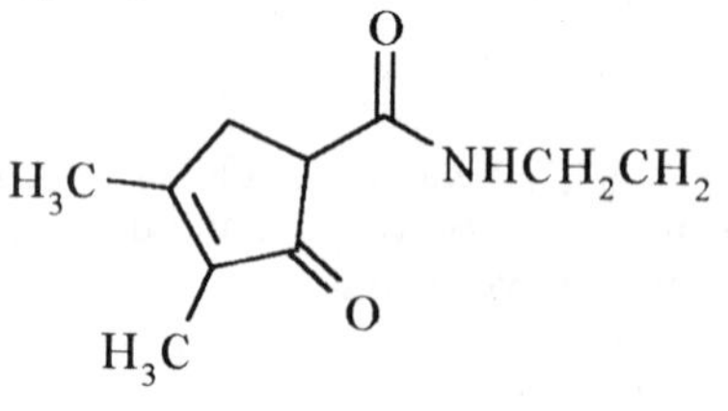	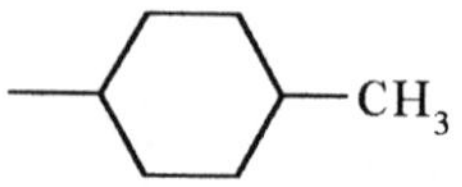

(4) Blood dyscrasias, such as leukopenia, thrombocytopenia, agranulocytosis, and hemolytic anemia

(5) Cholestatic jaundice

(6) Hyponatremia due to a potentiation of the effects of antidiuretic hormone (seen primarily with chlorpropamide)

b. **Biguanides** do not cause hypoglycemia but have been associated with the following adverse effects:

(1) Fatal lactic acidosis. Phenformin was withdrawn from the United States market in 1977 because of a high incidence of this serious adverse effect. The frequency of this

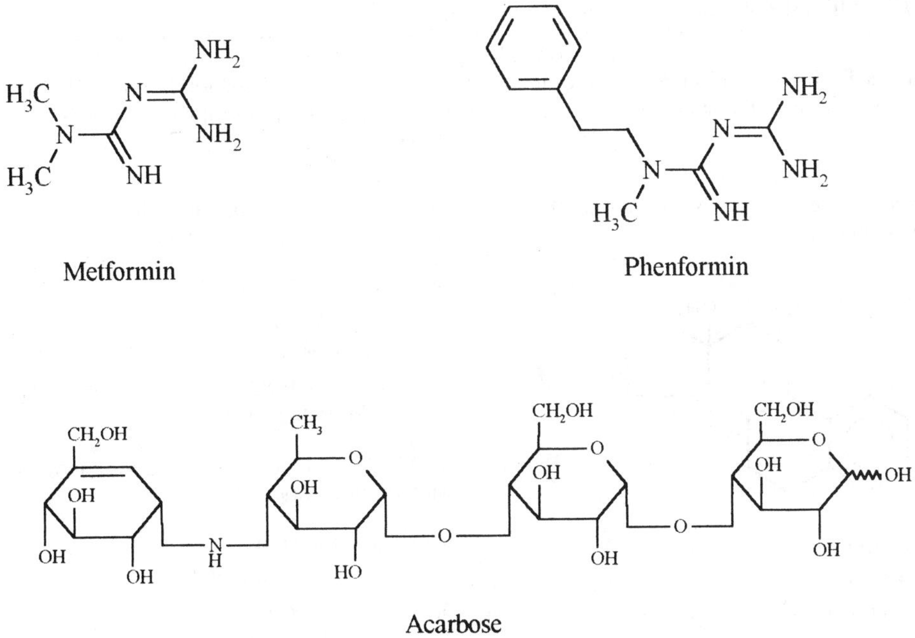

Figure 19-19. Structures of oral hypoglycemic agents: biguanides (metformin and phenformin) and α-glucosidase inhibitors (acarbose).

effect in metformin is considerably less than that seen with phenformin, and in most if not all reported cases, the lactic acidosis occurred in patients in which metformin was contraindicated.

(2) Metallic taste

(3) GI effects, such as epigastric distress, nausea, vomiting, diarrhea, and anorexia

c. **α-Glucosidase inhibitors** also do not cause hypoglycemia but have been associated with GI distress due to the presence of undigested carbohydrates in the lower GI tract.

STUDY QUESTIONS

Directions: Each of the numbered items or incomplete statements in this section is followed by answers or by completions of the statement. Select the **one** lettered answer or completion that is **best** in each case.

1. The following structure is a hormone. It would be classified best as

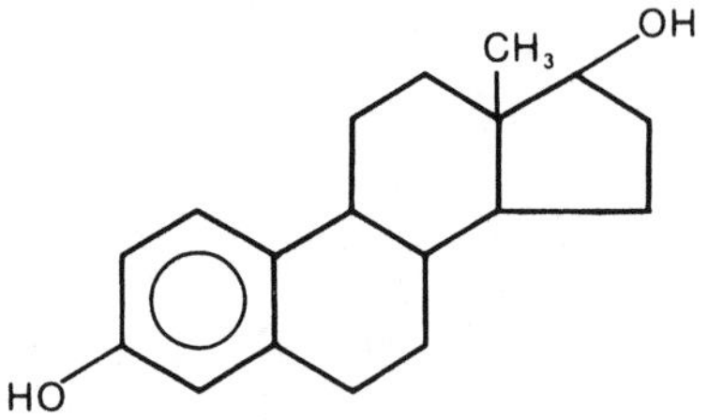

(A) an estrogen
(B) a progestin
(C) an androgen
(D) a gonadotropin
(E) an adrenocorticosteroid

2. All of the following substances are endogenous tropic hormones secreted by the pituitary gland EXCEPT

(A) somatotropin
(B) human chorionic gonadotropin (hCG)
(C) follicle-stimulating hormone (FSH)
(D) thyroid-stimulating hormone (TSH)
(E) corticotropin (ACTH)

3. Which of the following substances when present in urine is the most likely positive sign of pregnancy?

(A) Thyroid-stimulating hormone (TSH)
(B) Corticotropin (ACTH)
(C) Human chorionic gonadotropin (hCG)
(D) Interstitial cell-stimulating hormone (ICSH)
(E) Protamine zinc insulin (PZI)

4. All of the following hormonal drugs possess a steroidal nucleus EXCEPT

(A) ethinyl estradiol
(B) norethindrone
(C) liothyronine
(D) prednisolone
(E) fluoxymesterone

5. Which of the following glucocorticoids produces the least sodium retention?

(A) Cortisone
(B) Hydrocortisone
(C) Prednisolone
(D) Dexamethasone
(E) Fludrocortisone

6. Which of the following insulins can be administered intravenously?

(A) Regular insulin
(B) Isophane insulin (NPH)
(C) Protamine zinc insulin (PZI)
(D) Semilente insulin
(E) Ultralente insulin

7. In comparing levothyroxine to liothyronine, which of the following statements is NOT correct?

a. Both levothyroxine and liothyronine are naturally occurring thyroid hormones
b. Liothyronine can be converted in the peripheral circulation to levothyroxine
c. Liothyronine is more potent than levothyroxine
d. The plasma concentration of liothyronine is less than that of levothyroxine
e. Liothyronine has a shorter duration of action than levothyroxine

8. Which of the following classes of compounds stimulates the release of insulin from pancreatic β-cells?

a. Progestins
b. Biguanides
c. α-Glucosidase inhibitors
d. Thiourylenes
e. Sulfonylureas

Directions: Each question below contains three suggested answers of which **one or more** is correct. Choose the answer

- **A** if **I only** is correct
- **B** if **III only** is correct
- **C** if **I and II** are correct
- **D** if **II and III** are correct
- **E** if **I, II, and III** are correct

9. Hormones that form lipophilic esters without prior structural modifications include

I. hydrocortisone
II. testosterone
III. progesterone

10. Insulin preparations that contain a modifying protein include

I. lente insulin
II. regular insulin
III. isophane insulin (NPH)

Directions: Each group of items in this section consists of lettered options followed by a set of numbered items. For each item, select the **one** lettered option that is most closely associated with it. Each lettered option may be selected once, more than once, or not at all.

Questions 11–13

For each pharmacologic property, select the hormone that most closely relates to it.

(A) Testosterone
(B) Insulin
(C) Corticotropin
(D) Estradiol
(E) Vasopressin

11. Secreted by pancreatic β-cells to facilitate glucose and amino acid transport for normal cellular metabolic processes

12. Initiates and controls male sexual development and maintains the integrity of the male reproductive system

13. Promotes the resorption of water at the renal distal convoluted tubule

Questions 14–16

For each adverse effect, select the class of drug that most closely relates to it.

(A) Antithyroid agents
(B) Sulfonylurea oral hypoglycemics
(C) Adrenocorticosteroids
(D) Progestins
(E) Androgens

14. Peptic ulceration and gastrointestinal hemorrhage; hyperglycemia, hypertension, and edema; "buffalo hump" and "moon face"; psychological disturbances; and increased susceptibility to infection

15. Agranulocytosis and other blood dyscrasias; cholestatic jaundice; nausea and vomiting; hypoglycemia; and photosensitivity

16. Hepatotoxicity and jaundice; urinary retention and azoospermia; prostatic hypertrophy and priapism; and paradoxical gynecomastia

ANSWERS AND EXPLANATIONS

1. The answer is A *[III A 1 a; Figure 19-1].*
Ring A is aromatic. Because the only type of steroidal hormone that has an aromatic A ring is an estrogen, this structure represents an estrogen. Other structural characteristics of estrogens include the fact that the structure contains 18 carbon atoms; thus, it is an estrane and contains a β-alcohol group in position 17.

2. The answer is B *[II A 2 a, b].*
Human chorionic gonadotropin (hCG) is produced by placental tissue and serves to stimulate the secretion of progesterone during pregnancy. Growth hormone (somatotropin), follicle-stimulating hormone (FSH), thyroid-stimulating hormone (TSH), and corticotropin (ACTH) are all secreted by the anterior pituitary gland.

3. The answer is C *[II A 2 b (3)].*
Human chorionic gonadotropin (hCG) is a proteinaceous tropic hormone that is secreted by chorionic (e.g., placental) tissue. Thus, hCG is present in the urine only after conception has occurred.

4. The answer is C *[V A 1; Figures 19-3, 19-8, 19-17].*
Liothyronine is a thyroid hormone. Thyroid hormones consist of iodinated aromatic amino acids and are not steroidal in nature. Ethinyl estradiol is a steroidal estrogen, norethindrone is a steroidal 19-nor-progestin, prednisolone is an adrenocorticosteroid, and fluoxymesterone is a steroidal androgen.

5. The answer is D *[IV A 1 b (4); Figure 19-15].*
Glucocorticoids have varying degrees of mineralocorticoid activity. This mineralocorticoid activity, which can result in sodium and fluid retention, can be blocked by the introduction of a methyl or hydroxyl group in position 16 of the steroidal nucleus. Dexamethasone has a 16 α-methyl substituent.

6. The answer is A *[VI A 1 b].*
Most insulin preparations are suspensions; thus, they contain particulate matter. Only clear solutions may be administered intravenously. Regular insulin, which consists of water-soluble crystalline zinc insulin, is, therefore, suitable for intravenous administration. Insulin preparations normally are injected subcutaneously.

7. The answer is B *[V A 1 a, b]*
The thyroid gland produces both levothyroxine (T_4) and liothyronine (T_3). The natural ratio of these compounds is 4 to 1 in favor of levothyroxine; therefore, liothyronine is normally present at a lower concentration than levothyroxine. Liothyronine is more potent than levothyroxine, but has a shorter duration of action. Peripheral conversion involves deiodination, thus levothyroxine is converted to liothyronine. The reverse process is not possible.

8. The answer is E *[VI B 2 a–c]*
Of the five classes of compounds listed, only biguanides α-glucosidase inhibitors and sulfonylureas are oral hypoglycemic agents. Each of these classes of agents is useful for the treatment of non–insulin-dependent diabetes mellitus (NIDDM); however, each produces its beneficial effect via a different mechanism of action. Biguanides enhance the peripheral use of insulin and suppress gluconeogenesis. α-Glucosidase inhibitors decrease the absorption of glucose. Only the sulfonylureas stimulate the secretion of insulin.

9. The answer is C (I, II) *[III C 1; Figures 19-7, 19-13].*
Hydrocortisone has a 21-hydroxyl group, and testosterone has a 17-hydroxyl group; therefore, both of these agents can form esters (e.g., hydrocortisone acetate, testosterone propionate). Progesterone does not have any alcohol groups in its molecule; therefore, it cannot directly form any esters.

10. The answer is B (III) *[VI A 1 b].*
Regular insulin, which is a rapid-acting insulin preparation, contains only zinc insulin crystals. All lente insulins are free of modifying proteins, which contributes to their hypoallergenic properties. Isophane insulin is NPH insulin, which contains protamine, a strongly basic protein. The protamine reduces the water solubility of zinc insulin and lengthens its duration of action. Isophane insulin is classified as an intermediate-acting insulin preparation, having a duration of action of about 24 hours.

11–13. The answers are: 11-B *[VI B 1, 2],* **12-A** *[III C 2],* **13-E** *[II B 4].*
Insulin is required for the proper utilization of glucose and the transport of glucose and amino acids across cell membranes. Testosterone, which is produced principally from the Leydig cells of the testes, is responsible for male sexual characteristics. Vasopressin is secreted from the posterior pituitary and is sometimes referred to as an antidiuretic hormone.

14–16. The answers are: 14-C *[IV D],* **15-B** *[VI D 2],* **16-E** *[III D 3].*
Exogenously administered adrenocorticosteroids are effective anti-inflammatory agents but give rise to a wide range of metabolic and immunosuppressive effects that result in severe adverse effects. Oral antidiabetic agents of the sulfonylurea type can cause blood dyscrasias, impaired liver function, and photosensitivity. Exogenously administered androgens suppress sperm formation and cause paradoxical gynecomastia. Most significant is the hepatotoxicity produced by alkyl-substituted androgen compounds.

20
Drug Interactions

Leon Shargel

I. INTRODUCTION

A. Types of drug interaction

1. Drug interaction refers to an **adverse** drug response produced by the administration of a drug or co-exposure of the drug with another substance which modifies the patient's response to the drug. Some drug interactions are intentional in order to provide improved therapeutic response or to decrease adverse drug effects. A **precipitant** drug is the drug, chemical, or food element causing the interaction. An **object** drug is the drug affected by the interaction.

2. Drug interactions include:
   a. **Drug–drug** interactions
   b. **Food–drug** interactions (see II D)
   c. **Chemical–drug** interactions, such as the interaction of a drug with alcohol or tobacco (see II E)
   d. **Drug–laboratory test** interaction (an alteration in a diagnostic laboratory test results caused by the drug) [see Chapter 38]

B. Classification of drug interactions.
Drug interactions that occur in vivo are generally classified as **pharmacokinetic** or **pharmacodynamic** interactions.

1. **Pharmacokinetic** or **biopharmaceutic** interactions occur when the absorption, distribution (protein and tissue binding), or elimination (excretion and/or metabolism) of the drug is affected by another drug, chemical, or food element (see II).

2. **Pharmacodynamic** interactions occur when the pharmacodynamic effect of the drug is altered by another drug, chemical, or food element, producing an antagonistic, synergistic, or additive effect.

3. **Pharmaceutic** interactions are caused by a chemical or physical incompatibility when two or more drugs are mixed together. Pharmaceutic interactions can occur during the extemporaneous compounding of drugs, including the preparation of intravenous (IV) solutions. For example, an IV solution of aminophylline has an alkaline pH and should not be mixed with such drugs as epinephrine, erythromycin gluceptate, or cephalothin sodium, which decompose in alkaline pH. Phenytoin sodium will precipitate from a solution that has an acid pH. Pharmaceutic interactions are usually considered during the development, manufacturing, and marketing of the drug product. Only drug interactions causing pharmacokinetic or pharmacodynamic changes of the object drug will be considered in this chapter.

II. PHARMACOKINETIC INTERACTIONS

A. Absorption

1. Drug interactions can affect the **rate** and the **extent** of systemic drug absorption (bioavailability) from the absorption site, resulting in increased or decreased drug bioavailability.

2. The most common drug absorption **site** is in the **gastrointestinal (GI) tract.** However, drug bioavailability from other absorption sites, such as the skin, can be affected by drug interactions. For example, epinephrine, a vasoconstrictor, will decrease the percutaneous absorption of lidocaine, a local anesthetic agent.

Table 20-1. Drug Interactions that Affect the Bioavailability of the Drug from the Gastrointestinal (GI) Tract

Drug Interaction	Examples (Precipitant drugs)	Effect (Object drugs)
Complexation/chelation	Calcium, magnesium or aluminum and iron salts	Tetracycline complexes with divalent cations, causing a decreased bioavailability
Adsorption	Cholestyramine resin	Decreased bioavailability of Thyroxine, Digoxin
	Antacids	Decreased bioavailability of tetracycline
	Charcoal Antidiarrheal	Decreased bioavailability of many drugs
Increased GI motility	Laxatives, cathartics	Increases GI motility, decreases bioavailability for drugs that are absorbed slowly. May also affect the bioavailability of drugs from controlled-release products.
Decreased GI motility	Anticholinergic agents	Propantheline decreases the gastric emptying of acetaminophen (APAP) delaying APAP absorption from the small intestine.
Alteration of gastric pH	H-2 blockers and antacids	Both H-2 blockers and antacids increase gastric pH. The dissolution of ketoconazole is reduced, causing decreased drug absorption
Alteration of intestinal flora	Antibiotics (e.g., tetracyclines, penicillin)	Digoxin has better bioavailability after erythromycin. Erythromycin administration reduces bacterial inactivation of digoxin.
Inhibition of drug metabolism in intestinal cells	Monoamine oxidase inhibitors (MAO-I) (e.g., tranylcypromine, phenelzine)	Hypertensive crisis can occur in patients treated with MAO-I and foods containing tyramine.

3. Examples of drug interactions in the GI tract are shown in Table 20-1.
4. Other **potential** drug interactions that affect bioavailability in the GI tract could be due to:
   a. **Competition** for carrier-mediated drug absorption in which the participant drug (e.g., purine, pyrimidine) competes for the same carrier as the object drug (e.g., purine or pyrimidine antimetabolite).
   b. **Alteration** of intestinal blood flow caused by the precipitant drug. In congestive heart disease, the blood flow to the GI tract is poor and an orally administered drug can have a slower rate of bioavailability. After digoxin therapy, the perfusion of the GI tract is improved along with bioavailability of the object drug.

B. **Distribution.** The distribution of the drug may be affected by plasma protein binding and displacement interactions or tissue and cellular interactions.

1. **Plasma protein binding and displacement**
   a. **Valproic acid** displaces phenytoin from plasma protein-binding sites and reduces hepatic phenytoin clearance by inhibiting the liver's metabolism of phenytoin.
   b. **Aspirin** decreases protein binding and inhibits the metabolism of valproate.
2. **Tissue and cellular interactions.** Digoxin toxicity can be enhanced by concurrent administration of quinidine. Quinidine reduces digoxin clearance and displaces digoxin from tissue-binding sites, leading to a higher plasma digoxin concentration and a reduced distribution volume.

Table 20-2. Drug Interactions that Affect the Drug Metabolism

Drug Interaction	Examples (Precipitant drugs)	Effect (Objective drugs)
Enzyme induction	Smoking (polycyclic aromatic hydrocarbons)	Smoking increases theophylline clearance
	Barbiturates	Phenobarbital increases the metabolism of warfarin
Enzyme inhibition		
Mixed function oxidase	Cimetidine	Decreased theophylline clearance
Other enzymes	Monoamine oxidase inhibitors, MAO-I (e.g., pargyline, tranylcypromine)	Serious hypertensive crisis can occur following ingestion of foods with a high content of tyramine or other pressor substances (e.g., cheddar cheese, red wines).

C. Drug elimination and clearance

1. Drug metabolism and hepatic clearance

a. Drug metabolism (hepatic clearance) can be affected by enzyme induction, enzyme inhibition, substrate competition for the same enzyme, and changes in hepatic blood flow (Table 20-2).

b. Many drugs that share the same drug-metabolizing enzymes have a potential for a drug interaction. For example, fluconazole reduces the hepatic metabolism of various hypoglycemics (e.g., glyburide, tolbutamide, glipizide), causing clinically significant hypoglycemia. Fluconazole also inhibits the metabolism of phenytoin.

c. Phenytoin, carbamazepine, and phenobarbital elevate levels of glucuronyl transferase, increasing the clearance of valproate.

d. Nonhepatic enzymes can be involved in drug interactions. For example, serious drug interactions have been reported in patients receiving antidepressants similar to nefazodone HCl with a monamine oxidase inhibitor.

e. A decrease in the hepatic blood flow can decrease the hepatic clearance for high extraction drugs, such as propranolol and morphine.

2. Renal drug clearance and be affected by changes in glomerular filtration, tubular reabsorption, active drug secretion, and renal blood flow and nephrotoxicity (Table 20-3).

Table 20-3. Drug Interactions that Affect the Renal Clearance

Drug Interaction	Examples	Effect
Glomerular filtration rate (GFR) and renal blood flow	Methylxanthines (e.g., caffeine, theobromine)	Increased renal blood flow and GFR will decrease time for reabsorption of various drugs, leading to more rapid urinary drug excretion.
Active tubular secretion	Probenecid	Probenecid blocks the active tubular secretion of penicillin and some cephalosporin antibiotics
Tubular reabsorption and urine pH	Antacids, sodium bicarbonate	Alkalinization of the urine increases the reabsorption of amphetamine and decreases its clearance.
		Alkalinization of urine pH increases the ionization of salicylates, decreases reabsorption, and increases its clearance.
Nephrotoxicity	Aminoglycosides (e.g., gentamicin, tobramicin)	Nephrotoxicity interferes with the renal clearance of cephalothin.

Table 20-4. Affect of Food on Drug Bioavailability

Reduced or delayed	Increased	Not affected by food
NSAIDs (Non-Steroidal Anti-inflammatory Drugs) naproxen, naproxen sodium diclofenac, aspirin	Griseofulvin	Theophylline[1]
Acetaminophen	Metoprolol	Metronidazole
Antibiotics	Phenytoin	
Tetracycline, Penicillin	Propoxyphene	
Ethanol	Dicumarol	

[1]Food does not significantly affect drug absorption of theophylline in an immediate release dosage form. However, food may affect theophylline absorption from a controlled-release formulation.

D. Food–drug interactions

1. Food can increase, decrease, or not effect the absorption of drugs (Table 20-4).
2. Food can influence the bioavailability of a drug from a modified-release dosage form [e.g., controlled release, delayed release (enteric coated)] rather than from an immediate-release dosage form.
3. Complexation and adsorption of the drug in the GI tract with another food element is a common drug interaction that reduces the extent of drug absorption. For example, tetracycline complexes with calcium (found in milk products).

E. Chemical–drug interactions

1. **Smoking** by inhaling aromatic polycyclic hydrocarbons can increase the intrinsic clearance (enzyme induction) of drugs such as theophylline, diazepam, and tricyclic antidepressants.
2. **Alcohol** can increase or decrease the activity of hepatic drug metabolizing enzymes.
   a. **Chronic alcoholism** can increase the rate of metabolism of tolbutamide, warfarin, and phenytoin.
   b. **Acute alcohol intoxication** can inhibit hepatic enzymes in nonalcoholic individuals.

III. PHARMACODYNAMIC INTERACTIONS

A. Drugs that have similar pharmacodynamic actions may produce an excessive pharmacologic or **toxic response.** For example, central nervous system depressants, such as the combination of alcohol and antihistamines (e.g., diphenhydramine, chlorpheniramine) can produce increased drowsiness in the patient. Drugs having anticholinergic effects, such as promethazine and OTC antihistamines, can cause dryness of the mouth, blurred vision, and urinary retention.

B. The alteration of **electrolyte concentrations** produced by a diuretic, such as a thiazide derivative, will deplete potassium, resulting in sensitization of the heart to digoxin therapy. Depletion of sodium can also result in lithium toxicity.

C. By inhibiting platelet aggregation, aspirin increases the risk of bleeding in patients on anticoagulant (e.g., warfarin, dicumarol) therapy.

IV. CLINICAL SIGNIFICANCE AND MANAGEMENT OF DRUG INTERACTIONS

A. Potential drug interactions

1. **Multiple drug therapy** including both **prescription** and **nonprescription** (OTC) medication, can potentially lead to drug interactions. The more drugs used by a patient, the greater the potential for a drug interaction in the patient.
2. **Multiple prescribers.** Patients can be seen by different prescribers who prescribe interacting medication.

3. **Patient compliance.** Patients need to follow proper instructions for taking medications. For example, a patient might take tetracycline with food rather than before meals.

4. **Patient risk factors**
   a. Older patients are at more risk for drug interactions than younger patients. Older patients might have changes in their physiologic and pathophysiologic condition that lead to altered body composition, altered GI transit time and drug absorption, decreased protein binding, changes in body composition, and decreased drug clearance.
   b. Patients with predisposing illness (diabetes, asthma, AIDS) and patients who are clinically hypersensitive (atopic) are more at risk for drug interactions than nonatopic patients.

B. Clinical significance

1. Not all drug interactions are clinically significant or cause an adverse effect. In some cases, interacting drugs can be prescribed for patients as long as the patient is given proper instructions and is compliant. For example, cimetidine and an antacid might be prescribed to the patient, but the patient should be instructed not to take both medications at the same time.

2. Combination drug therapy can have beneficial effects. Drug combinations are used to improve the therapeutic objective or to decrease adverse events. Some examples include:
   a. Trimethoprim and sulfamethoxazole—a combination antibiotic for increased efficacy in urinary tract infections
   b. Amoxicillin and clavulanate potassium—a combination containing a β-lactamase inhibitor (clavulanate) to inhibit the breakdown of amoxicillin
   c. Hydrochlorothiazide and triamterene—a combination diuretic and antihypertensive to minimize potassium excretion

3. The determination of the clinical significance of a potential drug interaction should be documented in the literature. The likelihood of a drug interaction can be classified as follows:
   a. **Established**—a drug interaction supported by well-proven clinical studies
   b. **Probable**—a drug interaction that is very likely but might not be proven clinically
   c. **Suspected**—a drug interaction that might occur; some data might be available
   d. **Possible**—a drug interaction that could occur; limited data is available
   e. **Unlikely**—a drug interaction that is doubtful; no good evidence of an altered clinical effect is available

4. The clinical relevance of a potential drug interaction should also consider the:
   a. **Size** of the dose and the duration of therapy
   b. **Onset** (rapid, delayed) and **severity** (major, moderate, minor) of the potential interaction
   c. **Extrapolation** to related drugs

C. Management of drug interactions

1. Review the patient profile, including drug history and patient risk factors.

2. Avoid complex therapeutic drug regimens.

3. Determine the probability of a clinically significant drug interaction.

4. Suggest a different drug if there is a high probability for a clinically significant drug interaction. For example, acetaminophen can be used for headache instead of aspirin for a patient on anticoagulant therapy.

5. Carefully instruct the patient as to the timing of the medication. For example, the antacid and H-2 blocker should not be taken at the same time. The patient should use maximum spacing between drugs.

6. Monitor the patient for adverse events. Sulfonamides, such as sulfisoxazole and sulfamethoxazole, can prolong prothrombin time in patients given warfarin therapy. The prothrombin times should be monitored in these patients.

V. References.

A vast number of drug interactions are reported in the literature. Some general references that are updated periodically include:

A. *Drug Interaction Facts*, Facts and Comparisons, St. Louis, MO

B. *Drug Interactions & Updates,* Hansten, PD; Horn, JR, (ed) Applied Therapeutics, Inc., Vancouver, WA

C. *Evaluations of Drug Interactions,* Zucchero, FJ; Hogan, MJ; Schultz, CD (ed), Professional Drug Systems, St. Louis, MO

D. *PDR Guide to Drug Interactions, Side Effects, Indications,* Medical Economics Data, Montvale, NJ

STUDY QUESTIONS

Directions: Each question below contains three suggested answers of which **one or more** is correct. Choose the answer

- **A** if **I only** is correct
- **B** if **III only** is correct
- **C** if **I and II** are correct
- **D** if **II and III** are correct
- **E** if **I, II, and III** are correct

1. Drug interactions may be classed as

I pharmacokinetic interactions
II pharmacodynamic interactions
III pharmaceutic interactions

2. Situations that can potentially lead to drug interactions include

I multiple drug therapy
II multiple prescribers
III patient compliance

Directions: The question below is followed by five suggested answers. Select the **one** lettered answer that is the **best** response to the question.

3. Which of the following statements regarding drug interactions is true?

(A) All drug interactions can potentially cause an adverse response in the patient
(B) The clinical significance for each potential drug interaction must be considered individually
(C) A precipitant drug that inhibits the metabolism of the object drug causes a more serious drug interaction compared to a precipitant drug causing an increase in the bioavailability of the object drug
(D) If the patient is prescribed drugs that can potentially interact, the prescriber should be called, and a different precipitant drug should be suggested
(E) Food–drug interactions are unlikely to have clinical significance

ANSWERS AND EXPLANATIONS

1. The answer is E *[I B].*
Most drug interactions in vivo are caused by pharmacokinetic and pharmacodynamic interactions. Pharmaceutic interactions can occur during extemporaneous compounding, preparation of intravenous (IV) admixtures, and improper dosing, as in the case of giving aspirin with acidic juices (e.g., orange, cranberry).

2. The answer is E *[IV A 1–3].*
Patient profiles might not contain all the drug history information of the patient. Patients who take non-prescription (OTC) medications, go to several different physicians, or purchase drugs at various pharmacies may neglect to inform the pharmacist of all the medications being taken.

3. The answer is B *[IV B].*
Not all drug interactions are clinically significant. Some potential clinically significant drug interactions can be prevented by proper patient instruction and compliance. The potential for a clinically significant drug interaction should be documented before calling a physician concerning the prescribed medication.

21
Nuclear Pharmacy

Stephen C. Dragotakes
Ronald J. Callahan

I. INTRODUCTION

A. Overview

1. **Nuclear pharmacy** is defined by the *American Pharmaceutical Association's Nuclear Pharmacy Practice Standards,* as "patient-oriented service that embodies the scientific knowledge and professional judgment required to improve and promote health through the safe, and efficacious use of radioactive drugs for diagnosis and therapy."[1]

2. **Radiopharmaceuticals** are chemical entities that contain radioactive elements. Most radiopharmaceuticals are used in diagnostic medical imaging; however, they are also used in therapeutic applications, such as in the treatment of hyperthyroidism, thyroid cancer, polycythemia vera, and in the alleviation of bone pain.

3. **Nuclear pharmacy practice** entails the:
   - **a.** Procurement of radiopharmaceuticals
   - **b.** Compounding of radiopharmaceuticals
   - **c.** Performance of routine quality control procedures
   - **d.** Dispensing of radiopharmaceuticals
   - **e.** Distribution of radiopharmaceuticals
   - **f.** Implementation of basic radiation protection procedures and practices
   - **g.** Consultation and education of the nuclear medicine community, patients, pharmacists, other health professionals, and the general public regarding:
     - **(1)** Physical and chemical properties of radiopharmaceuticals
     - **(2)** Pharmacokinetics and biodistribution of radiopharmaceuticals
     - **(3)** Drug interactions and other factors that alter patterns of distribution

B. Properties of radiopharmaceuticals

1. **Pharmacologic effects.** Radiopharmaceuticals do not produce pharmacologic effects because the quantities range from picogram (pg) to nanogram (ng) per kilogram (kg) of administered dose.

2. **Route of administration.** Most radiopharmaceuticals are prepared as sterile, pyrogen-free intravenous solutions to be administered directly to the patient. Other routes of administration include oral, interstitial, and inhalation (e.g., radioactive gases, aerosols).

3. **Radionuclides**
   - **a.** The radioactive component of a radiopharmaceutical is referred to as a radionuclide. Nuclides are identified as atoms having a specific number of protons and neutrons in the nucleus. A nuclide is typically identified by the chemical symbol of the element with a mass number to the upper left superscript, indicating the sum of protons and neutrons [e.g., iodide 131 (^{131}I)]. When the atom is radioactive, it is called a radionuclide.
   - **b.** Radionuclides undergo spontaneous radioactive decay accompanied by the release of energy. The distribution, metabolism, and elimination of the radiopharmaceutical can be determined by measuring this energy with imaging equipment. There are **four major types of radiation** emitted through this process: **alpha, beta, gamma,** and **x-rays.** Alpha and beta radiations are not useful in medical imaging. Most radiopharmaceuticals use penetrating gamma radiation, which can be easily detected and converted into imaging data.

4. **Half-lives of radiopharmaceuticals**

a. **Physical half-life** of a radiopharmaceutical is the amount of time necessary for the radioactive atoms to decay to one-half their original number. Each nuclide is identified with a specific half-life.
b. **Biological half-life** of a radiopharmaceutical is the amount of time required for the body to eliminate one-half of the administered dose of any substance by the processes of biological elimination.
c. **Effective half-life** of a radiopharmaceutical is the time required for an administered radiopharmaceutical dose to be reduced by one-half due to both physical decay and biological elimination. It is defined as:

$$t_e \text{ (effective half-life)} = (t_p \times t_b)/(t_p + t_b),$$
where t_p = physical half-life and t_b = biological half-life.

C. Optimal radiopharmaceuticals

1. They should have a half-life short enough to minimize radiation exposure to the patient yet long enough to allow for collection of imaging information.
2. They should incorporate a gamma-emitting radionuclide, which decays with the emission of a photon energy between 100–300 kilo electron volts (keV), which is efficiently detected with current instrumentation.
3. Radiopharmaceuticals should localize rapidly in the organ system of interest and be metabolized or excreted from the nontarget tissues to maximize contrast and minimize absorbed doses of radiation.
4. They should be readily available and cost-effective.

II. SODIUM PERTECHNETATE TECHNETIUM 99m GENERATOR

A. Overview

1. **Technetium 99m (^{99m}Tc)** is the most commonly used radionuclide in diagnostic imaging today. This radionuclide is produced by the **radioactive decay of molybdenum 99** (^{99}Mo)
   a. ^{99m}Tc is obtained via commercially supplied sterile, pyrogen-free "generator" systems. A generator is a device used to separate a short half-life radionuclide from the longer-lived "parent" nuclide, while releasing the parent to produce more of the daughter nuclide. In this way, short half-life nuclides can be made available continuously at great distances from the sites of generator production.
   b. All of the commercially supplied generators currently use ^{99}Mo obtained from the tissue of uranium 235 (^{235}U). This ^{99}Mo parent is absorbed on an alumina (Al_2O_3) ion exchange column, and the ^{99m}Tc formed from its decay is exchanged for the chloride ion (Cl^-) available in the 0.9% saline eluate solution washed through the column, as the sodium pertechnetate $Na^+(^{99m}Tc\ O_4)^-$ form.
2. **The chemical valence state** of $Na^{+99m}TcO_4^-$ as it is eluted from the column is +7. Typically it must be reduced to a valence state of +3, +4, or +5 before it is able to react with other compounds. Although ^{99m}Tc can be reduced by many processes, the **stannous** ion (Sn^{2+}) **reduction method** is most commonly used in ^{99m}Tc radiopharmaceutical kits.
   a. A radiopharmaceutical kit consists of sterile, pyrogen-free vials containing a reducing agent, the compound to be labeled, and any additional adjuvants to effect the reaction or stabilize the labeled product. In most cases they are lyophilized.
   b. The contents of radiopharmaceutical kits are stored under a nitrogen atmosphere so as to minimize oxidation of Sn^{2+}.

B. Sodium pertechnetate ^{99m}Tc USP ($Na^+\ ^{99m}TcO_4^-$) as eluted from a generator in 0.9% sodium chloride (NaCl) solution is an isotonic, sterile, nonpyrogenic, diagnostic radiopharmaceuticals suitable for intravenous (IV) injection, oral administration, and direct instillation.

1. **Physical properties**
   a. The solution should be clear, colorless, and free of visible foreign material. The pH is 4.5–7.0.
   b. $Na^+\ ^{99m}TcO_4^-$ is used to radiolabel all other ^{99m}Tc radiopharmaceuticals.

2. **Biodistribution**
   a. Na^+ $^{99m}TcO_4^-$ is handled by the body in a fashion similar to ^{131}I; that is, it is taken up and released but not organified by the thyroid.
   b. After IV administration, Na^+ $^{99m}TcO_4^-$ concentrates in the choroid plexus, thyroid gland, salivary gland, and stomach, but remains in the circulation long enough for first-pass blood pool studies, organ perfusion, and major vessel studies.

3. **Decay data**
   a. Na^+ $^{99m}TcO_4^-$ decays by isomeric transition with a **physical half-life** of 6 hours.
   b. The primary **radiation emissions** are 140 keV gamma energy photons.

4. **Purity**
   a. **United States Pharmacopeia (USP) radionuclidic purity** requires a ^{99}Mo breakthrough limit of less than 0.15 μCi/mCi.
   b. **USP chemical purity** requires an aluminum ion (Al^{+3}) test result of less than 10 μg/ml.

5. **Administration and dosage.** All of the following imaging studies are administered via IV except nasolacrimal imaging, which is instilled into the lacrimal canal.
   a. Brain imaging: 10–20 mCi [370–740 megabecquerels (MBq)]
   b. Thyroid imaging: 1–10 mCi (37–370 MBq)
   c. Salivary gland imaging: 1–5 mCi (37–185 MBq)
   d. Placenta localization: 1–3 mCi (37–111 MBq)
   e. Blood pool imaging: 10–30 mCi (370–740 MBq)
   f. Urinary bladder imaging: 0.5–1 mCi (18–37 MBq)
   g. Nasolacrimal imaging: less than 100 μCi (less than 3.7 MBq)

III. RADIOPHARMACEUTICALS FOR CARDIOVASCULAR IMAGING

A. **Perfusion agents for cardiac imaging.** Radiopharmaceuticals are useful in cardiac imaging as agents that provide information of regional myocardial blood perfusion. They typically are administered as part of a stress test so as to provide information at peak cardiac output. Pharmacologic augmentation of treadmill exercise stress test perfusion imaging includes the use of IV coronary vessel dilating agents, such as dipyridamole, adenosine, and dobutamine.

1. **Thallous chloride ^{201}Tl USP** (^{201}Tl) is a radionuclide that is produced by cyclotron. It is used for myocardial perfusion imaging in the diagnosis of coronary artery disease and localization of myocardial infarction.
   a. **Biodistribution**
      (1) ^{201}Tl is a monovalent cation with distribution analogous to potassium ion (K^+); myocardial uptake is by active transport via the Na^+-K^+-adenosine triphosphatase (ATPase) pump.
      (2) Biodistribution is generally proportional to organ blood flow at the time of injection with blood clearance by myocardium, kidneys, thyroid, liver, and stomach. The remainder is distributed uniformly throughout the rest of the body.
      (3) ^{201}Tl is excreted slowly and equally in both urine and feces.
   b. **Decay data**
      (1) The **physical half-life** is 73 hours.
      (2) The **effective half-life** is 2–4 days.
      (3) The **biological half-life** is 11 days.
      (4) The **primary radiation emissions** are 68–80 keV x-rays and 167 keV and 135 keV gamma energy photons.
   c. **Administration and dosage.** ^{201}Tl is administered via IV 2–4 mCi (74–148 MBq).

2. **Technetium ^{99m}Tc sestamibi** (^{99m}Tc sestamibi) exists as a sterile, pyrogen-free IV injection after kit reconstitution with $Na^{+}$$^{99m}TcO_4^-$ and heating at 100°C for 10 minutes.
   a. **Biodistribution**
      (1) ^{99m}Tc sestamibi is a cation complex that has been found to accumulate in viable myocardial tissue similar to ^{201}Tl.
      (2) The major pathway for clearance of ^{99m}Tc sestamibi is the hepatobiliary system. This agent is excreted without any evidence of metabolism via urine and feces.
   b. **Decay data**
      (1) **The effective half-life** is 3 hours.
      (2) **Tl biologic half-life** is 6 hours.

c. **Administration and dosage.** IV, 10–30 mCi (370–1110 MBq)

3. **Technetium Tc 99m tetrofosmin USP** exists as a sterile, and pyrogen-free IV injection after kit reconstitution with sodium pertechnetate ^{99m}Tc injection USP.
   a. **Description.** ^{99m}Tc-Tetrofosmin is a lipophilic, cationic ^{99m}Tc complex that has been found to accumulate in viable myocardium.
   b. **Biodistribution.** The major pathways for clearance of ^{99m}Tc tetrofosmin are the renal system, and hepatobiliary system with 26% of the administered dose excreted in the feces, and 40% in the urine within 48 hours.
   c. **Physical Properties** (see II A 2 a, b; B 1,3 a, b)
   d. **Administration and dosage.** IV during exercise, 5–8 mCi (185–296 MBq); during rest, 15–24 mCi (555–1443 MBq)

4. **Technetium Tc 99m teboroxime (no longer available)**

5. **Rubidium chloride** (Rb 82 USP) is a generator-produced radiopharmaceutical obtained by the decay of its accelerator-produced parent (half-life is 25 days) adsorbed on a stannous oxide column.
   a. **Biodistribution**
      (1) When eluted with 0.9% NaCl at a rate of 50 ml/min, a solution of the short-lived daughter $^{82}Rb^+$ is eluted from the generator for direct IV administration.
      (2) After IV administration, $^{82}Rb^+$ rapidly clears from the blood and is extracted by the myocardial tissue in a manner analogous to K^+ .
      (3) Myocardial activity is visualized within 1 minute after administration.
   b. **Decay data**
      (1) The **physical half-life** is 75 seconds.
      (2) The **decay mode** is by positron emission.
      (3) The **primary radiation emissions** are annihilation 511 keV gamma energy photons.
      (4) Parent strontium (^{32}Sr) and contaminant ^{85}Sr breakthrough must be closely monitored. Acceptable levels of strontium breakthrough are less than 0.02 μCi ^{82}Sr/mCi $^{82}Rb^+$, and less than 0.2 μCi^{85}Sr/mCi $^{82}Rb^+$.
   c. **Administration and dosage.** IV, 30–60 mCi (1110–2220 MBq)

6. **Ammonia N 13 USP** exists under a USP monograph as an on-site-produced, sterile, IV, solution of $^{13}NH_4$ useful as a myocardial perfusion agent.
   a. **Decay Properties**
      (1) Physical half-life is 10 minutes.
      (2) Decay mode is positron emission with 511keV annihilation gamma photons.
   b. **Biodistribution**
      (1) After IV injection, it circulates as $^{13}NH_4$+ but localizes into the myocytes via diffusion as $^{13}NH_3$+. It is then metabolized to glutamine and retained by the myocytes.
      (2) After IV injection, it is cleared rapidly from the blood with less than 2% of the administered dose remaining after 5 minutes postinjection.
      (3) Predominately metabolized to $^{13}NH_3$ glutamine by different organs of the body.
      (4) Ten percent to twenty percent is excreted via the renal system.
   c. **Administration and dosage.** IV, 15–20 mCi (555–740 MBq)

B. **Agents used to measure cardiac function** (regional myocardial wall motion)

1. **^{99m}Tc-labeled** red blood cells (RBCs) are used for blood pool imaging, including cardiac first-pass and gated equilibrium imaging (regional cardiac wall motion).
   a. **Physical properties.** Autologous RBCs can be labeled by a number of techniques that use the Sn^{2+*} radiolabeling method with three general steps.
      (1) The cells are treated with Sn^{2+}($Sn^{2\ +}$: 10-20 μg/kg) to provide an intercellular source of the reducing agent.
      (2) Some procedures then allow for a removal of excess Sn^{2+} with scavenging agents.
      (3) All of the methods include the addition of Na^+ $^{99m}TcO_4^-$. This ^{99m}Tc, while in the +7 valence state, crosses the intact erythrocyte membrane and binds to intercellular hemoglobin (Hb) after being reduced by the available intercellular Sn^{2+}.
   b. **Biodistribution.** After IV injection, the labeling RBCs distribute within the blood pool and are well maintained in the blood pool with a **bi-exponential whole body clearance** of 2.5–2.7 hours and 75–176 hours (e.g., major route of excretion is via the urine).

c. **Administration and dosage.** IV, 10–20 mCi (370–740 MBq)

2. **Pyrophosphate injection USP and phosphates USP.** The major use for these agents in nuclear medicine is as convenient and stable sources of Sn^{2+} for the labeling of autologous RBCs. In this application, the kits are reconstituted with normal saline and injected via IV.

3. **Technetium ^{99m}Tc albumin (TcHSA) injection**
   a. **Biodistribution**
      (1) ^{99m}Tc albumin distributes initially within the intravascular space and leaves this space at a rate slow enough to permit imaging of the blood pool.
      (2) **Plasma clearance** is bi-exponential; a fast component clearing with a half-life of 2 hours and a slow component clearing with a half-life of 10–16 hours.
      (3) The major route of elimination is via the urine.
   b. **Administration and dosage.** IV, 20 mCi (740 MBq)

C. **Agents for imaging myocardial infarction** include **pyrophosphate injection USP** and phosphates USP.

1. **Mechanism of localization.** The skeletal localizing radiopharmaceutical pyrophosphate has been shown to accumulate also in zones of myocardial infarction. This localization is thought to be due to binding of the pyrophosphate to microcalcification with hydroxyapatite crystals found in infarcted tissue.

2. **Biodistribution** of labeled pyrophosphate depends on the ability of phosphates to become involved with calcium ion (Ca^{2+}) metabolism in necrotic cardiac tissue.

IV. SKELETAL IMAGING

A. Skeletal imaging agents

1. **Overview.** ^{99m}Tc-labeled bone agents are useful in the detection of bone lesions that are associated with metastatic neoplasms, metabolic disorders, and infections of the bone. The imaging advantages of ^{99m}Tc, coupled with the sensitivity of bone agent localization in skeletal bone hydroxyapatite, allows for detection of bone pathology before evidence is shown by conventional x-rays.

2. **^{99m}Tc bone agents.** There are many different forms of ^{99m}Tc bone agents with minor differences in their individual chemical structure. Currently used bone imaging agents are based on the P—C—P diphosphonate structure, including ^{99m}Tc medronate disodium, ^{99m}Tc oxidronate, and ^{99m}Tc pyrophosphate. These bone agents are Sn^{2+} reduction method kits, which exist as sterile, pyrogen-free IV radiopharmaceuticals after reconstitution with $Na^{+99m}TcO_4^-$.
   a. **Physical properties**
      (1) All of the ^{99m}Tc bone agents are susceptible to radiologic decomposition with reoxidation of the ^{99m}Tc to a higher valence state. These agents sometimes include antioxidants (e.g., ascorbic or gentisic acid) in their formulation.
      (2) Most agents should be used within 6 hours after formulation.
      (3) They should be stored at room temperature before and after reconstitution.
   b. **Biodistribution**
      (1) It is believed that the localization of the diphosphonates occurs on the hydroxyapatite mineral matrix of skeletal bone with uptake related to bone metabolic activity and bone blood flow.
      (2) For ^{99m}Tc medronate disodium and ^{99m}Tc oxidronate, approximately 50% of the administered dose localizes in the skeleton, and 50% is excreted by the kidneys within the first 4–6 hours after IV injection.
   c. **Administration and dosage.** IV, 10–20 mCi (370–740 MBq)

B. **Bone marrow imaging** (see VI B)

V. LUNG IMAGING. Radiopharmaceuticals are used to evaluate both pulmonary perfusion and pulmonary ventilation, to detect pulmonary embolism, and to assess pulmonary function before pneumonectomy.

A. Pulmonary perfusion imaging

1. **Technetium ^{99m}Tc albumin aggregated USP (TcMAA)**
   a. **Physical properties**
      (1) The ^{99m}Tc albumin aggregated kit contains human serum albumin that has been aggregated by heat denaturization.
      (2) This Sn^{2+} reduction method kit exists as a sterile, pyrogen-free suspension of radiolabeled aggregated particles after reconstitution with $Na^{+99m}TcO_4^-$.
      (3) It should be stored at 2°–8°C after reconstitution.
   b. **Biodistribution**
      (1) After IV administration of ^{99m}Tc albumin aggregated, 80% of the radiolabeled albumin particles become trapped by capillary blockade in the pulmonary circulation.
      (2) After trapping, the particles are cleared from the lungs mainly by mechanical breakup. These smaller particles are ultimately cleared from the circulation by the reticuloendothelial system.
      (3) Particle size should be controlled; that is, 90% of the particles should be between 10 and 90 μ, and none should be greater than 150 μ to ensure adequate trapping by the lung capillary bed but no occlusion of the large bore vessels.
      (4) Particle number should be between 200,000 and 700,000 particles per adult dose to obtain uniform imaging data without compromising capillary blood flow.
   c. **Decay data: Biologic half-life** in the lung is 2–3 hours.
   d. **Administration and dosage.** Intravenous, 1–4 mCi (37–148 MBq)

B. Pulmonary ventilation imaging. Pulmonary ventilation imaging with radioactive gases is a routine nuclear medicine procedure that can provide valuable information about regional lung ventilation. Radiopharmaceuticals that are used are either radioactive gases or radioaerosols.

1. **Xenon ^{133}Xe USP (^{133}Xe)** is supplied as a radioactive gas contained in glass septum vials to be administered by inhalation through a closed respiratory system or a spirometer. It is a byproduct of ^{235}U fission.
   a. **Biodistribution**
      (1) ^{133}Xe is a readily diffusible gas, which is neither used nor produced by the body. It passes through membranes and freely exchanges between blood and tissue, tending to concentrate more in body fat.
      (2) Inhaled ^{133}Xe distributes within the alveoli and enters the pulmonary venous circulation via the capillaries with most of the absorbed ^{133}Xe returned and exhaled from the lungs after a single pass through the peripheral circulation.
      (3) In concentrations used for diagnosis, the gas is physiologically inactive.
   b. **Decay data**
      (1) The **effective half-life** in the lung is 2 minutes.
      (2) The **physical half-life** is 5.2 days.
      (3) The **decay mode** is beta minus decay.
      (4) The **primary radiation emissions** are 100 keV beta energy and 81 keV gamma energy photons.
   c. **Administration and dosage.** Inhalation, 2–30 mCi (74–1110 MBq)

2. **Xenon ^{127}Xe USP (^{127}Xe)** is supplied as a radioactive gas contained in glass septum vials to be administered by inhalation through a closed respiratory system or a spirometer. It is produced by cyclotron.
   a. **Biodistribution.** Localization is the same as ^{133}Xe.
   b. **Decay data**
      (1) The **physical half-life** is 36.4 days.
      (2) The **decay mode** is by electron capture.
      (3) The **primary radiation emissions** are 203 keV, 190 keV, 172 keV, and 375 keV gamma energy photons.
   c. **Administration and dosage.** Inhalation, 5–10 mCi (185–370 MBq)

3. **Krypton ^{81m}Kr USP (^{81m}Kr)** is generator-produced by the decay of its parent radionuclide ^{81}Rb. It is supplied as a radioactive gas in the form of humidified oxygen eluted continuously through the generator and inhaled by the patient.
   a. **Decay data**
      (1) The **physical half-life** is 13 seconds.
      (2) The **parent** ^{81}Rb half-life is 4.6 hours.

(3) The **primary radiation emissions** are 190 keV gamma energy photons.

b. **Administration and dosage.** Inhalation, 1–10 mCi (37–370 MBq)

4. **Radioaerosols** have become increasingly used with the advent of nebulizers that produce particles of a consistent size necessary for uniform lung distribution.

a. **Biodistribution**

(1) ^{99m}Tc pentetate radioaerosols of approximately 0.25-μ mass median aerodynamic diameter are useful in determining lung ventilation.

(2) After deposition of the nebulized droplets within the airways, the ^{99m}Tc pentetate is absorbed into the pulmonary circulation.

(3) The material is subsequently excreted by the kidneys. Clearance from the lungs is sufficiently slow to allow for imaging of the lungs in multiple projections from a single administration.

b. **Physical properties** (see VII B 1 a)

c. **Administration and dosage.** Inhalation, 8 mCi (296 MBq)

VI. HEPATIC IMAGING

A. **Overview.** Hepatic imaging requires the use of two different classes of radiopharmaceuticals to evaluate the two cell types responsible for hepatic function.

1. **Reticuloendothelial system imaging.** The liver, spleen, and bone marrow are evaluated with radiolabeled colloidal material, ranging in size from 0.1–3.0 μ. These particles are rapidly cleared from the blood by the Küpffer cells.

2. **Liver-spleen imaging.** Radiopharmaceuticals are useful in imaging space-occupying primary tumors and metastatic neoplasms, as well as hepatic defects caused by abscesses, cysts, and trauma.

3. **Bone marrow imaging.** Images that localize in the bone marrow are useful in the evaluation of pathologies that affect bone marrow.

4. **Hepatobiliary imaging.** Hepatocyte function can be evaluated by substances meeting requirements of molecular weight, lipophilicity, and chemical structure, to be excreted by the polygonal cells into the hepatobiliary system. Hepatobiliary imaging radiopharmaceuticals are useful in the diagnosis of cystic duct obstruction in acute cholecystitis as well as defining postcholecystectomy anatomy and physiology.

B. **Reticuloendothelial imaging agents**

1. **Technetium ^{99m}Tc sulfur colloid (Tc_2S_7)** is a sterile, pyrogen-free IV radiopharmaceutical formed via a chemical reaction between $Na^{+}\ ^{99m}TcO_4^{-}$ and an acidified solution of sodium thiosulfate at 100°C.

a. **Physical properties**

(1) ^{99m}Tc sulfur colloid is thought to remain in the +7 valence state as the heptasulfide coprecipitate of elemental sulfur that occurs during the reaction.

(2) The use of $Na^{+}\ ^{99m}TcO_4^{-}$ with Al^{+3} levels over 10 μg/ml can lead to the formation of particles greater than 5 μm, which can result in lung uptake.

(3) Heating times should be controlled to preclude large particle formation.

b. **Biodistribution.** After administration, approximately 80%-90% of the dose is phagocytized by the Küpffer cells of the liver, 5%–10% by the spleen, and the balance by the bone marrow. The blood clearance half-life is approximately 2.5 minutes. Particles are not metabolized and reside in the reticuloendothelial system for a prolonged period.

c. **Administration and dosage.** IV, liver/spleen: 1–8 mCi (37–296 MBq); bone marrow: 3–12 mCi (111–444 MBq)

2. **^{99m}Tc albumin colloid** labeled with $Na^{+}\ ^{99m}TcO_4^{-}$ has been proposed as an alternative to ^{99m}Tc sulfur colloid. Possible advantages of this product include metabolism and clearance of the particle from the reticuloendothelial system and a single-step preparation, which does not require heating.

a. **Biodistribution.** After administration, approximately 80%–90% of the dose is phagocytized by the liver, 5%–10% by the spleen, and the balance by the bone marrow.

b. **Administration and dosage.** IV, 5–8 mCi (185–296 MBq)

C. Hepatobiliary imaging agents

1. **Overview**
   a. **Iminodiacetic acid (IDA) derivatives** are useful as hepatobiliary imaging agents because of their ability to be selectively cleared by a carrier-mediated hepatocyte pathway. Because these agents share the same excretion pathway as bilirubin, patients who have increased bilirubin levels exhibit decreased hepatic clearance and an increased renal clearance. Lack of gallbladder visualization is an abnormal finding suggestive of acute cholecystitis.
   b. **Cholecystokinetic agents,** such as sincalide, may be used to empty the contents of the gallbladder in fasting patients in an attempt to promote gallbladder filling and visualization.
   c. **Narcotic analgesics,** such as morphine, have been used to constrict the sphincter of Oddi to produce increased intraductal pressures to promote gallbladder filling.

2. **Technetium ^{99m}Tc disofenin (Tc-DISIDA)**
   a. **Physical properties** (see II A 2 a, b)
   b. **Biodistribution**
      (1) ^{99m}Tc disofenin is rapidly cleared from the blood with 8% remaining in the blood after 30 minutes.
      (2) Approximately, 9% of the administered activity is excreted in the urine during the first 2 hours. The remainder of the activity is cleared through the hepatobiliary system.
      (3) Peak liver uptake is within 10 minutes with peak gallbladder uptake by 30–40 minutes.
      (4) Gallbladder and intestinal visualization occurs within 60 minutes postadministration.
   c. **Administration and dosage.** IV, nonjaundiced patient: 1–5 mCi (37–185 MBq); jaundiced patient: 3–8 mCi (111–296 MBq)

3. **Technetium ^{99m}Tc lidofenin (Tc-HIDA)**
   a. **Physical properties** (see II A 2 a, b)
   b. **Biodistribution**
      (1) After administration, ^{99m}Tc lidofenin is rapidly cleared from the blood circulation with 7% remaining after 26 minutes.
      (2) Approximately 14%–22% of the administered activity can be excreted in the urine within the first 90 minutes with the remainder of the activity clearing through the hepatobiliary system.
      (3) Peak liver uptake occurs within 10–15 minutes with visualization of the hepatic duct and gallbladder within 20–30 minutes.
      (4) Intestinal activity can be visualized within 30 minutes.
   c. **Administration and dosage.** IV, nonjaundiced patient: 2–5 mCi (74–185 MBq jaundiced patient: 3–10 mCi (111–370 MBq)

4. **Technetium ^{99m}Tc mebrofenin (^{99m}Tc mebrofenin)**
   a. **Physical properties** (see II A 2 a, b)
   b. **Biodistribution**
      (1) ^{99m}Tc mebrofenin is rapidly cleared from the blood with 17% remaining after 10 minutes. Only 1% of the administered activity is excreted in the urine within the first hours, with the remainder of the activity clearing through the hepatobiliary system
      (2) Peak liver uptake occurs within 10 minutes with visualization of the hepatic duct and gallbladder within 10–15 minutes, then intestinal activity within 30–60 minutes.
   c. **Administration and dosage.** IV, nonjaundiced patient: 2–5 mCi (74–185 MBq jaundiced patient: 3–10 mCi (111–370 MBq)

VII. RENAL IMAGING

A. Overview

1. Radiopharmaceuticals are used in renal imaging to determine renal function, renal vascular flow, and renal morphology. They are also useful for the evaluation of renal transplant pa-

tients for complications such as obstruction, infarction, leakage, tubular necrosis, and rejection.

2. The use of radiopharmaceuticals to determine renal function or renal morphology is based on the two physiological mechanisms responsible for excretion: glomerular filtration and tubular secretion.

B. Agents cleared by glomerular filtration are useful in determining the glomerular filtration rate (GFR), renal artery perfusion, and the visualization of the collecting system.

1. **Technetium ^{99m}Tc pentetate USP (Tc-DTPA)**
   a. **Physical properties** (see II A 2 a, b)
   b. **Biodistribution**
      (1) After administration, ^{99m}Tc pentetate rapidly distributes throughout extracellular fluid space from which it is rapidly cleared by glomerular filtration.
      (2) Up to 10% may be protein bound, leading to a decrease in measured GFR.
      (3) After administration, 50% of the dose is cleared by the kidneys within 2 hours, and up to 95% is cleared by 24 hours.
   c. **Administration and dosage.** Intravenous 10–20 mCi (370–740 MBq)

2. **Sodium iothalamate ^{125}I injection** is a commercially supplied sterile, pyrogen-free injection containing 1 mg sodium iothalamate per milliliter.
   a. **Biodistribution**
      (1) Sodium iothalamate ^{125}I is used for determination of the GFR but not for imaging due to poor imaging emissions of ^{125}I.
      (2) Thyroid blockade with oral potassium iodide (KI) is suggested.
   b. **Decay data**
      (1) The **physical half-life** is 59 days.
      (2) The **decay mode** is by electron capture.
      (3) The **primary radiation emissions** are 35 keV gamma energy photons and x-rays.
   c. **Administration and dosage.** IV, 10–50 μCi (3.7–18.5 MBq)

C. Tubular secretion agents are used to evaluate renal tubular function and measure effective renal plasma flow.

1. **Iodohippurate ^{123}I hippuran and iodohippurate ^{131}I hippuran.** These are commercially supplied sterile, pyrogen-free, IV solutions. ^{123}I is produced by cyclotron and ^{131}I, by reactor.
   a. **Biodistribution**
      (1) Iodohippurate ^{123}I hippuran and ^{131}I hippuran are excreted 80% by tubular secretion and 20% by glomerular filtration.
      (2) Whole body biological half-life, excluding the bladder, is less than 1 hour.
      (3) Approximately 50% of an administered dose is excreted within 30 minutes, with 90% excreted within 8 hours.
      (4) Thyroid blockade with KI is suggested.
   b. **Decay data and dosage**
      (1) **Iodohippurate ^{123}I**
         (a) The **physical half-life** is 13 hours.
         (b) The **decay mode** is by electron capture.
         (c) The **primary radiation emissions** are 159 keV gamma energy photons.
         (d) **Administration and dosage.** IV, 100–400 μCi (3.7–14.8 MBq)
      (2) **Iodohippurate ^{131}I**
         (a) The **physical half-life** is 8 days.
         (b) The **decay mode** is by beta minus decay.
         (c) The **primary radiation emissions** are 197 keV beta energy and 364 keV gamma energy photons.
         (d) **Administration and dosage.** IV, 10–100 μCi (0.4–3.7 MBq)

2. **Technetium ^{99m}Tc mertiate (Tc-MAG3)**
   a. **Description**
      (1) Supplied as a sterile, pyrogen-free, lyophilized kit containing betiatide precursor of mertiatide, and chelation adjuvants.
      (2) On addition of $Na^+\ ^{99m}TcO_4^-$, this kit requires the addition of heat (100°C) to form ^{99m}Tc mertiatide from the betiatide precursor.

b. Biodistribution

(1) Renal elimination with 90% of administered dose excreted within 3 hours postinjection.

(2) Primarily cleared via active tubular secretion and to a small extent via glomerular filtration.

c. Physical properties (see II A 2 a,b; B 1 b, 3 a,b)

d. Administration and dosage: IV, 5–10 mCi (185–370 MBq)

D. Renal cortical imaging agents are used to evaluate renal anatomy because of their ability to accumulate in the kidney and provide anatomic imaging data.

1. Technetium ^{99m}Tc gluceptate (Tc-GLH)

a. Physical properties (see II A 2 a, b)

b. Biodistribution

(1) ^{99m}Tc gluceptate rapidly distributes throughout the body with rapid blood clearance via glomerular filtration and tubular secretion.

(2) Approximately 25% of the administered dose is excreted within the first hour, 65% within 6 hours, and 70% within 24 hours.

(3) After 3–6 hours, a maximum of 5%–15% of the dose administered is concentrated in the proximal renal tubular cells of the renal cortex.

c. Administration and dosage. IV, 10–20 mCi (370–740 MBq)

2. Technetium ^{99m}Tc succimer USP (Tc-DMSA)

a. Physical properties (see II A 2 a, b) ^{99m}Tc succimer complex must be allowed to incubate for 10 minutes postreconstitution and must be used within 30 minutes postincubation.

b. Biodistribution

(1) Within 3–6 hours postadministration, 40%–50% of the dose localizes in the renal cortex where it is taken up by the tubular cells.

(2) Excretion into the urine is slow with 5%–20% being excreted within the first 2 hours, 10%–30% by 6 hours, and less than 40% by 24 hours.

c. Administration and dosage. IV, 2–6 mCi (74–222 MBq)

VIII. THYROID IMAGING

A. Overview

1. The basic function of the thyroid gland is the production of thyroid hormone for the regulation of metabolism. The thyroid hormones are produced within the gland with the organification of iodine obtained from the oxidation of available iodide circulating in the blood. The inability of the body to distinguish between the isotopes of iodine provides a perfect metabolic tracer for the thyroid biochemical system.

2. The function of the thyroid gland can be evaluated by the uptake of ^{131}I, allowing the detection of hypothyroidism with decreased uptake and hyperthyroidism with increased uptake.

3. $^{99m}TcO_4^-$ is a monovalent ion with an ionic radius similar to iodide. As a result the pertechnetate ion is trapped by the thyroid gland in a fashion similar to iodide. The two species are sufficiently different that organification of the $^{99m}TcO_4^-$ does not occur, and it is subsequently released.

B. Thyroid imaging agents

1. **Sodium iodide ^{123}I** is a radiopharmaceutical available in either solution or capsule form for oral administration. It is produced by cyclotron.

a. Biodistribution

(1) Orally administered iodine is rapidly absorbed from the gastrointestinal (GI) tract with thyroid gland uptake evident within minutes.

(2) Sodium iodide ^{123}I is considered an ideal radiopharmaceutical for iodine uptake and imaging studies because of its short half-life and useful 159 keV primary gamma emissions.

b. Decay data

(1) The **physical half-life** is 13 hours.

(2) The **biological half-life** is 3.5 days.

(3) The **decay mode** is by electron capture.
(4) The **primary radiation emissions** are 159 keV, 27 keV, and 529 keV gamma energy photons.

c. **Administration and dosage.** Oral thyroid uptake: 10–20 μCi (0.37–0.74 MBq); thyroid image: 100–500 μCi (3.7–18.5 MBq)

2. **Sodium iodide ^{131}I** is a classic radioiodine used for thyroid uptake and imaging studies; however, it is now used less often because of the high radiation dose absorbed.

a. **Biodistribution**

(1) Orally administered iodine is rapidly absorbed from the GI tract with thyroid gland uptake within minutes.
(2) Sodium iodide ^{131}I is not considered an ideal radioiodine radiopharmaceutical for iodine uptake and imaging studies because of its long half-life and the high radiation dose to the thyroid from its beta decay component.
(3) The radiation dose from the high energy beta particle with the imaging potential of its gamma emissions make this radionuclide the agent of choice for therapeutic treatment of hyperthyroidism and thyroid cancer.

b. **Decay data**

(1) The **physical half-life** is 8.08 days.
(2) The **decay mode** is by beta decay.
(3) The **primary radiation emissions** are 606 keV and 333 keV beta energy and 364 KeV, 637 keV, and 284 keV gamma energy photons.

c. **Administration and dosage.** Sodium iodide ^{131}I is available as either a capsule or in solution for oral administration.

(1) **Diagnostics**
(a) **Thyroid uptake:** 2–15 μCi (0.074–0.555 MBq)
(b) **Thyroid image:** 30–50 μCi (1.11–1.85 MBq)
(c) **Whole body image:** 1–5 mCi (37–185 MBq)

(2) **Therapeutics**
(a) **Thyroid ablation:** 5–15 mCi (185–550 MBq)
(b) **Thyroid carcinoma:** 50–200 mCi (1850–7400 MBq)

3. **Na^+ ^{99m}**TcO_4^- (see II B)

4. **^{201}Tl (parathyroid imaging)**

a. **Biodistribution.** ^{201}Tl concentrates in the thyroid and also in parathyroid adenomas, which can be detected by a dual isotope subtraction technique of subtracting thyroid uptake counts from Na^+ $^{99m}TcO_4^-$ to unmask nonthyroid thallium uptake counts (see III A 1).

b. **Administration and dosage.** IV, 2 mCi (74 MBq)

IX. BRAIN IMAGING

A. **Cerebral perfusion brain imaging agents.** Radiopharmaceuticals for evaluating brain perfusion must possess a lipophilic partition coefficient sufficient to diffuse passively across the blood-brain barrier almost completely within one pass of the cerebral circulation, as well as being sufficiently retained to permit data collection. The regional uptake of these agents is proportional to cerebral blood flow. This class of radiopharmaceuticals is useful in the diagnosis of altered regional blood perfusion in stroke.

1. **Technetium Tc 99m exametazime (Tc-HMPAO)** exists as a sterile, and pyrogen-free IV injection after reconstitution with sodium pertechnetate ^{99m}Tc USP, which may be stabilized with the addition of a methylene blue/phosphate buffer stabilizing solution.

a. **Description**

(1) ^{99m}Tc Exametazime is a neutral, lipid soluble complex that freely crosses the blood-brain barrier (BBB). This is a relatively unstable complex, which rapidly converts to a secondary complex incapable of penetrating into the brain. The in vitro addition of a methylene blue/phosphate buffer stabilizing solution after preparing the ^{99m}Tc exametazime will stabilize the lipid soluble complex for 4 hours.
(2) Additional limitations on kit preparation parameters require the use of high mole fraction technetium generator elutes of less than 2 hours postelution from a generator previously eluted within 24 hours.

b. Biodistribution

(1) ^{99m}Tc Exametazime rapidly clears from the blood with a maximum brain uptake of 3.5%–7%, with up to 2.5% remaining after 24 hours.

(2) The activity is widely distributed throughout the body, with 30% distributing to the GI tract.

(3) Within 48 hours 40% of the dose is excreted through the urine and 15% eliminated via the feces.

c. Physical Properties (see II: A 2 a,b; B 1 b,3 a,b)

d. Administration and dosage. IV 10–20 mCi (370–740 MBq)

2. Technetium ^{99m}Tc bicisate (^{99m}Tc-ECD)

a. Description

(1) ^{99m}Tc bicisate exists as a sterile, and pyrogen-free IV injection after reconstitution with sodium pertechnetate ^{99m}Tc USP and the addition of a phosphate buffer.

(2) After reconstitution a stable lipophilic ^{99m}Tc bicisate complex is formed which is able to cross the BBB by passive diffusion.

b. Biodistribution

(1) ^{99m}Tc Bicisate is rapidly cleared from blood with a maximum of 6.5% of administered dose localized in the brain, and 5% left in the blood after 1 hour

(2) Once located in the brain cells, ^{99m}Tc bicisate is metabolized by endogenous enzymes to a polar compound that is unable to diffuse out of the brain cells.

(3) ^{99m}Tc Bicisate is primarily eliminated via the kidneys with 50% excreted within 2 hours, and 74% in 24 hours. Hepatobiliary excretion accounts for approximately 12.5% of the administered dose after 48 hours.

c. Radionuclide properties (see II A 2 a,b; B 1 b, 3 a,b)

d. Administration and dosage. IV, 10–30 mCi (370–1110 MBq)

3. Iofetamine hydrochloride ^{123}I is not commercially available.

a. Biodistribution

(1) Iofetamine hydrochloride ^{123}I rapidly distributes throughout the body with rapid uptake in the brain; 5%–7% of the dose localizes in 20–60 minutes after administration because of its high lipophilicity.

(2) After injection, iofetamine hydrochloride ^{123}I is rapidly metabolized with two major metabolites: p-iodoamphetamine and p-iodobenzoic acid.

(3) The primary route of elimination is via the urine with 20% excreted after 24 hours and 30% after 48 hours.

(4) Thyroid blockade with oral KI is suggested.

b. Decay data

(1) The **physical half-life** is 13 hours.

(2) The **decay mode** is by electron capture.

(3) The **primary radiation emissions data** are 159 keV and 27 keV gamma energy photons.

c. Administration and dosage. IV 3–6 mCi (111–222 MBq)

B. Carrier-mediated transport (cerebral metabolism) mechanisms. These are responsible for transporting glucose across the blood-brain barrier. Agents such as **^{18}F Fludeoxyglucose** aid in the evaluation of cerebral function by mapping the distribution of glucose metabolism. ^{18}F Fludeoxyglucose is produced by cyclotron.

1. Biodistribution. Currently, there is a USP monograph for on-site-produced ^{18}F Fludeoxyglucose, which is a glucose analogue. ^{18}F Fludeoxyglucose concentrates in the brain where it is phosphorylated but does not undergo subsequent metabolism because of the replacement of the hydroxyl group in the 2 position with a fluorine atom. It is then metabolically trapped for a sufficient time to allow imaging.

2. Decay data

a. The **physical half-life** is 109 minutes.

b. The **decay mode** is by positron emission.

c. The **primary radiation emissions** are 633 keV energy positrons and 511 keV gamma energy photons.

3. Administration and dosage. IV, 5–10 mCi (185–370 MBq)

C. Cerebral neurotransmitter imaging. Fluorodopa F 18 injection:

1. **Description**
   a. Cerebral neurotransmitter synthesis can be studied with Fluorodopa F 18 injection. The intracerebral distribution of this neurotransmitter tracer can be used in the assessment of neurogenerative diseases such as Parkinsonism.
   b. Fluorodopa F 18 injection exists under a USP monograph as an on-site-produced sterile IV solution of a levodopa analog in which a portion of the moleceule has been replaced with ^{18}F, a positron-emitting radionuclide.

2. **Biodistribution**
   a. After IV injection, plasma activity decreases to 10% of the administered dose within 5 minutes after injection.
   b. Fluorodopa F 18 injection is predominately metabolized in periphery via dopa decarboxylase, and catechol-O-methyl transferase. To maximize brain uptake, Carbidopa may be used to decrease peripheral metabolism.
   c. Rapid excreted via renal system as dopamine metabolites

3. **Radionuclide data** (see IX B 2)

4. **Administration and dosage.** IV 10–20 mCi (370–740 MBq)

D. Cerebrospinal fluid (CSF) dynamics. Radionuclide cisternography is useful in the evaluation of hydrocephalus and in detecting CSF leaks. In CSF imaging, the radiopharmaceutical **Indium ^{111}In pentetate (^{111}In-DTPA)** is introduced intrathecally into the spinal subarachnoid space, ascends through the basal cisterns, proceeds over the cerebral hemispheres, and drains eventually into the superior sagittal sinus. ^{111}In pentetate is commercially supplied as a sterile, pyrogen-free unit dose injection. It is produced by cyclotron.

1. **Biodistribution**
   a. After intrathecal injection, this radiopharmaceutical normally ascends to the parasagittal region within 24 hours.
   b. After absorption into the bloodstream via the arachnoid villi, the major route of elimination is by kidney with 65% of the dose excreted within 48 hours and 85% within 72 hours.

2. **Decay data**
   a. The **physical half-life** is 67 hours.
   b. The **CSF biological half-life** is 12 hours.
   c. The **effective half-life** is 10 hours.
   d. The **mode of decay** is by electron capture.
   e. The **primary radiation emissions** are 245 keV and 171 keV gamma energy photons.

3. **Administration and dosage.** Intrathecal, 500 μCi (18.5 MBq)

X. Infection and Inflammation.

Evaluation of sites of infection include the use of agents that can associate with components of the natural defense mechanisms, and accumulate where they localize.

A. Membrane/metabolic agents. Gallium citrate Ga 67 USP:

1. **Description**
   a. It is supplied as a sterile pyrogen-free radiopharmaceutical with preservatives.
   b. The mechanism of localization is thought to be dependent on the formation of a gallium tranferrin complex in the blood, and binding to tranferrin receptors associated with infection and inflammation.
   c. It accumulates in areas of WBC localization.

2. **Biodistribution**
   a. After administration, the highest concentration of ^{67}Ga citrate is in the renal cortex other than site of infection. After 24 hours, the maximum concentration shifts to bone and lymph nodes, but after 1 week, it is mainly concentrated in the liver and spleen.
   b. ^{67}Ga Citrate is excreted slowly from the body, with 26% via urine, and 9% via feces, and a whole body retention of 65% after 7 days.

3. **Radionuclide data**

a. Mode of production: cyclotron
b. Mode of decay: electron capture
c. Physical half-life: 78 hours
d. Decay emissions: 93 keV, 185 keV, 300 keV, 393 keV gamma photons

4. **Administration and dosage.** IV, for infection, 3–8 mCi (111–300 MMq)

B. **WBC labeling agents.** Radiolabeled WBCs are used in the detection of a wide variety of infectious and inflammatory processes. Current use includes the diagnosis of intra-abdominal abcesses, inflammatory bowel disease, appendicitis, fever of unknown origin, and osteomyelitis.

1. **Indium In 111 oxyquinolone solution (^{111}In-OXINE)**
   a. **Description**
      (1) ^{111}In-Oxyquinolone is supplied as a sterile preservative-free, pyrogen-free, radiopharmaceutical solution for use in the radiolabeling of autologous leukocytes.
      (2) ^{111}In forms a saturated (a ratio of 1 to 3) neutral lipophilic complex with oxyquinoline, which enables it to penetrate a cell membrane.
      (3) After incubation of ^{111}In oxyquinoline with a population of autologous leukocytes the ^{111}In is thought to become firmly bound to cytoplasmic components, thereby allowing the free oxine to be released by the cell.
   b. **Biodistribution**
      (1) After radiolabeling, the autologous leukocytes are reinjected, with 30% taken up by the spleen, and 30% taken up by the liver, reaching peak at 2–4 hours postinjection.
      (2) Pulmonary uptake is immediately evident postinjection, but it clears with minimal activity visible after 4 hours.
      (3) There is a bi-exponential blood clearance with 9%–24%, clearing with a biological half-life of 2–5 hours, and the remainder of 13%–18% clearing with a biological half-life of 64–116 hours.
      (4) Elimination is mainly through radioactive decay with less than 1% excreted in feces and urine during the first 24 hours.
   c. **Radionuclide data**
      (1) Mode of production: cyclotron
      (2) Mode of decay: electron capture
      (3) Physical half-life: 67 hours
      (4) Decay emissions: 245 keV, 171 keV
   d. **Administration and dosage.** IV, 200–500 μCi (7.4–18.5 MBq)

2. **Technetium Tc 99m exametazime.** As a sterile, and pyrogen-free IV injection after reconstitution with sodium pertechnetate, ^{99m}Tc may be used to radiolabel leukocytes.
   a. **Description**
      (1) ^{99m}Tc exametazime is a neutral, lipid soluble complex that is able to penetrate the WBC membrane. This lipophilic complex is relatively unstable, and rapidly converts to a secondary complex incapable of penetrating the WBCs.
      (2) The methylene blue/phosphate buffer stabilized solution is not able to radiolabel cells and should not be used.
      (3) Additional limitations on kit preparation parameters require the use of high mole fraction technetium generator elutes of less than 2 hours postelution from a generator previously eluted within 24 hours.
   b. **Biodistribution**
      (1) After IV injection, the radiolabeled cells localize in the lungs, liver, spleen, blood pool, bone marrow, and bladder.
      (2) Elimination is primarily via liver.
   c. **Radionuclide data: (see II A 2 a, b; B 1 b, 3 a, b)**
   d. **Administration and dosage.** IV, for infection, 7–25 mCi (260–925 MBq)

XI. TUMORS

A. **Membrane/metabolic agents.** The usefulness of radiopharmaceuticals in the detection of tumors varies in sensitivity, and specificity with differences in tumor location and type.

1. **Gallium citrate Ga 67 USP**

a. **Description**
   (1) Gallium citrate Ga 67 is supplied as a sterile pyrogen-free radiopharmaceutical with preservatives.
   (2) The mechanism of localization is thought to be dependent on the formation of a gallium transferrin complex, or binding to transferrin receptors on tumor cells.
   (3) It accumulates in primary metastatic tumor sites and may detect the presence of Hodgkin's disease, lymphoma, and bronchogenic carcinoma.

b. **Biodistribution**
   (1) After administration, the highest concentration of ^{67}Ga citrate is in the renal cortex other than site of infection. After 24 hours, the maximum concentration shifts to bone and lymph nodes, but after 1 week, it is mainly concentrated in the liver and spleen.
   (2) ^{67}Ga citrate is excreted slowly from the body, with 26% via urine, and 9% via feces, and a whole body retention of 65% after 7 days.

c. **Radionuclide data** (see X A 1 c (1)–(4)
   (1) Mode of production: cyclotron
   (2) Mode of decay: electron capture
   (3) Physical half-life: 78 hours
   (4) Decay emissions: 93 keV, 185 keV, 300 keV, 393 keV gamma photons

d. **Administration and dosage.** IV, for tumor, 10 μCi (370 MBq)

2. **Indium In 111 pentetreotide**

a. **Description**
   (1) It is supplied as a sterile pyrogen-free kit for the preparation of In-111 pentetreotide. The two-component kit consists of a reaction vial containing lyophilized mixture of pentetreotide with stabilizer adjuvants, and a second vial containing an indium In-111 chloride/ferric chloride solution.
      (a) The pentetreotide molecule is a conjugate of pentetate [diethylenetriamine-pentaacetic acid (DTPA)], and octroetide, a somatostatin analog.
      (b) In-111 penteteotide is prepared by adding the ^{111}In/Fe chloride solution to the vial containing the pentetreotide. The pentetate portion of the molecule acts as a bifunctional chelate linking the ^{111}In radionuclide to the biological active octreotide portion of the agent.
   (2) Indium ^{111}In pentetreotide is indicated for localization of primary and metastatic neuroendocrine tumors expressing somatostatin receptors.

b. **Biodistribution**
   (1) Within 1 hour after IV injection indium ^{111}In pentetreotide distributes from the plasma to extravascular space with less than one-third of the administered dose remaining in the plasma 10 minutes postinjection.
   (2) Indium ^{111}In pentetreotide localizes as a function of somatostatin receptor density with accumulation in normal pituitary, thyroid, liver, spleen, and the urinary bladder.
   (3) Elimination is primarily renal with 50% of the administered dose excreted within 6 hours postinjection, 85% after 24 hours, and less than 90% after 48 hours. Less than 2% of the administered dose is cleared via the feces within 72 hours postinjection.

c. **Radionuclide data**
   (1) Mode of production: cyclotron
   (2) Mode of decay: electron capture
   (3) Physical half-life: 67 hours
   (4) Decay emissions: 245 keV, 171 keV

d. **Administration and dosage.** IV, 3–6 mCi (111–222 MBq)

3. **Iobenguane I 131 injection**

a. **Description**
   (1) It is supplied as a sterile pyrogen-free radiopharmaceutical for use as an adjunctive diagnostic agent for the localization of primary and metastatic pheochromocytomas and neuroblastomas.
   (2) Iobenguane (meta-iodobenzylguanidine) labeled with ^{131}I acts as a physiological analog of norepinephrine and is transported and accumulated in the adrenal medulla. This allows for the detection of neuroendocrine tumors via the specific uptake of labeled iodobenguane.
   (3) Because of its physiological similarities to norepinephrine, many classes of drugs that interfere with catecholamine transport and function may affect the uptake and localization of labeled iobenguane.

b. **Biodistribution**
   (1) After IV injection, there is rapid uptake in the liver with lesser amounts accumulating in the lungs, heart, spleen.
   (2) Normal adrenal gland uptake is low, but for tumors such as pheochromocytomas and neuroblastomas, the uptake is relatively higher.
   (3) Elimination is renal with most of the drug excreted mainly unchanged. Forty percent to fifty percent of the administered dose is excreted within 24 hours, and 70%–90% is excreted within 4 days postinjection.
   (4) Administration of potassium iodide 1 day before and for 10 days after administration is suggested to reduce thyroid uptake of potential radioiodide contaminants.

c. **Physical data (VIII B1 b, 2 b)**

d. **Administration and dosage.** IV, 0.5–1 mCi (18.5–37 MBq)

4. **Thallous chloride T1 201 USP.** This agent has utility as a tumor-imaging agent because of its accumulation in the rapidly metabolizing cells of certain tumors in accordance with its mechanism of localization (see III A 1). **Administration and dosage** is via IV, 1.5–3 mCi (55–111 MBq).

5. **Fludeoxyglucose F 18 USP.** This agent has utility as a tumor-imaging agent because of an increased demand for glucose by tumors with advanced state of malignancy. Not only can F-18 FDG locate and differentiate tumors, but it can also help to distinguish between recurrent brain tumor from radiation necrosis in patients receiving radiation therapy (see IX B). **Administration and dosage** is via IV,5–10 mCi (185–370 MBq)

B. Antibodies. Indium In 111 satumomab pendetide USP:

1. **Description**

   a. It is supplied as a sterile pyrogen-free kit for the preparation of indium ^{111}In satumomab pendetide. The kit consists of a single dose reaction vial containing 1 mg of satumomab pendetide, a monoclonal antibody (MoAb) conjugate, in a sodium phosphate–bufferred saline solution. A second vial containing a sodium acetate solution is to be used for buffering an indium ^{111}In chloride solution used to label the satumomab pendetide.
      (1) Satumomab portion of the conjugate is a murine MoAb that binds specifically to the TAG-72 glycoprotein which is expressed at high levels on colorectal and ovarian adenocarcinomas. The pendetide portion of the conjugate is a linker chelator which is attached to the Fc carbohydrate portion of the satumomab antibody.
      (2) The agent is prepared by adding a buffered solution of indium ^{111}In chloride solution to the single dose vial and allowing the mixture to sit for 30 minutes to allow the labeling reaction to occur.

   b. Indium ^{111}In satumomab is indicated for determining the extent and location of extrahepatic malignant disease in patients who have known colorectal or ovarian cancer.

   c. As a foreign protein this product may produce human antimurine antibodies with accompanying potentially serious allergic reactions.

2. **Biodistribution**

   a. After IV injection, indium ^{111}In satumomab pendetide localizes in colorectal adenocarcinomas and ovarian epithelial carcinomas. It exhibits a slow plasma clearance and a monoexponential or bi-exponential clearance with a terminal phase half-life of 56 hours.

   b. Elimination is renal with 10% of the administered dose excreted within the first 72 hours postinjection as a small molecular weight product of the catabolized indium In-111 satumomab penditide.

3. **Radionuclide data**

   a. Mode of production: cyclotron
   b. Mode of decay: electron capture
   c. Physical half-life: 67 hours
   d. Decay emissions: 245 keV, 171 keV

4. **Administration and dosage.** IV (slow) 5 mCi (185 MBq)

XII. THERAPEUTIC AGENTS.

The therapeutic use of radiopharmaceuticals is based on the concept of selective localization of radiopharmaceuticals coupled with the lethality of the same because of the tissue damage resulting from highly ionizing particulate emissions such as beta particles.

A. Chromic phosphate P 32 suspension USP

1. **Description**. Available as a sterile pyrogen-free aqueous suspension used in treatment of peritoneal or pleural effusions caused by metastatic disease. Also used in the treatment of ovarian and prostate cancer

2. **Biodistribution**
   a. Colloidal suspension of P-32 is rapidly taken up by macrophages adhering to cavity wall thereby concentrating and localizing the irradiation effect of the P-32 radionuclide beta particulate emission.
   b. After infusion, the suspension rapidly distributes from within cavity and may locate in lungs, adrenal glands, kidneys, lymph nodes, liver, spleen bone marrow, plasma, erythrocytes, and leukocytes depending on colloidal particle size.
   c. Elimination is primarily renal

3. **Radionuclide data**
   a. Mode of production: reactor produced
   b. Mode of decay: beta
   c. Physical half-life: 14.3 days
   d. Decay emissions: 695 keV mean energy beta, 100% abundance

4. **Administration and dosage**
   a. Intraperitoneal instillation: 10–20 mCi (370–740 MBq)
   b. Intrapleural instillation: 6–12 mCi (222–444 MBq)
   c. Carcinoma interstitial: 0.1–0.5 mCi (3.7–18.5 MBq)
   d. Caution for visual inspection to prevent misadministration of the sodium phosphate form (clear, colorless) which is designated for intravascular use only.

B. Sodium phosphate P 32 solution USP

1. **Description**
   a. It is available as a commercially supplied sterile, pyrogen-free, radiopharmaceutical.
   b. It is primarily used as an antineoplastic for the treatment of polycythemia rubra vera, and selectively for the palliative treatment of metastatic bone pain.
   c. Its therapeutic effect is due to cell damage resulting from irradiation produced by beta particulate emission.

2. **Biodistribution**
   a. It concentrates as phosphate, within the DNA of rapidly dividing hematopoetic cells in the treatment of polycythemia rubra vera, and as phosphate in areas of increased bone formation.
   b. After IV administration, it diffuses rapidly into extracellular, and intracellular space; concentrating in the bone marrow, spleen, and liver.
   c. Elimination is primarily renal with 5%–10% excreted within 24 hours and 20% within 1 week.
   d. Whole body biological half-life is approximately 39 days.

3. **Radionuclide data**
   a. Mode of production: reactor produced
   b. Mode of decay: beta
   c. Physical half-life: 14.3 days
   d. Decay emissions: 695 keV mean energy beta, 100% abundance

4. **Administration and dosage**
   a. Polycythemia rubra vera: IV, 3–5 mCi (111–185 MBq)
   b. Metastatic bone lesions: IV, 10–21 mCi (370–777 MBq)
   c. Caution is advised for visual inspection to prevent misadministration of the chromic phosphate form (green, cloudy) which is designated for interstitial use only.

C. Sodium iodide I 131 USP—Therapeutic

1. **Description**
   a. It is indicated for treatment of hyperthyroidism, and thyroid carcinoma.
   b. Its therapeutic action is due to the accumulation and retention of iodine and its isotope 131 I.

2. **Biodistribution** (see VIII A,B 2). Biological half-life (thyroid); euthyroid, 80 days; hyperthyroid, 5–40 days
3. **Radionuclide data** (see VII B 2 b)
4. **Administration and dosage.** Oral capsule or oral solution:
   a. Antithyroid, 4–10 mCi (148 MBq–370 MBq)
   b. Antineoplastic, 30–200 mCi (1110–7400 MBq)

D. Strontium ^{89}Sr chloride

1. **Description**
   a. It is indicated for the alleviation of bone pain arising from metastatic bone disease from carcinomas.
   b. As a metabolic analog of calcium, ^{89}Sr concentrates selectively in areas of increased osteogenes, thus delivering a radiation dose sufficient to provide a palliative effect.
   c. Pain relief begins between 7 and 21 days after administration with maximum relief by 6 weeks and an average duration of 6 months.
   d. Reduction in patient analgesic usage occurs in up to 75% of patients treated with complete pain relief in 20% of treated patients, and 20%–25% experience no pain relief.
   e. Bone marrow suppression effects limits use to patients with initial WBC counts more than 2400, and platelet counts more than 60,000.
2. **Biodistribution**
   a. After administration clears rapidly from blood and localizes in bone hydroxyapatite.
   b. Initial biological half-life in normal bone is 14 days with longer retention in metastatic bone lesion. Between 12%–90% of administered dose is retained for up to 3 months after administration.
   c. Elimination is primarily renal with 66% of administered dose cleared via GFR within the first 2 days. 33% is excreted via feces.
3. **Radionuclide data**
   a. Method of production: accelerator produced
   b. Decay mode: beta decay
   c. Emission data: 1.46 MeV maximum beta energy, 100% abundance
   d. Physical half-life: 50.5 days
4. **Administration and dosage** is via IV, 4 mCi (148 MBq) 40–60 μCi/kg(1.5–2.2 Mbq/kg)

REFERENCES

1. *American Pharmaceutical Association's Nuclear Pharmacy Practice Standards.* Academy of Pharmacy Practices, 1978.

STUDY QUESTIONS

Directions: Each of the numbered items or incomplete statements in this section is followed by answers or by completions of the statement. Select the **one** lettered answer or completion that is **best** in each case.

1. Which of the following emissions from the decay of radionuclides is most commonly used in nuclear medicine imaging?

(A) X-ray
(B) Beta
(C) Alpha
(D) Gamma
(E) Positron

2. Which of the following radionuclides is most commonly used in nuclear pharmacy practice?

(A) ^{67}Ga
(B) ^{201}Tl
(C) ^{99m}Tc
(D) ^{123}I
(E) ^{133}Xe

3. Which of the following radionuclides is generator-produced?

(A) ^{99m}Tc
(B) ^{201}Tl
(C) ^{67}Ga
(D) ^{133}Xe
(E) ^{123}I

4. Which of the following radiopharmaceuticals can be used in skeletal imaging?

(A) Technetium ^{99m}Tc albumin aggregated
(B) Technetium ^{99m}Tc medronate disodium
(C) Xenon ^{133}Xe USP
(D) Thallous chloride ^{201}Tl USP
(E) Technetium ^{99m}Tc disofenin

5. Which of the following radiopharmaceuticals is used in the diagnosis of acute cholecystitis?

(A) Technetium ^{99m}Tc sulfur colloid
(B) Technetium ^{99m}Tc medronate disodium
(C) Technetium ^{99m}Tc albumin
(D) Technetium ^{99m}Tc exametazime
(E) Technetium ^{99m}Tc disofenin

6. Which of the following cyclotron-produced radiopharmaceuticals is used for assessing regional myocardial perfusion as part of an exercise stress test?

(A) Thallous chloride ^{201}Tl USP
(B) Sodium iodide ^{123}I
(C) Gallium citrate ^{67}Ga USP
(D) Indium ^{111}In pentetate
(E) Cobalt ^{57}Co cyanocobalamin

7. Glomerular filtration and the urinary collection system can best be evaluated, using which of the following agents?

(A) Technetium ^{99m}Tc sulfur colloid
(B) Technetium ^{99m}Tc albumin
(C) Technetium ^{99m}Tc sestamibi
(D) Technetium ^{99m}Tc disofenin
(E) Technetium ^{99m}Tc pentetate

Directions: Each item below contains three suggested answers of which **one or more** is correct. Choose the answer

A if **I only** is correct
B if **III only** is correct
C if **I and II** are correct
D if **II and III** are correct
E if **I, II, and III** are correct

8. The definition of the optimal radiopharmaceutical includes which of the following attributes?

I. Short half-life
II. Gamma photon with a 100–300 keV energy
III. Rapid localization in target tissue and quick clearance from nontarget tissue

9. Which of the following statements are true for sodium pertechnetate ^{99m}Tc USP?

I. It is used to radiolabel all other ^{99m}Tc radiopharmaceuticals.
II. The molybdenum 99 (^{99}Mo) breakthrough limit is less than 0.15 μCi ^{99}Mo/mCi ^{99m}Tc (less than 0.15 kBq/ MBq).
III. It has a physical half-life of 16 hours.

10. Which of the following organs can be imaged with technetium ^{99m}Tc sulfur colloid?

I. Liver
II. Spleen
III. Bone marrow

11. Which of the following radiopharmaceuticals may be used to image the thyroid gland?

I. Sodium iodide ^{131}I
II. Sodium pertechnetate ^{99m}Tc USP
III. Sodium iodide ^{123}I

Directions: The group of items in this section consists of lettered options followed by a set of numbered items. For each item, select the **one** lettered option that is most closely associated with it. Each lettered option may be selected once, more than once, or not at all.

Questions 12–16

Match each radiopharmaceutical with its mechanism of localization.

(A) Metabolic trapping
(B) Phagocytosis
(C) Capillary blockade
(D) Active transport
(E) Passive diffusion

12. Thallous chloride ^{201}Tl USP

13. Technetium ^{99m}Tc albumin aggregated USP

14. Technetium ^{99m}Tc sulfur colloid

15. Technetium ^{99m}Tc exametazime

16. ^{18}F fluorodeoxyglucose

ANSWERS AND EXPLANATIONS

1. The answer is D *[I B 3 b].*
Current camera technology most efficiently detects gamma radiation. Alpha and beta emissions are not useful in nuclear medicine imaging because of their harmful particulate emissions and low tissue penetration. Although x-ray emissions can be used as in the case of the mercury daughter of the thallous chloride ^{201}Tl parent, they are not efficiently detected. Annihilation radiation associated with positron decay can be imaged, but this technology is currently limited to a few specialized centers.

2. The answer is C *[I C; II A 1].*
Technetium 99m (^{99m}Tc) has become the radionuclide of choice in current nuclear pharmacy practice since its introduction in the mid-1960s. ^{99m}Tc fulfills all of the requirements of the optimal radiopharmaceutical with its physical half-life of 6 hours, 140 keV gamma energy emission, ready availability, cost, and ability to be radiolabeled to a wide variety of biologically active compounds.

3. The answer is A *[II A 1 a].*
Technetium 99m (^{99m}Tc) is obtained via commercially supplied sterile, pyrogen-free "generator" systems. A generator is a device used to separate a short half-life radionuclide from the longer-lived "parent" nuclide, while retaining the parent to produce more of the daughter nuclide. In this way, short half-life nuclides can be made available on a continuous basis at great distances from the sites of generator production.

4. The answer is B *[IV A 2].*
The technetium 99m (^{99m}Tc) diphosphonate compounds are the most popular bone imaging agents currently used in nuclear medicine imaging. They are rapidly taken up by skeletal bone with 50% of the administered dose adsorbed onto bone hydroxyapatite and with the remainder excreted by the kidneys. The imaging advantages of the ^{99m}Tc, coupled with the sensitivity of bone agent localization in skeletal bone hydroxyapatite, allows for detection of bone pathology before evidence of pathology can be shown by conventional x-ray.

5. The answer is E *[VI C 1, 2].*
Technetium ^{99m}Tc disofenin is an iminodiacetic acid derivative, which is useful for hepatobiliary imaging due to its ability to be selectively cleared by a carrier-mediated hepatocyte pathway. Lack of gallbladder visualization is an abnormal finding suggestive of acute cholecystitis.

6. The answer is A *[III A 1].*
Regional uptake of thallous chloride ^{201}Tl USP (^{201}Tl) is proportional to myocardial blood supply. The injection of ^{201}Tl in concert with a treadmill exercise stress test determines myocardial perfusion at maximum cardiac output when cardiac demand outstrips supply and the distribution of ^{201}Tl is less after affected by collateral blood supply within the myocardium. Regions that do not take up ^{201}Tl are interpreted as areas of infarct or ischemia. If these focal areas of decreased uptake subsequently fill in with redistributed ^{201}Tl, they are interpreted to be areas of ischemia in contrast to areas of infarct, which remain as diminished areas of activity.

7. The answer is E *[VII B 1].*
Technetium ^{99m}Tc pentetate is cleared through glomerular filtration in the same manner as inulin and can be used to determine the glomerular filtration rate (GFR) as well as in the evaluation of obstruction of vascular supply, and renal morphology.

8. The answer is E (all) *[I C].*
The optimal radiopharmaceutical has a half-life short enough to minimize radiation exposure to the patient yet long enough to allow for collection of imaging information. It should incorporate a gamma-emitting radionuclide, which decays with the emission of a photon energy between 100–300 keV, which is efficiently detected with current instrumentation. The radiopharmaceutical should localize rapidly in the organ system of interest and be metabolized, excreted, or both from the nontarget tissues to maximize contrast and minimize radiation absorbed dose.

9. The answer is C (I, II) *[II A, B].*
Sodium pertechnetate ^{99m}Tc USP decays by isomeric transition with a physical half-life of 6 hours. The emission of a gamma photon has the energy of 140 keV.

10. The answer is E (all) *[VI B 1].*
Technetium ^{99m}Tc sulfur colloid localizes within the reticuloendothelial system with approximately 80%–90% of the dose of phagocytized by the Küpffer cells of the liver, 5%–10% by the spleen, and the balance by the bone marrow.

11. The answer is E (all) *[VIII B].*
Although all of the listed agents accumulate in the thyroid gland, only sodium iodide ^{123}I possesses ideal imaging characteristics and organification into thyroid hormone. While the imaging properties of sodium pertechnetate ^{99m}Tc USP are good, the pertechnetate ion is only trapped by the thyroid and not organified, thus limiting the information provided by the image.

12–16. The answers are: 12-D *[III A 1],* **13-C** *[V A 1],* **14-B** *[VI B 1],* **15-E** *[IX A 1],* **16-A** *[IX B 1].*
Thallous chloride ^{201}Tl USP is a monovalent cation with distribution analogous to potassium ion (K^+). Myocardial uptake is by active transport via the Na^+-K^+-ATPase pump.

After IV administration of technetium ^{99m}Tc albumin aggregated USP, 80% of the radiolabeled albumin particles become trapped by capillary blockade in the pulmonary circulation.

After the administration of technetium ^{99m}Tc sulfur colloid, approximately 80%–90% of the dose is phagocytized by the Küpffer cells of the liver, 5%–10% by the spleen, and the balance by the bone marrow.

Technetium ^{99m}Tc exametazime is used for evaluating brain perfusion. It possesses a lipophilic partition coefficient sufficient to diffuse passively across the blood–brain barrier almost completely within one pass of the cerebral circulation, as well as being sufficiently retained to permit data collection.

^{18}F fluorodeoxyglucose is used in evaluating cerebral function by mapping the distribution of cerebral glucose metabolism. As an analogue of glucose, ^{18}F fluorodeoxyglucose is transported into the brain by carrier-mediated transport mechanisms responsible for transporting glucose across the blood-brain barrier. Because the presence of the F atom in the 2 position prevents metabolism beyond the phosphorylation step, ^{18}F fluorodeoxyglucose becomes metabolically trapped within the brain.

PART II

PHARMACY PRACTICE

22
Pharmaceutical Care and the Scope of Pharmacy Practice

Peggy C. Yarborough

I. INTRODUCTION

A. The **practice of pharmacy** embraces a variety of settings, patient populations, and specialist as well as generalist pharmacists. Central to the practice of pharmacy, however, is the provision of clinical services directly to, and for the benefit of, **patients.**

B. Definition. The term **pharmaceutical care** (sometimes called **pharmacist care**) describes specific activities and services through which an individual pharmacist "cooperates with a patient and other professionals in designing, implementing and monitoring a therapeutic plan that will produce specific therapeutic outcomes for the patient."[1]

II. SCOPE OF PRACTICE WITHIN PHARMACEUTICAL CARE

A. Role. Pharmaceutical care has evolved from an emphasis on prevention of drug-related problems (basically **drug management**) to the expanded roles of pharmacists in the **triage of patients, treatment of routine acute illnesses, management of chronic diseases,** and **primary disease prevention.**

B. Function. The provision of pharmaceutical care does not imply that the pharmacist is no longer responsible for dispensing functions. In many instances, however, implementation of pharmaceutical care services necessitates a redesign of the professional work flow (see VI), with assignment of technical functions to technical personnel under the direct supervision and responsibility of the pharmacist.

III. UNIQUENESS OF PHARMACEUTICAL CARE.

Provision of pharmaceutical care overlaps somewhat with other aspects of pharmacy practice (Table 22-1). However, pharmaceutical care is not the same as these other areas, which include:

A. Clinical pharmacy

B. Patient counseling

C. Pharmaceutical services; when the activities of a pharmacy or pharmacy department are performed for "faceless" patients or charts, the activity is one of pharmacy service, not pharmaceutical care (e.g., chart or drug profile reviews without input from the patient or care giver is not pharmaceutical care).

Table 22-1. Uniqueness of Pharmaceutical Care

	Traditional Pharmacy	Clinical Pharmacy	Pharmaceutical Care
Primary focus	Prescription order or OTC request	Physicians or other health professionals	Patient
Continuity	Upon demand	Discontinuous	Continuous
Strategy	Obey	Find fault or prevention	Anticipate or improve
Orientation	Drug product	Process	Outcomes

IV. ESSENTIAL COMPONENTS OF PHARMACEUTICAL CARE

A. Pharmacist—patient relationship. The importance of putting a face and personality with the clinical picture is a key component of pharmaceutical care. A pharmacist can have a caring relationship with a patient but not with a chart or drug profile. A pharmacist cannot have empathy for words on a page or on a computer screen. Pharmaceutical care is based upon a collaborative effort between pharmacist and patient.

B. Pharmacist's workup of drug therapy (PWDT). The provision of pharmaceutical care is often centered around a process described as the PWDT.[2] Although the forms or methods used for this process may vary, the components are essentially the same.

1. **Data collection.** Collect, synthesize, and interpret relevant information, such as:
   - a. Patient demographic data: age, race, sex
   - b. Pertinent medical information
     - (1) Current and past medical history
     - (2) Family history
     - (3) Social history
     - (4) Dietary history
     - (5) Medication history (prescription, OTC, social drugs; allergies)
     - (6) Physical findings (e.g., weight, height, blood pressure, edema)
     - (7) Laboratory or other test results (e.g., serum drug levels, potassium level, serum creatinine as relevant to drug therapy)
   - c. Patient complaints, symptoms, signs

2. Develop or identify the **CORE pharmacotherapy plan**[3]
   - a. **C = Condition** or patient need
   - b. **O = Outcome** desired for that condition
   - c. **R = Regimen** selected (prescribed) to achieve that outcome
   - d. **E = Evaluation** parameters to assess outcome achievement

3. Identify the **PRIME pharmacotherapy problems** or indications for pharmacist interventions.[3] The goal is to identify actual or potential problems that could compromise the desired patient outcomes (Table 22-2).
   - a. **P = Pharmaceutical-**based problems
   - b. **R = Risks** to patient
   - c. **I = Interactions**
   - d. **M = Mismatch** between medications and condition or patient needs
   - e. **E = Efficacy** issues

4. Formulate a **FARM progress note** to describe and document the interventions intended or provided by the pharmacist.[3]
   - a. **F = Findings:** the patient-specific information that gives a basis for, or leads to, the recognition of a pharmacotherapy problem or indication for pharmacist intervention.
   - b. **A = Assessment:** the pharmacist's evaluation of the findings, including a statement of:
     - (1) Any additional information that is needed to best assess the problem in order to make recommendations
     - (2) The severity, priority, or urgency of the problem
     - (3) The short-term and long-term goals of the intervention proposed or provided

Table 22-2. PRIME Pharmacotherapy Problem Types[3]

Pharmaceutical	. . . assess for incorrect • dose • form • route • timing • duration • frequency
Risks to patient	. . . *assess for* • known contraindication • patient medication allergy • drug-induced problem • improper utilization (i.e., risk if misused) • common/serious adverse effects • medication error considerations
Interactions	. . . *assess for* • drug–drug • drug–disease/condition • drug–food • drug–lab
Mismatch between medications and indications/conditions/complaints	. . . *assess for* • medication used without indication • indication, condition, or complaint untreated
Efficacy issues	. . . *assess for* • suboptimal selection of pharmacotherapy for indication • minimal or no evidence of therapeutic effectiveness • suboptimal utilization of pharmacotherapy (taking or receiving medications incorrectly) — patient preference considerations (e.g., undesirable prior experiences with medication, does not believe it works) — medication availability considerations — compliance or administration considerations (e.g., inability to pay, unable to administer correctly or at all)

(a) Examples of **short-term goals** include: eliminate symptoms, lower blood pressure (BP) to 140/90 within 6 weeks, manage acute asthma flare up without requiring hospitalization.

(b) Examples of **long-term goals** include: prevent recurrence, maintain BP at less than 135/80, prevent progression of diabetic nerve disease.

c. R = Resolution (including prevention): the intervention plan includes actual or proposed actions by the pharmacist or recommendations to other health care professionals. The rationale for choosing a specific intervention should be stated. Intervention options may include:

(1) Observing, reassessing, or following: no intervention necessary at this time. If no action was taken or recommended, the FARM note serves as a record of the event and should constitute part of the patient's pharmacy chart or database.

(2) Counseling or educating the patient or care giver

(3) Making recommendations to the patient or care giver

(4) Informing the prescriber

(5) Making recommendations to the prescriber

(6) Withholding medication or advising against use

d. M = Monitoring and follow-up: the parameters and timing of follow-up monitoring to assess the efficacy, safety, and outcome of the intervention. This portion of the FARM note should include:

(1) The parameter to be followed (e.g., pain, depressed mood, serum potassium level)

(2) The intent of the monitoring (e.g., efficacy, toxicity, adverse event)

(3) How the parameter will be monitored (e.g., interview patient, serum drug level, physical examination)

(4) Frequency of monitoring (e.g., weekly, monthly)

(5) Duration of monitoring (e.g., until resolved, while on antibiotic, until resolved then monthly for one year)

(6) Anticipated or desired finding (e.g., no pain, euglycemia, healing of lesion)

(7) Decision point to alter therapy when or if outcome is not achieved (e.g., pain still present after 3 days, mild hypoglycemia more than 2 times a week)

V. CLINICAL SKILLS AND PHARMACISTS ROLES IN PHARMACEUTICAL CARE.

The skills, activities, and services inherent in the provision of pharmaceutical care include, but are not limited to, the following:

A. Patient assessment

1. Physical assessment
2. Barriers to adherence
3. Psychosocial issues

B. Patient education and counseling

1. Interview skills
2. Communication skills (e.g., empathy, listening, speaking or writing at the patient's level of understanding)
3. Ability to motivate, inspire
4. Develop and implement patient education plan based on an initial education assessment
5. Identification and resolution of compliance barriers

C. Patient-specific pharmacist care plans (see IV B)

1. Recognition, prevention, and management of drug interactions
2. Pharmacology and therapeutics (innovative and conventional)
3. Interpretation of laboratory tests
4. Knowledge of community resources, professional referrals
5. Communication and rapport with community medical providers

D. Drug treatment protocols

1. Develop and maintain (update) protocols.
2. Follow protocols as a pharmacist clinician.
3. Monitor aggregate adherence to treatment protocols [e.g., drug-utilization evaluations (DUE)] especially for managed care or health system facility.

E. Dosage adjustment

1. Identify patients at risk for exaggerated or subtherapeutic response.
2. Apply pharmacokinetic principles to determine patient-specific dosing.
3. Order and interpret relevant tests at correct time intervals to assess dosage adjustment (e.g., plasma drug concentrations, blood glucose levels, blood pressure measurements).

F. Selection of therapeutic alternatives

1. Use drug information resources effectively.
2. Review and critique drug literature.
3. Construct comparative analyses to support therapeutic decisions.

G. Prescriptive authority in designated practice sites or positions

H. Preventive services

1. Immunizations

2. Screenings
3. Health and wellness education

I. Managerial skills

1. **Plan, direct,** and **implement** pharmaceutical care activities within various practice environments, such as community pharmacy, ambulatory care settings, managed or contractual care, home health services, long-term care facilities, inpatient hospital practice, and others.
2. **Allocate** resources.

VI. PHARMACEUTICAL CARE AS THE MODEL FOR PHARMACY PRACTICE. The concepts, activities, and services of pharmaceutical care form the basis for provision of clinical services directly to, and for the benefit of, patients in all pharmacy practice settings. These settings include home health, hospital, ambulatory care, primary care, consultation, long term care, and community pharmacy practice. Work flow, staffing patterns, processes, and pharmacy programs might differ, but the core approach to patient care remains pharmaceutical care in all settings. Figures 22-1 and 22-2 illustrate pharmaceutical care models in the institutional and community pharmacy settings.

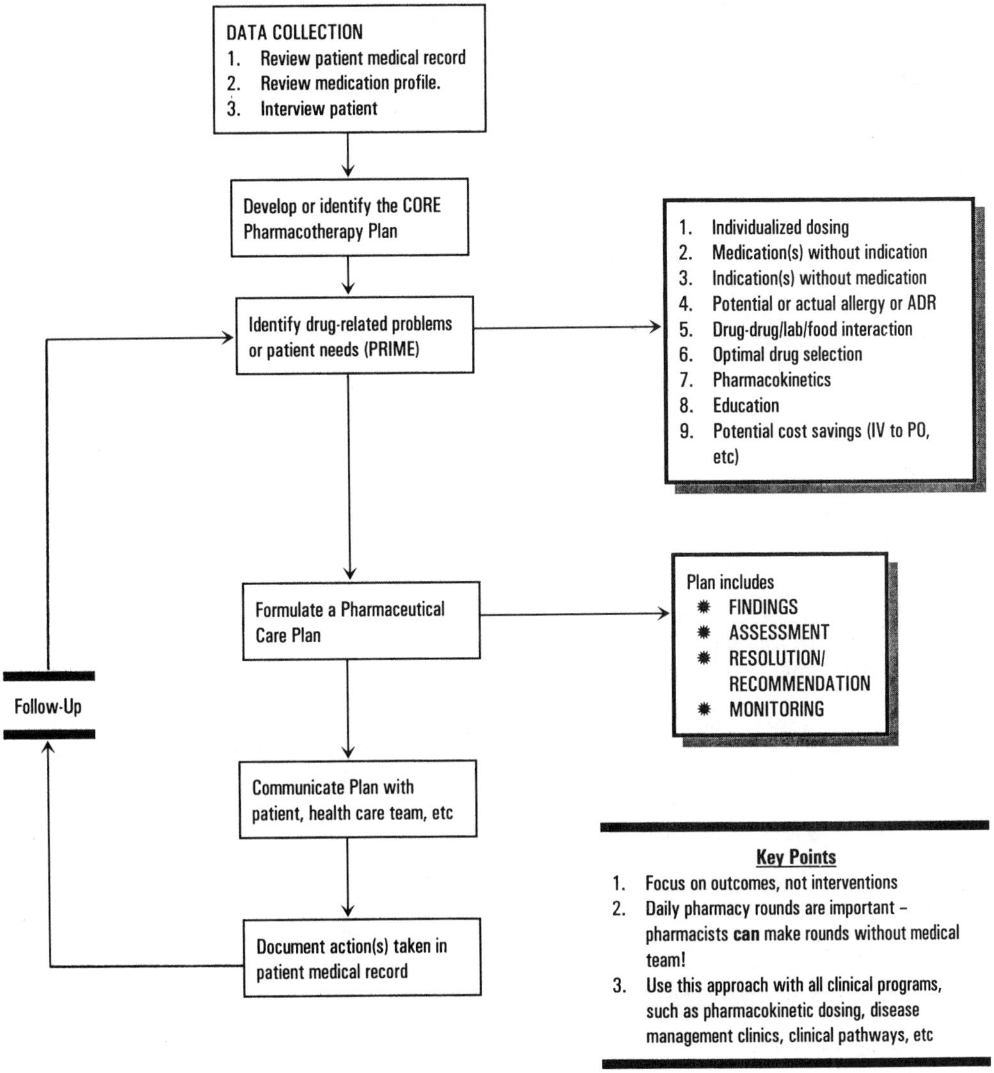

Figure 22-1. Template for pharmaceutical care: institutional practice.

Patient perceives problem or needs routine medical check-up

↓

1. Medical care provider
2. Diagnosis
3. Prescription/Treatment Plan

↓

Community Pharmacy

Pharmaceutical Care Component	**Prescription Processing Component**
1. Patient presents prescription to pharmacist or technician	
2. If new patient: fills out medical data information form	→ 2a. Technician enters standard information into software
3. Data collection: If new patient, pharmacist clarifies initial medical information (if needed), by interviewing patient. If established patient, pharmacist asks patient about a. recent changes in medical status b. recent OTC drug use c. drugs acquired at other facilities (e.g., physician samples; other pharmacies) d. drug concerns of patient or recent adverse effects	
4. CORE Pharmacotherapy plan: Pharmacist enters new data and prescription into software to integrate these with the existing CORE plan.	
5. PRIME pharmacotherapy problems: Pharmacist performs prospective drug utilization review (DUR), to identify problems or patient needs	→ 5a. If no therapeutic concerns are raised, technician proceeds to fill prescription
6. Pharmacist formulates FARM progress note to document care provided. Special attention should be given to a. RECOMMENDATIONS:	
1) If therapeutic concerns are raised, contact prescriber. Document resolution.	→ When therapeutic concerns are resolved, technician proceeds to fill prescription
2) If patient requires extensive counseling (e.g., beyond OBRA '90 requirements), document interventions provided. Example: instruction on use of insulin, actions of insulin, and recognition/prevention/treatment of hypoglycemia.	→ Technician processes claim form for submission to insurance company or prepares patient billing for expanded counseling
3) If patient is candidate for monitoring program or additional education services, recommend appropriate program and set up appointment for patient. Examples include: diabetes, hypertension, asthma, smoking cessation monitoring and/or education sessions. b. MONITORING: see section 9 below.	→ Technician maintains master schedule for pharmacist-patient appointments
7. Pharmacist counsels patient on prescription (or other interventions as determined in FARM note) while technician is completing dispensing process	
8. Prescription is checked by pharmacist when dispensing process is completed by technician 9. MONITORING a. Follow-up with patient on new prescriptions: e.g., 1) call 2 days after dispensing of antibiotic to ascertain improvement of symptoms 2) call 7 days after antihypertensive prescription to determine if side effects are so bothersome that compliance may be affected. b. Relay follow-up findings to prescriber, when appropriate. c. Confirm follow-up appointment with patient who enrolled in a monitoring or education program. d. Document follow-up. New problems uncovered during follow-up become the FINDING of subsequent FARM note.	→ Technician gives prescription to patient and concludes prescription processing by completing billing procedures (cash, charge, insurance billing, etc)

Figure 22-2. Template for pharmaceutical care: community practice.

VII. DOCUMENTATION OF PHARMACEUTICAL CARE.

"If it isn't documented, it isn't done!" Documentation of pharmaceutical care is integral to continuity of care, demonstration of clinician competence, communication among health care providers, evidence of contributions to patient care, and reimbursement of professional services.

A. Pharmaceutical care, including the pharmaceutical care plan process (CORE, PRIME, FARM), is a systematic method for recording the pharmacist's examination of a patient's pharmacotherapy and subsequent identification of medication-related problems (see IV).

B. In most practice settings, **computer software programs** maintain patient data and drug profile records. Thus, after documentation of the initial pharmaceutical care plan, patient data or drug regimens are included in subsequent FARM notes only if a change occurs that is relevant to the therapeutic issue being addressed in the note.

C. Forms that summarize pharmacists' interventions using a **unified coding system** are useful for processing reimbursement or billing forms, but these forms are not adequate documentation of pharmaceutical care. These forms do not communicate to other health professionals the depth and quality of pharmacist interventions or the pharmacist's plan for ongoing pharmaceutical care.

VIII. PHARMACEUTICAL CARE: AN ONGOING PROCESS.

The **patient profile** (database) is revised and re-assessed each time a new drug is added to or deleted from the medication regimen, a new disease or condition is diagnosed, or the patient undergoes other clinical intervention, such as surgery. When the patient returns to the pharmacy or is readmitted to the health system facility, the pharmacist uses the patient profile, PWDT, and FARM notes (maintained in the patient pharmacy chart or in the medical chart) as the basis for ongoing pharmacist–patient interactions.

IX. IMPORTANCE OF PHARMACEUTICAL CARE IN TODAY'S PHARMACY PRACTICE

A. The potential for **medication errors** is growing, and one professional group must assume a primary role in addressing this issue rather than fragmented efforts by various groups or individuals. The pharmacist is trained specifically to address these therapeutic issues.

1. The use of prescription and nonprescription medications is growing and now constitutes the primary therapeutic modality available to health care practitioners and patients.
2. The number, complexity, and potency of prescription and nonprescription drug products is increasing.

B. The need for pharmaceutical care secures an enduring role for the pharmacist in the American health care system. Every encounter with patients, regardless of practice setting, provides pharmaceutical care.

C. Pharmaceutical care activities integrate pharmacists into the health care system of the future.

REFERENCES

1. Hepler CD, Strand LM. Opportunities and responsibilities in pharmaceutical care. *Am J Hosp Pharm.* 1990;47:533–543.
2. Strand LM, Morley PC, Cipolle RJ, Ramsey R, Lamsam GD. Drug-related problems: their structure and function. *Ann Pharmacother.* 1990;24:1093–1097.
3. Canaday BR and Yarborough PC. Documenting Pharmaceutical Care: Creating a Standard. *Ann Pharmacother.* 1994; 28:1292–1296.

STUDY QUESTIONS

Directions: Each of the numbered items or incomplete statements in this section is followed by answers or by completions of the statement. Select the **one** lettered answer or completion that is **best** in each case.

1. Which of the following statements best describes FARM?

(A) Cultivation of a pharmacist's knowledge in order to better serve the public
(B) Findings, assessment, resolution, monitoring
(C) Findings, assessment, recognition, management
(D) The process by which an individual pharmacist interacts with a specific patient to attain pertinent medical information

2. An example of an expanded role of the pharmacist is

(A) community leader
(B) preparation of compounded prescriptions
(C) maintaining adequate inventory of orphan drugs
(D) triage of patients

3. What is the most important focus of pharmaceutical care?

(A) The pharmacist
(B) The patient
(C) The prescription
(D) The patient chart

4. Which of the following statements regarding pharmaceutical care is true? Pharmaceutical care

(A) usually does not overlap into other areas of heath care
(B) and clinical pharmacy are synonymous
(C) implies that the pharmacist is no longer responsible for dispensing functions
(D) is based on strategies to provide continuous patient care in order to attain desired outcomes

5. Essential components of pharmaceutical care include

(A) patient–pharmacist relationship, legible physician orders, and accurate data collection
(B) pharmacist–patient relationship and workup of drug therapy
(C) a software program that accesses medication history and prompts the pharmacist concerning questions to ask the patient
(D) maintenance of patient medication history for at least 2 years and a focus on acute illness

6. In the CORE pharmacotherapy plan, what does the "E" represent?

(A) Education of patient or care-giver
(B) Efficacy issues
(C) Elaboration
(D) Evaluation parameters

7. The most important reason for using the FARM note is to

(A) collect information for the physician
(B) document problem-solving and/or interventions performed by the pharmacist
(C) keep a log of all drug interactions
(D) create a uniform method of recording patient information

8. Which of the following topics would NOT be included in the assessment portion of the FARM note?

(A) Recommendations made to the patient or care-giver
(B) Severity, priority, or urgency of the problem
(C) Short-term and long-term goals of the intervention
(D) Additional information that is needed to best assess the problem

9. Immunizations, screenings, and wellness education are examples of which clinical skill?

(A) Community health overview
(B) Patient medication education and counseling
(C) Preventive services
(D) Managerial services

10. The pharmacist's role in the selection of therapeutic alternatives requires which of the following clinical skills?

(A) Review and critique drug literature
(B) Ability to motivate, inspire patients
(C) Perform drug utilization evaluations (DUE)
(D) Knowledge of community resources

ANSWERS AND EXPLANATIONS

1. The answer is B *[IV B 4].*
A FARM progress note is used to describe and document the interventions intended or provided by the pharmacist. The acronym FARM means Findings, Assessment, Resolution, and Monitoring and follow up.

2. The answer is D *[II A].*
Pharmaceutical care has evolved from an emphasis on prevention of drug-related problems to the expanded roles of pharmacists in the triage of patients, treatment of routine acute illnesses, management of chronic diseases, and primary disease prevention.

3. The answer is B *[IV A].*
Pharmaceutical care is based on a collaborative effort between pharmacist and patient.

4. The answer is D *[I B; VIII].*
The term pharmaceutical care describes specific activities and services through which an individual pharmacist cooperates with a patient and other professionals in designing, implementing and monitoring a therapeutic plan that will produce specific therapeutic outcomes for the patient. The patient profile (database) is revised and the potential for drug-related problems re-assessed each time a new drug is added to or deleted from the medication regimen, a new disease or condition is diagnosed, or the patient undergoes other clinical intervention (e.g., surgery).

5. The answer is B *[IV A, B].*
The essential components of pharmaceutical care are the pharmacist–patient relationship and the pharmacist's workup of drug therapy.

6. The answer is D *[IV B 2].*
The acronym CORE refers to the components of the pharmacotherapy plan, which is part of the pharmacist's workup of drug therapy. CORE stands for Condition or patient need; Outcome desired for that condition; Regimen selected to achieve that outcome; and Evaluation parameters to assess outcome achievement.

7. The answer is B *[IV B 4; VII C].*
The FARM note is the pharmacist's progress note, describing and documenting the interventions intended or provided by the pharmacist. This constitutes the progress note in the medical chart (in health system facilities) or in the pharmacy patient chart (in community pharmacy or sites without ready access to the medical chart).

8. The answer is A *[IV B 4].*
The assessment portion of the FARM note states the pharmacist's evaluation of the findings. Recommendations are made to the patient or care giver to resolve or prevent an actual or potential problem identified by the pharmacist. Thus, such recommendations would be included in the resolution portion of the FARM note.

9. The answer is C *[V H].*
Immunizations, screenings, and health and wellness education are examples of clinical skills used in a pharmacist's provision of preventive services.

10. The answer is A *[V F].*
For effective selection of therapeutic alternatives, a pharmacist would use certain clinical skills, including use of drug information resources, comparative analyses, and review and critique of drug literature.

23
Drug Information Resources

Paul F. Souney
Connie Lee Barnes

I. DEFINITION. Drug information is current, critically examined, relevant data about drugs and drug use in a given patient or situation.

A. Current information uses the most recent, up-to-date sources possible.

B. Critically examined information should meet the following criteria.

1. More than one source should be used when appropriate.
2. The extent of agreement of sources should be determined; if sources do not agree, good judgment should be used.
3. The plausibility of information, based on clinical circumstances, should be determined.

C. Relevant information must be presented in a manner that applies directly to the circumstances under consideration (e.g., patient parameters, therapeutic objectives, alternative approaches).

II. DRUG INFORMATION RESOURCES. There are three sources of drug information: journals (primary sources), indexing and abstracting services (secondary sources), and textbooks (tertiary sources).

A. Primary sources

1. **Benefits.** Journal articles provide the most current information about drugs and, ideally, should be the source for answering therapeutic questions. Journals enable pharmacists to:
   a. Keep abreast of professional news
   b. Learn how a second clinician handles a particular problem
   c. Keep up with new developments in pathophysiology, diagnostic agents, and therapeutic regimens
   d. Distinguish useful from useless or even harmful therapy
   e. Enhance communication with other health care professionals and consumers
   f. Obtain continuing education credits
   g. Share opinions with other health care professionals through letters-to-the-editor columns
   h. Prepare for the Board certification examination in pharmacotherapy, nutrition support, etc.
2. **Limitations.** Although publication of an article in a well-known, respected journal enhances the credibility of information contained in an article, this does not guarantee that the article is accurate. Many articles possess inadequacies that become apparent as the ability to evaluate drug information improves.

B. Secondary sources

1. **Benefits.** Indexing and abstracting services (Table 23-1) are valuable tools for quick and selective screening of the primary literature for specific information, data, citation, and articles. In some cases, the sources provide sufficient information to serve as references for answering drug information requests.
2. **Limitations.** Each indexing or abstracting service reviews a finite number of journals. Therefore, relying on only one service can greatly hinder the thoroughness of a literature search. Another important fact to remember is the substantial difference in lag time (i.e., the interval between publication of an article and citation of the article in an index) among various services. Several examples are given in Table 23-1.

Table 23-1. Examples of Abstracting/Indexing Services

Secondary References	Journals Indexed	Lag time
ClinAlert	150	1–6 weeks
Current Contents	1200	1–6 weeks
Drugs in Use	1000	6–24 months
Drugdex		3–6 months
Index Medicus	3700	3–12 months
Inpharma	1700	3 weeks–6 months
International Pharmaceutical Abstracts	800	6–14 months
Iowa Drug Information System	200	3–12 months
Pharmaceutical News Index		2–8 weeks
Reactions	1700	3 weeks–6 months
Science Citation Index	2000	3–12 months

a. Secondary sources usually **describe** only articles and clinical studies from journals. Frequently, readers respond to, criticize, and add new information to published articles and studies through letters. Services such as Index Medicus, Drugs in Use, or the Iowa Drug Information System generally do include pertinent letters to the editor within the scope of coverage.

b. Indexing and abstracting services are primarily used to **locate** journal articles. In general, abstracts should not be used as primary sources of information because they are generally interpretations of a study and may be a misinterpretation of important information. Pharmacists should obtain and evaluate the original article because abstracts might not tell the whole story.

C. Tertiary sources

1. Benefits. General reference textbooks can provide easy and convenient access to a broad spectrum of related topics. Background information on drugs and diseases is often available. Although a textbook might answer many drug-related questions, the limitations of these sources should not be overlooked.

a. It could take several years to publish a text, so information available in textbooks might not include the most recent developments in the field. Other resources should be used to update or supplement information obtained from textbooks.

b. The author of a textbook might not have done a thorough search of the literature, so pertinent data could have been omitted. An author also might have misinterpreted the primary or secondary literature. Reference citations should be available to verify the validity and accuracy of the data.

2. General considerations when examining and using textbooks as sources of drug information include:

a. The author, publisher, or both: What are the author's and publisher's track records?

b. The year of publication (copyright date)

c. The edition of the text: Is it the most current edition?

d. The presence or absence of a bibliography: If a bibliography is included, are important statements accurately referenced? When were the references published?

e. The scope of the textbook: How accessible is the information?

f. Alternative resources that are available (e.g., primary and secondary sources, other relevant texts)

III. ELECTRONIC BULLETIN BOARDS

A. Benefits. An electronic bulletin board (EBB) expands the ability to monitor therapies recently published or discussed in the media. The use of EBBs may prevent duplication of drug information searches by users.

B. Limitations

1. Unlike information published in journals or textbooks, information obtained from an EBB is generally not peer reviewed or edited before release.
2. Information from the EBB is only as reliable as the person who posted it and the users who read and comment on its contents.

C. Use. EBBs can be reached using a computer with a modem and communication software to access telephone communication lines. Specifics regarding modem settings required to access the EBB may be obtained via the EBB's system operator. Information obtained from the EBB should be used in the same way information obtained from a consultation with a colleague is handled. See Table 23-2 for a list of EBBs specific for pharmacists.

IV. STRATEGIES FOR EVALUATING INFORMATION REQUESTS. It is important to obtain as many clues as possible about drug information requests before beginning a literature search. Both time and money can be wasted doing a vast search. Below are important questions to ask the inquirer or evaluate before a manual or computerized search.

A. Talk with the inquirer. Before spending time searching for information, talk to the person who is requesting the information and acquire any necessary additional information.

1. **Determine the reason for the inquiry.** Find out where the inquirer heard or read about the drug. Is he or she taking the medication? If so, why? Because the search can be done by the drug or disease name, determine if the inquirer has a medical condition. Ascertaining the reason for the inquiry helps determine what additional information should be provided. For example, if the inquiry concerns a foreign drug, the inquirer might ask for a domestic equivalent.
2. **Clarify the drug's identification and availability.** Make sure that the drug in question is available and double check information about the drug, such as:
   a. The **correct spelling** of the drug's name
   b. Whether it is a **generic** or **brand-name drug**
   c. What **pharmaceutical company** manufactures the drug and in what **country** the drug is manufactured
   d. Whether the drug is **prescription** or **nonprescription**
   e. Whether the drug is still **under investigation** and, if it is on the market, **the length of time on the market**
   f. The **dosage form** of the drug
   g. The **purpose** of the drug (i.e., what medical condition or symptom is the drug intended to alleviate; this information helps narrow the search if products with similar names are found)

B. To **identify** or **assess product availability,** consider using **these resources** (see Appendix E).

1. For drugs manufactured in the **United States,** the following resources are available:

Table 23-2. Selected Pharmacy-Oriented Electronic Bulletin Boards (EBBs)/Internet Connections

EBB	Sponsor	Availability	Internet Address	Phone Number
ClinNet	American College of Clinical Pharmacy (ACCP)	For ACCP members only	http://www.accp.com	412-648-7893
F.I.X.	The Formulary Information Exchange	Annual subscription fee		800-262-8664
PharmNet	American Society of Health-System Pharmacists (ASHP)	For ASHP members only	http://www.ashp.com/pub/ashp	800-848-8980 (call for local number)
FDA	Food and Drug Administration (FDA)	Anyone can access; no fee	http://www.fda.gov	800-222-0185

a. *The American Drug Index,* which is updated annually
b. *Drug Facts and Comparisons,* which is updated monthly and bound annually
c. *Drug Topics Red Book* or *Blue Book,* which releases supplements and is updated annually
d. The *Physician's Desk Reference (PDR),*which is updated annually
e. The *American Hospital Formulary Service (AHFS) Drug Information,* which is supplemented quarterly and updated annually
f. *Martindale: The Extra Pharmacopoeia,* which is updated every 5 years

2. For drugs manufactured in **foreign countries,** the following resources are available:
   a. *Martindale: The Extra Pharmacopoeia*
   b. *Index Nominum*
   c. *United States Adopted Names (USAN)* and the *United States Pharmacopeia (USP) Dictionary of Drug Names*

3. For **investigational drugs,** the following resources are available:
   a. *Martindale: The Extra Pharmacopoeia*
   b. *Drug Facts and Comparisons*
   c. *Unlisted Drugs*
   d. *NDA Pipeline*

4. For **orphan drugs** [i.e., drugs that are used to prevent or treat a rare disease (affects less than 200,000 people in the United States, so the cost of development is not likely to be offset by sales) and for which the United States Food and Drug Administration (FDA) offers assistance and financial incentives to sponsors undertaking the development of the drugs], the following resources are available:
   a. *Drug Facts and Comparisons*
   b. The *National Information Center for Orphan Drugs and Rare Diseases (NICODARD)*
   c. *Drugdex*

5. For an **unknown drug** (i.e., one that is in hand but not identified) chemical analysis can be performed or the drug can be identified by physical characteristics, such as color, special markings, and shape. Consult the following sources for help:
   a. The *PDR, PDR Generics, PDR Drug I.D. System, Drug Facts and Comparisons, Drug Topics Red Book, Ident-A-Drug Handbook*
   b. *Identidex*
   c. The manufacturer
   d. A laboratory

V. SEARCH STRATEGIES.

To develop an effective search strategy for locating drug information literature, the following tactics should be followed after determining whether primary or secondary sources are desired.

A. Determine whether the question at hand is **clinical** or **research-related. Define the question** as specifically as possible. Also, identify appropriate index terms (also called key words or descriptors) with which to search for the information.

B. Determine the **type of information** and **how much** is needed (i.e., only one fact, the most recent journal articles, review articles, a comprehensive database search).

C. **Ascertain as much information as possible** about the drug being questioned and the **inquirer's association** with it. Remember that data on adverse drug effects or drug interactions are often fragmented and inadequately documented. See IV A 2 for the specific drug information that should be acquired, and also determine answers to the following questions.

1. What is the indication for the prescribed drug?

2. Is the drug's use approved or unapproved? This information can be found in the following resources (remember to check how often these resources are updated to ensure having the latest information):
   a. **Approved uses** of drugs can be checked in:
      (1) *AHFS Drug Information* for the current year and in the year's supplements
      (2) *Drug Facts and Comparisons*
      (3) The *PDR*

        (4) *USP DI*
        (5) *Drugdex*
    b. **Unapproved uses** of drugs can be found in:
        (1) *AHFS Drug Information*
        (2) *Drug Facts and Comparisons*
        (3) *Martindale: The Extra Pharmacopoeia*
        (4) Index Medicus or other computer programs (e.g., Medline, Paperchase)
        (5) *Drugdex*
        (6) *Inpharma*
        (7) *USPDI*

3. What is the age, sex, and weight of the patient in question?

4. Does the patient have any other medical conditions or renal or hepatic disease?

5. Is the patient taking any other medications?

6. What drugs has the patient taken during the past 6 months and what were the dosages?

7. Did the patient experience any signs or symptoms of a possible adverse drug reaction? If so:
    a. How severe was the reaction?
    b. When did the reaction appear?
    c. Has the patient (or any member of the patient's family) experienced any allergic or adverse reactions to medications in the past?
    d. Consult the following resources for more information:
        (1) Meyler's *Side Effects of Drugs* (SEDBASE online)
        (2) A general drug reference
        (3) *Reactions* (ADIS)
        (4) Index Medicus
    e. Also, the manufacturer of the drug may be a useful source for missing information. In exchange for information, most companies expect to receive an adverse drug reaction form.

8. Did the patient experience any signs or symptoms of a drug interaction? If so:
    a. What were the specific drugs in question?
    b. What were the respective dosages of the drugs?
    c. What was the duration of therapy?
    d. What was the length of the course of administration?
    e. What are the details of the events secondary to the suspected reaction?
    f. Consult the following resources for more information:
        (1) A drug interactions reference [e.g., *Drug Interaction Facts,* Hansten's *Drug Interaction and Updates, Evaluations of Drug Interactions (EDI)*]
        (2) A general drug reference (e.g., The *PDR*)
        (3) *Reactions*
        (4) Index Medicus

9. What is the patient's current medication status?

10. Does the patient have any underlying diseases?

11. How has the patient been managed so far?

12. What is the stability of the drug and how is compatibility of the drug with other drugs, the administration technique, and the equipment that holds it? Resources to check for this information include:
    a. Trissel's *Handbook on Injectable Drugs*
    b. King's *Guide to Parenteral Admixtures*
    c. Trissel's *Stability of Compounded Formulations*

D. Explore other possible information resources if necessary. For example, it may be useful to find background material in textbooks (tertiary references), and then go to the journal literature (primary references) for more current information.

VI. EVALUATING A CLINICAL STUDY. Resource identification is followed by a critical assessment of the available information. This step is critical in developing an appropriate response for the inquirer.

A. **Evaluate the objective of the study.** Determine the aim of the research that was performed.

1. What did the researchers intend to examine?
2. Is this goal stated clearly (i.e., is the objective specific)?
3. Was the research limited to a single objective, or were there multiple drugs or effects being tested?

B. **Evaluate the subjects of the study.** Determine the profile of the study population by looking for the following information.

1. Were healthy subjects or affected patients used in the study?
2. Were the subjects volunteers?
3. What were the criteria for selecting the subjects?
4. How many subjects were included and what is the breakdown of age, sex, and race?
5. If a disease was being treated, did any of the subjects have diseases other than that initially being treated? Were any additional treatments given? Were there any contraindications to the therapy?
6. What was the patient selection method and who was excluded from the study?
7. A patient selection review should be done. You will find that most groups of subjects are homogeneous (i.e., they all have comparable characteristics). If a disease state is studied, patients should exhibit similar severity of symptoms. Researchers wish to eliminate interpatient variability. By selecting patients with similar characteristics, researchers can avoid results that are caused by individual differences among patients. Strong individual differences can obscure the results of the experiment. If studying a group of patients that exhibit significant interpatient variability is necessary, researchers may divide the patients into groups according to the variables likely to be associated with responsiveness to therapy. This is known as stratification.

C. **Evaluate the administration of the drug treatment.** For each drug being investigated, determine the following information:

1. **Details of treatment** with the agent being studied:
   a. Daily dose
   b. Frequency of administration
   c. Hours of day when administered
   d. Route of administration
   e. Source of drug (i.e., the supplier)
   f. Dosage form
   g. Timing of drug administration in relation to factors affecting drug absorption
   h. Methods of ensuring compliance
   i. Total duration of treatment
2. **Other therapeutic measures** in addition to the agent being studied

D. **Evaluate the setting of the study.** Try to determine the environment of the study and the dates on which the trial began and ended. Look for the following information:

1. People who made the observations; various professionals who offer different and unique perspectives based on their backgrounds and interests (Were the same people making observations throughout the study?)
2. Whether the study was done on an inpatient or outpatient basis
3. Description of physical setting (i.e., hospital, clinic, ward)
4. Length of the study (i.e.,dates on which the trial began and ended)

E. **Evaluate the methods and design of the study.** The method section of the research paper explains how the research was conducted. The study design (i.e., retrospective, prospective, blind, crossover) and the methods used to complete the study are important in judging whether the study and the results are reliable and valid. From the study, try to determine answers to the following questions:

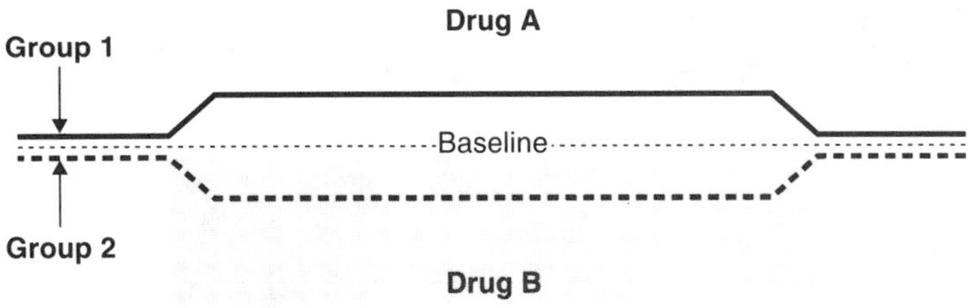

Figure 23-1. Parallel study design.

1. Are the methods of assessing the therapeutic effects clearly described?
2. Were the methods standardized?
   a. **Retrospective versus prospective**
      (1) **Retrospective** studies look at events that have already occurred to find some common link between them; require reliance on patient memories and accurate medical records; and are unable to show cause and effect. Retrospective studies are useful for studying rare diseases (or effects); can help to decide if enough information exists to warrant prospective examination of a problem.
      (2) **Prospective** studies look forward in time at a question the study seeks to answer. They can be observational or experimental (i.e., clinical trials).
   b. **Treatment allocation**
      (1) **Parallel** study design is a protocol in which two or more patient groups are studied concurrently. The groups are treated identically except for one variable, such as a drug therapy (Figure 23-1).
      (2) **Crossover** design may be used as an additional control for interpatient and intrapatient variability (Figure 23-2). In this type of design, each patient group undergoes each type of treatment. However, the sequence in which the subjects undergo treatment is reversed for one group. Crossover design reduces the possibility that the results were strongly influenced by the order in which therapy was given. And, because both groups of patients receive both types of treatment, any differences in responsiveness between the groups due to patient selection will be uncovered.
3. Were **control measures** used to reduce variation that might influence the results? Examples of such control methods include:
   a. Concurrent controls
   b. Stratification or matched subgroups
   c. A run-in period
   d. The patient as his or her own control (i.e., crossover design)
   e. Identical ancillary treatment
4. Were controls used to reduce bias? Examples of such controls include:
   a. **Blind assessment,** which means that the people observing the patients do not know who is a subject and who is a control

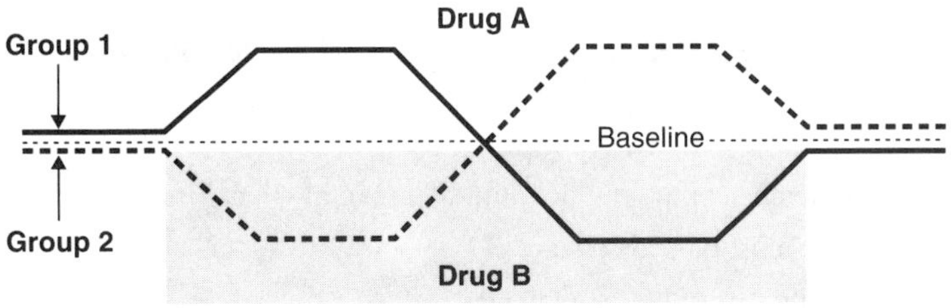

Figure 23-2. Crossover study design.

Table 23-3. Types of Blind Studies

Types of Blinds	Patient Aware of Treatment	Physician Aware of Treatment
Open label (non-blind)	X	X
Single-blind	—	X
Double-blind	—	—

b. **Blind patients,** which means that the patients do not know whether they received the substance being studied or a placebo [**double blind** combines points a and b] (Table 23-3)

c. **Random allocation,** which means that patients involved in the study have an even chance of being assigned to either the group of subjects receiving the active drug or the group receiving controls

d. **Matching dummies,** which are placebos that are physically identical to the active agent being studied

e. **Comparison** of a placebo or a therapy to a recognized standard practice

F. **Evaluate the analysis of the study.** After looking at specific areas of the study separately, gather the information together to determine whether the trial is acceptable and the conclusions are justified by determining answers to the following questions (Figure 23-3).

1. Were the subjects suitably selected in relation to the aim(s) of the study?
2. Were the methods of measurement valid in relation to the aim(s) of the study?
3. Were the methods adequately standardized?
4. Were the methods sufficiently sensitive?
5. Was the design appropriate?
6. Were there enough subjects?
7. Was the dosage appropriate?
8. Was the duration of treatment adequate?
9. Were carry-over effects avoided or were compensations made for them?
10. If no controls were used, were they unnecessary or overlooked?
11. If controls were used, were they adequate?
12. Was the comparability of treatment groups examined?
13. Are the data adequate for assessment?
14. If statistical tests were not done, were they unnecessary or overlooked?
15. If statistical tests are reported, assess the following:
    a. Is it clear how the statistical tests were done?
    b. Were the tests appropriately used?
    c. If results show no significant difference between test groups, were there enough patients (i.e., statistical power)?

VII. GENERAL GUIDELINES FOR RESPONSES TO DRUG INFORMATION REQUESTS

A. Do not guess!

B. Responses to a member of the public must take several ethical issues into account.

1. Patient privacy must be protected.
2. Professional ethics must be maintained.
3. The patient–physician relationship cannot be breached.

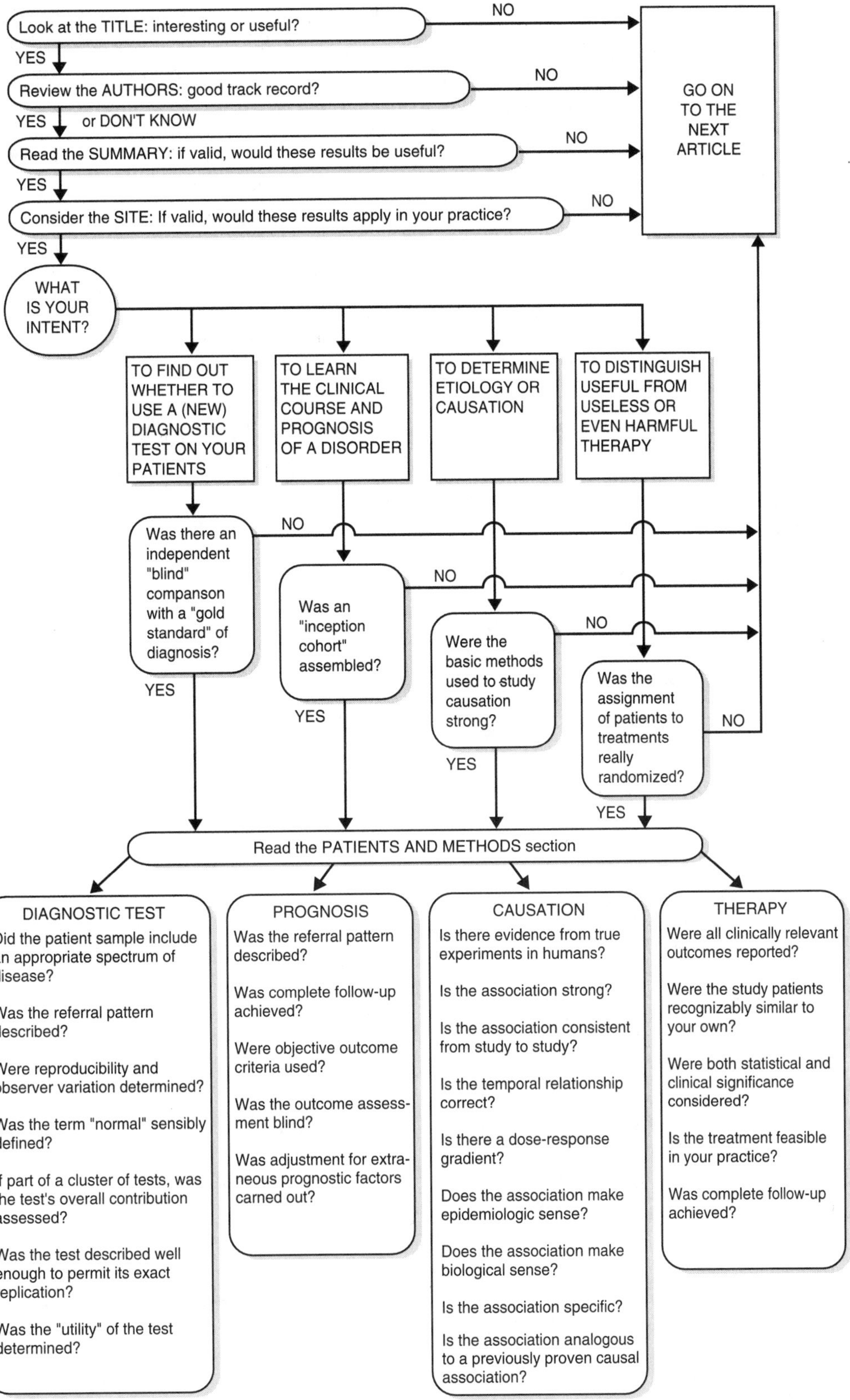

Figure 23-3. Evaluation of study analysis.

4. Response is not necessary if the inquirer intends to misuse or abuse information that is provided. The inquirer often admits intent or offers clues to potential abuse, such as in the following examples.
   a. A patient asks how a certain drug is dosed (i.e., how much the drug can be increased, when it can be increased, and what the maximum daily dose is). This kind of inquiry signals that the patient might be adjusting his or her own therapy.
   b. A patient asks a pharmacist to identify a tablet that is a prescription product known for a high rate of abuse.

C. Organize information before attempting to communicate the response to the inquirer. Anticipate additional questions.

D. Tailor the response to the inquirer's background. Also, consider the environment of the practice, institutional policy and procedure, and formulary.

E. Inform the inquirer where the information was found. Exercise caution with statements such as, "There are no reports in the literature."

F. Use **extreme** caution with statements such as, "I recommend ..." Do not hesitate to refer consumers to their physicians.

G. Use more than abstracts to answer drug information questions because they might be taken out of context and do not include all of the data available in the original article.

H. Alert the inquirer of a possible delay when it takes longer than anticipated to answer the question.

I. Ask if the information that is provided answers the inquirer's questions.

J. Ask if the inquirer wishes to have reprints of articles or a written response.

24
Federal Pharmacy Law

Robert C. Pavlan, Jr.

I. FEDERAL CONTROLLED SUBSTANCES ACT

A. Schedules of controlled substances. Certain drugs have a potential for abuse that lead to physical or psychological dependence. As a result, the federal government has placed these drugs into schedules (schedules I, II, III, IV, V) and refers to them as controlled substances. The Attorney General of the United States has the authority to add or remove a drug or substance from one of the federal schedules, or to transfer a drug from one federal schedule to another. The federal schedules are updated and published annually by the federal government.

1. **Schedule I (CI; C-I).** Schedule I drugs may not be kept in a pharmacy nor dispensed pursuant to a prescription (except for properly registered facilities for investigative or research purposes). A controlled substance analogue of a drug in any federal schedule, commonly referred to as a "designer drug," is considered a schedule I substance to the extent intended for human consumption. Required findings by the government for placement of a drug into schedule I include:
   - **a.** The drug or other substance has a high potential for abuse.
   - **b.** The drug or other substance has no currently accepted medical use in treatment in the United States.
   - **c.** There is a lack of accepted safety for use of the drug or other substance under medical supervision.

2. **Schedule II (CII; C-II).** Required findings for placement of a drug into schedule II include:
   - **a.** The drug or other substance has a high potential for abuse.
   - **b.** The drug or other substance has a currently accepted medical use in treatment in the United States or a currently accepted medical use with severe restrictions.
   - **c.** Abuse of the drug or other substance may lead to severe psychological or physical dependence.

3. **Schedule III (CIII; C-III).** Required findings for placement of a drug into schedule III include:
   - **a.** The drug or other substance has a potential for abuse less than the drugs or other substances in schedules I and II.
   - **b.** The drug or other substance has a currently accepted medical use in treatment in the United States.
   - **c.** Abuse of the drug or other substance may lead to moderate or low physical dependence or high psychological dependence.

4. **Schedule IV (CIV; C-IV).** Required findings for placement of a drug into schedule IV include:
   - **a.** The drug or other substance has a low potential for abuse relative to the drugs or other substances in schedule III.
   - **b.** The drug or other substance has a currently accepted medical use in treatment in the United States.
   - **c.** Abuse of the drug or other substance may lead to limited physical dependence or psychological dependence relative to the drugs or other substances in schedule III.

5. **Schedule V (CV; C-V).** Required findings for placement of a drug into schedule V include:
   - **a.** The drug or other substance has a low potential for abuse relative to the drugs or other substances in schedule IV.
   - **b.** The drug or other substance has a currently accepted medical use in treatment in the United States.
   - **c.** Abuse of the drug or other substance may lead to limited physical dependence or psychological dependence relative to the drugs or other substances in schedule IV.

B. Registration requirements. This Act regulates the use of controlled substances by requiring all entities who lawfully handle them to register with the federal government, specifically, the Drug Enforcement Administration (DEA).

1. Entities that must register

a. Manufacturers and **wholesalers** of controlled substances must register with the DEA initially and reregister every year thereafter.

b. Dispensers (practitioners and pharmacies) of controlled substances must register with the DEA initially and reregister every 3 years thereafter. Pharmacists, pharmacy interns, pharmacy technicians, and all other employees or agents of a pharmacy do not have to register, providing the pharmacy is properly registered and the employee or agent is acting in the usual course of employment or business.

c. All other entities that lawfully handle any controlled substance must register with the DEA, including researchers, clinics and laboratories, and teaching institutions.

2. Separate registration for separate activities. Every entity that engages in one of the following activities must register with the DEA. A separate registration is required for each activity, with certain exceptions (e.g., a manufacturer of a schedule of a controlled substance is allowed to distribute that schedule without being registered as a distributor).

a. Manufacturing controlled substances
b. Distributing controlled substances
c. Dispensing controlled substances listed in schedules II–V (e.g., practitioners, pharmacies)
d. Conducting research with controlled substances listed in schedules II–V
e. Conducting instructional activities with controlled substances listed in schedules II–V
f. Conducting a narcotic treatment program using any narcotic drug listed in schedules II, III, IV, or V
g. Conducting research and instructional activities with controlled substances listed in schedule I
h. Conducting chemical analysis with controlled substances listed in any schedule
i. Importing controlled substances
j. Exporting controlled substances
k. Participating in maintenance or detoxification treatment and mixing, preparing, packaging, or changing the dosage form of a narcotic drug listed in schedules II, III, IV, or V for use in maintenance or detoxification treatment by another narcotic treatment program.

3. Separate registrations for separate locations. Each principal place of business of a registrant having more than one location must have its own registration certificate. Each pharmacy, chain pharmacy, and hospital that dispenses controlled substances must have its own registration certificate. Registration is not required for an office that is used by a registrant where controlled substances are neither stored nor dispensed.

a. Warehouses. A warehouse where controlled substances are stored by or on behalf of a registrant are not required to register unless one of the following occur:

(1) Controlled substances are directly distributed from the warehouse to a registered location different than the location from which the substances were shipped.

(2) Controlled substances are directly distributed from the warehouse to a person or entity not required to register under the Act.

4. Registration procedure. Applications to become registered must be submitted to the DEA on the appropriate form with the required fee, information, and signature of one of the following:

a. The individual who owns and operates the entity, if doing business as an individual
b. A partner of the applicant, if a partnership
c. An officer of the applicant, if a corporation, corporate division, association, trust, or other entity
d. One or more individuals who have been granted a power of attorney by an applicant. A **power of attorney** allows one to lawfully act in place of another. The power of attorney must be signed by one of the individuals listed above in a–c and by the individual receiving the power of attorney. The power of attorney remains valid until revoked by the applicant.

5. Registration action by the DEA. If an application is complete, it will be accepted for filing. If it is defective, the DEA will return the application with a statement indicating the reason for its nonacceptance. The application may be corrected and resubmitted at any time.

a. **Issuance of certificate of registration.** A certificate of registration will be issued by the DEA when it determines that the registration is required by law in order to conduct such activity (e.g., manufacturing, distributing, dispensing a controlled substance). The certificate must be conspicuously maintained and readily retrievable at the registered location.
b. **Denial of registration.** If the DEA determines that a registration is not required by law, it will issue an Order To Show Cause why the registration should not be denied. The applicant may request a hearing and explain why the certificate of registration should be issued. After the hearing, the DEA may deny the application, or issue the certificate.

6. **Modification of registration.** A registrant may submit a letter of request to the DEA seeking to modify its registration. A modification may be sought when there is a change in the name or address that appears on the certificate, or when the pharmacy seeks DEA approval to dispense additional controlled substances (if initially authorized to only dispense a particular schedule(s) of controlled substances).

7. **Transfer of registration.** A registration to dispense controlled substances may not be transferred to any other person or entity except when the ownership of a pharmacy is being transferred from one entity to another. In such a case, controlled substances in schedules II–V must be properly disposed of or transferred to the new entity.

8. **Suspension or revocation of registration.** The DEA may suspend or revoke any registration. The DEA must first issue an Order To Show Cause (upon the registrant) why the registration should not be revoked or suspended. The registrant may request a hearing to explain why the registration should not be suspended or revoked. After a hearing, the DEA may suspend, revoke or take no action on the registration.
   a. **Order of suspension or revocation.** After a registrant has received an order suspending or revoking its registration, it must take the following action:
      (1) Immediately deliver its certificate of registration and any DEA 222 order forms in its possession to the nearest office of the DEA
      (2) As instructed by the DEA, either:
         (a) Deliver all controlled substances in its possession to the nearest office of the DEA or to authorized agents of the DEA
         (b) Place all controlled substances in its possession under seal
   b. **Imminent danger to public health or safety.** The DEA may serve on a registrant an order of immediate suspension when it finds that there is an **imminent danger** to the **public health** or **safety.** The immediate suspension remains in effect until the conclusion of all proceedings, either administrative proceedings by the DEA or judicial proceedings. After receiving an order of immediate suspension, the registrant must take the same action as outlined above under I B 8 a.

9. **Exemptions from registration.** Certain individuals are exempt from registration under the Act. The following are exempt:
   a. **Military officials.** Military officials, including Public Health Service and Bureau of Prisons officials, who are authorized to prescribe, dispense, or administer, but not to procure or purchase, controlled substances in the course of his official duties, are exempt from registering with the DEA. The individual must, however, obtain a registration for such activities conducted during any separate private practice.
   b. **Law-enforcement officials.** Federal and state law-enforcement personnel acting in the course of enforcing any law relating to controlled substances are exempt from registration.
   c. **Civil defense officials.** Civil defense and disaster relief organization officials are exempt from registration in order to maintain and dispense controlled substances during times of proclaimed emergencies or disasters.
   d. **Agents and employees of registrants.** Agents and employees, while acting lawfully in the usual course of their business or employment, are exempt from registration when the business or employment is conducted on behalf of a person (or business) who is registered under the Act. Delivery personnel (e.g., United Parcel Service, Federal Express) are therefore not required to register. Likewise, pharmacists working for a registered pharmacy are not required to register.

10. **Termination of registration.** The registration of any person or entity will terminate when the person dies, ceases legal existence (corporate dissolution, partnership dissolution), or discontinues business or professional practice. The DEA must be notified promptly when any

of these occurs. In such a case, all controlled substances in schedules II–V must be properly disposed.

C. Required inventories. The Act requires all pharmacies and hospitals (every separately registered location) to conduct an initial inventory and biennial inventory of all controlled substances in schedules II, III, IV, and V.

1. **Initial inventory.** The initial inventory must be taken on the date the entity commences business and begins dispensing controlled substances. If the entity has no controlled substances on hand, a record of this fact must be maintained as its initial inventory.

2. **Biennial inventory.** The biennial inventory must be taken every 2 years from the date of the initial inventory.
   a. **Biennial date.** The biennial date must be one of the following dates:
      (1) On the day of the year (2 years later) on which the initial inventory was taken (The DEA does not need to be notified if this date is used.)
      (2) On the registrant's regular general physical inventory date that is nearest to, and does not vary by more than 6 months from, the biennial date used under method (1) above (The registrant must first notify the DEA of this election and of the date on which the inventory will be taken.)
      (3) On any fixed date that does not vary by more than 6 months from the biennial date used under method (1) above (The registrant must first notify the DEA of this election and of the date on which the inventory will be taken.)
   b. **Four-day variance.** A registrant may take the inventory on a date within 4 days of the biennial inventory date, regardless of which method is chosen. The regional office of the DEA must first be notified of the exact date on which the inventory will be taken.

3. **Inventory procedures**
   a. All inventories must be maintained in a **written, typewritten,** or **printed form** and be conducted at either the opening of business or the close of business on the inventory date (which must be noted on the inventory).
   b. **Separate inventory record for schedule II controlled substances.** Because all records for schedule II controlled substances must be maintained separately from other records, schedule II inventories must be maintained separate from other controlled substance inventories.

4. **Inventory content.** All inventory records must contain the following:
   a. Date the inventory is taken
   b. Each finished form of the substance (dosage form and strength)
   c. Number of units or volume of each finished form in each commercial container (e.g., 100 tablet bottle). For opened commercial containers inventory must be taken as follows:
      (1) For schedule II controlled substances, an exact count or measure must be taken.
      (2) For schedule III, IV, and V controlled substances, an estimated count or measure may be taken, except that an exact count must be taken if the container holds more than 1,000 tablets or capsules.
   d. For each controlled substance maintained for extemporaneous compounding or for substances which are damaged, defective, or impure and awaiting disposal:
      (1) Name of the substance
      (2) Total quantity to the nearest metric unit weight or the total number of units of finished form
      (3) Reason the substance is being maintained and whether it is capable of use in the manufacture of any controlled substance in finished form

5. **Inventory record maintenance.** Every inventory record must be maintained at the registered location (e.g., pharmacy, hospital) for at least 2 years from the date of the inventory.
   a. Schedule II inventories must be maintained separately from all other records of the pharmacy.
   b. Schedule III, IV, and V inventory records must be maintained either separately from all other records of the pharmacy or in such a manner that the required information is readily retrievable from ordinary business records of the pharmacy. "Readily retrievable" means that the inventory records can be separated out from all other records in a reasonable time.

6. **Perpetual inventories.** The Act does not require a dispenser registrant (e.g., pharmacy, hospital) to maintain a perpetual inventory of any controlled substance.

7. **Newly controlled substances or changes in scheduling of a substance.** An inventory of a substance must be taken when, by order of the DEA, it becomes a newly controlled substance or it shifts into another schedule. The inventory of that particular controlled substance must be taken on the effective date of the change. A complete inventory of all controlled substances is not required, nor is an inventory required when a substance moves from a controlled-substance schedule to a non-federal schedule.
8. **Transfer of business activity.** An inventory of controlled substances II–V must be taken at the time a pharmacy or hospital undergoes a change in ownership. The inventory must be taken on the date of transfer and serves as the final inventory of the transferor and the initial inventory of the transferee.
9. **Inventory record submission.** The Act does not require the submission of inventory records to anyone, including the DEA. The records must be maintained at the registered location for inspection and copying by authorized agents of the DEA.

D. **Obtaining controlled substances.** Schedule II controlled substances must be obtained from a supplier (wholesaler, manufacturer) by using DEA Form 222. The Act does not require the use of any special form to obtain controlled substances in schedules III–V.

1. **DEA Form 222.** Only entities that are registered to dispense or handle schedule II controlled substances may obtain Form 222. The forms are serially numbered and issued by the DEA with the name, address, registration number, authorized activity, and schedules of the registrant. Each form contains an original, duplicate, and triplicate copy (Copy 1, Copy 2, and Copy 3, respectively).
   a. **Execution of Form 222.** Form 222 may be executed only on behalf of the registrant named on the form and only if the registration has not expired nor been revoked or suspended. The form must be prepared in triplicate as provided by the DEA by use of a typewriter, pen, or indelible pencil in the following manner:
      (1) Only one item may be ordered on each of the ten numbered lines on the form. The total number of items ordered must be noted on the form in the space provided.
      (2) One item may consist of one or more commercial or bulk containers of a product. A separate item must be made for different commercial or bulk containers of a product. For each item, the form must contain the following information:
         (a) Name of the article ordered
         (b) Finished or bulk form of the product (dosage form and strength)
         (c) Number of units or volume in each commercial or bulk container (e.g., 100 tablet bottle)
         (d) Number of commercial or bulk containers ordered
         (e) If the article is not in pure form, the name and quantity per unit of the controlled substance or substances contained in the article.
      (3) The supplier's name and address must be included on the form. Only one supplier may be listed on any one form.
      (4) Each form must include the date of the order, and no form is valid more than 60 days after its execution by the purchaser.
      (5) The form must be signed either by the person who signed the most recent application for registration or reregistration, or by a person authorized to obtain and execute order forms by a **power of attorney.**
         (a) Any purchaser may authorize one or more individuals (does not have to be an attorney at law), whether or not located at the registered location, to obtain and execute 222 Forms by executing a power of attorney for the individual(s).
         (b) The power of attorney must be signed by the person who signed the most recent application for registration or reregistration and by the individual(s) receiving the power of attorney. This form must be similar or identical to the DEA's "Power of Attorney for DEA Order Forms."
         (c) Once properly executed, the individual receiving the power of attorney may obtain and sign DEA Form 222 to the same extent as the individual who signed the most recent application for registration or reregistration.
         (d) The power of attorney must be filed with the executed 222 order forms of the purchaser and be retained for the same period as any order form bearing the signature of the attorney [see I D 1 a (8)]. The power of attorney does not have to be submitted to the DEA.

(6) Copy 1 and 2 must be submitted to the supplier. Copy 3 must be retained by the purchaser.
(7) When the ordered schedule II controlled substances are received by the pharmacy, the following information must be recorded on the retained Copy 3:
  (a) Number of commercial or bulk containers furnished on each item (or line)
  (b) Date on which the containers are received by the pharmacy
(8) DEA 222 Forms must be maintained at the registered location (pharmacy or hospital) for at least 2 years from its execution. The time of execution would be the date the last entry was made on Copy 3.

b. **Cancellation by purchaser.** A purchaser may cancel all or part of an order by notifying the supplier in writing. The supplier must indicate the cancellation on Copies 1 and 2 by drawing a line through the canceled items and printing the word "canceled" in the space provided for number of items shipped. Likewise, a supplier may void all or part of an order by notifying the purchaser in writing and printing the word "canceled" in the space provided for number of items shipped.

c. **Maintenance of DEA Form 222.** Executed Copy 3 forms and Copy 1 and 2 of each unaccepted or defective form and the statement of refusal from the supplier must be maintained by the purchaser. They must be kept separate from all other records and be available for inspection for at least 2 years. All forms must be maintained at the registered location pre-printed on the form, and not at a central location.

d. **Loss or theft of DEA Form 222.** Any used or unused form stolen from or lost by a purchaser or supplier must be reported immediately to the DEA. Such notification must include the serial number of each form lost or stolen.

2. **Obtaining schedule III–V controlled substances.** There is no special form for obtaining schedule III-V controlled substances. Each registrant must, however, maintain a complete and accurate record of receipt for each such substance. The record must be maintained at either the registered location of the pharmacy or hospital, or at a central location, for 2 years. If a central location is used, the pharmacy must first notify the DEA, indicating its intention to keep central records. Central records may then be maintained unless the DEA denies the request to keep such records. An invoice or packing slip will suffice as a record of receipt, providing the following information is included:
   a. The name of the controlled substance
   b. Finished form of the substance (dosage form and strength)
   c. Number of units or volume of the finished form in each commercial container (e.g., 100 tablet bottle)
   d. Number of commercial containers of each such finished form received from other persons
   e. Date of actual receipt of each commercial container
   f. Name, address and registration number of the person from whom the containers were received

E. **Storage of controlled substances.** All controlled substances in schedules II, III, IV, and V must be stored in one of the following ways:

1. In a securely locked, substantially constructed cabinet

2. Dispersed throughout the stock of unscheduled prescription medication to prevent any theft or diversion

F. **Theft or significant loss of schedule II–V controlled substances.** Every registrant must promptly notify the regional office of the DEA of the theft or significant loss of any controlled substance in schedules II–V. This report must be done using DEA **Form 106.**

G. **Disposal of controlled substances.** Every disposal of a controlled substance must be accomplished by submitting DEA **Form 41** to the DEA (except for disposals pursuant to a valid prescription, discussed below). The form must list the controlled substances earmarked for disposal. The DEA will authorize the disposal and instruct the registrant to dispose of the controlled substances in one of the following ways:

1. By the transfer to a person or entity registered with the DEA and authorized to possess the substance. Schedule II controlled substances must be transferred by use of the transferee's (another pharmacy or hospital, or the wholesaler or manufacturer) DEA Form 222. A writ-

ten record of the transfer of schedule III–V controlled substances must be kept for at least 2 years and include the following information:

a. Name of the controlled substance
b. Finished form of the substance (dosage form and strength)
c. Number of units or volume of the finished form in each commercial container (e.g., 100 tablet bottle)
d. Number of commercial containers of each finished form transferred
e. Date of the transfer
f. Name, address, and registration number of the transferree

2. By the delivery to an agent of the DEA or to the nearest office of the DEA

3. By the destruction in the presence of an agent of the DEA or other authorized person

4. By any other means that the DEA determines to assure that the substance does not become available to unauthorized persons or entities

H. Regular Disposals of controlled substances. If a registrant regularly disposes of controlled substances in schedules II–V (usually hospitals), the DEA may authorize disposals without prior approval in each instance. If the DEA grants this authority, the registrant must keep records of each disposal and file periodic reports to the regional office of the DEA summarizing the disposals. The DEA may place additional conditions on such disposal, including the method of disposal and the frequency and detail of reports.

I. Disposal of controlled substances pursuant to a valid prescription

1. Persons who may issue prescriptions for controlled substances. A controlled substance prescription may be issued only by a practitioner who is granted such authority by the state in which that practitioner is licensed. Although the Act is federal legislation, each state determines who will be authorized to dispense controlled substances. Most states allow the following individuals to prescribe: physicians, dentists, podiatrists, veterinarians. Some states allow the following individuals, referred to as mid-level practitioners, to prescribe (usually with certain restrictions): physician's assistant, nurse practitioner, certified nurse midwife, psychiatric nurse mental health clinical specialist. All prescribers must be registered with the DEA or exempted from registration (see I B 9).

a. DEA numbers and authenticity. After registering with the DEA, all registrants are assigned a DEA number by the DEA. A practitioner's DEA number consists of nine characters. The first two characters are letters. The first letter will be either A or B. The second letter will be the first letter of the practitioner's last name. The next six characters are randomly chosen numbers. The last character is a number often referred to as the "check digit." For example, Dr. Henry Jones may have a DEA number of AJ 4357782.

(1) Authentication of DEA number. The DEA assigns DEA numbers with a quick method of verification built into the number. This allows a dispensing pharmacist to make a cursory review of the number for authenticity. For example, using the above DEA number, the practitioner's last name must start with a J. Also, the following quick calculation can be made to verify that the "check digit" is correct:

(a) The digits in position 1, 3, and 5 are added together to reach a number. In the above example, that would be $4 + 5 + 7 = 16$.

(b) The digits in position 2, 4, and 6 are added together then multiplied by 2. In the above example, that would be $(3 + 7 + 8) \times 2 = 36$;

(c) These numbers above are added together: $16 + 36 = 52$. The far right digit becomes the check digit. The check digit must therefore be a 2. If the check digit is anything other than a 2 the number may not be a valid DEA number. In such a case, the DEA should be notified in order to verify the number.

(2) Mid-level practitioner DEA numbers. Mid-level practitioner DEA numbers are similar to practitioner DEA numbers except for the first character. Instead of the letter A or B, mid-level practitioners have the letter M as the first character in their DEA number. The mathematical method for verifying the authenticity of the number is the same.

2. Purpose of issuance of controlled substance prescriptions. A controlled substance prescription may be issued only in good faith for a legitimate medical purpose by a practitioner acting in the usual course of her professional practice. The practitioner and the dispensing pharmacist have the responsibility to ensure that a prescription is properly issued and dispensed (referred to as corresponding responsibility of the pharmacist).

a. **Legitimate medical purpose.** Legitimate medical purpose and good faith are prerequisites for all controlled substance prescriptions. With respect to a pharmacist, these requirements will be apparent from an objective point of view. As a general rule, if, from all the surrounding facts and circumstances, a reasonably prudent pharmacist would form the opinion that a prescription was issued for a legitimate medical purpose, then the pharmacist has fulfilled his responsibility under the Act and the prescription may be legally dispensed.

b. **Usual course of professional practice.** A **pracitioner–patient relationship** for the purpose of treating and caring for the patient must be present. Usually such a relationship includes the taking and recording of an appropriate medical history, and an appropriate physical exam. This limits a practitioner's ability to prescribe outside his or her course of professional practice (e.g., a veterinarian may not prescribe a controlled substance for a human). The notion of "usual course of practice" becomes more unclear with respect to medical doctors who specialize. Such specialists often issue prescriptions "outside" their specialty. Generally, all controlled substance prescriptions from medical doctors are deemed to be "in the usual course of professional practice" as long as it is issued for a human, regardless of whether the problem being treated is within the doctor's specialty.

c. **Restrictions on issuance of a controlled substance prescription**
   (1) A prescription may not be issued by a practitioner in order for that practitioner to obtain controlled substances for the purpose of **general dispensing** to her patients.
   (2) A prescription may not be issued for the dispensing of controlled substances for **detoxification** or maintenance treatment. Administration and direct dispensing of controlled substances are allowed only when conducted in properly registered treatment programs. A prescription for **methadone** is valid only when issued as an analgesic in cases of severe pain. Methadone may be dispensed in a hospital to maintain a patient's addiction as long as the patient is admitted and being treated for some other medical condition and is not administered methadone solely for detoxification purposes.

3. **Manner of issuance of a controlled substance prescription.** Schedule II controlled substance prescriptions must be written with ink or indelible pencil or typewritten (except in cases of oral emergency schedule II prescriptions). Schedule III–V controlled substance prescriptions may be orally ordered by the practitioner. Prescriptions may be prepared by either the practitioner or an agent of the practitioner, and communicated to the pharmacy by the practitioner or the agent. Authorization for the prescription (or refill) must, however, originate with the practitioner. Both the practitioner and dispensing pharmacist are responsible for the completeness of the prescription. All prescriptions for controlled substances must include the following information:
   a. Full name and address of the patient
   b. Date the prescription is issued and signed (one and the same)
   c. Drug name, strength and dosage form
   d. Quantity of drug prescribed
   e. Directions for use
   f. Name, address and DEA registration number of the practitioner
   g. The signature of the practitioner (no preprinted or stamped signatures) as she would sign any legal document (All schedule II controlled substance prescriptions must be manually signed by the practitioner.)

4. **Emergency dispensing of schedule II controlled substances**
   a. An oral schedule II controlled substance prescription may be received from a practitioner in an emergency situation. An emergency prescription must include all of the information required for any controlled substance prescription. An emergency situation exists when **all three** of the following factors are present:
      (1) The immediate administration of the controlled substance is necessary for proper treatment of the patient
      (2) No appropriate alternative treatment is available, including administration of a controlled substance which is not in schedule II
      (3) It is not reasonably possible for the practitioner to provide a written prescription to be presented to the person dispensing the controlled substance before the dispensing
   b. **Proper dispensing.** The quantity prescribed and dispensed must be limited to the amount necessary to adequately treat the patient during the emergency period. If the practitioner

is not known to the pharmacist, the pharmacist must make a reasonable good faith effort to determine that the oral authorization came from a registered practitioner.

(1) Delivery of written prescription. The practitioner who authorizes the emergency prescription must, within 72 hours of the oral authorization, deliver a written prescription to the dispensing pharmacist. The prescription must contain the information required of all controlled substance prescriptions, have written on its face the words "Authorization for Emergency Dispensing," and the date of the oral authorization. The prescription may be delivered in person or by mail; if delivered by mail, it must be postmarked within the 72-hour period. Upon receipt, the dispensing pharmacist must attach it to the oral emergency prescription, which was previously reduced to writing.

(2) Failure to deliver a written prescription. If a practitioner fails to deliver the written prescription as required, the dispensing pharmacist must notify the regional office of the DEA. Failure by the pharmacist to notify the DEA serves to void the pharmacist's authority to dispense an oral emergency schedule II prescription. The pharmacist will be deemed to have unlawfully dispensed a schedule II controlled substance.

5. Persons who may dispense controlled substance prescriptions. A **pharmacist** acting in the usual course of his professional practice in a DEA registered pharmacy (or hospital or other registered facility) may dispense a controlled substance pursuant to a prescription. A **pharmacy intern** acting under the direct supervision of his preceptor in a DEA registered facility may also dispense a controlled substance pursuant to a prescription.

6. Dispensing procedures of controlled substances pursuant to a prescription. Once a controlled substance prescription has been lawfully issued by a practitioner and presented to a pharmacist, it may de dispensed in accordance with the following:

a. Presentation to the pharmacist. Schedules III and IV controlled substance prescriptions are valid for 6 months from the date of issuance by the practitioner. Schedule II controlled substance prescriptions have no time limit for presentation under the Act, although they are often recognized to be valid for up to 6 months. Schedule V controlled substance prescriptions also have no set time limit for presentation under the Act. Regardless of which schedule of controlled substance is involved, the good faith and "legitimate medical purpose" limitation will always apply and may serve to otherwise limit the validity of a prescription.

b. Information that must be recorded on the prescription by the dispensing pharmacist. Under the Act, a filled prescription is considered to be a lawful record of disposition for a controlled substance. As a result, every prescription for a controlled substance must contain certain information. Some of the information will already be contained in the prescription, although the dispensing pharmacist is responsible to ensure that all of the following information is recorded (usually on the face of the prescription):

(1) Name of the controlled substance
(2) Finished form of the controlled substance (dosage form and strength)
(3) Name and address of the person to whom it was dispensed
(4) Date of dispensing
(5) Number of units or volume dispensed (quantity)
(6) Written or typewritten name or initials of the individual who dispensed the controlled substance
(7) Serial number of the prescription

c. Required information on prescription labels. Every prescription label for a controlled substance must include the following information:

(1) Name and address of the pharmacy
(2) Serial number assigned to the prescription
(3) Date of the initial filling of the prescription (For refills, the date originally filled)
(4) Name of the patient
(5) Name of the prescribing practitioner
(6) Directions for use, and cautionary statements, if any
(7) For schedule II, III, and IV controlled substances, the federal crime transfer warning must appear on the container: "Caution: Federal law prohibits the transfer of this drug to any person other than the patient for whom it was prescribed."

d. Allowable quantities that may be dispensed. The Act contains no limitation concerning the quantity of a controlled substance that may be dispensed pursuant to a prescription. All quantities are, of course, limited to the "good faith" and "legitimate medical purpose" standards.

e. Filing controlled substance prescriptions. Written controlled substance prescriptions must be maintained for a period of 2 years from the date of the original dispensing or last refill, whichever is later. They must be available for inspection and copying by employees and agents of the DEA and be filed **segregated** from all other records in one of the following ways (state law usually dictates the method to be used):

(1) Using **three separate files** as follows:

(a) One file for schedule II controlled substance prescriptions

(b) One file for schedule III, IV, and V controlled substance prescriptions

(c) One file for unscheduled prescription drugs

(2) Using **two separate files** as follows:

(a) One file for all controlled substance prescriptions (II–V), as long as schedule III, IV, and V prescriptions have the letter "C" stamped in red ink in the lower right corner no less than one inch high

(b) One file for unscheduled prescription drugs

(3) Using **two separate files** as follows:

(a) One file for schedule II controlled substance prescriptions

(b) One file for all other controlled substances (III–V) and unscheduled prescription drugs, as long as schedule III, IV, and V prescriptions have the letter "C" stamped in red ink in the lower right corner no less than one inch high

f. Refill dispensing of controlled substances. Prescriptions for schedule II controlled substances may not be refilled. Prescriptions for schedules III and IV controlled substances may be refilled up to five times within 6 months from the date of issue of the prescription. Schedule V controlled substance prescriptions have no limitations for refilling under the Act; however, once again, the "good faith" and "legitimate medical purpose" limitations apply here as well as to all controlled substance refills.

(1) Refill information may be maintained either manually or by use of a computer. The Act requires that the information be maintained one way or the other, but not both ways. If **computerized refill records** are maintained, the system must have certain capabilities and the dispensing pharmacist must follow certain procedures.

(a) The computer must be able to provide on-line retrieval of the original prescription information, provide on-line retrieval of the refill history, a refill-by-refill audit trail, and an auxiliary procedure in those cases where the system experiences down-time.

(b) The system must also allow the pharmacist who refills a prescription to document that the information he entered into the computer is correct.

(2) When dispensing a refill, the pharmacist must record, on the back of the original prescription or by computer, the following information:

(a) Date of the refill

(b) Name or initials of the refilling pharmacist

(c) Amount of the medication dispensed (If the amount is omitted, the refill will be deemed to have been for the full face amount prescribed by the practitioner.)

g. Partial dispensing of controlled substances. The Act does not prohibit the partial dispensing of controlled substances in schedules III–IV, providing each partial filling is recorded in the same manner as refills, the total quantity dispensed in all partial fillings does not exceed the total quantity prescribed, and no partial filling occurs after 6 months from the date of issuance of the prescription. Likewise, all partial fillings of a schedule V prescription must not exceed the total quantity prescribed.

(1) Partial dispensing of a schedule II controlled substance. The partial dispensing of a schedule II prescription is allowed if the pharmacist is unable to supply the full quantity or the prescription is for a terminally ill patient or a patient in a long-term care facility (LTCF). Under no other circumstance may a schedule II prescription be partially dispensed.

(a) Inadequate supply. In cases of an inadequate supply, the dispensing pharmacist must note on the face of the prescription the amount dispensed. The remaining balance of the schedule II prescription must be dispensed within 72 hours of the first partial filling. If, for any reason, the balance is not dispensed within the 72-hour period, the pharmacist must notify the prescribing practitioner of this fact. The pharmacist may not dispense any further amounts pursuant to this prescription beyond the 72-hour period.

(b) Terminally ill and patients in LTCFs. It is the pharmacist's responsibility to ensure that a patient has a medical diagnosis documenting a terminal illness or that the patient is in a LTCF. Before any partial dispensing, the pharmacist must record on the prescription whether the patient is "terminally ill" or a "LTCF patient." Any partial dispensing without one of these notations shall be deemed to be a dispensing in violation of the Act. The total amount of the schedule II substance dispensed in all partial fillings must not exceed the total quantity prescribed. Schedule II prescriptions for a terminally ill patient or a patient in a LTCF are valid up to 60 days from the date of issuance of the prescription by the practitioner. All of the following information must be recorded, either manually on the back of the prescription or via computer (with similar capabilities required for computerized refill record-keeping), when partially dispensing a schedule II prescription for a terminally ill patient or patient in a LTCF:

(1) Date of the partial filling
(2) Quantity of drug dispensed
(3) Remaining quantity authorized to be dispensed
(4) Identification of the dispensing pharmacist

h. Transfer of refill information for a controlled substance prescription. Refill information concerning schedules III, IV, and V controlled substances may be transferred to another pharmacy only once (if allowed by state law). The communication must be made directly between two licensed pharmacists. Both the original prescription and the transferred prescription must be maintained for 2 years from the date of the last refill. Certain information must be recorded as follows:

(1) The **transferring pharmacist** must:
- **(a)** Write the word "void" on the face of the original prescription
- **(b)** On the back of the prescription, record the name, address, and DEA registration number of the pharmacy to which it was transferred and the name of the pharmacist receiving the information
- **(c)** Record the date of the transfer and the name of the transferring pharmacist

(2) The **receiving pharmacist** must:
- **(a)** Write the word "transfer" on the face of the transferred prescription
- **(b)** Record all of the information required for any controlled substance prescription (see I I 3), and include the following:
  - **(i)** Date of issuance of the original prescription
  - **(ii)** Original number of refills authorized on the original prescription
  - **(iii)** Date the prescription was initially dispensed
  - **(iv)** Number of valid refills remaining and the date of the last refill
  - **(v)** Pharmacy's name, address, DEA registration number, and original prescription number from which the prescription information was transferred
  - **(vi)** Name of the transferring pharmacist

J. Disposal of controlled substances to a patient without a prescription. Controlled substances that are not prescription (or legend) drugs under federal law may be dispensed to a patient at retail without a prescription. These drugs do not have on the manufacturer's label the federal statement: "Caution: Federal law prohibits dispensing without a prescription." The substances may be dispensed without a prescription in accordance with the following:

1. The dispensing must be made only by a licensed pharmacist. The actual cash transfer or delivery may be made by a nonpharmacist.

2. Not more than 8 ounces of any substance containing opium, 4 ounces of any other controlled substance, 48 dosage units of any substance containing opium, or 24 dosage units of any other controlled substance may be dispensed to the same purchaser in any 48-hour period.

3. The purchaser is at least 18 years old.

4. Any purchaser not known to the pharmacist must furnish suitable identification.

5. A bound record book must be maintained for 2 years from the date of the last entry. The following information must be recorded for each purchase:
- **a.** Name and address of the purchaser
- **b.** Name and quantity of controlled substance purchased
- **c.** Date of each purchase
- **d.** Name or initials of the pharmacist who dispensed the substance to the purchaser

6. All dispensing of a controlled substance without a prescription must be done in good faith and not to evade the provisions of the Act.

K. Security considerations

1. **Controlled substance seals.** Manufacturers must package certain controlled substances in a container with a securely affixed seal to reveal any tampering. Every bottle, multiple dose vial, or other commercial container of any controlled substance listed in schedule II, or of any narcotic controlled substance listed in schedules III and IV, must be packaged with such a seal.

2. **Felony convictions.** No DEA registrant may employ an individual who has access to controlled substances if that individual had previously been convicted of a felony offense relating to controlled substances.

3. **Manufacturer's label.** Every commercial container of a controlled substance must have on its label the symbol designating the schedule in which the controlled substance is listed. The symbol must appear in the upper right corner of the label or be overprinted on the label.

L. Record maintenance. All records required to be maintained under the Act must be kept by the registrant for a period of 2 years. The records may be maintained at a central location (e.g., at a chain pharmacy's regional office) after notifying the DEA. However, executed DEA 222 Forms (Copy 3), all controlled substance prescriptions, and all inventories must be maintained at the pharmacy, not centrally. All schedule II controlled substance records must be maintained separately and readily retrievable from all other records.

M. DEA inspections. Inspections by the DEA of any registered facility may be conducted only in a reasonable manner and during regular business hours. Inspection may be conducted after obtaining consent of the registrant or after the DEA has obtained an administrative warrant from a judge. An application for an administrative warrant must state with specificity the nature, extent, and authority to conduct the requested inspection. The scope of an administrative inspection extends to any records required under the Act, equipment and containers used in the handling of controlled substances, and the verification of compliance with any requirement of the Act. If records are removed from the registrant by the DEA, a receipt given to the registrant will list the items taken.

II. Federal Food, Drug, and Cosmetic Act (FDCA). In 1937, sulfanilamide elixir containing deadly diethylene glycol (automobile antifreeze) was manufactured without any safety data. There were numerous deaths associated with its use which prompted the federal government to pass the 1938 FDCA. The FDCA requires that all new drug products intended for use as labeled by the manufacturer in the United States must be proven to the federal government to be safe and effective. Such proof is submitted to the Food and Drug Administration (hereinafter "FDA") by use of a New Drug Application.

A. Definition. Under the FDCA, the term *drug* is defined as including all of the following:

1. Articles recognized in the official *United States Pharmacopoeia (USP),* official *Homeopathic Pharmacopoeia of the United States,* or official *National Formulary,* or any supplement to these

2. Articles intended for use in the diagnosis, cure, mitigation, treatment, or prevention of disease in man or other animals

3. Articles (other than food) intended to affect the structure or any function of the body of man or other animals

4. Articles intended for use as a component of any article specified in 1, 2, or 3 above

B. Legend drugs. Legend drugs are those medications that have on their label from the manufacturer the following federally required statement: "Caution: Federal law prohibits dispensing without prescription." Such medications may be dispensed directly to the patient by means of a valid written or oral prescription from a practitioner or by a valid refill authorization of either. By law, these medications must bear a label with adequate directions for use, which can only be given by a licensed practitioner and, therefore, the requirement of a prescription. A drug, intended for use by humans, is considered a legend drug (and have the above caution on its label) if any of the following apply:

1. It is a **habit-forming** drug (or derivative) containing any quantity of the narcotic or hypnotic substance α-eucaine, barbituric acid, β-eucaine, bromal, cannabis, carbromal, chloral, coca, cocaine, codeine, heroin, marijuana, morphine, opium, paraldehyde, peyote, or sulfonmethane.

2. Because of the drug's toxicity or other potential for a harmful effect, or its method of use, or collateral measures necessary to its use, it is **not safe** for use **except under the supervision** of a practitioner licensed by law to administer such drug.

3. The drug is a **new drug** for which an approved New Drug Application (NDA) limits its use to the professional supervision of a practitioner licensed by law to administer such drug. A new drug is broadly defined as being one that generally is not recognized among experts as safe and effective for use under the conditions prescribed, recommended, or suggested in the labeling. It is also defined as being a drug that, as a result of investigations to determine its safety and effectiveness for use under such conditions, has become so recognized but that has not, other than in the investigations, been used to a material extent or for a material time under such conditions. Finally, a new drug may result from a change in the dosage form, labeling, indications, or any other change in a drug product which is already being marketed. The ultimate decision of whether a drug is a new drug lies with the FDA because of its expertise in resolving technical and scientific questions.
   a. **NDA.** Every new drug marketed in the United States must be safe and effective for its intended use as labeled by the manufacturer. Proof of safety and effectiveness must be submitted to the FDA by the manufacturer via the NDA. When a new chemical entity (NCE) is identified by a manufacturer, it must obtain an Investigational New Drug Application (IND) before conducting preclinical animal tests and clinical human investigations.
   b. **IND.** Because a NCE has not yet been approved by the FDA as a safe and effective drug, a manufacturer is required to file an IND with the FDA. The IND allows a manufacturer to conduct research with the NCE and exempts the drug from certain prohibitions of the FDCA in order to facilitate clinical investigations, hence INDs are referred to sometimes as an Investigational New Drug Exemption. Generally, clinical investigation of a NCE is divided into three phases, with each phase involving a greater number of human subjects.
      (1) **Phase 1.** A phase 1 investigation is the initial introduction of an investigational new drug into humans to determine the metabolism, pharmacology, side effects, mechanism of action, and early evidence on effectiveness.
      (2) **Phase 2.** A phase 2 investigation includes the well-controlled, closely monitored clinical studies in order to evaluate the effectiveness of the drug for a particular indication and to further determine side effects and risks.
      (3) **Phase 3.** A phase 3 investigation includes expanded clinical trials to gather additional information concerning safety, effectiveness, and the overall benefit–risk relationship associated with the drug's use. This phase also includes gathering information to provide an adequate basis for physician labeling.
   c. **Treatment INDs (or treatment protocols).** The FDA may allow treatment IND, which allows a researcher (physician) to use an investigational drug as treatment in serious and life-threatening diseases where no comparable or satisfactory alternative drug or other therapy is available.

C. **Over-the-Counter (OTC) Medications.** Certain medication may be dispensed OTC at retail without a prescription. The federal government has determined that these medications may be safely and properly self-administered without the supervision of a practitioner licensed by law to administer (or prescribe) such a drug. Generally, these medications are not habit-forming and have a low toxicity or other potential for a harmful effect. These medications do not have the federal caution statement on their label (see II B).

1. OTC preparations must have **adequate directions** for use on their label, and the product must comply with the applicable FDA monograph. The FDCA requires all drugs marketed in the United States to be generally recognized as safe and effective. As a result, it convened review panels to review OTC drug effectiveness and create monographs for each therapeutic class of OTC drugs. This review is referred to as the Drug-Efficacy (or Effectiveness) Study

Implementation (DESI). All OTC drugs must comply with the applicable drug monograph or be considered misbranded (see II I) and subject to FDA regulatory action.

2. OTC preparations must have the following information on its label:
   a. Identity, in bold face, of the OTC product on the principal display panel
   b. Adequate directions for use
   c. Ingredients (including inert or inactive ingredients) in the product
   d. Net quantity of contents
   e. Expiration date of the product
   f. Lot number of the product
   g. Name and place of business of the manufacturer, packer, or distributor
   h. Disclosure of certain contents and the declaration of certain warnings, including habit-forming ingredients and warnings, pregnancy/nursing warnings, and aspirin warnings

D. Generic drugs

1. **Definition.** The *generic name* of a drug has been defined as its chemical name, a common name, or an official name used in an official compendium. A manufacturer seeking approval from the FDA for a drug that has already been proven to be safe and effective may file an Abbreviated New Drug Application (ANDA).

2. **ANDA.** A filing of an ANDA allows the approval of a drug for which exhaustive safety and efficacy studies have already been performed. A drug is considered to be the same as an approved drug when the two are identical in active ingredient(s), dosage form, strength, route of administration, indications, and conditions of use. Rigorous animal and human data to determine safety and effectiveness is not required in the ANDA. However, information showing that the generic version of the drug is bioavailable and bioequivalent to the pioneer (original) drug is necessary. Such approved drugs are listed by the FDA in the "Approved Drug Products with Therapeutic Equivalence Evaluations," commonly referred to as the FDA Orange Book (because it comes from the FDA in an orange binder).

E. Proprietary drugs. The *proprietary name* of a drug is the name given by the manufacturer to designate the drug's source of manufacture and to differentiate it from the same or chemically similar drugs from other manufacturers. Another name for the proprietary name of a drug is its tradename.

F. Established names for drugs. The FDCA authorizes the Commissioner of the FDA to designate an official name for any drug if he determines that such action is necessary or desirable in the interest of usefulness and simplicity. The FDCA also requires that a drug's established name appear on the label and labeling of the drug. A drug's *established name* is defined as follows:

1. It may be an **official name** designated by the Commissioner of Food and Drugs. For NCEs, the name should be simple and useful. In this regard, the FDA recognizes the U.S. Adopted Names Council (USAN) in deriving names for NCEs. The USAN name is considered to be an official name recognized in an official compendium. The FDA may use another name if the USAN or common or usual name is unduly complex, misleading, or is not useful for any other reason.

2. If no official name has been designated for the drug and the drug is an article recognized in an official compendium, then the **official title** contained in the compendium may be the established name.

3. If neither of the above two apply, then the **common** or **usual name** of the drug may be its established name.

G. Dispensing a prescription drug. A prescription drug may be dispensed only by a practitioner or by a pharmacist pursuant to a written or oral prescription of a practitioner, or a refill of either. The prescription label on the container dispensed to the patient must contain certain information or it will be considered misbranded and dispensed in violation of the FDCA. This information is minimal under the FDCA and is usually supplemented by state laws, which require more information. So long as this information is in English, the dispensing pharmacist will be in compliance with the FDCA. If any of the required information is in another language, then all of the required information must be in that language. The prescription must also be packaged in a child-resistant container as required under the Poison Prevention Packaging Act (see III). The following information must appear on every prescription label:

1. Name and address of the pharmacy
2. Serial number of the prescription
3. Date of filling the prescription or the date of the prescription
4. Name of the prescriber
5. Name of the patient (if stated in the prescription)
6. Directions for use and any cautionary statements contained in the prescription

H. Drug recall. The FDCA allows the FDA to initiate regulatory actions to ensure that unsafe, unfit, or ineffective products do not reach the market, or to promptly remove those products that do reach the marketplace. The enforcement actions that may be initiated include the release of information to the general public and/or professional groups; administrative actions and inspections; the institution of recall; or seizure, injunction, or criminal prosecution.

1. **Voluntary action of the manufacturer.** After several unsuccessful attempts by the FDA to receive court ordered recalls, the FDA recognizes that recalls are voluntary actions of the manufacturers and distributors. As a result, a recall may be undertaken at any time, or upon request of the FDA. If the FDA is unsuccessful in persuading a company to recall a product, or when the FDA determines that a recall is or will be ineffective, it may seek a court order condemning the product and allowing the product's seizure.

2. **Drug recall classification.** After the FDA has evaluated the problem(s) associated with the product and the degree of health hazard has been determined, the FDA will assign the recall one of the following classifications:
   a. **Class I**—a situation in which there is a reasonable probability that the use of or exposure to a violative product will cause serious adverse health consequences or death
   b. **Class II**—a situation in which use of or exposure to a violative product may cause temporary or medically reversible adverse health consequences or where the probability of serious health consequences is remote
   c. **Class III**—a situation in which use of or exposure to a violative product is not likely to cause adverse health consequences

3. **Recall procedure.** A recall strategy will be developed that will consider the depth of the recall (consumer level, retail level, wholesale level), the need for public warnings, and the extent of effectiveness checks for the recall. Every recalling company is responsible for notifying each of its affected direct accounts by first class mail, mailgram, or telegram. Public notification is made by the FDA via the weekly FDA Enforcement Report, which publishes each recall according to its classification.

I. Misbranding and adulteration. A misbranding or adulteration of a drug is prohibited by the FDCA. Although the misbranding and adulteration provisions are mainly concerned with the manufacturing of a drug, a pharmacist may also misbrand or adulterate a drug. The purpose of the misbranding and adulteration statutes is to protect the public health of consumers who are largely unable to protect themselves where drugs are involved. The adulteration and misbranding statutes are criminal in nature and may subject a pharmacist to criminal proceedings in federal court, in addition to administrative proceedings.

1. **Adulteration.** In general, the term *adulteration* refers to a change or variation from official formulary standards or from the manufacturer's standards. A drug is considered adulterated if any of the following conditions occur.
   a. If the drug consists in whole or in part of any filthy, putrid, or decomposed substance
   b. If the drug has been prepared, packed, or held under unsanitary conditions where it may have been contaminated with filth or rendered injurious to health
   c. If the drug's container is composed, in whole or in part, of any poisonous or deleterious substance that may render the contents injurious to health
   d. If the drug contains, for purposes of coloring only, a color additive that is unsafe within the meaning of the FDCA

e. If the drug is a new animal drug, or an animal feed containing a new animal drug, that is unsafe within the meaning of the FDCA
f. If the drug is purported to be a drug that is recognized in an official compendium, and its strength differs from, or its quality or purity falls below, the standard set forth in the compendium, unless the deviation is plainly and specifically stated on its label
g. If the drug is not a compound recognized by name in an official compendium; if its strength differs from, or its purity or quality falls below, that which it purports or is represented to possess
h. If the drug has been mixed or packed with another substance so as to reduce the drug's quality or strength
i. If the drug has been substituted, wholly or partially, with another substance
j. If the drug is an OTC drug and it is not packaged in the required tamper-resistant packaging or properly labeled in conformity with the tamper-resistant regulations (see IV)
k. If the drug (or medical device) is an ophthalmic preparation offered or intended for ophthalmic use that is not sterile

2. Misbranding. In general, the term *misbranding* means that a drug is sold or dispensed with a label or labeling that is in violation of the FDCA. *Label* is defined as being a display of written, printed, or graphic matter upon the immediate container of any article (or drug). *Labeling* is more broadly defined to include the label as well as other written, printed, or graphic matter upon any article or any of its containers or wrappers, or accompanying the article (or drug). A drug is considered misbranded if any of the following conditions occur.
a. If the labeling is false or misleading in any particular
b. If the drug is an imitation of another drug, or if it is offered for sale under the name of another drug
c. If the drug is composed wholly or partly of insulin and it is not properly batch certified under the FDCA
d. If the drug is composed wholly or partly of an antibiotic and it is not properly batch certified under the FDCA
e. If the drug is dispensed by a name that is recognized in an official compendium and it is either not packaged or labeled in conformity with the official compendium
f. If the drug is determined by the federal government to be liable to deterioration and it is not packaged in a proper form and manner, and the label fails to bear a statement of proper precautions
g. If the drug is dispensed in a non–child-resistant container, when a child-resistant container is otherwise required (see III)
h. If the manufacturer fails to place on the label any of the following:
  (1) Fact that certain drugs may be habit forming
  (2) Name of each active ingredient
  (3) Name and place of business of the manufacturer, packer, or distributor
i. If a pharmacist fails to place on a prescription container label any of the following:
  (1) Name and address of the pharmacy
  (2) Serial number of the prescription
  (3) Date of filling the prescription or the date of the prescription
  (4) Name of the prescriber
  (5) Name of the patient
  (6) Directions for use and any cautionary statements contained in the prescription
j. If an oral contraceptive is dispensed without the required patient package insert
k. If an intrauterine device that must be dispensed with a patient package insert is dispensed without the insert
l. If an estrogen product is dispensed without the required patient package insert
m. If a progestogen-containing product is dispensed without the required patient package insert
n. If a legend drug is dispensed (or refilled) without a prescription (or refill authorization) of a licensed practitioner it is deemed to be misbranded by the dispensing pharmacist
o. If the drug is an OTC drug and it is not packaged in tamper-resistant packaging or properly labeled in conformity with the tamper-resistant regulations (see IV)
p. If the drug is an OTC drug and it is not properly labeled in conformity with the labeling requirements of the FDCA
q. If the drug (or medical device) is an ophthalmic preparation offered or intended for ophthalmic use that is not sterile

3. **Violations under the Act.** Any misbranding or adulteration of a drug may subject the individual (e.g., a pharmacist) to imprisonment, a fine, or both. A pharmacy and pharmacist will be exempt from criminal sanctions in either of the following cases:
   a. **Certain cases of good faith.** When adulterated or misbranded products are received from a manufacturer or wholesaler in good faith by the pharmacy, it may not be held responsible in certain situations. This exemption applies only if it is a first violation and, if requested, the pharmacy or pharmacist furnishes to the government the name and address of the person from whom he received the drug and copies of all documents pertaining to its delivery.
   b. **Receipt of drug with a signed, written guaranty.** A pharmacy and pharmacist will be exempt from misbranding and adulteration violations when a signed, written guaranty is received from the wholesaler or manufacturer. The guaranty must contain the name and address of the person residing in the United States from whom the drug was received in good faith and a statement that the drug is not adulterated or misbranded.

4. **Seizures.** Any adulterated or misbranded drug will be subject to condemnation and seizure by the United States government after a hearing in any district court of the United States (or Territory) with proper jurisdiction. A seizure may be done without a hearing if the federal government has probable cause to believe that the violation would be dangerous to health, that the labeling of the misbranded article is fraudulent, or would be materially misleading to the injury or damage of the purchaser or consumer.

5. **Investigations and inspections**
   a. The United States Secretary of Health and Human Services has the authority to conduct examinations and inspections through federal employees and by officers and employees of any State, Territory or political subdivision duly commissioned by the U.S. Secretary of Health and Human Services as an officer of the U.S. Department of Health and Human Services.
   b. **Scope of investigation.** An investigator may enter a pharmacy or other establishment where adulterated or misbranded drugs are held and inspect all drugs, materials, containers, and labeling. The inspection does not extend to financial data, sales data other than shipment data, pricing data, personnel data, and other records that have no bearing on adulteration and misbranding. The investigator must present appropriate credentials and a written notice to the owner, operator, or agent in charge that he is authorized to conduct an investigation. The inspection must be done at reasonable times, within reasonable limits, and in a reasonable manner.

6. **Current good manufacturing practice (CGMP).** Under the FDCA, a drug is considered adulterated if it is not manufactured "in conformity with current good manufacturing practice." FDA regulations state with particularity the minimum CGMPs for methods to be used in, and the facilities or controls to be used for, the manufacture, processing, packing, or holding of a drug. The CGMPs ensure that a drug meets the requirements of the FDCA as to safety and has the identity and strength and meets the quality and purity characteristics that it purports.

J. **Registration of producers of drugs**

1. Manufacturers and businesses that distribute a drug manufactured by another but sold under its own label or tradename must register their establishment with the FDA. They also must submit a list of every drug (prescription and OTC) in commercial distribution with updates every June and December.

2. Pharmacies properly licensed by state law that do not manufacture or possess drugs for sale other than in the regular course of the practice of pharmacy are not required to register with the FDA. A pharmacy engaged in manufacturing or processing activities that is considered beyond the normal practice of pharmacy must register with the FDA and supply a list of every drug in commercial distribution.

K. **Package inserts.** The federal government has determined that prescription medication information needs to be disseminated to health professionals and, in the case of certain drugs, to the patient.

1. **Manufacturer's insert.** An amendment to the FDCA required that all manufacturers provide "full disclosure" concerning prescription medication that they market. Full disclosure is accomplished by means of a package insert that is enclosed with every commercial container

of a drug product. The insert should contain essential scientific information needed for the safe and effective use of the drug and be informative and accurate. It must not be promotional in tone, false, or misleading.

2. **Patient package insert.** The FDA has determined that, because of certain side effects associated with the use of particular drug products, patient package inserts must be dispensed to the patient at the time of dispensing the medications. The following products must be dispensed with a patient package insert which is supplied with the product from the manufacturer:
   a. **Oral contraceptives.** Hospital inpatients or long-term care facility patients may receive the insert before administration of the first oral contraceptive and every 30 days thereafter, as long as the therapy continues.
   b. **Intrauterine devices** for human use in contraception. Every practitioner dispensing such a device must provide the patient with an informative insert.
   c. **Estrogen and estrogen containing products.** Hospital inpatients or long term care facility patients may receive the insert before administration of the first estrogen and every 30 days thereafter, as long as the therapy continues.
   d. **Progestational drug products.** Hospital inpatients or long term care facility patients may receive the insert before administration of the first progestational drug product and every 30 days thereafter, as long as the therapy continues.
   e. **Isoproterenol inhalation products** require the following warning statement on the immediate container label of such a product: "Warning: Do not exceed the dose prescribed by your physician. If difficulty persists, contact your physician immediately."
   f. **Miscellaneous drug products.** Certain drug products were approved by the FDA with the provision that they must be dispensed along with a patient package insert that includes a particular warning or statement of benefits and risks associated with the use of the drug. For example, isotretinoin was approved for dispensing with an insert warning about serious fetal harm when administered to pregnant women.

L. Prescription drug samples

1. An **amendment** to the FDCA (Prescription Drug Marketing Act) severely restricted the distribution of drug samples by manufacturers. Under the FDCA, no person may sell, purchase, trade or offer to sell, purchase, or trade any drug sample. Samples may only be distributed upon written request of a practitioner. Manufacturers must maintain records of every sample distribution for a period of three years. Pharmacies may not receive samples from a manufacturer except in certain situations where a practitioner requests storage of his samples in the pharmacy.

2. **Importation under FDCA.** The Prescription Drug Marketing Act prohibits the import of prescription drugs once exported. Importation is allowed after notification and approval of the FDA and in cases of an emergency.

M. Medical devices. An amendment to the FDCA in 1976 (Medical Device Amendments) required a device manufacturer to provide reasonable assurance of the safety and effectiveness of the device. The amendment required the FDA to categorize each device on the market in 1976 into one of three classes: Class I, Class II or Class III, depending on each device's safety and effectiveness. Generally, **Class I** devices are those that have a reasonable assurance of safety and effectiveness. **Class II** devices are those that do not have the reasonable assurance of safety and effectiveness, but there is sufficient information about the device to establish special controls to ensure its safety and effectiveness (and may be marketed with such controls). **Class III** devices are those where information is not sufficient to provide reasonable assurance of their safety and effectiveness. Class III devices may be marketed only if they are proven to be substantially equivalent to a device on the market before 1976, by approval of a premarket application, or by reclassification into Class I or II.

1. **Medical device tracking.** Manufacturers of medical devices whose failure would be reasonably likely to have a serious adverse health consequence must track the device down the chain of distribution to the patient. Such tracking allows the manufacturer to take appropriate action with respect to recalls, defects, or other relevant information concerning the device. Every final distributor such as a pharmacy, hospital, or home health-care company must report certain information to the manufacturer. Tracking information must be maintained by the manufacturer and distributor for the useful life of the device and be available for inspection by FDA personnel.

2. **Manufacturer's reports.** Every device manufacturer must report to the FDA information, when received or made aware of, that reasonably suggests that one of its marketed devices may have caused or contributed to a death or serious injury. Likewise, hospitals and other medical service facilities must provide reports on adverse reactions to, or malfunctioning of, medical devices.

3. **Misbranding and adulteration.** Medical devices may be misbranded or adulterated in the same way that drugs are misbranded or adulterated (see II I).

III. Poison Prevention Packaging Act (PPPA).

The PPPA of 1970 requires that drugs for human use in an oral dosage form must be packaged for the consumer in special packaging. All such federal controlled substances and drugs dispensed pursuant to a prescription must be dispensed to the consumer in special packaging. ***Special packaging,*** referred to as **child-resistant** containers, is defined as a container that is designed to be significantly difficult for children under 5 years of age to gain access within a reasonable time. The container must not be too difficult for normal adults (ones with no overt physical or mental handicaps) to use properly and does not include packaging that all such children cannot gain access within a reasonable time. The Consumer Products Safety Commission is responsible for interpreting, establishing rules and regulations for, and enforcing the provisions of the PPPA.

A. Exceptions. The following medications are exempt from the special packaging requirements:

1. Sublingual dosage forms of nitroglycerin—other dosage forms intended for oral administration, such as nitroglycerin sustained release preparations, must be packaged in child-resistant containers
2. Sublingual and chewable forms of isosorbide dinitrate in dosage strengths of 10 mg or less
3. Erythromycin ethylsuccinate granules for oral suspension and oral suspensions in packages containing not more than 8 g of the equivalent of erythromycin
4. Cyclically administered oral contraceptives in manufacturers' mnemonic (memory-aid) dispenser packages that rely solely on the activity of one or more progestogen or estrogen substances
5. Anhydrous cholestryamine in powder form
6. All unit dose forms of potassium supplements, including individually wrapped effervescent tablets, unit dose vials of liquid potassium, and powdered potassium in unit-dose packages, containing not more than 50 mEq of potassium per unit dose
7. Sodium fluoride drug preparations, including liquid and tablet forms, containing no more than 264 mg of sodium fluoride per package and containing no other prescription medication
8. Betamethasone tablets packaged in manufacturers' dispenser packages, containing no more than 12.6 mg betamethasone
9. Pancrelipase preparations in tablet, capsule, or powder form and containing no other prescription medication
10. Prednisone in tablet form, when dispensed in packages containing no more than 105 mg of the drug, and containing no other prescription medication
11. Mebendazole in tablet form in packages containing not more than 600 mg of the drug and no other prescription medication
12. Methylprednisolone in tablet form in packages containing not more than 84 mg of the drug and no other prescription medication
13. Colestipol in powder form in packages containing not more than 5 g of the drug and no other prescription medication
14. Erythromycin ethylsuccinate tablets in packages containing no more than the equivalent of 16 g erythromycin
15. Conjugated estrogens tablets, USP, when dispensed in mnemonic packages containing not more than 32 mg of the drug, and containing no other prescription medication

16. Norethindrone acetate tablets, USP, when dispensed in mnemonic packages containing not more than 50 mg of the drug and no other prescription medication

17. Medroxyprogesterone acetate tablets

B. Requests for a non–child-resistant container. A prescribing practitioner may make a request in the prescription that the medication be dispensed in a non–child-resistant container. A practitioner may not, however, make a blanket request that all prescriptions issued by him be dispensed in non–child-resistant containers. The purchaser, or patient, may also make a request that the medication be dispensed in a non child-resistant container. The request of the purchaser, or patient, does not (under the PPPA) have to be in writing. The purchaser, or patient, may make a blanket request that none of his medications be dispensed in a child-resistant container. A dispensing pharmacist may never make the decision to use non–child-resistant containers.

C. Reuse of child-resistant containers. Reuse of child-resistant containers are prohibited by regulation of the federal Consumer Products Safety Commission. However, the Commission has indicated that glass containers may be reused as long as a new safety closure is used.

D. Manufacturer's packaging. Packaging from the manufacturer that is intended to be dispensed directly to the patient must be in child-resistant packaging. Bulk packaging intended to be repackaged by the pharmacist for each prescription does not have to be in special packaging from the manufacturer. Unit packaging from the manufacturer that will be dispensed directly to the consumer, or patient, must comply with the child-resistant requirements of the PPPA (unless specifically exempted; see III A).

E. Exemptions for easy access. Special packaging is not required in cases where OTC medication needs to be readily available to the elderly or handicapped persons. A manufacturer may supply a single size of a drug product in non–child-resistant packaging, as long as it also supplies the medication in packages that use the special packaging. Additionally, the package must be conspicuously labeled with the statement: "This package for households without young children." For those packages too small for this statement, the statement "Package not child-resistant" may be used.

F. Hospitals and institutions. The special packaging requirements of the PPPA of 1970 apply to household substances. *Household substance* is defined as "any substance which is customarily produced or distributed for sale for consumption or use, or customarily stored, by individuals in or about the household. . ." As long as the medication is administered by institutional personnel and is not directly dispensed to the consumer (patient), child-resistant containers are not required.

G. Miscellaneous products requiring special packaging. The PPPA of 1970 requires that certain household substances be distributed to the consumer in special packaging. Examples of these substances include furniture polish containing petroleum distillates, drain pipe cleaners, turpentine, paint solvents, and lighter fluid.

IV. Anti-Tampering Act.

The United States Congress passed the Anti-Tampering Act in 1984 due to a number of deaths that occurred in the early 1980s from OTC medication capsules contaminated with cyanide.

A. Violations. Unlawful acts involving a consumer product can be broken down into one of the following listed violations. The term *consumer product* includes any food, drug, device, or cosmetic, as well as any article, product, or commodity that is customarily used by individuals for purposes of personal care or to perform services ordinarily done within a household.

1. Tampering. Any individual who tampers or attempts to tamper with any consumer product that affects interstate or foreign commerce, or its labeling or container, may be in violation of the statute. A violation occurs when the individual acts (or threatens to act) with reckless disregard for the risk that another person will be placed in danger of death or bodily injury. Any individual who taints any consumer product or causes its labeling or container to be materially false or misleading is in violation of the statute if done with intent to cause serious injury to the business of another.

2. **False communications.** Knowingly communicating false information that a consumer product has been tainted may be a violation. If such tainting, had it occurred, would create a risk of death or bodily injury to another person, then the false communication is deemed a violation.

3. **Conspiracy.** An agreement between two or more persons to do (or further) either of the above acts is considered a violation.

B. **OTC tamper-resistant packaging.** Certain OTC products must be packaged, by FDA regulation, in tampering-resistant packaging. Examples include contact lens solutions and ophthalmic solutions. A **tamper-resistant package** is one having one or more indicators or barriers to entry which, if breached or missing, can reasonably be expected to provide visible evidence to consumers that tampering has occurred. To reduce tampering, the package must have **one** of the following characteristics:

1. Be distinctive by design so that the product cannot be duplicated by commonly available materials or processes

2. Use one or more indicators or barriers to entry that employ an identifying characteristic

C. **OTC tamper-resistant labeling.** The OTC product must be labeled with a prominently placed statement alerting consumers to the specific tamper-resistant feature of the package. The statement must be place so that it will be unaffected if the tamper-resistant feature is breached or missing.

D. **Medical devices and cosmetics.** Certain medical devices and cosmetics must be packaged in tamper-resistant packaging. The packaging requirements are similar to the requirements outlined above for OTC drug products.

V. Mailing prescription medication.

A. All prescription medication, including controlled substances and narcotics in schedules II–V, may be mailed from a physician, or pharmacist pursuant to a prescription, to the patient. Flammable substances (e.g., acetone) and alcoholic beverages may not be sent to a patient through the United States mail.

B. The medication must be placed in a plain outer container or be securely overwrapped in plain paper. There must be no markings of any kind on the outside wrapper or container that would indicate the nature of the contents.

VI. Ominibus Budget Reconciliation Act of 1990 (OBRA '90).

Under the Constitution of the United States, the federal government has no power or authority to directly regulate the practice of pharmacy. Such power rests with each state. The federal government can, however, indirectly regulate, or affect, the practice of pharmacy by attaching conditions of participation and reimbursement for federally funded programs.

A. **Medicaid prescriptions.** With respect to prescriptions dispensed to Medicaid patients (paid in part by the federal government along with the state government), the federal government has attached certain conditions for reimbursement. Such conditions were deemed necessary to stem the always increasing cost of the Medicaid programs. It was believed that improved medication compliance by Medicaid recipients would, in the long run, reduce the cost of the programs by reducing subsequent hospitalizations and other subsequent utilization of health care. As a result, pharmacists are required to do the following in the course of dispensing a Medicaid prescription:

1. Make a reasonable good faith effort to obtain and maintain a history of the patient, including a medication history

2. Conduct a review of every prescription for appropriateness and to screen for potential drug therapy problems

3. Make an offer to counsel each medicaid recipient concerning the drug (If the offer is accepted, the counseling must include the drug's proper administration; common adverse or severe side effects; techniques for self-monitoring; and proper storage.)

B. Manufacturer's best price. OBRA '90 requires manufacturers that wish to participate in the Medicaid program to offer the federal government its best price for prescription drugs. *Best price* is defined as the lowest price at which any purchaser is purchasing that drug product.

VIII. Narcotic treatment programs. Methadone use is currently allowed as part of a total treatment program for narcotic addiction. It is the only narcotic drug that has been approved by the FDA for use in the treatment of narcotic addiction. Regulations concerning methadone treatment programs have been jointly established by the DEA and FDA. Narcotic-dependent individuals are those who physiologically need heroin or a morphine-like drug to prevent the onset of signs of withdrawal.

A. Definition. A narcotic treatment program is an organization that administers or dispenses a narcotic drug to a narcotic addict for maintenance or detoxification treatment, and provides, when appropriate or necessary, a comprehensive range of medical and rehabilitative services. The program must be:

1. Approved by the FDA
2. Approved by the appropriate state agency, usually the state's Department of Public Health or equivalent
3. Registered under the Federal Controlled Substances Act with the DEA to use a narcotic drug for the treatment of narcotic addiction

B. Detoxification treatment is defined as dispensing of narcotic drugs in decreasing doses to an individual to alleviate adverse physiologic or psychologic effects incident to withdrawal of narcotic drug use. Detoxification is for a period not in excess of 180 days.

C. Maintenance treatment is the dispensing of a narcotic drug, at relatively stable dosage levels, in the treatment of an individual for dependence on heroin or other morphine-like drug.

D. Requirements to admit patients into a program. In general, for a patient to be admitted into a comprehensive maintenance program the following requirements must be met:

1. A program physician must determine that the person is currently physiologically dependent upon a narcotic drug and became physiologically dependent at least 1 year before admission to the program.
2. The patient must have voluntarily chosen to participate in the program, and must sign a "Consent to Methadone Treatment" (provided by the FDA) after being clearly and adequately informed about the use of methadone.

E. Take-home methadone. Take-home methadone may be given only to patients who, in the clinical judgment of the program physician, are responsible in handling narcotic drugs. The patient must come to the clinic for observation daily or at least 6 days a week. Over time, the program physician may reduce clinical observations to once weekly. Methadone for take-home use must be dispensed similarly to the dispensing of any schedule II controlled substance and include the treatment center's name, address, and telephone number on its label.

STUDY QUESTIONS

Directions: Each of the numbered items or incomplete statements in this section is followed by answers or by completions of the statement. Select the **one** lettered answer or completion that is **best** in each case.

1. All of the following prescription medications may be delivered by mail to the patient via the United States Postal Service EXCEPT

(A) Procainamide
(B) Ampicillin
(C) Hydromorphone
(D) Diazepam
(E) all of the above may be delivered by mail

2. Which of the following narcotic drugs has been approved by the FDA for use in the treatment of narcotic addiction?

(A) Morphine
(B) Codeine
(C) Methadone
(D) Hydrocodone
(E) None of the above

3. For the United States government to place a drug into Schedule III, which of the following findings must be made concerning the drug?

(A) The drug or other substance has a high potential for abuse
(B) Abuse of the drug or other substance may lead to limited physical dependence or psychologic dependence relative to the drugs or other substances in schedule IV
(C) The drug or other substance has no currently accepted medical use in treatment in the United States
(D) Abuse of the drug or other substance may lead to moderate or low physical dependence or high psychological dependence
(E) There is a lack of accepted safety for use of the drug or other substance under medical supervision

4. Under the Federal Controlled Substances Act, all of the following items must appear on a controlled substance prescription label EXCEPT the

(A) name, address and DEA number of the pharmacy
(B) name of the patient
(C) name of the prescribing practitioner
(D) serial number assigned to the prescription
(E) date of the initial filling of the prescription

5. Under the Federal Controlled Substances Act, all of the following entities must register with the DEA EXCEPT

(A) prescribers of controlled substances
(B) pharmacists who dispense controlled substances
(C) distributors of controlled substances
(D) importers of controlled substances
(E) universities conducting instructional activities with controlled substances listed in schedules II–V

6. Under the Federal Controlled Substances Act, which of the following statements concerning the emergency dispensing of a schedule II controlled substance is true?

(A) The practitioner who authorizes the oral prescription must, within 72 hours, cause a written prescription to be delivered to the dispensing pharmacist
(B) The quantity prescribed and dispensed must be limited to the amount necessary to adequately treat the patient during the emergency period
(C) It is not reasonably possible for the practitioner to provide a written prescription to be presented to the person dispensing the controlled substance prior to the dispensing
(D) No appropriate alternative treatment is available, including administration of a controlled substance which is not in schedule II
(E) All of the above statements are true

7. Under the Federal Controlled Substances Act, the crime transfer warning, "Caution: Federal law prohibits the transfer of this drug to any person other than the patient for whom it was prescribed," must appear on the prescription container label of all controlled substances EXCEPT

(A) Schedule II controlled substances
(B) Schedule III controlled substances
(C) Schedule IV controlled substances
(D) Schedule V controlled substances

8. Which of the following statements concerning drug recall classification is true?

(A) A Class I recall is a situation in which use of, or exposure to, a violative product is not likely to cause adverse health consequences
(B) A Class I recall is a situation in which use of, or exposure to, a violative product may cause temporary or medically reversible adverse health consequences or where the probability of serious health consequences is remote
(C) A Class I recall is a situation in which there is a reasonable probability that the use of, or exposure to, a violative product will cause serious adverse health consequences or death
(D) A Class II recall is a situation in which use of, or exposure to, a violative product is not likely to cause adverse health consequences
(E) A Class III recall is a situation in which there is a reasonable probability that the use of, or exposure to, a violative product will cause serious adverse health consequences or death

9. Under the Federal Food, Drug, and Cosmetic Act, all of the following statements are considered a misbranding of a drug EXCEPT if

(A) the labeling is false or misleading in any particular
(B) an oral contraceptive is dispensed without the required patient package insert
(C) the drug is an imitation of another drug, or if it is offered for sale under the name of another drug
(D) the drug consists in whole or in part of any filthy, putrid, or decomposed substance

10. All of the following oral medications are exempt from child-resistant packaging EXCEPT

(A) anhydrous cholestyramine in powder form
(B) nitroglycerin preparations in sustained release form
(C) cyclically administered oral contraceptives in manufacturers' mnemonic (memory-aid) dispenser packages that rely solely upon the activity of one or more progestogen or estrogen substances
(D) pancrelipase preparations in tablet, capsule, or powder form and containing no other prescription medication

ANSWERS AND EXPLANATIONS

1. The answer is E *[V].*
Narcotics and controlled substances in schedules II–V may be delivered to the patient by mail. The United States Postal Service no longer prohibits the mailing of narcotics by a physician or pharmacist (pursuant to a prescription) to the patient.

2. The answer is C *[VIII, VIII A, I I 2 c (2)].*
Methadone is the only narcotic drug that is approved by the FDA for use in the treatment of narcotic addiction. Only a properly registered narcotic treatment program may dispense methadone for maintenance or detoxification treatment. Pharmacies that are not so registered may only dispense methadone for severe pain.

3. The answer is D *[I A 3].*
To place a drug into schedule III the United States government must make the following findings concerning the drug: 1) it has a potential for abuse less than the drugs or other substances in schedules I and II; 2) it has a currently accepted medical use in treatment in the United States; and 3) abuse of the drug may lead to moderate or low physical dependence or high psychologic dependence.

4. The answer is A *[I I 6 c (1)–(7)].*
A pharmacy's DEA number is not required to appear on the medication container label dispensed to the patient.

5. The answer is B *[I B 2 a–k, I B 9 d].*
Agents and employees of DEA registrants, such as pharmacists, are exempt from registering with the DEA. Pharmacies must register with the DEA, not the individual pharmacists.

6. The answer is E *[I I 4 a, b].*
Emergency dispensing of an oral schedule II controlled substance prescription must be done in strict compliance with law. Before dispensing such a prescription, the pharmacist must make the threshold determination that ALL three factors are present which define an emergency situation (see I I 4 a). If any one of the three factors are absent the prescription is not for an emergency situation and a written prescription must be presented to the pharmacist.

7. The answer is D *[I I 6 c (7)].*
The federal crime transfer warning label is not required to appear on the prescription container label of schedule V controlled substances.

8. The answer is C *[II H 2 a–c].*
A Class I recall is a situation in which there is a reasonable probability that the use of, or exposure to, a violative product will cause serious adverse health consequences or death.

9. The answer is D *[II I 1,2].*
The Federal Food, Drug, and Cosmetic Act states that a drug is considered adulterated if it consists in whole or in part of any filthy, putrid, or decomposed substance. The terms "misbranding" and "adulteration" are often referred to in literature and case law as being the same or similar violations under the law. However, the Act sets forth specific instances of adulteration and specific instances of misbranding.

10. The answer is B *[III A 1].*
Only sublingual dosage forms of nitroglycerin are exempt from child-resistant packaging.

25
Reviewing and Dispensing Prescription and Medication Orders

Todd A. Brown

I. DEFINITIONS

A. Prescriptions are orders for medications, nondrug products, and services that are written by a licensed or mid-level practitioner who is authorized by statute to prescribe (see Appendix A). Prescriptions may be written or presented orally (by telephone) or presented electronically (i.e., via fax) to the pharmacist. The requirements of the prescription form may vary with state regulations. The prescription serves as a vehicle for communication from the licensed practitioner to the pharmacist about the pharmaceutical care needs of the patient. The following information should be included on a prescription:

1. **Patient information,** including name, age, and local address
2. **Date** on which the prescription was written
3. **Name and dosage form of the product.** The name of the product can be any of the following:
   - **a.** Proprietary (brand)
   - **b.** Nonproprietary (generic)
   - **c.** Chemical
4. **Product strength.** The strength of the product is not required if only one strength is commercially available or if the product contains a combination of active ingredients. It is advisable to include the strength to reduce the chance of misinterpreting the prescription. The strength of the product dispensed can be decided by the pharmacist after calculating the patient's dose.
5. **Quantity to be dispensed.** This should include the amount and the units of measure (e.g., grams, ounces, tablets). If the amount is not specified, the directions should specify the dose to be taken and the duration of therapy so that the pharmacist can calculate the quantity required for the patient.
6. **Directions for the pharmacist.** Directions may be required for:
   - **a.** Preparation (e.g., compounding)
   - **b.** Labeling (information to be put on the prescription label)
7. **Directions for the patient.** These should include explicit instructions on the quantity, schedule, and duration for proper use. "As Directed" should be avoided. If the directions vary, a minimum and maximum dose can be used.
8. **Refill information.** If refill information is not supplied, it is generally assumed that no refills are authorized. "As needed" [pro re nata (prn)] refills are not acceptable.
9. **Prescriber information.** This should include the name, office address, telephone number, Drug Enforcement Administration (DEA) number, state controlled-substance number, and signature of the prescriber. In some circumstances prescriptions may be written by a mid-level practitioner (not licensed to prescribe alone) under the supervision of a licensed prescriber. In these cases, both the mid-level practitioner writing the prescription and the supervising licensed prescriber's name should be included.

B. Medication orders are orders for medications, nondrug products, and services that are intended for use by patients in an institutional setting. The medication order generally includes:

1. **Patient information** (e.g., name, age, identification number)
2. **Any known allergies**
3. **Date and time** the order was written

4. **Prescriber information** (e.g., name, signature)
5. **Name and dosage form of the product.** This may include any of the following names:
   a. Proprietary (brand)
   b. Nonproprietary (generic)
   c. Chemical
6. **Product strength, dose, and route of administration.** The strength of the product is not required if only one strength is commercially available or if the product contains a combination of active ingredients. It is advisable to include the strength to reduce the chance of misinterpreting the prescription. The strength of the product dispensed may be decided by the pharmacist after calculating the patient's dose. The dosage and route of administration should be included to reduce the chance of misinterpreting the order and to allow for correct administration to the patient.
7. **Directions for the pharmacist.** These can be used for:
   a. Preparation (e.g., compounding)
   b. Labeling (i.e., information to be put on the prescription label)
8. **Instructions for administration,** including quantity schedule and duration of use
9. **Ancillary services** (e.g., radiologic procedures, laboratory tests, diet)

II. UNDERSTANDING THE PRESCRIPTION OR MEDICATION ORDER AND EVALUATING ITS APPROPRIATENESS

A. Understanding the order. A complete understanding of all information contained in a prescription or medication order is required. Each piece of information should be appropriate and consistent with the remaining information (i.e., the instructions for use should be appropriate for the medication being ordered). The pharmacist should read the entire prescription or medication order carefully to determine the prescriber's intent by interpreting the following information:

1. The patient's disease or condition requiring treatment
2. The reason the order is indicated, relative to the medical need of the patient (e.g., an antibacterial for an infection)
3. All terminology, including units of measure (apothecary, metric, or English) and Latin abbreviations (see Appendix A)
4. The name of the product, the quantity prescribed, and instructions for use
5. The name and address of both the patient and the prescriber

B. Evaluating the appropriateness. Complete information is required on the prescription or medication order to allow the pharmacist to evaluate the appropriateness. When it is incomplete, the pharmacist should obtain the required information from the patient or the prescriber. The following should be considered during an evaluation:

1. The patient's disease or condition requiring treatment
2. The patient's allergies or hypersensitivities
3. The pharmacologic or biologic action of the prescribed product
4. The prescribed route of administration
5. Whether the prescribed product might result in a drug–drug, drug–disease, or drug–food interaction
6. Whether the dose, dosage form, and dosage regimen are safe and likely to meet the needs of the patient
7. Whether the patient will have any difficulties adhering to the regimen and what the potential impact on the patient's outcome will be
8. Whether the total quantity of medication prescribed is sufficient to allow proper completion of a course of therapy

9. Whether a physical or chemical incompatibility might result (i.e., if the product requires extemporaneous compounding)

10. Whether the prescription was issued in good faith, for a legitimate medical purpose, by a licensed practitioner, acting in the course and scope of practice

C. **Discovering inappropriate prescriptions or medication orders.** Pharmacists are required to review medication profiles to ensure the appropriateness of prescriptions or medication orders. This is commonly called **drug utilization review.** Pharmacists should not fill prescriptions or medication orders that they have concerns with or that are considered inappropriate but should contact the prescriber. The process of calling a prescriber to discuss concerns is called **therapeutic intervention.**

1. When performing a therapeutic intervention, the following information should be provided:
   a. A brief description of the problem
   b. A reference source that documents the problem
   c. A description of the clinical significance of the problem
   d. A suggestion of solution to the problem

2. The following resolutions are possible to solve the problem or concern:
   a. The prescription or medication order will be dispensed as written.
   b. The prescription or medication order will not be dispensed.
   c. The prescription or medication order will be altered and dispensed.

3. If the pharmacist feels that, in his professional judgment, an order is inappropriate and could harm the patient, the pharmacist should not process the order. The pharmacist may also be required to explain the situation to the patient. If, after a therapeutic intervention, the pharmacist believes the order is still inappropriate, the guidelines of the institution should be followed.

III. **PROCESSING PRESCRIPTIONS AND MEDICATION ORDERS** requires that the pharmacist follow appropriate guidelines. An environment that limits distractions and disruptions during these activities will assist in increasing the accuracy of this process. Automation and the use of pharmacy technicians allow the pharmacist to oversee these functions but spend less time performing these activities. The time saved allows the pharmacist greater time for patient-focused activities, such as dispensing and counseling.

A. The following **information should be recorded on the prescription:**

1. The prescription number (for initial filling)

2. The date of filling or refilling

3. The product and quantity dispensed

4. The pharmacist's initials

B. **Product selection.** Generic substitution statutes as well as formulary and therapeutic substitution policies might provide direction in product selection.

C. **Product preparation** for use by the patient. The following might be necessary for preparation:

1. Obtaining the proper amount of medication to be dispensed

2. Reconstitution (the addition of liquid to make a solution or suspension)

3. Extemporaneous compounding (see Chapter 5)

4. Assembly of the medication delivery unit

D. **Selection of the proper package or container** is required to ensure product stability, to promote patient compliance, and to comply with legal requirements.

E. **Labeling the prescribed product**

1. The **prescription label** must contain the following information:
   a. Name and address of the pharmacy
   b. Patient's name
   c. Original date of filling
   d. Prescription number
   e. Directions for use
   f. Product's generic and/or brand name
   g. Product strength (if available in more than one strength)
   h. Quantity of medication dispensed
   i. Prescriber's name
   j. Lot number and expiration date
   k. Pharmacist's initials

2. **Unit-dose packages** contain one dose or one unit of medication. For a medication order that is dispensed in **unit-dose packages,** the label should identify the product's brand or generic name, strength, lot number, and expiration date.

3. **Auxiliary and cautionary labels.** To ensure proper medication use, storage, and compliance with applicable statutes, and to reinforce information provided during counseling, auxiliary and/or cautionary labels should be affixed when appropriate (see Appendix A).

4. For medication in schedules II–IV (see Chapter 24), a federal transfer warning is required.

F. **Record keeping.** The pharmacist should maintain **prescription files** and **records** in accordance with standards of sound practice and statutory requirements (see Chapter 24). These records should include a **patient profile system,** containing patient demographic information and a complete chronologic record of all medication use and services provided in the delivery of pharmaceutical care.

1. The patient profile should contain the following **patient information:**
   a. Patient's name
   b. Patient's address or room number (in institutional settings)
   c. Any known allergies, sensitivities, or history of idiosyncratic reactions to previous medications
   d. Birth date (i.e., to assess the appropriateness of the dose)
   e. Clinical condition(s) [i.e., to assist in ascertaining the appropriateness of the medication order and to prevent drug-disease interactions]
   f. Weight (i.e., to assess the appropriateness of the dose)
   g. Occupation (i.e., to detect conditions associated with a particular occupation and to assist in determining if the patient will be able to comply regimen)
   h. Nonprescription medication use (i.e., to prevent drug–drug interactions, drug–disease interactions, to assess medication effectiveness, and to detect possible adverse effects)

2. In addition, the patient profile should contain the following information from each prescription or medication order:
   a. Name of the medication
   b. Medication strength
   c. Dosage form
   d. Quality dispensed
   e. Directions for use
   f. Prescription number
   g. Dispensing date
   h. Number of refills authorized and remaining
   i. Prescriber's name
   j. Pharmacist's initials

IV. DISPENSING MEDICATION AND COUNSELING.

The dispensing of medication requires that the pharmacist verify that patients have the necessary knowledge and ability to adhere to the prescribed treatment. This will increase the likelihood of obtaining the desired outcomes.

A. **Counseling patients.** The pharmacist should evaluate the patient's understanding of each medication and supply additional information when the patient's information is incorrect or insufficient. The pharmacist might need to advise patients regarding the proper dosage, appearance, and name of the medication. Information about the route of administration, instructions for use, duration for use, and the reason the product was prescribed may also be needed. In addition, the following topics might also be appropriate during the counseling session:

1. **Special procedures.** As appropriate, the pharmacist should advise patients on how to take the medication (e.g., on an empty stomach, with plenty of water) and instruct the patient on foods to avoid while taking the medication (e.g., alcoholic beverages or dairy products).

2. **Potential adverse effects.** The pharmacist should ensure that patients are aware of the possible adverse effects associated with the medication. Patients should understand:
   a. The **frequency** of an adverse effect. This will assist patients in looking for common adverse effects and not being concerned with those that are rare.
   b. The **severity** of an adverse effect. This will assist patients in focusing on those adverse effects that are severe and not those that are inconsequential.
   c. What action should be taken to **manage** or **minimize** the adverse effect. This will assist patients in dealing with possible adverse effects in the appropriate manner.

3. **Proper storage.** The pharmacist should counsel patients on how to store medications properly to ensure stability and potency.

4. **Over-the-counter (OTC) products.** The pharmacist should instruct patients about the use of OTC products that might or might not be appropriate when taking a prescribed product.

B. **Counseling health professionals.** Medications may be administered to patients by health professionals (i.e., in an institutional setting). In these cases, the pharmacist should ensure that the health professional has sufficient knowledge to administer the product. Information that health professionals would need to administer medications safely and effectively include:

1. The choice of a particular product
2. The proper dosage, dosage regimen, and route of administration
3. The cost of the prescribed product and the costs associated with its use (i.e., administration costs and costs of treating possible adverse effects)
4. The availability of commercially made products
5. Potential adverse effects
6. Drug interactions
7. Physical incompatibilities
8. Safe handling and disposal procedures
9. Nutritional interactions or requirements
10. Drug interference with laboratory tests

V. PATIENT MONITORING.

The provision of pharmaceutical care requires a **pharmaceutical care plan.** Monitoring the impact of drug therapy should be performed on a regular basis. A pharmaceutical care plan maximizes the benefits of the prescribed therapy by increasing desired outcomes and decreasing undesired outcomes. Undesired outcomes associated with drug therapy are frequently called **drug-related problems.**

A. **Desired outcomes.** To increase the frequency and the benefits of desired outcomes, a pharmaceutical care plan should include the following:

1. **Therapeutic parameters.** To ensure that the patient achieves the maximum benefit from the prescribed product, the pharmacist should monitor for desired effects. This might require feedback from the patient about the reduction of signs and symptoms associated with the condition. This monitoring also might involve laboratory or other tests to measure the changes in patients. When a medication does not produce the desired outcome, it is commonly called **therapeutic failure.** Signs of therapeutic failure include:
   a. No change in the patient's clinical condition after an appropriate trial of medication
   b. A desire by the patient for nonprescription medication that has similar effects, or is used to treat the same condition as the prescribed medication

2. **Adherence.** A prerequisite of obtaining desired outcomes is that patients take the correct amount of medication in the correct way. This is commonly called **adherence.** Pharmacists can impact adherence by focusing on individual patient needs and resolving issues that are influencing the patient's behavior. The following situations should alert the pharmacist to possible adherence problems:
   a. Late refills in maintenance products. Patients who need to take medication on a long-term basis might forget to take their medication. Pharmacists can assist these patients by recommending products or activities that assist patients with these activities.
   b. Acute conditions for which completion of therapy of essential (i.e., completing the last 5 days of a 10-day course of antibiotic therapy). When patients do not receive enough medication to complete a course of therapy, pharmacists should ensure that patients obtain the remainder needed for successful completion.
   c. Early refills on medications that have abuse potential. Some medications can have addictive properties that can be abused by patients. Pharmacists can detect these problems by reviewing the amount of medication being dispensed to the patient and the frequency of requested refills.

B. **Drug-related problems.** The therapeutic drug-monitoring plan should attempt to detect drug-related problems with the goal of minimizing the frequency of these problems and decreasing the impact of those that continue. The plan should include monitoring for the following:

1. **Adverse effects.** Treatment of adverse effects that impact the patient increase the likelihood of positive outcomes by assisting the patient in compliance to the prescribed therapy. It also decreases the negative impact on quality of life.

2. **OTC interactions.** Monitoring for OTC interactions is important to ensure that patients do not take nonprescription medications that could interact with the prescribed therapy.

3. **Additive effects** consist of similar pharmacologic or physiologic effects from two different medications, which, when given together, cause unwanted effects in the patient.

STUDY QUESTIONS

Directions: Each of the numbered items or incomplete statements in this section is followed by answers or by completions of the statement. Select **one** lettered answer or completion that is **best** in each case.

1. Medication orders differ from prescriptions in which of the following ways? They

(A) are intended for ambulatory use
(B) contain only the generic name of the medication
(C) contain nonmedication instructions from the prescriber
(D) contain refill information
(E) contain the quantity of medication to be dispensed

2. If a therapeutic intervention is necessary, all of the following information should be communicated to the prescriber EXCEPT

(A) a declaration that "a mistake was made"
(B) a brief description of the problem
(C) a reference source that documents the problem
(D) an alternative or suggestion to resolve the problem
(E) a description of the clinical significance of the problem

3. The following information should be recorded on a prescription EXCEPT the

(A) prescription number
(B) date of filling
(C) expiration date
(D) product and quantity dispensed
(E) pharmacist's initials

4. A prescription label should contain all of the following EXCEPT the

(A) quantity dispensed
(B) lot number
(C) patient's diagnosis
(D) expiration date
(E) prescriber's name

5. Auxiliary and cautionary labels should be utilized for all of the following purposes EXCEPT to

(A) substitute for verbal consultation
(B) ensure proper usage
(C) inform of storage requirements
(D) comply with regulatory requirements
(E) warn against the concomitant use of certain drugs or foods

6. The following items are essential for a patient profile system EXCEPT

(A) the patient's name
(B) the prescriber's DEA registration number
(C) the patient's allergies
(D) the patient's birth date
(E) instructions for medication use

ANSWERS AND EXPLANATIONS

1. The answer is C *[I B].*
Because they are written for the care of inpatients, medication orders often contain laboratory, radiologic, and other nonmedication orders. Both medication orders and prescriptions may contain the brand or generic name of the drug. Only prescriptions contain the quantity of medication to be dispensed.

2. The answer is A *[II C 1].*
Information provided to the prescriber during a therapeutic intervention should include a description of the problem, reference source, description of the clinical significance, and an alternative. Informing the prescriber that a mistake was made does not encourage cooperation and resolution of the problem.

3. The answer is C *[III A].*
The prescription number, date of filling, product and quantity dispensed, and pharmacist's initials should be recorded on the prescription. The expiration date of the product being dispensed is not required.

4. The answer is C *[III E 1].*
The quantity of medication dispensed, lot number, expiration date of the product, and prescriber's name should be included on the label. The patient's diagnosis, although listed in the patient's profile, is not included on the prescription label.

5. The answer is A *[III E 3; IV A 1].*
Auxiliary and cautionary labels are an adjunct to verbal consultation, not a replacement. Appropriate uses for such labels include assuring for proper use, storage requirements, and compliance with statutory requirements; and warning against food and drug interactions.

6. The answer is B *[III F 1-2].*
The patient's name is required to identify each patient. Often the address or room number is required to identify patients with similar names. The patient's allergies, birth date, and instructions for use are required to prevent drug allergies and to assess the appropriateness of the prescription or medication order. The prescriber's DEA registration number is not necessary for a patient profile system.

26
Sterile Products

Ernest R. Anderson, Jr.

I. INTRODUCTION

A. Sterility, an absolute term, means the absence of living microorganisms.

1. **Sterile products** are pharmaceutical dosage forms that are sterile. Such products include parenteral preparations, irrigating solutions, and ophthalmic preparations (see Chapter 29).
2. **Aseptic technique** refers to the procedures used to maintain the sterility of pharmaceutical dosage forms.
3. **Parenteral preparations** are pharmaceutical dosage forms that are injected through one or more layers of skin. Because the parenteral route bypasses the protective barriers of the body, parenteral preparations must be sterile. The pH of a solution may markedly influence the stability and compatibility of parenteral preparations (see V B).
4. **Pyrogens** are metabolic by-products of live or dead microorganisms that cause a pyretic response (i.e., a fever) upon injection.
5. **Tonicity** refers to the tone of a solution and is directly related to the osmotic pressure exerted by the solute.
   a. **Hypotonic solutions** have a lower osmotic pressure than blood or 0.9% sodium chloride solution. Because these solutions cause cells to expand, administration can lead to pain and hemolysis.
   b. **Isotonic solutions** exert the same osmotic pressure as blood or 0.9% sodium chloride solution.
   c. **Hypertonic solutions** have a greater osmotic pressure than blood or 0.9% sodium chloride solution. These solutions are administered through a central vein to avoid the pain caused by red blood cell shrinkage (resulting from water loss).

B. Design and function of sterile product areas

1. **Clean rooms.** These areas are specially constructed, filtered, and maintained to prevent environmental contamination of sterile products during the manufacturing process. Clean rooms must meet several **requirements:**
   a. **High-efficiency particulate air (HEPA) filters** are used to cleanse the air entering the room. These filters remove all airborne particles size 0.3 μm or larger with an efficiency of 99.97%. In addition, HEPA-filtered rooms generally are classified as Federal Class 10,000, which means that they contain no more than 10,000 particles size 0.5 μm or larger per cubic foot of air.
   b. **Positive-pressure air flow** is used to prevent contaminated air from flowing into the clean room. In order to achieve this, the air pressure inside the clean room is greater than the pressure outside the room, so that when a door to the clean room is opened, the air flow is outward.
   c. **Counters** in the clean room are made of stainless steel or other nonporous, easily cleaned material.
   d. **Walls** and **floors** are free from cracks or crevices and have rounded corners. If walls or floors are painted, epoxy paint is used.
   e. **Air flow.** As with the HEPA filters used in clean rooms, the air flow moves with a uniform velocity along parallel lines. The velocity of the air flow is 90 (+ or − 20) feet per minute.
2. **Laminar flow hoods.** These clean-air work benches are specially designed, like clean rooms, to ensure the aseptic preparation of sterile products. Laminar flow hoods generally are used in conjunction with clean rooms. However, not all pharmacies involved in preparing sterile

products have clean rooms; in these instances, laminar flow hoods are vital to ensure aseptic preparation.

a. **HEPA filter requirement.** Like clean rooms, laminar flow hoods use HEPA filters, but the hoods use a higher-efficiency air filter than do clean rooms. Laminar flow hoods are classified as Federal Class 100, meaning that they contain no more than 100 particles size 0.3 μm or larger per cubic foot of air with an **efficiency of 99.99%.**

b. **Types of laminar flow hoods**

(1) **Horizontal** laminar flow hoods were the first hoods used in pharmacies for the preparation of sterile products. Air flow in horizontal hoods moves across the surface of the work area, flowing first through a prefilter and then through the HEPA filter. The major **disadvantage** of the horizontal hood is that it offers no protection to the operator, which is especially significant when antineoplastic agents are being prepared (see V D 2).

(2) **Vertical** laminar flow hoods provide **two major advantages** over horizontal flow hoods.

(a) The air flow is vertical, flowing down on the work space. This air flow pattern protects the operator against potential hazards from the products being prepared.

(b) A portion of the HEPA-filtered air is recirculated a second time through the HEPA filter. The remainder of the filtered air is removed through an exhaust filter, which may be vented to the outside to protect the operator from chronic, concentrated exposure to hazardous materials.

3. **Inspection and certification.** Clean rooms and laminar flow hoods are inspected and certified when they are first installed, at least every 6–12 months thereafter, and, in the case of hoods, when moved to a new location.

a. **Inspections** are conducted by companies with the sensitive equipment needed for testing procedures and with personnel who are specially trained in these procedures.

b. The **dioctyl phthalate (DOP) smoke test** ensures that no particle larger than 0.3 μm passes through the HEPA filter. In addition, an anemometer is used to determine air flow velocity, and a particle counter is used to determine the particle count.

II. STERILIZATION METHODS AND EQUIPMENT.

Sterilization is performed to destroy or remove all microorganisms in or on a product. Sterilization can be achieved through thermal, chemical, radioactive, or mechanical methods.

A. **Thermal sterilization** involves the use of either moist or dry heat.

1. **Moist heat sterilization** is the **most widely used** and reliable sterilization method.

a. Microorganisms are destroyed by **cellular protein coagulation.**

b. The objects to be sterilized are exposed to saturated steam under pressure at a minimum temperature of **121°C** for at least **15 minutes.**

c. An **autoclave** commonly is used for moist heat sterilization.

d. Because it does not require as high a temperature, moist heat sterilization causes **less product damage** compared to dry heat sterilization.

2. **Dry heat sterilization** is appropriate for materials that cannot withstand moist heat sterilization. Objects are subjected to a temperature of at least **160°C** for **120 minutes** (if higher temperatures can be used, less exposure time is required).

B. **Chemical (gas) sterilization** is used to sterilize surfaces and porous materials (e.g., surgical dressings) that other sterilization methods may damage.

1. In this method, **ethylene oxide** is used generally in combination with heat and moisture.

2. **Residual gas** must be allowed to dissipate after sterilization and before use of the sterile product.

C. **Radioactive sterilization** is suitable for the industrial sterilization of contents in sealed packages that cannot be exposed to heat (e.g., prepackaged surgical components and some ophthalmic ointments).

1. This technique involves either **electromagnetic** or **particulate radiation.**

2. Accelerated drug decomposition sometimes results.

D. **Mechanical sterilization (filtration)** removes but does not destroy microorganisms and clarifies solutions by eliminating particulate matter. For solutions rendered unstable by thermal, chemical, or radiation sterilization, filtration is the preferred method. A depth filter or screen filter may be used.

1. **Depth filters** usually consist of fritted glass or unglazed porcelain (i.e., substances that trap particles in channels).

2. **Screen (membrane) filters** are films measuring 1–200 μm thick made of cellulose esters, microfilaments, polycarbonate, synthetic polymers, silver, or stainless steel.
   a. A **mesh** of millions of microcapillary pores of identical size filter the solution by a process of physical sieving.
   b. **Flow rate.** Because pores make up 70%–85% of the surface, screen filters have a higher flow rate than depth filters.
   c. **Types of screen filters**
      (1) **Particulate filters** remove particles of glass, plastic, rubber, and other contaminants.
         (a) **Other uses.** These filters also are used to reduce the risk of phlebitis associated with administration of reconstituted powders. Filtration removes any undissolved powder particles that may cause venous inflammation.
         (b) The **pore size** of standard particulate filters ranges from 0.45–5 μm. Consequently, particulate filters cannot be used to filter blood, emulsions (e.g., fat emulsions), or suspensions because these preparations have a larger particle size. Special filters are available for blood filtration.
      (2) **Microbial filters,** with a pore size of 0.22 μm or smaller, ensure complete microbial removal or sterilization that is referred to as cold sterilization.
      (3) **Final filters,** which may be either particulate or microbial, are in-line filters used to remove particulates or microorganisms from an intravenous (IV) solution before infusion.

III. PACKAGING OF PARENTERAL PRODUCTS.

Parenteral preparations and other sterile products must be packaged in a way that maintains product sterility until the time of use and prevents contamination of contents during opening.

A. **Types of containers**

1. **Ampules,** the oldest type of parenteral product containers, are made entirely of **glass.**
   a. Intended for **single use only,** ampules are opened by breaking the glass at a score line on the neck.
   b. **Disadvantages.** Because glass particles may become dislodged during ampule opening, the product must be filtered before it is administered. Their unsuitability for multiple-dose use, the need to filter solutions before use, and other safety considerations have markedly reduced ampule use.

2. **Vials** are glass or plastic containers closed with a rubber stopper and sealed with an aluminum crimp.
   a. Vials have several **advantages** over ampules.
      (1) Vials can be designed to hold multiple doses (if prepared with a bacteriostatic agent).
      (2) The product is easier to remove from vials than from ampules.
      (3) Vials eliminate the risk of glass particle contamination during opening.
   b. However, vials also have certain **disadvantages.**
      (1) The rubber stopper can become cored causing a small bit of rubber to enter the solution.
      (2) Multiple withdrawals (as with multiple-dose vials) can result in microbial contamination.
   c. Some drugs that are unstable in solution are packaged in vials unreconstituted and must be **reconstituted** with sterile water or sterile sodium chloride for injection before use.
      (1) To accelerate the dissolution rate and permit rapid reconstitution, many powders are lyophilized (freeze dried).
      (2) Some of these drugs come in vials that contain a double chamber.
         (a) The top chamber, containing sterile water for injection, is separated from the unreconstituted drug by a rubber closure.

(b) To dislodge the inner closure and mix the contents of the compartments, external pressure is applied to the outer rubber closure. This system eliminates the need to enter the vial twice, thereby reducing the risk of microbial contamination.

3. Some drugs come in vials that may be attached to an IV bag for reconstitution and administration (**Add-Vantage** by Abbott).
   a. The Add-Vantage vial is screwed into the top of an Add-Vantage IV bag, and the rubber diaphragm is dislodged from the vial allowing the IV solution to dissolve the drug.
   b. The reconstituted Add-Vantage vial and IV bag are ready for administration when hung.

4. **Prefilled syringes** and **cartridges** are designed for maximum convenience.
   a. **Prefilled syringes.** Drugs administered in an emergency (e.g., atropine, epinephrine) are available for immediate injection when packaged in prefilled syringes.
   b. **Prefilled cartridges** are ready-to-use parenteral packages that offer improved sterility and accuracy. They consist of a plastic cartridge holder and a prefilled medication cartridge with a needle attached. The medication is premixed and premeasured.

5. **Infusion solutions** are divided into two categories: **small volume parenterals** (SVP), those having a volume less than 100 ml; and **large volume parenterals** (LVP), those having a volume of 100 ml or greater. Infusion solutions are used for the intermittent or continuous infusion of fluids or drugs (see VIII B).

B. Packaging materials. Materials used to package parenteral products include glass and plastic polymers.

1. **Glass,** the original parenteral packaging material, has superior clarity, facilitating inspection for particulate matter. Compared to plastic, glass less frequently interacts with the preparation it contains.

2. **Plastic polymers** used for parenteral packaging include polyvinylchloride (PVC) and polyolefin.
   a. **PVC** is flexible and nonrigid.
   b. **Polyolefin** is semi-rigid; unlike PVC, it can be stored upright.
   c. Both types of plastic offer several **advantages** over glass including durability, easier storage and disposal, reduced weight, and improved safety.

IV. PARENTERAL ADMINISTRATION ROUTES.

Parenteral preparations may be given by a variety of administration routes.

A. Subcutaneous administration refers to injection into the subcutaneous tissue beneath the skin layers, usually of the arm or thigh. Insulin is an example of a subcutaneously administered drug.

B. Intramuscular administration means injection into a muscle mass. The mid-deltoid area and gluteus medius are common injection sites.

1. No more than 5 ml of a solution should be injected by this route.

2. Drugs intended for prolonged or delayed absorption (e.g., methylprednisolone) commonly are administered intramuscularly.

C. IV administration is the most important and most common parenteral administration route. It allows an immediate therapeutic effect by delivering the drug directly into the circulation. However, this route precludes recall of an inadvertent drug overdose. Antibiotics, cardiac medications, and many other drugs are given intravenously.

D. Intradermal administration involves injection into the most superficial skin layer. Because this route can deliver only a limited drug volume, its use generally is restricted to skin tests and certain vaccines.

E. Intra-arterial administration is injection directly into an artery. It delivers a high drug concentration to the target site with little dilution by the circulation. Generally, this route is used only for radiopaque materials and some antineoplastic agents.

F. **Intracardiac** administration is injection of a drug directly into the heart.

G. **Hypodermoclysis** refers to injection of large volumes of a solution into subcutaneous tissue to provide a continuous, abundant drug supply. This route occasionally is used for antibiotic administration in children.

H. **Intraspinal** administration refers to injection into the spinal column.

I. **Intra-articular** administration means injection into a joint space.

J. **Intrasynovial** administration refers to injection into the joint fluid.

K. **Intrathecal** administration is injection into the spinal fluid; it sometimes is used for antibiotics.

V. PARENTERAL PREPARATIONS

A. **IV admixtures.** These preparations consist of one or more sterile drug products added to an IV fluid, generally dextrose or sodium chloride solution alone or in combination. IV admixtures are used for drugs intended for continuous infusion and for drugs that may cause irritation or toxicity when given via direct IV injection.

B. **IV fluids and electrolytes**

1. **Fluids** used in the preparation and administration of parenteral products include sterile water and sodium chloride, dextrose, and Ringer's solutions, all of which have multiple uses. For example, these fluids serve as vehicles in IV admixtures, provide a means for reconstituting sterile powders, and serve as the basis for correcting body fluid and electrolyte disturbances and for administering parenteral nutrition.
   a. **Dextrose (D-glucose) solutions** are the most frequently used glucose solutions in parenteral preparations.
      (1) **Uses.** Generally, a solution of 5% dextrose in water (D5W) is used as a vehicle in IV admixtures. D5W may also serve as a hydrating solution. In higher concentrations (e.g., a 10% solution in water), dextrose provides a source of carbohydrates in parenteral nutrition solutions.
      (2) **Considerations.** Because the pH of D5W ranges from 3.5 to 6.5, instability may result if it is combined with an acid-sensitive drug.
         (a) Dextrose concentrations greater than 15% must be administered through a central vein.
         (b) Dextrose solutions should be used cautiously in patients with diabetes mellitus.
   b. **Sodium chloride** usually is given as a 0.9% solution. Because it is isotonic with blood, this solution is called normal saline solution (NSS). A solution of 0.45% sodium chloride is termed half-normal saline.
      (1) **Sodium chloride for injection,** which is a solution of 0.9% sodium chloride, is used as a vehicle in IV admixtures and for fluid and electrolyte replacement. In smaller volumes, it is suitable for the reconstitution of various medications.
      (2) **Bacteriostatic sodium chloride for injection,** which is also a 0.9% solution, is intended solely for multiple reconstitutions. It contains an agent that inhibits bacterial growth (e.g., benzyl alcohol, propylparaben, methylparaben), which allows for its use in multiple-dose preparations.
   c. **Waters** are used for reconstitution and for dilution of such IV solutions as dextrose and sodium chloride. Waters suitable for parenteral preparations include sterile water for injection and bacteriostatic water for injection.
   d. **Ringer's solutions,** which are appropriate for fluid and electrolyte replacement, commonly are administered to postsurgical patients.
      (1) **Lactated Ringer's injection** (i.e., Hartmann's solution, Ringer's lactate solution) contains sodium lactate, sodium chloride, potassium chloride, and calcium chloride. Frequently, it is combined with dextrose (e.g., as 5% dextrose in lactated Ringer's injection).
      (2) **Ringer's injection** differs from lactated Ringer's injection in that it does not contain sodium lactate and has slightly different concentrations of sodium chloride and cal-

cium chloride. Like lactated Ringer's injection, it may be combined in solution with dextrose.

2. **Electrolyte preparations.** With ions present in both intracellular and extracellular fluid, electrolytes are crucial for various biologic processes. Surgical and medical patients who cannot take food by mouth or who need nutritional supplementation require the addition of electrolytes in hydrating solutions or parenteral nutrition solutions.
   a. **Cations** are positively charged electrolytes.
      (1) **Sodium** is the chief extracellular cation.
         (a) **Importance.** Sodium plays a key role in interstitial osmotic pressure, tissue hydration, acid—base balance, nerve-impulse transmission, and muscle contraction.
         (b) **Parenteral sodium preparations** include sodium chloride, sodium acetate, and sodium phosphate.
      (2) **Potassium** is the chief intracellular cation.
         (a) **Importance.** Potassium participates in carbohydrate metabolism, protein synthesis, muscle contraction (especially of cardiac muscle), and neuromuscular excitability.
         (b) **Parenteral potassium preparations** include potassium acetate, potassium chloride, and potassium phosphate.
      (3) **Calcium**
         (a) **Importance.** Calcium is essential to nerve-impulse transmission, muscle contraction, cardiac function, and capillary and cell membrane permeability.
         (b) **Parenteral calcium preparations** include calcium chloride, calcium gluconate, and calcium gluceptate.
      (4) **Magnesium**
         (a) **Importance.** Magnesium plays a vital part in enzyme activities, neuromuscular transmission, and muscle excitability.
         (b) **Parenteral preparation.** Magnesium is given parenterally as magnesium sulfate.
   b. **Anions** are negatively charged electrolytes.
      (1) **Chloride** is the major extracellular anion.
         (a) **Importance.** Along with sodium, it regulates interstitial osmotic pressure and helps to control blood pH.
         (b) **Parenteral chloride preparations** include calcium chloride, potassium chloride, and sodium chloride.
      (2) **Phosphate** is the major intracellular anion.
         (a) **Importance.** Phosphate is critical to various enzyme activities. It also influences calcium levels and acts as a buffer to prevent marked changes in acid–base balance.
         (b) **Parenteral phosphate preparations** include potassium phosphate and sodium phosphate.
      (3) **Acetate**
         (a) **Importance.** Acetate is a bicarbonate precursor that may be used to provide alkali to assist in the preservation of plasma pH.
         (b) **Parenteral acetate preparations** include potassium acetate and sodium acetate.

C. **Parenteral antibiotic preparations** are available as sterile unreconstituted powders, which must be reconstituted with sterile water, normal saline, or D5W, or as a sterile liquid parenteral.

1. **Administration methods.** Parenteral antibiotics may be given intermittently by direct IV injection, short-term infusion, intramuscular injection, or intrathecal injection.

2. **Uses.** Parenteral antibiotics are used to treat infections that are serious and require high blood levels or when the gastrointestinal tract is contraindicated, such as in ileus.

3. **Dosing frequencies** of parenteral antibiotics vary from once daily to as often as every 2 hours depending on the kinetics of the drug, seriousness of the infection, and patient's disease or organ status (e.g., renal disease).

D. **Parenteral antineoplastic agents.** These medications can be toxic to the personnel who prepare and administer them, necessitating special precautions to ensure safety. In addition, patients receiving antineoplastics can experience various problems associated with drug delivery.

1. **Administration methods.** Parenteral antineoplastics may be given by direct IV injection, short-term infusion, or long-term infusion. Some are administered by a nonintravenous route, such as the subcutaneous, intramuscular, intra-arterial, or intrathecal route.

2. **Safe antineoplastic handling guidelines.** All pharmacy and nursing personnel who prepare or administer antineoplastics should receive special training in the following guidelines to reduce the risk of injury from exposure to these drugs.
   a. A **vertical laminar flow hood** should be used during drug preparation, with exhaust directed to the outside.
   b. All syringes and IV tubing should have **Luer-Lok fittings** (see VII B 1, 4).
   c. **Clothing.** Personnel should wear closed-front cuffed surgical gowns and double-layered latex surgeon's gloves.
   d. **Negative-pressure technique** should be used during withdrawal of medication from vials.
   e. **Final dosage adjustment** should be made into the vial, ampule, or directly into an absorbent gauze pad.
   f. **Priming equipment.** Special care should be taken when IV administration sets are primed.
   g. Proper procedures should be followed for **disposal** of materials used in the preparation and administration of antineoplastics.
      (1) **Needles** should not be clipped or recapped.
      (2) **Preparations** should be discarded in containers that are puncture-proof, leak-proof, and properly labeled.
      (3) **Hazardous waste** should be incinerated at a temperature sufficient to destroy organic compounds (1000°C).
   h. After removal of gloves, personnel should **wash hands** thoroughly.
   i. Personnel and equipment involved in the preparation and administration of antineoplastic agents should be **monitored** routinely.

3. **Patient problems.** Infusion phlebitis and extravasation are the most serious problems that may occur during the administration of parenteral antineoplastics.
   a. **Infusion phlebitis** (inflammation of a vein) is characterized by pain, swelling, heat sensation, and redness at the infusion site. Drug dilution and filtration can eliminate or minimize the risk of phlebitis.
   b. **Extravasation** (infiltration of a drug into subcutaneous tissues surrounding the vein) is especially harmful when antineoplastics with vesicant properties are administered. Measures must be taken immediately if extravasation occurs.
      (1) Depending on the drug involved, emergency measures may include stopping the infusion, injecting hydrocortisone or another anti-inflammatory agent directly into the affected area, injecting an antidote (if available), and applying a cold compress (to facilitate a drug–antidote reaction).
      (2) A warm compress may then be applied to increase the flow of blood, and thus the vesicant, away from damaged tissue.

E. **Parenteral biotechnology products** are created by the application of biologic processes to the generation of therapeutic agents, such as monoclonal antibodies, various vaccines, and colony-stimulating factors.

1. **Potential uses** of these agents include cancer therapy, septic shock, infections, transplant rejection and vaccines against cancer, HIV infection, hepatitis B, herpes, and malaria.

2. **Characteristics.** Protein and peptide biotechnology drugs have a shorter half-life, often require special storage such as refrigeration or freezing, and must not be shaken vigorously lest the protein molecules be destroyed.

3. **Administration.** Many biotechnology products require reconstitution with sterile water or normal saline and may be parenterally administered by direct IV injection or infusion, or by intramuscular or subcutaneous injection.

VI. IRRIGATING SOLUTIONS.

Although these sterile products are manufactured by the same standards used to process IV preparations, they are **not intended for infusion into the venous system.**

A. **Topical administration.** Irrigating solutions for topical use are packaged in pour bottles so that they can be poured directly onto the desired area. These solutions are intended for such purposes as irrigating wounds, moistening dressings, and cleaning surgical instruments.

B. Infusion of irrigating solutions. This procedure, using an administration set attached to a Foley catheter, is commonly used for many surgical patients. Surgeons performing urologic procedures often use irrigating solutions to perfuse tissues in order to maintain the integrity of the surgical field, remove blood, and provide a clear field of view. To decrease the risk of infection, 1 ml of Neosporin G.U. Irrigant, an antibiotic preparation, often is added to these solutions.

C. Dialysis. Dialysates are irrigating solutions used in the dialysis of patients with such disorders as renal failure, poisoning, and electrolyte disturbances. These products remove waste materials, serum electrolytes, and toxic products from the body.

1. In **peritoneal dialysis,** a hypertonic dialysate is infused directly into the peritoneal cavity via a surgically implanted catheter. The dialysate, which contains dextrose and electrolytes, removes harmful substances by osmosis and diffusion. After a specified period of time, the solution is drained. Antibiotics and heparin may be added to the dialysate.

2. In **hemodialysis,** the patient's blood is transfused through a dialyzing membrane unit that removes the harmful substances from the patient's vascular system. After passing through the dialyzer, the blood reenters the body through a vein.

VII. NEEDLES AND SYRINGES

A. Hypodermic needles are stainless steel or aluminum devices that penetrate the skin for the purpose of administering or transferring a parenteral product.

1. **Needle gauge** is the outside diameter of the needle shaft; the larger the number, the smaller the diameter. Gauges in common use range from 13 (largest diameter) to 27. Subcutaneous injections usually require a 24-gauge or 25-gauge needle. Intramuscular injections require a needle with a gauge between 19 and 22. Needles between 18 gauge and 20 gauge are commonly used for compounding parenterals.

2. **Bevels** are slanting edges cut into needle tips to facilitate injection through tissue or rubber vial closures.
   a. **Regular-bevel needles** are the most commonly used type, and they are suitable for subcutaneous and intramuscular injections and hypodermoclysis.
   b. **Short-bevel needles** are used when only shallow penetration is required (as in intravenous injections).
   c. **Intradermal-bevel needles** are designed for intradermal injections and have the most bevelled edges.

3. **Needle lengths** range from 1/4 inch to 6 inches. Choice of needle length depends on the desired penetration.
   a. For **compounding parenteral preparations,** $1\frac{1}{2}$ inch-long needles are commonly used.
   b. **Intradermal injection** necessitates a needle length of 1/4 inch to 5/8 inch.
   c. **Intracardiac injection** requires a needle length of $3\frac{1}{2}$ inches.
   d. **IV infusion** requires needles that range in length from $1\frac{1}{4}$ inches to $2\frac{1}{2}$ inches.

B. Syringes are devices for injecting, withdrawing, or instilling fluids. Syringes consist of a glass or plastic barrel with a tight-fitting plunger at one end; a small opening at the other end accommodates the head of a needle.

1. The **Luer syringe,** the first syringe developed, has a universal needle attachment accommodating all needle sizes.

2. **Syringe volumes** range from 0.3 to 60 ml. Insulin syringes have unit gradations (100 units/ml) rather than volume gradations.

3. **Calibrations,** which may be in the metric or English system, vary in specificity depending on syringe size; the smaller the syringe, the more specific the scale.

4. **Syringe tips** come in several types.
   a. **Luer-Lok tips** are threaded to ensure that the needle fits tightly in the syringe. Antineoplastic agents should be administered with syringes of this type (see V D 2).
   b. **Luer-Slip tips** are unthreaded so that the syringe and needle do not lock into place. Because of this, the needle may become dislodged.

c. Eccentric tips, which are set off center, allow the needle to remain parallel to the injection site and minimize venous irritation.
d. Catheter tips are used for wound irrigation and administration of enteral feedings. They are not intended for injections.

VIII. INTRAVENOUS DRUG DELIVERY

A. Injection sites

1. **Peripheral vein injection** is preferred for drugs that do not irritate the veins, administration of isotonic solutions, and patients who require only short-term IV therapy. Generally, the dorsal forearm surface is chosen for venipuncture.

2. **Central vein injection** is preferred for administration of irritating drugs or hypertonic solutions, patients requiring long-term IV therapy, and situations in which a peripheral line cannot be maintained. Large veins in the thoracic cavity, such as the subclavian, are used.

B. Infusion methods

1. **Continuous-drip infusion** is the slow, primary-line infusion of an IV preparation to maintain a therapeutic drug level or provide fluid and electrolyte replacement.
   a. Flow rates must be carefully monitored. Generally, these rates are expressed as volume per unit of time (e.g., ml/hr or drops/min) and sometimes as μg/min for certain drugs.
   b. Administration. Such drugs as aminophylline, heparin, and pressor agents typically are administered by this method.

2. **Intermittent infusion** allows drug administration at specific intervals (e.g., every 4 hours) and is most often used for antibiotics.
   a. Three different techniques may be used.
      (1) Direct (bolus) injection rapidly delivers small volumes of an undiluted drug. This method is used to:
         (a) Achieve an immediate effect (as in an emergency)
         (b) Administer drugs that cannot be diluted
         (c) Achieve a therapeutic serum drug level quickly
      (2) Additive set infusion, using a volume-control device, is appropriate for the intermittent delivery of small amounts of IV solutions or diluted medications. The fluid chamber is attached to an independent fluid supply or placed directly under the established primary IV line.
      (3) The **piggyback method** is used when a drug cannot be mixed with the primary solution. A special coupling for the primary IV tubing permits infusion of a supplementary secondary solution through the primary system.
         (a) This method eliminates the need for a second venipuncture or further dilution of the supplementary preparation.
         (b) Admixtures in which the vehicle is added to the drug are known as manufacturers' piggybacks. Admixtures in which a special drug vial is attached to a special IV bag are known as the Add-Vantage system.
   b. In some cases, **intermittent infusion injection devices** are used. Also called scalp-vein, heparin-lock, or butterfly infusion sets, these devices permit intermittent delivery while eliminating the need for multiple venipunctures or prolonged venous access with a continuous infusion. To prevent clotting in the cannula, dilute heparin solution or normal saline solution may be added. Benefits of intermittent infusion injection devices include the following.
      (1) This method is especially suitable for patients who do not require, or would be jeopardized by, administration of large amounts of IV fluids (e.g., those with congestive heart failure).
      (2) Because intermittent infusion injection devices do not require continuous attachment to an IV bottle or bag and pole, they permit greater patient ambulation.

C. Pumps and **controllers** are the electronic devices used to administer parenteral infusions when the use of gravity flow alone might lead to inaccurate dosing or risk patient safety. Pumps and controllers are used to administer parenteral nutrition, chemotherapy, cardiac medications, and blood products.

1. **Pumps** are used to deliver IV infusions with accuracy and safety.
   a. Two **types of mechanisms** are used in infusion pumps.
      (1) **Piston-cylinder mechanisms** use a piston in a cylinder or a syringe-like apparatus to pump the desired volume of fluid.
      (2) **Linear peristaltic mechanisms** use external pressure to expel the fluid out of the pumping chamber.
   b. **Types of pumps**
      (1) **Volumetric pumps** are used for intermittent infusion of medications such as antibiotics. They are also used for continuous infusion of IV fluid, parenteral nutrition, anticoagulants, and anti-asthma medications.
      (2) **Syringe pumps** are used to administer intermittent or continuous infusions of medications (e.g., antibiotics, opiates) in concentrated form.
      (3) **Mobile infusion pumps** are small infusion devices designed for ambulatory and home patients, and are used for administering chemotherapy and opiate medications.
      (4) **Implantable pumps** are infusion devices surgically placed under the skin to provide a continuous release of medication, typically an opiate. The reservoir in the pump is refilled by injecting the medication through a latex diaphragm in the pump. This type of pump allegedly has a lower incidence of infection.
      (5) **Patient-controlled analgesia pumps** are used to administer narcotics intermittently or on demand by the patient within the patient-specific parameters, which are ordered by the physician and programmed into the pump.
   c. **Benefits.** Despite their extra costs and the training required by personnel, pumps provide a number of important benefits. They maintain a constant, accurate flow rate; they detect infiltrations, occlusions, and air. Pumps also may decrease the amount of time a nurse spends dispensing medication.

2. **Controllers,** unlike pumps, exert no pumping pressure on the IV fluid. Rather, they rely on gravity and control the infusion by counting drops electronically, or they infuse the fluid mechanically and electronically (e.g., volumetric controllers). In **comparison to pumps,** the following are characteristics of controllers.
   a. Controllers are less complex and generally less expensive.
   b. They achieve reasonable accuracy.
   c. Controllers are very useful for uncomplicated infusion therapy but cannot be used for arterial drug infusion or for infusion into small veins.

D. IV incompatibilities. When two or more drugs must be administered through a single IV line or given in a single solution, an undesirable reaction can occur. Although such incompatibilities are relatively rare, their consequences may be significant. A patient who receives a preparation in which an incompatibility has occurred could experience toxicity or an incomplete therapeutic effect.

1. **Types of incompatibilities**
   a. A **physical incompatibility** occurs when a drug combination produces a visible change in the appearance of a solution.
      (1) An **example** of physical incompatibility is the evolution of carbon dioxide when sodium bicarbonate and hydrochloric acid are admixed.
      (2) Various **types** of physical incompatibilities may occur:
         (a) Visible color change or darkening
         (b) Formation of precipitate, which may result from the combination of phosphate and calcium
   b. A **chemical incompatibility** reflects the chemical degradation of one or more of the admixed drugs, resulting in toxicity or therapeutic inactivity.
      (1) The degradation is not always visible. **Nonvisible chemical incompatibility** may be detected only by analytical methods.
      (2) Chemical incompatibility occurs in several **varieties.**
         (a) **Complexation** is a reaction between products that inactivates them. For example, the combination of calcium and tetracycline leads to formation of a complex that inactivates tetracycline.
         (b) **Oxidation** occurs when one drug loses electrons to the other, resulting in a color change and therapeutic inactivity.
         (c) **Reduction** takes place when one drug gains electrons from the other.

(d) **Photolysis** (chemical decomposition caused by light) can lead to hydrolysis or oxidation, with resulting discoloration.

c. A **therapeutic incompatibility** occurs when two or more drugs, IV fluids, or both are combined and the result is a response other than that intended. An example of a therapeutic incompatibility is the reduced bactericidal activity of penicillin G when given after tetracycline. Because tetracycline is a bacteriostatic agent, it slows bacterial growth; penicillin, on the other hand, is most effective against rapidly proliferating bacteria. To prevent therapeutic incompatibility in this case, penicillin G should be given before tetracycline.

2. **Factors affecting IV compatibility**

a. **pH.** Incompatibility is more likely to occur when the components of an IV solution differ significantly in pH. This increased risk is explained by the chemical reaction between an acid and a base, which yields a salt and water; the salt may be an insoluble precipitate.

b. **Temperature.** Generally, increased storage temperature speeds drug degradation. To preserve drug stability, drugs should be stored in a refrigerator or freezer, as appropriate.

c. **Degree of dilution.** Generally, the more diluted the drugs are in a solution, the less chance there is for an ion interaction leading to incompatibility.

d. **Length of time in solution.** The chance for a reaction resulting in incompatibility increases with the length of time that drugs are in contact with each other.

e. **Order of mixing.** Drugs that are incompatible in combination, such as calcium and phosphate, should not be added consecutively when an IV admixture is being prepared. This keeps these substances from pooling, or forming a layer on the top of the IV fluid, and, therefore, decreases the chance of an incompatibility. Thorough mixing after each addition is also essential.

3. **Preventing or minimizing incompatibilities.** To reduce the chance for an incompatibility, the following steps should be taken.

a. Solutions should be administered promptly after they are mixed to minimize the time available for a potential reaction to occur.

b. Each drug should be mixed thoroughly after it is added to the preparation.

c. The number of drugs mixed together in an IV solution should be kept to a minimum.

d. If a prescription calls for unfamiliar drugs or IV fluids, compatibility references should be consulted.

E. **Hazards of parenteral drug therapy.** A wide range of problems can occur with parenteral drug administration.

1. **Physical hazards**

a. **Phlebitis,** which is generally a minor complication, may result from vein injury or irritation. Phlebitis can be minimized or prevented through proper IV insertion technique, dilution of irritating drugs, and a decreased infusion rate.

b. **Extravasation** may occur with administration of drugs with vesicant properties (see V D 3 b).

c. **Irritation** at the injection site can be reduced by varying the injection site and applying a moisturizing lotion to the area.

d. **Pain** from infusion is most common with peripheral IV administration of a highly concentrated preparation. Switching to central vein infusion and diluting the drug might alleviate the problem.

e. **Air embolism,** potentially fatal, can result from entry of air into the intravenous tubing.

f. **Infection,** a particular danger with central IV lines, may stem from contamination during IV line insertion or tubing changes. Infection may be local or generalized (septicemia). The infection risk can be minimized by following established protocols for the care of central lines.

g. **Allergic reactions** can result from hypersensitivity to an IV solution or additive.

h. **Central catheter misplacement** may lead to air embolism or pneumothorax. To prevent this problem, catheter placement should always be verified radiologically.

i. **Hypothermia,** possibly resulting in shock and cardiac arrest, might stem from administration of a cold IV solution. This problem can be prevented by allowing parenteral products to reach room temperature.

j. **Neurotoxicity** may be a serious complication of intrathecal or intraspinal administration of drugs containing preservatives. Preservative free drugs should be used in these circumstances.

2. **Mechanical hazards**
   a. **Infusion pump** or **controller failure** can lead to runaway infusion, fluid overload, or incorrect dosages.
   b. **IV tubing** can become kinked, split, or cracked. It also may produce particulates, allow contamination, or interfere with the infusion.
   c. **Particulate matter** may be present in a parenteral product.
   d. **Glass containers** may break, causing injury.
   e. **Rubber vial closures** may interact with the enclosed product.

3. **Therapeutic hazards**
   a. **Drug instability** may lead to therapeutic ineffectiveness.
   b. **Incompatibility** may result in toxicity or reduced therapeutic effectiveness.
   c. **Labeling errors** can cause administration of an incorrect drug or improper dosage.
   d. **Drug overdose** can be caused by runaway IV infusion, failure of an infusion pump or controller, or nursing or pharmacy errors.
   e. **Preservative toxicity** can be a serious complication, especially in children. For example, premature infants receiving parenteral products containing benzyl alcohol can develop a fatal acidotic toxic syndrome, which is referred to as the **gasping syndrome.**

IX. QUALITY CONTROL AND QUALITY ASSURANCE

A. Definitions

1. **Quality control** is the day-to-day assessment of all operations from the receipt of raw material to the distribution of the finished product, including analytic testing of the finished product.

2. **Quality assurance,** an oversight function, involves the auditing of quality control procedures and systems, with suggestions for changes as needed.

B. Testing procedures. Various types of tests are used to ensure that all sterile products are free of microbial contamination, pyrogens, and particulate matter. In addition, ampules are subjected to a leaker test to ensure that the container is completely sealed.

1. **Sterility testing** ensures that the process used to sterilize the product was successful.
   a. The **official *United States Pharmacopeia (USP)* standard** for sterility testing calls for the following:
      (1) A 10-test sample for batches of 20–200 units
      (2) A minimum of two test samples for batches of less than 20 units
   b. The **membrane sterilization method** is often used to conduct sterility testing. Test samples are passed through membrane filters and a nutrient medium is then added to promote microbial growth. After an incubation period, microbial growth is determined.

2. **Pyrogen testing**, by means of qualitative fever response test in rabbits and an in vitro limulus lysate test, is often difficult to conduct because of a lack of facilities. Therefore, people handling sterile products should attempt to avoid problems with pyrogens by purchasing pyrogen-free water and sodium chloride for injection from reputable manufacturers and by using proper handling and storage procedures. Commercial laboratories are available to perform these tests.

3. **Clarity testing** is used to check sterile products for particulate matter. Before dispensing a parenteral solution, pharmacy personnel should check it for particulates by swirling the solution and looking at it against both light and dark backgrounds, using a clarity testing lamp or other standard light source.

C. Practical quality assurance programs for noncommercial sterile products include training, monitoring the manufacturing process, quality control check, and documentation.

1. **Training of pharmacists and technicians** in proper aseptic techniques and practices is the single most important aspect of an effective quality assurance program. Training should impart a thorough understanding of departmental policies and procedures.

2. By **monitoring the manufacturing process,** a supervisor can check adherence to established policies and procedures and take corrective action as necessary.

3. **Quality control** checking includes monitoring the sterility of a sample of manufactured products. The membrane sterilization method is practically employed using a commercially available filter and trypticase soy broth media.

4. **Documentation** of training procedures, quality control results, laminar flow hood certification, and production records are required by various agencies and organizations.

STUDY QUESTIONS

Directions: Each of the numbered items or incomplete statements in this section is followed by answers or by completions of the statement. Select the **one** lettered answer or completion that is **best** in each case.

1. Parenteral products with an osmotic pressure less than that of blood or 0.9% sodium chloride are referred to as

(A) isotonic solutions
(B) hypertonic solutions
(C) hypotonic solutions
(D) iso-osmotic solutions
(E) neutral solutions

2. Sterilization of an ophthalmic solution could be achieved in a community pharmacy by

(A) using a 5 -μm filter
(B) cold sterilization
(C) incorporating the drug into an already sterile vehicle
(D) radiation sterilization
(E) heat sterilization

3. Which needle has the smallest diameter?

(A) 25-gauge × 3/4″
(B) 24-gauge × 1/2″
(C) 22-gauge × 1″
(D) 20-gauge × 3/8″
(E) 26-gauge × 5/8″

4. Intrasynovial injection refers to injection into the

(A) muscle mass
(B) subcutaneous tissue
(C) spinal fluid
(D) superficial skin layer
(E) joint fluid

5. Advantages of the intravenous route include

(A) ease of removal of the dose
(B) a depot effect
(C) low incidence of phlebitis
(D) rapid onset of action
(E) a localized effect

6. The peripheral vein may be considered a suitable route for intravenous administration in which of the following situations?

(A) When an irritating drug is given
(B) When hypertonic drugs are given
(C) For long-term therapy
(D) For administering dextrose 15% as parenteral nutrition
(E) For postoperative short-term therapy

7. The formation of an insoluble precipitate as a result of admixing calcium and phosphate is an example of what type of incompatibility?

(A) Chemical
(B) Physical
(C) Pharmacologic
(D) Medicinal
(E) Therapeutic

8. Parenteral drug products in ampules undergo what type of testing to ensure the integrity of this parenteral container?

(A) Clarity testing
(B) Leaker testing
(C) Pyrogen testing
(D) Sterility testing
(E) Solubility testing

9. Which of the following drugs should NOT be prepared in a horizontal laminar flow hood?

(A) Ampicillin
(B) Dopamine
(C) CisPlatinum
(D) Nitroglycerin
(E) Bretylium tosylate

10. All of the following statements about D5W are true EXCEPT

(A) its pH range is 3.5–6.5
(B) it is hypertonic
(C) it is a 5% solution of D-glucose
(D) it should be used with caution in diabetic patients
(E) it is often used in intravenous admixtures

11. All of the following are potential hazards of parenteral therapy EXCEPT

(A) hypothermia
(B) phlebitis
(C) extravasation
(D) allergic reactions
(E) ileus

12. Procedures for the safe handling of antineoplastic agents include all of the following EXCEPT

(A) use of Luer-Lok syringe fittings
(B) wearing double-layered latex gloves
(C) use of negative-pressure technique when medication is being withdrawn from vials
(D) wearing closed-front, surgical-type gowns with cuffs
(E) use of horizontal laminar flow hood

ANSWERS AND EXPLANATIONS

1. The answer is C *[I A 5 a].*
Hypotonic solutions have an osmotic pressure less than that of blood (or 0.9% saline), whereas hypertonic solutions have an osmotic pressure greater than that of blood, and isotonic or iso-osmotic solutions have an osmotic pressure equal to that of blood.

2. The answer is B *[II D 2 c (2)].*
The use of a microbial 0.22 μm or smaller filter or cold sterilization is necessary to achieve sterilization. The addition of a nonsterile drug to a sterile vehicle will not accomplish this. Radiation sterilization is an industrial technique and is not suitable for use in a community pharmacy. Heat sterilization might degrade the ophthalmic drug, making it unsafe to use.

3. The answer is E *[VII A 1].*
The gauge size refers to the outer diameter of the needle. The lower the gauge size number, the larger the needle.

4. The answer is E *[IV J].*
Intrasynovial injection refers to an injection into the joint fluid. This administration route generally is used for certain types of corticosteroids to reduce inflammation.

5. The answer is D *[IV C].*
The intravenous route of drug administration allows for rapid onset of action and, therefore, immediate therapeutic effect. There can be no recall of the administered dose, and phlebitis, or inflammation of a vein, can occur. In addition, a depot effect (i.e., accumulation and storage of the drug for distribution) cannot be achieved by administering a drug intravenously. Delivering a drug intravenously results in a systemic rather than a localized effect.

6. The answer is D *[V B 1 a].*
Irritating drugs, hypertonic drugs, long-term therapy, and Dextrose 15% are best given by central intravenous (IV) administration. Peripheral vein injection is used for postoperative hydration, administration of nonirritating drugs, or isotonic solutions and for short-term IV therapy.

7. The answer is B *[VIII D 1 a].*
Physical incompatibilities occur when two or more products are combined and produce a change in the appearance of the solution, such as the formation of a precipitate.

8. The answer is B *[IX B].*
Leaker testing ensures that ampules are completely sealed during the manufacturing process. Pyrogen testing checks products for the presence of pyrogens, clarity testing tests for the presence of particulates, and sterility testing ensures that parenteral products are free from microbial contamination. Solubility testing may be done to determine the maximum soluble concentration of a drug.

9. The answer is C *[I B 2 b 1].*
CisPlatinum is an antineoplastic agent and, consequently, should be prepared only in a vertical laminar flow hood because of the potential hazard of these toxic agents to the operator.

10. The answer is B *[V B 1 a].*
D5W [dextrose (D-glucose) 5% in water] is acidic, its pH ranges from 3.5 to 6.5, and it is isotonic. It is often used in intravenous admixtures and should be used with caution in diabetic patients.

11. The answer is E *[VII E 1].*
Parenteral therapy is often a treatment for ileus. Hypothermia, phlebitis, extravasation, and allergic reactions can be hazards of parenteral therapy.

12. The answer is E *[V D 2].*
In order to prevent drug exposure a verticle flow laminar hood (not horizontal) should be used when an antineoplastic agent is prepared. The other precautions mentioned in the question are important safety measures for handling parenteral antineoplastics. All pharmacy and nursing personnel who handle these toxic substances should receive special training.

27 Parapharmaceuticals, Home Diagnostics, and Medical Devices

Todd A. Brown

I. AMBULATORY AIDS

A. Canes. These simple ambulatory aids provide balance and allow for the transfer of weight off a weakened limb.

1. **Use.** A cane is usually used by the strong side of a body to allow for a shifting of weight from the weakened side. The height of the cane must be adjusted to the individual patient. A cane that is correctly fitted allows for maximum weight transfer without allowing the patient to lock the elbow. The correct height should provide a 25° angle at the elbow or the top of the cane should come to the crease of the wrist while the patient is standing erect.

2. **Types of canes.** Canes may be made of wood or metal.
   a. **Wooden canes** come in varying thicknesses. The thicker ones are intended for males and the thinner ones are for females. Canes must be cut to the correct height for the patient.
   b. **Metal canes** are usually adjustable to fit the individual patient.
   c. **Folding canes** will fold into three sections to allow for easy transport when not in use.
   d. A **quad cane** is a metal cane that has a quadrangular base with four legs. This allows for greater weight transfer. The base of the quad cane comes in two sizes. The larger base is more stable but is more difficult to manipulate because of the size and weight.

B. Crutches may be used by patients with temporary disabilities (e.g., sprains fractures) or by those with chronic conditions.

1. **Use.** Crutches are used to take all the weight off an injured or weakened leg. The crutches are used in place of the leg. Crutch sizes range to fit from toddler to adult. Accessories that are used with a crutch include a tip to prevent slipping, hand grip cushion, and arm pad (for axillary crutch).

2. **Types of crutches**
   a. An **axillary crutch,** the **most commonly used** crutch, is typically used for temporary disabilities. The top of the crutch should be 2 inches below the axilla to prevent "crutch paralysis" (i.e., injury to the axillary nerves, blood vessels, and lymph nodes). The height of the hand grip should be set so that the elbow forms a 25° angle.
   b. A **forearm crutch** (also called a **Canadian** or **Lofstrand** crutch) supports the wrist and elbows, attaching to the forearm by a collar or cuff. It is commonly used by patients who need crutches on a long-term basis.
   c. A **quad crutch** is a forearm crutch with a quadrangular base that has four legs. The base is attached to the crutch with a flexible rubber mount. This allows for more stability and constant contact with the ground.

C. Walkers are lightweight devices that are made of metal tubing and have four widely placed legs.

1. **Use.** Walkers are used by patients who need more **support** than a cane or crutch but have reasonably good arm, hand, and wrist function. The patient holds onto the walker and takes a step, then moves the walker and takes another step.

2. **Types of walkers.** Walkers come in two sizes: **adult** and **child.** Some walkers are adjustable in height. Some walkers will fold to make storage or transporting easier. Walkers can have wheels on the legs. This allows the user to move the walker by rolling it instead of having to pick it up. Patients with loss of arm, wrist, or hand function on one side might use a **hemi-walker** or a **side-walker.**

a. A **hemiwalker** is similar to a standard walker except that it has one handle in the center of the walker for manipulation.

b. A **side walker** is placed on the side of the patient instead of in front of the patient.

D. Wheelchairs. Many different types of wheelchairs are available. The patient's disabilities, size, weight, and activities are the main considerations in wheelchair selection. The following options should be considered when selecting a wheelchair.

1. **Seat size.** The standard chair width is 16–18 inches, with widths available up to 48 inches. The chair should be 2 inches wider than the widest part of the patient's body (usually around the buttocks or thighs).
2. **Arms** can be fixed, detachable, half length, full length, or tilt back. The armrest and padding must also be considered.
3. **Tires** can be hard rubber or pneumatic (i.e., air filled).
4. **Wheels** can be reinforced with spokes or can be composite based.
5. **Leg rests** can be of different sizes and are available with padding.
6. **Footrests** can be of different sizes and are available with or without heel loops.
7. **Casters** (i.e., **front wheels**) can be hard rubber or pneumatic.
8. **Calf rests** can be of different sizes and are available with padding.
9. **Seat drapery** can be made of mesh or vinyl.
10. **Back drapery** can be made of mesh or vinyl.
11. **Cross braces** add stability and durability to the chair.
12. **Weight.** Standard wheelchairs weigh 35–50 pounds. Lightweight wheelchairs (25–35 pounds) are available for those who are unable to manipulate a standard chair and for ease of transport.

E. Sports chairs are wheelchairs that are lightweight and durable. They are designed for people who are very active.

F. Powered wheelchairs are designed for people who cannot wheel themselves. This type of wheelchair is powered by a motor and battery.

II. BATHROOM EQUIPMENT.

This equipment is used for patients who cannot get to the bathroom or to provide assistance to patients using the toilet or bathtub.

A. Elevated toilet seats are used to increase the height at which the patient sits over the toilet. This assists patients with limited mobility in getting on and off the toilet. Additional support can be provided with **toilet safety rails.** These rails allow the patient to transfer weight from the feet to the hands and they help to prevent the patient from falling when getting on or off the toilet.

B. Commodes are portable toilets that are used by patients who cannot get to the bathroom. Commodes contain a frame (with or without a backrest), a seat, and a bucket. Some are adjustable in height and have arms that drop to facilitate transfer to and from the commode. Folding commodes are available to make storage easier.

C. Three-in-one commodes function as combination commode, elevated toilet seat, and toilet safety rails. These are beneficial for patients requiring varying assistance during recuperation.

D. Bath benches are seats that fit in the bathtub and allow the patient to sit while taking a shower.

E. Transfer benches are placed over the outside of the bathtub. A transfer bench assists the patient in getting into the bathtub and serves as a bath bench while the patient takes a shower.

III. BLOOD PRESSURE MONITORS.

Patients with hypertension use this equipment to monitor blood pressure so that appropriate therapeutic decisions can be made. The type of monitor that is recommended should be determined by the patient's ability to use the product correctly. Types of monitors include:

A. **Mercury sphygmomanometer.** This model is the **most accurate** and does not need calibration. It does require the use of a stethoscope, which is difficult for some patients. Mercury in a graduated column rises in response to pressure applied to the cuff. The blood pressure is determined by reading the column of mercury and listening for the Korotkoff's sounds in the stethoscope.

B. **Aneroid sphygmomanometer.** This is similar to a mercury sphygmomanometer, except that instead of a column of mercury, it has a dial to be read. Aneroid models have the advantage of being **less expensive** than mercury models; however, they do require regular calibration to ensure proper results.

C. **Electronic or digital monitor.** This model detects blood pressure by using a microphone or by oscillometric technology, which converts movement of vessels into blood pressure. This type is easier to use than a sphygmomanometer and does not require the use of a stethoscope. These models are more **expensive** and need to be calibrated on a regular basis, but they represent an alternative for those patients who cannot use a sphygmomanometer.

D. **Finger monitors.** These detect blood pressure by compressing the finger and converting blood vessel movement into blood pressure by oscillometric technology. Many environmental conditions and medications can interfere with the results of these monitors, which are the **least accurate** and should be used only as a last resort.

IV. **HEAT AND COLD THERAPY.** For musculoskeletal disorders (e.g., sprains, strains, arthritis), treatment may include the application of heat or cold to specific areas of the body.

A. **Heat** can be applied in a dry or moist form. **Dry** heat is less effective than moist heat but is tolerated better and, thus, its clinical effectiveness is similar. **Moist** heat has an advantage of not causing as much perspiration and is often recommended. The application of heat produces vasodilatation and muscle relaxation. This facilitates pain relief and healing. Products that can deliver heat include:

1. A **hot water bottle,** a rubber container, should be half-filled with hot water. The remaining air is squeezed out of the container, which is then capped. This results in a flexible container that can be shaped to the area of the body for which it is being used to provide dry heat.
2. A **heating pad,** is an electrically powered pad that can produce moist or dry heat. Moist heat is supplied by inserting a wet sponge in a pocket that is next to the pad. Patients should be instructed to place the pad on top of the body instead of lying on the pad in order to prevent burning.
3. A **moist heat pack** (also called a hydrocollator) contains silica beads, which absorb heat when placed in boiling water. The heated pack is wrapped in a towel and applied to the body to provide moist heat. A moist heat pack must be kept moist to retain its absorbent properties. The pack should be wrapped in plastic and stored in the refrigerator if use is anticipated or in the freezer if long term storage is required.
4. A **gel pack** provides dry heat after it is heated in boiling water or in the microwave. It is reusable by repeating the heating process.
5. **Chemical hot packs** provide dry heat by mixing chemicals from two compartments. The chemicals undergo an exothermic reaction. Some packs are reusable by reheating in boiling water or in the microwave.
6. **Paraffin baths** provide moist heat by covering the body with heated paraffin. Once the wax cools and hardens it is removed. This method is commonly used for patients with arthritis in the hands and fingers.

B. **Cold** application is indicated mainly as acute therapy to decrease circulation to a local area and to provide pain relief. Cold is contraindicated in patients with circulatory stasis or lacerated tissue. Products that can deliver cold include:

1. An **ice bag** is a flexible plastic container designed to hold ice. The bag is then applied to the body.
2. A **gel pack** can be used to apply cold by freezing and then applying to the body.
3. **Chemical packs** can be used to apply cold. Chemicals from two compartments are mixed together, resulting in a chemical reaction that produces cold. These packs are used once and then disposed of.

V. HOME DIAGNOSTIC AIDS

A. Self-care tests or **kits** are used as screening tests or for monitoring. Many factors can affect the accuracy of the tests. The most common factor is the patient not following directions or having poor technique. Pharmacists should be prepared to counsel patients on the proper use and interpretation and to refer patients to appropriate medical follow-up if necessary.

B. Types of self-care tests

1. **Urine tests**
   a. The **urine glucose test** detects sugar in the urine. Patients with diabetes can use this to evaluate glucose control. Blood glucose testing is preferred, however, as it is more accurate and gives a better description of current glycemia.
   b. The **ketone test** detects the presence of ketones in the urine. This is used by patients with diabetes as an indicator of glucose control.
   c. **Ovulation prediction tests** predict when ovulation occurs to increase the chance of conception. These tests detect the presence of **luteinizing hormone (LH)** in the urine. Its presence means that ovulation should occur within 12–24 hours. When the patient performs the test is dependent on the length and regularity of the menstrual cycle.
   d. **Pregnancy tests** detect pregnancy by the presence in the urine of **human chorionic gonadotropin (hCG),** which is secreted after implantation of the embryo in the uterus. Many pregnancy test kits can detect hCG one day after missed menses. Patients taking hCG (e.g., as part of infertility therapy) could get false positive results. Patients should be referred to appropriate medical follow-up if they receive a positive result or two negative results 7 days apart and have not had menses.
   e. The **urinary bacteria test** detects the presence of nitrite in the urine. The presence of nitrite is used as an indicator of a **urinary tract infection (UTI)** because the most common bacteria associated with UTIs are gram-negative bacteria, which convert nitrate to nitrite. Because this test is not specific for bacteria, false results can occur. This test is used by patients who have chronic UTIs, as one indicator of a possible infection.

2. **Blood tests**
   a. The **cholesterol test** determines a patient's total cholesterol. The patient supplies a large drop of blood, and the test separates and then measures the total cholesterol. The measurement of the amount of cholesterol is then converted to a number via a chart that is provided with the test. This test can be useful for patients who want to monitor therapy; it is also useful as a screening test. It is not useful in determining appropriate therapy because more information about the patient is required. Patients with results that are borderline or higher should be referred to appropriate medical follow-up.
   b. The **blood glucose test** measures the concentration of glucose in the blood. Patients with diabetes use this information, along with diet, exercise, and medication, to keep glucose levels within a target range. Some blood glucose tests can be read visually by comparing the color change to a chart provided with the test. Visually read tests give an approximation of the blood glucose. Other tests are designed to be used with **blood glucose meters,** which read the test and display the actual blood glucose value. Patients using blood glucose tests must perform the test properly and understand appropriate actions to take when values are outside the desired range.

3. **Fecal occult blood tests** detect the presence of blood in the stool as a screening test for colorectal cancer. Patients drop a pad into the toilet after defecation. The pad will change color if blood is present. Patients should eat high fiber foods during the testing period and are instructed to test three consecutive stool samples. Patients with a positive result should be referred to appropriate medical follow-up. Certain conditions (gastrointestinal bleed,

nosebleed, menstruation), foods (red meat), medications (NSAIDs), and toilet bowl cleaners can produce false positive results.

VI. HOSPITAL BEDS AND ACCESSORIES.

Hospital beds are used by patients who are confined to bed for long periods of time or who require elevation of the head or feet as part of their treatment. Hospital beds may be manually or electrically operated.

A. Types of hospital beds

1. A **manual** hospital bed has no electrically powered motors; the head, foot, and bed height are adjusted manually.
2. A **semi-electric** hospital bed contains two motors that raise the head and foot of the bed. The patient can usually adjust the bed's position with a hand-held control. The height of the bed is adjusted manually. The semi-electric bed can usually be adjusted manually in case of loss of electricity.
3. A **fully electric** hospital bed contains three motors that can change the height of the bed as well as raise the head and foot via electrically powered motors. The fully electric hospital bed can usually be adjusted manually in case of loss of electricity.

B. Accessories

1. **Bed rails** keep the patient in the bed and assist in position changes.
2. A **trapeze** is a triangular-shaped object that hangs above the patient and is used to change position.
3. **Alternating pressure pads** are used by patients to prevent decubitus ulcers (i.e., bed sores). As a preventative measure, these pads inflate and change the areas of the body that receive pressure.

VII. INCONTINENCE AND INCONTINENCE PRODUCTS

A.

Urinary incontinence is a condition in which involuntary urine loss is a social or hygienic problem and is objectively demonstrable. Incontinence is a common problem in the elderly. Types of incontinence include:

1. **Urge** incontinence, which is the uncontrolled contractions of the bladder
2. **Stress** incontinence, a weakness of the sphincter that causes leakage when intra-abdominal pressure increases (i.e., laughing, coughing, sneezing); common in pregnancy
3. **Overflow** incontinence, which is caused by obstruction of urine flow from the bladder; common in elderly men due to prostrate enlargement
4. **Functional incontinence**, which is related to physical or psychologic problems that impair the patient's ability to get to the bathroom
5. **Iatrogenic incontinence,** caused by drugs or surgery

B. Incontinence products

1. **Shields** are disposable, absorbent pads that are placed in the underwear and held with an adhesive strip on the back of the pad. These pads are used for light incontinence problems.
2. **Undergarments** are disposable absorbent garments that are worn under the underwear and held in place with elastic straps that go around the hips. They are designed for moderate incontinence problems.
3. **Briefs** look like adult-sized diapers that are kept in place with adhesive strips. They are designed for heavy incontinence problems.
4. **Underpads** are absorbant pads to be placed on the bed underneath a patient with incontinence. These pads have a barrier to protect the bedding.
5. **Waterproof sheets** are plastic or vinyl sheets that protect the mattress. They may be lined with a soft material to prevent friction against the skin.

6. **Incontinence systems** are garments that look like underwear but have a pouch or pocket designed for a disposable or reusable pad.

VIII. ORTHOPEDIC BRACES AND SURGICAL FITTINGS.

These products promote proper body alignment and support injured areas. Pharmacists should have additional training before attempting to fit an orthopedic device.

A. **Abdominal supports** are elastic and are used to support and hold surgical dressings in place. Abdominal supports come in different widths.

B. **Arm slings** are used to provide comfort and support during recuperation from fractures, sprains, and surgery. The elbow should form a 90° angle in an arm sling to allow for proper circulation.

C. **Back supports** are worn by patients to provide support or promote proper alignment. The support is named to describe the area of the spine in which it is worn.

1. A **sacral belt** (also called **sacral cinch** or **sacroiliac belt**) supports the lower back.
2. A **lumbosacral support** supports the lower and middle back.
3. A **thoracolumbar support** supports the middle and higher areas of the back.

D. **Cervical collars** support or limit the range of motion of the neck. Cervical collars should be of sufficient length so that the patient can adjust the degree of compression. The width of the cervical collar should be the measurement from the chin to the sternum when the patient is standing straight, looking ahead.

1. **Soft** or **foam** cervical collars provide mild support and remind the wearer to keep the neck straight.
2. **Hard** or **rigid** cervical collars provide more support and limit movement to a greater degree.
3. A **Philadelphia** or **extrication** collar is used to immobilize the neck and is commonly used in emergency situations.

E. **Clavicle supports** are used as aids for the reduction and stabilization of the clavicle (i.e., collarbone). These supports are sometimes called **figure-eight straps** because of their appearance.

F. **Knee braces** (also called **knee cages**) are used to support the knee. Some braces have metal stays on the side to prevent the lateral movement of the knee. Those with metal stays may also have hinges to allow for movement of the knee. Some knee braces have a cut-out hole and padding around the patella (i.e., knee cap) to prevent its movement.

G. **Knee immobilizers** extend from the thigh to the ankle to prevent any motion of the knee and are used for severe injuries and fractures.

H. **Rib belts** are used to stabilize rib fractures. Female rib belts are cut down in the front to go under the breasts.

I. **Shoulder immobilizers** prevent movement of the shoulder and arm. The elbow should be at a 90° angle to allow for healing without affecting circulation.

J. **Tennis elbow supports** apply pressure to the forearm to provide for pain relief and decrease inflammation from tennis elbow (i.e., epicondylitis).

IX. OSTOMY APPLIANCES AND ACCESSORIES

A. **Definitions.** An **ostomy** is a surgical procedure in which an artificial opening is created in the abdominal wall for the purpose of eliminating waste. The opening is called a **stoma.** Each procedure is named to describe the anatomical location involved.

1. In a **colostomy,** part of the colon is cut and attached to the abdominal wall. This procedure is done mainly in patients with colon or rectal cancer, lower bowel obstruction, or

diverticulitis. A colostomy may be temporary or permanent, the discharge may be liquid or semisolid (as with an **ascending** colostomy), or it may be solid (as with a **descending** or **sigmoid** colostomy). Patients with an ascending colostomy and some patients with a transverse colostomy have gastric enzymes present in the discharge. These patients must take extra care to ensure that the discharge does not come into contact with the skin.

2. In an **ileostomy,** the ileum is attached to the abdominal wall. This procedure is performed in patients with ulcerative colitis or Crohn's disease.

3. A **urostomy** is performed in patients with bladder cancer. In this procedure, an **ileal conduit** is created by attaching the ureters to the ileum and the distal end of the ileum to the abdominal wall.

B. Ostomy appliances. The selection of an ostomy appliance (a device used to collect stomal discharge) depends on the type of discharge produced. In addition to size, flexibility, and size of the stoma, appliances may have detachable pouches and be able to be drained by releasing a clip at the bottom of the appliance.

C. Ostomy accessories

1. **Washers, powder paste,** and **barriers** are designed to protect the skin around a stoma.
2. **Cement, elastic belts,** and **tape** are used to hold the appliance in place.
3. **Deodorizers** help control fecal odor. **External** deodorizers can be placed into the appliance, systemic deodorizers (e.g., bismuth subgallate, chlorophyll, charcoal) can be ingested as **internal** deodorizers.
4. **Moisturizers** and **disinfectants** can be used to treat the skin and prevent complications.

D. Special considerations for ostomy patients. Drug therapy can present unique problems for ostomates. Absorption of enteric-coated or sustained-release products may not be possible. Antibiotics, sulfa drugs, laxatives, and diuretics are some of the common problem medications in these patients.

X. RESPIRATORY EQUIPMENT

A. Continuous positive airway pressure is used in patients with sleep apnea. The pressure supplied from this machine keeps the airway open. It is worn typically while sleeping to allow the patient to sleep without disturbance.

B. A **humidifier** puts moisture into the air by breaking water into small particles and blowing them into the air to be evaporated. Humidifiers are sometimes called "cool mist vaporizers." An **ultrasonic humidifier** contains a transducer, which produces a finer mist. It is commonly used to promote expectoration in patients with upper respiratory infections. Both types of humidifiers need to be cleaned regularly to prevent the growth of mold or bacteria.

C. A **nebulizer** is used to deliver medication to the mouth or throat. Patients with a sore throat may use a nebulizer to deliver a topical anesthetic to the throat. An **ultrasonic nebulizer** is used to deliver medication into the lungs. The medication is diluted with normal saline and then inhaled. An ultrasonic nebulizer is used by patients with respiratory infections, asthma, or chronic obstructive pulmonary disease (COPD).

D. Oxygen is administered for a variety of conditions. Oxygen can be stored as a gas or a liquid or can be extracted from the air via a **concentrator.** The amount of oxygen required by the patient is measured in liters per minute (L/min). Before oxygen is delivered to the patient, moisture is added to reduce irritation to the respiratory tract. A **registered respiratory therapist** can be consulted for information on the correct procedures, cautions, and laws regarding oxygen use.

E. A **peak flow meter** is used by patients with asthma to detect constriction of the airways before symptoms appear. Early detection of an upcoming attack allows for therapy designed to stop or minimize the severity of the disease. Patients exhale as much as possible into a peak flow meter to obtain the expiratory flow rate. If this rate is below a predetermined baseline, patients might be instructed to change therapy.

F. Vaporizers are similar to humidifiers because they are used to deliver moisture to the air. These devices produce moisture by heating water to produce steam. They are commonly used to promote expectoration in patients with upper respiratory infections.

XI. THERMOMETERS.

These instruments measure body temperature and are **most commonly used** to detect or evaluate the treatment of infections.

A. A **mercury fever thermometer** has a sealed glass constriction chamber that contains liquid mercury. Responding to temperature changes, the mercury expands or contracts. It remains at the maximum temperature registered until shaken back into the reservoir at the bottom. Mercury fever thermometers are graduated from 96° F to 106° F in two-tenths of a degree increments. Mercury thermometers should be cleaned and sterilized with alcohol after each use.

1. The **oral** thermometer has a long slender reservoir. It is placed under the tongue, and the lips are sealed around the thermometer for 3 minutes.
2. The **rectal** thermometer has a blunt, pear-shaped bulb to prevent breakage and aid in retention. It is inserted 1 inch into the rectum and left for at least 2 minutes. A lubricant should be used to aid insertion. Rectal temperature is 1° higher than oral temperature.
3. The **security** thermometer (also called a **stubby** thermometer) has a short, stubby bulb to prevent it from breaking. It can be used as an oral or rectal thermometer.
4. Any of the three types of mercury thermometers can be used to take the **axillary temperature** if an oral or rectal temperature cannot be taken. An axillary temperature is taken by holding the thermometer snugly under the arm for 3–4 minutes. Axillary temperature is 1° lower than oral temperature.

B. The **basal thermometer** is used to measure basal body temperature. The basal body temperature is used to predict ovulation to increase or decrease the chance of conception. Basal body temperature is usually taken orally but can also be taken rectally.

C. Electronic thermometers register temperature quickly. Heat alters the current running through a resistor and the temperature is displayed via a digital readout. The current is supplied by a battery, some of which are rechargeable. Electric thermometers can be used orally or rectally and generally require placing a plastic sheath over the tip of the thermometer before using.

D. Tympanic thermometers use infrared technology to detect the temperature of the tympanic membrane. The temperature is determined within seconds and is less invasive than other thermometers. These thermometers use disposable tips that are inserted into the ear.

E. Liquid crystal strips are placed directly on the skin (usually the forehead) to calculate body temperature. This method is not as accurate as others and should be reserved for situations in which other methods are not possible.

XII. URINARY CATHETERS.

These devices allow for the **collection** and **removal of urine** from the bladder.

A. External catheters are used for **heavy incontinence** problems or complete loss of urine control. They are attached to a stationary collection device or a leg bag to allow for ambulation. Types of external catheters include:

1. The **male** external catheter, which is also called a **condom** catheter because of its appearance. Some have adhesive to assist in keeping the catheter secure.
2. The **female** external catheter, which is a contoured device that fits snugly in the vagina. It is connected to a stationary collection device or a leg bag as with the male external catheter.

B. Internal catheters are used during **surgery** or when external catheters are inappropriate. Internal catheters can be used at home, but the patient must be taught proper insertion techniques to prevent infection. The catheter is inserted through the urethra into the bladder and is attached to a stationary collection device or leg bag. Catheters are sized by the **French scale:** the larger the number, the larger the diameter of the catheter. Types of catheters include:

1. The **straight** catheter, which is used for **intermittent catheterization** to drain the bladder. It consists of a rubber tube in which one end has a hole to allow the drainage of urine; the other end connects to the collection device.

2. The **Foley** catheter, an indwelling catheter that can be used for **up to 30 days before changing.** The end that is inserted into the bladder contains a balloon that is inflated with sterile water or saline. The inflated balloon holds the catheter in place. The balloon is deflated before removal.

STUDY QUESTIONS

Directions: Each of the numbered items or incomplete statements in this section is followed by answers or by completions of the statement. Select the **one** lettered answer or completion that is **best** in each case.

1. When a patient is fitted with an axillary crutch, how far below the underarm should the top of the crutch rest?

(A) 0.5 inch
(B) 1 inch
(C) 2 inches
(D) 3 inches
(E) 4 inches

2. What angle should the elbow form when a cane is the correct height?

(A) 10°
(B) 25°
(C) 45°
(D) 60°
(E) 90°

3. A product that delivers moisture to the air by heating water to produce steam is called a

(A) nebulizer
(B) humidifier
(C) ventilator
(D) peak flow meter
(E) vaporizer

4. An absorbant product designed for patients with light incontinence problems is a

(A) brief
(B) shield
(C) undergarment
(D) underpad
(E) catheter

5. When an oral temperature is taken, the thermometer should be placed into the mouth for

(A) 1 minute
(B) 2 minutes
(C) 3 minutes
(D) 4 minutes
(E) 5 minutes

6. The diameter of urinary catheters is measured by which of the following scales?

(A) Leur
(B) English
(C) French
(D) Gauge
(E) Metric

7. A cervical collar that immobilizes the neck is called a

(A) soft cervical collar
(B) hard cervical collar
(C) foam cervical collar
(D) extrication collar
(E) rigid cervical collar

8. Incontinence that is caused by an obstruction of the bladder is called

(A) overflow incontinence
(B) urge incontinence
(C) stress incontinence
(D) functional incontinence
(E) iatrogenic incontinence

9. A colostomy or ileostomy could be performed for all of the following conditions EXCEPT

(A) lower bowel obstruction
(B) malignancy of the colon or rectum
(C) ulcerative colitis
(D) duodenal ulcer
(E) Chrohn's disease

10. Pregnancy test kits are designed to detect which substance?

(A) Luteinizing hormone (LH)
(B) Progesterone
(C) Human chorionic gonadotropin (hCG)
(D) Estrogen
(E) Follical-stimulating hormone

ANSWERS AND EXPLANATIONS

1. The answer is C *[I B 2].*
When a patient is fitted for an axillary crutch, the top of the crutch should be 2 inches below the axilla (underarm).

2. The answer is B *[I A 1].*
When a patient is properly fitted for a cane, the elbow should form a 25° angle. This allows for maximum weight transfer.

3. The answer is E *[X F].*
A vaporizer produces moisture by heating water to produce steam. A humidifier also produces moisture; however, it works by mechanically creating small water particles. A nebulizer is used to deliver liquid to the mouth and throat. A ventilator is used to assist in breathing. A peak flow meter is used to detect airway constriction.

4. The answer is B *[VII B 1].*
Shields are pads that are placed in the underwear and held with adhesive strips. They are used for patients with light incontinence problems.

5. The answer is C *[XI A 1].*
Oral temperature is taken by inserting the bulb of the thermometer under the tongue and sealing the lips around the thermometer for 3 minutes.

6. The answer is C *[XII B].*
The French scale is used to measure the diameter of a urinary catheter. The Leur scale is used to measure syringe tip size. The gauge scale is used to measure needle diameter. The metric scale is a general system of measurement.

7. The answer is D *[VIII D 3].*
An extrication collar (also known as a Philadelphia collar) is used to immobilize the neck. It is commonly used in emergency situations. Soft or foam cervical collars provide mild support and remind the patient to keep the neck straight. Hard or rigid cervical collars provide moderate support but allow some movement.

8. The answer is A *[VII A 3].*
Overflow incontinence is caused by obstruction of the bladder. Urge incontinence is caused by uncontrolled bladder contractions. Stress incontinence is caused by increases in intra-abdominal pressure. Functional incontinence is related to physical or psychologic problems. Iatrogenic incontinence is caused by drugs or surgery.

9. The answer is D *[IX A 1–2].*
Lower bowel obstruction, malignancy of the colon or rectum, and diverticulitis may all require a colostomy. Ulcerative colitis and Chrohn's disease may require an ileostomy. The treatment of a duodenal ulcer would not include a colostomy or an ileostomy.

10. The answer is C *[V B 1 d].*
Pregnancy tests detect human chorionic gonadotropin (hCG) in the urine. This is secreted after the embryo has implanted in the uterus. Ovulation prediction tests detect luteinizing hormone (LH). Progesterone, estrogen, and follicle stimulating hormone are all involved in controlling the menstrual cycle.

28
Nonprescription Medication: An Overview

Larry N. Swanson

I. OVER-THE-COUNTER DRUGS

A. Over-the-counter (OTC) drugs. Under current law, there are only two classes of drugs available on the market: OTC drugs—those safe for consumers to use on the basis of their labeling alone—and prescription drugs—those that cannot be used safely without a physician's or other authorized prescriber's prescription. Generally, OTC drugs pose minimum risk and possess a higher safety profile than prescription drugs. Another important distinction between the two classes of drugs is that OTC drugs are used to treat complaints or illnesses for which users recognize their own symptoms and level of relief; conditions treated by prescription drugs are usually more difficult to self-assess. OTC drugs can treat or cure about 400 different common health complaints. According to the **Food and Drug Administration (FDA) regulations,** a drug must be safe and effective in order to be sold over the counter.

1. An OTC drug is **safe** if it has a low incidence of adverse reactions or significant side effects under adequate directions for use as well as low potential for harm, which may result from abuse under conditions of widespread availability.
2. An OTC drug is **effective** if there is a reasonable expectation that for a significant portion of the target population the drug, when used under adequate directions for use, with warnings against unsafe use, provides clinically significant relief of the type claimed.

B. OTC drug labels. Whereas prescription drug labels for the patient have minimal information, the FDA requires that OTC drug labels be much more detailed so the consumers can properly use the products without the advice of a health professional.

1. The label on each nonprescription medicine includes:
   - **a.** Product name and statement of identity
   - **b.** Active ingredients
   - **c.** Inactive ingredients
   - **d.** Name and location of the manufacturer, distributor, or packer
   - **e.** Net quantity of contents
   - **f.** Description of tamper resistant features
   - **g.** Indications for use
   - **h.** Directions and dosage instructions
   - **I.** Warnings, cautionary statements, and drug interaction precautions (if any)
   - **j.** Expiration date and lot or batch code
2. Despite labeling regulations, some labeling issues, such as **label clarity** continue to cause concern. Studies show that about 90% of consumers read OTC drug labels (96% in the case of children's medicine labels). Nonetheless, about 10% of consumers say that OTC labels are too difficult to understand. Although many OTC drug labels are written on a ninth-grade level, the average consumer reads at only the eighth-grade level, and 20% of Americans are functionally illiterate. Label readability can also be affected by such factors as poor vision and inadequate lighting in retail settings, particularly for the elderly. The FDA has been moving toward a more simplified label approach on OTC medications. The prototypes deliver information in "bullet" rather than paragraph form and highlight active ingredients, uses, directions, and consumer warnings.

C. OTC drug market. The OTC drug market is approximately $13 billion, an amount that increases 8% to 10% annually. With more medications being transferred from prescription to OTC status in years to come, it is estimated that by the year 2000 the OTC drug market may be as large as

$20 billion per year, and by 2010, OTC drug sales are expected to reach $28 billion, more than double today's volume.

1. The OTC drug market is a very important component in the nation's overall health care. One study estimated that if 2% of the OTC drug consumers chose to visit a physician rather than selecting an OTC drug for their particular health problems, physician office visits would increase by 62%.

2. One of the main benefits of OTC drugs is their relatively low cost, a factor that has contributed greatly to their success and growing popularity in the market place. In fact, a typical OTC drug costs the consumer less than $4.00, compared with $24.00 for an average prescription drug.

3. Growth of the OTC drug market is fueled in part by three important trends: heightened interest among consumers in their own care (the "self-care movement") an increase in the number of OTC products, mainly through prescription to OTC drug switches (see II) and product line extensions, and a national health care agenda geared toward controlling cost.
   a. The process of **switching prescription drugs to OTC drug status** makes entire new categories of treatments available to consumers without a prescription. Many proposed OTC drug switches are already in process and may be granted OTC drug status in the near future. The availability of these medications will give consumers an even greater degree of control over their own care, and at a low price. By the year 2000, in fact, it is estimated that switches will have saved the United States $34 billion in health care costs.
   b. One important sales trend gaining momentum—and providing consumers with even more OTC drug alternatives—is **the private label.** These are OTC products sold under a store name and generally offered at competitive prices.
   c. **Line extensions** are another important strategy that drug makers are using to bring new products to the shelves of the nations 750,000 OTC drug outlets, pharmacies, super markets, convenient stores, and mass merchandisers. This is the practice of extending an established brand name to an entire line of nonprescription products. OTC product manufacturers do not introduce totally new trade names, but rely on existing trade names whenever possible. In marketing terms, this type of product is referred to as a "line-extension." The manufacturer hopes that recognition of one trade name and corresponding loyalty to that trade name will be perpetuated across other products bearing the same trade name.

D. **OTC drug therapy.** Therapy using OTC drugs requires a very definite role for the pharmacist both professionally and economically.

1. **The importance of OTC medications** is especially apparent with the increasing number of prescription **agents moving to nonprescription status.** There are many conditions in which an OTC medication can or should be the primary therapy. Head lice, acne, vaginal candidiasis, constipation, and dysmenorrhea are a few examples.

2. OTC agents have the potential for significant **interactions** with prescription medications (e.g., aspirin and warfarin, antihistamines and alcohol, cimetidine and several drugs). Additionally, some OTC agents used by people who are affected by certain diseases may cause serious problems (e.g., oral decongestants should be avoided generally by patients with hypertension, arrhythmias, or ischemic heart disease).

3. Because of the abundance of nonprescription medications available, helping a person select an OTC medication for that patient's particular need is one of the most professionally rewarding activities of the community pharmacist.

4. The pharmacist is the most accessible health care practitioner, and a pharmacist's advice about OTC medications is very important. In one study, the following data were produced. Of those surveyed:
   a. Ninety-five percent would purchase a pharmacist-recommended product.
   b. Ninety-two percent were satisfied with previous pharmacist-recommended products.
   c. Ninety percent would consult with a physician if a pharmacist said to do so.
   d. Seventy-six percent would take a pharmacist's advice over the advice of a friend.
   e. Seventy-eight percent would buy a product recommended by a pharmacist over one they had picked up on a display.

5. Many consumers prefer buying their OTC drugs in a pharmacy because a pharmacist is on hand to provide counseling. There are, for instance, more than 750,000 OTC drug outlets,

and only about 10% of these are pharmacies (65,000). Yet, about 45% of all the nation's OTC drugs are bought in drug stores. Consumers clearly go out of their way to purchase OTC drugs in a pharmacy. OTC drugs are a crucial element in pharmacy practice with about 30% of pharmacy revenues coming from OTC drug sales.

6. The **"self-care movement"** of recent years has also increased the role that pharmacists can play in nonprescription medication use. This movement has been stimulated by the following:
   a. Rising educational levels of the general population
   b. Greater dissemination of health care information via print (e.g., newspapers, magazines) and electronic (e.g., television, radio) media
   c. A lack of available medical services to some individuals
   d. A greater awareness of the limitations of medicine
   e. A general increase in consumerism
   f. Personal focus on health and fitness
   g. Increasing health care costs

II. THE FDA OTC DRUG REVIEW

A. History

1. In 1938, Congress enacted the **Federal Food, Drug, and Cosmetic Act (FFDCA),** which required manufacturers to market safe products.
2. In 1951, the **Durham-Humphrey Amendment** to the FFDCA was passed. For the first time, medications were separated into **two distinct classes: prescription (legend) products and nonprescription, or OTC products.** The Durham-Humphrey Amendment established a consumer's right to self-treatment with safe and effective OTC drugs. It also stated that if a drug is safe and effective, and its labeling can be written so that the consumer may use it without professional supervision, it must be available over the counter. Prescription drugs, on the other hand, were defined by the 1951 amendment as:
   a. Certain habit-forming drugs
   b. Drugs not safe for use except under a physician's supervision because of toxicity or other potential harmful effects, the method of use, or other measures necessary to use
   c. Drugs limited to prescription use under a new drug application
3. In **1962,** Congress passed the **Kefauver-Harris Amendment** to the FFDCA. This act required manufacturers to prove that their products were not only safe but also truly effective.
   a. **Implementation of the amendment.** To implement the Kefauver-Harris Amendment, the FDA contracted the National Academy of Sciences/National Research Council to assess drug efficacy for agents marketed between 1938 and 1962. This was followed by the FDA's implementation procedure, which is called the Drug Efficacy Study Implementation (DESI).
   b. **Drugs reviewed for efficacy.** Of the approximately 4000 drugs that were reviewed, about 500 were OTC medications. Of these, about 300 were considered to be ineffective, which made it clear to the FDA that a comprehensive OTC drug review was necessary.
   c. **Official start of the FDA OTC drug review.** The FDA OTC drug review officially began in 1972 and was expected to be completed within approximately 5 years. To date, the review is still not complete, but the process should be essentially finished in 1997.

B. Focus. The principal focus of the review was to establish the safety, effectiveness, and proper labeling of OTC medications. Originally, 17 advisory review panels were established to study 70 product categories. Because of the large number of OTC products available (approximately 300,000), the OTC drug review focused on active ingredients, which ultimately totalled approximately 800.

1. **Original panels.** The original panels reviewed medications in various product categories and classified the ingredients into **three categories:**
   a. **Category I.** Ingredients are generally recognized as safe and effective for the claimed therapeutic indication.
   b. **Category II.** Ingredients are not generally recognized as safe and effective or have unacceptable indications.

c. **Category III.** Because of insufficient data, the FDA cannot classify these ingredients into category I or II.

2. **Completed reports.** Once the advisory panels completed their reports, they submitted information to the FDA, which was published in the *Federal Register* as Advanced Notices of Proposed Rulemaking (ANPRs). After FDA evaluation of this material, the FDA published its findings as a tentative final monograph and gave manufacturers and others an opportunity to incorporate additional information into the final monograph.

3. **Final monographs.** Once final monographs are published, manufacturers must comply with the requirements for marketing only those agents that are considered to be category I (monograph condition; original categories II and III are nonmonograph conditions). Manufacturers may petition the FDA with new supportive data for their product to amend a monograph, or they may submit a new drug application (NDA) for OTC use for the desired agent.

4. **OTC drug switching procedures.** The process of switching a prescription drug to nonprescription status also establishes its safety and efficacy as an OTC drug. There were six switches approved by the FDA in 1995, bringing the total number of prescription to OTC drug switches to 58 since 1975. There are a number of mechanisms used to switch a prescription product:
   a. The FDA advisory panels for OTC drug review may recommend that a drug be switched. This type of review is responsible for about 40 of the switches to date, including hydrocortisone, diphenhydramine, and oxymetazoline.
   b. A full NDA can be submitted for a current Rx drug in a new dosage or formulation. This mechanism, which deals with products rather than ingredients, is behind the approval of new OTC products including ibuprofen, loperamide, permethrin, miconazole, and clotrimazole.
   c. A supplemental NDA may be filed by a holder of an approved original or abbreviated application for a closely related product.
   d. An abbreviated NDA may be submitted for products that are identical to an existing prescription product. This is used mainly for near duplicates of a prescription drug.

C. **Implications to pharmacists**

1. **Pharmacists are now able to recommend products that contain ingredients that have been reviewed by a panel of experts and the FDA.** There has been a trend away from multiple drug combination products. Because many OTC agents were found to be ineffective, many products in a particular therapeutic category now contain identical active ingredients. Most OTC products contain only one category I (monograph) agent (with the exception of cough and cold products).

2. **Pharmacists need to stay current on product ingredients.** A trade name for a product may remain the same although there is a change in the ingredients. For example, Kaopectate, which previously contained kaolin and pectin, now contains attapulgite, based on the final recommendations of the FDA after review of the available OTC antidiarrheal agents. To stay competitive, manufacturers have increasingly relied on product "line extensions" to market their various products. The FDA, however, has expressed concern about whether the proliferation of products confuses consumers. Although the manufacturer may make the trade name slightly different (e.g., adding a qualifier such as "plus" or "II") the seeds of confusion have been sewn. Examples include:
   a. The original Unisom contains doxylamine, whereas the recently introduced Unisom Sleep Gels contain diphenhydramine.
   b. Kaopectate contains attapulgite but Kaopectate II contains loperamide.
   c. The trade name Robitussin has been associated many years with guaifenesin. However, products bearing the Robitussin name have been introduced that do not contain guaifenesin. Robitussin Pediatric Cough Suppressant, and Robitussin Maximum Strength Cough and Cold contain only dextromethorphan.
   d. Bayer has been associated with aspirin for many years. However, a line of products known as Bayer Select includes products for sinus pain relief and several other conditions. The line of products often includes pain relievers such as acetaminophen or ibuprofen, usually combined with cough suppressants, decongestants and/or antihistamines, caffeine, guaifenesin, or diuretics.
   e. Tylenol has traditionally been identified with the agent acetaminophen. Many other Tylenol products contain other agents in addition to acetaminophen.

f. Chlor-Trimeton has for many years been the trade name for chlorpheniramine. Chlor-Trimeton Non-Drowsy contains only the decongestant pseudoephedrine.

3. **Pharmacists need to stay current on what prescription drugs are given OTC status.** During the FDA OTC review process, many of the panels recommended that certain prescription drugs be switched to OTC drug status.
   - **a.** Examples of **OTC drugs that had been prescription drugs** include topical hydrocortisone, oxymetazoline, chlorpheniramine in higher strengths, diphenhydramine, miconazole, tolnaftate, and ibuprofen.
   - **b. Prescription drugs that are possible candidates to become OTC drugs** include a long list of agents (e.g., terfenadine, nitroglycerin, and tretinoin).

III. A "PHARMACIST-ONLY" CLASS OF DRUGS.

These are also referred to as the third class of drugs. "Pharmacist-only" drugs have been advocated for many years, the principal impetus being to protect the public from improperly using some of the OTC medications. Countries that have a "pharmacist-only" drug class include Canada, France, Germany, and Switzerland.

A. Benefits

1. The public would have some measure of **protection against misdiagnosing and self-prescribing,** but those who need the drugs could still obtain them without prescription.
   - **a.** According to the National Council on Patient Information and Education, 50% of all medications are taken incorrectly.
   - **b.** The patient counseling required for a third class of drugs could significantly improve drug use outcomes.
2. The pharmacist has patient profiles for prescription drugs, so possible **incompatibilities** with **prescription medication could be checked** and OTC drug sales could be entered onto the patient profile.
3. This class of drugs would provide consumers with **monitoring and follow-up,** which is not available when patients select certain drugs themselves.
4. The designation of an additional class of drugs could also help in **monitoring drugs that are switched from prescription to nonprescription status.**
5. The advocated change might **save money** for patients both by preventing inappropriate drug selections and reducing the need for some office visits.

B. Opposition.

Opposition to the creation of such a class of drugs focuses primarily on the restrictions to consumer access to these agents.

1. **Fewer hours and areas of availability.** OTC drugs are currently sold to consumers in more than 750,000 retail outlets, whereas the proposed third class of drugs would be available only in an estimated 65,000 pharmacies. This may limit the access of consumers to these drugs, particularly at night and in rural areas.
2. **Increased prices due to decreased competition.** Another objection to moving to a third class of drugs focuses on the concern that prices would increase if competition from other retail outlets is eliminated.

C. Government report.

A recent United States General Accounting Office report (August 1995) "Nonprescription Drugs—Value of a Pharmacist-Controlled Class Has Yet to Be Demonstrated," concluded that "little evidence supports the establishment of a pharmacy or pharmacist class of drugs in the United States at this time, as either a fixed or a transition class," and "experience in Florida with a class of drugs similar to a pharmacist class has not been successful: pharmacists have not regularly prescribed these drugs, and record keeping requirements have not been followed."

IV. THE FDA OFFICE OF OTC DRUG EVALUATION.

This office was established in 1991 because of an increase in the creation, categorizing, and use of OTC drugs.

A. Purpose. This office was established to insure the regulation of OTC medications and is on the same operational level as the office responsible for regulation of prescription drugs.

B. Functions. The office has nine functions:

1. Coordinating and/or reviewing and deciding on the appropriate action, including approval or disapproval of all applications for OTC drug products, prescription drug switches to OTC status, and applications for other related drug products with the exception of new molecular entities and generic drug applications
2. Overseeing the development and implementation of standards for the safety and effectiveness of OTC drugs
3. Formulating, implementing, and publishing OTC drug monographs
4. Developing policy and procedures for the development of OTC drug reviews
5. Coordinating research activities throughout the FDA on all OTC drug issues
6. Serving as the primary agency contact for OTC drug information, regulation, and status
7. Maintaining a document control system for OTC drug submissions and a management information system for the office
8. Initiating actions based on recommendations made by OTC advisory panels, public comments, and new data
9. Participating in agency-sponsored consumer and professional educational programs on OTC drugs

C. Responsibility. The OTC Drugs Advisory Committee was also created as part of the FDA's efforts to expand and reorganize the office of OTC Drug Evaluation in response to the increasing demand for OTC products. The OTC Drugs Advisory Committee is responsible for the following functions:

1. Reviewing and evaluating available data concerning the safety and effectiveness of OTC drugs for use and treatment of a broad spectrum of human symptoms and diseases
2. Advising the commissioner on the approval of new drug applications
3. Serving as a forum to discuss the potential for some drug products to be switched from prescription to nonprescription status
4. Advising the commissioner on the promulgation of monographs establishing conditions under which OTC drugs are generally recognized as safe and effective and not misbranded
5. Conducting peer review and extramural scientific biomedical programs in support of the FDA's mission and regulatory responsibilities.

STUDY QUESTIONS

Directions: Each of the numbered items or incomplete statements in this section is followed by answers or by completions of the statement. Select the **one** lettered answer or completion that is **best** in each case.

1. Which one of the following statements regarding the Food and Drug Administration's (FDA's) Over-the-Counter (OTC) Drug Review process is correct?

(A) In the FDA OTC Drug Review process, individual products on the market were reviewed rather than individual ingredients
(B) Patients were found to be reluctant to follow a pharmacist's advice regarding OTC products
(C) The FDA OTC Drug Review began in 1972
(D) Approximately 500 OTC drugs were found to be ineffective

2. All of the following statements concerning over-the-counter (OTC) drugs are correct EXCEPT

(A) category I OTC agents are now referred to as monograph agents
(B) the 1938 Federal Food, Drug, and Cosmetic Act (FFDCA) required medications to be safe
(C) the Durham-Humphrey Amendment created prescription and nonprescription categories of medications
(D) the Kefauver-Harris Amendment requires pharmacists to counsel patients on all OTC medications
(E) category III OTC agents do not have sufficient data to be classified as category I or II agents

3. All of the following are required on the label of an over-the-counter (OTC) medication EXCEPT

(A) the name and address of the store selling the product
(B) the directions and dosage instructions
(C) the expiration date
(D) a list of inactive ingredients
(E) the net quantity of the contents

4. All of the following results stem from the Food and Drug Administration's (FDA's) Over-the-Counter (OTC) Drug Review EXCEPT

(A) many products that required prescriptions were made available as OTC products
(B) a third class of drugs was created in addition to prescription and nonprescription
(C) many products in a particular therapeutic class have the same active ingredient(s)
(D) pharmacists can recommend products more confidently because of the rigorous review of the ingredients in each product
(E) trade names of many products have remained the same while the ingredients have changed

ANSWERS AND EXPLANATIONS

1. The answer is C *[II A 3 c, B].*
The Food and Drug Administration's (FDA's) review of over-the-counter (OTC) drugs began in 1972, was expected to take 5 years, and is now expected to be essentially finished in 1997. Approximately 4000 drugs were reviewed as a result of implementing the Kefauver-Harris Amendment to the Federal Food, Drug, and Cosmetic Act (FFDCA). Of those 4000 drugs, 500 were OTC products and 300 of them were found to be ineffective. This finding reinforced the need for a comprehensive OTC drug review. The complete review focused on approximately 800 active ingredients, which are found in approximately 300,000 OTC products. The large number of OTC products rendered a complete review of all products infeasible.

2. The answer is D *[II A 3].*
The 1962 Kefauver-Harris Amendment to the 1938 Federal Food, Drug, and Cosmetic Act (FFDCA) required that manufacturers of pharmaceuticals prove the effectiveness, as well as safety, of their products. It does not require pharmacists to counsel patients on all OTC medications.

3. The answer is A *[I B 1].*
There are 10 items that are required to be on the labels of OTC medications; however, there is no requirement to have the name and address of the store selling the product.

4. The answer is B *[II c, III].*
The third class of drugs, which does not require a prescription but can only be sold by the pharmacist (not off the shelf), has been frequently discussed but does not presently exist in the United States.

29
OTC Otic, Dental, and Ophthalmic Agents

Larry N. Swanson
Connie Lee Barnes
Constance A. McKenzie

I. OTIC OVER-THE-COUNTER (OTC) PRODUCTS

A. The ear structure

1. The **external ear** consists of the **auricle (pinna),** which is the visible outer structure of the ear that serves to funnel sounds into the ear canal.
2. The **ear canal,** also known as the external auditory meatus, is a channel that is about 1 inch in length, points downward, and ends in a cul-de-sac at the **tympanic membrane (eardrum).**
   a. The **skin lining the ear canal** is very thin and tightly stretched. The slightest degree of inflammation elicits a significant amount of pain. This canal is also lined with glands that secrete substances that form **cerumen (earwax),** which lubricates the lining of the ear canal and aids the removal of organisms and other foreign debris.
   b. The **tympanic membrane** vibrates when hit by sound waves and it transmits that sound into the middle ear.
3. The **middle ear** is a small chamber about the size of a pea and contains the three small bones known as the **ossicles,** which amplify and transmit the sound waves farther into the inner ear.
   a. The middle ear is normally filled with air. The **eustachian tubes,** which are about the size of a pencil lead, connect the middle ear with the nasopharynx and equilibrate air pressure between the middle ear and the outer atmosphere. The "popping" (or "clicking") sensation that is heard upon swallowing is the sound of air bubbles passing through these tubes, which then open.
   b. In the presence of a cold or allergy, these eustachian tube walls may swell, which prevents air from passing through. A pressure drop in the middle ear may create a vacuum, which draws fluid into the middle ear. Bacteria may then grow in this fluid and produce a condition known as **otitis media** (middle ear infection).
4. The **inner ear** consists of the **cochlea** (the organ of hearing) and the **vestibular apparatus,** which is involved with maintaining balance and equilibrium.

B. Common ear disorders.

Table 29-1 differentiates the symptoms of the common otic disorders encountered by pharmacists. There are three ear-related conditions for which pharmacists may recommend OTC medications: earwax softening, pressure due to altitude changes, and prevention of otitis externa (i.e., swimmer's ear).

1. **Excessive earwax**

Table 29-1. Symptoms of Otic Disorders

	Boil	Bacterial External Otitis	Impacted Cerumen	Suppurative Otitis Media
Pain*	Often	Often	Rarely	Usually
Hearing deficit	Rarely	Possibly	Often	Possibly
Purulent discharge	Rarely	Often	Rarely	Occasionally, when present, it indicates perforation
Bilateral symptoms	Rarely	Possibly	Rarely	Occasionally
Appropriateness of self-medication	Auricle only	Never	Never	Never

*Pain is increased with chewing, traction on the auricle, and medial pressure on the tragus, except in otitis media, where it is knife-like and steady.

a. **Functions** of cerumen include:
   (1) Lubrication of the lining of the ear canal
   (2) Aiding in the removal of organisms and debris by its outward movement, which is caused by movement of the jaw during chewing and talking. The healthy ear is "self-cleaning" through this process.
   (3) Helping to protect the ear canal through its bacteriostatic and possibly fungistatic properties

b. There are primarily **four reasons why earwax accumulates:**
   (1) Overactive ceruminous glands, which are rare
   (2) An anatomically narrowed ear canal
   (3) A large amount of hair in the canal, which occurs often in the elderly
   (4) Inefficient or insufficient chewing or talking, which may also occur in the elderly

c. **Improper removal methods.** Attempts should not be made to remove earwax by using cotton-tipped applicators, match sticks, or hairpins, as this usually pushes the earwax down further in the canal and makes it more difficult to remove.

d. **Earwax-softening agents** include:
   (1) **Carbamide peroxide** [urea hydrogen peroxide (e.g., Debrox, Murine Ear)] is the only approved monograph agent for earwax removal (not impacted earwax).
      (a) **Action.** Carbamide peroxide releases oxygen and, via a mechanical action of effervescence, loosens the wax debris and aids in its removal.
      (b) To **prevent vertigo,** one should warm the vial of this medication in the hands and put 5–10 drops in the ear.
      (c) **Use.** Carbamide peroxide should be used twice a day for 4 days, and the ear canal may be irrigated with the use of an ear syringe.
      (d) **Cautions**
         (i) Do not use if ear drainage, discharge, pain, or irritation or rash occurs.
         (ii) Do not use if injury or perforation of the ear drum exists.
         (iii) If the patient feels pain or a severe fullness in the ear when instilling drops into the ear, this might indicate the presence of a ruptured tympanic membrane.
   (2) **Cerumenolytics** such as triethanolamine polypeptide oleate (Cerumenex) may be used for **impacted earwax.** This is available by prescription and must be administered under the supervision of a physician.
   (3) Other agents that have been used for earwax softening include: olive oil (sweet oil), mineral oil, glycerin, diluted hydrogen peroxide solution, propylene glycol, and baking soda solution (1/2 teaspoonful baking soda in 2 ounces of warm water).

2. **Altitude and ear pressure.** During situations such as airplane descent when there are rapid changes in air pressure, the **eustachian tubes** may not function properly. Traveling from low atmospheric pressure to a higher air pressure causes a vacuum to form in the middle ear. As a result, the eardrum retracts and cannot vibrate, which creates a muffled sound and some pain. Patients with a cold or allergy might be more susceptible to this problem.
   a. The act of **swallowing** (induced by chewing gum or letting hard candy dissolve in the mouth), activates the muscles that pull open the eustachian tubes and helps to unblock the ears. Giving a baby a bottle of milk or juice upon airplane descent helps prevent ear pain.
   b. **Yawning** is also effective in opening the eustachian tubes.
   c. Another effective method of unblocking the ears is pinching the nostrils and, using the cheek and throat muscles, **forcing air into the back of the nose** as if trying to blow off the thumb and fingers from the nostrils.
   d. The use of **decongestant** medication may be recommended, either in the form of an oral agent such as pseudoephedrine (e.g., Sudafed) which should be taken about an hour before descent, or a topical decongestant such as oxymetazoline (e.g., Afrin), which should be administered 10–15 minutes before descent.

3. **Otitis externa** (also called **swimmer's ear** or **hot weather ear**) usually occurs during the summer months.
   a. **Pathophysiology**
      (1) Typically, this condition develops when water accumulates in the external ear canal after swimming. The combination of heat and humidity results in softening and swelling of the ear wax, which interferes with the normal protective function of the ear wax. The pH in this area then increases and sets the stage for bacterial invasion.
      (2) The resulting itching makes affected patients scratch the area [with fingers or cotton-tipped applicators (Q-tips)], which further interferes with the integrity of the ear canal.

(3) In more than 50% of cases, the microorganism that is involved is *Pseudomonas aeruginosa*.
(4) The infection is commonly unilateral.

b. Symptoms
(1) Itching
(2) Pain that is accentuated by moving the ear (i.e., pulling upward on the auricle or pressing on the tragus)
(3) A fluid discharge from the canal (in severe cases)
(4) A decrease or loss of hearing (if the ear canal is completely blocked)

c. Treatment
(1) There is **no OTC treatment** for this condition.
(2) Prescription treatment usually includes an antibiotic/steroid combination, such as neomycin, polymyxin, hydrocortisone (e.g., Cortisporin Otic), or an acetic acid and hydrocortisone combination (e.g., Vosol-HC Otic).

d. Prevention
(1) After swimming or showering, the head should be turned to the side to drain water out of the ear. If otitis externa is a frequent occurrence, **wax stopples,** which are placed in the ear before swimming, may be recommended.
(2) To dry the ear after swimming, several drops of a **50/50 solution of isopropyl alcohol and white vinegar,** which contains acetic acid and restores the acid pH to the external auditory canal, can be instilled in the ear. Other methods for prevention of otitis externa include **2% acetic acid prescription eardrop** (e.g., Vosol Otic)**,** one of the **OTC boric acid products** (e.g., Auro-Ari), or a product such as Swim-Ear (95% isopropyl alcohol and 5% anhydrous glycerin).

4. Boils (i.e., **furuncles**) are infected hair follicles in the ear canal that usually involve the organism *Staphylococcus aureus*. This condition is usually self-limiting and is best treated by the application of warm compresses, which brings the boil to a head.

5. Otitis media is an infection of the middle ear, with *S. pneumoniae* and *Haemophilus influenzae* being the **most frequent** organisms encountered. With the exception of colds, this is the most common infection in young children.
a. The **symptoms** include pain in the ear, fever, fluid discharge from the ear, and possibly decreased hearing.
b. The **treatment** involves the use of oral antibiotics, which are available on prescription.
c. Bottle feeding infants in a supine position should be avoided because this allows milk to drain down the eustachian tubes into the middle ear. Infants have relatively short eustachian tubes and horizontal configuration. Occasionally, when an infant is bothered by middle ear infections, a physician may choose to insert tympanostomy tubes into the ear drum for drainage and pressure equalization purposes.

C. Administration of ear medication

1. When administering ear drops, pull the earlobe up and back to straighten the canal for adults and down and back to straighten in children.

2. Avoid touching the ear dropper tip to the ear; this prevents recontamination of the external ear if treating external otitis.

3. One should instruct patients using a bulb syringe for ear irrigation to direct the solution up against the upper portion of ear canal and not directly against the tympanic membrane.

4. The adult ear canal can hold about 17 drops (~0.85 ml.) of fluid.

5. Warm ear drops in hands to body temperature for 1–2 minutes. Too cold or too warm drops may cause vertigo (dizziness).

6. Tilt the head sideways with affected ear upward when applying the drops.

II. DENTAL OTC PRODUCTS

A. Dental anatomy. Anatomically, the teeth are divided into two parts: the **crown** (above the gingival line) and the **root** (below the gingival line).

1. **Enamel** is the crystalline calcium salts (hydroxyapatite) that cover the crown to protect the underlying tooth structure.
2. **Dentin** is the largest part of the tooth structure located beneath the enamel. It protects the dental pulp.
3. **Cementum** is a bone-like structure that covers the root and provides the attachment of the tooth with the periodontal ligaments.
4. **Pulp** consists of free nerve endings.

B. Common dental problems and OTC products

1. **Dental caries** (i.e., **cavities**) are formed by the growth and implantation of cariogenic microorganisms.
   a. **Causes**
      (1) **Bacteria** (primarily *Streptococcus mutans* and *Lactobacillaceae*) produce acids (e.g., lactic acid) that demineralize enamel. Initially, demineralized enamel appears as a white, chalky area and becomes bluish-white and eventually brown or yellow.
      (2) **Diet** is another factor in the development of dental caries. Foods with a high concentration of refined sugar (i.e., sucrose) increase the risk of dental caries. Sucrose is converted by bacterial plaque into volatile acids that destroy the hydroxyapatite.
         (a) **Fructose** and **lactose** are less cariogenic than sucrose.
         (b) **Noncariogenic sugar substitutes** are xylitol, sorbitol, and aspartame.
   b. **OTC products** for dental caries include products that can alleviate the pain and sensitivity until the patient can get to the dentist. Examples of ingredients that are beneficial in this regard include eugenol, benzocaine (e.g., Anbesol, Orajel), or an oral analgesic (e.g., aspirin, acetaminophen).
2. **Plaque and calculus**
   a. **Causes**
      (1) **Plaque** is a sticky substance formed by the attachment of bacteria to the pellicle, which is a thin, acellular, glycoprotein (a mucoprotein coating that adheres to the enamel within minutes after cleaning a tooth).
      (2) **Calculus** (or **tartar**) is the substance formed when plaque is not removed within 24 hours. The plaque begins to calcify into calculus when calcium salt precipitates from the saliva. Calculus can be removed only by a professional dental cleaning.
   b. **OTC products**
      (1) **Toothbrushes.** Soft, rounded, nylon bristles are preferred by dentists because hard bristles can irritate the gingival margins and cause the gums to recede. Electric toothbrushes can benefit patients who require someone to clean their teeth for them or patients who have orthodontic appliances.
      (2) **Irrigating devices** direct a high-pressure stream of water through a nozzle to the hard-to-clean areas by gently lifting the free gingiva to rinse out crevices. Two types are available: **pulsating** (i.e., intermittent low- and high-pressure water streams) and **steady** (i.e., constant and consistent water pressure), neither of which has shown superior irrigating ability.
         (a) Irrigating devices should serve as adjuncts in maintaining oral hygiene.
         (b) **Examples** include Dento-Spray, Hydro Pik, Propulse 7618, and the Water Pik Oral Irrigator.
   c. **Dental floss** is available waxed, unwaxed, thick, thin, flavored, or unflavored. There are no differences between dental flosses in terms of plaque removal and prevention of gingivitis. There is no evidence of a residual wax film with the use of waxed dental floss.
      (1) The selection of dental floss depends upon characteristics of the patient, such as tooth roughness or tightness of tooth contacts (e.g., waxed floss is recommended for tight-fitting teeth because it can pass easily between the teeth without shredding).
      (2) The American Dental Association (ADA) recognizes the following brands as safe and effective: Butler, Johnson & Johnson, Dr. Flosser, and Oral-B.
   d. **Dentifrices** are products that enhance the removal of stains and dental plaque by the toothbrush. These include toothpastes, antiplaque and anticalculous mouthwashes, cosmetic whiteners, desensitizing agents, and disclosing agents.
      (1) **Toothpastes** are beneficial in decreasing the incidence of dental caries, reducing mouth odors, and enhancing personal appearance. **Ingredients** include the following.

(a) **Abrasives** are responsible for physically removing plaque and debris. Examples include silicates, sodium bicarbonate, dicalcium phosphate, sodium metaphosphate, calcium pyrophosphate, calcium carbonate, magnesium carbonate, and aluminum oxides. Mentadent contains sodium bicarbonate, whereas Peroxi-Care has sodium bicarbonate and peroxide.

(b) **Surfactants** are foaming agents that are incorporated into most dentifrices because their detergent action aids in removing debris. The **most frequently used** surfactants are **sodium lauryl sulfate** and **sodium dodecyl benzenesulfonate.** Recent reports say that sodium lauryl sulfate-containing dentifrices might increase the occurrences of canker sores.

(c) **Humectants** prevent the preparation from drying. Examples include sorbitol, glycerin, and propylene glycol.

(d) **Suspending agents** add thickness to the product. Examples include methylcellulose, tragacanth, and karaya gum.

(e) **Flavoring agents** include sorbitol or saccharin.

(f) **Pyrophosphates** are found in tartar-control toothpastes. These products retard tartar formation; however, they form an alkaline solution that may irritate the skin. Some patients might experience a rash around the outside of the mouth. These patients should use regular toothpaste with only occasional uses of tartar-control toothpaste.

(g) **Fluoride** is anticariogenic because it replaces the hydroxyl ion in hydroxyapatite with the fluoride ion to form fluorapatite on the outer surface of the enamel. Fluorapatite hardens the enamel and makes it more acid resistant. Fluoride also has demonstrated antibacterial activity.

(i) Fluoride is **most beneficial** if used from birth through **age 12 or 13** because unerupted permanent teeth are mineralizing during that time. Whether or not a patient receives fluoride depends upon the concentration in their drinking water (Table 29-2).

(ii) **Common fluoride compounds** in toothpaste include 0.24% sodium fluoride and 0.76% or 0.80% sodium monofluorophosphate (e.g., Aim, Crest, Aqua-Fresh, Colgate). Crest Gum Care contains a reformulated version of stannous fluoride (0.454%), which might reduce gingivitis and bleeding of the gums by an average of 20% and 33%, respectively.

(2) **Antiplaque** dentifrice ingredients include micronized silica abrasives and sodium bicarbonate. To date, no antiplaque dentifrices have been accepted by the ADA as efficacious.

(3) **Anticalculous dentifrices** include zinc chloride, zinc citrate, and 33% pyrophosphate as ingredients to prevent calculus formation. To date, anticalculous products have not been evaluated by the ADA, therefore they do not carry the seal of acceptance.

(4) **Cosmetic whitening agents.** The **most common ingredient** in these products that is responsible for whitening the teeth is **10% carbamide peroxide** (e.g., in Rembrandt). This ingredient is a white crystal that reacts with water to release hydrogen peroxide, which in turn liberates free oxides. Some cosmetic whiteners may contain calcium peroxide (e.g., EpiSmile).

Table 29-2. Daily Fluoride Supplement Requirements for Infants and Children Based on Concentration of Fluoride in Drinking Water

Water Concentration	Age	Fluoride Supplement Required
>0.7 ppm of fluoride	6 months to 3 years	0
	3–6 years	0
0.3 to 0.7 ppm of fluoride	6 months to 3 years	0
	3–6 years	0.25 mg per day
	6–16 years	0.50 mg per day
<0.3 ppm of fluoride	6 months to 3 years	0.25 mg per day
	3–6 years	0.50 mg per day
	6–16 years	1.00 mg per day

(a) **Possible risks** associated with using whitening products include alteration of normal flora, tissue irritation, teeth sensitivity, and gingivitis.
(b) **Antiseptics** have been used as whiteners, (e.g., Gly-Oxide, Proxigel).

(5) **Desensitizing agents** reduce the pain in sensitive teeth caused by cold, heat, or touch. These products should be nonabrasive and should not be used on a permanent basis unless directed by a dentist.
(a) Examples of **5% potassium nitrate compounds** include Denquel, Promise, and Fresh Mint Sensodyne.
(b) An example of **10% strontium chloride hexahydrate product** is Original Formula Sensodyne.
(c) An example of a **dibasic sodium citrate product** is Protect.

(6) **Disclosing agents** aid in visualizing where dental plaque has formed. These products are for occasional use only and should not be swallowed. The FDA-approved products are D&C red No. 28 and FD&C Green No. 3. Following use, the consumer should rinse the mouth with water and expectorate.

(7) **Mouthwashes** may contain astringents, demulcents, detergents, flavors, germicidal agents, and fluoride. They can be used for cosmetic purposes, reducing plaque, or supplementing fluoride consumption.
(a) **Cosmetic mouthwashes** freshen the breath. They are nontherapeutic and are not effective as an antiseptic agent. These mouthwashes are classified by their active ingredients, alcohol content, and appearance. The most popular products are those that contain medicinal phenol and mint. The higher the percent of alcohol, the higher the impact of flavor within the mouth.
(b) **Antiplaque mouth rinses.** Products that have received the ADA seal are Kmart Antiseptic Mouthrinse, Listerine Antiseptic, and Peridex Oral Rinse.
(c) **Fluoridated mouthwashes** are used after cleaning the teeth and should be expectorated. Nothing should be put into the mouth for 30 minutes after using these mouthwashes. The ADA has approved the following products: ACT Anti-Cavity Dental Rinse, ACT for Kids, Fluorigard Anti-Cavity Dental Rinse, and Reach Fluoride Dental Rinse.

3. **Gingivitis** is inflammation of the gingiva. The gingiva may appear larger in size with a bluish hue caused by engorged gingival capillaries and a slow venous return.
   a. **Cause.** Gingivitis is caused by microorganisms that eventually damage cellular and intercellular tissues. **Chronic gingivitis** may be localized or generalized. The gums readily bleed when probed or brushed, and the patient should seek dental assistance.
   b. **OTC products** include anesthetics containing eugenol or benzocaine (e.g., Orajel) to relieve the pain. Mouthwashes may freshen the breath; however, it is important to consider the potential of these products to disguise and delay treatment of pathologic conditions (e.g., gingivitis) before use. Also, acetaminophen (Tylenol) can be recommended. The patient should seek the advice of a dentist.

4. **Periodontal disease** is the result of chronic gingivitis left untreated. The periodontal ligament attachment and alveolar bone support of the tooth deteriorate.

5. **Acute necrotizing ulcerative gingivitis (ANUG)** is also called **trench mouth** and is characterized by necrosis and ulceration of the gingival surface with underlying inflammation. This condition is usually seen in teens and young adults.
   a. **Signs** and **symptoms** of ANUG include severe pain, halitosis, bleeding, foul taste, and increased salivation.
   b. The **cause** of ANUG is unknown. It is postulated that it might be associated with the overgrowth of spirochete and fusiform organisms.
   c. **Risk factors** include anxiety, stress, smoking, malnutrition, and poor oral hygiene.
   d. **Treatment** consists of local debridement. Also, penicillin VK (penicillin V is a derivative of penicillin G, however it is more stable in an acidic medium and, therefore, is better absorbed from the gastrointestinal tract; K stands for potassium) or metronidazole may be used in certain cases (e.g., widespread lesions).
   e. **OTC products** include acetaminophen and products with benzocaine (not eugenol because it may cause soft-tissue damage). The patient should be advised to see a dentist. The use of salicylates is not recommended if the patient is predisposed to bleeding. Also, adequate nutrition, high fluid intake, and rest are essential. Rinsing the mouth with warm normal saline or 1.5% peroxide solution might be helpful for the first few days.

6. **Temporomandibular joint (TMJ) syndrome** is caused by an improper working relationship between the chewing muscles and the TMJ.
   a. **Signs** and **symptoms** include a dull, aching pain around the ear, headaches, neck aches, limited opening of the mouth, and a clicking or popping noise upon opening the mouth.
   b. **Risk factors** include bruxism (i.e., grinding the teeth) and occlusal (i.e., bite) abnormalities.
   c. **Treatment** consists of moist heat applied to the jaw, muscle relaxants, bite plates or occlusal splints, a diet of soft foods, correcting the occlusion, or surgery.
   d. **OTC products** that can help relieve the pain include oral analgesics (e.g., acetaminophen, ibuprofen).

7. **Teething pain.** The ADA has not accepted any product for teething pain. A **frozen teething ring** can provide symptomatic relief. Persisting pain may be treated with a local anesthetic such as benzocaine (found in Baby Anbesol and Baby Orajel). If a teething child presents with a fever, a physician should be contacted.

8. **Xerostomia** (i.e., dry mouth) is caused by improper functioning of the salivary glands (as in Sjögren's syndrome). **Artificial saliva** is available as an OTC product. The ADA has approved the following artificial saliva products: Moi-Stir, Salivart, Xero-Lube, and Saliva Substitute.

C. Common oral lesions and OTC products

1. **Canker sores** (also called **recurrent aphthous ulcers** or **recurrent aphthous stomatitis**)
   a. The **cause** of canker sores is unknown. Recent studies suggest that the cause may be dysfunction of the immune system initiated by minor trauma.
   b. **Lesions** can occur on any nonkeratinized mucosal surface in the mouth (i.e., tongue, lips) and usually appear gray-to-yellow with an erythematous halo of inflamed tissue surrounding the ulcer. Most lesions persist for 10–14 days and heal without scarring.
   c. **OTC products** can control the pain of canker sores, shorten the duration of current lesions, and prevent new lesions. Products include **protectants** and **local anesthetics.**
      (1) **Protectants** include Orabase, denture adhesives (see II F 2), and benzoin tincture. Denture adhesives are not approved for this use by the FDA.
      (2) **Local anesthetics,** such as benzocaine or butacaine, are the **most common anesthetics** found in these OTC products.
         (a) The FDA has approved the following ingredients:
            (i) Benzocaine (5%–20%)
            (ii) Benzyl alcohol (0.05%–0.1%)
            (iii) Dyclonine (0.05%–0.1%)
            (iv) Hexylresorcinol (0.05%–0.1%)
            (v) Menthol (0.04%–2%)
            (vi) Phenol (0.5%–1.5%)
            (vii) Phenolate sodium (0.5%–1.5%)
            (viii) Salicyl alcohol (1%–6%)
         (b) Examples of OTC local anesthetics for oral use include Anbesol, Blistex, Campho-Phenique, Orajel, Orajel CoverMed, Zilactin-B, Benzodent, and Viractin.
         (c) The use of products containing substantial amounts of menthol, phenol, camphor, and eugenol should be discouraged due to their ability to irritate tissue.
         (d) Aspirin should not be retained in the mouth or placed on an oral lesion in an attempt to provide relief.
         (e) **Investigational products** include thalidomide, which is being studied for the treatment of AIDS-associated oral canker sores. Amelexanox (Apthasol) has approvable status for the treatment of the signs and symptoms of canker sores.

2. **Cold sores** (also called **fever blisters**) are caused primarily by the herpes simplex type I virus. An outbreak may be provoked by stress, minor infection, fever, or sunlight. Cold sores usually occur on the lips and are recurrent, often arising in the same location.
   a. **Presentation.** An outbreak is preceded by burning, itching, or numbness. Red papules of fluid-containing vesicles then appear, and these eventually burst and form a crust. These sores are typically self-limited and heal in 10–14 days without scarring.
   b. **OTC products** for cold sores include products that contain softening compounds (e.g., emollient creams, petrolatum, protectants), which keep the cold sore moist to prevent it from drying and fissuring. Local anesthetics in nondrying bases (e.g., Orabase, with benzocaine) decrease pain. Highly astringent bases should be avoided. The ADA con-

traindicates caustic agents (e.g., phenol, silver nitrate), camphor and other counterirritants, and hydrocortisone for the treatment of cold sores.

(1) If a **secondary infection** develops, bacitracin or neomycin ointments should be recommended. If necessary, the patient should consult a physician for a systemic antibiotic prescription.

(2) A lip **sunscreen** should be used for patients whose cold sores appear to be due to sun exposure.

(3) The essential amino acid L-lysine has been used in oral doses of 300–1200 mg daily to accelerate recovery or suppress recurrence of cold sores. However, studies have produced conflicting data regarding L-lysine and its effect on the duration, severity, and recurrence rate of cold sores.

c. **Prescription products.** Acyclovir 400 mg orally twice a day has been studied for delaying recurrence and reducing the frequency of cold sores. Also, **acyclovir 5%** in a modified aqueous cream applied four times daily significantly reduced the healing time of cold sores and the number of recurrent sores. One study of **famciclovir** 125 mg, 250 mg, 500 mg administered three times a day for five days reduced the size of lesions and decreased the pain and healing time of cold sores.

D. Common oral infections and OTC products

1. **Candidiasis** (also called **thrush**) is caused by the fungus *Candida albicans,* which is the most common opportunistic pathogen associated with oral infections. Thrush has a milky curd appearance, and affected patients should contact a physician.

2. **Oral cancer.** The most common oral cancer is **squamous cell carcinoma,** which can appear as red or white lesions, ulcerations, or tumors.

a. **Signs** and **symptoms** include a color change in the tongue, a sore throat that does not heal, and persistent or unexplained bleeding. Patients with any of these signs should contact a physician or a dentist.

b. **Risk factors** include smoked and smokeless tobacco as well as alcohol.

c. **Treatment** consists of eliminating use of tobacco and alcohol in any form (e.g., alcoholic beverages, mouth rinses with alcohol). Also, treatment generally includes **wide local excision** for small lesions and **en bloc excisions** for larger lesions (in continuity with radical neck dissection if lymph nodes are involved). Radiation, alone or combined with surgery, may be appropriate. Chemotherapy may be used as palliation or as an adjunct to surgery and radiation.

d. **OTC medications** should not be administered until after checking with a physician. For example, OTC medication used for inflammation can increase the effects of methotrexate. Chemotherapeutic agents can produce many possible side effects that require immediate medical attention (e.g., chest pain, inflammation, unusual bleeding). Some examples of side effects that usually do not require medical attention include nausea, vomiting, loss of appetite or hair, and trouble sleeping. OTC medications can be useful in these cases; however, nausea and vomiting are treated by prescription medications such as ondansetron or metoclopramide. Nonpharmacologic measures, such as avoiding disturbing environmental odors and vestibular disturbances, might be helpful in minimizing nausea and vomiting.

E. Recommended standard prophylaxis for prevention of endocarditis

1. **Amoxicillin** 3.0 g orally 1 hour before procedure, then 1.5 g 6 hours after initial dose is the recommended standard prophylactic regimen for all dental, oral, and upper respiratory tract procedures.

2. For patients who are allergic to **amoxicillin or penicillin,** the recommended **alternative oral regimens** include **erythromycin ethylsuccinate,** 800 mg, or **erythromycin stearate,** 1.0 g, orally 2 hours before procedure; then half the dose 6 hours after initial dose or **clindamycin** 300 mg orally 1 hour before procedure and 150 mg 6 hours after initial dose.

F. OTC denture products

1. **Denture cleansers** are either **chemical** or **abrasive** in respect to their cleansing ability.

a. **Chemical** denture cleansers include alkaline peroxide, alkaline hypochlorite, or dilute acids.

(1) **Alkaline peroxide** is the **most commonly used** chemical denture cleanser and is available as tablets or powder. It causes oxygen to be released, which creates a

cleansing effect. Alkaline peroxide does not damage the surface of acrylic resins; however, it may bleach them.

(2) **Alkaline hypochlorite** (i.e., bleach) dissolves the matrix of plaque but has no effect on calculus. It is both bactericidal and fungicidal. A **disadvantage** of alkaline hypochlorite is that it **corrodes metal denture components.** It can also bleach acrylic resin, therefore, it should not be used more than once a week.

b. **Abrasive** denture cleansers are available as gel, paste, or powder (e.g., silicates, sodium bicarbonate, dicalcium phosphate, calcium carbonate).

(1) Dentures should not be soaked in hot water because the heat could distort or warp the appliances.

(2) The ADA accepts the following denture cleansers as safe and effective: Complete, Dentu-Gel, Dentu-Creme, Efferdent, Polident, and Fresh 'N' Brite.

2. **Denture adherents** contain materials (e.g., karaya gum, pectin, methylcellulose) that swell, gel, and become viscous in order to promote adhesion, which increases the denture attachment to underlying soft tissues.

a. **Disadvantages.** As the use of denture adherents increases, the soft tissue deteriorates. Denture adherents can also provide a medium for bacterial and fungal growth. Daily use of denture adherents is not recommended.

b. The ADA accepts the following denture adherents as safe and effective: Co-Re-Ga, Perma-Grip, Effergrip, Firmdent, Wernet's products, Orafix, and Secure.

G. Pharmacists' responsibilities to the patient using OTC oral products

1. **Refer** a patient to a dentist if the oral complaint involves an abscess with fever, swelling, malaise, lymphadenopathy, or purulent exudate.

2. **Remind** patients that cold and canker sores, with appropriate treatment, are usually a self-limiting problem.

3. Patients should be informed about **how to use recommended products,** the duration of use, the expectations of using the product, and the procedure to follow if the product is ineffective.

4. If a nonprescription product does not improve a condition, or if the condition worsens, use of the product should be discontinued and a physician or dentist should be contacted.

III. OPHTHALMIC PRODUCTS

A. Anatomy

1. **Eyelids** are folds of tissue that protect the eye and distribute tears.

2. The **external eye** is formed by the lacrimal apparatus and the conjunctival cul-de-sac.

3. **Internal eye**

a. The **sclera** is the outer coating over the eyeball.

b. The **iris** is the colored membrane that regulates the entrance of light through the pupil.

c. **Aqueous humor** is the fluid derived from the blood by a process of secretion and ultrafiltration.

d. The **lens,** which is a transparent refracting membrane, focuses rays to form an image on the retina.

e. The **retina** receives the image formed by the lens.

f. The **conjunctiva** is the mucous membrane that lines the eyelids.

g. The **trabecular meshwork** and **Schlemm's canal** serve as exit pathways for aqueous humor.

B. Eye disorders

1. **Conditions affecting the eyelid** include irritation, inflammation, and infections [e.g., contusions (black eyes), styes].

a. **Symptoms of a stye** include pain, tenderness, redness, and swelling. A stye is defined as a localized, purulent, inflammatory infection of one or more sebaceous glands of the eyelid. Styes cannot be treated with OTC medications. Often, hot compresses applied four times a day are helpful. However, some patients may require treatment with an antibiotic.

b. Inflammation of the eyelid (blepharitis) can be detected by redness of the lids, and burning, itching, and scaly skin. The underlying problem (e.g., seborrheic dermatitis, *Staphylococcus aureus*) should be treated, which often requires an antibiotic.

c. Black eyes may be treated with cold compresses for the first 24 hours then warm compresses. Damage to the eyelid itself should be referred to a physician.

2. External ocular disorders include chemical burns, conjunctivitis, and lacrimal system disorders.

a. Symptoms of conjunctivitis include redness, itching, and discharge.

(1) Familiar types of conjunctivitis include bacterial, chlamydial, viral, and allergic.

(2) Treatment. Antihistamines and decongestants can be used for symptomatic relief for allergic and bacterial conjunctivitis.

b. Dacryoadenitis (i.e., swelling of the lacrimal gland) should be referred to a physician. Symptoms include red, burning eyes and the sensation of a foreign body in the eye.

c. Corneal edema is the result of an underlying cause (e.g., damage to the eye). Hypertonic solutions and decongestants can be helpful treatments. However, if edema persists for more than 24 hours, a physician should be contacted.

d. Insufficient tearing (e.g., Sjögren's syndrome) is generally successfully treated with artificial tear products (see III D 5).

e. Chemical burns should be referred to a physician.

3. Internal ocular disorders include glaucoma (i.e., an increase in intraocular pressure), cataracts (i.e., opacity of the crystalline lens of the eye or its capsule), and uveitis (i.e., inflammation of the uvea). These internal ailments should be diagnosed and treated by a physician.

C. Treatment. The following **pharmaceutical agents** are included in ophthalmic products for the specific purposes listed below.

1. Antioxidants and **stabilizers** are used to delay or prevent deterioration of the drug. Examples include edetic acid, sodium bisulfite, sodium metabisulfite, sodium thiosulfate, and thiourea.

2. Buffers are designed to keep products within the appropriate pH range, which is 6.0–8.0 (tears are 7.4). Buffers include: acetic acid, boric acid, hydrochloric acid, phosphoric acid, potassium bicarbonate, potassium borate, potassium tetraborate, potassium bicarbonate, potassium citrate, the potassium phosphates, sodium acetate, sodium bicarbonate, sodium biphosphate, sodium borate, sodium carbonate, sodium citrate, sodium hydroxide, and sodium phosphate.

3. Clarifying or wetting agents reduce surface tension of the lens. Examples include polysorbate 20, polysorbate 80, poloxamer 282, and tyloxapol.

4. Preservatives destroy or inhibit the development of microorganisms. Examples of these agents are benzalkonium chloride and benzethonium chloride.

5. Tonicity adjusters include dextrose, glycerine (1%), potassium chloride, propylene glycol (1%), and sodium chloride. Agents considered to be isotonic should equal 0.9%±0.2% sodium chloride. When applied to the eye, these agents pull water from the middle of the cornea. Nonisotonic agents used in the eye may produce excessive blinking or cause damage.

6. Viscosity-increasing agents are used to increase the retention time for ophthalmic medications. These agents include cellulose derivatives, dextran 70, gelatin (0.01%) and liquid polyols.

D. Medicinal agents. There are no FDA-approved anti-infective products available for OTC ophthalmic use. The following compounds are medicinal agents used for ophthalmic therapy.

1. Astringents. The only FDA-recommended astringent is zinc sulfate (0.25%). This agent is relatively mild but still provides some relief from eye irritation because it decreases inflammation. The recommended dose is 1–2 drops four times a day.

2. Demulcents are relatively free of side effects and are used to protect and lubricate the eye from dryness and irritation from sun exposure. Demulcents include carboxymethylcellulose sodium, dextran 70, gelatin, glycerin, hydroxyethyl cellulose, hydroxypropyl methylcellulose, methylcellulose, polyethylene glycol 300, polyethylene glycol 400, polysorbate 80, polyvinyl alcohol, povidone, and propylene glycol.

3. **Decongestants and vasoconstrictors**
   a. **Mechanism of action.** These agents work by producing a temporary constriction of the blood vessels located in the conjunctiva.
   b. **Products** include naphazoline hydrochloride (e.g., Clear Eyes), phenylephrine hydrochloride (e.g., Isopto Frin), tetrahydrozoline hydrochloride (e.g., Murine Plus), and oxymetazoline hydrochloride (OcuClear). Combination decongestant and antihistamine products include Naphazoline Plus Solution, Naphcon-A, and Opcon-A.
   c. **Rebound congestion** can occur with a long duration of use.
   d. **Contraindication.** The available OTC agents are useful in relieving eye redness and irritations and are contraindicated in angle-closure glaucoma patients.

4. **Hypertonic agents** (e.g., sodium chloride 2%–5%) are used for the relief of corneal swelling. Although they are available as nonprescription products, these products should be used under the supervision of a physician because of their concentration.

5. **Artificial tears** (combination of hypertonic agent, buffer, viscosity agent, and preservative) are used to lubricate the eye for relief of dry eyes or irritation.

E. General patient information

1. Patients should be counseled regarding appropriate administration of individual products. They also should be told to wash hands thoroughly before applying these products.

2. If a patient presents with a headache or vision abnormalities, has had symptoms persisting for more than 3 days, or a recommended OTC product has not abated symptoms during this time, a physician should be contacted. In general, OTC ophthalmic products should not be used for more than 3 days without physician supervision.

F. Contact lenses. Wearing contact lenses successfully depends on adequate tear production.

1. **General considerations**
   a. **Indications** include keratoconus (protrusion of the central part of the cornea), aphakia (absence of lens), visual aberrations, myopia (nearsightedness), hyperopia (farsightedness), astigmatism (improper focus of light rays), presbyopia (diminution of the accommodation of the lens), and monovision.
   b. **Contraindications** include occupations with exposure to excessive dust, wind, or smoke; chronic conjunctivitis or blepharitis; and recurrent bacterial, fungal, or viral infections.
   c. **Caution** should be taken by patients suffering from diseases that can affect the normal eye (e.g., epilepsy, high blood pressure, heart disease, diabetes mellitus). Similar cautions should be taken by patients using medications that can alter the eye (e.g., oral contraceptives). Certain diseases and drugs may have direct effects on the eye. For example, high blood pressure can produce retinal hemorrhage; diabetes mellitus produces an outgrowth of vessels in the iris and anterior chamber of the eye; and oral contraceptives have numerous possible effects on the eye (e.g., increased corneal sensitivity, color changes, decreased visual acuity).

2. **Types of contact lenses**
   a. **Hard lenses** are rigid, hydrophobic products. The **most common plastic used** is polymethylmethacrylate (PMMA), better known as **Lucite** or **Plexiglas.**
      (1) **Advantages** include the ability to mark the contact lens to identify for which eye the contact is intended. Cost compared to soft lenses could be considered an advantage.
      (2) **Disadvantages** include minimal wetability and limited oxygen permeability, which limits the length of patient wear and the ability to adapt to the lens.
   b. **Soft lenses** contain a hydroxyl group or a combination of hydroxyl and lactam groups, which allows the lens to hold water.
      (1) **Advantages.** Soft contact lenses are easier to apply, more comfortable to wear, and more difficult to dislodge than hard lenses.
      (2) **Disadvantages** include the potential to absorb compounds (e.g., chemicals) from products, cost, the necessary extended care to keep the lens from deteriorating, and altered visual acuity due to hydration of the lens.

(3) With the exception of a small number of rewetting solutions, patients should be advised against the application of ophthalmic products when wearing soft lenses.

c. **Gas-permeable lenses** combine soft lens material and PMMA.

(1) **Advantages** of the combined products include increased visual acuity and more comfort than with hard lenses.

(2) **Disadvantages** to gas-permeable lenses are that they accumulate protein and lipid deposits and are made of hydrophobic materials.

3. **Adverse effects of lenses**

a. **Corneal edema** can result from inadequate oxygenation.

b. **Medications** can affect the eye and potentiate problems (e.g., edema of the cornea). Examples include oral contraceptives, decongestants, antihistamines, tricyclic antidepressants, and diuretics.

4. **Contact lens care**

a. **Hard lens care** includes cleaning to remove oils and debris, soaking in a storage medium, wetting to produce a hydrophobic surface, and rewetting (cleaning and rewetting of lens).

b. **Soft lens care** includes cleaning (with surface-active or enzymatic cleaners), disinfecting (thermal and chemical), and rewetting.

c. **Gas-permeable lens care** involves cleaning, wetting, and soaking. Some of these lenses contain more silicone agents, requiring conditioning solutions, which are made especially for rewetting purposes.

d. **Solution ingredients**

(1) **Cleaning products** generally contain nonionic or amphoteric surfactants, which dislodge mucus, lipids, and proteins from the lens. Contact lenses should be rinsed following the cleansing step to prevent eye irritation.

(2) **Wetting solutions** are applied directly to the lens before insertion into the eye. Wetting solutions are intended to lubricate, decrease lens surface tension, and change the lens surface from hydrophobic to hydrophilic.

(3) **Soaking** and **storage solutions** are used to provide an aseptic environment and to hydrate the lens.

(4) **Preservatives** used in these solutions include: benzalkonium chloride, thimerosal, phenylmercuric nitrate, sorbic acid, and sodium edetate. Thimerosal causes a great deal of irritation to many soft contact lens wearers.

STUDY QUESTIONS

Directions: Each of the numbered items or incomplete statements in this section is followed by answers or by completions of the statement. Select the **one** lettered answer or completion that is **best** in each case.

1. Ophthalmic agents contraindicated in glaucoma patients include which of the following substances?

(A) Antioxidants
(B) Antipruritics
(C) Decongestants
(D) Emollients

2. Which of the following is the only FDA-recommended astringent?

(A) Benzalkonium chloride
(B) Sodium chloride
(C) Zinc sulfate
(D) Edetic acid

3. Abrasives, ingredients in dentifrices, are noted for which of the following actions?

(A) Providing flavor
(B) Cleansing via a foaming detergent action
(C) Removing plaque and debris
(D) Preventing dental caries
(E) Adding thickness to the product

4. The appropriate pH range for ophthalmic products is

(A) 2.0–3.0
(B) 4.0–6.0
(C) 6.0–8.0
(D) 8.0–10.0

5. Which type of contact lens can most easily be ruined by the absorption of chemicals?

(A) Hard lenses
(B) Soft lenses
(C) Gas-permeable lenses

6. All of the following statements concerning the use of alkaline peroxide as a denture cleanser are true EXCEPT

(A) it may bleach the denture
(B) it is available as tablets or powders
(C) it acts by releasing oxygen
(D) it is fungicidal and bactericidal
(E) it does not damage the surface of acrylic resins

7. All of the following statements concerning teeth-whitening products are true EXCEPT

(A) possible risks include tissue irritation and gingivitis
(B) most products contain 10% carbamide peroxide
(C) most products contain zinc to prevent calculus formation
(D) antiseptics (e.g., Proxigel) have been used as bleaching agents
(E) calcium peroxide and sodium monofluorophosphate are teeth-whitening agents

8. All of the following desensitizing agents are recommended for sensitive teeth EXCEPT

(A) 10% carbamide peroxide
(B) 5% potassium nitrate
(C) dibasic sodium citrate
(D) 10% strontium chloride hexahydrate

9. Which of the following statements is NOT correct?

(A) The "clicking" sound you hear when you swallow is caused by the air movement in the eustachian tubes
(B) Giving a baby a bottle of milk can help prevent ear pain during aircraft descent
(C) Chewing and talking actually aid in the natural outward movement of ear wax
(D) The pain of otitis media is usually made worse by pressing on the tragus
(E) The product Swim-Ear could be recommended to prevent otitis externa

10. Carbamide peroxide appears to soften earwax by

(A) causing oxygen to be released, which loosens the wax
(B) stimulating fluid secretion in the ear canal
(C) actually dissolving the ear wax
(D) decreasing lipid content of the wax
(E) none of the above

11. All of the following statements are true regarding otitis externa EXCEPT

(A) One of the other names for this condition is "swimmers ear"
(B) Heat and humidity are considered contributing factors in the pathogenesis of this condition
(C) Although there are no OTC agents available to treat this condition, Debrox is considered a useful preventive agent
(D) This condition may require prescription topical antibiotic ear drops
(E) The use of cotton-tipped applicators (e.g., Q-tips) in the ear canal may predispose a person to this condition

12. A common oral problem caused by herpes simplex type I virus (HSV-1) is

(A) aphthous ulcers
(B) canker sores
(C) aphthous stomatitis
(D) fever blisters
(E) thrush

13. Mrs. Smith enters a pharmacy and says, "I think I've picked up one of my grandchildren's colds and have developed painful cold sores." The pharmacist would offer all of the following statements as advice for the treatment of cold sores EXCEPT

(A) lesions should be kept clean by gently washing with mild soap solutions.
(B) factors that delay healing (e.g., wind, sunlight, fatigue) should be avoided
(C) cold sores should be kept moist to prevent drying and fissuring by using Orabase cream
(D) hydrocortisone should be placed directly on the lesion
(E) application of a topical antibiotic (e.g., Neomycin) 3–4 times daily may be warranted if there are signs and symptoms of secondary bacterial infection

14. The definition of a surfactant (an ingredient in toothpaste) can best be described by which of the following statements? Surfactant

(A) prevents drying of the preparation
(B) removes debris by its detergent action and causes foaming, which is usually desired by the patient
(C) physically removes plaque and debris
(D) determines the texture, dispersiveness, and appearance of the product
(E) adds flavor to the preparation which makes it more appealing to the patient

15. A sixteen-year-old girl stops by a pharmacy on her way home from school. She says to the pharmacist, "I have been using Proxigel daily to bleach my teeth in preparation for my spring formal. However, my teeth are becoming very sensitive." All of the following statements are advice that the pharmacist might suggest EXCEPT

(A) there is a possibility that you may damage the gingival tissue and tooth pulp
(B) oxidizing agents may have the potential for mutating or enhancing the carcinogenic effects of other agents (e.g., tobacco)
(C) discouraging the girl from attempting tooth bleaching without dental supervision
(D) Proxigel is an antiseptic that contains zinc and has not been used for cosmetic whitening of the teeth
(E) the most common ingredient in products responsible for teeth whitening is 10% carbamide peroxide and it can cause sensitivity

16. All of the following products may be recommended by a pharmacist for the treatment of canker sores EXCEPT

(A) Benzocaine
(B) Zilactin-B
(C) Bayer aspirin should be placed on the oral lesion
(D) Anbesol
(E) Orajel

17. A FDA-approved ingredient for protection against painful sensitivity of the teeth due to cold, heat, acids, sweets, or contact is

(A) dicalcium phosphate
(B) sodium lauryl sulfate
(C) 5% potassium nitrate
(D) Zinc chloride
(E) Calcium carbonate

Directions: Each item below contains three suggested answers of which **one or more** is correct. Choose the answer

- **A** if **I only** is correct
- **B** if **III only** is correct
- **C** if **I and II** are correct
- **D** if **II and III** are correct
- **E** if **I, II, and III** are correct

18. Which of the following compounds are considered a suspending agent (an ingredient in dentifrices)?

    I. Dicalcium phosphate
    II. Karaya gum
    III. Methylcellulose

19. Cold-sore treatment might include which of the following ingredients?

    I. Benzocaine
    II. Dyclonine
    III. Camphor

20. Pharmacists can recommend OTC drug treatment for which of the following ear conditions?

    I. Treatment of accumulated ear wax
    II. Prevention of "blocked ears" due to altitude changes
    III. Prevention of "Swimmer's ear"

ANSWERS AND EXPLANATIONS

1. The answer is C *[III D 3].*
Decongestants can cause a slight pupillary dilation. Although this is not significant in open-angle glaucoma, these agents should be avoided in angle-closure patients. In angle-closure glaucoma, the blockage to outflow is more severe and directly involves the anterior chamber.

2. The answer is C *[III C 1, D].*
Zinc sulfate is the only ophthalmic astringent recommended by the FDA. Sodium chloride is a hypertonic agent. Benzalkonium chloride is a preservative used in contact lens solutions. Edetic acid is an antioxidant used to slow or prevent deterioration of ophthalmic drugs.

3. The answer is C *[II B 2 d (1) (a)].*
Abrasives are components in dentifrices that are responsible for physically removing plaque. Patients should use the least abrasive dentifrice, unless directed otherwise by the dentist.

4. The answer is C *[III C 2].*
The appropriate pH range for ophthalmic agents is 6.0–8.0, which is similar to the pH of tears (7.4).

5. The answer is B *[III F 2 b].*
Soft lenses allow for easier product absorption, and the absorption of chemicals from ophthalmic products can ruin the lenses. They also contain hydroxyl or hydroxyl and lactam groups, all of which are chemically reactive.

6. The answer is D *[II E 1 a (1)].*
The mechanism of action of alkaline peroxide is the release of oxygen for a mechanical cleaning effect. It can be used safely on acrylic appliances; however, it may bleach the appliance. It is available in tablet or powder form. Alkaline hypochlorite, not alkaline peroxide, is both bactericidal and fungicidal.

7. The answer is C *[II B 2 d (4)].*
Teeth-whitening agents usually contain 10% carbamide peroxide, which is a white crystal that reacts with water to release hydrogen peroxide and, therefore, liberates free oxides. Cosmetic agents can alter the normal flora or cause tissue irritation, gingivitis, and teeth sensitivity. Antiseptics (e.g., Gly-Oxide, Proxigel) and calcium peroxide (e.g., calprox in EpiSmile) have been used as teeth whitening agents. In addition, sodium monofluorophosphate is found in EpiSmile.

8. The answer is A *[II B 2 d (5)].*
Desensitizing agents should not be abrasive or used on a chronic basis unless directed by a dentist. The products approved by the American Dental Association include the ingredients 5% potassium nitrate, 10% strontium chloride hexahydrate, and dibasic sodium citrate 2% in pluronic gel. The ingredient 10% carbamide peroxide is a whitening agent that can cause teeth sensitivity and, therefore, should not be used by a patient with sensitive teeth.

9. The answer is D *[I B 3 b (2)].*
The pain of otitis externa (not media) is made worse by moving the ear (pulling upward on the auricle or pressing the tragus). Because otitis media involves the middle ear, this pain is not affected by movement of the external ear structure.

10. The answer is A *[I B 1 c (1) (a)].*
Carbamide peroxide releases oxygen and, via a mechanical action of effervescence, loosens the wax debris and aids in its removal.

11. The answer is C *[I B 3].*
Debrox, a trade name for carbamide peroxide, is used to soften ear wax, not as a preventive agent for otitis externa. Prevention includes the instilling of ear drops containing either a 50:50 solution of isopropyl alcohol and white vinegar, boric acid solution, acetic acid solution, or an isopropyl alcohol/anhydrous glycerin solution.

12. The answer is D *[II C 2].*
Cold sores (also called fever blisters) are primarily caused by the herpes simplex type I virus.

13. The answer is D *[II C 2].*
Stress, minor infection, fever, or sunlight may provoke and delay healing of cold sores. OTC products for the treatment of cold sores include products that contain softening compounds (e.g., emollient creams, petrolatum, protectants), which keep the cold sore moist to prevent it from drying and fissuring. If a secondary infection develops, bacitracin or neomycin ointments should be recommended.

14. The answer is B *[II B 2 d (1)(b)].*
Sodium lauryl sulfate is used frequently as a surfactant in most dentifrices. Its detergent action aids in the removal of debris and the foaming is usually desired by the patient. There is no evidence that surfactants possess anticaries activity or decrease periodontal disease. The FDA considers surfactants an inactive ingredient in dentifrices.

15. The answer is D *[II B 2 d (4)].*
Teeth-whitening agents usually contain 10% carbamide peroxide, which is a white crystal that reacts with water to release hydrogen peroxide and, therefore, liberates free oxides. Cosmetic agents can alter the normal flora or cause tissue irritation, gingivitis, and teeth sensitivity. Antiseptics have been used as cosmetic whiteners (e.g., Gly-Oxide, Proxigel) along with calcium peroxide (e.g., calprox in EpiSmile). EpiSmile also contains sodium monofluorophosphate.

16. The answer is C *[II C 1 c (2)].*
Local anesthetics can provide relief of pain for canker sores. The most common local anesthetics found in OTC products include benzocaine and butacaine. Some examples are Anbesol, Zilactin-B, and Orajel. Aspirin should not be retained in the mouth before swallowing or placed in the area of the oral lesions because of the high risk for chemical burn with necrosis.

17. The answer is C *[II B 2 d (5)].*
Desensitizing agents should not be abrasive or used on a chronic basis unless directed by a dentist. The products approved by the American Dental Association include the ingredients 5% potassium nitrate, 10% strontium chloride hexahydrate, and dibasic sodium citrate 2% in pluronic gel.

18. The answer is D (II, III) *[II B 2 d (1) (c)].*
Suspending agents are products that add thickness to the dentifrices. Examples are tragacanth, karaya gum, and methylcellulose. Dicalcium phosphate is categorized as an abrasive product.

19. The answer is C (I, II) *[II C 1 c].*
Cold-sore treatment involves keeping the lesion moist with emollient creams, petrolatum, or protectants. In addition, local anesthetics (e.g., benzocaine, dyclonine, salicyl alcohol) may be used. Topical counterirritants (e.g., camphor) and caustics or escharotic agents (e.g., phenol, menthol, silver nitrate) are not recommended because they may further irritate the tissue. Cold sores are usually self-limiting and heal within 10–14 days without scarring.

20. The answer is C *[I B].*
OTC drug treatment can be recommended for all of these ear conditions.

30 OTC Agents for Pediculosis, Acne, Sun Protection, and Contact Dermatitis

Larry N. Swanson

I. PEDICULOSIS AND PEDICULICIDES

A. Introduction. Pediculosis is a skin infestation produced by blood-sucking lice. Lice are small, flat, wingless insects with stubby antennae and three pairs of legs that end in sharp, curved claws. Three **types of lice infest humans:**

1. *Pediculus humanus capitis* (i.e., the head louse)
2. *Pediculus humanus corporis* (i.e., the body louse)
3. *Phthirus pubis* (i.e., the pubic, or crab, louse)

B. Life cycles. The lice that infest humans pass through similar life cycles.

1. **Location.** All lice need human warmth to survive.
   a. **Head** and **pubic lice** spend their entire cycle on the skin of the human host.
   b. **Body lice** live in clothing, coming to the skin surface only to feed.
2. **Development**
   a. Each type of louse develops from **eggs (nits)** that incubate for about 1 week. When the small, grey-white, tear-shaped eggs hatch, the nymphs appear.
   b. In about 3 weeks, the **nymphs** mature; then, the females start to lay eggs.
   c. Each type of louse survives about 1 month as a **mature adult.** During this time, the female head lice can produce 7–10 eggs a day over her 40 day lifespan.
3. **Egg deposit**
   a. **Body lice** deposit their eggs on fibers of clothing, particularly in the seams. These lice can survive without food up to 10 days, and the eggs may remain viable for about 1 month.
   b. **Head** and **pubic lice** deposit their eggs on hair strands, about 1/4 inch from the skin.

C. Incidence. The incidence of lice infestations increases each year.

1. As many as 12 million cases of head lice occur each year in the United States.
2. The bulk of these cases occur between September and November, when students are back in school.
3. In outbreaks of head lice, 70% of cases occur in children younger than age 12 years.
4. Infestations tend to be more common in girls, presumably because of their greater tendency to share grooming items.
5. Unlike the other two forms of lice, body lice are associated with improper hygiene and are often present in homeless people. This infestation is rare in the United States, especially when people follow proper hygiene routines.

D. Medical problems

1. Both adult and nymph lice are blood-sucking; they feed on humans by piercing the skin and introducing a small amount of saliva (which contains an **anticoagulant**) into the feeding area.
   a. The attachment of lice to the body causes the **erythematous papule,** which may **itch.**
   b. The female louse produces a sticky **cement-like secretion** that holds the eggs in place on the hair shaft so securely that ordinary shampooing does not remove it.

2. Neither head nor crab lice transmit infections, but body lice transmit **typhus, relapsing fever,** and **trench fever.**

3. Lice and humans have a true **parasitic relationship;** lice depend on the human host for shelter, food, and reproductive success. Once hatched, nymphs must have access to the human host within the first 12- to 24-hour period, if they are to survive.

E. Methods of transmission

1. **Head lice** are most commonly spread by head-to-head contact with an infested person through hats, caps, scarves, pillowcases, communal combs and brushes, or clothing that is hung close together (e.g., on a coat rack).

2. **Pubic lice** are transmitted primarily through sexual contact, but also through shared undergarments, towels, or toilet seats.
   - **a.** The lice affect teens and young adults most often through sexual contact.
   - **b.** Lice frequently coexist with other sexually transmitted diseases.
   - **c.** Scratching in the genital areas may transmit pubic lice to other hairy regions, such as the eyelashes, eyebrows, sideburns, and mustaches.

F. Signs and symptoms

1. **Head lice**
   - **a.** Most patients have fewer than 10 lice.
   - **b.** The most common symptom is head-scratching.
   - **c.** Skin redness around the nape (i.e., back) of the neck and above the ears is usually seen.
   - **d.** The lice can be identified by direct examination using wooden applicator sticks or a comb to part the hair, then looking at the hair through a magnifying glass.
   - **e.** The lice appear as tiny brownish grey spots, that are often difficult to see. The shiny, whitish-silver eggs, which appear almost as grains of sugar, are more likely to be seen than the lice. The nits usually reside about one-fourth inch from the scalp on the hair shaft, and they may be confused with dandruff or hair spray droplets.

2. **Pubic lice.** The primary symptom is scratching in the genital area.

3. **Body lice.** The most common symptoms are bites and itching, which are commonly seen as vertical excoriations on the trunk area.

G. Treatment

1. There are **two goals** in the treatment of lice:
   - **a.** To kill the lice and nits
   - **b.** To control the symptoms of itching in order to prevent secondary infection

2. **Itching.** Pharmacists should advise patients that even after the causative organism and nits have been killed, itching may persist for several days. This aspect is very important because patients may decide to use pediculicides excessively, thinking that they have been ineffective when the itching continues. Excessive use of pediculicides may result in excessive drying, which can cause further itching.

3. **Home remedies.** Because of the social stigma attached to lice infestation, some individuals may resort to harmful home remedies. Examples of such uncomfortable, ineffective, and potentially dangerous approaches include:
   - **a.** Shaving the head and pubic area
   - **b.** Applying heat to the infested area with a hair dryer
   - **c.** Soaking the head in hot water for several minutes
   - **d.** Soaking the area of infestation with gasoline or kerosene

4. **Over-the-counter (OTC) pediculicide products** include:
   - **a. Pyrethrins 0.17%–0.33% with piperonyl butoxide 2%–4%.** This product is safe and effective for the treatment of head, pubic, and body lice. The combination of ingredients is an example of **pharmacologic synergism.**
     - **(1) Pyrethrins** kill by disrupting ion transport mechanisms at the nerve membranes. These natural insecticides are derived from a mixture of substances obtained from the flowers of the chrysanthemum plant. Because not all eggs may be killed with a

single application of this agent or removed with a nit comb, it may be necessary to reapply the pyrethrin product within 7–10 days of the first application (because the usual hatching time of eggs is 7–10 days).

(2) **Piperonyl butoxide** enhances the pediculicide effect of pyrethrins by suppressing the oxidative degradation mechanisms of the lice. Therefore, the length of time that the pyrethrins contact the lice is increased.

(3) **Side effects** from either agent are **uncommon.**

(a) **Contact dermatitis** (see IV) is the most frequently reported side effect.

(b) **Allergic reactions.** Because pyrethrins are derived from a plant (chrysanthemum), they may produce hay fever (i.e., allergic rhinitis) and asthma attacks in susceptible individuals. Thus, patients who have known allergies to ragweed or chrysanthemum plants should use this product with caution.

(4) Common **trade names** for this product include A-200 Pyrinate Shampoo, R and C, and RID.

(5) **Directions for use**

(a) Apply the product, undiluted, to the infested area until it is entirely wet.

(b) Allow the product to remain on the area for 10 minutes.

(c) Wash the area thoroughly with warm, soapy water or shampoo.

(d) Dry the area, preferably with a disposable cloth.

(e) Comb hair in the previously infested area with a fine-toothed comb to remove dead lice and eggs.

(f) Do not exceed two applications within 24 hours.

b. Permethrin (Nix) is a pyrethroid (i.e., a synthetic version of a pyrethrin). It is indicated only for head lice.

(1) **Mechanism of action.** Permethrin has the same mechanism of action as the pyrethrins.

(2) **Application.** Permethrin comes in the form of a creme rinse and should be applied like a conventional hair conditioner after the hair has been shampooed, rinsed, and towel-dried. The hair should be thoroughly saturated with permethrin, which should remain on the hair for 10 minutes then rinsed.

(3) **Effectiveness.** A single application is 97%–99% effective in killing lice and eggs.

(a) Because the agent is retained on the hair shaft, the product provides **protection** for up to 14 days. This 2-week therapeutic effect persists regardless of normal shampooing.

(b) **Re-treatment** is required in less than 1% of cases.

(c) Because of this prolonged effect, **nits do not need to be removed.** However, for cosmetic reasons or school policy, they should be.

(d) Many people consider permethrin to be the **agent of choice** in treating head lice infestations.

c. OTC pediculicide treatment failure. The National Pediculosis Association has received some reports of treatment failure with the use of the preceding agents. Speculations as to the cause of this treatment failure include failure to follow product instructions, noncompliance with nit removal, and possible head-lice drug resistance.

5. Prescription products

a. Malathion (Ovide) is an organophosphate cholinesterase inhibitor that has been widely used as a lawn and garden insecticide. It is indicated only for head lice. Malathion kills both lice and nits in vitro.

(1) **Mechanism of action.** Sulfur atoms in the malathion bind with sulfur groups on the hair, giving a residual protective effect against reinfestation.

(2) **Application.** Malathion is prepared as a lotion in 78% alcohol; therefore, caution should be used near an open flame or a hair dryer. The product should be sprinkled on dry hair and left for 8–12 hours before rinsing. A fine-toothed comb should be used to remove the dead lice and eggs.

(3) No systemic **adverse effects** have been reported with topical use of this medication.

(a) The alcoholic vehicle may produce stinging.

(b) Although this agent is very effective, its unpleasant odor (due to sulfhydryl compounds) and the required time of 8–12 hours on the scalp represent two main drawbacks.

b. Lindane, or gamma-benzene hexachloride has fallen into disfavor because of the potential for toxicity and the fact that its efficacy is less than the other agents available (both prescription and OTC products). It is available as a shampoo, cream, or lotion. It is indicated for head, pubic, and body lice.

(1) Mechanism of action. Lindane is neurotoxic to head lice and their eggs.

(2) Application. For head lice, the lindane shampoo should be applied to dry hair and thoroughly worked into the hair and scalp of the infested individual.

(a) The area should **be shampooed for 4 minutes,** then rinsed and towel dried.

(b) The nits should **be removed** with a fine-toothed comb designed for this purpose.

(3) It has **neurotoxicity potential** because of percutaneous absorption; therefore, its use should be avoided in infants, pregnant and nursing women, and anyone with a neurologic disorder. Severe **central nervous system (CNS) toxicity** has occurred in infants, with seizures and deaths reported, particularly when the lotion is used or when the agent is ingested. Toxicity has been minimal when the shampoo is used properly to treat head lice.

6. Adjunctive therapy

a. Nit removal

(1) The pediculicide products mentioned vary in their ability to kill the lice nits. To ensure successful therapy, after pediculicide application, the nits should be removed with a **fine-toothed comb.** Many schools have a **"no nit" policy;** that is, a child's hair and scalp must be free of nits before he or she is allowed to return to the classroom.

(2) Although various substances have been used in an effort to dislodge the nits from the hair shafts, most have been unsuccessful. A **formic acid formulation** (e.g., Step 2 Creme Rinse) softens the strong adhesive that binds the nits to the hair shaft. Indicated for use after pediculicide shampoo treatments, it comes packaged with a special fine-toothed comb. A mixture of 50% vinegar and 50% water applied and left on the hair for 1 hour has been recommended. A lice egg remover containing various enzymes comes as part of a kit in the Clear Total Lice Elimination System.

b. Treatment of other household members. Once a lice infestation has been identified in one member of the household, all other members should be examined carefully. Everyone who is infested should be treated at the same time.

c. Adjunctive methods for controlling lice infestations

(1) Washable material items should be machine-washed in hot water (130°F) for 5–10 minutes.

(2) Nonwashable material goods should be dry-cleaned or sealed in a plastic bag for 35 days.

(3) Personal items (e.g., comb, brushes) should be soaked in hot water (130°F) for 5–10 minutes.

(4) Furniture and household items (e.g., carpets, chairs, couches, pillows) should be vacuumed thoroughly. OTC spray products that contain pyrethrins are no more effective than vacuuming in terms of removing the risk of reinfestation.

d. Pediculicides should not be used around the eyes. For **eyelash pubic lice infestations, petrolatum** applied five times a day asphyxiates lice, or gentle removal with baby shampoo may be helpful.

H. Head lice myths are numerous. The following additional facts may reassure and inform patients and parents of patients.

1. No significant difference in incidence occurs among the various socioeconomic classes or races.

2. Hygiene and hair length are not contributing factors.

3. Head lice do not fly or jump from person to person.

4. Head lice do not carry other diseases.

5. Head lice cannot be contracted from animals, and pets are not susceptible to *Pediculus humanus capitis.*

6. The head does not have to be shaved to get rid of lice.

7. Washing hair with "brown" soap is not effective.

8. Head lice are unrelated to ticks.

9. Hair does not fall out as a consequence of infestation.

10. Head lice infestations can occur at any time of the year.

II. ACNE AND ITS REMEDIES

A. Overview

1. Definition. *Acne vulgaris* is a disorder of the pilosebaceous units, mainly of the face, chest, and back. The lesions usually start as open or closed comedones and evolve into inflammatory papules and pustules that either resolve as macules or become secondary pyoderma, which results in various sequelae.

2. Incidence

a. Acne vulgaris is the **most common** skin disease of adolescence; it affects about 90% of all adolescents.

b. It affects primarily adolescents in junior high and senior high, then decreases in adulthood.

3. Importance

a. Acne vulgaris is usually **self-limiting.**

b. However, the condition is significant to adolescents because of heightened self-consciousness about appearance.

c. A great majority of people do not consult a physician for treatment of acne; therefore, a pharmacist can play a significant role.

B. Etiology and pathophysiology

1. The **pathogenesis** of acne vulgaris involves **three events.**

a. Increased sebum production

(1) Sebum secretion is regulated primarily by **androgens,** which are actively secreted in both sexes beginning at puberty.

(2) One of these androgens, testosterone, is converted to **dihydrotestosterone (DHT).**

(3) DHT levels induce the sebaceous glands to increase in size and activity, resulting in increased amounts of sebum.

b. Abnormal clumping of epithelial horny cells within the pilosebaceous unit

(1) Normally, keratinized horny cells are sloughed from the epithelial lining of the pilosebaceous duct in the hair follicles and are carried to the skin surface with a flow of sebum.

(2) In the patient with acne, the keratinization process is abnormal, characterized by increased adherence and production of follicular epithelial cells. This process is called **retention hyperkeratosis,** and it results in obstruction of the outflow of the pilosebaceous unit.

c. Presence of *Propionibacterium acnes* (a gram-positive anaerobe)

(1) People with acne have skin colony counts of *P. acnes* that are significantly higher than the counts of those without acne.

(2) *P. acnes* produces several enzymes, including lipases, that break down sebum triglycerides to short-chain free fatty acids (FFAs), which are irritating, cause comedones, and result in inflammation.

2. Sequence of acne lesion development

a. Mechanical blockage of a pilosebaceous duct by clumped horny cells results in a closed comedo (i.e., a whitehead).

b. When a closed comedo develops, it can form either a papule or an open comedo (i.e., a blackhead). The color is attributed to melanin or oxidized lipid, not to dirt.

c. The lesion may enlarge and fill with pus, which is then termed a pustule.

d. In more severe cases of acne, papules may develop into nodules or cysts.

e. The term "pimple" nonspecifically refers to whiteheads, blackheads, papules, and pustules.

C. Clinical features

1. Location. Acne vulgaris lesions usually occur on the face, neck, chest, upper back, and shoulders. Any or all types of lesions may be seen on a single patient.

2. **Symptoms.** This condition is usually asymptomatic; however, some patients may have pruritus or pain if large, tender lesions are present.

3. **Classification.** It is important to differentiate **noninflammatory** from **inflammatory** acne to determine the best treatment approach. There have been many rating or grading scales for acne severity. One can further classify inflammatory acne as seen in Table 30-1. **Cystic acne** is present when the follicular wall ruptures occur deeper in the dermis and nodules and cysts are seen. Because of the potential for scarring, cystic acne patients should be referred to a physician for treatment. Scarring occurs with hypertrophic ridges, keloids, or atrophic "ice pick" pits.

D. **Complicating factors.** Other factors have been implicated in the exacerbation of acne.

1. **Drugs and hormones**
   a. Many topical and systemic medications (e.g., bromides, iodides, topical coal tar products, androgens, phenytoin, progestins, lithium, corticosteroids) can be comedogenic and can make acne worse or can induce acne-like eruptions (i.e., acneiform lesions).
   b. **Acneiform eruptions** differ from true acne lesions in that apparently no comedo forms, eruptions are usually acute, and the lesions usually are all in the same stage of development.

2. **Stress.** Despite rare individual exceptions, psychological stress is generally not thought to contribute to severity or exacerbations of acne.

3. **Diet.** There is very little evidence to support a relationship between diet and acne. Many different foods have been blamed for acne, from chocolates and sweets to shellfish to nuts and other fatty foods. Several studies have demonstrated that **chocolate does not affect acne.** The majority of dermatologists today make the following recommendations regarding diet:
   a. The patient should be eating a well-balanced diet. As with most other diseases, and as a matter of good health, excess fats and carbohydrates should be avoided.
   b. The patient who insists that certain foods cause exacerbation of acne should probably avoid those foods.

4. **Physical trauma** or **irritation** can promote the rupture of plugged follicles, which can produce more inflammatory reactions. Scrubbing the face, wearing headbands, cradling the chin with the hand, and picking at the pimples can contribute to the primary inflammation process. **Gentle** regular **washing** with soap and water can be beneficial.

5. **Cosmetics.** Some cosmetic bases and certain cosmetic ingredients are comedogenic (e.g., lanolins, petroleum bases, cocoa butter). Preparations such as cleansing creams, suntan oils, and heavy foundations should be avoided.

6. **Menstrual cycle.** Some women may notice flare-ups of acne during the premenstrual part of the cycle. Fluctuations in the level of progesterone are the probable cause.

7. **Environmental factors.** Very humid environments or heavy sweating lead to keratin hydration, swelling, and a decrease in the size of the pilosebaceous follicle orifice, which results in duct obstruction. The sun, as well as artificial ultraviolet (UV) light, can help acne by drying and peeling the skin, but both also can aggravate acne.

E. **Treatment and care**

1. **General**
   a. Most patients can be treated successfully with either topically or systemically administered medications or both. Acne often improves when patients reach their early twenties.

Table 30-1. Severity Grading of Inflammatory Acne Lesions

Severity	Papules/Pustules	Nodules
Mild	Few to several	None
Moderate	Several to many	Few to several
Severe	Numerous and/or extensive	Many

Adapted from *Handbook of Nonprescription Drugs,* 11th ed. Washington, D.C., American Pharmaceutical Association, 1996, p. 572.

b. Even the most effective treatment programs may take several weeks to produce any clinical improvement. This aspect must be emphasized.
c. People affected with acne should avoid anything that seems to worsen the condition (e.g., cosmetics, clothing, cradling the chin with the hand)
d. The number and type of lesions should be roughly determined to assess further therapeutic responses.

2. **Cleansing recommendations**
   a. Because many acne patients have oily skin, **gentle cleansing** two to three times daily is recommended for removing excess oil.
   b. Acne lesions cannot be scrubbed away. Compulsive scrubbing may actually worsen the acne by disrupting the follicular walls and, thus, setting the stage for inflammation.
   c. Mild facial soaps, such as Dove, Neutrogena, and Purpose, should be used to cleanse the skin.
   d. Medicated soaps containing sulfur, resorcinol, or salicylic acid are of little value because the medication rinses away rather than penetrating the follicle.
   e. Patients with mild comedonal acne might find benefit from cleansers containing pumice, polyethylene, or aluminum oxide particles (e.g., Brasivol). However, patients with inflammatory acne or sensitive skin should avoid these products.

3. **Approaches** to treatment depend on the severity of the condition. Although acne cannot be cured, most cases can be managed successfully with topical treatment alone. Based on the pathogenesis of the condition, potential methods include:
   a. **Unblocking** the sebaceous duct so that the contents can be easily expelled
   b. **Decreasing** the amount of sebum that is secreted
   c. **Changing** the composition of the **sebum** to make it less irritating by decreasing the population of *P. acnes*

4. **Nonprescription topical medications**
   a. **Benzoyl peroxide** (e.g. Oxy, Exact) (Category III; 2.5%–10%) has traditionally been recognized as the most effective topical OTC agent for acne, and many OTC acne products contain it. However, the final monograph from the Food and Drug Administration (FDA) changed the status of benzoyl peroxide from Category I to Category III, indicating that more data are needed to prove its safety with regards to long-term photocarcinogenic effects. (see Chapter 28 II B for category descriptions).
      (1) **Effects.** Benzoyl peroxide has irritant, drying, peeling, comedolytic, and antibacterial effects. The clinical response shows only minimal differences among the 2.5%, 5%, and 10% concentrations.
         (a) A **beneficial effect** should be noticed within about 2 weeks, but the usual length of a therapeutic trial is 6–8 weeks.
         (b) As for **adverse effects,** benzoyl peroxide may cause a burning or stinging sensation, which gradually disappears. Most of the adverse effects from this agent relate to its therapeutic effect of irritating and drying the skin. For this reason, the lowest concentration available should be chosen initially. From 1% to 3% of patients may be hypersensitive to benzoyl peroxide.
         (c) The vehicle for the benzoyl peroxide is also important in its overall activity. The alcohol gel vehicle tends to be more effective than the lotion or cream formulations.
         (d) Benzoyl peroxide can discolor certain types of fabric or clothing material and can also bleach hair.
      (2) **Mechanism of action.** Benzoyl peroxide has a dual mode of action, so it is effective against both inflammatory and noninflammatory acne.
         (a) Benzoyl peroxide decomposes to release oxygen, which is lethal to the *P. acnes* anaerobe.
         (b) As an irritant, it increases the turnover rate of epithelial cells, resulting in increased sloughing and promoting of resolution of comedones.
      (3) **Application**
         (a) The affected area should be washed with mild soap and water, then gently patted dry.
         (b) The product should be massaged gently into the skin, avoiding the eyes, mouth, lips, and inside of the nose.
         (c) The product can be applied at night, left on for 15 or 20 minutes to test sensitivity, then washed off.

(d) If no excessive irritation develops, apply once daily for the first few days.
(e) If drying, redness, or peeling does not occur in 3 days, increase application to twice daily.
(f) If patients have to use benzoyl peroxide during the day, advise them to use a sunscreen and avoid unnecessary sun exposure.

b. **Salicylic acid** (Category I; 0.5%–2%), an irritant keratolytic agent, results in increased turnover of the epithelial lining. Through this effect, salicylic acid probably promotes the penetration of other acne products.

c. **Sulfur (3%–8%), sulfur 3% to 8% combined with resorcinol 2%** or **resorcinol monoacetate 3%** (Category I; Clearasil Adult Care, Acnomel).
(1) Sulfur is a keratolytic agent and has antibacterial actions.
(2) Sulfur traditionally has been recognized as a less desirable product because it may be acnegenic with continued use, and it has an offensive color and odor.

d. **Resorcinol** (Category II; as a single agent) is a keratolytic agent that has been recognized as effective against acne when the agent is combined with sulfur.

F. **Prescription medications, both topical and systemic,** are included here to put into perspective how OTC agents fit into acne therapy.

1. **Topical prescription agents**

a. **Tretinoin** (Vitamin A acid, retinoic acid, Retin-A) increases the turnover rate of nonadhering horny cells in the follicular canal, which results in comedo clearing and inhibits new comedo development.
(1) **Effectiveness.** Tretinoin is probably the most effective topical agent for acne, especially acne characterized by comedones. It is best used for **noninflammatory** acne. Tretinoin also may be used in combination with antibiotics or benzoyl peroxide for management of severe inflammatory acne.
(2) **Side effects.** Because of its irritant properties, tretinoin can cause **excessive irritation, erythema, peeling,** and increased risk for **severe sunburn.** There may be an initial exacerbation of the acne, and a total of 12 weeks may be necessary to fully assess treatment efficacy.
(3) **Application.** The cream formulation of tretinoin, which is less irritating than the gel form (which in turn is less irritating than the solution form), should be used initially. Because of the irritant properties, tretinoin should be applied 30 minutes after washing. Initially, it should be applied every other day, then daily. Other irritating substances, such as strong abrasive cleaners and astringents, should be avoided during treatment with tretinoin.

b. **Antibiotics: tetracycline** (Topicycline), **meclocycline sulfosalicylate** (Meclan), **erythromycin** (T-Stat, Eryderm), **clindamycin** (Cleocin-T). Combination products containing benzoyl peroxide and erythromycin are also available (Benzamycin).
(1) **Mechanism of action.** The mechanism of action apparently involves suppression of the *P. acnes* organism, which in turn minimizes the inflammatory response due to the acne.
(2) **Application.** These antibiotics are applied directly to acne sites, thus minimizing serious sides effects from oral administration.
(3) **Side effects.** There are **minimal** side effects to these topically applied antibiotics. **Mild burning** or **irritation** may occur. Tetracycline may discolor the skin and fluoresce in black light. Clindamycin can be absorbed to result in pseudomembranous colitis.

c. **Azelaic acid 20% cream (Azelex)** is a new topical agent on the United States market, and it appears to be **as effective** as benzoyl peroxide or tretinoin for the treatment of mild to moderate inflammatory acne. This agent has both antibacterial and antikeratinizing activity. It inhibits the growth of *P. acnes* and has an antiproliferative effect on keratinocytes. It seems to be less irritating than benzoyl peroxide or tretinoin. **Stinging, burning, tingling, pruritus,** and **erythema** have been reported in a low number of patients. It also decreases pigmentation in the areas of increased pigmentation but apparently does not affect freckles, nevi, or normal skin.

2. **Systemic prescription agents**

a. **Oral antibiotics** are the most effective against inflammatory lesions because they suppress *P. acnes.* Oral antibiotics have an onset of action of 3–4 weeks. Antibiotics do not affect existing lesions, but prevent future lesions through this effect.
(1) **Tetracycline** is the **most frequently used** oral antibiotic for acne.

(a) **Initial doses** are 250 mg, two to four times daily, gradually reduced to a maintenance dose of about 250 mg per day.
(b) **Side effects.** The more common adverse effects include upset stomach, vaginal moniliasis, and photosensitivity.

(2) **Erythromycin** may be used as an alternative to tetracycline.
(a) **Initial doses** range from 500 mg to 2000 mg per day in divided doses. A maintenance dose ranges from 250 mg to 500 mg per day.
(b) **Side effects.** The primary side effect associated with erythromycin is gastrointestinal distress.

(3) **Clindamycin.** Rare cases of pseudomembranous colitis limit the use of clindamycin.

(4) **Minocycline.** Side effects including dizziness or vertigo and headache limit the use of this agent.

b. **Isotretinoin** (Accutane) is a vitamin A derivative indicated for **severe recalcitrant nodulocystic acne.** A single course of therapy can result in a complete and prolonged remission period.

(1) **Mechanism of action.** Although the exact mechanism is unknown, isotretinoin decreases sebum production and keratinization, and it reduces the population of *P. acnes.*

(2) **Dosage.** Doses range from 0.5 mg/kg/day to 2 mg/kg/day given twice daily for 15–20 weeks.

(3) **Side effects** include:
(a) **Mucocutaneous dryness.** Cheilitis (i.e., inflammation of the lips), dryness of the nasal mucosa, and facial dermatitis may occur with isotretinoin use. These effects can be treated with topical lubricants. Dryness of the eye can also occur, so people using isotretinoin should not wear contact lenses.
(b) **Elevated serum levels.** Isotretinoin may elevate serum triglycerides and cholesterol, as well as liver enzymes.
(c) **Birth defects.** Isotretinoin is a **potent teratogen** and should not be given to pregnant women.

c. **Antiandrogens and hormones**

(1) **Estrogens** can decrease sebum production through an antiandrogenic effect.

(2) Some **progestin agents** in oral contraceptives (e.g., norethindrone, norgestrel) have androgenic activity that can stimulate sebum secretion. **Norethynodrel** has the least androgenic activity among the available progestins. Therefore, it is favored as an ingredient in combination oral contraceptives used in women with acne.

(3) **Corticosteroids.** Although corticosteroids have been implicated as causing acne, they also can be used to treat severe acne. Intralesional injections of triamcinolone and systemic corticosteroids have been used for severe inflammatory acne and severe cystic acne respectively. Prednisone (or its equivalent) in doses of 20 mg per day or higher may be used for a short period of time to quickly improve acne for important events like a wedding. Topical corticosteroids are not effective.

(4) **Spironolactone (Aldactone)** is an androgen antagonist that may be used on a limited basis.

III. SUNLIGHT, SUNSCREENS, AND SUNTAN PRODUCTS

A. **Introduction.** Overexposure to sunlight damages skin. A suntan, which has traditionally been associated with health, is actually a response to injury. Of the three types of solar radiation, only the ultraviolet (UV) spectrum produces sunburn and suntan.

1. The **UV spectrum** ranges from 200 to 400 nanometers (nm). Natural and artificial UV light is further subdivided into three bands.

a. **UVA** (320–400 nm) can cause the skin to tan and it tends to be weak in causing the skin to redden. UVA is about 1000 times less potent than a comparable dose of UVB in causing erythema, but it is only slightly blocked out by the ozone layer and reaches the earth's surface in 10–100 times the amount of UVB. Some have proposed that UVA be further subdivided into UVA I (340–400 nm) and UVA II (320–340 nm). UVA I is less erythrogenic and melanogenic than UVA II or UVB. UVA II is similar in effect to UVB.

(1) **Uses.** UVA is often used in tanning booths and in psoralen plus UVA (PUVA) treatment of psoriasis.

(2) **Disadvantages.** UVA is responsible for many photosensitivity reactions, photoaging, and photodermatoses. UVA rays can also penetrate deeply into the dermis and augment the cancerous effects of UVB rays.

b. **UVB** (290–320 nm) causes the usual sunburn reaction and stimulates tanning. It has long been associated with sunlight skin damage, including the various skin cancers. It is the **most erythrogenic** and **melanogenic** of the three UV radiation bands. Small amounts of this radiation are required for normal **vitamin D synthesis** in the skin.

c. **UVC** (200–290 nm) does not reach the earth's surface because most of it is absorbed by the ozone layer. Artificial UVC sources (e.g., germicidal and mercury arc lamps) can emit this radiation.

2. The **visible spectrum** (400–770 nm) produces the "brightness" of the sun.

3. The **infrared spectrum** (770–1800 nm) produces the "warmth" of the sun.

B. Sunburn and suntanning

1. **Sunburn** is generally a superficial burn involving the epidermis. This layer is rapidly repaired while old cells are being sloughed off in a process called **peeling.** The newly formed skin is thicker and offers protection for the lower dermal layers.

   a. **Normal sequence after mild-to-moderate sunlight (UVR) exposure**

      (1) Erythema occurs within 20–30 minutes as a result of oxidation of bleached melanin and dilation of dermal venules.

      (2) The initial erythema rapidly fades, and true sunburn erythema begins 2–8 hours after initial exposure to the sun.

      (3) Dilation of the arterioles results in increased vascular permeability, localized edema and pain, which become maximal after 14–20 hours and last 24–72 hours.

   b. **Manifestations** range from mild (a slight reddening of the skin) to severe (formation of blisters and desquamation). If the effect is severe, the patient may experience pain, swelling, and blistering. Fever, chills, and nausea may also develop, as well as prostration, which is related to excessive synthesis and diffusion of prostaglandins.

2. **Suntan** is the result of two processes:

   a. **Oxidation of melanin,** which is already present in the epidermis

   b. **Stimulation of melanocytes** to produce additional melanin, which is subsequently oxidized upon further exposure to sunlight

      (1) With increased melanin production, the melanocytes introduce the pigment into keratin-producing cells, which gradually become darkened keratin and a full suntan in 2–10 days.

      (2) Tanning increases tolerance to additional sunlight and reduces the likelihood of subsequent burning. However, dark skin is not totally immune to sunburn.

C. Factors affecting exposure to UV radiation (UVR)

1. **Time of day and season.** The greatest exposure to harmful UVB rays occurs between 10 A.M. and 2 P.M. in midsummer. UVA rays are fairly continuous throughout the day and season.

2. **Altitude.** Sunburn is more likely to occur at high altitudes. UVB intensity increases 4% with each 1000-foot increase in altitude.

3. **Environmental factors.** Atmospheric conditions (e.g., smog, haze, smoke) may affect (i.e., decrease) the amount of UVR reaching the skin. Although direct sunlight greatly reduces the amount of UV exposure needed to produce a burn, sunburn can occur without it. For example, a sunburn can also develop on a cloudy day due to the percentage of UVR penetration through cloud layers (60%–80%). However, the **reflection of light rays** (e.g., by snow, sand, water) greatly **increases** the amount of UV **exposure to sunlight.**

4. **Predisposing factors.** People with fair skin and light hair are at greater risk for developing sunburn and other UVR skin damage than their darker counterparts (Table 30-2).

D. Other reactions to sunlight (UVR) exposure

1. **Actinic keratosis** is a precancerous condition and may occur after many years of excessive exposure to sunlight. Typically arising during middle age or later, this disorder manifests as a sharply demarcated, roughened, or hardened growth, which may be flat or raised and it may progress to **squamous cell carcinoma.**

Table 30-2. Recommended Sunscreen Product Guide[1]

Skin type	Patient characteristics[2]	Suggested product SPF
I	Always burns easily; rarely tans	20 to 30
II	Always burns easily; tans minimally	12 to <20
III	Burns moderately; tans gradually	8 to <12
IV	Burns minimally; always tans well	4 to <8
V	Rarely burns; tans profusely	2 to <4
VI[3]	Never burns; deeply pigmented (insensitive)	None indicated

[1]Based on the FDA's tentative final monograph (TFM) for sunscreen products.

[2]Based on first 45–60 minutes sun exposure after winter season or no sun exposure.

[3]This skin type not included in TFM.

©1996 by Facts and Comparisons. Used with permission from *Drug Facts and Comparisons. 1996 ed.* St. Louis: Facts and Comparisons.

2. **Skin cancer.** Chronic overexposure to sunlight may lead to **squamous cell carcinoma, basal cell carcinoma,** or **malignant melanoma.**
   a. **Squamous cell carcinoma.** Lesions usually appear as thickened, rough, scaly patches which can bleed and most commonly develops from actinic keratosis. It accounts for about 15% of skin cancers.
   b. **Basal cell carcinoma.** This is the most common of all skin cancers and accounts for about 80% of skin cancers. It may appear as pearly or translucent bumps and originates in the basal cells.
   c. **Malignant melanoma.** Malignant melanoma originates from melanocytes and is the deadliest form of skin cancer, and its incidence has been increasing. Moles should be watched for indications of malignancy—the ABCDs are **a**symmetrical shape, **b**order irregularity, nonuniform **c**olor, and **d**iameter over 6 mm. Malignant melanoma formation may be associated with intense, intermittent overexposure to the sun (sunburning).

3. **Drug-induced photosensitivity reactions**
   a. **Types**
      (1) **Photoallergy reactions** occur when light makes a drug become antigenic or act as a hapten (i.e., a photoallergen). These reactions also require previous contact with the offending drug. Photoallergy reactions are relatively **rare** and are associated more frequently with topically applied agents than with oral medications.
         (a) **Occurrence** of these reactions is not dose-related. The patient is usually cross-sensitive with chemically related compounds.
         (b) **Rashes** are most prominent on light-exposed sites (i.e., face, neck, forearms, back of hands), and they usually occur, after an incubation period of 24–48 hours of combined drug and sun exposure, as an intensely pruritic eczematous dermatitis (a severe rash).
      (2) **Phototoxic reactions** occur when light alters a drug to a toxic form, which results in tissue damage that is independent of an allergic response.
         (a) **Occurrence.** These reactions are usually dose-related, and the patient usually has no cross-sensitivity to other agents.
         (b) **Rashes** often appear as an exaggerated sunburn and are usually confined to areas of combined chemical and light exposure.
      (3) **Implicated drugs.** Many drugs have been implicated in causing photoallergy and phototoxic reactions: thiazides, tetracyclines, phenothiazines, sulfonamides, and even sunscreens. Some drugs may produce both types of reactions.
   b. **Prevention.** Standard sunscreens do not always prevent photosensitivity reactions caused by drugs. UV light above 320 nm (i.e., UVA light) has been implicated in inducing photosensitivity reactions, so a chemical or physical sunscreen must cover this spectrum [see III E 2].

4. **Photodermatoses** are skin conditions that are triggered or worsened by light within specific wavelengths. These conditions include polymorphous light eruption (PMLE), lupus erythematosus, and solar urticaria.

5. **Photoaging** is a skin condition that is not merely an acceleration of normal aging. UVA radiation is thought to be involved. The skin appears dry, scaly, yellow, and deeply wrinkled; it is also thinner and more fragile.

E. **Sunscreen agents.** People can protect their skin from harmful UVR by avoiding exposure to sunlight and other sources of UVR, wearing protective clothing, and applying sunscreen.

1. **Application and general information.** All exposed areas should be covered evenly with sunscreen, optimally 30 minutes to 2 hours (for PABA & PABA esters) before sun exposure to allow for penetration and binding to the skin.
   a. **Substantivity.** Perspiration, swimming, sand, towels, and clothing tend to remove sunscreen and may increase the need for reapplication.
      (1) Substantivity is the ability of a sunscreen formulation to adhere to the skin while swimming or perspiring.
      (2) Labeling a product as "waterproof" indicates that the product formula maintains sunburn protection after the patient has been in the water up to 80 minutes.
      (3) "Water resistant" labeling indicates that the formula maintains protection after being in the water up to 40 minutes.
   b. **Protection.** Sunscreen products vary widely in their ability to protect against sunburn; the sun protection factor (SPF) and UVA/UVB ray protection should be noted to determine the level of protection. Moreover, baby oil, mineral oil, olive oil, and cocoa butter are not sunscreens (but are often used to attain a tan).
      (1) **SPF** gives the consumer a guide for determining how the product will protect the skin from UV rays, principally UVB rays. An SPF of 30 blocks ~97% of the UVB rays. The FDA is proposing an upper limit for SPF values of 30. Scientific evidence shows a point of diminishing returns at levels more than 30; any benefits that might be derived from using sunscreens with SPFs more than 30 are negligible. An SPF of at least 15 for most individuals is recommended by the Skin Cancer Foundation.
         (a) **Derivation.** SPF is defined as the **minimal erythema dose (MED)** of protected skin divided by the MED of unprotected skin. MED is the amount of solar radiation needed to produce minimal skin redness.
         (b) **Example.** A person who usually gets red after 20 minutes in the sun and wants to stay in the sun for 2 hours (120 minutes) should apply a sunscreen with an SPF of 6 (120 minutes divided by 20 minutes = SPF 6). An SPF 6 product should provide adequate coverage provided it is not washed off (as from swimming) or dissolved by sweat. An SPF of 15 blocks ~93% of the UVB rays.
         (c) There is no generally accepted comparable term that measures UVA protection, although a few have been proposed. One major concern is that people may be staying out in the sun longer as they use sunscreen products that have high SPF values. If inadequate UVA protection is provided in that product, these individuals may be exposing themselves to very high amounts of UVA with the potential for significant overexposure to this form of UV radiation.
   c. **Sensitivity.** Some people may be hypersensitive to sunscreen agents.

2. The two basic **types of sunscreen agents** are physical sun blocks and chemical sunscreens (Table 30-3).
   a. **Physical sun blocks** are opaque formulations that reflect and scatter up to 99% of light in both the UV and visible spectrums (290–700 nm). Examples include titanium dioxide and zinc oxide. These sun blocks are less cosmetically acceptable than chemical sunscreens because they have a greasy appearance, but they may be useful for protecting small areas (e.g., the nose). These sun blocks are also useful for photosensitization protection. Newer, more dilute versions of titanium dioxide products are more cosmetically appealing. Red petrolatum covers a lesser spectrum (290–365 nm).
   b. **Chemical sunscreens** act by absorbing a specific portion of the UV light spectrum to keep it from penetrating the skin. They can be categorized on the basis of their spectra of UVR blockage and basic chemical classification. Five main groups of chemical sunscreens are available.
      (1) **PABA** and **PABA esters** primarily absorb UVB rays. Examples are *p*-aminobenzoic acid, padimate O, and glyceryl PABA.
      (2) **Cinnamates** primarily absorb UVB rays. Examples are cinoxate and octyl methoxycinnamate.

Table 30-3. Sunscreen Ingredients

	Sunscreens	UV spectrum (nm)	Concentrations (%)
	Benzophenones	UVA and UVB	
	Oxybenzone	270–350	2–6
	Dioxybenzone	260–380[1]	3
	PABA and PABA esters	UVB	
	p-aminobenzoic acid	260–313	5–15
	Ethyl dihydroxy propyl PABA	280–330	1–5
	Padimate O (octyl dimethyl PABA)	290–315	1.4–8
	Glyceryl PABA	264–315	2–3
Chemical			
	Cinnamates	UVB[2]	
	Cinoxate	270–328	1–3
	Ethylhexyl p-methoxycinnamate	290–320	2–7.5
	Octocrylene	250–360	7–10
	Octyl methoxycinnamate	290–320	–
	Salicylates	UVB[3]	
	Ethylhexyl salicylate	280–320	3–5
	Homosalate	295–315	4–15
	Octyl salicylate	280–320	3–5
	Miscellaneous	UVB	
	Menthyl anthranilate	260–380[4]	3.5–5
	Digalloyl trioleate	270–320	2–5
	Avobenzone (butyl-methoxy-dibenzoylmethane; Parsol 1789)	UVA 320–400	3
Physical			
	Titanium dioxide	290–700	2–25
	Red petrolatum	290–365[5]	30–100
	Zinc oxide	290–700	–

[1]Values available when used in combination with other screens.

[2]Some UVA spectrum.

[3]Primarily UVB, but has about $^1/_3$ the absorbency of PABA.

[4]Values are concentrations higher than normally found in nonprescription drugs.

[5]At 334 nm, 16% UV radiation is transmitted; at 365 nm, 58% is transmitted.

©1996 by Facts and Comparisons. Used with permission from *Drug Facts and Comparisons. 1996 ed.* St. Louis: Facts and Comparisons.

(3) **Salicylates** primarily absorb UVB rays. Examples are ethylhexyl salicylate and homosalate.

(4) **Benzophenones** absorb UVB rays and sometimes extend into the UVA range. Examples are oxybenzone and dioxybenzone. Because of their extension into the UVA range, they are somewhat protective against photosensitivity reactions.

(5) **Miscellaneous.** The newest agent, butylmethoxydibenzoylmethane (Parsol 1789, Avobenzone), provides coverage over the entire UVA range. In combination with oxybenzone and octyl methoxycinnamate, this product (Shade UVA Guard) offers the greatest protection in both the UVA and UVB ranges.

c. **OTC sunscreen products.** Most sunscreen products on the market contain combinations of two or more of the classes of chemical sunscreen agents noted in the preceding paragraphs.

F. Special agents of interest

1. Dihydroxyacetone (DHA) is a chemical agent that darkens the skin by interacting with keratin in the stratum corneum to produce an artificial suntan. It provides no protection against UV rays and may not produce a natural-looking tan. DHA must be applied evenly. If an artificial suntan is achieved with this chemical, it wears off in a few days. In addition, it can discolor hair and clothing.

2. **Beta-carotene,** a vitamin A precursor, may produce skin coloration when ingested orally. While beta-carotene is protective against some forms of abnormal photosensitivity (e.g., ery-

thropoietic protoporphyria), it has not been shown to protect against sunburn in normal individuals.

3. **Canthaxanthine** is a carotenoid (provitamin A). It has been used as a food coloring agent but has not been approved by the FDA for use as an oral tanning agent. It does not produce a true suntan, but is deposited into fatty tissues under the skin. It probably does not protect the skin from sunburn.

4. **Tyrosine** has been promoted as a tan accelerator or tan magnifier. Because melanin pigment is eventually synthesized from tyrosine, the theory is that topically applied tyrosine will enhance the formation of melanin. However, studies have not confirmed an enhanced tanning effect from this agent.

IV. CONTACT DERMATITIS AND ITS TREATMENT

A. Introduction

1. **Types of contact dermatitis.** Contact dermatitis is one of the **most common** dermatologic conditions encountered in clinical practice. It has traditionally been divided into **irritant contact dermatitis** and **allergic contact dermatitis** on the basis of the etiology and immunologic mechanism.
   a. **Irritant contact dermatitis** is caused by direct contact with a primary irritant. These irritants can be classified as absolute or relative primary irritants.
      (1) **Absolute primary irritants** are intrinsically damaging substances that injure, on first contact, any person's skin. Examples include strong acids, alkalis, and other industrial chemicals.
      (2) **Relative primary irritants** cause most cases of contact dermatitis seen in clinical practice. These irritants are less toxic than absolute primary irritants, and they require repeated or prolonged exposure to provoke a reaction. Examples of relative primary irritants include soaps, detergents, benzoyl peroxide, and certain plant and animal substances.
   b. **Allergic contact dermatitis.** Many plants, and almost any chemical, can cause allergic contact dermatitis. Poison ivy is a classic example of allergic contact dermatitis, which is classified as a type IV hypersensitivity reaction. This type of allergic reaction is T—cell-mediated, and the following **sequence of events** must occur to provoke it.
      (1) The epidermis must come in **contact** with the hapten (i.e., the specific allergen).
      (2) The **hapten–epidermal protein complex** (i.e., the complete antigen) must form.
      (3) The antigen must **enter the lymphatic system.**
      (4) **Immunologically competent lymphoid cells,** which are selective against the antigen, must form.
      (5) On **re-exposure** to the hapten, the typical, local delayed hypersensitivity reaction (i.e., contact dermatitis) occurs.
      (6) The **induction period,** during which sensitivity develops, usually requires 14–21 days but may take as few as 4 days or more than several weeks. **Once sensitivity is fully developed:**
         (a) Re-exposure to even minute amounts of the same material elicits an eczematous response, typically with an onset of 12 hours and a peak of 48–72 hours after exposure.
         (b) Sensitivity usually persists for life.
            (i) Most contact allergens produce sensitization in only a small percentage of exposed persons.
            (ii) Allergens or substances such as poison ivy, however, produce sensitization in more than 70% of the population (50%–95% are sensitive to the poison ivy plant)

2. **General phases of contact dermatitis**
   a. **Acute stage.** "Wet" lesions, such as blisters or denuded and weeping skin, are evident in well-outlined patches. Also evident are erythema, edema, vesicles, and oozing.
   b. **Subacute stage.** In this phase, crusts or scabs form over the previously wet lesions. Allergic contact dermatitis and irritant contact dermatitis caused by absolute primary irritants produce both the acute and subacute stages.

c. **Chronic stage.** In this phase, the lesions become dry and thickened (i.e., lichenified). Initially, dryness and fissuring are the signs. Later, erythema, lichenification, and excoriations appear. The chronic phase of contact dermatitis usually occurs more often with irritant contact dermatitis caused by relative primary irritants.

B. Toxic plants. Poison ivy and poison oak are the **most common causes** of allergic contact dermatitis in North America. These plants were formerly known as the *Rhus* genus, but they are now properly referred to as the *Toxicodendron* genus.

1. **Poison ivy** (*Toxicodendron radicans*) grows as a vine or as a bush. It is found in most parts of the United States, but is especially prevalent in the northeastern part of the country. Poison ivy is often identified by its characteristic growth pattern, described by the saying, "Leaves of three, let it be."
2. **Poison oak** (*T. diversilobum*) is found in the western United States and Canada. It grows as an upright shrub or a woody vine. *T. quercifolium* is found in the eastern United States.
3. **Poison sumac** (*T. vernix*) grows in woody or swampy areas as a coarse shrub or tree and is prevalent in the eastern United States and southeastern Canada.

C. Toxicodendron dermatitis. In order for dermatitis to develop, previous sensitization (a 5- to 21-day incubation period) caused by direct contact with a sensitizing agent is required (see IV A 1 b). An oleoresin, **urushiol oil,** which is a pentadecacatechol, is the active sensitizing agent in poison ivy, poison oak, and poison sumac. There are slight differences in the chemical structures of the sensitizing agent in each of these plants, but the three agents cross react.

1. **Release of the urushiol oil.** The plants must be bruised or injured to release the oleoresin. It is present in the roots, stems, leaves and fruit. The urushiol oil may remain active on tools, toys, clothes, and pets, and under fingernails if those items have had contact with the broken plants.
   a. Urushiol oil does not volatilize, so one cannot get dermatitis from just being near a poison ivy plant; direct contact is necessary. **Burning plants,** however, can cause droplets of oil carried by smoke to enter the respiratory system, which can cause significant respiratory distress.
   b. A cut or damaged poison ivy, poison oak, or poison sumac plant yields a milky sap containing the oleoresin, which turns black within a few minutes. This change can be a means for confirming identification of these plants.
   c. Because the oleoresin can rapidly penetrate the skin, the affected area must be washed with soap and water within 10–15 minutes after exposure to prevent the dermatitis eruption.
2. If an individual has been **previously sensitized,** the lesions usually occur within 6–48 hours after contact with the allergen. If the patient becomes initially sensitized as a result of this contact, the lesions may not appear for 9–14 days.
3. Typically, the **initial eruption** exists as small patches of erythematous papules (usually streaks). Pruritus (itching) is the primary symptom.
   a. Papules may progress to vesicles, which may then ooze and bleed when they are scratched. Secondary infection may then develop. Often, the inflammation is severe, and a significant amount of edema occurs over the exposed area.
   b. The lesions may last from a few days to several weeks. Left untreated, the condition rarely persists longer than 2–3 weeks.
4. **Poison ivy dermatitis does not spread.** New lesions, however, may continue to appear for several days despite lack of further contact with the plant. This reaction may be due to the following facts.
   a. Skin that has been minimally exposed to the antigen begins to react only as the person's sensitivity heightens.
   b. Antigen is absorbed at varying rates through the skin of different parts of the body.
   c. The person inadvertently touches contaminated objects or may have residual oleoresin underneath the fingernails, for instance.
5. **Poison ivy is not contagious.** The serous fluid from the weeping vesicles are not antigenic. No one can "catch" poison ivy from another person.

D. Treatment. The treatment of irritant and allergic contact dermatitis focuses on therapy for the specific symptomatology.

1. A pharmacist should **refer a patient** with a poison ivy eruption to a physician if:
   a. The eruption involves more than 15% of the body
   b. The eruption involves the eyes, genital area, mouth, or respiratory tract (some patients may experience respiratory difficulties if they inhale the smoke of burning poison ivy plants)

2. The **severity of the eruption** depends on:
   a. The quantity of allergen that the patient has been exposed to
   b. The individual patient's sensitivity to the allergen

3. **For severe eruptions,** a patient should consult a physician, who may prescribe **systemic corticosteroids.**
   a. Systemic corticosteroids are the cornerstone of therapy. One should use sufficiently high doses to suppress this inflammation. Generally, it is recommended that prednisone be given in the dose of 60 mg/day for 5 days, then reduced to 40 mg/day for 5 days, then 20 mg/day for 5 days, then discontinued.
   b. Some blisters may be drained at their base. The skin on top of the blister should be kept intact. Draining the blister allows more topical medication to penetrate for an antipruritic effect. Baths and soaks [see IV D 4 b 1 (b)] may be beneficial as well.

4. **For a less severe eruption,** the principal goals are to relieve the itching and inflammation and to protect the integrity of skin.
   a. Several therapeutic classes of agents can be used **to relieve itching.**
      (1) The application of **local anesthetics** [e.g., benzocaine (5%–20%)] may relieve itching. Relief may be of short duration (30–45 minutes), but application of benzocaine may be especially useful at bedtime, when pruritus is most bothersome. There is some question about the frequency of the sensitizing ability of benzocaine (0.17%–5%). Certainly, treatment should be discontinued if the rash worsens.
      (2) **Oral antihistamines** may be helpful in alleviating pruritus mainly due to their sedating effect rather than a specific antipruritic effect. The principal concern with these agents involves the effect of CNS depression (drowsiness) and possible anticholinergic effects.
      (3) **Topical antihistamines** [e.g., diphenhydramine (Benadryl cream or spray)] provide relief of mild itching principally through a topical anesthetic effect rather than any antihistamine effect. The main concern with topical antihistamines is that they may also have a significant sensitizing potential and in children with varicella infections (integrity of skin compromised) systemic absorption has occurred with symptoms of anticholinergic toxicity produced.
      (4) **Counterirritants** include camphor (0.1%–3%), phenol (0.5%–1.5%), and menthol (0.1%–1%). These agents have an analgesic effect due to depression of cutaneous receptors. The exact antipruritic mechanism is not fully known, but a placebo effect may result from the characteristic "medicinal" odors of these agents.
      (5) **Astringents** are mild protein precipitants that result in contraction of tissue, which in turn decreases the local edema and inflammation.
         (a) The principal agent used is **aluminum acetate** (Burow's solution).
         (b) **Calamine** (zinc oxide with ferric oxide) is also used sometimes. Calamine contracts tissue and helps dry the area, but the formation of the thick dried paste may not be acceptable to some people. This agent is not considered effective by the FDA.
      (6) **Topical hydrocortisone,** (e.g., Cortaid), which is available in concentrations up to 1%, is useful for its antipruritic and anti-inflammatory effects. The antipruritic effect, however, may not be seen for 1–2 days.
   b. **Basic treatment**
      (1) **Acute (weeping) lesions** (see IV A 2 a)
         (a) **Wet dressings** work on the principle that water evaporating from the skin cools it and, thus, relieves itching. Wet dressings have an additional benefit of causing gentle debridement and cleansing of the skin.
         (b) **Burrow's solution** (Domeboro) in concentrations of 1:20–1:40 as a wet dressing or a cool bath of 15–30 minutes, three to six times per day provides a significant antipruritic effect.
         (c) **Colloidal oatmeal baths** (e.g., Aveeno) may also provide an antipruritic effect.
         (d) **Topical therapy that may hinder treatment**
            (i) **Local anesthetics and topical antihistamines** may sensitize
            (ii) **Calamine** may "make a mess" without doing much good!

(2) **Subacute dermatitis** (see IV A 2 b). A thin layer of hydrocortisone cream or lotion (0.5%–1%) may be applied three or four times a day to treat subacute dermatitis. Supplemental agents, such as oral antihistamines or topical anesthetics, may be used as well.

(3) **Chronic dermatitis** (see IV A 2 c) is best treated with hydrocortisone ointment. This stage is observed more frequently in forms of contact dermatitis that involve continuous exposure to the irritant or allergen.

E. Prevention

1. The best treatment for poison ivy contact dermatitis is to **prevent contact** with the offending cause. This approach involves avoiding the plant and wearing protective clothing.
2. **Barrier preparations.** Linoleic acid dimers (e.g., Stoko Gard) and organic clays have been used, with limited success, to prevent urushiol from binding to the dermis. Quaternium-18 bentonite (Ivy Block) is expected to be marketed beginning in early 1997 as a lotion that should be applied at least 15 minutes before contact with the plant and then every 4 hours for continued protection against urushiol.
3. **Hyposensitization** using plant extracts of poison ivy has had mixed success. Maximal hyposensitization requires 3–6 months to develop, and it diminishes rapidly when administration of the extract ceases.

STUDY QUESTIONS

Directions: Each of the numbered items or incomplete statements in this section is followed by answers or by completions of the statement. Select the **one** lettered answer or completion that is **best** in each case.

1. A woman, who has not been in the sun for 4 months, develops redness on her chest after lying in the sun for 20 minutes. The next day, she applies a suntan lotion and develops the same degree of redness on her back in 2 hours and 20 minutes. What is the sun protection factor (SPF) of the lotion she is using?

(A) 14
(B) 10
(C) 12
(D) 9
(E) 7

2. Which of the following cleansing products would a pharmacist recommend for a patient with inflammatory acne?

(A) An abrasive facial sponge and soap used four times daily
(B) Aluminum oxide particles used twice daily
(C) Sulfur 5% soap used twice daily
(D) Mild facial soap used twice daily

3. If a patient needs a second application of an OTC pyrethrin pediculicide shampoo, how many days after the first application should this be done?

(A) 4–5
(B) 6
(C) 7–10
(D) 14–21
(E) 15–17

4. All of the following treatments for personal articles infested with head lice would be effective EXCEPT

(A) placing woolen hats in a plastic bag for 35 days
(B) using an aerosol of pyrethrins with piperonyl butoxide to spray all bathrooms
(C) machine-washing clothes in hot water and drying them using the hot setting on the dryer
(D) dry-cleaning woolen scarves
(E) soaking hair brushes in hot water for 5–10 minutes

5. All of the following sunscreen agents or combinations of agents would likely help prevent a drug-induced photosensitivity reaction EXCEPT

(A) titanium dioxide
(B) glyceryl *p*-aminobenzoic acid (PABA) plus homosalate
(C) oxybenzone and padimate O
(D) zinc oxide
(E) padimate O plus butylmethoxydibenzoylmethane

6. All of the following would be appropriate recommendations for a patient in the acute stage (i.e., blistering, weeping) of poison ivy contact dermatitis EXCEPT

(A) two 25-mg capsules of diphenhydramine at night for itching
(B) 60 mg per day of prednisone initially, then tapered over 15 days
(C) Burow's solution; 1:20 wet dressing to area for 15–30 minutes, four times per day
(D) two soaks per day in Aveeno Bath Treatment
(E) two applications of Stoko Gard

7. All of the following nonprescription agents have been classified by the FDA as safe and effective (Category I) for acne EXCEPT

(A) sulfur
(B) salicylic acid
(C) sulfur-resorcinol combination
(D) benzoic acid

8. Pharmacists educating patients about acne should mention all of the following EXCEPT

(A) eliminating all chocolate and fried foods from the diet
(B) cleansing skin gently two to three times daily
(C) using water-based noncomedogenic cosmetics
(D) not squeezing acne lesions
(E) keeping in mind that acne usually resolves by one's early twenties

9. A 15-year-old male patient has been using benzoyl peroxide 5% cream faithfully every day for the past 2 months with no apparent side effects. All of the following can be said about this patient EXCEPT

(A) he has been using this product for a long enough time to determine if the dose and dosage form are going to have any benefit
(B) he should use this product no more frequently than every other day because of its irritating properties
(C) this starting dose and dosage form are useful, especially if he has dry skin or it is wintertime
(D) his scalp hair may look bleached if the product comes in contact with it
(E) the product would sting if it got into his eyes

10. All of the following descriptions match the therapeutic agent for poison ivy EXCEPT

(A) Calamine—phenolphthalein gives it the pink color
(B) Stoko Gard—it contains linoleic acid dimer and has some effect in preventing poison ivy dermatitis
(C) Benzocaine—data regarding incidence of hypersensitivity are conflicting
(D) hydrocortisone—it may take 1–2 days for an antipruritic effect

11. All of the following statements related to sun protection are true EXCEPT

(A) the sun's intensity increases 20% when going from sea level to an altitude of 5000 feet
(B) a patient with skin type II should use a product with an SPF of 12 to 19
(C) baby oil is not a sunscreen, but its application to the skin after tanning causes melanin to rise to the surface
(D) products now have SPFs greater than 20, but 30 is probably the highest SPF necessary
(E) the SPF is really only a measure of ultraviolet B (UVB) protection

12. All of the following statements about sunscreens are true EXCEPT

(A) malignant melanoma formation may be associated with intense, intermittent overexposure to the sun (sunburning)
(B) dihydroxyacetone (DHA) will not prevent sunburn
(C) canthaxanthine provides only minimal protection against sunburn in normal patients
(D) *p*-aminobenzoic acid (PABA) is best applied within 10 minutes before sun exposure
(E) tyrosine has been marketed as a tan accelerator

ANSWERS AND EXPLANATIONS

1. The answer is E *[III E 1].*
The sun protection factor (SPF) is the minimal erythema dose (MED) of protected skin divided by the MED of unprotected skin. Thus, 2 hours and 20 minutes (140 minutes) divided by 20 minutes equals an SPF of 7.

2. The answer is D *[II E 2 c, e].*
For patients with inflammatory acne, the best product is a mild facial soap used twice daily. The soap should be gently rubbed into the skin with only the fingertips. Cleansing products that irritate already inflamed skin should be avoided.

3. The answer is C *[I G 4 a (1)].*
Reapplication of pyrethrins with piperonyl butoxide should be within 7–10 days of the first application. Any lice nits that were not killed on the first application would have time to hatch and then be killed with the second application.

4. The answer is B *[I G 4 a, 6 c].*
Pyrethrins with piperonyl butoxide in an aerosol form can be sprayed directly on inanimate objects (e.g., chairs, headrests) to kill head lice, but the combination should not be sprayed in the air like an aerosol deodorizer. Moreover, vacuuming the furniture would probably be as effective as spraying it. The other selections are appropriate for personal articles infested with head lice.

5. The answer is B *[III E 2 b (1)].*
Glyceryl *p*-aminobenzoic acid (PABA) and homosalate protect against only ultraviolet B (UVB) exposure. Because photosensitivity reactions are often associated with UVA radiation exposure, people also need sunscreen protection for this portion of the UV radiation band. The other agents listed cover at least part of both UVA and UVB spectra.

6. The answer is E *[IV D 4 b].*
Stoko Gard is used as a barrier protectant for the prevention of poison ivy dermatitis, not for the treatment of an acute eruption. The other options are appropriate to recommend to someone suffering from the acute stage of poison ivy dermatitis.

7. The answer is D *[II E 4].*
Benzoic acid has not been shown to be effective for acne treatment. The other agents—sulfur, salicylic acid, and a sulfur-resorcinol combination—are all safe and effective products for treating acne.

8. The answer is A *[II D 3].*
Evidence does not show that acne worsens from any particular type of food, including chocolate or fried foods. The other choices are pieces of information that the pharmacist should convey to a patient with acne.

9. The answer is B *[II E 4 a].*
Although the irritating properties of benzoyl peroxide would indicate applying it only every other day upon initiating treatment, this patient has tolerated the agent on a daily basis for 2 months. Thus, there would be no need to decrease the application frequency. All of the other choices do apply to this patient's use of benzoyl peroxide.

10. The answer is A *[IV D 4 a].*
Ferric oxide provides the pink color of calamine. All of the other descriptions match their associated agents.

11. The answer is C *[III C 2, E 1 b, c; 2 b; 3; Table 30-2].*
Baby oil is not a sunscreen, and it has no effect on melanin. SPF does measure ultraviolet B (UVB) protection, and an SPF higher than 30 is probably not necessary. People with skin type II (that is, very fair or fair) should use a product with an SPF of 12 to 19. The intensity of the sun does increase by 4% with each 1000-feet elevation.

12. The answer is D *[III D 2, E 1, 2 b (1); F 1, 3, 4].*
Optimally, sunscreens should be applied 1–2 hours before exposure to the sun. This allows time for the product to bind to the stratum corneum, which provides better protection. The other responses are correct.

31
OTC Weight Control and Sleep Aids

Larry N. Swanson

I. WEIGHT CONTROL

A. Obesity

1. **Definition.** Obesity has been defined generally as surplus body fat that results in a weight that exceeds a person's ideal body weight by more than 20%.

2. **Types**
   a. Overweight people with large abdomens are generally in worse health than equally obese people who have fat distributed around their hips and limbs.
   b. Waist measurement to hip measurement ratios of greater than 0.95 for men and 0.80 for women are associated with higher death rates.
   c. See Table 31-1 for healthy weights.

3. **Cause.** Although many hypotheses, theories, and proposed mechanisms have been discussed, no uniform cause of obesity has been determined. Patients can become obese because they consistently ingest more calories than their body is able to metabolize. Observations about the cause of obesity include the following.
   a. Patients may have an **elevated body weight "set point."** When these patients lose weight, compensatory adjustments in metabolism result in their regaining the weight, even with a decreased caloric intake.
   b. **Heredity** is accepted as an important factor in the etiology of obesity. Studies of identical twins raised apart show that each twin's weight does not vary significantly, which in-

Table 31-1. Healthy Weights—An Update

The chart below is used as the government's 1995 guidelines for healthy weight. The two sexes are combined in this one table. The higher weights generally apply to men or people with more muscle and bone; the lower weights to women.

Suggested Weight (without clothes or shoes)

Height	**Weight (lbs.)**
5′0″	97–128
5′1″	101–132
5′2″	104–137
5′3″	107–141
5′4″	111–146
5′5″	114–150
5′6″	118–155
5′7″	121–160
5′8″	125–164
5′9″	129–169
5′10″	132–174
5′11″	136–179
6′0″	140–184
6′1″	144–189
6′2″	148–195
6′3″	152–200
6′4″	156–205

dicates that genetics has a more important role than environmental factors in determining obesity.

c. Obese patients may be **more responsive to external food cues** (e.g., taste, smell, sight of food).

4. Statistics

a. Obesity afflicts more people in the United States than does any disease. As much as **one third of the United States population over age 30 years** may be obese, and a recent study suggests that one in three adults in the United States is attempting to lose weight.

b. Yearly, more than **10 billion dollars** is spent on the treatment of obesity, yet less is known about its cause than is known about the cause of most other medical conditions.

c. The **medical management** of obesity is almost universally unsuccessful. An estimated 90% of all patients who lose more than 25 pounds in a diet program regain that weight within 3 years.

5. Medical consequences

a. Numerous studies have shown that a significant number of patients with hypertension, non–insulin-dependent diabetes mellitus, and osteoarthritis can significantly control their conditions through weight loss. According to a recent study, it now appears that **even a modest weight gain as one ages** puts middle-aged women at **a higher risk of heart disease.** Women who gained 12–18 pounds after age 18 had a 25% greater chance of suffering a heart attack than their leaner counterparts. People who are 20% or more over their ideal body weight are more likely to suffer from the following diseases or disorders:

(1) Amenorrhea
(2) Cancer of the cervix, colon, endometrium, gallbladder, prostate, and uterus
(3) Congestive heart failure
(4) Coronary heart disease
(5) Diabetes mellitus
(6) Fatty liver
(7) Gallbladder disease
(8) Hirsutism
(9) Hypertension
(10) Hypertriglyceridemia
(11) Respiratory tract infections and other problems
(12) Varicose veins

b. While being overweight can raise the risk of disease, especially cardiovascular disease, the risk is only partially determined by body weight. The **body mass index (BMI)** is used as a parameter to assess the overall risk of developing heart disease when patients are overweight.

$$\text{BMI} = \frac{\text{Weight (kg)}}{\text{Height}^2\text{ (meters)}} \textbf{ or } \frac{\text{Weight (lbs)} \times 700}{\text{Height (inches)}}\text{, then divide by the height again.}$$

Long-term studies show that the overall risk of developing heart disease is generally related to the BMI as follows:

(1) BMI of 25 or less—-risk is very low to low.
(2) BMI between 25 and 30—-risk is low to moderate.
(3) BMI of 30 or more—-risk is moderate to very high.
(4) Some believe that a BMI of 27 or above is the cut-off for significant concern for the need for weight loss.

B. Management. Weight reduction involves an integrated program of diet, correct eating habits, exercise, patient follow-up, and, sometimes, medication. An approximate **weight loss goal** should be set when the patient and physician are establishing ideal body weight. Realistic goals about the frequency of weight loss should be established.

1. A weight loss goal of 1–2 pounds per week is appropriate.

2. To lose 1 pound in a week, a person must expend 3500 calories through physical work or decrease caloric intake by 3500 calories during that week.

3. For example, a patient who normally consumes 3000 calories per day must decrease that intake by 500 calories per day in order to lose 1 pound in 1 week (500 x 7 days = 3500 calories).

C. Diets are specific eating plans that provide a certain number of calories per day.

1. **Balanced diets** with calories derived from protein, carbohydrate, and fat are optimal. The caloric intake of fat should be minimized (i.e., less than 30% of total calories, less than 10% saturated fat) for general health reasons (e.g., incidence of ischemic heart disease, certain types of cancer). Also, fat contains 9 calories per gram; carbohydrate or protein contains 4 calories per gram.

2. **Fad diets** do not teach patients how to eat properly for long-range benefits. Weight maintenance is the key.

3. **Very low-calorie diets,** which provide 300–800 calories per day, can be useful in severely obese patients under strict medical supervision.
   - **a.** Adequate protein must be present in these diets in order to preserve lean body mass.
   - **b.** Patients must be monitored carefully for electrolyte imbalances, postural hypotension, and electrocardiogram (ECG) abnormalities.
   - **c. Formula diets**
     - **(1)** The **"Last Chance Diet,"** a liquid protein diet marketed over the counter in the mid-1970s, resulted in several deaths from cardiovascular problems, which were probably caused by a negative nitrogen balance due to the poor-quality protein in these products.
     - **(2)** **Optifast, Medifast, and Health Management Resources (HMR)** are available through physicians or hospitals as part of a packaged weight-reduction program (approximately 400–800 calories per day) that uses high-quality (i.e., milk or egg, not vegetable) protein and variable proportions of carbohydrate and fat. These products appear to be safe, but maintenance of weight loss over the long term is still the main issue.
     - **(3)** **Slimfast** and **Ultra Slimfast** are high-quality protein, over-the-counter (OTC) variations to formula diets. The consumer is instructed to mix the formula with milk (approximately 200 calories) and use it to replace one or two meals. For the third meal, the patient eats regular food.

D. Eating habits. Patients need to be trained in gaining self-control of their eating behavior if they are planning to lose weight and maintain the weight loss.

1. **Behavior modification programs,** which seek to eliminate improper eating behaviors (e.g., eating while watching television, eating too rapidly, eating when not hungry), may be beneficial.

2. **Self-help groups** (e.g., Weight Watchers, Nutri-System, Jenny Craig) use a program of diet, education, and positive emotional support to help patients lose weight.

E. Exercise. Because 3500 calories of work must be expended to lose 1 pound, exercise is clearly a difficult way to lose weight. However, an effective weight loss program incorporates exercise.

1. **Benefits**
   - **a.** Exercise burns calories [e.g., walking (2 mph) burns 200 calories per hour; running (5.3 mph) burns 570 calories per hour].
   - **b.** Exercise raises body metabolism, which can have an extended effect on weight loss.
   - **c.** Exercise can decrease appetite.
   - **d.** Patients usually feel better (mentally and emotionally) when they exercise regularly.
   - **e.** Exercise helps to prevent the loss of muscle mass.

2. **Effective exercise expends energy.** Vibrating belts, continuous passive motion machines, and similar products do not result in increased weight loss because using them does not expend energy.

F. Prescription weight-loss products

1. **Overview.** Despite the interest in pharmacotherapy, there had been no new drugs approved for weight control in the United States for more than 20 years until dexfenfluramine came on the market in 1996. This has been due to a combination of factors, but an important one has been the manner in which the Drug Enforcement Agency (DEA) has classified these drugs.
   - **a.** The initial drugs used for appetite suppression, **amphetamine, methamphetamine,** and **phenmetrazine** (Preludin) are classified as Schedule II because they have a high potential for abuse. These drugs are no longer used for weight control.

b. Drugs that were marketed later, **phendimetrazine** (Plegine), **diethylpropion** (Tenuate), **phentermine** (Ionamin), and **fenfluramine** (Pondimin), have shown little evidence of abuse potential but have still been classified as controlled substances and are only recommended for short-term use (usually no more than a few weeks).

2. Indication. Prescription weight-loss drugs have been justified for someone who has lost weight on a diet and then reaches a plateau or, more rarely, for someone who is beginning a diet. These agents traditionally have been used for short-term therapy (8–12 weeks), and their use results in small, but statistically significant weight loss (~0.5 lb per week more than with placebo).

3. The **mechanism of action** apparently involves suppression of the satiety center in the hypothalamic ventromedial nucleus. Most suppressants augment brain catecholamine action, with the exception of agents such as fenfluramine, which acts specifically on serotonin. Other mechanisms may be involved as well.

4. Drug selection and side effects. No superiority has been shown for the appetite suppressant effects of any of these agents. Patients often tolerate one agent better than another. Restlessness, insomnia, tremors, tachycardia, nausea, diarrhea, constipation, dry mouth, and mydriasis are commonly reported side effects. In susceptible patients, elevated blood pressure and cardiac arrhythmias may occur. There is the potential for dependence and abuse of some of these agents. Agents acting on serotonin (i.e., fenfluramine, fluoxetine) are an exception, producing sedation and hypotension.

5. Long-term use. There is a growing interest in treating obesity as a **long-term chronic disease** in the same manner that we view hypertension and diabetes mellitus. A fairly recent 4 year study that used two of these agents, **phentermine** (Ionamin) and **fenfluramine** (Pondimin), concluded that prescription appetite suppressants can enable people to lose and keep off weight as long as they were continuing to use the medication. In 1996, **dexfenfluramine (Redux),** the dextro isomer of fenfluramine, became the first new diet pill to be cleared for marketing by the FDA in more than 20 years.

a. This drug suppresses appetite and carbohydrate cravings by increasing the availability of serotonin. It is indicated only for those who are at least 20%–30% overweight and who show benefit during the first four weeks of use.

b. The most common **side effects** are drowsiness, diarrhea, and dry mouth. As with any of the prescription appetite suppressants used for longer than 3 months, there is an increased risk of **primary pulmonary hypertension,** which can be fatal. The safety and effectiveness of Redux beyond one year have not been determined at this time.

G. OTC weight-loss products

1. Benzocaine and **phenylpropanolamine (PPA)** are two OTC agents that have been considered Category I for weight control. However, considerable controversy has developed about the true effectiveness of these agents.

a. Benzocaine appears to act topically on nerve endings in the oral cavity to decrease the ability to detect different degrees of sweetness. Through this numbing effect, the desire for food can be decreased in some people.

(1) The **dosage form** must be a substance that remains in the mouth for an extended period of time, such as gum, a lozenge, or candy.

(2) The **dose** is 3–15 mg just before food consumption.

(3) The principal **adverse effect** with this medication is hypersensitivity.

(4) Examples of products that contain benzocaine in this form include Diet Ayds and Slim-Mint.

b. PPA, which is the active ingredient in Dexatrim, Acutrim, and Prolamine, is a sympathomimetic agent that is chemically related to amphetamines. It appears to have an appetite-suppressing effect similar to that of the amphetamines and amphetamine-related agents found in prescription medications for obesity.

(1) Dose and dosage form. The approved dose is 37.5 mg in an immediate-releasing dosage form, which should be taken about 30 minutes before a meal. The approved dose for the sustained-release form is 75 mg, which is the maximum daily dose.

(2) Safety. Because of its sympathomimetic properties, PPA should be used cautiously by patients with heart disease, hypertension, diabetes, and hyperthyroidism. When used in therapeutic doses, PPA has only minimal cardiovascular effects.

(a) **Central nervous system (CNS) stimulation** might be a problem, producing such symptoms as insomnia, nervousness, and headache.

(b) **Drug interactions.** Patients should exercise caution when using other OTC products containing PPA (e.g., cold and allergic rhinitis medications). PPA can antagonize the effects of antihypertensive agents through various mechanisms. Concurrent use of PPA and other sympathomimetic agents can also result in additive CNS and cardiovascular effects.

(3) **Efficacy.** PPA-containing products show minimal efficacy, but modest weight loss is achieved. For example, in a 4-week, double-blind study, a group treated with PPA (combined with caffeine) had an average weight loss of 5.5 pounds versus 4 pounds in the placebo group. The OTC panel that originally reviewed these agents stated that each of the double-blind, placebo-controlled studies available at the time were defective in one way or another.

2. **Additional agents.** A number of other OTC agents have been proposed for the treatment of obesity, but support for their effectiveness is weak. For example, the bulk-producing laxatives have been proposed to create a feeling of fullness in the stomach. However, x-ray studies have shown that the bulk leaves the stomach within 30 minutes.

II. SLEEP AIDS

A. Normal sleep and sleep requirements

1. **Length.** Sleep time and quality of sleep vary widely among individuals. The usual range of sleep time per night is 5–10 hours, with an average of about 7 1/2 hours.

2. **Sleep requirements** change as a person ages. Newborns may sleep up to 18 hours. Preteens usually fall asleep within 5 or 10 minutes, sleep for 9 1/2 hours, and spend 95% of their time in bed in solid, continuous, deep sleep. By adulthood, 7 or 8 hours of sleep usually provide adequate rest. In old age, 6 hours may suffice.

3. **Polysomnography** uses electroencephalogram (EEG), electro-oculogram (EOG), and electromyogram (EMG) recordings to note changes that occur during sleep.

   a. **Stages.** Using polysomnography, researchers have discovered five stages of sleep.

      (1) **One rapid eye movement (REM) stage** occupies about 25% of normal total sleep time.

      (2) **Four non-rapid eye movement (NREM) stages** make up the remaining 75% of normal total sleep time. Stages three and four of NREM sleep are considered to be the deepest sleep and are often referred to collectively as **delta sleep** or **restorative sleep.**

   b. Most **dreaming** occurs during the REM stage of sleep, and the degree of "restfulness" of sleep is associated with the amount of REM sleep.

   c. Most of the **medications** used to treat insomnia, including the OTC agents, interfere with some component of the sleep stages, especially the REM sleep.

B. Insomnia

1. **Definition.** Insomnia is an interruption of the natural sleep cycle that results in impaired daytime performance. Insomnia must be defined not only in terms of the amount of sleep but also with attention to the perceived quality of sleep.

2. **Diagnosis.** Daytime performance deficits, not the number of hours slept, should be the primary determinant of an insomnia diagnosis.

   a. An occasional night of inadequate or no sleep is of little concern in healthy individuals. Apart from **extreme sleepiness** and the occurrence of **"microsleeps,"** remarkably little **pathology** is associated with extended sleeplessness.

   b. As long as patients awake each morning feeling fully refreshed and do not need an afternoon nap, they should be reassured that they do not have insomnia and that the full 8-hour sleep pattern at night is not absolutely necessary. Oftentimes, simple **reassurance** may be all that is needed to "cure" insomnia.

3. **Categories.** Insomnias can generally be divided into three categories.

a. **Transient** insomnia, which accounts for approximately 15% of insomnia cases, generally lasts less than 7 days. Causes of transient insomnia include **jet lag, shift work,** or **acute anxiety.**
b. **Short-term** insomnia lasts from 1–3 weeks. Causes of short-term insomnia include usually identifiable, often self-limiting problems, such as **grief, pain, noise,** or an **anxiety-provoking situation.**
c. **Long-term** insomnia (or chronic insomnia) lasts longer than 3 weeks, indicates an underlying pathology, and requires a thorough assessment of the patient's physical and emotional health. Long-term insomnia may stem from an underlying medical condition such as **hyperthyroidism** or **arthritis.** Often, treatment strategies that relieve the underlying physical disorder resolve the insomnia complaint.

4. **Causes.** Patients who experience insomnia have different causes for this condition.
   a. **Intrinsic sleep disorders**
      (1) **Psychophysiologic insomnia** is a conditioned form of sleep loss in which the patient associates increased wakefulness with the bedroom and the bedtime routine.
      (2) **Restless legs syndrome** is characterized by extremely uncomfortable sensations in leg muscles at rest, which are relieved only by getting up and moving around.
      (3) **Sleep apnea** can be obstructive or centrally mediated. The hallmark is breathing that stops for short periods during sleep. Patients with sleep apnea should not use hypnotics or OTC sleep aids.
      (4) **Sleep-related myoclonus** is the periodic, rhythmic curling or jumping of the feet during sleep.
   b. **Extrinsic sleep disorders**
      (1) **Adjustment sleep disorder** is prompted by a stressful life change.
      (2) **Inadequate sleep hygiene** is caused by a lifestyle that reduces the amount of quality sleep.
      (3) **Hypnotic-, stimulant-,** or **alcohol-dependent** sleep disorder is caused by dependence, tolerance, or over reliance on a given agent.
   c. **Circadian sleep disorders**
      (1) **Delayed sleep phase syndrome** occurs in people whose natural sleep times are altered due to work. For instance, a person who must be at work at 8 A.M., but naturally gets tired after 2 A.M. and wakes after 10 A.M., would be affected by this type of disorder.
      (2) **Jet lag** is primarily a problem for people who travel across several time zones.
   d. **Psychiatric disorders,** such as **major depressive disorder,** result in poor sleep that usually improves with specific antidepressant medication.

5. **Treatment** of insomnia is highly dependent on the type of insomnia. It is very important to distinguish among transient insomnia, short-term insomnia, and long-term insomnia (see II B 3).
   a. **Nondrug intervention** and **sleep-hygiene measures** include the following lifestyle and environmental recommendations:
      (1) Establishing a regular bedtime
      (2) Going to bed when tired and ready to sleep
      (3) If unable to sleep, getting out of bed
      (4) Shortly before bedtime, engaging in a relaxing activity, such as taking a warm bath, eating a light snack, or doing relaxation exercises
      (5) Avoiding strenuous exercise or other stimulating activity for several hours before bedtime
      (6) Avoiding alcohol because it could produce fragmented sleep
      (7) Making sure that the bedroom and the bed are comfortable for sleeping
      (8) Avoiding stimulants (e.g., caffeine, nicotine, PPA, pseudoephedrine) late in the day
      (9) Avoiding naps during the day
   b. **Drug treatment of transient and short-term insomnia.** Wakefulness and sleep are antagonistic states competing for control of brain activity. Several neurotransmitters play a role in arousal. Their actions help explain why medications that mimic or counteract their effects can influence sleep. **Serotonin** and **γ-aminobutyric acid (GABA)** are believed to promote slow-wave sleep. **Acetylcholine** regulates REM sleep. **Norepinephrine, epinephrine,** and **dopamine** stimulate wakefulness. Individuals vary greatly in their natural levels of neurotransmitters and their sensitivity to these chemicals. Hypnotics exert their

effects by modulating brain neurotransmitters and neuropeptides such as serotonin, norepinephrine, acetylcholine, histamine, adenosine, and GABA.

(1) The **goal of therapy** for transient and short-term insomnia is:

(a) Restoring daytime functioning

(b) Avoiding the self-reinforcing pattern that may develop into chronic insomnia

(2) **Therapeutic contract.** A wise strategy for using hypnotics is to enter into a therapeutic contract with patients, limiting hypnotic use to no more than two or three nights in succession, followed by one or more medicine-free nights. In this way, hypnotics can serve as a safety net, and patients can be assured that they will have no more than one night of sleeplessness without obtaining relief.

(3) **Prescription hypnotic agents** are reserved primarily for this type of insomnia. Sedative hypnotic agents should be used only as part of a plan that makes use of good sleep-hygiene techniques.

(a) **Benzodiazepines** have been considered to be the drugs of choice for symptomatic relief of insomnia, and they are the closest to an ideal hypnotic sleep aid.

(i) **Mechanism of action.** The benzodiazepines work by enhancing the activity of the inhibitory neurotransmitter GABA, which calms brain activity.

(ii) **Selection** of a benzodiazepine is based on the specific pharmacokinetic profile that matches the particular sleep problem (Table 31-2).

(b) **Zolpidem** (Ambien) is the newest hypnotic on the United States market. It is a nonbenzodiazepine with the structure of an imidazopyridine. Although it is not a benzodiazepine, it acts on the benzodiazepine receptor (ω-1 subtype). It has a minimal effect on sleep stages and, therefore, is reputed to promote a more natural sleep.

(i) **Advantages** over the benzodiazepines include lack of withdrawal effects, no rebound insomnia and little or no tolerance demonstrated. It has a rapid onset of action and is useful for both initiating and maintaining sleep.

(ii) **Adverse effects** of zolpidem include nightmares, agitation, headaches, gastrointestinal (GI) upset, dizziness, and daytime drowsiness.

(c) **Barbiturates** are prescribed less commonly for management of insomnia because of the risk of excessive CNS depression. The **early nonbarbiturate nonbenzodiazepine** sedative hypnotics were originally thought to be superior to the barbiturates, but they were found to share many disadvantages in addition to having disadvantages of their own. **Chloral hydrate** might be considered an exception, but it still has some issues of concern (displaces some highly protein-bound drugs, some GI irritation).

(4) **OTC drug therapy**

(a) The Food and Drug Administration (FDA) has deemed two antihistamines, **diphenhydramine** (e.g., Nytol, Sleep-Eze, Sominex II, Compoz) and **doxylamine** (e.g., Unisom), safe and effective sleep aids. They are both ethanolamine antihistamines, which possess the highest sedative effects and the lowest GI side effects of the various antihistamines.

(i) The **therapeutic use** of these agents capitalizes on the drowsiness side effect.

(ii) **Indications.** These OTC products are indicated for mild situational insomnia.

(iii) The usual **dose** for adults is 25 mg for doxylamine and 50 mg for diphenhydramine. Increasing the dose of diphenhydramine does not produce a linear increase in hypnotic effect. However, it does produce greater anticholinergic side effects, particularly in elderly people.

Table 31-2. Examples of Short-, Intermediate-, and Long-acting Benzodiazepines

Agent	Rate of Elimination	Onset of Action (minutes)	Usual Adult Dose (mg)
Triazolam (Halcion)	Rapid	15–30	0.125–0.25
Estazolam (Prosom)	Intermediate	15–30	1–2
Temazepam (Restoril)	Intermediate	45–60	15–30
Flurazepam HCl (Dalmane)	Slow	15–30	15–30
Quazepam (Doral)	Slow	15–30	7.5–15

(iv) The most common **side effects** include dizziness, dry mouth, blurred vision, and upset stomach. Both doxylamine and diphenhydramine cause REM suppression and, therefore, some REM rebound after discontinuation. Anticholinergic effects include constipation and urinary retention. Central anticholinergic effects that also affect the elderly include confusion, disorientation, impaired short-term memory, and, at times, visual and tactile hallucinations.

(v) **Contraindications.** These agents should not be used by individuals under age 12 and should not be taken longer than 2 weeks. In addition, they should be used cautiously by patients who have asthma, narrow-angle glaucoma, and prostate enlargement.

(vi) **Efficacy.** Diphenhydramine and doxylamine are considered to be roughly equivalent in efficacy.

(b) **Melatonin** (e.g., Melatonex) has been prominently featured in the media because of various therapeutic claims. Among these has been the recommendation to use this agent to treat insomnia and jet lag. It has **not** been approved by the FDA for this use. This hormone is produced in a predictable daily rhythm by the pineal gland, which is located deep in the brain between the two hemispheres. Levels of melatonin climb after dark and ebb after dawn. Older people, who often suffer from insomnia, have lower serum concentrations of melatonin. Melatonin might turn out to be an effective hypnotic and could have some beneficial effect on jet lag. But large controlled trials have not been done. The purity of the products sold in health food stores and the adverse effects of taking the hormone are unknown.

STUDY QUESTIONS

Directions: Each of the numbered items or incomplete statements in this section is followed by answers or by completions of the statement. Select the **one** lettered answer or completion that is **best** in each case.

1. Based on the calorie decrease necessary to lose 1 pound of body fat, how many pounds will a woman likely lose in 20 days if she cuts her caloric intake from 2200 per day to 1600 per day but does not increase her physical activity?

(A) 10 pounds
(B) Approximately 5 pounds
(C) Approximately 3.5 pounds
(D) Slightly less than 2 pounds
(E) Not enough data to calculate

2. All of the following statements about diphenhydramine are true EXCEPT

(A) a 50-mg dose that is ineffective should be doubled for the elderly patient
(B) it suppresses rapid eye movement (REM) sleep
(C) it should not be taken with alcohol
(D) it is similar to doxylamine in efficacy as a sleep aid

3. All of the following statements about sleep stages are true EXCEPT

(A) a normal, young, healthy adult spends about 20%–25% of total sleep time in rapid eye movement (REM) sleep
(B) the degree of restfulness of sleep is associated with the amount of REM sleep
(C) dreaming appears to occur most often in the first stage of non-rapid eye movement (NREM) sleep
(D) stages three and four of NREM sleep are often referred to as delta sleep

4. All of the following would be useful sleep hygiene measures EXCEPT

(A) exercising intensely just before bedtime
(B) taking a warm bath just before bedtime
(C) reading until drowsy
(D) keeping the bedroom somewhat cool
(E) establishing a regular bedtime

5. All of the following statements about obesity are true EXCEPT

(A) an obese patient is generally defined as a person who has surplus body fat and is above their ideal body weight by at least 20%
(B) very low-calorie diets initially result in a significant amount of water loss, as glycogen and protein are metabolized
(C) fad diets do not teach patients how to eat for long-term maintenance of the decreased weight
(D) a bulk laxative such as Metamucil has been proven to be an effective weight loss agent

ANSWERS AND EXPLANATIONS

1. The answer is C *[I A 6].*
The woman would lose about 3.5 pounds. To lose 1 pound of fat, caloric intake must decrease by 3500 calories. This woman decreased her caloric intake from 2200 calories per day to 1600 calories per day, a decrease of 600 calories. Six hundred calories multiplied by 20 days equals a decrease of 12,000 calories. Twelve thousand divided by 3500 equals 3.43 pounds, or approximately 3.5 pounds.

2. The answer is A *[II 8 5 b (4) (a)].*
Increasing the dose of diphenhydramine does not automatically bring a linear increase in hypnotic effect. However, it does produce greater anticholinergic side effects, which are particularly troublesome in the elderly. Diphenhydramine, which suppresses rapid eye movement (REM) sleep, produces a sedation more unpleasant than that of alcohol or benzodiazepines. Diphenhydramine should not be taken with alcohol. As a sleep aid, it is similar in efficacy to doxylamine.

3. The answer is C *[II A 3].*
Most dreaming appears to occur during rapid eye movement (REM) rather than non-REM (NREM) sleep. The average, young, healthy adult spends about one-quarter of the time sleeping in REM sleep. The amount of REM sleep is associated with the degree of restfulness. Delta sleep consists of stages three and four of NREM sleep.

4. The answer is A *[II B 5 a].*
Exercising intensely just before going to bed will usually have a stimulating effect. Taking a warm bath shortly before bedtime, reading until drowsy, keeping the bedroom cool, and establishing a regular bedtime are considered appropriate sleep hygiene measures.

5. The answer is D *[I A 1, C 1–3].*
Bulk laxatives produce a feeling of fullness, but x-ray studies show that the bulk leaves the stomach within 30 minutes. They may decrease appetite somewhat, but the effectiveness of bulk laxatives as a weight loss agent is weak. Obese people are those who have surplus body fat and are at least 20% above their ideal body weight. Very low-calorie diets result in initial significant water loss, as glycogen and protein are metabolized. Fad diets do not teach people how to eat to maintain any achieved weight loss. Consequently, many people who follow fad diets regain weight.

32
OTC Agents for Fever, Pain, Cough, Cold, and Allergic Rhinitis

Gerald E. Schumacher
Larry N. Swanson

I. ANALGESIC, ANTI-INFLAMMATORY, AND ANTIPYRETIC AGENTS. Over-the-counter (OTC) analgesics and antipyretics relieve mild-to-moderate pain and reduce inflammation and fever. These agents are effective for somatic pain (e.g., musculoskeletal pain in the joints, pain from headache, myalgia, dysmenorrhea, and discomfort resulting from generalized inflammation), but they are not effective in reducing discomfort from the visceral organs (e.g., stomach, lungs, heart). Salicylates and nonsteroidal anti-inflammatory drugs (NSAIDs) reduce pain, inflammation, and fever, but acetaminophen generally is effective for only pain and fever.*

A. Pathogenesis of pain. Intense stimulus (e.g., tissue injury) releases substances that sensitize pain receptors to mechanical, thermal, and chemical stimulation. This triggers pain receptors to send pain impulses over afferent nerve fibers to the central nervous system (CNS).

1. **Awareness** of pain occurs in the thalamus.
2. Pain **recognition** and **localization** occur in the cortex.
3. **Mechanism of analgesic, anti-inflammatory, and antipyretic action.** These agents inhibit (centrally, peripherally, or both) the biosynthesis of various **prostaglandins,** substances involved in the development of pain and inflammation as well as in the regulation of body temperature.

B. Salicylates

1. **Therapeutic uses.** Salicylates are used to relieve mild-to-moderate pain and reduce inflammation and fever. Aspirin (acetylsalicylic acid), specifically, is also used to reduce the incidence of:
   a. **Strokes** in men at risk
   b. **Myocardial infarction** in men and women who have had a previous infarction, stable and unstable angina pectoris, or coronary artery bypass surgery
2. **Mechanism of action**
   a. **Analgesic and anti-inflammatory actions.** The action of aspirin results from both the acetyl and the salicylate portions of the drug. Actions of other salicylates (e.g., sodium salicylate, salicylsalicylic acid, choline salicylate) results only from the salicylate portion of the agents.
      (1) These drugs **inhibit cyclooxygenase,** the enzyme that is responsible for the formation of precursors of prostaglandins and thromboxanes from arachidonic acid (Figure 32-1).
      (2) Analgesia is produced mainly by **blocking the peripheral generation of pain impulses** mediated by prostaglandins and other chemicals. Analgesia probably secondarily involves a reduction in the awareness of pain in the CNS.
   b. **Antipyretic action.** The principal antipyretic action occurs in the CNS. Salicylates act on the hypothalamic heat-regulating center to produce peripheral vasodilation, which results from the inhibition of prostaglandin synthesis.
   c. **Antiplatelet and antithrombotic actions**

---

*In some instances, aspirin is considered to be a nonsteroidal anti-inflammatory drug (NSAID), whereas in other instances it is not. For the purpose of demonstrating different information, aspirin and NSAIDs are discussed separately in this chapter.

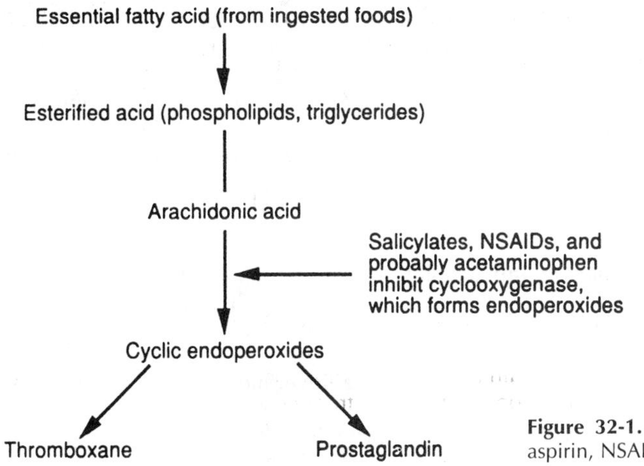

Figure 32-1. Inhibition of prostaglandin formation by aspirin, NSAIDs, and acetaminophen.

(1) **Antiplatelet.** Aspirin (but not other salicylates, acetaminophen, or NSAIDs) **irreversibly inhibits cyclooxygenase in platelets,** which prevents the formation of the aggregating agent thromboxane A_2.

(2) **Antithrombotic.** Aspirin also **reversibly inhibits the formation of prostacyclin** [prostaglandin I_2 (PGI_2)], which is an aggregation inhibitor in blood vessels.

3. **Administration and dosage**

a. For **analgesia** or **antipyresis in adults,** 325–650 mg every 4 hours or 650–1000 mg every 6 hours should be administered as needed. The maximum daily dose is 4000 mg for no longer than 10 days for pain or 3 days for fever, without consulting a physician.

b. **Child dosage** depends on age. The dosages are 160 mg every 4 hours for children 2–4 years of age, 400–480 mg every 4 hours for children 9–12 years of age. Salicylates should be given for no longer than 5 days for pain, 3 days for fever, and 2 days for sore throat, without consulting a physician.

c. The **antirheumatic dosage for adults** is 3600–4500 mg daily in divided doses.

d. For patients with **ischemic heart disease,** a 325-mg dose given daily. Every other day is recommended for individuals with stable angina, unstable angina, and evolving myocardial infarction. For patients without clinically apparent ischemic heart disease, the hemorrhagic complications associated with routine aspirin use may outweigh its benefit, unless subjects have established risk factors for atherosclerotic disease.

e. **Anti-inflammatory dosages.** Although antipyretic and analgesic effects should appear within the first few doses, the anti-inflammatory effect may take 2 or more weeks to appear, even at high doses. The usual anti-inflammatory dosage of aspirin is 4000–6000 mg per day. The usual anti-inflammatory dosage of ibuprofen is 1200–3200 mg per day.

4. **Precautions**

a. **Hypersensitivity** to aspirin occurs in up to 0.5% of the population.

(1) Allergic reactions resulting in bronchoconstriction occur most frequently in people with **nasal polyps.**

(2) **Cross-reactivity** with other NSAIDs occurs in more than 90% of people. Cross-reactivity with acetaminophen occurs in 5% of people.

b. **Contraindications.** Aspirin is contraindicated in patients with bleeding disorders or peptic ulcers. Also, aspirin should not be given to children or teenagers with a viral illness, because Reye's syndrome (i.e., fatty liver degeneration accompanied by encephalopathy) may occur.

c. **Pregnancy.** Salicylates in chronic high doses are recommended with extreme caution during the last trimester of pregnancy because of:

(1) Potential bleeding problems in the mother, fetus, or neonate

(2) Prolonging or complicating delivery

d. **Gastrointestinal (GI) disturbances** resulting from the inhibition of the gastric prostaglandins occur in 10%–20% of people at analgesic and antipyretic dosages. Anti-inflammatory regimens affect up to 40% of people. These percentages decrease by using enteric-coated dosage forms and taking salicylates with food or large doses of antacids. Buffered aspirin products contain insufficient "buffers" to counteract the adverse GI effects of aspirin.

e. **CNS disturbances** such as tinnitus, dizziness, or headache may occur at anti-inflammatory doses in some patients.

f. **Salicylism** (salicylate toxicity) may occur at anti-inflammatory doses. In addition to the CNS disturbances above, respiratory alkalosis, nausea, hyperthermia, confusion, and convulsions may occur.

5. **Significant interactions**
   a. Salicylates potentiate the effect of **anticoagulants** and **thrombolytic agents.**
   b. Salicylates potentiate (at anti-inflammatory doses) the effect of **hypoglycemics.**
   c. Salicylates potentiate the adverse gastrointestinal reaction resulting from chronic **alcohol** or **NSAID** use.
   d. Aspirin may competitively inhibit the metabolism of **zidovudine,** resulting in potentiation of zidovudine or aspirin toxicity.
   e. **Caffeine** taken in conjunction with salicylates appears to enhance the analgesic effect.

C. Acetaminophen

1. **Therapeutic uses.** Acetaminophen is used to relieve mild-to-moderate pain and reduce fever. Guidelines from the American College of Rheumatology now recommend it as first-line therapy for osteoarthritis of the knee and hip. Because it has minimal anti-inflammatory activity, it cannot be used to treat the swelling or stiffness resulting from rheumatoid arthritis.

2. **Mechanism of action.** The analgesic and antipyretic actions of acetaminophen are the same as those for aspirin (see I B 2 a–b).

3. **Administration and dosage.** Available dosage forms are 325 mg and 500 mg.
   a. For **analgesia** or **antipyresis in adults,** the dosage is 500–1000 mg three times daily as needed. The maximum daily dose is 4000 mg for no longer than 10 days for pain or 3 days for fever, without consulting a physician. For osteoarthritis, 1000 mg four times daily is recommended.
   b. For **children age 6 years or older,** 325 mg is administered every 4–6 hours as needed. The maximum daily dose is 1600 mg for no longer than 5 days for pain, 3 days for fever, and 2 days for sore throat, without consulting a physician.
   c. **Routine use.** Acetaminophen is routinely used in patients who are:
      (1) Sensitive to the GI disturbances caused by salicylates and NSAIDs
      (2) Prone to bleeding disorders
      (3) Are hypersensitive to salicylates

4. **Precautions.** Patients with active alcoholism, hepatic disease, or viral hepatitis are at risk from chronic administration of acetaminophen. Toxicity is rare, but chronic daily ingestion of 5 g or more for longer than 1 month is likely to result in liver damage. Acute doses of 10 g or more are hepatotoxic.

5. **Significant interactions.** Acetaminophen may competitively inhibit the metabolism of **zidovudine,** resulting in potentiation of zidovudine or acetaminophen toxicity.

D. NSAIDs.

Currently, **ibuprofen, naproxen,** and **ketoprofen** are the only NSAIDs available without a prescription.

1. **Therapeutic uses.** NSAIDs are used to relieve mild-to-moderate pain and reduce inflammation and fever. OTC drug use largely focuses on the analgesic and antipyretic indications of these agents. Maximum OTC drug dosage is generally recommended for osteoarthritis.

2. **Mechanism of action**
   a. **Analgesic and anti-inflammatory actions.** NSAIDs inhibit prostaglandin synthesis both peripherally and centrally. Like salicylates, these drugs inhibit cyclooxygenase (see Figure 32-1). NSAIDs produce analgesia mainly by blocking the peripheral generation of pain impulses that are mediated by prostaglandins and other chemicals. Secondarily, analgesia probably involves a reduction in the awareness of pain in the CNS.
   b. **Antipyretic action.** The principal antipyretic action is central. NSAIDs act on the hypothalamic heat-regulating center to produce peripheral vasodilation, which results from the inhibition of prostaglandin synthesis.

3. **Administration and dosage.** The available OTC dosage forms of ibuprofen are a 200 mg tablet and a 100 mg per 5 ml oral suspension. Naproxen sodium OTC is available as a 220 mg (200 mg of naproxen) tablet. Ketoprofen OTC is a 12.5 mg tablet.
   a. For **analgesia** or **antipyresis in adults,** the dosage of **ibuprofen** is 200–400 mg every 4–6 hours as needed. The maximum daily dose is 1200 mg for no longer than 10 days for pain or 3 days for fever, without consulting a physician. For **naproxen sodium,** the recommended dose is 220 mg every 8–12 hours as needed. The maximum daily dose is 660 mg. **Ketoprofen** is recommended as 12.5 mg every 4–6 hours as needed, with a maximum daily dose of 75 mg. Both naproxen and ketoprofen caution about the same limitations on the duration of treatment without consulting a physician as recommended for ibuprofen.
   b. For **rheumatoid arthritis dosage in adults, ibuprofen** is recommended to a maximum daily dosage of 3200 mg (administered on a 4–6 hours basis), **naproxen sodium** to a daily maximum of 1100 mg (divided in doses every 8–12 hours), and **ketoprofen** to a maximum of 300 mg per day (administered every 4–6 hours).
   c. **Naproxen sodium** and **ketoprofen** are not recommended for children under 12 years of age. **Ibuprofen** is available as a suspension for children 2–11 years of age.

4. **Precautions**
   a. NSAIDs are contraindicated in patients with **bleeding disorders** or **peptic ulcers.**
   b. NSAIDs are recommended with extreme caution during the last trimester of **pregnancy** because of:
      (1) Potential adverse effects on fetal blood flow
      (2) The possibility of prolonging pregnancy
   c. **GI disturbances** resulting from the inhibition of the gastric prostaglandins occur in 5%–10% of people at analgesic and antipyretic doses. Anti-inflammatory regimens (i.e., higher doses) affect up to 20% of people. These percentages decrease by taking NSAIDs with food or large doses of antacids. Ibuprofen is often preferred to aspirin by patients because ibuprofen causes fewer GI disturbances and bleeding events.
   d. **Renal toxicity** during chronic administration is a significant concern and may occur in the form of nephrotic syndrome, hyperkalemia, or interstitial nephritis.

5. **Significant interactions**
   a. NSAIDs potentiate the effect of **anticoagulants** and **thrombolytic agents.**
   b. NSAIDs potentiate (at anti-inflammatory doses) the effect of **hypoglycemics.**
   c. NSAIDs potentiate the adverse GI reactions resulting from chronic **alcohol** or **salicylate** use.
   d. **Caffeine** taken in conjunction with ibuprofen appears to enhance the analgesic effect.
   e. Hypersensitivity to **aspirin** can occur with NSAID use.
   f. OTC labeling for these agents cautions against use of an NSAID with other NSAIDs.

II. THE COMMON COLD

A. General

1. The common cold has been described as the **most expensive illness** in the United States. It is estimated that **30 million days** are lost from work or school each year due to the common cold.

2. In the United States, **100 million cases** are reported annually. Generally adults will have between two and four colds per year; children will have between six and ten colds per year.

3. There is probably no other category of self-medication that requires more of the pharmacist in terms of time, advice, and patient counseling.

B. Etiology

1. There are **between 120 and 200 identified viral strains** that invade the nasal and bronchial epithelial cells to cause the common cold.

2. The viruses **most commonly responsible** for the common cold are the **rhinoviruses** (about 30%–35% of cases) followed by the **coronaviruses.**

3. In order to produce infection, a rhinovirus must penetrate the protective mucus blanket that covers the nasal epithelium.

4. Mucus in the nasal passages traps and removes most contaminants, but the rhinovirus remains attached to the **nasal mucus membranes** via a specific receptor.

5. **Rhinovirus infection** leads to the release of various inflammatory mediators. Mediators like prostaglandins, leukotrienes, and kinins are involved in symptoms such as nasal congestion, runny nose, and sore throat.

6. **Histamine** is not involved in the inflammation associated with rhinovirus infection, but it is associated with the immediate phase of allergic response (sneezing and itching). Now that the importance of chemical mediators in the common cold is understood, new therapies can be developed to relieve symptoms. Because inflammation plays a dominant role, anti-inflammatory therapy may emerge as an appropriate course of action (Figure 32-2).

7. Scientists believe that the common cold is actually **200 different infections** caused by 200 viruses. Each infection may result in lifetime immunity or at least long-term immunity so that each cold endured means one less virus to worry about. Indeed, people generally get fewer colds as they get older. Immunity is partly responsible, but less contact with children as people age may be an even more important factor.

C. Pathogenesis

1. Experts disagree on how colds are transmitted. Some say through the air (i.e., in the mist created by a sneeze). Evidence favors **direct contact,** such as shaking hands with a cold sufferer who has just blown his nose, as the main route of transmission.

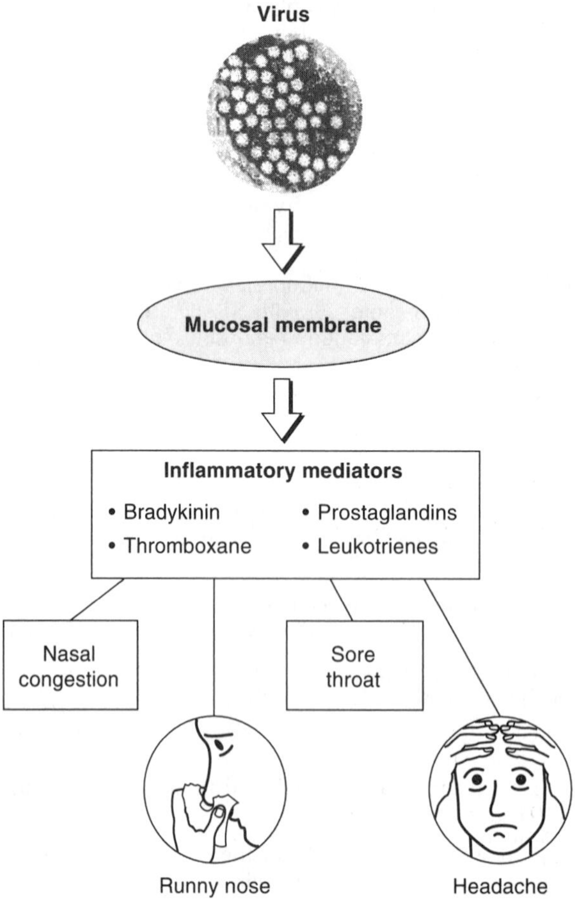

Figure 32-2.

2. On the skin, certain fabrics, and hard non-porous materials such as stainless steel and wood, self-inoculation occurs readily. These viruses can survive up to 3 hours outside the body. For example, a susceptible person picks up the virus from a contaminated surface and then, when fingers rub the nose or eyes, transfers the virus to the nasal mucus membranes (a favorite nesting spot of the cold virus).
3. Shaking hands, opening a door, picking up a toy, and rubbing noses are more frequent infection routes than sneezing, coughing, and even kissing. It is probably easier to catch a cold by shaking hands than by kissing. Cold viruses are present in very low amounts in saliva. Studies of kissing couples (one with a cold, one without) found that kissing seldom led to inoculation.
4. "Catching" a cold occurs most probably by having contact with the hands of an infected person as well as objects that the infected person has touched.
5. To **avoid infection,** experts advise:
   - **a.** Keeping hands away from the eyes and nose
   - **b.** Washing hands frequently with soap and hot water
   - **c.** Washing contaminated objects
   - **d.** Using disposable tissues instead of a handkerchief
   - **e.** Covering a cough or a sneeze
6. Getting chilled or wet will not cause a cold. Viruses, not weather, cause colds. Studies have shown that people exposed to bone-chilling temperatures, icy baths, and drafts with or without wet feet or hair do not catch colds unless they are exposed to viruses. Colds are more common in winter because people (especially kids in school) spend more time indoors and thus are exposed to more viruses.
7. Several factors affecting susceptibility and transmission of viruses have been identified. **Poor nutritional state, fatigue,** and **emotional stress** are all associated with decreased resistance to viral infection.
8. Children's noses have been called "the chief reservoirs for infectious rhinoviruses." Preschoolers have the most colds (between six and ten per year), and young parents often catch the virus from their children.

D. Symptoms

1. The common cold is usually benign and self limiting. Typically cold symptoms begin slowly, 18–48 hours after exposure to a virus.
2. The first symptoms are usually a scratchy, sore throat followed by a runny nose, watery-itchy eyes, sneezing, and feeling of general fatigue. Patients note an increase in the secretions found in the nose, throat and bronchial tubes, and a cough may develop.
3. With time, the watery discharge is transformed to a thick, tenacious consistency. Generally, the most annoying and troublesome symptoms of the cold last approximately 4–5 days, with symptoms gradually diminishing and disappearing completely after 10 days or so.
4. There are five symptom areas where a pharmacist can recommend treatment: stuffy or runny nose, sore or scratchy throat, cough, headache, and a general feeling of malaise.

E. Treatment

1. **Decongestants**. **Nasal** decongestants are **sympathomimetic amines.** They stimulate the α-adrenergic receptors of vascular smooth muscle, which constrict dilated arterioles. Vessels that are located within the nasal mucosa become smaller and less engorged with blood. This decreases edema and, thus, increases nasal ventilation and drainage. Headache caused by congested sinuses may also be relieved. **Excessive nose blowing,** which irritates the nostrils and mucous membranes, is decreased with the use of decongestants. Too much nose blowing can further spread the virus and cause discomfort to the patient due to the possibility of pushing infected fluids into nasal sinuses or into the eustachian tubes. Decongestants may be applied to the nasal mucosa or taken orally.
   - **a. Topical decongestants**
     - **(1)** Topical decongestants induce prompt and profound vasoconstriction with relief of congestion.

(2) The major disadvantage for topical decongestants is the potential to develop a **rebound congestion** (rhinitis medicamentosa). Rebound congestion may be expected whenever topical decongestants are used longer than 3–5 days. This effect is more common with the short-acting agents [see II E 1 a (7)].
   (a) The **mechanism** for rebound congestion is not completely known. If the patient truly has a cold, a duration of 3–5 days for the use of topical decongestants is all that will usually be necessary.
   (b) **Treatment** of rebound congestion
      (i) The simplest but least comfortable therapy for rebound congestion is to completely withdraw the topical vasoconstrictor.
      (ii) As this action above promptly results in bilateral vasodilation with total nasal obstruction, a more acceptable method is to initially discontinue the medication in only one nostril. The patient can use as much medication as desired in the other side. When the rebound condition subsides in the drug-free nostril (normally 1–2 weeks), a total withdrawal from the other side is undertaken.
      (iii) An alternative approach is to D/C the topical decongestant and give a systemic decongestant.
      (iv) The patient can use saline drops or spray (i.e., Ocean, Ayr, NaSal). A saline product has the dual function of keeping the nasal mucosa moist while providing psychologic assistance to the individual. ("We're doing something for the nose.")

(3) These topical agents have varying durations of action. Selection of these agents can be administered in a convenient every 12-hour dosage form [e.g., oxymetazoline (Afrin)].

(4) These topical agents usually are not absorbed to any significant extent to cause problems with the patient who has high blood pressure. Because of the short duration of any blood pressure elevating effect, the short-acting agents should be used if a topical decongestant is needed in a hypertensive patient. Some of these products may not be used for young children (e.g., topical naphazoline has resulted in CNS depression in young children). (See note* below)

(5) These agents are similarly effective in equipotent doses with duration of action varying. The addition of aromatic vapors (e.g., menthol, camphor, eucalyptol) does not add any therapeutic benefit.

(6) Topical saline decongestants are recommended for children less than age 2 years and pregnant women (concern of possible harm to the fetus by sympathomimetic agents).

(7) These are the nasal decongestants approved by the FDA:
   (a) Ephedrine (topical) 0.5% (q 4–6h)—**not less than (NLT) age 6 years**
   (b) Naphazoline (topical) 0.025%–0.05% (Privine) (q 4–6h)—**NLT age 12 years**
   (c) Phenylephrine (topical) 0.125%–1%, (Neo-Synephrine, Nostril) (q 4–6h)
   (d) Propylhexedrine (inhaled) (Benzedrex) (q2h)—**NLT age 6 years**
   (e) 1-Desoxyephedrine (Inhaled) (Vicks Inhaler) (q 2h)—**NLT age 6 years**
   (f) Xylometazoline (topical) 0.05%–0.1% (Otrivin) (q 8–10h)
   (g) Oxymetazoline (topical) 0.025%–0.05% (Afrin Neo-Synephrine 12 Hour, Nostrilla) (q 12h)

(8) See Table 32-1 for patient counseling information.

b. Oral decongestants

(1) An oral decongestant may be useful in reaching deep into the **nasopharyngeal** and **sinus passages** where topical solutions may not be accessible. Because oral agents induce less intense vasoconstriction locally, they have not been associated with rebound congestion.

(2) Oral agents also may be favored for use in **small children** when topical application of a sympathomimetic amine may sometimes prove difficult.

(3) Because these agents are administered orally, potential systemic **side effects** may be more likely. CNS stimulation is the most common.

(4) Oral decongestants should be avoided (or used cautiously) in patients with problems such as heart disease, hypertension, diabetes, hyperthyroidism, benign prostatic hypertrophy, and narrow angle glaucoma. (Pseudoephedrine may have the least effect on blood pressure in the controlled hypertensive population.)

(5) Decongestants are contraindicated in patients taking MAO inhibitors.

Table 32-1. Patient Counseling Information on Nasal Decongestants

Drops	Spray (Atomizer)	Inhalers	Metered Dose Pump (Spray)
• Blow your nose. • Squeeze rubber bulb on dropper and withdraw medication from bottle. • Recline on a bed and hang head over the side (preferred) OR tilt head back while standing or sitting. • Place drops into each nostril and gently tilt the head from side to side to distribute the drug. • Keep head tilted back for several minutes after instilling the drops. • Rinse the dropper with hot water.	• Blow your nose. • Remove cap from spray container. • For best results, do not shake the squeeze bottle. • Administer one spray with head in upright position. • Sniff deeply while squeezing the bottle. • Wait 3–5 minutes and blow nose. • Administer another spray if necessary. • Rinse the spray tip with hot water taking care not to allow water to enter the bottle. • Replace cap.	• Blow your nose. • Warm inhaler in your hand to increase volatility of the medication. • Remove the protective cap. • Inhale medicated vapor in one nostril while closing off the other nostril, repeat in other nostril. • Wipe the inhaler clean after each use. • Replace cap immediately. • Note: Inhaler loses its potency after 2–3 months even though the aroma may linger.	• Blow your nose. • Remove the protective cap. • Prime the metered pump by depressing several times (for first use), pointing away from the face. • Hold the bottle with the thumb at the base and nozzle between first and second fingers. • Insert pump gently into the nose with the head upright. • Depress pump completely and sniff deeply. • Wait 3–5 minutes and then blow nose. • Administer another spray if necessary. • Rinse the spray tip with hot water taking care not to allow water to enter the bottle. • Replace cap.

(6) Oral decongestants include:
  (a) Phenylephrine 10 mg q 4h
  (b) Phenylpropanolamine 25 mg q 4h or 50 mg q 8h
  (c) Pseudoephedrine 60 mg q 6h (Sudafed)

(7) General **guidelines** for dosages for **children** regarding decongestants (Note: this also applies to antihistamines, guaifenesin, and antitussives.)
  (a) Ages 6–12 years—1/2 the adult dose
  (b) Ages 2–6 years—1/4 the adult dose
  (c) Under age 2 years—not specified

c. Nasal strips (e.g., Breathe Right). This is an adhesive bandage device that pulls open the nostrils and might relieve nasal congestion and decrease snoring. This device might be useful in persons who need to avoid the sympathomimetic agents (e.g., pregnant women).

2. Antihistamines

a. Overview. A common cold is an infection caused by a virus that results in the release of chemicals called **kinins.** Kinins cause inflammation in the lining of the nose. This inflammation results in sneezing, runny nose, and stuffiness.

b. Use. Although antihistamines have been prescribed by physicians for colds for decades (presumably because the symptoms are similar to those caused by allergies), scientific studies have conclusively demonstrated that these symptoms are **not** caused by **histamine.** Therefore, it is generally viewed that there is questionable rational for the use of antihistamines for the common cold (may rely on anticholinergic effect of these agents). The use of antihistamines to treat the common cold is **controversial.** Some studies show no effect, whereas others have shown a decrease in sneezing and nasal secretions with specific antihistamines (e.g., chlorpheniramine, doxylamine, clemastine). These studies' results should not be extrapolated to all of the available antihistamines.

c. Side effects

(1) Because of its anticholinergic properties, antihistamines may cause **dry mouth ("cotton mouth"), blurred vision, difficulty in urination, constipation, irritability,** and **dizziness** (see III B 1).

(2) Patients with narrow angle glaucoma and benign prostatic hypertrophy should avoid antihistamines because of the anticholinergic activities may exacerbate their condition.
(3) It has long been thought that asthma suffers should not take antihistamines because their anticholinergic properties would exacerbate asthma; however, the FDA recently found no evidence that the mucous drying action is harmful in asthmatic patients.
(4) Other side effects of antihistamines include nausea, vomiting, and GI upset. CNS stimulation rather than drowsiness may occur in children; therefore, caution should be noted in hyperactive children receiving antihistamines.
(5) The newer, **second generation antihistamines,** which are currently only available by prescription, have difficulty crossing the blood–brain barrier. Consequently, they tend to cause less unwanted CNS side effects.

d. Antihistamines are divided into several classes.
(1) **Alkylamines**
(a) Brompheniramine—4 mg q 4–6h (Dimetane)
(b) Dexbrompheniramine—6 mg q 12h (time release in Drixoral)
(c) Chlorpheniramine—4 mg q 4–6h (Chlor-Trimeton, Teldrin)
(d) Pheniramine—12.5–25 mg q 4–6h
(e) Triprolidine—2.5 mg q 6–8h (in Actifed)
(2) **Ethylenediamines**
(a) Pyrilamine—25–50 mg q 6–8h
(b) Thonzylamine—50–100 mg q 6–8h
(3) **Ethanolamines**
(a) Diphenhydramine—25–50 mg q 4–6h (Benylin, Nytol)
(b) Doxylamine—7.5 mg q 4–6h
(c) Clemastine—1.34 mg q 12h (in Tavist)
(4) **Piperidines** (e.g., Phenindamine—25 mg q 4–6h)

e. OTC antihistamines vary in the degree of drowsiness produced. All OTC antihistamines have sedative effects, but **ethanolamines** cause the **most sedation.** Among the most potent H1 antagonists is the chemical class of alkylamines, which include chlorpheniramine (Chlor-Trimeton) and brompheniramine (Dimetane). These agents have a lower incidence of drowsiness and may cause CNS stimulation (usually in children).

f. GI upset is more common with the ethylenediamines

3. Expectorants and antitussives. Cough is a physiologic protective reflex that assists in clearing the respiratory tract of mucus, inhaled irritants, and other foreign debris. Coughing from the common cold usually is caused by stimulation of cough receptors located within the **epithelial lining** of the **tracheobronchial tree.** The cough center in the **medulla** coordinates a series of events which leads to the cough response. A cough may be nonproductive or productive. **Nonproductive** coughs can be suppressed with **antitussives. Productive** coughs respond best to increased fluid intake and an OTC **expectorant.** Productive coughs generally should not be suppressed because they are essential to the removal of accumulated debris.

a. Antitussives
(1) Patients with dry, nonproductive coughs are candidates for therapeutic cough suppression. Such coughs, if persistent, bothersome, or sleep disrupting, may be suppressed with an antitussive.
(2) The nonproductive cough, if not treated, may become self-perpetuating as rapid air expulsion via the cough (up to 75 mph) may cause further irritation of the tracheal and pharyngeal mucosa.
(3) Antitussives inhibit or suppress coughing. Most act centrally to depress the medullary cough center and thus elevate the threshold for incoming cough impulses. Examples include **narcotics,** such as **codeine** and the nonnarcotic antitussive **dextromethorphan**.
(4) Antitussives may act peripherally on sensory nerve receptors within the respiratory tract. These agents are exemplified by the volatile agents such as **camphor** and **menthol** (e.g., Vicks Vaporub)
(5) **Demulcents,** such as hard candy or cough drops, soothe an irritated throat and bronchial passageway and may produce an antitussive action.
(6) Antitussives include:

(a) Codeine. Codeine and its salts are widely employed cough suppressants and the standard against which all other antitussives are measured. (Dose = 10–20 mg q 4–6h.)

(i) The potential for codeine **abuse** is negligible but has been observed.

(ii) Because codeine in this dosage form is schedule C-V, its OTC sale in cough syrups may be restricted in some states.

(iii) Adverse effects include drowsiness, lightheadedness, excitement, loss of appetite, nausea and vomiting, headache, abdominal discomfort, and constipation.

(iv) Children under 6 years of age are most vulnerable to serious adverse effects of codeine.

(v) Respiratory depression usually occurs with prescription analgesic doses of this drug. Respiratory arrest, coma, and death have been reported in the less than 6 years of age group following single doses of 5–12 mg/kg.

(b) Dextromethorphan. Dextromethorphan is a synthetic non-narcotic agent, having no analgesic or addictive properties. (Dose = 10–20 mg q 4h or 30 mg q 6–8h.)

(i) As a cough suppressant, it is as effective as codeine on a milligram-to-milligram basis.

(ii) Dextromethorphan may be indicated in persons for whom adverse effects of codeine are particularly bothersome.

(iii) Usual therapeutic doses do not cause a significant effect on either respiratory or cardiovascular functions.

(iv) Adverse effects include drowsiness, GI upset, nausea, and dizziness.

(c) Diphenhydramine. Diphenhydramine is an antihistamine and antitussive agent. Its antitussive effects are due to its central acting mechanism through the medullary cough center. (Dose = 25 mg q 4h.)

(i) Diphenhydramine **acts centrally** on the cough center similarly to codeine, rather than by generalized depression of the CNS.

(ii) Part of diphenhydramine's antitussive action may be mediated through **anticholinergic activity.**

(iii) As an ethanolamine antihistamine, this agent may produce **sedation** and symptoms of anticholinergic action (e.g., dry mouth, blurred vision).

(d) Camphor and menthol. A 4.7%–5.3% camphor and a 2.6%–2.8% menthol concentration in petrolatum (e.g., Vick's Vaporub) rubbed on the chest or neck effectively reduces coughing. Likewise, camphor and menthol used in a hot steam vaporizer at a concentration of 0.1% camphor or 0.05% menthol in water are safe and effective antitussives.

(i) Menthol, in doses of 5–10 mg in a lozenge (e.g., Hall's Mentho-Lyptus) or a compressed tablet dissolved in the mouth is safe and effective as an antitussive

(ii) These agents produce a sensation of coolness on the respiratory tract, presumably by stimulating cold sensory receptors. This engenders a **local anesthetic effect** on respiratory passageways, which produces an antitussive affect.

b. Expectorants

(1) Expectorants purportedly facilitate removal of mucus and other irritants from the respiratory tract. This supposedly produces formation of less tenacious secretions and/or decreases the viscosity of thickened secretions. Some clinicians believe that an expectorant action is best obtained by pushing fluids (i.e., 8–10 glasses of water per day).

(2) Their major pharmacologic action is to irritate receptors in the gastric mucosa. This promotes increased output from secretory glands of the GI system and reflexively increases flow of fluids from glands lining the respiratory tract. The outcome is increased volume and decreased viscosity of bronchial secretions.

(a) Guaifenesin (e.g., Robitussin)

(i) Guaifenesin is the only expectorant that has demonstrated safety and efficacy for self administration per the FDA. There is still controversy as to whether this agent is truly effective. (Dose = 200–400 mg q 4h.)

(ii) Guaifenesin occasionally causes gastric disturbance, nausea, and vomiting. Taking it with a full glass of water may reduce gastric irritation.

(iii) Because of the conflicting therapeutic endpoints, some clinicians question the rationale for combined use in the same product of an antitussive and an expectorant (e.g., Robitussin DM).

4. **Demulcents.** Demulcents are used to relieve dry or sore throat. Sucking on hard candy works by promoting salivary flow, which is soothing. Often, **lozenges** and **gargles** containing analgesics may help soothe a sore throat, though relief is only short term because the antiseptics and topical anesthetics found in these products are not powerful enough to fight off a virus. If demulcents or gargles do not relieve discomfort to a tolerable level, local **anesthetic sprays** (e.g., Chloraseptic) or lozenges such as benzocaine may be administered to provide short term comfort. These remedies should be given every 3–4 hours.

5. **Analgesics.** Early symptoms of the common cold include **mild malaise** and **headaches.** OTC products available to relieve these symptoms include aspirin, acetaminophen, ibuprofen, naproxen sodium, and ketoprofen.

6. **Combination products**
   a. It is best to treat a specific symptom that is causing the patient most difficulty, as opposed to recommending a "shotgun" product with a large number of ingredients that may not be necessary. Such a product may expose the patient to the possibility of side effects for medications that are not needed (e.g., Nyquil).
   b. There are a large number of combination cough and cold products on the market. Certain product name designations help to identify the ingredients (Table 32-2).
      (1) **"Night Time"** or **"PM"** usually signifies product contains **diphenhydramine.**
      (2) **"Sinus"** usually signifies a **decongestant** (pseudoephedrine) and/or an **analgesic** (acetaminophen)
      (3) **"Cough"** usually signifies that product contains **dextromethorphan.**
      (4) **"No Drowsiness"** on the label usually indicates that the product contains a **decongestant** (pseudoephedrine) and does not contain an antihistamine.

7. **Vitamin C and zinc.** Several controlled studies have failed to validate earlier reports that high-dose vitamin C and zinc lozenges are effective in preventing the common cold.

F. Patients with the following signs or symptoms should be referred for medical follow-up as these may indicate the presence of strep throat, bacterial pneumonia, or other more serious infections.

1. A **fever** greater than 101°F (38.3°C) accompanied by shaking chills, and coughing up thick phlegm (especially if greenish or foul smelling)
2. Sharp chest pain when taking a deep breath
3. Cold-like symptoms that do not improve after 7 days
4. Any fever greater than 103°F or 39.4°C
5. Coughing up blood
6. Any significant throat pain in a child
7. A painful throat in addition to any of the following:
   a. Pus (yellowish-white spots) on the tonsils or throat
   b. Fever greater than 101°F or 38.3°C
   c. Swollen or tender glands or bumps in the front of the neck
   d. Exposure to someone who has a documented case of strep throat
   e. A rash that appears during or after a sore throat
   f. A history of rheumatic fever, rheumatic heart disease, kidney disease, or chronic lung disease, such as emphysema or chronic bronchitis

III. ALLERGIC RHINITIS (Table 32-3)

A. **Introduction.** Approximately 20% of Americans suffer symptoms of allergic rhinitis, which can be seasonal or perennial. **Seasonal** outbreaks are cyclic and associated with pollination patterns of offending allergens. Although seasonal rhinitis is commonly called **"hay fever,"** the term is inappropriate. Hay is not a causative agent, and fever is not a symptom. **Perennial** rhinitis is

Table 32-2. Tylenol Products and Other Selected Combination Cough/Cold Products

Children's Tylenol	— Acetaminophen
Tylenol	— Acetaminophen
Tylenol Extra-Strength	— Acetaminophen
Tylenol Extended Relief	— Acetaminophen
Tylenol Headache Plus	— Acetaminophen, calcium carbonate
Tylenol Sinus	— Acetaminophen, pseudoephedrine
Tylenol Cough	— Acetaminophen, dextromethorphan
Tylenol Extra-Strength PM	— Acetaminophen, diphenhydramine
Children's Tylenol Cold	— Acetaminophen, pseudoephedrine, chlorpheniramine
Tylenol Allergy Sinus	— Acetaminophen, pseudoephedrine, chlorpheniramine
Tylenol Cold Effervescent	— Acetaminophen, phenylpropanolamine, chlorpheniramine
Tylenol Allergy Sinus NightTime	— Acetaminophen, pseudoephedrine, diphenhydramine
Tylenol Flu NightTime	— Acetaminophen, pseudoephedrine, diphenhydramine
Tylenol Cold NightTime	— Acetaminophen, pseudoephedrine, diphenhydramine
Tylenol Flu	— Acetaminophen, pseudoephedrine, dextromethorphan
Tylenol Cough with decongestant	— Acetaminophen, pseudoephedrine, dextromethorphan
Tylenol Cold No Drowsiness	— Acetaminophen, pseudoephedrine, dextromethorphan
Tylenol Cold & Flu No Drowsiness	— Acetaminophen, pseudoephedrine, dextromethorphan
Children's Tylenol Cold *MS* + cough	— Acetaminophen, pseudoephedrine, chlorpheniramine, dextromethorphan
Tylenol Cold & Flu Powder	— Acetaminophen, pseudoephedrine, chlorpheniramine, dextromethorphan
Multi-Symptom Tylenol Cold	— Acetaminophen, pseudoephedrine, chlorpheniramine, dextromethorphan
Advil Cold & Sinus	— Ibuprofen, pseudoephedrine
Alka-Seltzer Plus Cold & Cough	— Aspirin, phenylpropanolamine, chlorpheniramine, dextromethorphan
Thera Flu—Flu & Cold	— Acetaminophen, pseudoephedrine, chlorpheniramine
Thera Flu—Flu, Cold, & Cough	— Acetaminophen, pseudoephedrine, chlorpheniramine, dextromethorphan
Sudafed Cold & Cough	— Pseudoephedrine, acetaminophen, dextromethorphan, guaifenesin
Actifed Plus *Sev.* Cold & Sinus	— Pseudoephedrine, triprolidine, acetaminophen
Motrin IB Sinus	— Ibuprofen, pseudoephedrine

MS = Multi-Symptom; *Sev.* = Severe

chronic and is caused by antigens such as house dust or animal protein that are not linked to the changing seasons.

1. There are **three separate allergy seasons.**
   a. Spring (trees)
   b. Late spring-early summer (grasses)
   c. Late summer to the first killing frost (weeds, most commonly **ragweed**)
2. **Symptoms** include sneezing episodes, nasal pruritus with congestion, clear rhinorrhea, itching of the palate, conjunctival erythema and itching, and ear fullness with popping and pressure on the cheeks and forehead. Constitutional feelings of weakness, malaise, and fatigue may also be seen.
   a. Symptoms are similar and overlap with those of the common cold. For this reason consumers often refer to allergic rhinitis as a **"summer cold."**

Table 32-3. How Do the Common Cold and Allergic Rhinitis Differ?

Sign	Common Cold	Allergic Rhinitis
Sneezing	Occurs	Common
Nasal discharge	Mucopurulent; occurs especially during days 1–3	Watery; common, occurs anytime
Itchy nose and eyes	Occurs	Common
Watering and redness of eyes	Common	Common
Nasal congestion	Common	Common
Cough	Common, especially in later phase	Uncommon
Fever	Rare	Absent
Pruritus	Uncommon	Common
Inciting cause	Virus	Allergen
Occurrence	Anytime	Seasonal (seasonal type); anytime (perennial type)

b. The symptoms associated with allergic rhinitis are due to an **immunoglobulin E** (IgE)-mediated immunologic reaction.

3. Pathophysiology

a. Released from its storage sites in response to its allergen challenge, histamine binds with and activates specific receptors on cell membranes. There are at least two types of receptors. Histamine-1 (H1) receptors are associated with vascular dilation, edema, and the inflammatory process and are the cause of the allergic response and symptoms.

b. Other physiologic substances involved in the allergic response are also released along with the histamine from the mast cells and basophils. These include serotonin, heparin, eosinophil and neutrophil chemotactic factors, leukotrienes, and various proteolytic enzymes.

B. Treatment. The best treatment for allergic rhinitis although not always practical, is to avoid the allergen or allergens that trigger the allergic symptoms. For example, if a patient is allergic to ragweed, counsel him/her to stay in an air conditioned environment as much as possible. Air conditioning, with frequent filter changes, helps reduce the pollen count in the room. If the patient is allergic to dust mites, removing rugs, furniture, or mattresses that harbor dust mites is helpful. Incasing items such as mattresses in an air tight plastic can also decrease mites.

1. Antihistamines

a. The **primary nonprescription medication** used to treat allergic rhinitis is an oral antihistamine. Antihistamines cause competitive blockade of the actions of histamine at receptor sites.

b. If possible, antihistamine therapy should be started 1–2 weeks before a known allergy season or several hours before exposure to a known allergen. Regular, rather than PRN, dosing of antihistamines is more effective.

c. These drugs stimulate their own metabolism, so tolerance with reduced therapeutic response may follow continued administration.

d. Whereas there are variations in potency, duration of action, and extent of adverse effects, there are no major therapeutic differences in the various OTC antihistamines.

e. Drowsiness is common to all OTC antihistamines and the most troublesome to allergy suffers. Drowsiness is often transient and tolerance to this effect may occur after 5–7 days of therapy.

f. Antihistamines should be taken uninterrupted throughout the pollen season. To be effective, they must combine with the specific histamine receptor and block histamine binding. This is a dynamic competition between the antihistamine and histamine.

g. Antihistamines are useful for treating the sneezing, rhinorrhea, pruritus, lacrimation, and irritated itchy eyes. They do not work to correct nasal congestion.

h. The **first generation** (mostly the OTC antihistamines) and **second generation** [e.g., prescription products such as terfenadine (Seldane)] antihistamines are roughly of equal efficacy in their ability to relieve symptoms of histamine release.

i. Because the peripheral H1 histamine blockade may last longer than the presence of the antihistamine in the serum, these agents may not have to be dosed as frequently to get the desired effect.

2. **Decongestants**
   a. Antihistamines are less effective in reversing nasal and ocular congestion. Decongestants counter congestion and help reverse drowsiness associated with antihistamines.
   b. Systemic decongestants are preferred when a decongestant action is required for longer than 3–5 days, because of the rebound congestion that occurs with topical decongestants.
   c. If the patient does not respond adequately to antihistamines alone, the next step would be to add an oral decongestant.

3. **Prescription treatment**
   a. **Cromolyn sodium**
      (1) The proposed mechanism of action is stabilization of mast cells, interfering with calcium transport and induction of degranulation.
      (2) This agent is effective in treating seasonal and perennial allergic rhinitis in some patients.
      (3) To be maximumly effective, cromolyn sodium (Nasalcrom) must be started 2–4 weeks before the exposure of the offending allergens and continued throughout the contact period.
      (4) Dosed 4–6 times per day in each nostril initially, administration frequency may be decreased when the symptoms are under control.
      (5) To be effective, it must be used on a regular basis.
   b. **Corticosteroids**
      (1) Intranasal steroids have emerged as the most effective treatment of allergic rhinitis, relieving sneezing, nasal pruritus, congestion, and rhinorrhea associated with the inflammation.
      (2) Intranasal steroids are ineffective in the treatment of ocular tearing or ocular pruritus.
      (3) Symptom relief is thought to be related to the ability of steroids to inhibit the activity of multiple cell types (e.g., mast cells, basophils, eosinophils, neutrophils, macrophages, lymphocytes) and mediators of the inflammatory response.
      (4) Decreased capillary permeability and decreased nasal mucus secretion also contribute to the effectiveness achieved by intranasal steroids.
      (5) The more recently developed formulations of beclomethasone (Vancenase, Beconase), budesonide (Rhinocort), flunisolide (Nasalide), fluticasone (Flonase), and triamcinolone (Nasacort) avoid the adrenal suppression at recommended doses.
      (6) Major **adverse effects** of intranasal steroids are local dryness or irritation as evidenced by stinging, irritation, nose bleeds, sore throat, or burning and irritation.
      (7) It may take up to 3 weeks for the peak effects of clinical improvement to occur.
      (8) Treatment with these medications should start at the first signs of clinical symptoms and is usually continued throughout the allergen season.
   c. **Immunotherapy**
      (1) Immunotherapy is usually begun only when the patient does not show a response to environmental modification and pharmacotherapy or cannot tolerate the medications.
      (2) Routine injections of the diluted antigen are administered initially, with the concentration of the antigen increasing over time.
      (3) Although the precise mechanism is not known, serum IgE levels specific to the antigens given tend to decrease during the course of immunotherapy. Conversely, there is an increase in serum IgG levels. A blocking antibody is thought to compete with mast cell-bound IgE for antigen binding.
      (4) Because of the **time** and the **expense** involved, immunotherapy is usually reserved for moderate to **severe cases** of chronic allergic rhinitis.

STUDY QUESTIONS

Directions: Each of the numbered items or incomplete statements in this section is followed by answers or by completions of the statement. Select the **one** lettered answer or completion that is **best** in each case.

1. Which statement concerning the use of OTC analgesic agents is true?

(A) Aspirin is indicated for mild to moderate analgesia, inflammatory diseases, antipyresis, and prophylaxis for patients with ischemic heart disease
(B) Ibuprofen is indicated for mild to moderate analgesia, reduction of fever, and prophylaxis for patients with ischemic heart disease, but not for inflammatory disorders
(C) Acetaminophen is indicated for mild to moderated analgesia but not for reduction of fever and arthritis
(D) Naproxen sodium is indicated for mild to moderate analgesia, antipyresis, and prophylaxis for patients with ischemic heart disease

2. Which statement concerning drug interactions with OTC analgesic agents is true?

(A) Aspirin potentiates the effects of antihypertensives, cardiac glycosides, and anticoagulants
(B) Ibuprofen potentiates the effect of zidovudine, hypoglycemics, and aminoglycosides
(C) Acetaminophen potentiates the effect of zidovudine
(D) For naproxen sodium, the OTC dosage recommendations are similar to the prescription dosage

3. All of the following statements concerning contraindications with **chronic** use of OTC analgesic agents are correct EXCEPT

(A) aspirin, ibuprofen, naproxen sodium, and ketoprofen are contraindicated in patients with bleeding disorders, peptic ulcer, and the third trimester of pregnancy
(B) aspirin, acetaminophen, and ibuprofen are implicated in Reye's syndrome
(C) acetaminophen is contraindicated in patients with active alcoholism, hepatic disease, or viral hepatitis

4. Which statement concerning dosage recommendations for OTC analgesic agents is true?

(A) Aspirin for analgesia or antipyresis in adults is 325–650 mg every 4 hours or 650–1000 mg every 6 hours, with a maximum daily dose of 4000 mg for no longer than 10 days for pain and 3 days for fever, without consulting a physician; the antirheumatic dosage for adults is 3600–4500 mg daily in divided doses; and patients with ischemic heart disease take 325 mg daily or every other day
(B) Ibuprofen for analgesia or antipyresis in adults is 300–600 mg every 6–8 hours, with a maximum daily dose of 1800 mg for no longer than 10 days for pain and 3 days for fever, without consulting a physician; and the anti-inflammatory dosage for adults is 1800–3600 mg daily in divided doses
(C) Acetaminophen for analgesia or antipyresis in adults is 325 mg every 8–12 hours, with a maximum daily dose of 2000 mg for no longer than 10 days for pain and 3 days for fever, without consulting a physician; and patients with ischemic heart disease take 325 mg daily or every other day

5. A 57-year-old male with hypertension has a dry, irritating, nonproductive cough due to a "cold." He is feeling better on the fifth day of having common cold symptoms, and the cough is the only current problem. Of the following choices, the best recommendation for this patient would be

(A) a product that contains pseudoephedrine and chlorpheniramine
(B) a product that preferably contains only guaifenesin
(C) a product that contains dextromethorphan to be given at bedtime
(D) Nyquil (dextromethorphan, acetaminophen, doxylamine, pseudoephedrine)
(E) Sudafed (pseudoephedrine) long-acting tablets to be taken twice daily

6. A 32-year-old woman with perennial allergic rhinitis asks a pharmacist's advice for the treatment of her symptoms. She has never used any product for this condition and informs the pharmacist that she is hyperthyroid. Which of the following medicines would be the best recommendation?

(A) Sudafed 30 mg tablets—usual dose and frequency per directions on package
(B) Afrin nasal spray—two sprays in each nostril bid
(C) Drixoral tablets (pseudoephedrine and dexbrompheniramine)—per directions on the package
(D) Chlor-Trimeton 12 mg sustained action tablets—one tablet p.o. q 12 hr
(E) Neo-synephrine nasal spray—two sprays q 6 hr

7. A patient with seasonal allergic rhinitis comes into a pharmacy and asks the pharmacist to recommend a product for him. He has been taking Chlor-Trimeton 12 mg tablets bid with some significant relief, but he is still complaining of some nasal congestion. What would be the best recommendation for this patient?

(A) Switch to another antihistamine
(B) Afrin nasal spray—2 sprays in each nostril bid for 10 days
(C) Neo-Synephrine nasal spray—2 sprays in each nostril q 4 h until congestion goes away
(D) Recommend a product like Drixoral (pseudoephedrine & dexbrompheniramine) tablets: take as directed on the label
(E) Ocean nasal spray as required for nasal stuffiness

8. All of the following statements regarding the common cold are true EXCEPT

(A) about 75% of common colds are caused by rhinoviruses
(B) histamine is not involved in the inflammation associated with the common cold
(C) there is no vaccine available to prevent the common cold because there are so many viral strains involved in causing this condition
(D) when you are infected with a particular cold virus strain, lifetime or long-term immunity develops to that specific virus
(E) the incidence of colds is highest in children, followed next by mothers of young children

9. All of the following statements about topical nasal decongestants are true EXCEPT

(A) the menthol present in some of these products results in an antitussive action in addition to the decongestant effect
(B) the metered dose pump dosage form prevents "back flow" of nasal secretions that may occur with the atomizer spray dosage form
(C) after it is opened, the inhaler dosage form loses its potency after 2–3 months
(D) ideally, one should restrict the use of a topical decongestant spray to one individual in the family to prevent spread of the cold virus from person to person
(E) a second administration of the nasal decongestant metered dose pump can be given about 3–5 minutes after the first dose—the patient should blow his/her nose prior to this second administration

10. All of the following statements regarding Breathe-Right nasal strips are true EXCEPT they

(A) might relieve nasal congestion
(B) might decrease snoring
(C) might be useful for pregnant women where there is concern about the use of sympathomimetic decongestants
(D) have been proven to increase athletic performance
(E) look like a Band-aid that is worn across the nose

11. All of the following measures would be useful in preventing the spread of the cold virus EXCEPT

(A) cover a cough or sneeze
(B) keep hands away from your eyes and nose
(C) make sure that person with a cold is kept warm
(D) use disposable tissues rather than a cloth handkerchief
(E) wash hands frequently with soap and water

ANSWERS AND EXPLANATIONS

1. The answer is A *[I B].*
Aspirin is the only analgesic agent with an approved labeling for analgesia, antipyresis, inflammation, and prophylaxis for ischemic heart disease.

2. The answer is C *[I C].*
Acetaminophen may competitively inhibit the metabolism of zidovudine, resulting in potentiation of zidovudine or acetaminophen toxicity. As for the other choices, OTC dosage levels are generally one-half the prescription dosage; aspirin is not commonly recognized to interact with antihypertensives or cardiac glycosides; nor is acetaminophen expected to interact with aminoglycosides.

3. The answer is B *[I B 4 b].*
Aspirin is the only analgesic agent associated with the development of Reye's syndrome.

4. The answer is A *[I B 3, C 3, D 3].*
The aspirin dosage OTC recommendations are correct, the levels for acetaminophen are too low, and for ibuprofen too high. In addition, acetaminophen does not carry an ischemic heart disease prophylaxis recommendation.

5. The answer is C *[II E 3 a].*
It appears that this patient's cold is resolving. The only bothersome symptom is a nonproductive cough. An antitussive should be given at bedtime to permit the patient to get some sleep. A product containing the safe and effective dextromethorphan is indicated. The patient has hypertension and usually should not take an oral decongestant. A single ingredient product aimed at the specific symptom is best.

6. The answer is D *[III A, B].*
The patient should try to identify the cause of her allergic rhinitis and avoid the allergen if possible. Perennial allergic rhinitis is caused by things like animal dander and house dust mites. Keeping a pet outdoors, encasing pillows, etc. might be useful. Pharmacologic treatment is usually begun with an antihistamine. The patient does not have any contraindications to this agent. Oral decongestants should usually be avoided when hyperthyroidism is present. Because of rebound congestion, topical agents are not indicated for long term use in allergic rhinitis.

7. The answer is D *[III B 1, 2].*
The first line of pharmacologic therapy is the antihistamines. These agents will correct most of the symptoms, but may not completely alleviate the symptoms of nasal congestion. The addition of an oral decongestant would be the next therapeutic intervention. Tolerance to the therapeutic benefit may develop to the antihistamines with continued use, but in this patient significant relief has been obtained; only the congestion remains. Topical decongestants can only be used for a few days, so they have limited value in allergic rhinitis.

8. The answer is A *[II B].*
Approximately 30%–35% of colds are caused by rhinoviruses. Histamine is not believed to be a chemical mediator that is released in response to viral invasion. There are up to 200 different viral strains that have been identified as causing the common cold; it is, therefore, virtually impossible to develop a vaccine that would be able to cover such as large spectrum of viruses. Immunity (oftentimes, lifetime) does develop to the specific strain that infects a person. And colds are most common in children because they have not had time to develop immunity to many of these agents. Women in their twenties and thirties are the next most commonly infected group because many of these women are mothers of the children who become infected with the cold virus and then end up having the virus transmitted to them.

9. The answer is A *[II E 3 a (6) (d)].*
In the appropriate concentration as a lozenge, compressed tablet, or topical ointment, menthol is an effective antitussive. Small amounts of aromatic vapors (i.e., menthol, camphor, eucalyptol) do not add any therapeutic benefit to the topical sympathomimetic decongestants. The metered dose pump dosage form does prevent "back flow" of nasal secretions. The inhaler dosage form does lose its potency after 2–3 months after it is opened and it is appropriate to administer a second dose of decongestant after 3–5 minutes and after blowing the nose to insure the appropriate spread of the medication into the nasal passages.

10. The answer is D *[II E 1 c].*
Nasal strips have been used by professional athletes with the thought that this might improve athletic performance because the nostrils are more "open" and, therefore, able to take in more oxygen. There is no proof of this, however. The FDA approved use of this agent for nasal congestion and snoring. It may be especially useful in patients who should not use topical or oral sympathomimetic amines (i.e., the pregnant patient).

11. The answer is C *[II C].*
The most likely route of transmission of the cold virus from one patient to the next is via nasal secretions from the infected person to the hands of the noninfected person who then puts their fingers in the eye or nose. The virus is also spread via sneezing and coughing. Efforts should, therefore, be directed towards measures to break these transmission pathways. Covering a cough or sneeze, washing the hands frequently, using disposable tissues versus a handkerchief, and keeping one's fingers away from the eyes or nose are all appropriate methods to decrease transmission. Patients do not "catch a cold" simply by being exposed to a chilly or drafty environment; the cold virus must be present. Thus, keeping a patient warm has no bearing on the transmission of the common cold.

33
OTC Agents for Constipation, Diarrhea, Hemorrhoids, and Heartburn

Stephen H. Fuller
Larry N. Swanson
Julianne B. Pinson

I. CONSTIPATION

A. General information

1. **Definition.** Constipation is the difficult or infrequent passage of stool. Normal stool frequency ranges from two to three times daily to two to three times per week. Patients may experience abdominal bloating, headaches, or a sense of rectal fullness from incomplete evacuation of feces.

2. **Causes.** Constipation can be caused by many factors, including:
   a. **Insufficient dietary fiber**
   b. **Lack of exercise**
   c. **Poor bowel habits,** such as failure to respond to the defecatory urge or hurried bowels (i.e., incomplete evacuation)
   d. **Medications,** such as narcotics, antacids, or anticholinergics (e.g., antidepressants, antihypertensives, antihistamines, phenothiazines, antispasmodics)
   e. **Organic problems,** such as intestinal obstruction, tumor, inflammatory bowel disease, diverticulitis, hypothyroidism, or hyperglycemia

3. **Practitioners should question the patient about the following:**
   a. Normal stool frequency
   b. Duration of the constipation
   c. Frequency of constipation episodes
   d. Exercise routine
   e. Amount of dietary fiber consumed
   f. Presence of other symptoms
   g. Medications used currently
   h. Medications used to relieve constipation and their effectiveness

B. Treatment

1. **Nonpharmacologic**
   a. Increase intake of fluids and fiber (e.g., cereals, green vegetables, fruit, potatoes)
   b. Increase exercise to increase and maintain bowel tone
   c. Bowel training to increase regularity

2. **Pharmacologic.** Therapeutic agents are classified according to their mechanism of action. Laxatives should not be taken if nausea, vomiting, or abdominal pain is present.
   a. **Bulk-forming laxatives.** These medications are natural or synthetic polysaccharide derivatives that adsorb water to soften the stool and increase bulk, which stimulates peristalsis. Bulk-forming laxatives work in both the small and large intestines. The onset of action of these agents is slow (12–24 hours and up to 72 hours), which is why they are best used to prevent constipation rather than to treat severe acute constipation. There are both natural and synthetic products. All bulk-forming agents must be given with at least 8 ounces of water to minimize the possible constipation experienced by some patients. Some bulk-forming medications may contain sugar, so diabetics should use sugar-free products. Bulk-forming agents should not be used if patients have an obstructing bowel lesion, intestinal strictures, or Crohn's disease because they can make this situation worse and possibly result in bowel perforation.
      (1) **Natural bulk-forming laxatives**

(a) **Psyllium** (e.g., Metamucil, Konsyl, Fiberall Natural). An **adult dosage** is 3.5–7 g one to three times per day. A **child's dosage** is half the adult dosage one to three times per day.

(b) **Malt soup extract** (e.g., Maltsupex). An **adult dosage** is 16 g two to four times per day. A **child's dosage** is 16 g one to two times per day.

(2) **Synthetic bulk-forming laxatives**

(a) **Methylcellulose** (e.g., Citrucel). An **adult dosage** is 1–2 g one to three times per day. A **child's dosage** is 0.5 g one to three times per day.

(b) **Polycarbophil** (e.g., Konsyl Fiber, Fiber Con, Fiberall). An **adult dosage** is 1 g one to four times per day. A **child's dosage** is 0.5 g one to three times per day. Calcium polycarbophil may impair the absorption of tetracyclines if the drugs are taken concurrently.

b. **Saline** and **osmotic laxatives** work by creating an osmotic gradient to pull water into the small and large intestine. This increased volume results in distention of the intestinal lumen, causing increased peristalsis and bowel motility. These laxatives also increase the activity of cholecystokinin-pancreozymin, which is an enzyme that increases the secretion of fluids into the gastrointestinal (GI) tract. The **onset of action varies** depending upon the ingredient and dosage form. Rectal formulations (e.g., enemas, suppositories) have an onset of action of 5–30 minutes, whereas oral preparations work within 4 hours.

(1) **Saline laxatives** include sodium and magnesium salts. As much as 20% of magnesium may be absorbed from these products, which may lead to hypermagnesemia in patients with preexisting renal impairment. Patients with hypertension or congestive heart failure should not receive saline laxatives on a prolonged basis due to fluid retention from sodium absorption. Products include:

(a) **Magnesium citrate or** citrate of magnesia

(b) **Magnesium hydroxide** (e.g., Phillips' Milk of Magnesia)

(c) **Magnesium sulfate** or Epsom salt

(d) **Sodium phosphate** (e.g., Fleet Phospho-Soda)

(2) **Osmotic laxatives**

(a) **Glycerin** is available in rectal products in suppository or liquid form (e.g., Fleet Babylax). Rectal burning may occur with glycerin products. In addition to the osmotic effect, sodium stearate in these products can produce a local irritant effect. An **adult dose** is 3 g in suppository form or 5–15 ml as an enema. A **child's dose** is 1.5 g in suppository form or 2–5 ml as an enema.

(b) **Lactulose** (e.g., Chronulac) is available only by prescription and is used to decrease blood ammonia levels in hepatic encephalopathy. It may cause flatulence and cramping and should be taken with fruit juice, water, or milk to increase the palatability. An **adult dosage** is 15–30 ml two to three times daily. A **child's dosage** is 2.5–5 ml two to three times daily.

(c) **Sorbitol,** a nonabsorbable sugar, is similar in efficacy to lactulose, which can be administered orally (70% solution) or rectally (25% solution). The **adverse effects** are the same and include flatulence, cramping, and abdominal pain over the first few days. An **adult dose** is 15 ml orally (70% solution) or 120 ml rectally (25% solution). A **child's dose** is 15 ml orally (70% solution) or 30–60 ml of a rectal solution (25%).

c. **Stimulant laxatives.** These medications work in the small and large intestine to stimulate bowel motility and increase the secretion of fluids into the bowel. All stimulant laxatives can cause abdominal cramping. Also, chronic use of stimulant laxatives can lead to **cathartic colon,** which results in a poorly functioning colon and resembles the symptoms of ulcerative colitis. However, most cases of cathartic colon were published before 1960 when more toxic ingredients (e.g., podophyllin) were used in laxative products. The oral preparations usually have an onset of action within 6–10 hours. Rectal preparations usually have an onset of action within 30–60 minutes.

(1) **Anthraquinone laxatives** include senna, cascara sagrada, and casanthranol. **Melanosis coli,** which is a dark pigmentation of the colonic mucosa, can result with long-term use of anthraquinone laxatives. This usually disappears 6–12 months after discontinuing the medication. In addition, there is no indication that melanosis results in adverse consequences. Discoloration (pink/red, yellow, or brown) of the urine may occur. Cascara sagrada is excreted into breast milk. Anthraquinone products include:

(a) **Senna** (e.g., Senokot, Fletcher's Castoria) is considered to be more potent than cascara products; however, senna causes more abdominal cramping.
(i) An **adult dosage** is 300–1200 mg/day.
(ii) A **child's dosage** is 100–600 mg/day.
(b) **Cascara sagrada.** Liquid preparations of cascara are more reliable than solid dosage forms. An **adult dosage** is 300–1000 mg/day.
(c) **Casanthranol** is considered to be a mild stimulant laxative and is present in Peri-Colace, which also contains docusate.
(2) **Diphenylmethane derivatives** include the following:
(a) **Phenolphthalein** preparations (e.g., Ex-Lax, Feen-a-mint, Modane) have caused allergic reactions in some patients (e.g., a rash of pink-purple eruptions, itching, burning), which necessitates discontinuation of phenolphthalein products. An **adult dosage** is 60–200 mg/day. Alkaline urine may be discolored pink/red, red/violet, or red/brown.
(b) **Bisacodyl** (e.g., Dulcolax). The tablet formulations of bisacodyl are enteric coated, so they should not be crushed or chewed. Also, bisacodyl-containing products should not be taken within 1 hour of ingesting antacids or milk.
(3) **Castor oil** (e.g., Purge) has an onset of action within 2–6 hours. Castor oil works primarily at the small intestine, which can result in strong cathartic effects (e.g., excessive fluid and electrolyte loss). These cathartic effects can lead to dehydration. Castor oil should not be used in pregnant patients because it may induce premature labor. An **adult dose** is 15 to 60 ml; a **child's dose** is 5–15 ml.

d. **Emollient laxatives** act as surfactants by allowing absorption of water into the stool, which makes the softened stool easier to pass. These medications are particularly useful in patients who must avoid straining to pass hard stools, such as those who recently had a myocardial infarction or rectal surgery. However, clinical trials evaluating emollient "stool-softening" laxatives show that these products, when compared to placebo, do not affect the weight or water content of the stool or the frequency of stool passing.
(1) **Onset of action.** Emollient laxatives have a slow onset of action (24–72 hours), which is why they are not considered the drug of choice for severe acute constipation, and they are more useful for preventing constipation.
(2) **Products.** Emollient laxatives are salts of the surfactant **docusate.** These products contain insignificant amounts of calcium, sodium, or potassium, and there are no specific guidelines for the selection of any one product. The products include:
(a) **Docusate sodium** (e.g., Colace, Doxinate)
(b) **Docusate calcium** (e.g., Surfak)
(c) **Docusate potassium** (e.g., Dialose)
(3) **Dosage information.** The **adult dosage** is 100–300 mg per day. A **child's dosage** is 50–150 mg per day. Each dose must be taken with at least 8 ounces of water. Liquid preparations should be taken in fruit juice or infant formula to increase palatability. Docusate products may facilitate the systemic absorption of mineral oil, so these agents should not be used concurrently.

e. **Lubricant laxative (mineral oil).** Mineral oil works at the colon to increase water retention in the stool to soften the stool. It has an **onset of action** of 6–8 hours
(1) **Dosage information.** An **adult dosage** is 15–45 ml per day. A **child's dosage** is 10–15 ml per day.
(2) **Warnings**
(a) Mineral oil can **decrease absorption of fat-soluble vitamins** (i.e., vitamins A, D, E, K), so it should not be used on a chronic basis.
(b) Elderly, young, debilitated, and dysphagic patients are at the greatest risk of **lipid pneumonitis** from mineral oil aspiration.
(c) Emollients (e.g., docusate) may increase the systemic absorption of mineral oil, which can lead to **hepatotoxicity.**
(d) Mineral oil products may cause anal seepage, which results in itching (i.e., pruritus ani) and perianal discomfort.
(e) Mineral oil should be taken on an empty stomach.

C. Special patient issues

1. **Pediatric patients.** The bowel patterns of pediatric patients varies. During the first weeks of life, infants pass approximately four stools per day. As children get older, approximately 1–3

stools are passed per day. Constipation should be expected if there is a drastic change from a child's baseline bowel function.

   a. **Nonpharmacologic methods,** such as increasing the amount of fluid or sugar in a child's formula in younger children or increasing the bulk content of the child's diet (fruit, fiber cereals, vegetables), should be tried before the use of medications.
   b. **If nonpharmacologic methods do not work,** rectal stimulation may be useful. Pharmacologic agents that can be used for acute relief include glycerin suppositories and magnesium laxatives. Stimulant laxatives should be administered as a last resort, but enemas should not be used in children less than 2 years of age and with extreme caution in children between 2 and 5 years of age (see I C 4). Bulk-forming agents and stool softeners can be used if the constipation does not need immediate relief.

2. **Pregnant patients.** Constipation in pregnancy is common and is often due to compression of the colon by the enlarged uterus. Pregnant patients should avoid any preparation that may be absorbed systemically (e.g., stimulant laxatives), any preparation that can interfere with vitamin absorption (e.g., mineral oil), or any preparation that can induce premature labor (e.g., castor oil). Pregnant patients should use bulk-forming agents or stool softeners.

3. **Geriatric patients** tend to be at risk for constipation due to insufficient dietary (fiber) and fluid ingestion, failure to establish a regular bowel time habit, and abuse of stimulant laxatives resulting in a loss of smooth muscle tone in the bowel promoting constipation (see I C 5). These causes should be investigated in addition to primary disease states (e.g., hypothyroidism) and medications (opiates, anticholinergics) that may lead to constipation in elderly patients.
   a. **Contraindications.** A major concern with geriatric patients is the possible loss of fluid that can be induced by aggressive laxative treatment (e.g., enemas and high-dose saline laxatives). Geriatric patients should not use stimulant laxatives on a chronic basis, and patients with renal impairment should not use magnesium products.
   b. **Treatment of acute constipation** can include glycerin suppositories with bulk-forming agents and Metulese (available by prescription) used on a chronic basis.

4. **Use of enemas.** Enemas are useful for evacuation of the bowel before surgery, child birth, and for the treatment of acute constipation that has not responded to other medications (e.g., bisacodyl suppositories). An enema is the dosage route with the enema fluid determining the mechanism of evacuation (stimulant, osmotic). When administered correctly, an enema evacuates only the distal colon similar to a normal bowel movement. This is accomplished by having the patient lie on his/her side with the knees tucked toward the chest. While in this position, one pint (500 ml) of enema solution should be slowly squeezed into the rectum. This should be retained up to 1 hour or until definite lower abdominal cramping is felt. At this point the bowel movement is ready for expulsion. Although all enemas cause abdominal cramping, some may have more serious **adverse effects** than others. Soap sud enemas can cause much rectal irritation and have been reported to cause anaphylaxis and rectal gangrene. The popular sodium phosphate enemas (e.g., Fleet) are very effective but have resulted in hyperphosphatemia, hypocalcemia(tetany), hypokalemia, metabolic acidosis, and cardiac death usually due to conduction abnormalities in very small children. This has mainly occurred in children less than 2 years of age or between 2 and 5 years of age with predisposing factors. These factors include chronic renal disease, anorectal malformations, and/or Hirschprung's disease, which allow phosphate blood concentrations to become abnormally high and potassium and calcium to become low predisposing these patients to cardiac arrhythmias and potentially death. Therefore, the use of enemas is highly discouraged in children under 5 years of age.

5. **Laxative abuse** is a term to describe the routine, chronic use of laxatives on a daily basis (e.g., elderly patients) to the administration of high doses several times daily by patients with anorexia nervosa or bulimia for weight control. Excessive use of laxatives can lead to excessive diarrhea and vomiting resulting in fluid and electrolyte abnormalities. In addition to the risks to patients from hypokalemia (metabolic alkalosis, cardiac conduction problems), patients can also develop osteomalacia, liver disease, and cathartic colon. Cathartic colon results from superficial ulcerations in the colon as well as damage to the muscularis mucosa and submucosa. This results in a loss of tone of the smooth and striated muscle and causes poor bowel function.

II. DIARRHEA. Diarrhea is an abnormal increase in the frequency and looseness of stools. The overall weight and volume of the stool is increased (more than 200 g or ml/day), and the water content is increased to 60%–90%. In general, diarrhea results when some factor impairs the ability of the intestine to absorb water from the stool, which causes excess water in the stool. **Antidiarrheals** may serve to prevent an attack of diarrhea or to relieve existing symptoms.

A. Classification. Diarrhea can be classified based on mechanisms or etiology.

1. **Classification by mechanism**
   a. **Osmotic diarrhea** occurs when a nonabsorbable solute pulls excess water into the intestinal tract.
      (1) Ingestion of large meals or certain osmotic substances (e.g., sorbitol, glycerin) can lead to diarrhea.
      (2) Disaccharidase deficiency, which is a lack of enzymes needed to break down disaccharides in the gut for absorption (e.g., lactase deficiency), results in an increase in osmotic sugars (i.e., lactose, sucrose) in the intestinal tract.
      (3) Medications that can induce osmotic diarrhea include lactulose and magnesium-containing antacids and laxatives.
   b. **Secretory diarrhea** occurs when the intestinal wall is damaged, resulting in an increased secretion rather than absorption of electrolytes into the intestinal tract. Common sources include:
      (1) **Bacterial endotoxins** (e.g., *Escherichia coli, Vibrio cholerae, Shigella, Staphylococcus aureus*)
      (2) **Bacterial infections** (e.g., *Shigella, Salmonella*)
      (3) **Viral infections** (e.g., rotavirus, Norwalk virus)
      (4) **Protozoal infections** (e.g., *Giardia lamblia, Entamoeba histolytica*)
      (5) **Miscellaneous causes**—inflammatory bowel disease and medications (e.g., prostaglandins, antibiotics, colchicine, chemotherapeutic agents)
   c. **Motility disorders.** Diarrhea induced by motility disorders results from decreased contact time of the fecal mass with the intestinal wall, so less water is absorbed from the feces.
      (1) **Motility disorders** include irritable bowel syndrome, scleroderma, diabetic neuropathy, gastric/intestinal resection, and vagotomy.
      (2) **Medications** that can induce motility disorders include parasympathomimetic agents that enhance the effects of acetylcholine (e.g., metoclopramide, bethanechol), digitalis, quinidine, and antibiotics.
         (a) Antibiotics cause diarrhea by causing intestinal irritation, increased bowel motility, and altered bowel microbial flora.
         (b) Most antibiotic-induced diarrhea can be minimized by taking the agent with food.

2. **Classification by etiology**
   a. **Acute diarrhea** (lasts less than 2 weeks)
      (1) **Infection. Most common** sources include viral and bacterial, but protozoal diarrhea also occurs. Organisms include:
         (a) **Viruses** that commonly cause diarrhea include rotaviruses and the Norwalk virus.
            (i) **Rotaviruses** usually affect children under 2 years of age. The virus has an onset of 1–2 days and lasts 5–8 days. Patients usually have vomiting, a mild fever, and may experience severe dehydration. There is usually no blood or pus in the stool.
            (ii) The **Norwalk virus** affects older children and adults. It has an onset of 1–2 days and lasts 24–48 hours (the "24-hour bug"). As with rotaviruses, there is mild fever but no blood or pus in the stool.
         (b) **Bacteria.** Most bacterial diarrhea results from consumption of contaminated water or food with an onset of diarrhea in 8 hours to several days. Diarrhea due to consumption of contaminated food or water that occurs in a foreign country (e.g., Mexico, third world countries) is referred to as turista or traveler's diarrhea.
            (i) **Toxigenic bacteria.** Diarrhea caused by toxigenic *E. coli, S. aureus, V. cholerae,* and *Shigella* results from the secretory effects of enterotoxins released by these organisms in the small intestine. Patients usually experience large-volume stools that are watery or greasy.
            (ii) **Invasive bacteria.** Diarrhea caused by invasive *E. coli, Shigella, Salmonella, Campylobacter,* and *Clostridium difficile* results from mucosal inva-

sion of the colon. This results in a dysentery-like diarrhea, which is characterized by an extreme urgency to defecate, abdominal cramping, tenesmus, fever, chills, and small-volume stools that contain blood or pus.

(c) **Protozoa.** *G. lamblia, E. histolytica,* and *Cryptosporidium* cause explosive, foul-smelling, large-volume, watery stools. This is thought to be caused by invasion of the small intestine, which causes damage to the microvilli and, therefore, decreases absorption of fluids. This type of diarrhea can result in large fluid losses, and patients are at risk for dehydration. Although protozoan-induced diarrhea is self-limiting, it may persist for several months, so therapy should be considered to eradicate the organism.

(2) **Diet-induced diarrhea.** Diarrhea induced by foods results from food allergies, high-fiber diets, fatty or spicy foods, large amounts of caffeine, or milk intolerance. The best treatment is prevention, by avoiding troublesome foods.

(3) **Drug-induced diarrhea** (see II A 1 a–c)

b. **Chronic diarrhea** (lasts longer than 2 weeks). If a patient suffers from diarrhea for long periods of time, or from recurrent episodes of diarrhea, the following causes must be considered: protozoal organisms, food-induced diarrhea (e.g., lactose intolerance), irritable bowel syndrome, malabsorption syndromes (e.g., celiac sprue, diverticulosis, short bowel syndrome), inflammatory bowel disease, pancreatic disease, and hyperthyroidism.

B. Patient evaluation

1. Pharmacists who are consulted by patients should ask the patient for the following information before recommending a therapy:
   a. **Age** of the patient
   b. **Onset and duration** of the diarrhea
   c. **Description of stool** (i.e., frequency, volume, blood, pus, watery)
   d. **Other symptoms** (e.g., abdominal cramping, fever, nausea, vomiting, weight loss)
   e. **Medications** recently started or medications used to relieve the diarrhea
   f. **Recent travel** (where and how long ago)
   g. **Medical history** (history of GI disorders)

2. **Referrals to a physician** should be made by the pharmacist who encounters a patient with diarrhea that meets the following criteria:
   a. **Younger than 3 years** of age or **older than 60 years** of age (with multiple medical problems)
   b. **Bloody stools**
   c. **High fever** (greater than 101°F or 38°C)
   d. **Dehydration or weight loss** greater than 5% of total body weight; signs of dehydration—dry mouth, sunken in eyes, crying without tears, dry skin that is not elastic like normal skin
   e. **Duration of diarrhea longer than 5 days**
   f. **Vomiting**

C. Treatment

1. **Nonpharmacologic**
   a. **Food/breast feeding.** There has been much controversy regarding the decision "to feed" or "not to feed" children during acute episodes of diarrhea. Originally, parents were told that children should not receive food, milk-products, or breast feed for 6–48 hours after the onset of diarrhea. Recent information shows that children should remain on their normal diet or breast feeding during bouts of diarrhea because these do not make the diarrhea worse and may actually improve the diarrhea.
   b. **Fluids.** The most important part of treating acute diarrhea is the replacement of lost fluids. If patients experience mild to moderate fluid loss this can be done with oral rehydration solutions. If fluid loss is severe (more than 10% loss of body weight) and/or severe vomiting persists, then patients may need intravenous rehydration before oral maintenance fluids can be administered. Oral rehydration solutions can be easily made at home (Table 33-1) or purchased ready-to-use (Pedialyte, Ricelyte, Infalyte, Rehydralyte, Resol). Because the secretory and absorptive mechanisms of the bowel function separately, this allows these oral rehydration solutions to be absorbed during acute episodes of diarrhea preventing severe dehydration and complications.

Table 33-1. Guidelines for Oral Replacement Therapy Established by the World Health Organization (WHO)

Ingredients	Dose
Sodium chloride (table salt)	90mEq (0.5 teaspoon)
Potassium chloride (potassium salt)	20 mEq (0.25 teaspoons)
Sodium bicarbonate (baking soda)	30 mEq (0.5 teaspoons)
Glucose (sugar)	20g (2 tablespoons)
Water	Enough to make 1 liter of solution

(1) **Fluid and electrolyte replacement.** Fluid and electrolyte therapy is aimed at replacing what the body has lost. During this situation, the patient's fluid input and output as well as weight should be monitored. The World Health Organization has established guidelines for oral replacement therapy (see Table 33-1). Recommended doses are given in Table 33-2.

(2) **Fluids to be avoided** include hypertonic fruit juices and drinks (e.g., apple juice, powdered drink mixes, gelatin water) or carbonated beverages, which can make diarrhea worse and do not contain needed electrolytes (i.e., Na^+, K^+). Gatorade diluted in water (1:1) is adequate and provides the necessary combination of glucose, sodium, and potassium.

2. **Pharmacologic.** Based on the Food and Drug Administration (FDA) review of the various antidiarrheal products, three agents have been identified as Category I (i.e., safe and effective) ingredients: activated attapulgite, calcium polycarbophil, and loperamide. Several other agents are still marketed as Category III agents, pending final assessment of their status by the FDA. Antidiarrheal agents are classified in different categories on the basis of their chemical class or pharmacologic mechanism of action.

a. **Antiperistaltic drugs**

(1) **Mechanism of action.** Antiperistaltic drugs act directly on the circular and longitudinal musculature of the small and large intestine to normalize peristaltic intestinal movements. They slow intestinal motility and affect water and electrolyte movement through the bowel. The frequency of bowel movements is decreased, and the consistency of stools is increased.

(2) **Contraindication.** Antiperistaltic medications have always been restricted in patients with acute bacterial diarrhea because of the potential for these drugs to decrease clearance of the organism and enhance systemic invasion of the organism. Most information shows that this is not significant and probably will cause no harm. However, these medications should not be used in patients with colitis (potential for the development of toxic megacolon) or in children less than 2 years of age.

(3) **Prescription agents** in this class include the opiate and opiate-related agents including diphenoxylate/atropine (e.g., Lomotil) and difenoxin/atropine (e.g., Motofen).

(4) **Nonprescription agents. Loperamide** (e.g., Imodium A-D, Kaopectate II, Pepto Diarrhea Control) provides effective control of diarrhea as quickly as 1 hour after ad-

Table 33-2. Guidelines for Fluid and Electrolyte Replacement Therapy

Age Group	Dose
Adults ($\geq$ 10 years)	2000–3000 ml/day
Children (5 to 10 years)	1000–2000 ml/day
Children ($<$ 5 years)	40-75 ml/kg for the first 6 hours **or** 5–10 ml every 10 to 15 minutes for 30 minutes then 15–20 ml every 10 to 15 minutes for 30 minutes then 30 ml (1 ounce) every 30 minutes to complete the first 6 hours 60 ml (2 ounces; 1/4 cup) every 30 minutes for the next 12 hours Fluids as tolerated for the next 24 hours

ministration. Antiperistaltic drugs should not be used for more than 48 hours in acute diarrhea.

(a) **Side effects.** At recommended doses, loperamide is generally well tolerated. Side effects are infrequent and consist primarily of abdominal pain, distention, or discomfort; drowsiness; dizziness; and dry mouth.

(b) **Dosage information.** An **adult dosage** is 4 mg followed by 2 mg after each unformed stool not to exceed 16 mg/day. A **child's dosage** is 1–2 mg up to three times per day, depending on weight and age.

b. Adsorbents. These medications adsorb toxins, bacteria, gases, and fluids. They are not absorbed systemically, so they produce **few adverse effects.** There are several products available; some are more effective than others, but none are very effective for severe acute diarrhea. These products are given for symptomatic relief, and are usually administered in large doses immediately following a loose stool.

(1) **Activated attapulgite** (e.g., Kaopectate Maximum Strength, Donnagel, Diar-Aid). Attapulgite is a naturally occurring aluminum magnesium silicate that absorbs eight times its weight in water. It is considered to be safe and effective in reducing the number of bowel movements, improving stool consistency, and relieving cramps associated with diarrhea.

(a) **Dosage information.** An **adult dose** is 1200 mg after each loose stool. A **child's dose** is 300–600 mg after each loose stool.

(b) **Adverse effects.** Because activated attapulgite is inert and is not absorbed systemically, **side effects** are essentially nonexistent.

(2) **Calcium polycarbophil** (e.g., FiberCon, Mitrolan, Fiberall, Fiber-Lax) is a synthetic, hydrophilic polyacrylic resin that has the potential to absorb up to 60 times its weight in water. Polycarbophil has been shown to be safe and effective for the symptomatic treatment of diarrhea.

(a) **Side effects.** As with attapulgite, calcium polycarbophil is not systemically absorbed. It is metabolically inactive and essentially does not produce systemic side effects.

(b) **Dosage information.** An **adult dosage** is 1 gram one to four times daily. A **child's dosage** is 0.5 grams one to four times daily.

c. Miscellaneous agents

(1) **Bismuth subsalicylate** (e.g., Pepto-Bismol). Bismuth salts work as adsorbents but also are believed to decrease secretion of water into the bowel. Bismuth preparations have moderate effectiveness against traveler's diarrhea, but doses required for relief are large and must be administered frequently so these preparations may be inconvenient.

(a) **Dose.** An **adult dosage** is two tablets or 30–60 ml (524 mg) every hour as needed to a maximum of eight doses in a 24-hour period. A **child's dosage** is 1/3 to 1/2 the adult dose. Bismuth subsalicylate can prevent traveler's diarrhea when two tablets are taken four times per day.

(b) **Adverse effects** may include harmless grayish-black stools or tongue and ringing in the ears, if high doses are taken or if the patient is simultaneously taking other salicylate products.

(c) **Contraindication.** Bismuth subsalicylate should not be given to children or teenagers during or after recovery from chicken pox or flu because of the possible association of salicylates with Reye syndrome.

(2) **Lactobacillus** (e.g., Bacid, Lactinex) products are intended to replace the normal bacterial flora that is lost during the administration of oral antibiotics. However, there is little information to show that these products are useful for antibiotic-induced diarrhea, so most clinicians do not recommend their use.

(3) **Lactase** (e.g., LactAid, Lactrase, Dairy Ease) is indicated for individuals who have insufficient amounts of lactase in the small intestine. Lactose (a disaccharide present in dairy products) must be broken down to glucose and galactose to be fully digested. If it is not, lactose draws water into the GI tract and diarrhea results. Lactase is the enzyme responsible for digesting lactose. The dose is one to two capsules taken with milk or dairy products or added to milk before drinking. Titration of doses to higher levels may be required in some cases.

(4) **Anti-infectives.** Depending upon the suspected etiology of the infectious diarrhea, prescription antibiotics and antiprotozoal medications can be used to eradicate the organisms and decrease the duration of symptoms (Table 33-3). If antibiotics are

Table 33-3. Drugs and Doses Used to Treat Infectious Diarrhea

Antibacterials	Antiprotozoals	Dose
Ciprofloxacin	N/A	500 mg twice daily
Doxycycline	N/A	100 mg twice daily
Norfloxacin	N/A	400 mg twice daily
Tetracycline	N/A	250 mg four times a day
Trimethoprim/Sulfamethoxazole DS	N/A	1 tablet twice daily
N/A	Metronidazole	250 mg three times a day
N/A	Quinacrine	100 mg three times a day

used to prevent traveler's diarrhea, therapy should be started 1 day before arrival in high-incidence regions and continue until 2 days after departure. If diarrhea has occurred, antibiotic treatment should last for 7 days.

(5) **Anticholinergics** (e.g., atropine, hyoscyamine) decrease bowel motility, which results in an increase of fluid absorption from the intestinal tract and a decrease in abdominal cramping. These products are found in combination with adsorbents or opiates. However, the amount of anticholinergic found in most products is not considered to be enough to alter the course of severe acute diarrhea. **Adverse effects** include dry mouth, blurred vision, and tachycardia. These products should not be used in patients with narrow-angle glaucoma.

III. HEMORRHOIDS traditionally have been defined as clusters of dilated blood vessels in the lower rectum (internal hemorrhoids) or anus (external hemorrhoids). It has been determined that hemorrhoids simply represent downward displacement of anal cushions that contain arteriovenous anastomoses. Hemorrhoids are common, and, although they are considered a minor medical problem, they may cause considerable discomfort and anxiety. A proper diagnosis is important because there are a number of conditions that may produce symptoms that mimic those of hemorrhoids (see III D). For example, colorectal cancer may cause bleeding, which is a common symptom of hemorrhoids. Fortunately, patient reassurance and the proper administration of a few simple treatments usually improve the condition.

A. Types of hemorrhoids are determined by their anatomic position and vascular origin.

1. An **internal** hemorrhoid is an exaggerated vascular cushion with an engorged internal hemorrhoidal plexus located above the dentate line and covered with a mucous membrane.

2. An **external** hemorrhoid is a dilated vein of the inferior hemorrhoidal plexus located below the dentate line and covered with squamous epithelium.

B. Causes. Although heredity may predispose a person to hemorrhoids, the exact cause is probably related to acquired factors.

1. Situations that result in **increased venous pressure** in the hemorrhoidal plexus (e.g., chronic straining during defecation; small, hard stools; prolonged sitting on the toilet; occupations that routinely require heavy lifting; pregnancy) can transform an asymptomatic hemorrhoid into a problem.

2. The hemorrhoidal veins are pushed downward during defecation or straining, and, with increased venous pressure, they **dilate** and **become engorged.** Over time, the **fibers** that anchor the hemorrhoidal veins to their underlying muscular coats **stretch,** which results in **prolapse.**

C. Symptoms

1. The **most common** symptom of hemorrhoids is **painless bleeding** occurring during a bowel movement. The blood is usually bright red and may be visible on the stool, on the toilet tissue, or coloring the water in the toilet.

2. **Prolapse** is the **second most common** symptom of hemorrhoids. A temporary protrusion may occur during defection, and it may need to be replaced manually. A permanently prolapsed hemorrhoid may give rise to chronic, moist soiling of the underwear and these patients may complain of a dull aching feeling.

3. **Pain** is unusual unless **thrombosis** involving external tissue is present, and then the pain can be excruciating.

4. **Discomfort, soreness, pruritus, swelling,** and **discharge** may also occur with hemorrhoids.

D. **Other conditions** that may **mimic** hemorrhoids include the following, which usually require a physician's intervention.

1. An **anal abscess,** usually a *Staphylococcus* infection

2. **Cryptitis,** which is inflammation of the crypts (the small indentations at the mucocutaneous junction)

3. **Anal fissure,** which is a small tear in the lining of the anus

4. An **anal fistula,** which is an abnormal communication between the mucosa of the rectum and the skin adjacent to the anus

5. A **polyp,** which is a tumor of the large intestine

6. **Colorectal cancer**

E. **Internal** hemorrhoids are graded and classified into one of **four groups.**

1. A **first-degree** hemorrhoid (grade 1) does not descend, or prolapse, during straining when defecating.

2. A **second-degree** hemorrhoid (grade 2) descends but returns spontaneously with relaxation.

3. A **third-degree** hemorrhoid (grade 3) requires manual replacement into the rectum after prolapse.

4. A **fourth-degree** hemorrhoid (grade 4) is permanently prolapsed.

F. **Treatment.** The symptoms of hemorrhoids are produced by a cycle of events: the protrusion of the vascular submucosal cushion through a tight anal canal, which becomes further congested and hypertrophic, which causes the cushion to protrude further. All treatments of hemorrhoids aim to break this cycle, and they fall into a number of broad groups.

1. For **first-** and **second-degree internal** hemorrhoids that bleed minimally, a conservative approach can usually be taken.
   a. To **reduce straining** and **downward pressure** on the hemorrhoids, patients should be told to avoid straining when defecating and to avoid sitting on the toilet longer than necessary.
   b. **Correction of constipation is paramount importance.** This can be accomplished by eating a high-fiber diet and increasing the intake of water. Bulk-forming laxatives, such as psyllium, and stool softeners, such as docusate, may be helpful.
   c. **Sitz baths** taken several times a day can soothe the anal mucosa. Warm (not hot) water should be used, and prolonged bathing should be avoided. Epsom salts (magnesium sulfate) added to the bath or the application of an ice pack can help reduce the swelling of an edematous or clotted hemorrhoid.
   d. **OTC hemorrhoidal ointments, creams, foams,** and **suppositories** may also help relieve symptoms (see III G).

2. **Higher-grade internal hemorrhoids** usually require physician expertise and specialized procedures for treatment.
   a. Symptomatic grades 2 or 3 hemorrhoids are usually best treated with **hemorrhoid banding** (rubber band ligation). This procedure is performed through a anoscope; a rubber band ligature is placed on the rectal mucosa above the hemorrhoid, well above the dentate line to avoid excessive discomfort. The ligated area sloughs off in a few days.
   b. **Infrared coagulation** can be used for grade 2 hemorrhoids; it is less effective than banding with large hemorrhoids.
   c. **Sclerotherapy** (injection of a sclerosing agent into the hemorrhoid) or cryotherapy ("freezing" the hemorrhoid) are older therapies that have been used.
   d. **Surgical hemorrhoidectomy** should be undertaken only for grades 3 or 4 hemorrhoids. Whether the procedure is done **traditionally** or with a **laser,** most patients have significant discomfort and a period of postoperative disability.

3. An **external, thrombosed hemorrhoid** can be completely excised in an office setting, clinic, or operating room.

G. **Nonprescription medication for hemorrhoidal and other anorectal diseases (Table 33-4).** The FDA has identified several ingredients as safe and effective to alleviate burning, discomfort, inflammation, irritation, itching, pain, and swelling. These products are simply palliative; they are not meant to cure hemorrhoids or other anorectal disease. If these products do not improve symptoms within 7 days, a physician should be consulted. A physician should also be consulted if there is bleeding, prolapse of the hemorrhoid, seepage of feces or mucus, thrombosis, or severe pain.

1. **Ointments versus suppositories.** Generally, the ointment or cream dosage form is believed to be superior to a suppository, which may bypass the affected area. Patients should be advised to wash the anorectal area with mild soap and warm water and pat (not wipe) the area dry before applying a product. Alternatively, patients can use an OTC anal cleansing pad (e.g., Tucks). Some ointments come with rectal pipes (pile pipes) that allow the patient to insert and apply the medication in the rectum. The openings in the rectal pipe allow the ointment to cover large areas of the rectal mucosa unreachable with the finger. The rectal pipe should be lubricated by spreading ointment around the tip of the pipe before insertion. Some clinicians advise against the use of the rectal pipe because the anal canal could be traumatized if the pipe is not inserted properly.

2. **Local anesthetics** work by blocking nerve impulse transmission. They should be used for symptoms of pain, itching, burning, discomfort, and irritation in the perianal region or lower anal canal (not in the rectum).
   a. **Agents** deemed safe and effective include benzocaine 5%–20% (e.g., Americaine), pramoxine HCl 1% (e.g., Tronolane, Anusol), benzyl alcohol 1%–4%, dibucaine and dibucaine HCl 0.25%–1%, dyclonine HCl 0.5%–1%, lidocaine 2%–5% (e.g., Xylocaine), tetracaine and tetracaine HCl 0.5%–1%.
   b. **Adverse effects.** These agents may produce a hypersensitivity reaction with burning and itching similar to that of anorectal disease.

3. **Vasoconstrictors** have been shown to decrease mucosal perfusion in the anorectal area after topical application. However, because bleeding in this area may be a sign of more serious disease, vasoconstrictors are not approved for control of minor bleeding. For temporary relief of itching and swelling, these agents have a local anesthetic effect of unknown mechanism.
   a. **Agents** deemed safe and effective (although none of these agents are commercially available in the dosage forms below) include ephedrine sulfate 0.1%–0.125% in aqueous solution, epinephrine HCl 0.005%–0.01% in aqueous solution, and phenylephrine HCl 0.25% in aqueous solution These agents are present in various ointments (e.g., Pazo) and suppositories (e.g., Medicone).
   b. **Contraindications** apply to people with cardiovascular disease, high blood pressure, hyperthyroidism, diabetes, and prostate enlargement because of the possibility of systemic absorption.

4. **Protectants** provide a **physical barrier,** forming a protective coating over skin or mucous membranes, for temporary relief of itching, irritation, discomfort, and burning. They prevent

Table 33-4. Guide to Hemorrhoidal Therapy Based on Approved Indication for OTC Anorectal Drug Products

	Burning	Discomfort	Irritation	Itching	Pain	Soreness	Swelling
Analgesic, Anesthetic, Antipruritic	Yes	Yes		Yes	Yes	Yes	
Astringent	Yes	Yes	Yes	Yes			
Keratolytic		Yes		Yes			
Local anesthetic	Yes	Yes		Yes	Yes	Yes	
Protectant	Yes	Yes	Yes	Yes			
Vasoconstrictor		Yes	Yes	Yes			Yes
Hydrocortisone		Yes		Yes			Yes

irritation of anorectal tissue and prevent water loss from the stratum corneum. Protectants are often the bases or vehicles for the other agents used for anorectal disease. Products include aluminum hydroxide gel, cocoa butter, kaolin, lanolin, hard fat, mineral oil, white petrolatum, petrolatum, glycerin (external use only), calamine, topical starch, cod liver oil, shark liver oil, and zinc oxide. When protectants are incorporated into the formulation of an OTC product, they should make up at least 50% of the dosage unit. If two to four protectants are used, their total concentration should represent at least 50% of the whole product. When calamine, cod liver oil, shark liver oil, and zinc oxide are used as protectants, they must be combined with other protectant active ingredients.

a. **Absorbents** take up fluids that are on or secreted by skin or mucous membranes.
b. **Adsorbents** attach to substances secreted by skin or mucous membranes.
c. **Demulcents** combine with water to form a colloidal solution, which protects the skin in a way similar to mucus.
d. **Emollients,** which are derived from animal or vegetable fats or petroleum products, soften or protect internal or external body surfaces.

5. **Astringents** lessen mucus and other secretions and protect underlying tissue through a local and limited protein coagulant effect. Action is limited to surface cells, but astringents provide temporary relief of itching, discomfort, irritation, and burning. Products considered to be safe and effective include calamine 5%–25% (internal and external), witch hazel 10%–50% (external), and zinc oxide 5%–25%.

6. **Keratolytics** cause desquamation and debridement of the surface cells of the epidermis and provide temporary relief of discomfort and itching. It is theorized that keratolytics help expose underlying tissue to other therapeutic agents. Products considered to be **safe** and **effective** include aluminum chlorhydroxyallantoinate (alcloxa) 0.2%–2.0% and resorcinol 1%–3%.

7. **Analgesics, anesthetics,** and **antipruritics** provide temporary relief of burning, discomfort, itching, pain, and soreness. The FDA has redesignated several ingredients into this category that were formerly classified as counterirritants. Ingredients considered to be **safe** and **effective** for external use in the anorectal area include menthol (0.1%–1%), juniper tar (1%–5%), and camphor (0.1%–3%).

8. **Wound-healing agents.** There are a few ingredients that have been claimed to be effective in promoting wound healing or tissue repair in the anorectal region. Live yeast cell derivative (LYCD) [skin respiratory factor], which is a water-soluble extract of brewer's yeast, was present in Preparation H in the past. LYCD has recently been removed from the list of "safe and effective" active ingredients by the FDA as it determined that this agent was not proven effective as per the studies submitted to it. Preparation H products have been reformulated without LYCD. Preparation H Ointment now contains the protectants (petrolatum, mineral oil, shark liver oil) and the vasoconstrictor, phenylephrine.

9. **Hydrocortisone (0.25%–1%)** works by causing vasoconstriction, stabilization of lysosomal membranes, and antimitotic activity. These agents have the potential to reduce itching, inflammation, and discomfort in the anorectal area.

IV. GASTROESOPHAGEAL REFLUX DISEASE (HEARTBURN)

A. General information

1. **Definition.** The reflux of gastric contents into the esophagus, or gastroesophageal reflux, is generally a benign physiologic process that occurs in normal individuals multiple times throughout the day. However, patients with gastroesophageal reflux disease (GERD) may experience esophageal tissue damage (reflux esophagitis) and/or symptoms of heartburn when the acidic gastric contents stay in prolonged contact with the esophagus.

2. **Symptoms.** Heartburn typically is described as a burning sensation or pain located in the lower chest. Because the pain may radiate up into the chest, heartburn may be confused with pain associated with myocardial infarction. Symptoms usually occur soon after meals and when lying down at bedtime. Pain on swallowing (odynophagia) may suggest severe mucosal damage in the esophagus.

3. **Complications.** Patients with severe, uncontrolled GERD may suffer bleeding from esophageal ulcers and pulmonary complications resulting from the aspiration of refluxed

material into the upper airways and lungs. Patients who describe difficulty swallowing (i.e., dysphagia) may have an esophageal stricture, cancer, or a motility disorder.

4. **Causes.** Many patients with GERD have a weak lower esophageal sphincter (LES). As a result, the high pressure in the stomach creates enough force to overcome the weak squeeze of the LES and allows reflux to occur. Numerous factors may promote reflux by reducing LES tone, delaying gastric emptying, increasing acid secretion, or impairing the gastroesophageal pressure gradient (see I B 1). Drugs that reduce LES tone include:
   a. Calcium channel antagonists (e.g., nifedipine, verapamil, diltiazem)
   b. Nitrates
   c. Anticholinergic agents (e.g., tricyclic antidepressants, antihistamines)
   d. Oral contraceptives and estrogen

5. Pharmacists who are consulted by patients should ask for the following information before recommending a therapy:
   a. Duration and frequency of symptoms
   b. Severity of the pain and symptoms
   c. Timing of the symptoms (especially in relation to meals and at bedtime)
   d. Presence of other symptoms (nausea, vomiting, bloody stools, weight loss)
   e. Use of alcohol or tobacco
   f. Amount of high-fat foods, caffeine-containing products, chocolate, and tomato-based foods consumed
   g. Medications used currently, including nonprescription medications
   h. Medications used to relieve heartburn and their effectiveness

6. Patients with the following symptoms or conditions should be referred to a physician for evaluation rather than treated with nonprescription agents.
   a. Severe abdominal or back pain
   b. Unexplained weight loss
   c. Chest pain that is indistinguishable from ischemic pain
   d. Difficulty or pain on swallowing
   e. Presence or history of vomiting blood
   f. Black tarry bowel movements (if not taking iron or bismuth subsalicylate)
   g. Children younger than 12 years of age
   h. Possibility of being pregnant
   i. Symptoms not responding to antacids or nonprescription histamine$_2$-receptor antagonists (H_2RAs) within 2 weeks or recurring soon after stopping

B. Treatment

1. **Nonpharmacologic.** Nonpharmacologic interventions for GERD attempt to reduce or eliminate dietary and lifestyle factors that promote reflux. Specific recommendations include:
   a. Elevate the head of the bed about 6 inches with blocks or by placing a foam wedge under the patient's head. This position improves esophageal clearance and reduces the duration of reflux.
   b. Eat evening meals at least 3 hours before going to bed to allow adequate time for gastric emptying.
   c. Avoid foods that reduce LES tone.
      (1) Chocolate
      (2) Mints
      (3) High-fat foods
   d. Avoid foods that irritate the esophagus.
      (1) Tomato-based products
      (2) Coffee
      (3) Citrus juices
   e. Reduce the size of meals.
   f. Avoid lying down after meals.
   g. Stop smoking.
   h. Limit alcohol intake.
   i. Lose weight if appropriate.
   k. Avoid wearing tight-fitting clothing.

2. **Pharmacologic.** The management of GERD may be viewed as a stepped-care approach, with antacids, nonprescription H_2RAs, and nondrug measures forming the basis for the first step (Figure 33-1). These measures may help to alleviate symptoms in patients with mild to moderate GERD but cannot be expected to heal damaged esophageal mucosa or prevent complications.
   a. **Antacids.** Antacids neutralize gastric acid, which increases the pH of refluxed gastric contents and LES pressure. As a result, the refluxed contents are not as damaging to the esophageal mucosa. Antacids generally relieve heartburn within 5–15 minutes of administration. The duration of relief ranges from 1–3 hours. Because of their short duration, patients may need to take 4–5 doses throughout the day for adequate symptom relief. Antacids will not provide sustained neutralization of acid throughout the night. An **adult dose** is 40–80 mEq acid neutralizing capacity (ANC) taken as needed for symptoms. If necessary, these doses may be titrated to a scheduled regimen, such as 40–80 mEq after meals and at bedtime.
      (1) **Sodium bicarbonate** (e.g., Alka-Seltzer, Bromo-Seltzer) should be used only for short-term relief of symptoms. Because each gram of sodium bicarbonate contains 12 mEq of sodium, it is contraindicated in patients with edema, congestive heart failure, renal failure, cirrhosis, and patients on low-salt diets.
      (2) **Calcium carbonate** (e.g., Tums) is useful for GERD but may cause constipation or diarrhea.
      (3) **Aluminum hydroxide** (e.g., Amphojel, Alternagel) often causes constipation and should be avoided in patients with hemorrhoids or constipation, which is common in the elderly.
      (4) **Magnesium hydroxide** (e.g., Milk of Magnesia) rarely is used alone for heartburn because it frequently causes diarrhea.
      (5) **Magnesium–aluminum** combination antacids (e.g., Maalox, Mylanta) provide the highest ANC per volume of antacid and are used most frequently. The predominant adverse effect of these combinations is diarrhea.

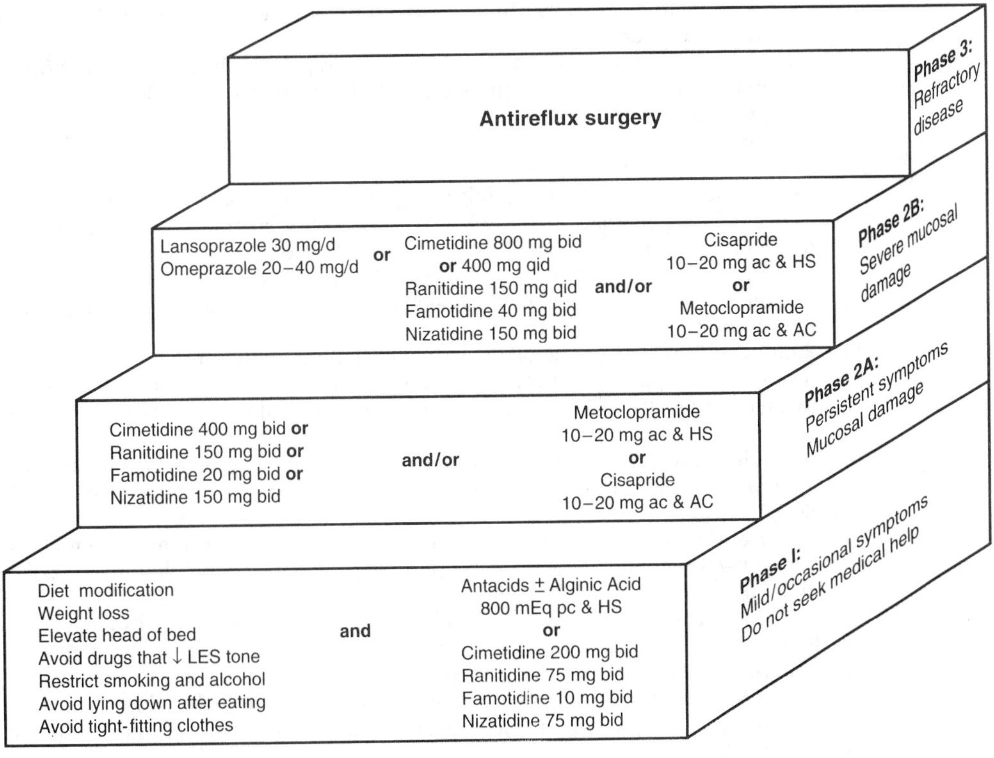

Figure 33-1. Step-Wise Progression of Therapy for GERD.
ac = before meals HS = bedtime bid = twice daily qid = four times daily ANC = acid neutralizing capacity

(6) **Patient information**

(a) Patients with renal failure should avoid the use of all antacids. Potassium and magnesium content of antacids should be considered for patients with cardiac disease.

(b) Patients should not take more than 500–600 mEq ANC of antacid per day.

(7) Antacids can interfere with the absorption of many drugs. In general, antacids should be spaced at least two hours apart from the administration of interacting drugs. Important clinical interactions with antacids may occur with the following drugs.

(a) Tetracycline antibiotics

(b) Quinolone antibiotics (e.g., ciprofloxacin, ofloxacin)

(c) Iron supplements

(d) Digoxin

b. **Alginic acid**

(1) **Mechanism of action.** Alginic acid works by reacting with sodium bicarbonate and saliva to form a viscous solution of **sodium alginate.** This viscous solution floats on the surface of gastric contents so that, when reflux occurs, sodium alginate rather than acid is refluxed, and irritation is minimized.

(2) **Patient information**

(a) Alginic-acid tablets must be chewed to be effective and should be followed by a full glass of water so that the viscous foam can float on it in the stomach.

(b) Alginic acid products work best when patients are in the upright position. Thus, these products should not be taken at bedtime or just before lying down.

c. **Nonprescription H_2RAs.** These medications inhibit gastric acid secretion by competitively blocking H_2-receptors on the parietal cell. By decreasing gastric acid secretion, the refluxed material is less damaging to the esophagus. The onset of symptom relief with H_2RAs is approximately 1–2 hours.

(1) **Cimetidine (Tagamet-HB)**

(a) The **adult dosage** of nonprescription cimetidine is 200 mg as needed for symptoms, up to twice daily. Cimetidine 200 mg suppresses gastric acid for approximately 6 hours.

(a) Nonprescription doses of cimetidine may **impair** the **hepatic metabolism** and thus increase serum concentrations and the pharmacologic effects of:

(i) Warfarin

(ii) Phenytoin

(iii) Theophylline

(2) **Famotidine (Pepcid-AC).** The **adult dosage** of nonprescription famotidine is 10 mg as needed for symptoms, up to twice daily. Patients who anticipate heartburn or indigestion may take one famotidine 10 mg tablet 1 hour before eating, with a maximum of two tablets within a 24-hour period. Famotidine 10 mg suppresses acid secretion for 8–10 hours. Unlike cimetidine, famotidine does not impair hepatic metabolism of other drugs.

(3) **Ranitidine (Zantac75).** The **adult dosage** of nonprescription ranitidine is 75 mg as needed for symptoms, up to twice daily. Ranitidine inhibits hepatic metabolism five to ten times less than cimetidine, therefore, the potential for drug interactions is very small.

(4) **Nizatidine (Axid-AR).** The adult dosage of nizatidine is 75 mg as needed for symptoms up to twice daily. Nizatidine does not impair hepatic metabolism of other drugs.

(5) **Adverse effects.** These agents are extremely well tolerated. The **most common** adverse effects reported with nonprescription doses are headache, diarrhea, dizziness, and nausea.

d. **Prescription H_2RAs.** Patients with moderate to severe symptoms and/or esophageal mucosal lesions require higher doses of H_2RAs than are available over the counter. Unlike patients with peptic ulcer disease, patients with GERD respond best to multiple daily doses of H_2RAs rather than to single bedtime doses. At these higher doses, cimetidine may cause mental confusion and depression in elderly patients, especially those with poor renal function.

e. **Prokinetic agents.** Patients with moderate to severe GERD may benefit from the addition of these medications which stimulate esophageal motility and increase LES tone. Prokinetic agents are available only by prescription.

(1) **Metoclopramide (Reglan, generic). Adverse effects** limit the usefulness of this agent for many patients. Such effects include sedation, depression, and extrapyramidal effects.

(2) **Cisapride** (Propulsid) may relieve GERD symptoms and heal esophageal damage. Drugs that inhibit certain isoenzymes of the cytochrome p450 system can increase cisapride levels and cause serious cardiac arrhythmias and even death. Concomitant administration of cisapride with the following drugs is contraindicated:

(a) Ketoconazole (Nizoral)
(b) Itraconazole (Sporanox)
(c) Miconazole (Monistat) intravenous
(d) Fluconazole (Diflucan)
(e) Erythromycin (various)
(f) Clarithromycin (Biaxin)
(g) Troleandomycin (TAO)

f. Proton pump inhibitors. These prescription-only agents provide complete acid suppression by inhibiting the hydrogen-potassium ATPase pump on the surface of the parietal cell. The duration of acid suppression with these agents is about 3 days. Proton pump inhibitors are the most potent and effective agents available for relieving severe GERD symptoms and healing esophageal lesions.

(1) **Omeprazole (Prilosec).** Omeprazole may inhibit hepatic metabolism and thus increase serum concentration/pharmacologic effects of the following drugs:

(a) Phenytoin
(b) Warfarin
(c) Diazepam

(2) **Lansoprazole** (Prevacid)

C. Special patient populations

1. Pediatric patients. Gastroesophageal reflux occurs commonly in infants and children. Signs and symptoms in pediatric patients include vomiting, chest pain, irritability, feeding refusal, belching, and apnea. Serious complications (e.g., failure to thrive, esophageal strictures) can occur in infants and children.

a. Antacids, with or without alginic acid, have been widely used in infants and children, but their safety has not been clearly established.

b. H_2RAs have been used safely in children under the supervision of health care providers. However, the nonprescription H_2RAs are not approved for use in children younger than 12 years of age unless directed by a physician.

2. Pregnant patients. Heartburn occurs commonly during pregnancy because of increased abdominal pressure due to the expanding uterus as well as reduced LES pressure resulting from high concentrations of estrogen and progesterone. Nearly half of pregnant women experience GERD, especially during the third trimester.

a. Antacids are generally considered safe in pregnancy as long as chronic high doses are avoided. It is best to avoid sodium bicarbonate because of the risks of systemic alkalosis and the sodium load leading to edema and weight gain.

b. Data regarding the **safety** of **alginic acid** during pregnancy are not available.

c. Controlled data regarding the **safety** of **H_2RAs** in pregnancy are limited. Pregnant women seeking a nonprescription H_2RA for GERD should be directed to use antacids, unless a physician has instructed her otherwise.

3. Elderly patients. Antacids and nonprescription H_2RAs may be safely used in elderly patients without any dosage adjustments.

a. Dosage reduction of prescription H_2RAs may be necessary in elderly patients with reduced renal function.

b. Elderly patients are more likely to be taking drugs that interact with antacids, H_2RAs, omeprazole, and/or cisapride.

STUDY QUESTIONS

Directions: Each of the numbered items or incomplete statements in this section is followed by answers or by completions of the statement. Select the **one** lettered answer or completion that is **best** in each case.

1. Which laxative should NOT be used to treat acute constipation because of its slow onset of action?

(A) Glycerin
(B) Bisacodyl suppository
(C) Psyllium
(D) Phenolphthalein

2. Which is NOT a risk factor for hyperphosphatemia and death from sodium phosphate enemas when used in children?

(A) Renal insufficiency
(B) Hirschprung's disease
(C) Anorectal malformations
(D) Children between the ages of 6 and 12 years

3. All of the following statements about emollient "stool softeners" laxatives are true EXCEPT

(A) they are not good for acute constipation
(B) they are good for patients who should not strain by passing a hard stool (e.g., post-surgical patients)
(C) they never have been found to be better than placebo for long-term use
(D) they are more effective than placebo for long term use

4. Which of the following statements adequately describes bulk-forming laxatives?

(A) Can cause diarrhea if not taken with water
(B) Are derived from polysaccharides and resemble fiber (bran) in mechanism of action
(C) Onset of action is in 4–8 hours
(D) Produce much more complete evacuation of constipation than stimulant products

5. Which of the following statements about non-drug therapies for acute diarrhea is NOT correct?

(A) Breast feeding should be continued as normal
(B) Food should be withheld for 6–12 hours
(C) Fluids can be given to patients who experience vomiting, but small amounts of fluid should be used
(D) Replacement fluids mainly consist of water, sugar, potassium, sodium, and bicarbonate

6. Which of the following products should NOT be used to replenish lost fluids from acute diarrhea?

(A) Pedialyte solution
(B) Kool-Aid
(C) Gatorade (half strength diluted with water)
(D) The World Health Organization (WHO) solution

7. Which of the following statements about adsorbent drugs used for diarrhea is true?

(A) Useful for treatment of severe diarrhea
(B) Very safe because not absorbed systemically
(C) In general, small doses are needed to relieve diarrhea
(D) Kaolin and pectin is considered to be a very effective (category I) adsorbent

8. Which of the following statements concerning traveler's diarrhea (TD) is true?

(A) TD can usually be avoided by not eating raw vegetables, seafood, or eggs when traveling to third-world countries
(B) TD can be prevented by taking one dose of antibiotic one day before a trip
(C) A specie of *Helicobacter pylori* is the primary pathogen responsible for TD
(D) Phillip's Milk of Magnesia is used to prevent/treat TD

9. All of the following items are part of a standard conservative approach to the treatment of a first- or second-degree internal hemorrhoid EXCEPT

(A) Epsom salt sitz baths
(B) psyllium bulk laxatives
(C) avoiding prolonged sitting on the toilet
(D) a topical anesthetic (hemorrhoidal ointment)
(E) injection sclerotherapy

10. All of the following agents are considered close to ideal laxatives EXCEPT

(A) emollient laxatives
(B) bulk-forming laxatives
(C) fiber
(D) stimulant laxatives

11. All of the following rectal symptoms can be treated by over-the-counter (OTC) anorectal products EXCEPT

(A) bleeding
(B) itching
(C) burning
(D) discomfort
(E) irritation

12. All of the following statements about stool softeners are true EXCEPT

(A) there is minimal systemic absorption
(B) the onset of action is usually 1–2 days
(C) they are useful in patients with constipation who have experienced an acute myocardial infarction
(D) they can be taken with little or no water

13. All of the following statements adequately describe bulk-forming laxatives EXCEPT

(A) they produce a much more complete evacuation of constipation than stimulant products
(B) they can cause constipation if not taken with water
(C) they are derived from polysaccharides and resemble fiber (bran) in the mechanism of action
(D) the onset of action is 24–72 hours

14. A patient suffering from acute infectious diarrhea caused by *Shigella* can be managed in all of the following ways EXCEPT

(A) no treatment because signs and symptoms usually resolve in 48 hours
(B) use of glucose solutions (e.g., soda, apple juice) to settle the stomach and decrease the number of stools
(C) avoiding food for at least 6 hours, then slowly increasing fluid intake
(D) using antibiotics (e.g., Bactrim, Doxycycline) for 7 days

Directions: Each item below contains three suggested answers of which **one or more** is correct. Choose the answer

A if **I only** is correct
B if **III only** is correct
C if **I and II** are correct
D if **II and III** are correct
E if **I, II, and III** are correct

15. Which of the following drugs most commonly causes constipation?

I. Ampicillin
II. Narcotic analgesics
III. Drugs possessing anticholinergic properties

16. Which of the following statements about stimulant laxatives is correct?

I. They produce a stool quicker than any other type of laxative
II. They are associated with more adverse effects than any other type of laxative
III. They work by irritating the lining of the colon wall to increase peristalsis and produce a stool

17. When should a patient experiencing diarrhea be referred to a physician by a pharmacist?

I. If the patient has pus or blood in the stool
II. If the patient also suffers from vomiting
III. If the patient has a fever

18. Which of the following statements about adsorbent drugs used for diarrhea are true?

I. They are safe because they are not absorbed systemically
II. Polycarbophil has been found to be the most effective agent
III. In general, small doses are enough to relieve diarrhea

19. A rational conservative treatment of hemorrhoids would include all of the following EXCEPT

(A) sitz baths 15 minutes three times a day
(B) docusate sodium 100 mg BID p.o.
(C) Maalox 30 ml q 4 h p.o.
(D) Vaseline (petrolatum) to area b.i.d.
(E) avoid prolonged sitting on the toilet

20. Patients with anorectal symptoms should sometimes be referred to a physician for further evaluation. Which symptom set below best describes the needs for referral?

(A) Prolapse, severe pain, bleeding
(B) Severe pain, irritation, burning
(C) Bleeding, burning, prolapse
(D) Itching, thrombosis, seepage
(E) Swelling, discomfort, bleeding

21. A 42-year-old man comes into the pharmacy complaining of swelling from his hemorrhoids. Which of the following agents or products would be the pharmacist's best recommendation to treat the patient's complaint?

(A) A hemorrhoidal product containing pramoxine
(B) Vaseline
(C) Hydrocortisone ointment
(D) Preparation H
(E) Either hydrocortisone ointment or Preparation H

22. All of the following symptoms associated with gastroesophageal reflux disease (GERD) may be treated with nonprescription agents EXCEPT

(A) burning sensation located in the lower chest
(B) pain that is worse after meals
(C) pain or difficulty when swallowing
(D) pain that is worse upon lying down at bedtime

23. All of the following are appropriate nonpharmacologic recommendations for patients with gastroesophageal reflux disease (GERD) EXCEPT

(A) avoid foods that irritate the esophagus, such as tomato-based products
(B) eat evening meals immediately before going to bed
(c) stop smoking
(D) lose weight, if appropriate

24. All of the following statements regarding antacid use in gastroesophageal reflux disease (GERD) are correct EXCEPT

(A) The onset of symptom relief with antacids is 1–2 hours
(B) Antacids will relieve symptoms for 1–3 hours
(C) Sodium bicarbonate should not be used in patients with edema, congestive heart failure, and those on low-salt diets
(D) The most frequent side effect of aluminum-magnesium combination antacids is diarrhea

25. All of the following statements regarding use of nonprescription H_2RAs in gastroesophageal reflux disease (GERD) are correct EXCEPT

(A) the most common adverse effects of nonprescription H2RAs are headache, diarrhea, dizziness, and nausea
(B) cimetidine may increase serum concentrations of warfarin, theophylline, and phenytoin
(C) the onset of symptom relief with these agents is 1–2 hours
(D) nonprescription H_2RAs will heal severely damaged esophageal mucosa

26. All of the following statements regarding use of nonprescription products for gastroesophageal reflux disease (GERD) in special populations are correct EXCEPT

(A) nonprescription H_2RAs are not approved for use in children younger than 12 years of age
(B) antacids may be safely used in pregnant patients as long as chronic high doses are avoided
(C) sodium bicarbonate is the preferred antacid in pregnant patients
(D) doses of nonprescription H_2RAs do not need to be reduced in elderly patients

ANSWERS AND EXPLANATIONS

1. The answer is C *[1 B].*
Glycerin, bisacodyl suppository, and phenolphthalein all produce stools in one-half hour to a few hours, whereas psyllium, a bulk-forming laxative, produces stool in 24–72 hours in the same manner as a normal bolus of food or fiber.

2. The answer is D *[1 C 4].*
The popular sodium phosphate enemas (e.g., Fleet) are very effective but have resulted in hyperphosphatemia, hypocalcemia (tetany), hypokalemia, metabolic acidosis, and cardiac death usually due to conduction abnormalities in very small children. This has mainly occurred in children younger than 2 years of age or between 2 and 5 years of age with predisposing factors. These factors include chronic renal disease, anorectal malformations, and/or Hirschprung's disease, which allow phosphate blood concentrations to become abnormally high and potassium and calcium to become low. These conditions predispose these patients to cardiac arrhythmias and potentially death. Therefore, the use of enemas is highly discouraged in children under 5 years of age.

3. The answer is D *[I B 2 d].*
These agents have a long onset of action (24–48 hours); thus, they should never be used for acute constipation but mainly for patients who should not strain to pass hard bowels (e.g., pregnant patients, post-surgical patients, post-MI). However, they have never been found to be more effective than placebo in long-term use.

4. The answer is B *[I B 2 c].*
Stimulant products result in a quicker, more complete, and often more violent evacuation of the bowel than do the bulk-forming agents. Bulk-forming agents are developed from complex sugars, similar to fiber, that provide bulk to increase gastrointestinal motility and water absorption into the bowel. However, patients must take plenty of water to facilitate this absorption of water into the bowel or patients may become more constipated.

5. The answer is B *[II C 1 b].*
The most important part of treating acute diarrhea is the replacement of lost fluids. If patients experience mild-to-moderate fluid loss, replacement can be done with oral rehydration solutions. If fluid loss is severe (more than 10% loss of body weight) and/or severe vomiting, then patients may need intravenous rehydration before oral maintenance fluids can be administered. Oral rehydration solutions can be easily made at home (see Table 33-1) or purchased ready to use (e.g., Pedialyte, Ricelyte, Infalyte, Rehydralyte, Resol). Because the secretory and absorptive mechanisms of the bowel function separately, this allows these oral rehydration solutions to be absorbed during acute episodes of diarrhea, preventing severe dehydration and complications. There has been much controversy regarding the decision to feed or not feed children during acute episodes of diarrhea. Originally, parents were told that children should not receive food, milk-products, or breast milk for 6–48 hours after the onset of diarrhea. Recent information shows that children should remain on their normal diet or breast feeding during episodes of diarrhea because these do not make the diarrhea worse and may actually improve the diarrhea.

6. The answer is B *[II C 1 b].*
Replacement fluids for diarrhea should contain the appropriate amount of electrolytes (K^+, Na^+, Cl^-, citrate) and glucose per specified amount of water, as found in commercially available oral rehydration solutions such as Pedialyte, Rehydralyte. The World Health Organization (WHO) solution can be made easily at home to provide the necessary ingredients. In addition, one-half strength Gatorade will provide the necessary electrolytes and glucose to replenish lost fluids. Kool-Aid does not contain potassium, and carbonated beverages are low in potassium and some too high in glucose.

7. The answer is B *[II C 2 b].*
Adsorbents are not effective for severe diarrhea because they simply cannot adsorb enough water and do not reverse the cause of the diarrhea. Large doses may decrease symptoms slightly, but overall they are not very effective. Of all the adsorbents, polycarbophil is the most effective probably because it can adsorb more water than the other products. However, kaolin and pectin have not been found to be effective (category I) by the FDA. All adsorbents are safe because they are not adsorbed systemically.

8. The answer is A *[II A 2 (1)].*
Traveler's diarrhea (TD) primarily is caused by bacteria (mainly enterotoxin *Escherichia coli*). Prophylaxis and treatment regimens include oral antibiotics (fluoroquinolones, sulfonamides, doxycycline) and bismuth subsalicylate (Pepto-Bismol). *Helicobacter pylori* is the organism shown to contribute to refractory peptic ulcer disease.

9. The answer is E *[III F 1-2].*
A conservative approach to treatment includes sitz baths, the use of bulk laxatives to prevent straining when passing a stool, the avoidance of prolonged sitting on the toilet (as well as other good bowel habits), and the use of an anesthetic hemorrhoidal preparation. If improvement is not seen, more aggressive therapy may need to be pursued (e.g., injection sclerotherapy).

10. The answer is D *[I B 2].*
The ideal laxative is natural (i.e., similar to food) and produces stool on a regular basis. The product produces stool quickly (i.e., in several hours) without adverse effects such as abdominal cramping or the formation of a hard stool, which may be difficult to pass. Products such as fiber or bulk-forming agents produce a stool similar to a bolus of food, without adverse effects. Emollient laxatives (i.e., stool softeners) produce soft stools without difficult defecation. Stimulants produce a stool quickly, but patients often experience severe abdominal cramping and hard stools.

11. The answer is A *[III G 3].*
Because of the possibility that a serious anorectal condition (e.g., anorectal cancer) may cause bleeding, patients with this symptom should be referred to a physician for assessment. The vasoconstrictor agents that are present in some anorectal products may decrease bleeding, but these products cannot be labeled as doing so. Itching, burning, discomfort, and irritation may be abated by various over-the-counter products.

12. The answer is D *[I B 2 d].*
Stool softeners are safe and do not produce any adverse systemic effects. Because stool softeners work as surfactants, they allow absorption of water into the stool, which makes the stool softer and easier to pass. These products are useful in patients who should avoid straining to pass hard stools (e.g., post-myocardial infarction patients) because straining may be stressful to the patient. Each dose must be taken with 8 ounces of water.

13. The answer is A *[I B 2 a, c].*
Stimulant products result in a quicker, more complete, and often more violent evacuation of the bowel than do the bulk-forming agents. Bulk-forming agents are developed from complex sugars similar to fiber, which provide bulk to increase gastrointestinal motility and increase water absorption into the bowel. However, patients must drink plenty of water to facilitate the absorption of water into the bowel, or they may become more constipated.

14. The answer is B *[II C; Table 33-3].*
Giving highly osmotic solutions of glucose (e.g., soda, fruit juice) can result in more water absorbed into the intestinal tract and, thus, further diarrhea. Many cases of diarrhea resolve within 48 hours without treatment. People with diarrhea can avoid food for at least 6 hours, then increase their fluid intake slowly. Severe cases of infectious diarrhea can be treated with antibiotics or antiprotozoals, depending on the organism that caused the episode.

15. The answer is D (II, III) *[I A 2 d].*
Opiate analgesics (e.g., narcotics) and drugs with anticholinergic properties decrease bowel motility, which results in increased water absorption from the intestinal tract. This can cause a harder, drier stool, which results in constipation. Ampicillin in often poorly absorbed from the intestinal tract and can alter the flora of the intestinal bowel. This destruction of bowel organisms causes increased secretions into the bowel, which results in diarrhea.

16. The answer is D (II, III) *[I B 2 c].*
Stimulant laxatives do have a quick onset of action but not any quicker than the saline laxatives, which usually work in 4–6 hours. The mechanism of action for stimulant laxatives is that they irritate the lining of the colon wall, which increases peristalsis and produces a stool. These laxatives are associated with more adverse effects than other laxatives.

17. The answer is E (all) *[II B 2].*
Patients with pus or blood in the stool, vomiting, or fever may be suffering from severe bacterial diarrhea and may lose large amounts of fluid, which could result in severe dehydration.

18. The answer is C (I, II) *[II C 2 b].*
Large doses of adsorbents are needed to decrease symptoms slightly, but overall these agents are not very effective. Adsorbents are not effective for severe diarrhea because they cannot adsorb enough water and do not eliminate the cause. Of all the adsorbents, polycarbophil has been found to be the most effective, probably because it can adsorb more water than other products. All adsorbents are safe because they are not adsorbed systemically.

19. The answer is C *[III F 1].*
Sitz baths can be soothing to the patient's anal mucosa. Docusate as a stool softener helps prevent the patient from straining at defecation. Petrolatum is a safe and effective protectant to treat minor hemorrhoidal symptoms. Prolonged sitting on the toilet increases pressure on the hemorrhoidal tissue. Maalox is an antacid that may relieve stomach distress from a peptic ulcer, but this will not effect the hemorrhoids.

20. The answer is A *[III G].*
Symptoms in the anorectal area that are amenable to treatment with OTC agents and that may be caused by hemorrhoids include discomfort, burning, swelling, pain, itching, irritation, and soreness. Symptoms of bleeding, prolapse, seepage, thrombosis, and severe pain require an evaluation by a physician.

21. The answer is E *[III G; Table 33-1].*
The only safe and effective ingredients available OTC to treat swelling are the vasoconstrictor agents and hydrocortisone. Pramoxine is a local anesthetic. Vaseline contains petrolatum, which is a protectant. Hydrocortisone is effective for swelling in addition to itching and discomfort. Preparation H contains three protectants and a vasoconstrictor and is, therefore, useful for swelling also.

22. The answer is C *[1 A 2–3, 6].*
Pain on swallowing often suggests severe esophageal mucosal damage, which would require prescription medications for healing. Difficulty on swallowing may indicate an esophageal stricture, cancer, or motor disorder. All of these conditions require diagnosis and treatment by a health care provider.

23. The answer is B *[I B 1 a–k].*
Patients should be instructed to eat evening meals at least 3 hours before going to bed. This allows sufficient time for gastric emptying, so that the volume of refluxed material will be smaller and less irritating to the esophagus.

24. The answer is A *[I B 2 a].*
One of the major advantages of antacid use in heartburn is its quick onset of action. Most patients with mild gastroesophageal reflux disease (GERD) will experience relief from antacids within 5–15 minutes of administration.

25. The answer is D *[I B 2 c–d]*
Nonprescription doses of H_2RAs are too low to heal esophageal damage. Esophageal mucosal damage is very difficult to heal and requires very high doses of H_2RAs that are available only by prescription. Alternatively, proton pump inhibitors, which completely suppress acid secretion, may be used to heal esophageal mucosal damage.

26. The answer is C *[I C 2].*
Sodium bicarbonate should be avoided in pregnant patients because the high sodium load may cause systemic alkalosis, edema, and/or weight gain.

34
OTC Menstrual, Vaginal, and Contraceptive Agents

Constance A. McKenzie
Larry N. Swanson

I. MENSTRUATION AND MENSTRUAL PRODUCTS

A. Introduction. Menstruation is a cyclic, physiologic discharge of blood and mucus through the vagina of a nonpregnant woman. The menstrual cycle eliminates a mature, unfertilized egg and prepares the endometrium for the possible implantation of a fertilized egg the following month. The **average duration** of the menstrual cycle is 28 days. The duration of menstrual flow is 3–7 days.

B. Menstrual abnormalities

1. **Dysmenorrhea** is painful menstruation.
   a. **Types**
      (1) **Primary dysmenorrhea** is pain associated with menstruation with the absence of identifiable pelvic disease. It is prompted by increased levels of prostaglandins in the menstrual fluids.
      (2) **Secondary dysmenorrhea** is associated with an underlying pelvic disorder.
   b. **Symptoms** of dysmenorrhea often include nausea, vomiting, diarrhea, headache, dizziness, and lower abdominal cramping.
   c. **Treatment**
      (1) **Recommendation of therapy** should be based on the patient's assessment of the degree of pain. Pain associated with dysmenorrhea generally tapers within 2 days. Prolonged pain may be associated with an underlying problem, and patients should be referred to a physician.
      (2) **Agents** for the relief of dysmenorrhea include:
         (a) **Analgesics** are used as primary treatment of dysmenorrhea and for relief of cramping associated with premenstrual syndrome (PMS) [see I B 4]. Analgesic treatment with aspirin or acetaminophen may begin at the onset of the menstrual period and continue throughout the menstrual flow. Nonsteroidal anti-inflammatory drugs (NSAIDs) also are approved for treatment. The dosage of ibuprofen (e.g., Advil, Midol IB, Nuprin) is 200 mg every 4–6 hours with the maximum not exceeding 1200 mg per day. Other NSAIDS include ketoprofen (e.g., Orudis-KT, Actron) 12.5 mg every 4–6 hours not to exceed 25 mg in a 4–6 hour period or 75 mg in 24 hours and naproxen (Aleve) 200 mg every 8–12 hours not to exceed 600 mg per day.
         (b) **Diuretics** are **recommended** by the Food and Drug Administration (FDA) for use in eliminating water during premenstrual and menstrual periods. When administered approximately 5 days before menses, diuretics help relieve bloating, excess water, cramps, and tension. Included in this category are ammonium chloride, caffeine, and pamabrom.
            (i) **Ammonium chloride** (NH_4Cl) is an acid-forming salt often used in combination with caffeine. Up to 3 grams of NH_4Cl per day can be administered in three divided doses per day. Larger doses are often associated with gastrointestinal (GI) symptoms. Over-the-counter (OTC) products include Aqua Ban and Aqua Ban Plus, which contains NH_4Cl and caffeine.
            (ii) **Caffeine,** a xanthine derivative, promotes diuresis by inhibiting tubular reabsorption of sodium and chloride. The **recommended dosage** is 100–200 mg every 3–4 hours. **Side effects** associated with caffeine use are GI disturbances and CNS stimulation.

(iii) **Pamabrom** (Midol PMS, Pamprin) is a theophylline derivative often used in combination with analgesics and antihistamines. Dosages should not exceed 200 mg per day.

2. **Amenorrhea** is an absence of menstruation. The development of primary or secondary amenorrhea requires physician evaluation.

3. **Intermenstrual pain** and **bleeding** generally occur at midcycle and may last from several hours to days. Pain is often associated with ovulation (mittelschmerz). Therapy consists of non-prescription analgesics. Patients with pain lasting longer than 2 days should be referred to a physician.

4. **Premenstrual syndrome (PMS)**
   a. **Symptoms** (e.g., marked mood swings, fatigue, appetite changes, bloating) begin 1–7 days before the onset of menses.
   b. **Nonpharmacologic therapy** includes regular exercise and reduction of stress factors. Patients experiencing symptoms abnormal to their cycle should be referred to a physician.
   c. **Pharmacologic treatment.** The efficacy and safety of pharmacologic treatment of PMS are aimed at the proposed etiologies (e.g., a drop in progesterone concentrations, high levels of prolactin, elevated estrogen concentrations, deficiencies of vitamins A or B_6, or an underlying disorder) and are not well studied. Although clinical trials do not support the efficacy of vitamins A and B_6, both have been used for the treatment of PMS. Nonprescription diuretics are commonly used to reduce fluid accumulation associated with PMS. Prescription drug products that have been studied in the management of PMS include benzodiazepines, monoamine oxidase inhibitors, tricyclic antidepressants, and fluoxetine.

C. **Toxic shock syndrome (TSS)** is a rare but sometimes fatal disease often associated with menstruation.

1. TSS can be categorized either as menstrual or nonmenstrual with approximately two-thirds of cases associated with menstruation. TSS is known to occur in both men and women.

2. This condition usually affects women under 30 years of age who use tampons. Women between the ages of 15 and 19 years are at the highest risk.

3. TSS is characterized by an abrupt onset (8–12 hours) of flulike symptoms (e.g., high fever, myalgia, vomiting, diarrhea).

4. TSS results from an exotoxin produced by staphylococcus aureus.

5. The **primary risk factor** for TSS is the **use of tampons.** Additional risk factors include barrier contraceptives (e.g., diaphragms, cervical sponges).

6. When TSS is suspected, patients should be hospitalized immediately. To lower the risk of TSS, women should use lower-absorbency tampons and alternate the use of tampons with feminine pads.

II. VAGINAL PRODUCTS

A. Yeast infections

1. **General considerations**
   a. **Occurrence.** Approximately 75% of women will experience a yeast infection at least once, whereas 15%–20% may have a recurrence.
   b. **Cause.** The **most common cause** of this type of vaginitis is *Candida albicans.*
   c. **Predisposing factors** for vaginal candidiasis include antibiotics, diabetes, pregnancy, and sexual intercourse.
   d. **Symptoms** include vaginal burning, discomfort, itching, or abnormal vaginal discharge.

2. **Pharmacologic treatment**
   a. **Physical exam** by a physician is recommended for initial diagnosis.
   b. **Nonprescription agents** are recommended only for patients who have had a prior yeast infection and who can potentially diagnose and self-medicate.

c. Available nonprescription therapy includes the imidazole antifungal agents Gyne Lotrimin (clotrimazole), Monistat 7 (miconazole nitrate), and Femstat 3 (butoconazole nitrate).
d. Infections should be treated for 7 consecutive days when using Gyne Lotrimin or Monistat 7. Femstat 3 is the only imidazole indicated for 3 days of therapy.
e. Patients should refrain from intercourse during therapy.
f. If medication causes burning, if patient presents with a fever, lower abdominal, back or shoulder pain, if symptoms worsen, if there is no response to treatment, or with frequent recurrence (2 months), a physician should be contacted.
g. Pregnant women should consult their physician and not self-medicate.

B. **Feminine hygiene products.** There are a variety of feminine hygiene products available for cleansing and controlling the odor associated with vaginal discharge.

1. Vaginal douches irrigate the vagina and can be used for cleansing, soothing and refreshing, as an astringent, or to produce a mucolytic effect.

2. Vaginal suppositories are used for soothing and refreshing, to relieve minor irritations, and to reduce the number of pathogenic microorganisms.

III. OTC CONTRACEPTIVES

A. **Introduction.** The **efficacy** and **pregnancy rates** for various means of contraception depend greatly upon the **degree of compliance.** Table 34-1 gives ranges of pregnancy rates reported for various means of contraception.

Table 34-1. Pregnancy Rates for Various Means of Contraception (%)[1]

Method of contraception	Lowest expected[2]	Typical[3]
Oral Contraceptives		3
Combined	0.1	nd
Progestin only	0.5	nd
Mechanical/Chemical		
Levonorgestrel implant	0.2	0.2
Medroxyprogesterone injection	0.3	0.3
IUD		
Progesterone	2	nd
Copper T 380A	0.8	nd
Condom		
Without spermicide	2	12
With spermicide[4]	1.8	4–6
Spermicide alone	3	21
Diaphragm (with spermicidal cream or gel)	6	18
Female condom	2–4	12–25
Periodic abstinence (i.e., rhythm; all methods)	1–9	20
Sterility		
Vasectomy	0.1	0.15
Tubal ligation	0.2	0.4
No contraception	85	85

nd = no data.

[1]During first year of continuous use.

[2]Best guess of percentage expected to experience an accidental pregnancy among couples who initiate a method and use it consistently and correctly.

[3]A "typical" couple who initiate a method and experience an accidental pregnancy.

[4]Used as a separate product (not in condom package).

Adapted from Facts and Comparisons, St. Louis, April 1995, p. 535.

B. Methods of contraception that may make use of nonprescription products or devices include:

1. **Periodic abstinence,** also referred to as the **rhythm method, natural family planning,** or **ovulation detection method.** The various natural family planning methods allow the patient to monitor the natural physiologic signs that can in many women predict the fertile period (periovulatory phase of the menstrual cycle), enabling the couple to avoid coital exposure at that time. These methods are based on reproductive anatomy and physiology and are applied according to the signs and symptoms naturally occurring in the menstrual cycle. Calculations of the period of fertility take into account the **sperm viability** in the female reproductive tract, which is estimated to average **2–3 days** (with a range of 2–7 days), and the **fertile period of the ovum,** which is estimated to be **24 hours.** Thus, the span of fertility may be from **7 days before ovulation to 3 days after. Disadvantages** to the rhythm method (but necessary to ensure efficacy) include both the **long periods of abstinence** and the **charting of menses** that is required. Methods of natural family planning and periodic abstinence include temperature method, calendar method, Billings method, and symptothermal method.
   a. **Temperature method.** Basal temperature determination makes use of a **basal thermometer,** which can be purchased without a prescription. The thermometer covers the range of temperature from 96°F to 100°F, with 0.1°F gradations.
      (1) The significance of basal temperature determination lies in the fact that within 24 hours preceding ovulation, there is a **moderate drop in the basal temperature** followed by a **noticeable rise in the body temperature,** usually about 24 hours after ovulation. This rise is usually maintained for the remainder of the cycle and is thought to be due to the thermogenic properties of **progesterone,** the hormone indicative of the transition from the ovulatory phase to the luteal phase. Therefore, ovulation is represented by the transition of the falling temperature to the rising temperature.
      (2) For many women, **abstinence** should be practiced from approximately 5 days after the onset of menses until 3 days after the transition in temperature.
      (3) To minimize any fluctuation nonreflective of basal temperature, the thermometer should be **shaken down** the evening before and kept at bedside. Because the basal temperature reflects the amount of heat radiation when the body is at its metabolic low, the temperature should be taken first thing in the morning (i.e., before any activity). The thermometer may be placed on the tongue, in the rectum, or in the vagina (the temperature should always be taken from the same place) and should be left undisturbed for at least 5 minutes. Infection, tension, a restless night, or any type of excessive movement can cause variations nonreflective of the basal temperature.
   b. The **calendar method** estimates the possible day of ovulation. **Abstinence** should be practiced during the period around ovulation when there may be a fertilizable egg present. Whereas the calendar rhythm method was used for several decades, it has not been promoted as a method of natural family planning for many years. Although women who have regular menstrual cycles are able to use the calendar rhythm method successfully, women with irregular cycles, women who are breast feeding, or women with postponed ovulation cannot depend on the calendar rhythm method.
      (1) For a span of **approximately 1 year,** the patient records her menstruation dates on a calendar.
      (2) Calendar charting allows women to calculate the onset and duration of their fertile period—the time during which a viable egg is available for fertilization by sperm. Calculation of the fertile period rests on three assumptions:
         (a) **Ovulation** occurs on day **14 (plus or minus 2 days) before the onset of the next menses**
         (b) **Sperm remain viable for 2–3 days**
         (c) **The ovum survives for 24 hours**
      (3) The calendar is then reviewed to determine the length of her shortest and longest cycle.
         (a) Eighteen days should be subtracted from the number of days of the shortest cycle. This number should correspond with the first possible fertile day in any given cycle —14 + 2 = 16 days; 16 + 2 = 18 days (viability of sperm) [see III B 1 b].
         (b) Eleven days should be subtracted from the number of days of the longest cycle. This number should correspond with the last possible fertile day in any given cycle—14 − 2 = 12 days; 12 − 1 = 11 days (viability of ova) [see III B 1 b].
      (4) **Abstinence** should be practiced from the first possible fertile day through the last possible fertile day.

(5) **Example.** Assume the shortest number of days between two consecutive menses is 25 and the longest number of days between two consecutive menses is 32. Eighteen days subtracted from 25 days (the shortest cycle) equals 7 (or day 7). Eleven days subtracted from 32 days (the longest cycle) equals 21 (or day 21). Therefore, abstinence should be practiced from day 7 through and including day 21 of each cycle.

c. The **Billings** method of rhythm is based on the principle that the normal, thick, creamy white vaginal mucus becomes clear and tenacious around the time of ovulation—much like a raw egg white.

(1) The woman should watch for this change in mucus consistency and practice abstinence around the time of ovulation.

(2) The woman should consider herself fertile for 3–4 days after the peak change.

d. The **symptothermal** method, rather than relying on a single physiologic index, uses several indices to determine the fertile period.

(1) The **most common** calendar calculations and **changes in the cervical mucus** are used to estimate the **onset of the fertile period.**

(2) Changes in the mucus or basal temperature are used to estimate the end of the fertile period.

(3) Because several indices need to be monitored, this method is more difficult to learn than the single-index method, but it is more effective than the cervical-mucus method (i.e., Billings method) alone.

2. **Spermicidal agents** are composed of an **active spermicidal chemical,** which immobilizes or kills sperm, and an **insert base** (e.g., foam, cream or jelly), which localizes the spermicidal chemical in proximity to the cervical os.

a. **Mode of action.** These agents work by disrupting the sperm membrane and by decreasing the ability of sperm to metabolize fructose.

b. **Active ingredients** include **nonoxynol-9** or **octoxynol-9.**

(1) Both are considered safe and effective by the FDA.

(2) Side effects (e.g., sensation of warmth, rare allergic reactions) are minimal.

(3) There are no significant differences in birth-defect rates between users and nonusers.

c. **Effects against sexually transmitted diseases (STDs).** Nonoxynol-9 helps to inhibit a variety of sexually transmissible organisms, including those responsible for gonorrhea, chlamydial infection, candidiasis, genital herpes, syphilis, trichomoniasis, and AIDS.

d. **Dosage forms. Contraceptive spermicides** offer the greatest variety within one specific method of contraception, being available in various forms, including the following. (Table 34-2).

(1) **Creams** and **jellies** are used with a diaphragm. The concentration of spermicide is less than the necessary 8% to be employed as a single contraceptive method.

Table 34-2. Spermicides

Representative Products (Brand Names)	Spermicidal Agent	Comments
Film		
VCF (Vaginal Contraceptive Film)	Nonoxynol-9	Contraceptive protection begins 15 minutes after insertion; remains effective no more than 1 hour.
Foam		
Delfen, Emko, Koromex	Nonoxynol-9	Contraceptive protection is immediate; remains effective for at least 1 hour.
Emko Because, Emko Prefil	Nonoxynol-9	
Jellies and Creams		
Conceptrol, Delfen, Koromex Jel, Ortho Gynol II, Ramses	Nonoxynol-9	Contraceptive protection is immediate. When used alone remains effective at least 1 hour; used with diaphragm or cap remains effective at least 6–8 hours.
Koromex Cream, Ortho Gynol	Octoxynol	
Conceptrol Jel	Nonoxynol-9	
Suppositories and Tablets		
Encare, Intercept, Koromex Inserts, Semicid	Nonoxynol-9	Contraceptive protection begins 10–15 minutes after insertion; remains effective no more than 1 hour.

Adapted from Hatcher RA: *Contraceptive Technology 1994–1996,* 16th ed. NY, Irvington Publishers, 1994, p. 180.

(2) **Foams** disperse better into the vagina and over the cervical opening. They usually contain a higher concentration of spermicide (i.e., the optimal concentration of 8% or higher). Volume differences among brands may require various dosage amounts. If vaginal or penile irritation develops, another brand should be tried.

(a) The can should be shaken vigorously 20 times before use.

(b) The foam should be inserted intravaginally about two-thirds the length of the applicator, and the contents should be discharged.

(c) Foam should be reapplied during prolonged intercourse (e.g., that lasting longer than 1 hour) and before every subsequent act of intercourse.

(d) In order to ensure efficacy, at least 8 hours should pass before douching because this may dilute the spermicide effect or even "force" sperm into the cervix.

(3) **Suppositories and foaming tablets.** These agents are both small and convenient. Although solid at room temperature, suppositories melt at body temperature, whereas foaming tablets effervesce.

(a) The tablets should be wetted before insertion, which may create a sensation of warmth.

(b) The tablet or suppository should be inserted high into the vagina, and approximately 10–15 minutes should pass before intercourse.

(c) Intercourse must occur within 1 hour, or the dose must be repeated.

(d) Another tablet or suppository should be inserted before each repeated act of intercourse.

(e) In order to ensure efficacy, 6–8 hours after the last act of intercourse should pass before douching.

(4) **Sponges.** The nonprescription vaginal contraceptive sponge containing one gram of nonoxynol-9 (Today) was moistened in water and inserted into the vagina near the cervix. The only manufacturer of sponges in the United States (Whitehall-Robins) **discontinued production in early 1995** because of the costliness of upgrading its manufacturing plant to comply with the FDA's stringent air and water purity rules.

(5) **Film** comes as small paper-thin sheets (e.g., VCF). It is inserted into the vagina; 15 minutes must pass before intercourse.

(6) **Bioadhesive contraceptive gel** (Advantage 24 Bioadhesive Gel) contains nonoxynol-9 enmeshed in a matrix of carbofil polymer. The adhesive properties of this polymer enable the product to adhere more readily than other dosage forms to the cervix. The product may be applied up to 24 hours before intercourse, which may increase spontaneity. It must be reapplied, however, for each act of intercourse.

3. **Condoms** are used to prevent transmission of sperm into the vagina.

a. **Types.** They are made of latex rubber, processed collagenous lamb caecum sheaths (lambskin), or polyurethane.

(1) **Latex** condoms may help prevent the transmission of many STDs. They are usually packaged with the following label "when used properly, the latex condom may prevent the transmission of many STDs such as syphilis, gonorrhea, chlamydia infections, genital herpes, and AIDS."

(a) Latex affords greater elasticity than lambskin, and latex condoms are more likely to remain in place on the penis.

(b) Various types are available (e.g., lubricated, ribbed, colored), including some with spermicide. There is a standard size, but recently smaller and larger versions were put on the market.

(i) Latex condoms are available with a plain end or with a reservoir tip (sometimes designated as "enz"). The reservoir tip provides room for the ejaculate; however, a space may be left when using the plain-end condom, which accommodates the fluid just as effectively.

(ii) The **prelubricated condom** helps prevent dyspareunia in a couple with insufficient natural lubrication. Prelubrication decreases the risk of tearing the condom. However, the extra lubrication may be excessive, to the extent of lessening sexual fulfillment in a couple who have adequate natural lubrication or when contraceptive foam is also used.

(iii) Latex rubber may cause an allergic reaction, especially with continued exposure.

(2) **Lambskin** condoms are **not** considered as effective as latex condoms (and cannot be labeled as such) in preventing the transmission of STDs, including AIDS. The

lambskin condoms are structured to consist of membranes that reveal layers of fibers crisscrossing in various patterns. This gives the lambskin strength, but also allows for an occasional pore. Therefore, lambskin may allow HIV, which is smaller than a sperm, to pass through.

(a) Lambskin has less elasticity than latex, and lambskin condoms may slip off the penis.

(b) Lambskin affords greater sensitivity than latex.

(c) Lambskin condoms are more expensive than latex condoms.

(3) A **polyurethane condom** (Avanti) is available for men and is marketed for individuals who are allergic to latex. The effectiveness of this condom in terms of prevention of pregnancy and STD is unclear at this time.

b. Advantages and disadvantages. The relative accessibility, ease of transport, and low cost make condoms an attractive method of contraception. However, the coital act must be interrupted to apply the condom, and often one or both partners complain of a partial or complete decrease in sensation.

c. Use

(1) The female external genitalia should not be touched with the exposed penis, and the vagina should not be penetrated, until the condom is unrolled onto the erect penis.

(2) The condom should be unrolled onto the penis as far as it will go. With the plain-end condom, a space between the tip of the penis and the tip of the condom should be allowed to catch the ejaculate.

(3) With either reservoir-tip or plain-end condoms, the tip of the condom must be held between the thumb and index finger to avoid trapping air while unrolling the condom onto the penis. (The space will decrease the likelihood of both rupture secondary to pressure and regurgitation of the ejaculate onto the external genitalia.)

(4) Proper lubrication to minimize the possibility of tearing can be ensured by using either a lubricated condom or by applying K-Y jelly, spermicidal cream, or jelly to either the condom or the woman's genitalia. [Petroleum jelly (Vaseline) should never be used because it causes deterioration of the rubber and is a poor lubricant.] Spermicidal foam, cream, or jelly is an excellent adjunctive contraceptive.

(5) **Before the penis becomes flaccid,** it must be withdrawn from the vagina and the condom eased off. The **condom** should be handled with special care so as not to lose it into the vagina or spill any of the ejaculatory fluid onto the external genitalia.

(6) A condom should never be reused.

(7) Condoms should not be stored near excessive heat.

(8) If the condom should break or leak, spermicide foam should be immediately inserted vaginally.

(9) Do not buy or use condoms that have passed their expiration date.

(10) Be sure to store condoms in a cool, dry place, out of direct sunlight. The glove compartment of a car is not a good place to store condoms. Do not store condoms in pockets, purses, or wallets for more than a few hours.

4. The **female condom** (Reality) is a **disposable polyurethane sheath** that fits into the vagina and **provides protection from pregnancy and STDs.** The sheath resembles a plastic vaginal pouch and consists of an **inner ring,** which is inserted into the vagina near the cervix much like a diaphragm, whereas the **outer ring** remains outside the vagina, covering the labia. The condom is prelubricated, and additional lubricant is provided for use if needed. The polyurethane sheath is **stronger** and probably **less likely to tear or break** than the latex sheath of male condoms. Theoretically, it might be more effective than the male condom in preventing transmission of diseases such as herpes because it protects the labia and the base of the penis from contact with each other.

5. The diaphragm is a contraceptive device that is self-inserted into the vagina to block access of sperm to the cervix. It requires a prescription but must be used in conjunction with a nonprescription spermicide to seal off crevices between the vaginal wall and the device.

a. The diaphragm is held in place by the spring tension of a wire rim encased by rubber. When positioned properly, the diaphragm forms a flexible dome to cover the cervix, the sides pressing against the vaginal muscle wall and the pubic bone.

b. There are **four types** of diaphragms including the **coil spring,** the **flat spring,** the **arcing spring,** and a **wide-seal rim.** The tone of vaginal muscles as well as the position of the uterus and adjacent organs usually determine the type of diaphragm necessary.

c. Sizes of the diaphragm range from 50 mm to 95 mm in diameter, in 5-mm gradations

d. Use

(1) The diaphragm plus spermicide can be inserted as long as 6 hours before coitus. The device should be left in place for at least 6 hours after intercourse, but no longer than 24 hours. Additional spermicide is required for repeated intercourse.

(2) Before inserting the diaphragm, one teaspoonful (2–3 inch ribbon) of spermicidal cream or jelly is spread over the inside of the rubber dome.

(3) Also, spermicide is spread around the rim to permit a good seal between the diaphragm and the vaginal wall. (For added protection, it is applied outside of the dome.)

(4) To ensure efficacy, the diaphragm should not be removed for 6–8 hours after intercourse.

e. Proper care

(1) The diaphragm should be washed with soap and water, rinsed thoroughly, and dried with a towel.

(2) It should be dusted with cornstarch and kept in its original container (away from heat).

6. The **cervical cap** is the prescription rubber device smaller than a diaphragm, that fits over the cervix like a thimble. It is more difficult to fit than the diaphragm.

   a. It remains effective for more than one episode of intercourse, without adding more spermicide.

   b. The cap should be filled one-third full of spermicide cream or jelly; the spermicide is then applied to the rim.

   c. The cervical cap may be left in place for a maximum of 48 hours and should be left in place at least 8 hours after intercourse.

STUDY QUESTIONS

Directions: The numbered items in this section are followed by answers or by completions of the statement. Select the **one** lettered answer or completion that is **best.**

1. For how many consecutive days should a yeast infection be treated?

(A) 3
(B) 5
(C) 7
(D) 10

2. All of the following statements regarding contraceptives are correct EXCEPT

(A) using the basal temperature method, intercourse should be avoided for a full 6 days after the noted temperature transition
(B) if a condom should break or leak, one could recommend immediate insertion of a vaginal spermicide foam
(C) vaginal spermicides may kill many of the causative agents of sexually transmitted disease
(D) latex condoms are the type that can be labeled for the prevention of HIV transmission
(E) nonoxynol-9 and octoxynol-9 are the two safe and effective United States-marketed vaginal spermicides

3. All of the following statements concerning the vaginal spermicides are correct EXCEPT

(A) used without a condom or diaphragm, it is recommended that the nonoxynol-9 concentration should be at least 8%
(B) foams probably disperse the spermicide throughout the vaginal canal better than cream or jelly forms
(C) douching should not occur for 6–8 hours after the last intercourse since this may dilute the spermicide effect or even "force" sperm into the cervix
(D) evidence to date shows no definite link between these agents and birth defects
(E) none; all of the above statements are correct

4. All of the following statements concerning contraception or contraceptive agents are correct EXCEPT

(A) progesterone is apparently responsible for the increase in basal temperature after ovulation
(B) Vaseline should not be used as a lubricant with latex condoms
(C) using a condom alone is more effective as a contraceptive than taking a combination oral contraceptive
(D) according to Billings method, vaginal mucus appears like raw egg white at around the time of ovulation
(E) sperm may be viable for up to 7 days in the female reproductive tract with the right conditions

Directions: Question 5 below contains three suggested answers of which **one or more** is correct. Choose the answer

A if **I only** is correct
B if **III only** is correct
C if **I and II** are correct
D if **II and III** are correct
E if **I, II, and III** are correct

5. Which of the following statements about nonprescription treatment of vaginal infections are true?

I. Physical exam by a physician is recommended for initial diagnosis
II. Pregnant women should consult their physician and not self medicate
III. Patients need not refrain from intercourse

Directions: The group of items in this section consists of lettered options followed by a set of numbered items. For each item, select the **one** lettered option that is most closely associated with it. Each lettered option may be selected once, more than once, or not at all.

Questions 6–7

Match the following primary nonprescription treatments with the correct drug.

(A) Diuretics
(B) Salicylates
(C) Nonsteroid anti-inflammatory drugs (NSAIDs)
(D) Narcotic analgesics

6. The primary nonprescription pharmacologic treatment for pain associated with dysmenorrhea

7. Recommended by the FDA for elimination of water before and during menstruation

ANSWERS AND EXPLANATIONS

1. The answer is C *[II A 2].*
The recommended length of therapy with imidazole antifungal agents, which are the primary treatment for yeast infections, is 7 days. A physician should be contacted for those patients who do not respond to nonprescription therapy.

2. The answer is A *[III B 1 b (1)].*
Intercourse should be avoided for a full 3 days after the noted temperature transition. All of the other statements are correct.

3. The answer is E *[III B 2].*
Statements A–D are correct.

4. The answer is C *[Table 34-1].*
The most effective contraceptive product available today is the combination oral contraceptive. All of the other statements (A, B, D, and E) are correct.

5. The answer is C *[II A].*
Physical exam by a physician is always recommended for initial diagnosis. Nonprescription agents are recommended only for patients who have had a prior yeast infection and who can potentially accurately diagnose and self-medicate. Pregnant women should also consult their physician and not self-medicate. Patients should refrain from intercourse during therapy.

6–7. The answers are: 6-C *[I B 1 c (2) (b)],* **7-A** *[I B 1 c (2) (a)].*
Nonsteroidal anti-inflammatory drugs (NSAIDs) are approved by the FDA for the treatment of primary dysmenorrhea. For premenstrual and menstrual relief of water retention, bloating, and tension, the FDA has approved OTC diuretics.

35
Clinical Toxicology

John J. Ponzillo

I. OVERVIEW

A. This chapter is intended to provide the reader with an overview of the management of various toxic exposures. Emergency medical services (EMS) should be immediately contacted to provide advanced life support for patients with unstable vital signs resulting from a poisoning exposure. Additionally, these patients should be referred to a hospital for follow up.

B. Definitions

1. **Clinical toxicology**—focuses on the effects of substances in patients caused by accidental poisonings or intentional overdoses of medications, drugs of abuse, household products, or various other chemicals
2. **Intoxication**—toxicity associated with any chemical substance
3. **Poisoning**—a clinical toxicity secondary to accidental exposure
4. **Overdose**—an intentional exposure with the intent of causing self-injury or death

C. Epidemiology

1. Annually, approximately 8 million people are poisoned; 600,000 attempt suicide, accounting for 11,894 deaths and 218,500 hospitalizations.
2. In 1992, more than 1.8 million accidental and intentional poisonings were reported to the American Association of Poison Control Centers (AAPCC). A single substance was implicated in 93.3% of reports. The majority of poison exposures (87.1%) were accidental.

D. Information resources

1. **Computerized databases**
   a. **Poisindex** is a computerized CD-ROM database that is updated quarterly and is a primary resource for poison control centers.
   b. **TOMES** (Toxicologic, Occupational Medicine and Environmental Series) provides information on industrial chemicals.
2. **Printed publications.** Textbooks and manuals provide useful information regarding the assessment and treatment of patients exposed to various substances, although their usefulness is limited by the lag time of information published in the primary literature reaching updated editions.
   a. Ellenhorn MJ, Barecloux DG, eds. *Medical Toxicology: Diagnosis and Treatment of Human Poisonings.* 1st ed. New York: Elsevier Science Publishing Co., 1988.
   b. Haddad LM, Winchester JF, eds. *Clinical Management of Poisoning and Drug Overdose.* 2nd ed. Philadelphia: WB Saunders, 1990.
   c. Goldfrank L, ed. *Toxicologic Emergencies.* 5th ed. Norwalk, CT: Appleton and Lange: 1995.
   d. Grant WM. *Toxicology of the Eye.* 33rd ed. Springfield, IL: Charles C Thomas, 1986.
3. **Poison control centers.** Poison control centers accredited by the AAPCC provide information to the general public and health care providers. These centers are the most reliable and up-to-date sources of information and as such, their phone number should be readily available.

II. GENERAL MANAGEMENT

A. Supportive care and "ABCs." Evaluating and supporting vital functions (airway, breathing, circulation) are the mandatory first steps in the initial management of drug ingestions, and only after stabilization is begun should the specific issue of poisoning be addressed.

B. Treatment for patients with **depressed mental status** includes:

1. To rule out or treat hypoglycemia, 50 ml of 50% dextrose in adults and 1 ml/kg in children, intravenously
2. Thiamine 100 mg intravenous (IV) push (Glucose can precipitate the Wernicke-Korsakoff syndrome in thiamine-deficient patients.)
3. Naloxone 0.8–1.2 mg IV push, if opiate ingestion is suspected

C. Obtaining a history of exposure

1. **Identify** the substance(s) ingested, the route of exposure, quantity ingested, time since ingestion, signs and symptoms of overdose, and any associated illness or injury. **Corroborate** history and other physical evidence (e.g., pill containers) from prehospital providers.
2. **Neurologic examination** evaluates any seizures, alterations in consciousness, confusion, ataxia, slurred speech, tremor, headache, or syncope.
3. **Cardiopulmonary examination** evaluates any syncope, palpitations, cough, chest pain, shortness of breath, burning or irritation of the upper airway.
4. **Gastrointestinal (GI) examination** evaluates any abdominal pain, nausea, vomiting, diarrhea, or difficulty in swallowing.
5. **Past medical history includes:**
   a. Medications including nonprescription substances
   b. Alcohol or drug abuse
   c. Psychiatric history
   d. Allergies
   e. Occupational or hobby exposures
   f. Travel
   g. Prior ingestions
   h. Social history with potential for domestic violence or neglect
   i. Last normal menstrual period or pregnancy

D. Routine laboratory assessment

1. Complete blood cell count (CBC)
2. Serum electrolytes
3. Blood urea nitrogen (BUN); serum creatinine (SCr)
4. Blood glucose
5. Urinalysis
6. Electrocardiogram (ECG)
7. Chest roentgenogram

E. Toxicology laboratory tests

1. **Advantages**
   a. Can help confirm or **determine** the presence of a particular agent
   b. **Predict** the anticipated toxic effects or severity of exposure to some poisons
   c. Confirm or **distinguish** differential or contributing diagnosis
   d. Occasionally help **guide therapy**
2. **Disadvantages**
   a. These tests cannot provide a specific diagnosis for all patients.
   b. All possible intoxicating agents cannot be screened.

c. In critically ill patients, supportive treatment is needed before laboratory results of the toxicology screen are available.
d. Laboratory drug-detection abilities differ.
e. In general, only a **qualitative determination** of a substance or substances is necessary; however, **quantitative levels** of the following drugs are necessary to guide therapy:
(1) Acetaminophen
(2) Arsenic
(3) Carboxyhemoglobin
(4) Digoxin
(5) Ethanol
(6) Ethylene glycol
(7) Iron
(8) Lead
(9) Lithium
(10) Mercury
(11) Methanol
(12) Methemoglobin
(13) Phenobarbital
(14) Phenytoin
(15) Salicylates
(16) Theophylline

F. Skin decontamination should be performed when percutaneous absorption of a substance may result in systemic toxicity or when the contaminating substance may produce local toxic effects (e.g., acid burns). The patient's clothing is removed, and the areas are irrigated with copious quantities of water. **Neutralization should not be attempted.** For example, neutralizing acid burns with sodium bicarbonate will produce an exothermic chemical reaction, thereby exacerbating the patient's condition.

G. Gastric decontamination may be attempted when supportive care is begun. GI decontamination involves removal of the ingestant with emesis or lavage, the use of activated charcoal potentially to bind any ingestants, and the use of cathartics to hasten excretion and thereby limit absorption.

1. Emesis

a. Contraindications
(1) Children less than age 9 months
(2) Patients with central nervous system (CNS) depression or seizures
(3) Patients who have ingested a strong acid, alkali, or a sharp object
(4) Patients with loss of the gag reflex
(5) Patients who have ingested some types of hydrocarbons or petroleum distillates
(6) Patients who have ingested substances with an extremely rapid onset of action
(7) Patients with emesis following the ingestion

b. Syrup of ipecac may be useful up to 12 hours after ingestions.
(1) Mechanism of action. The onset of emesis usually occurs within 30 minutes after syrup of ipecac. The effects last for approximately 2 hours and produce approximately three episodes of emesis in 60 minutes.
(2) Dosages. Patients ages 9–11 months, 10 ml; patients ages 1–10 years, 15 ml; patients older than age 10 years, 30 ml. Each dose of syrup of ipecac should be followed with 120–240 ml of water. The patient should be upright to avoid accidental aspiration and should be supervised.

2. Gastric lavage

a. Use. Gastric lavage is used in patients who are not alert or have a diminished gag reflex. This procedure should also be considered in patients who are seen early following massive ingestions or in individuals who have a contraindication to syrup of ipecac.
b. Procedure. Patients are placed in the left lateral decubitus position. Lavage is performed after a cuffed endotracheal tube is in place to protect the airway. After aspiration of the gastric contents, 250–300 ml of tap water or saline is instilled and then aspirated. The sequence should be repeated until the return is continuously clear for at least 2 liters.

3. Activated charcoal adsorbs almost all commonly ingested drugs and chemicals and usually is administered to most overdose patients as quickly as possible. Commonly ingested substances not adsorbed include: **ethanol, iron, lithium, cyanide, ethylene glycol, lead, mercury, methanol, organic solvents, potassium, strong acids,** and **strong alkalis.**

a. **Dosage.** Activated charcoal is available as a premade colloidal dispersion with water or sorbitol. In **adults,** the dose of activated charcoal is 1 g/kg with a maximum dose of 50 g; the dose in **children** is 1 g/kg. A single dose of cathartic usually is administered with activated charcoal to speed GI transit and prevent charcoal aspiration. **Multiple doses** of any cathartics should be avoided because they can cause electrolyte imbalances and/or dehydration. Toxic ingestions with drugs having an enterohepatic circulation (e.g., theophyllines, phenobarbital, tricyclic antidepressants, phenothiazines, digitalis) generally require that the charcoal be readministered every 6 hours to prevent reabsorption during recirculation.

b. **Adverse effects.** Charcoal aspiration and empyema have been reported in the literature. As such, charcoal should be withheld if patients are vomiting. Bowel obstruction may occur with multiple doses of activated charcoal and/or patients who are receiving concomitant therapy with neuromuscular-blocking drugs.

H. **Whole-bowel irrigation** has been shown to be effective under certain conditions, particularly when activated charcoal lacks efficacy. An isosmotic cathartic solution such as polyethylene glycol (Golytely, Colyte) is used. The dosage is 1–2 L/hr given orally or by nasogastric tube until the rectal effluent is clear.

I. **Forced diuresis** and **urinary pH manipulation** may be used to enhance the elimination of substances whose elimination is primarily renal, if the substance has a relatively small volume of distribution with little protein binding.

1. **Alkaline diuresis** promotes the ionization of weak acids, thereby preventing their reabsorption by the kidney, which facilitates the excretion of these weak acids. This procedure has been used in the management of patients who have ingested long-acting barbiturates such as phenobarbital or salicylic acid. Patients are given 50–100 mEq of sodium bicarbonate IV push, followed by a continuous infusion of 50–100 mEq of sodium bicarbonate in 1 liter of 0.25%–0.45% normal saline, maintaining a urine pH of 7.3–8.5. Urine output should be 5–7 ml/kg/hr. **Complications** include metabolic alkalosis, hypernatremia, hyperosmolarity, and fluid retention.

2. **Acid diuresis** may promote the elimination of weak bases such as amphetamines, phencyclidine, and quinidine derivatives. This may be accomplished by administering ascorbic acid 500 mg to 1 gram orally or intravenously every 6 hours to maintain a urine pH of approximately 4.5–5.5. Alternatively, ammonium chloride is given 4 grams every 2 hours via nasogastric tube or a 1%–2% solution is given in normal saline intravenously. Serum electrolytes and pH should be monitored frequently.

J. **Dialysis.** In patients who fail to respond to the above measures of decontamination, hemodialysis, and to a lesser extent peritoneal dialysis, may enhance drug elimination. Substances that are removed by hemodialysis generally are water soluble, have a small volume of distribution (less than 0.5 L/kg), have a low molecular weight (less than 500 daltons), and are not significantly bound to plasma proteins. Hemodialysis usually is indicated for life-threatening ingestions of ethylene glycol, methanol, or paraquat. This technique also has been used to enhance the elimination of ethanol, theophylline, lithium, salicylates, and long-acting barbiturates.

K. **Hemoperfusion** is a technique where anticoagulated blood is passed through (perfused) a column containing activated charcoal or resin particles. This method of elimination clears substances from the blood more rapidly than hemodialysis, but it does not correct fluid and electrolyte abnormalities as does hemodialysis. Hemoperfusion, while more effective in removing phenobarbital, phenytoin, carbamazepine, methotrexate, and theophylline than hemodialysis, is less effective in removing ethanol or methanol. **Complications** of hemoperfusion include thrombocytopenia, leukopenia, hypocalcemia, hypoglycemia, and hypotension.

III. MANAGEMENT OF SPECIFIC INGESTIONS

A. **Acetaminophen** is an antipyretic-analgesic that can produce fatal hepatotoxicity in untreated patients through the generation of a toxic metabolite.

1. **Available dosage forms.** Acetaminophen is available in a variety of over-the-counter (OTC) and prescription drug products.

2. **Toxicokinetics.** Acetaminophen is well absorbed from the GI tract, has a half-life between 2 and 3 hours, and has less than 5% excreted unchanged in the urine, with the remainder metabolized in the liver by the cytochrome p-450 system.

3. **Clinical presentation**
   a. **Phase I** (12–24 hours post ingestion)—nausea, vomiting, anorexia, and diaphoresis
   b. **Phase II** (1–4 days post ingestion)—asymptomatic
   c. **Phase III** (2–3 days in untreated patients)—nausea, abdominal pain, progressive evidence of hepatic failure, coma, and death

4. **Laboratory data**
   a. **Serum acetaminophen levels.** Patients with levels greater than 150, 70, or 40 μg/ml at 4, 8, or 12 hours after ingestion require antidotal therapy with n-acetylcysteine (NAC) according to the Rumack-Matthews nomogram.
   b. Baseline liver function tests should be done in all patients.
   c. Renal function tests, including a BUN and Scr, should be done.
   d. Coagulation studies include prothrombin time (PT), partial thromboplastin time (PTT), and bleeding time.

5. **Treatment**
   a. Adult patients who have ingested more than 7 grams or children who have ingested more than 100 mg/kg require treatment. Elderly or alcoholic patients have an increased susceptibility to acetaminophen hepatotoxicity.
   b. The recommended treatment is GI decontamination with syrup of ipecac or gastric lavage for patients presenting within 2 hours of ingestion.
   c. Antidotal therapy with NAC is indicated for patients with toxic blood levels of acetaminophen.
      (1) **NAC dosage** is 140 mg/kg as a loading dose followed by 70 mg/kg every 4 hours for a total of 17 doses. NAC is administered either orally or via a nasogastric tube. NAC (Mucomyst) 20% contains 200 mg/ml. Each dose must be diluted 1:3 in either cola or fruit juice to mask the unpleasant taste and smell. The dose of NAC should be repeated if the patient vomits within one-half hour of administration. Patients with severe nausea secondary to NAC may be pretreated with IV metoclopramide 10 mg q 6 hours. Metoclopramide acts as an antiemetic and increases the rate of NAC absorption.
      (2) **IV NAC** is currently investigational for patients who are intolerant to oral NAC. Despite a shorter treatment period, IV NAC has produced a higher incidence of anaphylactoid reactions.

B. Alcohols

1. **Ethylene glycol**
   a. **Available forms.** Ethylene glycol commonly is used in antifreeze and windshield de-ice solutions. This form is sometimes colorless and has a sweet taste.
   b. **Toxicokinetics.** Ethylene glycol is hepatically metabolized by alcohol dehydrogenase to glycolaldehyde, which is metabolized by aldehyde dehydrogenase to glycolic acid. Glycolic acid is converted to glyoxylic acid, whose most toxic metabolite is oxalic acid.
   c. **Clinical presentation**
      (1) **Stage I** (0.5–12 hours post ingestion)—ataxia, nystagmus, nausea and vomiting, decreased deep tendon reflexes, and severe acidosis (more severe overdoses—hypocalcemic tetany and seizures, cerebral edema, coma, and death)
      (2) **Stage II** (12–24 hours post ingestion)—tachypnea, cyanosis, tachycardia, pulmonary edema, and pneumonitis.
      (3) **Stage III** (24–72 hours post ingestion)—flank pain and costovertebral angle tenderness; oliguric renal failure.
   d. **Laboratory data** may reveal severe metabolic acidosis, hypocalcemia, and calcium oxalate crystals in the urinalysis.
   e. **Treatment**
      (1) **Gastric lavage** is performed within 30 minutes of ingestion, followed by one dose of activated charcoal and a cathartic.

(2) **IV ethanol (EtOH)**
   (a) **Indications** include an ethylene glycol level more than 20 mg/dl, suspicion of ingestion pending level, or an anion gap metabolic acidosis with a history of ingestion, regardless of the level.
   (b) **EtOH dosage.** An EtOh level of at least 100 mg/dl should be maintained. Loading dose is 7.5–10 ml/kg of a 10% ethanol in d5w over 1 hour followed by a maintenance infusion of 1.4 ml/kg/hr. Infusion rates may need to be increased in patients receiving hemodialysis.

(3) **Pyridoxine** (100 mg i.v. q day) and **thiamine** (100 mg i.v. q day) are cofactors that may convert glyoxylic acid to nonoxalate metabolites.

(4) **Sodium bicarbonate** is used as needed to correct the acidosis.

(5) **Hemodialysis.** EtOH infusion must be continued, and the rate of administration may need to be increased. **Indications** include ethylene glycol level more than 50 mg/dl, congestive heart failure, renal failure, or severe acidosis.

2. Methanol

a. **Available forms** include gas-line antifreeze, windshield washer, and some sterno.

b. **Toxicokinetics.** Alcohol dehydrogenase converts methanol to formaldehyde, which is then converted to formic acid.

c. **Clinical presentation**
   (1) **Stage I**—euphoria, gregariousness, and muscle weakness for 6–36 hours depending on the rate of formation of formic acid
   (2) **Stage II**—vomiting, upper abdominal pain, diarrhea, dizziness, headache, restlessness, dyspnea, blurred vision, photophobia, blindness, coma, cerebral edema, cardiac and respiratory depression, seizures, and death

d. **Laboratory data** include severe metabolic acidosis, hyperglycemia, and hyperamylasemia.

e. **Treatment**
   (1) **Gastric lavage,** single-dose charcoal, and cathartic administration are used as treatment.
   (2) **IV EtOH**
      (a) **Indications** include any peak methanol level more than 20 mg/dl, a suspicious ingestion with a positive history, or any symptomatic patient with an anion gap acidosis.
      (b) **Administration** is the same as per ethylene glycol (see III B 1).
   (3) **Folinic acid** administered at 1 mg/kg (maximum 50 mg) IV q4h for 6 doses increases the metabolism of formate.
   (4) **4-Methylpyrazole** is an investigational alcohol dehydrogenase antagonist that is not yet available in the United States.
   (5) **Sodium bicarbonate** is used for severe acidosis.
   (6) **Hemodialysis** is used for methanol levels greater than 50 mg/dl, severe and resistant acidosis, renal failure, or visual symptoms.

C. Anticoagulants

1. Heparin

a. **Available dosage forms** include parenteral dosage forms for IV and subcutaneous administration.

b. **Toxicokinetics.** Heparin has a half-life of 1–1.5 hours and is primarily metabolized in the liver.

c. **Clinical presentation.** Look for any signs or symptoms of bleeding or bruising.

d. **Laboratory data.** Obtain PTT, bleeding time, and platelet counts.

e. **Treatment**
   (1) **Mild over-anticoagulation** can be reversed by stopping heparin administration for 1–2 hours and restarting therapy at a reduced dose.
   (2) **Severe overdoses** may require the administration of **protamine.** Protamine combines with heparin and neutralizes it. **One milligram of protamine neutralizes 100 units of heparin.** Protamine should be administered slowly, intravenously over 10 minutes.

2. Warfarin

a. **Available dosage forms** include oral tablets and a solution for parenteral administration.

b. **Toxicokinetics.** Warfarin is well absorbed following oral administration. Its mean half-life is 35 hours, protein binding is 99% with a 5-day duration of activity. Vitamin K-dependent clotting factors begin to decline 6 hours after administration, but therapeutic anticoagulation may require several days.

c. **Clinical presentation** includes minor bleeding, bruising, hematuria, epistaxis, and conjunctival hemorrhage. More serious bleeding includes GI, intracranial, retroperitoneal, and wound site.

d. **Laboratory data** include PT, INR, and bleeding time.

e. **Treatment**

(1) If **PT** or **INR** is **slightly elevated,** withhold warfarin for 24–48 hours, then reinstitute therapy with a reduced dosage.

(2) If **PT** or **INR** is **elevated** and **bleeding,** administer 10 mg of phytonadione (vitamin K) over 30 minutes. Patients who are bleeding may require the administration of blood products that contain clotting factors.

D. Antidepressants

1. **Tricyclic antidepressants (TCAs)**

a. **Available dosage forms** include amitriptyline, nortriptyline, imipramine, desipramine, doxepin, protriptyline, and clomipramine.

b. **Toxicokinetics.** The compounds are hepatically metabolized, undergo enterohepatic recirculation, are highly bound to plasma proteins, and have an elimination half-life of approximately 24 hours.

c. **Clinical presentation.** Anticholinergic effects include mydriasis, ileus, urinary retention, and hyperpyrexia. **Cardiopulmonary toxicity** exhibits tachycardias, conduction blocks, hypotension, and pulmonary edema. **CNS manifestations** range from agitation and confusion to hallucinations, seizures, and coma.

d. **Laboratory data.** Blood-level monitoring does not correlate well with clinical signs and symptoms of toxicity. Some authors suggest that electrocardiographic monitoring is a better guide to assessing the severity of ingestion.

e. **Treatment**

(1) **GI decontamination.** Ipecac syrup is not recommended because patients may quickly become comatose and increase the risk of aspiration. **Activated charcoal** is given at 1 mg/kg (up to 50 grams) every 6 hours.

(2) **Alkalinization** with sodium bicarbonate 1–2 mEq/kg to maintain an arterial pH of 7.45–7.55 decreases the free fraction of the absorbed toxins, while reversing some of the cardiac abnormalities.

(3) **Phenytoin** and/or **benzodiazepines** may be required to control seizures. Phenytoin must be administered at a rate not exceeding 25 mg/min due to hypotensive side effects.

(4) **Physostigmine** 2 mg IV over 1 minute is used to reverse **severe** anticholinergic toxicity due to these drugs. Because this antidote may exacerbate heart block in these patients, its use for TCA overdoses is declining.

2. **Selective serotonin reuptake inhibitors (SSRIs)**

a. **Available dosage forms** (non-tricyclic agents) include fluoxetine, sertraline, and paroxetine.

b. **Toxicokinetics.** SSRIs are well absorbed following oral administration. Peak levels within 2 to 6 hours. Hepatically metabolized with a half-life between 8 and 30 hours.

c. **Clinical presentation** includes mild symptomatology. Patients may become agitated, drowsy, or confused. Seizures and cardiovascular toxicity are rare.

d. **Laboratory data.** ECG monitoring is recommended. Blood-level monitoring is not recommended.

e. **Treatment** includes gastric lavage and supportive treatment.

E. Benzodiazepines

1. **Available dosage forms** include chlordiazepoxide, diazepam, flurazepam, midazolam, lorazepam, alprazolam, and triazolam.

2. **Toxicokinetics.** These drugs are hepatically metabolized.

3. **Clinical presentation** includes drowsiness, ataxia, and confusion. Fatalities are rare.

4. **Laboratory data.** Drug-level monitoring is not indicated.

5. **Treatment**
   a. **Supportive** treatment includes gastric emptying, activated charcoal, and a cathartic.
   b. **Flumazenil** is given 0.2 mg IV over 30 seconds; repeat doses of 0.5 mg over 30 seconds at 1-minute intervals for a maximum cumulative dose of 5 mg.
      (1) Flumazenil has a **short elimination half-life.**
      (2) **Careful observation** for **resedation** is necessary, especially for ingestions of long-acting benzodiazepines.
      (3) Flumazenil is **contraindicated** in mixed overdose patients (particularly involving tricyclic antidepressants) in whom seizures are likely.

F. β-Adrenergic antagonists

1. **Available dosage forms.** Class examples include propranolol, metoprolol, and atenolol. Oral and parenteral dosage forms are available.

2. **Toxicokinetics.** All of the members within this class differ with regard to renal versus hepatic elimination, lipid solubility and protein binding. Patients may become toxic due to changes in organ function.

3. **Clinical presentation** includes hypotension, bradycardia, and atrioventricular block. Bronchospasm may occur, particularly with noncardioselective agents.

4. **Laboratory data** include serum electrolytes and blood glucose (patients may become hypoglycemic).

5. **Treatment**
   a. **GI decontamination** includes gastric lavage and activated charcoal.
   b. **Glucagon** is given 50–150 μg/kg as a loading dose over 1 minute followed by a continuous infusion of 1–5 mg/hour.
   c. **Epinephrine** should be used cautiously in β-blocker overdoses. Unopposed α-receptor stimulation in the face of complete β-receptor block may lead to profound hypertension.

G. Calcium channel antagonists

1. **Available dosage forms** include verapamil, diltiazem, and the dihydropyridine class (nifedipine derivatives).

2. **Toxicokinetics.** Onset of action is approximately 30 minutes, whereas the duration is 6–8 hours. Several compounds are available as sustained-release dosage forms, which may contribute to prolonged toxicity.

3. **Clinical presentation.** Hypotension is common to all classes. Bradycardia and atrioventricular block more commonly are seen with ingestions of verapamil or diltiazem. Pulmonary edema and seizures (verapamil) are also seen.

4. **Laboratory data** include ECG and serum electrolytes.

5. **Treatment**
   a. **GI decontamination** includes gastric lavage, activated charcoal, and whole bowel irrigation (especially for ingestions with sustained release products).
   b. **Calcium.** Calcium chloride 10% (10–20 ml) IV push is given for the management of hypotension, bradycardia, or heart block.
   c. **Glucagon** dosage is the same as for β-blocker overdose.

H. Cocaine

1. **Available forms** include alkaloid obtained from *Erythroxylon coca.*

2. **Toxicokinetics.** Cocaine is well absorbed following oral, inhalational, intranasal, and IV administration. Cocaine is metabolized in the liver and excreted in the urine.

3. **Clinical presentation** includes CNS and sympathetic stimulation (e.g., hypertension, tachypnea, tachycardia, nausea, vomiting, seizures). Death may result from respiratory failure, myocardial infarction, or cardiac arrest.

4. **Laboratory data** include cocaine and cocaine metabolite urine screens.

5. **Treatment** is **supportive;** benzodiazepines for seizures, labetalol for hypertension, and neuroleptics for psychosis.

I. Corrosives

1. **Available forms** include strong acids or alkalis.
2. **Toxicokinetics.** Corrosives are well absorbed following oral and inhalational administration.
3. **Clinical presentation.** These compounds produce burns on contact.
4. **Laboratory data.** ABGs, chest radiographs, and at least 6 hours of observation are required for inhalation exposure.
5. **Treatment** is **decontamination.** Exposed skin must be irrigated with water. **Neutralization** should be **avoided** because these reactions are exothermic and will produce further damage.

J. Cyanide

1. **Available forms** include industrial chemicals and some nail polish removers.
2. **Toxicokinetics.** The drug is rapidly absorbed following oral or inhalational exposure.
3. **Clinical presentation** includes headache, dyspnea, nausea, vomiting, ataxia, coma, seizures, and death.
4. **Laboratory data** include cyanide levels, ABGs, electrolytes, and an ECG.
5. A cyanide **antidote kit** is used for **treatment.**
   a. **Amyl nitrite**—pearls are crushed and held under the patient's nostrils
   b. **Sodium nitrite** 10 ml IV push—converts hemoglobin to methemoglobin, which binds the cyanide ion
   c. **Sodium thiosulfate** 50 ml of a 25% solution IV push—may be repeated if there is no response
   d. **Oxygen**
   e. **Sodium bicarbonate—**as needed for severe acidosis
   f. **Hyperbaric oxygen**—for patients not responding to above

K. Digoxin

1. **Available dosage forms** include oral and parenteral.
2. **Toxicokinetics.** Digoxin is well absorbed, is primarily renally eliminated, and has a half-life of 36–48 hours. Its volume of distribution is 7–10 L/kg. Equilibration between serum level and myocardial binding requires approximately 6–8 hours.
3. **Clinical presentation** includes confusion, anorexia, nausea, and vomiting in mild cases. In more severe cases, cardiac dysrhythmias are seen.
4. **Laboratory data** include serum digoxin levels, electrolytes, particularly serum potassium levels, and an ECG.
5. **Treatment**
   a. **Decontamination** by ipecac or activated charcoal is recommended.
   b. **Supportive therapy** includes managing hyper or hypokalemia and inotropic support as needed.
   c. **Digoxin-specific fab antibodies.** To determine the dosage, use the formula dose (vials) = [ingested digoxin (mg) x 0.8]/0.6. Each vial contains 40 mg of digoxin antibodies (Digibind) and should be reconstituted with 4 ml of sterile water.

L. Electrolytes

1. **Magnesium**
   a. **Available dosage forms** include oral, rectal, and parenteral. Magnesium-containing cathartics (e.g., magnesium citrate) have been reported to produce hypermagnesemia in patients receiving repetitive doses with activated charcoal.
   b. **Toxicokinetics.** Magnesium is found intracellularly and is renally eliminated.
   c. **Clinical presentation**
      (1) **Mild**—deep tendon reflexes may be depressed, lethargy, and weakness

(2) **Severe**—respiratory paralysis and heart block; prolonged PR, QRS, and QT intervals

d. **Laboratory data**

(1) **Mild**—more than 4 mEq/L

(2) **Severe**—more than 10 mEq/L

e. **Treatment** is **10% calcium gluconate** to temporarily antagonize the cardiac effects of magnesium. In severe cases, **hemodialysis** may be required.

2. **Potassium**

a. **Available dosage forms** are oral and parenteral.

b. **Toxicokinetics.** Potassium is primarily an intracellular cation. Changes in acid–base balance produce shifts in serum potassium values (e.g., a 0.1 unit increase in serum pH produces a 0.1–0.7 mEq/L decrease in serum potassium values).

c. **Clinical presentation** includes cardiac irritability and peripheral weakness with minor increases. Cardiac dysrhythmias, including bradycardia, may progress to asystole.

d. **Laboratory data.** ECG data include **peaked T waves** and prolongation of the QRS complex.

e. **Treatment**

(1) **Calcium.** Administer calcium gluconate 10% 10 ml to antagonize the cardiac effects of hyperkalemia.

(2) **Sodium bicarbonate.** 50 mEq IV increases serum pH and causes an intracellular shift of potassium.

(3) **Glucose and insulin.** 50 ml of 50% dextrose and 5–10 units of regular insulin are administered via IV push to shift potassium from the extracellular fluid into the cells.

(4) **Cation exchange resins** bind potassium in exchange for another cation (sodium). **Sodium polystyrene sulfonate** (Kayexalate) is given 15 g/60 ml with 23.5% sorbitol in doses 15–30 g PO q 3–4 hours as needed until the hyperkalemia resolves. Alternatively, 50 g of sodium polystyrene sulfonate can be given rectally in 200 ml of sodium chloride as a retention enema.

(5) **Hemodialysis** is reserved for life-threatening hyperkalemia that does not respond to the above measures.

M. Iron (Fe)

1. **Available dosage forms.** Numerous OTC products are available. Toxicity is based on the amount of elemental iron ingested: sulfate salt = 20% elemental Fe; fumarate salt = 33% elemental Fe; and gluconate salt = 12% elemental Fe.

2. **Toxicokinetics.** Iron is absorbed in the duodenum and jejunum.

3. **Clinical Presentation**

a. **Phase I**—nausea, vomiting, diarrhea, GI bleeding, hypotension

b. **Phase II**—clinical improvement seen 6–24 hours after ingestion

c. **Phase III**—metabolic acidosis, renal and hepatic failure, sepsis, pulmonary edema, and death

4. **Laboratory data** include serum Fe levels, total iron-binding capacity (TIBC), ABGs, LFTs, hemoglobin, and hematocrit. Radiologic evaluation of the abdomen notes the presence of radiopaque pills.

5. **Treatment**

a. **Decontamination.** For ingestions greater than 30 mg/kg, ipecac emesis may be used. Gastric lavage uses sodium bicarbonate to facilitate the conversion to ferrous carbonate, which is poorly absorbed.

b. **Supportive treatment**

c. **Deferoxime** is used to chelate iron. Administer 25–50 mg/kg up to a dose of 1 gram, and observe for a red color in the urine. Then administer at a rate of 15 mg/kg/hr up to a maximum dose of 6 g/day. Continue until serum iron is less than TIBC.

N. Isoniazid (INH)

1. **Available dosage forms** include oral and parenteral.

2. **Toxicokinetics.** INH is well absorbed PO. Peak levels are within 1–2 hours after ingestion. Isoniazid is hepatically metabolized.

3. **Clinical presentation** includes nausea, vomiting, slurred speech, ataxia, generalized tonic-clonic seizures, and coma.

4. **Laboratory data** include severe lactic acidosis, hypoglycemia, mild hyperkalemia, and leukocytosis.

5. **Treatment**
   a. **Decontamination.** Avoid emesis because patients are at high risk for developing seizures; otherwise use gastric lavage.
   b. **Pyridoxine,** which reverses INH-induced seizures, is given in gram doses equivalent to the amount of pyridoxine ingested. Pyridoxine is mixed as a 10% solution in d5w and infused over 30–60 minutes.
   c. **Sodium bicarbonate** corrects the acidosis.

O. Lead

1. **Available forms** include lead-containing paint or gasoline fume inhalation.

2. **Toxicokinetics.** Lead has slow distribution with a half-life of approximately 2 months.

3. **Clinical presentation** includes nausea, vomiting, abdominal pain, peripheral neuropathies, convulsions, and coma.

4. **Laboratory data** include anemia and an elevated blood-lead level.

5. **Treatment**
   a. **Calcium EDTA** is given 50–75 mg/kg/day IM or slow IV in 4 divided doses.
   b. **Dimercaprol** is given 4 mg/kg IM q 4 h for up to 7 days.

P. Opiates

1. **Available dosage forms** include oral immediate-release and sustained-release preparations as well as parenteral agents.

2. **Toxicokinetics.** Some agents have prolonged elimination half-lives (e.g., heroin, methadone).

3. **Clinical presentation** includes respiratory depression and a decreased level of consciousness. Rare effects include hypotension, bradycardia, and pulmonary edema.

4. **Laboratory data** include baseline ABGs and toxicology screens.

5. **Treatment**
   a. **Naloxone** is given 0.8–2 mg every 5 minutes up to 10 mg and 0.03–0.1 mg/kg in pediatric patients. Naloxone has a very short half-life, and resedation is a concern in patients overdosing on long-acting opioids or sustained-release dosage forms.
   b. **Nalmefene** has a half-life of approximately 10 hours. Initial dosages are 0.5 mg/70 kg. A follow up dose 2–5 minutes later is 1 mg/70 kg.

Q. Organophosphates

1. **There are various available forms.**

2. **Toxicokinetics.** Organophosphates are absorbed through the lungs, skin, GI tract, and conjunctiva.

3. **Clinical presentation** includes excessive cholinergic stimulation.

4. **Laboratory data** include red blood cell acetylcholinesterase activity.

5. **Treatment**
   a. **Decontamination**
   b. **Atropine** is given 1–2 mg IV to reverse the peripheral muscarinic effects.
   c. **Pralidoxime (2-PAM)** is given 1 g IV over 2 minutes and repeated in 20 minutes as needed.

R. Salicylates

1. **Available dosage forms** include a variety of OTC products; oral, rectal, and topical products.

2. **Toxicokinetics.** Salicylates are well absorbed following oral administration. The half-life is 6–12 hours at lower doses. In overdose situations, the half-life may be prolonged to more than 20 hours.

3. **Clinical presentation** includes nausea, vomiting, tinnitus, and malaise (mild toxicity). Lethargy, convulsions, coma, and metabolic acidosis appear in more severe overdoses.

Potential **complications** from therapeutic and toxic doses include GI bleeding, increased prothrombin time, hepatic toxicity, pancreatitis, and proteinuria.

4. **Laboratory data** for the following 6-hour post-ingestion levels are:
   a. 40–60 mg/dl—tinnitus
   b. 60–95 mg/dl—moderate toxicity
   c. More than 95 mg/dl—severe toxicity
   d. With the presence of acidemia and aciduria, evaluate ABGs.
   e. Additionally, laboratory evaluation may show leukocytosis, thrombocytopenia, increased or decreased serum glucose and sodium, hypokalemia, and increased serum BUN, creatinine, and ketones.
5. **Treatment**
   a. **Decontamination** includes emesis with syrup of ipecac and activated charcoal every 6 hours with 1 dose of cathartic for all patients ingesting greater than 150 mg/kg. Whole-bowel irrigation for large ingestions.
   b. **Alkaline diuresis** is given as above to enhance salicylate excretion. This is indicated for levels greater than 40 mg/dl.
   c. **Hemodialysis** is used for severe intoxications when serum levels are greater than 100 mg/dl
   d. **Fluid** and **electrolyte** replacement is used as needed.
   e. **Vitamin K** and **fresh frozen plasma** are used to correct any coagulopathy.

STUDY QUESTIONS

Directions: Each of the numbered items or incomplete statements in this section is followed by answers or by completions of the statement. Select the **one** lettered answer or completion that is **best** in each case.

1. A physician receives a call from the parent of a 2-year-old child who has ingested an unknown quantity of morphine controlled-release tablets and is now unconscious. The physician's initial recommendation is

(A) to call EMS and have the child taken to the hospital emergency department
(B) administer 1 g/kg of activated charcoal with sorbitol
(C) administer syrup of ipecac 15 ml P.O. to induce vomiting
(D) suggest that the child receive emergency hemodialysis
(E) suggest that the child receive acid diuresis with ammonium chloride

2. A 3-year-old child ingests an unknown quantity of Draino, which is a liquid caustic. The patient's parents question the physician as to whether to administer the syrup of ipecac. The physician recommends which of the following treatments?

(A) Administer 15 ml of the syrup of ipecac
(B) Give the child some water or juice to drink
(C) Administer thiamine 100 mg IV push

3. An unconscious patient is brought into the emergency department. The patient is given 50 ml of 50% dextrose in water, thiamine 100 mg IV, followed by naloxone 0.8 mg at which point he awakens. This patient most likely has overdosed on which of the following substances?

(A) Methanol
(B) Amitriptyline
(C) Cocaine
(D) Haloperidol
(E) Heroin

4. Contraindications to the administration of syrup of ipecac include which of the following?

(A) An unconscious patient
(B) A patient who is experiencing a generalized tonic-clonic seizure
(C) A patient who has ingested a caustic substance
(D) All of the above
(E) None of the above

5. An unconscious patient is brought to the emergency department with a history of an unknown drug overdose. Which of the following actions should the physician perform?

(A) Administer 50 ml of 50% dextrose, thiamine 100 mg IV push, and naloxone 0.8 mg IV push
(B) Protect the patient's airway and ensure that vital signs are stable
(C) Perform gastric lavage
(D) Order the following laboratory tests: CBC, electrolytes, and a toxicology screen
(E) All of the above

6. A patient who overdoses on acetaminophen is admitted to the hospital for antidotal therapy with *N*-acetylcysteine. The patient has the following medication orders: *N*-acetylcysteine 140 mg/kg loading dose followed by 70 mg/kg for a total of 17 doses, ranitidine 50 mg IV q 8 hours, prochlorperazine 10 mg I.M. q 6 hours prn nausea, thiamine 100 mg IV q day for 3 doses, and Darvocet N-100 1–2 tablets every 4 hours prn headache. What is the best course of action?

(A) Call the physician to increase the dosage of ranitidine to 50 mg IV q 6 h
(B) Call the physician and have the Darvocet-N 100 discontinued
(C) Call the physician to initiate hemodialysis therapy
(D) Have the patient prophylactically intubated to protect the airway
(E) Administer ethanol 10% at a loading dose of 7.5 ml/kg over 1 hour followed by a continuous infusion of 1.4 ml/kg/hr for 48 hours

7. Ethyl alcohol (EtOH) is administered to patients who have ingested either ethylene glycol or methanol because EtOH

(A) helps to sedate patients
(B) increases the metabolism of ethylene glycol and methanol
(C) blocks the formation of the toxic metabolites of ethylene glycol and methanol.
(D) increases the renal clearance of ethylene glycol and methanol
(E) is not an antidote for ethylene glycol or methanol overdoses

8. A patient has inadvertently received 30,000 units of intravenous heparin during a coronary artery bypass graft (CABG) procedure, instead of sodium chloride for the intravenous flush. Which of the following treatments is recommended 1 hour later?

(A) Protamine 300 mg slow IV push over 10 minutes
(B) Phytonadione (vitamin K) 10 mg IV over 30 minutes
(C) Protamine 150 mg slow IV over 10 minutes
(D) The physician should contact the blood bank for immediate transfusion replacement therapy
(E) None of the above

9. A patient with renal failure is inadvertently given three doses of intravenous potassium chloride 40 mEq in 100 ml of 0.9% sodium chloride over a 3-hour period. This error is immediately discovered and a STAT serum potassium level is 8.0 mEq/L and the patient is bradycardic with a markedly prolonged QRS complex. The patient should receive which of the following?

(A) Calcium gluconate 10% 10 ml IV push
(B) Sodium bicarbonate 50 mEq IV push
(C) Insulin 10 units and dextrose 50% 50 ml IV push
(D) Sodium polystyrene sulfonate 30 grams PO q 3 h for 4 doses
(E) None of the above

10. Parenteral calcium is used as an antidote for which of the following situations?

(A) Verapamil overdoses
(B) Hyperkalemia
(C) Cocaine intoxication
(D) Verapamil overdoses and hyperkalemia

ANSWERS AND EXPLANATIONS

1. The answer is A *[I A].*
Patients with unstable vital signs should be taken to an emergency department for immediate treatment.

2. The answer is B *[II F].*
Vomiting should not be induced in patients who have ingested caustic substances because these chemicals can induce further burning when they come up in the emesis.

3. The answer is E *[III P 5].*
Naloxone reverses the effects of opioid receptor agonists, such as heroin, morphine, and propoxyphene.

4. The answer is D *[II G 1].*
Contraindications to ipecac include "the three C's": caustics, conscious, convulsions.

5. The answer is E *[I].*
The management of unconscious overdose patients involves aggressive support of vital signs, the administration of empiric antidotal therapy, while obtaining various laboratory tests to determine the nature of the overdose.

6. The answer is B *[III A].*
Darvocet N-100 is an acetaminophen-containing product that should not be given to a patient with documented acetaminophen toxicity. Be aware particularly of OTC products containing acetaminophen.

7. The answer is C *[III B].*
Ethanol saturates alcohol dehydrogenase and prevents the formation of the toxic metabolites of either ethylene glycol or methanol.

8. The answer is C *[III C 1].*
The elimination half-life of heparin is short. As a result, 1 hour after the overdose, 50% of the heparin has been eliminated, and only 50% of the required dose of protamine is necessary.

9. The answer is A *[III L 2].*
All of the selections are used to manage hyperkalemia, although in an unstable patient, the cardiac effects of hyperkalemia must first be reversed with intravenous calcium. There is a delay in the onset of action with sodium bicarbonate, insulin and dextrose, and sodium polystyrene sulfonate.

10. The answer is D *[III L 2].*
Parenteral calcium is used to reverse the cardiac effects of calcium channel blocker overdose and hyperkalemia.

36
Therapeutic Drug Monitoring

Lyndon D. Braun

I. INTRODUCTION

A. Basic pharmacokinetic terms

1. **Bioavailability** is the fraction of an administered dose that reaches the systemic circulation.
2. **Volume of distribution** is the amount of drug in the body relative to the concentration of drug in the blood (or plasma).

$$V_D = D/C_P$$

   where V_D is the apparent volume of distribution, D is the drug dose, and C_P is the plasma concentration of the drug.

3. **Clearance** is the volume of blood (or plasma) that can be completely cleared of a drug per unit of time (units = volume/time).
4. **Half-life** is the time required for the drug concentration in the plasma to be reduced by 50%, provided no drug absorption occurs during the decline. Half-life is also a measure of the time required for the drug concentration in the plasma to reach a steady-state concentration with a new dosing regimen.
5. **Steady-state concentration** is the drug concentration at which the body is in equilibrium (i.e., the rates of drug absorption and elimination are equal).
6. **Loading dose** is the amount of drug that must be administered to bring the drug concentration in the blood (or plasma) into the therapeutic range rapidly when initiating therapy or when increasing the dosing rate after subtherapeutic dosing.
7. **Maintenance dose** is the amount of drug that must be regularly administered to maintain a steady-state concentration.
8. **Dosing interval** is the amount of time between consecutive doses of a regularly administered drug. This is usually a multiple of 24 hours or a number that is easily divided into 24 hours.
9. **Trough or minimum concentration** is the lowest concentration of a drug within a dosing interval. It is typically reached at the end of the dosing interval, immediately before the next dose is administered.
10. **Peak or maximum concentration** is the highest drug concentration within a dosing interval. Peak concentration is usually reached within 2 hours of dose administration, but it depends on the route of administration.

B. Drug criteria for therapeutic drug monitoring (Tables 36-1 and 36-2)

1. **Serum drug concentration** and the **concentration at the receptor site** must be in equilibrium.
2. **Intensity** and **duration of the pharmacodynamic effect (efficacy** and **toxicity)** must be correlated with the timing of the sampling and drug concentration at the receptor site.

C. Benefits of therapeutic drug monitoring

1. When starting drug therapy where rapid and effective treatment is needed, as in antibiotic therapy or anticonvulsant therapy, drug monitoring quickly determines the optimal dose and dosing rate.

Table 36-1. Drugs Commonly Monitored Through Plasma Levels

Antibiotics	**Cardiovascular Agents**
Amikacin	Digoxin
Chloramphenicol	Disopyramide
Gentamicin	Lidocaine
Tobramycin	Procainamide
Vancomycin	Quinidine
Anticonvulsants	**Other Drugs**
Carbamazepine	Cyclosporine
Ethosuximide	Lithium
Phenobarbital	Salicylic acid
Phenytoin	Theophylline
Primidone	
Valproic acid	

2. During maintenance therapy in stable, chronically ill patients, such as those requiring antiarrhythmic therapy or antimanic therapy, drug monitoring determines the best possible dosage regimen—one that provides a therapeutic outcome while avoiding toxicity.

3. When interacting drugs are added to or removed from a dosage regimen, drug monitoring maintains optimal therapy.

4. Patients with altered physiologic and pharmacokinetic parameters may benefit from therapeutic drug monitoring.

a. Impaired renal function

(1) Dosages may need to be modified, depending on the extent of renal impairment and the amount of drug normally excreted unchanged that is in the urine.

(2) Renal function normally declines with increasing age; therefore middle-aged and older patients, in addition to patients with nephrotoxicity or acute or chronic renal failure, may require therapeutic monitoring.

(3) Measuring creatinine clearance can estimate renal function, using the **Cockcroft and Gault equation:**

$$\frac{(140 - \text{age in years})(\text{body weight in kg})(0.85 \text{ for females})}{(72)(\text{serum creatinine in mg/dl})} = \text{creatinine clearance in ml/min.}$$

b. Impaired hepatic function

(1) Dosage modification may be necessary in patients with impaired hepatic function, depending on the:

(a) Extent of hepatic impairment, which is often difficult to determine

Table 36-2. Drugs Occasionally Monitored Through Plasma Levels

Anticonvulsants	**Cardiovascular Agents**
Clonazepam	*N*-acetylprocainamide
Mephenytoin	Amiodarone
	Encainide
Antidepressants	Flecainide
Amitriptyline	Mexiletine
Doxepin	Propranolol
Fluoxetine	Tocainide
Imipramine	Verapamil
Maprotiline	
Trazodone	**Other Drugs**
	Fluphenazine
Toxic Agents	Methotrexate
Acetaminophen	
Ethanol	
Cocaine	

(b) Amount of drug normally metabolized

(c) Contribution of metabolites to therapeutic efficacy or toxicity

(2) Impaired hepatic albumin production may require a dosage change for drugs that are highly protein-bound.

(3) Unlike renal function tests, liver function tests measure the presence of hepatic injury, not the extent of hepatic function.

c. **Congestive heart failure** (CHF) can impair absorption, distribution, and elimination of many drugs.

d. Disease states and other **changes that affect protein binding** are discussed in IV D.

II. ROUTES OF DRUG ADMINISTRATION

A. **Intravenous (IV) administration.** This route delivers 100% of the drug directly into the circulation (bioavailability = 100%).

1. **Bolus.** The entire dose is administered rapidly, producing a high plasma concentration and, usually, the most rapid effect. **Injection volume** is limited only by the patient's size (i.e., plasma volume) and the properties (i.e., toxicities) of the drug or fluid administered.

2. **Infusion.** The drug is administered at a constant rate. At steady state, the rate of drug administration is equal to the rate of drug elimination. After 1 half-life, plasma concentration is 50% of the way to steady-state concentration; after 2 half-lives, 75%; and after 3.3 half-lives, 90%. **Injection volume** is unlimited.

B. **Subcutaneous administration.** The drug is injected into subcutaneous tissue (bioavailability ≤ 100%).

1. **Entry of the drug** into the circulation is slower than with IV administration and is limited by drug solubility, drug lipophilicity, and subcutaneous circulation.

2. The **peak effect** is generally much less than with IV administration; however, the **duration of effect** is generally longer than with IV administration, owing to slower release into the circulation.

3. The **maximum injection volume** is approximately 1 ml.

C. **Intramuscular administration.** The drug is administered into muscle tissue, usually deep muscle, such as the gluteus or deltoid (bioavailability ≤ 100%).

1. **Entry of the drug** into the circulation is slower than with IV administration and is limited by drug solubility, drug lipophilicity, and muscular circulation.

2. The **peak effect** is generally much less than with IV administration; however, the **duration of effect** is generally longer than with IV administration, owing to slower release into the circulation.

3. **Administration into a depot site** of a minimally soluble drug or vehicle can produce therapeutic levels of some drugs for up to 2–4 weeks.

4. The **maximum injection volume** is approximately 2–5 ml.

D. **Intradermal administration.** The drug is injected into dermal tissue. This route is generally used for local effects (e.g., allergy testing) and only rarely, if ever, for systemic effects, because of poor distribution into the systemic circulation. The **maximum injection volume** is approximately 1 ml.

E. **Subdermal administration.** The drug is injected into the subdermal tissues. This route is used for inserting a depot delivery system, such as levonorgestrel (Norplant®). The limited blood flow and sustained release capsules permit slow leaching of the drug from its delivery system, thus administering the drug over an extended period. The **duration of action** may last up to 5 years or longer.

F. **Oral administration.** The drug is swallowed (bioavailability ≤ 100%). **Entry of the drug** into the circulation is slower than with IV administration and limited by many factors.

1. **First-pass effect.** Orally administered drugs must pass through the portal circulation and the liver before entering the systemic circulation. Bioavailability of many drugs is reduced because they are significantly metabolized before reaching the bloodstream. Some drugs must be administered in much larger doses orally than intravenously (e.g., propranolol requires an oral dose 20–40 times larger than its IV dose).

2. **Metabolic activation.** Some drugs are activated as they pass through the liver before entering the systemic circulation. Drugs administered in an inactive form (e.g., clorazepate, sulindac) must be metabolically altered to a physiologically active and available form. This type of drug would have a much smaller effect if administered intravenously because only a small fraction of the systemic circulation passes through the liver. This situation contrasts with gastrointestinal absorption in which virtually all of the portal circulation passes through the liver.

G. **Sublingual administration.** The drug is administered by placing it under the tongue **(bioavailability ≤ 100%** but often greater than with oral administration). The advantages of this route include rapid absorption, owing to the vascularity of sublingual tissues, and increased bioavailability, because sublingual circulation passes directly into the systemic circulation rather than into the portal circulation. The usual form is a tablet but some agents are commercially available in a spray.

H. **Rectal administration.** The drug is administered rectally, usually in suppository form, but otherwise as a liquid **(bioavailability ≤ 100%). Absorption** is slow, erratic, and often incomplete. Bioavailability may be greater than with oral administration because only one (the superior hemorrhoidal vein) of the three rectal veins empties into the portal circulation.

I. **Vaginal administration.** The drug is administered vaginally as a suppository, tablet, cream, or foam. **Drug effects** are usually local, but systemic absorption does occur through the vaginal mucosa. Systemic effects are usually side effects rather than the desired therapeutic goal.

J. **Topical administration.** The drug is applied to the skin and absorbed into the systemic circulation after passing through all five layers of the stratum corneum (the outermost epidermis).

1. **Bioavailability** varies, depending on the thickness of the skin surface, circulation in the local area, drug lipophilicity, and skin condition (see III D).

2. **Advantages** of topical drug administration include a long duration of action and the ability to remove the dosage form when it is no longer needed.

3. **Absorption** is generally slower than with most other routes of administration.

K. **Inhalation.** The drug is inhaled into the lungs, where the site of action may be local (e.g., beclomethasone) or systemic (e.g., enflurane, other inhalational anesthetics).

1. **Absorption** is generally rapid, because of the vascular nature of the pulmonary capillary system, but it also depends on drug lipophilicity, droplet or particle size, pulmonary function, and respiratory status.

2. **Excretion.** Most systemic inhaled drugs are generally short-acting (minutes to hours) and may be eliminated by the lungs. Locally acting inhaled drugs generally have longer **durations of action** and may last from 2 to 12 hours or more.

L. **Buccal administration.** The drug is absorbed through the oral mucosa, after being placed between the cheek and the gums. **Absorption** is usually rapid, and bioavailability is similar to that of sublingual administration (see II G).

M. **Intranasal administration.** The drug is inhaled nasally and then absorbed through the nasal mucosa. Onset is generally rapid, but **bioavailability** can be variable and depends on the condition of nasal membranes. Drugs may be administered for a local (e.g., phenylephrine) or systemic (e.g., desmopressin) effect. The **duration of action** may be from minutes to hours, depending on the drug.

N. **Ophthalmic administration.** The drug is administered onto the conjunctiva. The effect is usually local with systemic side effects occasionally occurring. **Absorption** into the central nervous system (CNS) is sometimes a problem because of the proximity of the eyes to the brain and the lipophilic nature of ophthalmically active medications.

O. Otic administration. The drug is administered into the auditory canal, usually for local results, such as an anti-inflammatory or anti-infective effect.

III. DRUG ABSORPTION

A. Dissolution. Drugs administered in solid dosage forms must be dissolved so that they can be absorbed across membranes. The dissolution rate is determined by particle size, coating, or protective layer (e.g., tablets), and drug solubility. Some tablets owe their sustained-release properties to slow dissolution. Most highly bioavailable oral dosage forms are readily soluble in gastric juices.

B. Membrane transport. Drug molecules must cross the membrane of absorption to enter the systemic circulation.

1. Most drugs cross the membrane by **simple diffusion,** which depends on the lipophilicity of the drug molecule (i.e., highly lipophilic drugs cross the membrane more rapidly and more easily) and the drug concentration gradient existing across the membrane (i.e., a larger gradient causes faster transport).
2. Some drugs (e.g., vitamins) are carried across the absorption membrane by enzymes; such **carrier-mediated transport** may be passive or active and can move drugs against a concentration gradient as well as with the gradient.

C. Blood flow to the absorbing organ. Rapid and extensive blood flow to the organ or membrane of absorption:

1. Facilitates rapid and complete absorption of the drug
2. Reduces the drug concentration on the systemic side of the absorption membrane, thereby increasing the concentration gradient across which the drug molecule is absorbed
3. Facilitates more rapid drug entry into the systemic circulation, enabling the drug to exert its effect at the intended site of action

D. Skin condition is a concern only for topically administered medications. Highly vascular skin (e.g., scrotum, eyelid), broken skin (e.g., burned, eczematous), or hydrated skin (e.g., occluded) leads to a more rapid and complete systemic absorption of topically applied drugs. Thick and highly keratinized skin areas (e.g., calluses, soles of feet) are poor sites for systemic drug absorption because the thickened stratum corneum retards the passage of drug molecules. Drugs applied to such sites should be intended for local, not systemic, effects.

E. pH-Dependence. Some drugs (e.g., weak acids, weak bases) carry a molecular charge at different pHs. Weak bases become positively charged at low pH, such as that in the stomach. Charged molecules cannot cross the lipid membranes easily. Such molecules can be absorbed only when they are unchanged, as occurs lower in the gastrointestinal tract, where the pH is higher. Weak acids are more easily absorbed in acidic environments, where they are uncharged.

F. Bioavailability. Some drugs are incompletely absorbed from the administration site. Oral drugs are most commonly mentioned, but intramuscular, topical, and rectal administration sites are also common sites where incomplete absorption occurs. In addition to the first-pass effect discussed in II F 1, incomplete absorption is the other primary cause of low bioavailability.

1. Some sustained-release tablets may pass through the gastrointestinal tract and leave the body before their enteric coatings dissolve.
2. Sustained-release tablets may also retain some active drug in their wax matrices.

G. Compliance. If drugs are not actually taken in prescribed amounts or at prescribed (or recommended) intervals, plasma levels may be subtherapeutic or supratherapeutic. Therapeutic drug monitoring is sometimes used to monitor patient compliance.

H. Food co-administration. Many oral agents are incompletely absorbed if they are taken with food. Food can increase the gastric pH and hinder the dissolution of some medications.

1. Although high plasma levels are usually achieved with most drugs (particularly antibiotics) when taken on an empty stomach, many drugs can achieve therapeutic concentrations if taken with food.
2. Certain foods contain specific products that interfere with absorption. Tetracycline, for example, chelates calcium ions if taken with dairy products and forms a complex that cannot be absorbed.

IV. DRUG DISTRIBUTION

IV. DRUG DISTRIBUTION to various body tissues and compartments is affected by many factors, such as body composition and binding propensities. Measuring drug concentrations (most commonly in plasma) assesses drug distribution, a key element in therapeutic effect. Plasma concentrations may or may not reflect drug concentration at the site of action or the site of toxicity.

A. Therapeutic concentration and therapeutic index

1. For many drugs, the concentrations at which most patients begin to experience therapeutic effects (**minimum effective concentration** [MEC]) and toxic effects (**minimum toxic concentration** [MTC]) are known. These concentrations are generally used as the upper and lower limits of the therapeutic concentration range, or window. The science of clinical pharmacokinetics is concerned with designing dosage regimens to keep a specific patient's drug concentration within the therapeutic window.
2. The **therapeutic index** of a drug is the **ratio of the MTC to the MEC.**
   - **a.** If the **therapeutic index is small,** the patient is more likely to experience toxicity or ineffective therapy.
   - **b.** If the **therapeutic index is large,** the therapeutic window is usually larger, and it is easier to achieve an effective, nontoxic dosage regimen.

B. Tissue binding. Some drugs are bound to extravascular tissues, such as muscle or fat. Such drugs have low concentrations in the plasma compartment and a large apparent V_D. Some drugs preferentially distribute to specific body tissues, depending on blood flow, pH conditions, and the lipophilicity of the tissue. Other drugs remain largely in the plasma compartment, have a small apparent V_d, and produce a higher C_p for any given dose of drug.

C. Body composition. The composition of the body, which changes with certain disease states and with age, is an important consideration for how certain drugs are distributed. The examples of obesity and edema are discussed here, but similar principles are true for other abnormal physiologic conditions.

1. **Obesity.** The apparent V_d is usually based on a patient's weight.
   - **a.** In addition to increased adipose tissue, obese patients have excess fluid as compared with patients with a lean body mass.
   - **b.** Some drugs preferentially leave the plasma in favor of adipose tissue; thus, C_ps for these drugs are lower, resulting in a larger V_d in obese patients.
   - **c.** Drugs that have a low solubility in fat remain in the plasma and produce higher C_ps. In obese patients, therefore, the V_d is smaller (per weight unit) than in thinner patients. Doses for drugs that distribute poorly to adipose tissues (e.g., aminoglycosides) are usually based on a patient's lean body weight, rather than total body weight. This consideration is important because the relative proportion of adipose and lean tissue mass changes with age, with fat comprising a larger percentage of the body weight as the patient ages.
2. **Edema.** Some hydrophilic drugs (e.g., lithium, aminoglycosides) remain largely in the plasma compartment. Patients with edema or ascites may distribute a large proportion of such drugs into the extravascular tissues rather than into the target tissue (e.g., infected muscle tissue). If doses of such drugs are based on the patient's weight, the C_p is lower because of the large plasma compartment relative to the patient's weight, and the observed concentration, as well as the concentration at the target site, may be subtherapeutic.

D. Protein binding

1. **Free and bound concentrations.** Many drugs are bound to plasma proteins. In the plasma, these drugs exist in a state of equilibrium with some of the drug free (unbound) and some bound to proteins. Protein-bound drug is referred to as a **drug-protein complex**.
   a. Only the free drug can cross membranes to enter body tissues, and only the free drug can interact with receptors to produce therapeutic or toxic effects.
   b. Clinical laboratories generally report total C_ps (free plus bound drug). For most patients and most drugs, this information is sufficient because standard therapeutic concentrations reflect such factors as drug affinity for protein and free-drug concentrations. Special circumstances exist, however, in which data on total drug concentrations prove insufficient or misleading. Information about the free-drug concentration in a blood sample can be obtained for some drugs—notably phenytoin—but the test is expensive, difficult to perform, and not always available.

2. **Displacement.** Drugs are generally considered highly protein-bound when over 90% of the total drug in plasma is protein-bound. These drugs can sometimes be displaced by other substances that bind to the same protein. In such instances, the second drug competes with the first drug for a limited number of binding sites on the protein. Because there is more drug than available protein-binding sites, this causes a much higher free-drug concentration of the first drug while the total concentration remains unchanged.
   a. **Example.** If a patient has been stabilized on aspirin, which binds albumin, and then begins taking phenylbutazone, which also binds albumin, the phenylbutazone may displace some salicylic acid and increase the free salicylate concentration. This previously stable patient may now experience some symptoms of salicylate toxicity because of an increased C_p of free salicylate, despite an apparently normal concentration of salicylic acid (free plus bound). Eventually, the higher free salicylic acid concentration causes more salicylic acid to be excreted, and a new equilibrium (steady state) is reached.
   b. **Albumin**
      (1) The main plasma and drug-binding protein, albumin, is an abundant protein that occurs in a concentration of 3.5–5.5 g/dl (0.6 mmol) in the plasma.
      (2) Most drugs bound to albumin are acidic, including those listed in Table 36-3; some of them can also displace drugs bound to albumin.
      (3) For a drug to be an effective displacer, it must occupy a large number of binding sites on albumin (i.e., it must accumulate to high concentrations or be given in large doses).
      (4) Drugs such as aspirin, phenylbutazone, and sulfa drugs are the most common displacers. Other substances, such as bilirubin, may bind albumin and may be displaced. For example, sulfa drugs displace albumin-bound bilirubin, which can cause free bilirubin to increase to toxic concentrations. Because kernicterus can result, **sulfa drugs should not be administered to neonates,** who lack the hepatic capability to metabolize bilirubin.
      (5) Albumin levels may also be altered by certain disease states listed in Table 36-4. Increases in albumin concentration decrease the free concentration of drugs that bind to albumin; conversely, decreases in albumin concentration increase the free concentration of albumin-binding drugs.
   c. **Alpha$_1$-acid glycoprotein (AAG)**
      (1) After albumin, AAG is the second most important drug-binding plasma protein. AAG occurs in much smaller concentrations (2–4 mg/L [0.01–0.02 mmol]) than albumin and primarily binds the basic drugs listed in Table 36-5.
      (2) Circumstances affecting AAG concentrations are listed in Table 36-6.
      (3) The same basic protein-binding principles discussed for albumin are true for AAG. Conditions that increase AAG concentrations decrease free concentrations of drugs that bind AAG; those that decrease AAG increase free-drug concentrations. One no-

Table 36-3. Some Drugs That Bind to Albumin

Clofibrate	Salicylic acid
Ethacrynic acid	Sulfa drugs
Flufenamic acid	Sulfinpyrazone
Oxyphenbutazone	Warfarin
Phenylbutazone	

Table 36-4. Conditions That May Change Plasma Albumin Concentrations

Decrease Plasma Albumin	Increase Plasma Albumin
Acute infection	Benign tumor
Bone fractures	Gynecologic disorders
Burns	Myalgia
Cystic fibrosis	Schizophrenia
Inflammatory disease	
Liver disease	
Malnutrition	
Myocardial infarction	
Neoplastic disease	
Nephrotic syndrome	
Pregnancy	
Renal disease	
Surgical procedures	

table exception, however, is that few drugs are nearly totally bound to AAG, as some are to albumin. AAG exists in much smaller concentrations in the blood and is therefore unlikely to bind most of a drug, unless that drug is given in very small doses.

(4) Drug binding to AAG is not likely to be as clinically significant as drug-albumin binding.

E. Sample timing. Objectives of monitoring include assessing a drug in its steady state and anticipating drug clearance (particularly for toxic agents); thus, sampling should take into account approximate distribution time and the half-life of the drug.

1. Distribution. The rate and pattern of distribution vary widely among drugs and should be estimated when developing or considering a monitoring plan.

a. Certain drugs, such as aminoglycosides, reside in the plasma compartment before they are distributed to target tissues. This initial residence may last up to 30 minutes for an aminoglycoside. Therefore, a plasma aminoglycoside sample should not be drawn within 30 minutes of administration; the drug concentration would appear to be too high be-

Table 36-5. Some Drugs That Bind to Alpha$_1$-Acid Glycoprotein (AAG)

Amitriptyline	Lidocaine
Chlorpromazine	Meperidine
Dipyridamole	Nortriptyline
Disopyramide	Propranolol
Erythromycin	Quinidine
Imipramine	

Table 36-6. Circumstances That May Change Plasma Alpha$_1$-Acid Glycoprotein (AAG) Concentrations

Decrease Plasma AAG	Increase Plasma AAG
Nephrotic syndrome	Burns
	Chronic pain
	Inflammatory disease (e.g., Crohn's disease, rheumatoid arthritis)
	Myocardial infarction
	Neoplastic disease
	Surgical procedures
	Trauma injury

cause the drug would not have distributed to the tissues.

b. The probable location of receptor sites for specific drugs is important for sample planning. Digoxin, for example, exerts its therapeutic and toxic effects through receptor sites that reside in the tissue compartments of the heart. Thus, concentrations only become relevant after the drug has had a chance to redistribute from the plasma to the tissue compartment (about 6 hours for digoxin). Samples should not be drawn within 6–8 hours after an IV dose of digoxin is administered (longer for an oral dose).

2. Half-lives. When considering a change in administration rate, the patient should be at or near steady state when the sample is taken for evaluation. Steady state is usually achieved after the passage of four half-lives at a constant dosing rate.

a. If the sample is taken before steady state has been reached and the infusion rate is raised based on the results of the premature sample, the patient begins to accumulate drug from the new infusion while continuing to accumulate drug from the initial dose. This accumulation could result in toxic concentrations.

b. When administering toxic agents (or those with narrow therapeutic indices), it is prudent to sample sooner than usual (e.g., after one half-life). In this way, progress toward steady state can be determined while it is still possible to exert control, such as by reducing the dosage rate.

V. DRUG ELIMINATION

A. Metabolism. The liver is the site of metabolism for most drugs, but other organs and tissues (e.g., lungs, kidneys, intestines) may also metabolize drugs. Lipophilic drugs, for example, require chemical modification (e.g., acetylation, conjugation) by the liver to render them more water-soluble and thus more readily removable by renal filtration.

1. Extraction ratio

a. Drugs that are extensively metabolized during a single pass through the liver are said to have a high extraction ratio (i.e., the proportion of extracted drug to total drug that entered the liver is high). If a significant proportion of the drug has been extracted (rendered inactive) before entering systemic circulation—the **first-past effect** (see II F 1)—then the amount of active drug left to produce the desired effect is significantly reduced.

b. The difference in extraction ratios among drugs accounts for the differences in magnitude of the first-pass effect from drug to drug.

c. Oral agents traverse the liver before entering the systemic circulation. If a drug is administered orally and has a high extraction ratio (e.g., propranolol), then most of the drug is eliminated before reaching the systemic circulation. Therefore, the effective dose for such a drug given orally may be much higher than if given intravenously.

2. Hepatic blood flow changes

a. Changes in hepatic blood flow affect the rate at which the liver is presented with a drug. Because the liver effectively processes drugs as they arrive, a change in the presentation rate changes the rate at which drugs with a high extraction ratio are metabolized. (Most drugs with low extraction ratios are affected only minimally or not at all by changes in hepatic flow rate.)

b. Some drugs [e.g., most histamine$_2$ (H_2)-antagonists] reduce hepatic blood flow. Therefore, close monitoring of plasma drug concentrations is required if H_2-antagonists are administered to a patient already stabilized on a drug with a high extraction ratio (e.g., theophylline, propranolol, lidocaine).

3. Changes in enzyme activity

a. Metabolic enzyme activity, rather than hepatic blood flow, determines the removal rate of drugs with low extraction ratios.

b. Drugs and other substances can affect this activity, enhancing or inhibiting it, by altering the amount of enzymes or influencing their function.

(1) Inducing enzyme metabolism

(a) Phenobarbital can stimulate hepatic enzymes to speed metabolism and change the effect of other drugs metabolized by the liver. Thus a patient who has been stabilized on rifampin (a drug with a low extraction ratio) may experience subtherapeutic rifampin concentrations once phenobarbital is added to the regimen.

(b) Smoking can also increase enzyme activity, because the theophylline clearance rate is higher in smokers than in nonsmokers.

(2) **Inhibiting enzyme metabolism** may allow drug concentrations to build up to toxic levels. For example, less theophylline is removed if cimetidine is added to the regimen because cimetidine inhibits cytochrome P-450, a key element of the oxidative enzyme system.

4. **Metabolites.** Many metabolites are inactive and are simply removed by the kidneys. In some circumstances, however, drug metabolites must be considered in therapeutic drug monitoring. Like their parent drugs, metabolites may contribute both therapeutic and toxic effects.
   a. **Efficacy.** Some metabolites actually contribute to the therapeutic effectiveness of a drug. For instance, *N*-acetylprocainamide has antiarrhythmic properties that contribute to the effectiveness of procainamide, the parent drug. Other drugs with metabolites that enhance their therapeutic effectiveness include primidone, diazepam, flurazepam, imipramine, and nefazodone.
   b. **Toxicity.** Some metabolites may be more toxic than the parent drug. An example of a toxic metabolite is normeperidine, which is produced from meperidine. In most patients, normeperidine is quickly removed, but in patients with impaired renal function, it may build up to toxic levels and produce seizures. Other drugs with toxic metabolites include ethanol and acetaminophen.
   c. **Prodrugs.** Some drugs are inactive when they are administered and must be *activated,* usually by the metabolic process, to be effective. Examples include sulindac, clorazepate, and aspirin.
   d. **Assay interference.** Drug metabolites may be misinterpreted as active drugs. Most clinical laboratories and commercially available assays distinguish between parent drugs and metabolites, but mistakes occur. This is particularly relevant if a patient has impaired renal function and metabolites have built up to significant levels. If necessary, C_p for drug metabolites, such as *N*-acetylprocainamide or desipramine, can be obtained from the clinical laboratory.

B. Excretion

1. **Urinary excretion.** Most drugs are removed by the kidneys, either as unchanged drug or as metabolites; therefore, renal function greatly influences drug concentration and thus figures prominently in adjustments of drug regimens.
   a. **Renal function** is usually estimated using the **Cockcroft and Gault equation** [see I C 4 a (3)]. Generally, all aspects of renal function are assumed to rise or fall together; filtration, secretion, and reabsorption are considered impaired to the same degree in a patient with renal failure. However, the effect of an individual drug may rely more heavily on one of these three aspects. The individual processes are discussed in VI.
   b. **Dose adjustment.** Many nomograms have been developed to determine dosage adjustments (i.e., amount or frequency) in given circumstances. Generally, as the degree of renal impairment increases and the size of the fraction of the drug excreted remains unchanged, a greater dosage adjustment is needed to maintain drug concentrations in the plasma within the therapeutic range.

2. **Biliary and fecal excretion**
   a. Some drugs undergo biliary excretion and enterohepatic recycling. These drugs may be eliminated in the feces, even though they were administered intravenously. This is an important consideration for some drugs. For example, a patient who has taken an overdose of theophylline may be saved if activated charcoal is administered. The charcoal works, even if the theophylline was not given orally, because it adsorbs the theophylline on contact in the gastrointestinal tract, promotes gastrointestinal trapping of the theophylline, and hastens its elimination.
   b. Biliary elimination is only a consideration if a patient has impaired biliary function because some drugs may accumulate.

3. **Other routes.** Several other minor routes of drug elimination exist, but these are insignificant for purposes of therapeutic drug monitoring.
   a. Some volatile anesthetics (e.g., halothane) are eliminated primarily on exhalation.
   b. A few drugs are eliminated through perspiration, saliva, tears, and breast milk.

VI. PHARMACOKINETIC DRUG INTERACTIONS. Co-administering drugs can enhance, inhibit, or negate the effect each drug achieves when administered alone. These interactions occur when one drug alters, opposes, or potentiates the basic pharmacokinetics of the other drug.

A. Absorption

1. Rate

a. The **absorption rate decreases** when drugs are administered in a way that decreases local blood flow (e.g., topically), or that slows stomach emptying (e.g., orally).

(1) With co-administering propantheline and acetaminophen, propantheline slows stomach emptying; therefore, acetaminophen is absorbed more slowly.

(2) Vasoconstriction caused by epinephrine when it is co-administered with lidocaine for topical anesthesia reduces blood flow to and from the affected area, prolonging the effect of lidocaine and reducing the need for subsequent injections.

b. The **absorption rate increases** if the drug that speeds stomach emptying is co-administered. For example, metoclopramide, which speeds stomach emptying, increases the absorption rate of co-administered oral acetaminophen.

2. Extent. Co-administration can affect drug availability.

a. Increased bioavailability of digoxin, for example, is achieved by orally administering digoxin and propantheline together. The propantheline slows stomach emptying and improves the availability of the slow-dissolving digoxin tablets.

b. Decreased absorption (bioavailability) results from co-administration in many instances. Heavy metal ions and tetracyclines administered together result in the formation of nonabsorbable complexes; kaolin-pectin adsorbs co-administered digoxin and results in lower digoxin absorption.

c. Only nonionized molecules cross lipid absorption membranes. For this reason, drugs that alter the ionic status of other drug molecules affect their absorption. For example, ketoconazole is only absorbed from an acidic stomach; co-administered antacids greatly impair ketoconazole absorption.

B. Volume of distribution. Changes in protein binding (see IV D) are generally the cause of altered V_ds. For example, the V_d increases for salicylic acid when co-administered with phenylbutazone because the concentration of free (unbound) salicylic acid is the same as it was before phenylbutazone administration; however, the total concentration (free plus bound) is lower. Because the V_d is based upon total concentration, a lower salicylic acid concentration produces a larger apparent V_d.

C. Clearance

1. Metabolic clearance. Several factors influence metabolic clearance (see V A).

a. For drugs with a high extraction ratio, metabolism is inhibited by co-administering a drug that reduces hepatic blood flow. For example, co-administering lidocaine and cimetidine inhibits the elimination of lidocaine (a drug with a high extraction ratio) and produces higher than expected lidocaine concentrations.

b. Metabolic clearance may be increased for a drug with a low extraction ratio by co-administering an enzyme inducer. For example, warfarin (a drug with a low extraction ratio) metabolism is increased when phenobarbital is also administered. If a patient has been stabilized on warfarin and phenobarbital is introduced, close monitoring is required to maintain the appropriate coagulation status.

2. Renal clearance. Drugs eliminated by glomerular filtration are affected only by drugs that modify renal function, a pharmacodynamic interaction (e.g., nephrotoxic cisplatin impairs renal elimination of gentamicin). Secretion and reabsorption are subject to pharmacokinetic interactions.

a. Secretion. Some drugs, such as penicillins, are actively secreted. Co-administering a drug that competes for secretion may be used to improve the therapeutic outcome in patients with a history of poor compliance. For example, probenecid inhibits the secretion of penicillin and results in sustained blood levels of penicillin.

b. Reabsorption. Drugs that are filtered or secreted and then reabsorbed are also subject to drug interactions.

(1) If a drug becomes ionized in the renal tubule owing to a change in pH, it is impossible for it to be reabsorbed because only nonionized molecules can cross biologic membranes. For example, ammonium chloride decreases urinary pH. Amphetamine becomes positively charged at the lower pH and cannot be reabsorbed. More amphetamine is thus eliminated.

(2) Urine acidification or alkalinization is often used in cases of overdoses and poisonings.

STUDY QUESTIONS

Directions: The numbered item or incomplete statement in this section is followed by answers or by completions of the statement. Select the **one** lettered answer or completion that is **best.**

1. All of the following statements about intramuscular drug administration are true EXCEPT

(A) entry of the drug into the circulation is affected by the drug's degree of lipophilicity
(B) peak effect is generally less than with intravenous administration
(C) bioavailability equals 100%
(D) maximum injection volume is 2–5 ml
(E) drug effects generally last longer than with intravenous administration

Directions: Each item below contains three suggested answers of which **one or more** is correct. Choose the answer

A if **I only** is correct
B if **III only** is correct
C if **I and II** are correct
D if **II and III** are correct
E if **I, II, and III** are correct

2. True statements about protein binding include which of the following?

I. Only bound drug can interact with receptors to produce therapeutic or toxic effects
II. Drugs are considered highly protein-bound when over 90% of the total drug in plasma is protein-bound
III. Albumin is the main plasma protein that binds drugs

3. Which of the following patients should have therapeutic drug monitoring?

I. An 80-year-old man with congestive heart failure
II. A 6-year-old boy with kidney disease
III. A 3-month-old girl with acute gastroenteritis

4. Conditions that may decrease plasma albumin include

I. malnutrition
II. pregnancy
III. myalgia

5. True statements about therapeutic monitoring include which of the following?

I. Two patients with identical plasma drug levels within the therapeutic range will both experience the same benefit from the drug therapy being monitored.
II. Measurement of plasma drug levels is the best measure of a drug's effectiveness.
III. The same patient may have 2 samplings indicating the same total plasma concentration of a specific drug, but that patient may experience markedly different results at the 2 times of sampling.

ANSWERS AND EXPLANATIONS

1. The answer is C *[II C].*
With intramuscular administration, bioavailability is not always 100%. Only IV administration consistently provides 100% bioavailability. The other statements listed in the question are correct. The entry of an intramuscularly injected drug into the circulation is limited by the drug's solubility and lipophilicity and by the blood supply in the muscle. Because an intramuscular drug enters the blood more slowly and gradually than an IV drug, the peak effect of an intramuscular drug is not as great, but its duration of action is generally longer than with IV administration. Not more than 2–5 ml should be injected into any one intramuscular site.

2. The answer is D (II, III) *[IV D].*
Only free drug can interact with receptors to produce a therapeutic (or toxic) effect. A drug that is bound to plasma protein cannot cross membranes to enter body tissues and cannot interact with receptors to produce an effect. Albumin, one of the major proteins of blood plasma, is the main plasma protein that binds drugs. The second most important drug-binding plasma protein is $alpha_1$-acid glycoprotein (AAG). Albumin binds acidic drugs; AAG binds basic drugs.

3. The answer is E (all) *[I C 1, 4].*
Patients who need rapidly effective treatment and patients with altered physiologic and pharmacokinetic parameters would benefit from therapeutic drug monitoring. Also, extremes of age affect drug absorption, distribution, metabolism, and excretion, so that elderly patients and very young patients require special care when determining dosage. Congestive heart failure can impair absorption, distribution, and elimination of many drugs. Impaired renal function often requires modifying dosages. Acute gastroenteritis in an infant can rapidly cause dehydration and electrolyte imbalance and therefore calls for rapid, effective treatment and close monitoring.

4. The answer is C (I, II) *[Table 39-4].*
Albumin levels may be altered by a variety of disease states. Infections, malnutrition, myocardial infarction, and renal disease are among the numerous diseases that can lower the plasma albumin levels. Pregnancy can also cause a decrease in plasma albumin. Conditions that may increase plasma albumin levels include myalgia and some gynecologic disorders. A decrease in plasma albumin increases the free concentration of a drug that binds to albumin and thus increases the effects of the drug. Conversely, an increase in plasma albumin lowers the concentration of free drug and thus reduces its effects.

5. The answer is C (III) *[I B-C, IV A-D]*
For many drugs, the interpatient variability in response is very large; a concentration that is effective in one patient may be toxic or subtherapeutic in another patient. Measuring plasma drug levels is only one tool to assess effectiveness of pharmacotherapy. The best way to gauge a drug's effectiveness is to monitor the condition being treated and to monitor the patient for adverse effects resulting from pharmacotherapy. A patient's condition may change over time. As a disease progresses, higher plasma levels of a drug may be required to obtain the same effect. In addition, a patient's total drug concentration may be the same, but the free (unbound) drug concentration may be different; because effectiveness and toxicity are related to the unbound (in contrast to the total) drug concentration, the effect on the patient may be markedly different.

37
Drug Use in Special Patient Populations: Pediatric, Pregnant, Geriatric

Alan H. Mutnick
H. William McGhee

I. DRUG THERAPY IN PEDIATRIC PATIENTS

A. General considerations

1. Pediatric drug therapy challenges the pharmacist, because children are uniquely different from adults. Many of the assumptions made in adult drug therapy do not apply to children. For example, in contrast to the relatively stable pharmacokinetic profile that characterizes most of the adult years, **pharmacokinetic parameters in children change as they mature from birth to adolescence.** Complex processes relating to drug absorption, distribution, metabolism, and elimination are not fully developed at birth and mature at varying rates throughout childhood.

2. Drug selection, doses, and dosage intervals change throughout childhood, making **drug therapy monitoring** essential. The outline below describes pharmacokinetic differences in childhood that influence drug therapy. Then follows a discussion of problems inherent to pediatric drug monitoring as well as some brief comments on adverse drug reactions. Finally, some cautions are suggested concerning drug dosing in children.

B. Pharmacokinetic considerations

1. **Absorption.** Oral drug absorption is a complex and variable process. Many drug- and patient-related factors influence absorption, although drug-related factors are generally fixed and patient-related factors change. These include gastric pH, gastric emptying time, an underlying disease state, bile salt production, and pancreatic enzyme function.
   a. **Gastric pH.** Neonates are relatively achlorhydric. Increases in acid production correlate with starting enteral feedings. Acid production rises steadily from age 7 days to 1 month but is variable. Relative achlorhydria (i.e., pH > 4) is present in approximately 20% of neonates at 1 week of age, 15% at 2 weeks, and 8% at 3 weeks. By 6 weeks of age, gastric acid production is comparable to that in older infants and reaches adult values at 2 years of age. Relative achlorhydria may explain the increased bioavailability of basic drugs and the unpredictable, slower absorption of acidic agents.
   b. **Gastric emptying.** The rate of gastric emptying is important in determining the rate and extent of drug absorption. Gastric emptying is highly variable in neonates and is affected by gestational and postnatal ages and the type of feeding administered. At 6 to 8 months of age infants acquire the same rate of gastric emptying as adults.
      (1) Because most drugs are absorbed in the small intestine, a **reduced rate of emptying** slows the rate of absorption, which can reduce peak drug concentrations. **Prematurity** slows gastric emptying from an already reduced rate in term neonates (half-life [$t_{1/2}$] of gastric emptying is 90 minutes) as compared with adults ($t_{1/2}$ is 65 minutes).
      (2) An **increased rate of emptying** may reduce the extent of absorption, because contact time with absorptive surfaces in the small intestine is reduced.
      (3) **Breast-fed infants** empty their stomachs twice as fast as formula-fed infants, in whom gastric emptying is slower when given formula feedings of increasing caloric density.
   c. **Underlying disease state**
      (1) Disease states that can significantly **prolong gastric emptying** include pyloric stenosis, gastroesophageal reflux, respiratory distress syndrome, and congenital heart disease.
      (2) Short bowel syndrome greatly **reduces the total surface area available for drug absorption.**

(3) Cholestatic liver disease, biliary obstruction, and distal ileum resection can **interfere with bile acid excretion or reabsorption and reduce the absorption of lipid-soluble substances** including vitamins A, D, and E.

d. **Bile salt production.** The bile salt pool and the rate of bile salt synthesis are reduced approximately 50% in premature and young term infants as compared with adults. Decreased fat absorption from enteral feedings, as well as decreased drug absorption, can occur. For example, when vitamin D (i.e., calcifediol, also called 25-hydroxycholecalciferol) is administered to neonates, absorption is only 30% as compared with 70% in adults.

e. **Pancreatic enzyme function.** The absorption of lipid-soluble drugs is also affected by gastrointestinal concentrations of pancreatic enzymes. Neonates have low levels of lipases, and, when combined with reduced bile acid production, lipid-soluble drugs may be left insoluble and thus unabsorbed in the intestine. Oral suspensions, such as chloramphenicol palmitate, which require intraluminal hydrolysis by pancreatic lipases before being absorbed, have been associated with unreliable absorption of the active moiety in premature and term infants.

2. **Distribution.** How a drug distributes in the body is important in both the selection and dosage of a drug. Volume of distribution is affected by many age-dependent factors including the degree of protein binding, the sizes of various body compartments, and the presence of various endogenous substances.

a. **Protein binding.** Acidic drugs bind to **albumin** while basic substances bind primarily to **alpha$_2$-acid glycoprotein.** Both of these proteins are reduced in neonates, which allows greater amounts of free drug in the serum and tissues. This has been demonstrated for phenytoin, phenobarbital, chloramphenicol, penicillin, propranolol, lidocaine, and several other substances. The increase in the free fraction of certain drugs in neonates and infants challenges the reliability of serum concentration monitoring, which uses parameters derived from adult populations. Adult levels for albumin and alpha$_1$-acid glycoprotein occur at approximately 10 to 12 months of age.

b. **Size of body compartments.** At birth, extracellular fluid volume constitutes approximately 40% of total body weight, decreasing to 25% by 6 months, and 20% by 12 years. For polar compounds, such as the aminoglycosides that distribute into extracellular spaces, **loading doses** (i.e., the approximate amount of drug contained in the body during steady state) are required in neonates to achieve therapeutic concentrations. Loading doses are not necessary in older infants and children.

c. **Endogenous substances.** In neonates, various endogenous substances can bind to plasma proteins and reduce the degree of drug-protein binding. The two most important substances are **free fatty acids** and **unconjugated bilirubin,** which, when present in high concentrations, can increase the unbound:bound drug ratio in the plasma.

(1) The serum concentration of these two substances normalizes in early infancy.

(2) Caution is urged, however, in evaluating bilirubin- or free fatty acid-induced drug displacement reactions, because significant increases in the plasma concentrations of the drug occur only when the displaced drug is more than 90% bound and its metabolism is rate-limited.

(3) Usually, increases in unbound concentrations are only transient, because hepatic metabolism for most drugs is not rate-limited.

d. Because **bilirubin** competes with certain drugs for albumin binding sites, it can be displaced, which presents a **theoretical** concern for the development of **drug-induced kernicterus** in neonates. **Hyperbilirubinemia** develops because heme catabolism is accelerated and the conjugating ability of the liver is reduced.

(1) Unconjugated bilirubin normally binds noncovalently to plasma albumin, but the binding affinity is reduced in neonates, not approaching **adult values** until 6 months of age. Thus, it potentially can be displaced when certain highly bound acidic compounds are administered.

(2) The concern for drug-induced bilirubin displacement is theoretical, because it is derived from in vitro studies. It may be that drug-induced displacement of bilirubin and the development of clinical kernicterus are unlikely because the affinity of bilirubin for albumin greatly exceeds that of most drugs. This remains controversial, however, and requires further study.

3. **Metabolism.** Drug metabolism occurs primarily in the liver, with additional biotransformation occurring in the intestine, lung, adrenal gland, and skin. In the liver, metabolism involves

a series of **phase I and phase II reactions,** both of which are susceptible to enzyme-inducing (e.g., phenytoin, phenobarbital, carbamazepine, rifampin) and enzyme-inhibiting (e.g., cimetidine, erythromycin) agents.

a. **Phase I reactions** are nonsynthetic reactions (i.e., oxidation, reduction, hydrolysis, and hydroxylation) that result either in inactive compounds or in metabolites with equal, lesser, or, rarely, greater pharmacologic action.

(1) The major **enzymes** responsible for phase I oxidation reactions are those in the cytochrome P_{450} monooxygenase system, which at birth are at approximately 50% of adult levels.

(2) Consequently, the **metabolism of many drugs** (e.g., phenobarbital) **is reduced** and **drug serum half-lives are prolonged** correspondingly.

(a) The **ability to oxidize** drugs increases with increasing postnatal age so that by several weeks of postnatal life metabolic rates generally are equal to or greater than adult rates.

(b) **Metabolic rates** remain high for 1–5 years and gradually decline to adult levels at puberty.

b. **Phase II reactions** are synthetic reactions (i.e., conjugation with glycine, glucuronide, or sulfate) that result in polar, water-soluble, inactive compounds for renal and bile elimination.

(1) The underlying **enzyme systems** are unevenly depressed at birth and mature at varying rates.

(2) For example, the **ability to conjugate drugs with glucuronide** (e.g., chloramphenicol) is greatly reduced at birth and does not reach adult values until 3 to 4 years of age.

(3) Also, the **acetylation of sulfonamides** is significantly reduced at birth.

(4) However, the **ability to conjugate sulfate groups** (e.g., acetaminophen) is well-developed at birth.

(5) The **ability to conjugate carboxyl groups with glycine** apparently is only slightly reduced at birth and adult levels are achieved by about 6 months of age.

4. **Elimination.** The kidney is the major route of drug elimination for both water-soluble drugs and water-soluble metabolites of lipid-soluble drugs. Three basic processes contribute to renal elimination: glomerular filtration, tubular secretion, and tubular reabsorption. Both glomerular filtration and secretion promote the renal elimination of drugs, whereas reabsorption reduces it. All three processes display age-dependent changes in maturity.

a. At birth, **glomerular filtration in full-term neonates** is 30%–50% of the adult value and matures quickly, approaching 85% of adult values by 3–5 months of age. **Premature infants** (i.e., less than 34 weeks) at birth have glomerular filtration rates that are further reduced and do not obtain rates comparable to those of full-term infants until 4 to 6 weeks of age.

b. **Tubular function**

(1) **Tubular secretion** is an active process, using separate protein carriers for acids and bases. In contrast to glomerular filtration, secretion matures at a slower rate. At birth, **full-term infants** have secretory rates of approximately 20% of adult values and do not achieve adult rates until 6–7 months of age. Before secretion is fully mature, some drugs (e.g., penicillin) may stimulate their own secretion, leading to decreased efficacy unless the dosage is increased.

(2) **Tubular reabsorption** can be an active or passive process. It increases with postconceptional age and is reduced in neonates. Unlike tubular secretion, its development remains poorly understood.

c. **Two other considerations** in renal elimination include renal blood flow and drug-protein binding.

(1) **Renal blood flow** is the driving force underlying glomerular filtration. As cardiac output increases and renal vascular resistance decreases, renal blood flow increases, and adult values are attained by 6 to 12 months.

(2) **Protein binding** significantly affects glomerular filtration because only unbound drug is filtered.

C. **Problems in pediatric drug monitoring.** Several problems are inherent to pediatric pharmacotherapy and lack of recognition or concern for them may lead to greater morbidity or drug-related toxicity.

1. As previously discussed, children display unique **age-dependent changes** in pharmacokinetic parameters. Absorption, distribution, metabolism, and elimination of a drug can vary

greatly between different age groups. Lack of proper clinical monitoring can lead to underdosage, overdosage, therapeutic failure, or drug-related toxicity.

2. **Therapeutic drug monitoring** assumes a correlation exists between serum drug concentrations and therapeutic effects (see Chapter 36). Many of these correlations have been displayed in adult patients but not in children. Extrapolating target serum drug concentrations, which are derived from adults, to children may not always be justified. Drug-protein binding differences, different metabolite patterns, and other factors can change the amount of free drug availability at the receptor site and alter the therapeutic effects of a drug.
   a. A potential complication in interpreting serum drug levels is the **presence of endogenous substances,** which may cross-react with analytical drug assays. This has been demonstrated for digoxin in neonates and infants, and the potential exists that it may be applicable to other drugs.
   b. **Drug levels are not constant** (except when administered by continuous infusion) in the serum and may fluctuate greatly during dosage intervals. Accurate timing of drawing blood is essential to correctly interpret drug concentrations.

3. **Technical problems** may interfere with proper drug delivery. Pediatric drug doses often are in small fluid volumes, which may greatly prolong drug delivery when given through certain intravenous (IV) administration sets. Microbore tubing and infusion pumps can help prevent this problem. Enteral feeding tubes present similar problems.

D. **Adverse drug reactions.** Adverse drug reactions are not uncommon in children. Antibiotics (especially vancomycin, cephalosporins, and penicillins), anticonvulsants, narcotics, antiemetics, and contrast agents are leading causes of reactions in children. The majority of these are mild (e.g., red-man syndrome with IV vancomycin) and are treated relatively simply.

1. However, approximately **3 out of every 10 reactions prolong or require hospitalization** (e.g., syndrome of inappropriate antidiuretic hormone [SIADH] with carbamazepine) and approximately 1 out of 10 is considered severe (i.e., the reaction is life-threatening, or fatal, requires a prolonged recovery time, or is permanently disabling).

2. Examples of severe reactions include anaphylaxis after administering a cephalosporin or respiratory arrest, following the combined IV use of diazepam and phenobarbital.

E. **Dosing considerations in pediatric patients.** Paracelsus' (1493–1541) statement concerning drug dosages is applicable to children: "All substances are poisons, there is none which is not a poison. The right dose differentiates a poison from a remedy."

1. **Drug dosages** for adults cannot be extrapolated to children. This is especially true in neonates and infants and for drugs with a narrow therapeutic index. As previously reviewed, children differ considerably pharmacokinetically from adults, and various rules for dosing children based upon age or weight are unreliable and are not recommended. Pediatric dosages rarely need to be calculated. If a pediatric dosage needs to be calculated, using the body surface area (BSA) is recommended, and it can be determined by using a BSA nomogram or the following equation:

$$\text{BSA (in m}^2\text{)} = \sqrt{\frac{\text{height (cm)} \times \text{weight (kg)}}{3600}}$$

2. Pediatric drug dosages for nearly all drugs can be obtained from standard **pediatric references,** such as the *Harriet Lane Handbook, The Pediatric Drug Handbook,* or the *Manual of Pediatric Therapeutics.* Dosages are based primarily upon weight and occasionally upon BSA.

3. **Dosing intervals** are often different for children. For example, because of reduced renal and hepatic function, neonates generally require a longer dosing interval compared with children and adults. Older infants and children may require a shorter interval because of their enhanced elimination of drugs.

4. **Underlying disease states** may also affect pediatric doses and dosage intervals. For example, patients with cystic fibrosis and cancer often require larger doses and shorter dosing intervals for aminoglycoside antibiotics.

5. **Errors in dosage calculations or drug preparation** are more likely to occur in pediatric patients than in adults. Arithmetic errors are prone to occur when extemporaneously preparing pediatric dosage forms or when calculating dosages.

II. DRUG USE IN PREGNANT PATIENTS. Pregnant women may require drug therapy for preexisting medical conditions or for problems associated with their pregnancy. This patient population may be exposed to drugs or environmental agents that have adverse effects on the unborn. Clinical situations also exist where the fetus may be pharmacologically treated when the mother takes medication. It is important to understand the principles of drug use in these patients because any drug administered to a pregnant woman may directly harm the developing fetus or adversely influence her pregnancy. Furthermore, pharmacotherapy in such a patient population requires knowledge of drug clearance as well as latent effects that are unique in pregnancy.

A. Fetal development. The effects of drug therapy in pregnancy depend largely upon the **stage of fetal development** during which exposure occurs. Limited information exists regarding the effects of drugs in the period of conception and implantation. However, it is suggested that women who are at risk of conceiving or who wish to become pregnant should withdraw all unnecessary medication 3–6 months before conception.

1. **Blastogenesis.** During this stage (the first 15–21 days after fertilization), cleavage and germ layer formation occur. The embryonic cells are in a relatively undifferentiated state.

2. **Organogenesis** (14–56 days). All major organs start to develop during this period. Exposing the embryo to certain drugs at this time may cause major congenital malformations. Organogenesis is the most critical period of development.

3. **Fetal period** (ninth week to birth). At the ninth week the embryo is referred to as a fetus. Development during this time is primarily maturation and growth. Exposure to a drug during this period is generally not associated with major congenital malformations. However, the developing fetus may be at risk from exposure to the pharmacologic effects of a variety of fetotoxic drugs and microorganisms.

B. Placental transfer of drugs. The placenta, a product of conception, is the functional unit between the fetal body and the maternal blood.

1. The **functions** of the placenta include nutrition, respiration, metabolism, excretion, and endocrine activity to maintain fetal and maternal well-being. In conjunction with the fetus, the placenta produces a number of pregnancy-related hormones that are mainly secreted into the maternal circulation. In order for a drug to cause a teratogenic or pharmacologic effect in the embryo or fetus, it must cross from the maternal circulation to the fetal circulation or tissues. Generally, this passage occurs via the placenta.

2. The **placenta is not a protective barrier.** Previously, the placenta was considered to be a protective barrier that isolated the fetus from drugs and toxins present in the maternal circulation. However, the protective characteristics of the placenta are, in fact, limited. The concept that a placental barrier exists should be disregarded. The transfer of most nutrients, oxygen, waste products, drugs, and other substances occurs via **passive diffusion** primarily driven by the concentration gradient. A few compounds, however, are actively transported across the placental membranes.

3. **Factors affecting placental drug transfer.** Generally, the principles that apply to drug transfer across any lipid membrane can be applied to placental transfer of a drug. Most substances administered for therapeutic purposes have, by design, the ability to cross the placenta to the fetus. The critical factor is whether the rate and extent of transfer are sufficient to cause significant drug concentrations in the fetus. There are many factors that affect the rate and extent of placental drug transfer.
   a. **Molecular weight.** Low molecular weight drugs (i.e., less than 500 daltons [d]) diffuse freely across the placenta. Drugs of a higher molecular weight (500–1000 d) cross less easily. Drugs comprised of very large molecules (e.g., heparin) do not cross the placental membranes.
   b. **pH.** The pH gradient between the maternal and fetal circulation and the pH of the drug itself affect the degree of placental transfer. Weakly acidic and weakly basic drugs tend to rapidly diffuse across the placental membranes.
   c. **Lipid solubility.** Moderately lipid-soluble drugs easily diffuse across the placental membranes. It is important to note that many drugs that have been formulated for oral administration, and hence gastrointestinal absorption, are designed for optimal lipid membrane transfer. Generally, these drugs can cross the placenta.

d. Drug absorption. During pregnancy, gastric tone and motility are decreased, which results in delayed gastrointestinal emptying time. This may affect oral drug absorption. Nausea and vomiting, which are common in the first trimester, may also affect oral drug administration and absorption.

e. Drug distribution. The volume of distribution increases significantly during pregnancy and increases with advancing gestational age. The alteration in volume of distribution is the result of a combination of changes associated with pregnancy, including increased plasma volume and increased cardiac output secondary to an increase in stroke volume and heart rate. Total body fluid (i.e., both intravascular and extravascular volume) increases, as does fat content.

f. Plasma protein binding. Placental transfer of plasma protein-bound drug is unlikely, because only the free unbound drug crosses the placenta. During pregnancy, a reduction in the levels of two major drug-binding proteins is observed, namely albumin and alpha$_1$-acid glycoprotein.

(1) The reduction of these two important proteins potentially alters the free fraction of a drug.

(2) When these plasma protein concentrations are decreased there are fewer binding sites available for acidic drugs, and an increase in free drug concentration may result.

(3) However, concomitant increases in drug catabolism in the liver, renal clearance, increased tissue uptake, and altered receptor activity may counteract the effect of changes in plasma protein binding.

g. Physical characteristics of the placenta. As pregnancy progresses, the placental membranes become progressively thinner, resulting in a decrease in diffusion distance.

h. The pharmacologic activities of the drug. Drugs with vasoactive properties may affect maternal and placental blood flow, and therefore influence the amount of drug reaching the fetus.

i. Co-existent disease states. Maternal hypertension or diabetes may reduce or enhance placental drug transfer, as a result of alterations in placenta permeability.

j. Rate of maternal and placental blood flow. Factors that influence maternal blood flow (e.g., exercise, meals, vasoactive medications) may affect drug absorption, maternal drug concentration deliverable to the placenta, and ultimately the fetus.

4. Embryotoxic drugs are drugs that harm the developing embryo, resulting in termination of pregnancy or shortening of gestational length.

a. Many drugs (e.g., hormones, antidepressants, angiotensin-converting enzyme [ACE] inhibitors, and certain antibiotics) administered in early pregnancy may be embryotoxic.

b. Because the placenta has not quite fully formed by organogenesis (see II A 2), the embryo risks damage from a variety of compounds.

c. Some drugs may result in miscarriage by causing a severe chemical insult to the products of conception.

5. Teratogenic drugs cause physical defects in a developing fetus. This risk of teratogenesis is highest during the first trimester.

a. Teratogenesis may lead to physical malformation and/or mental abnormalities.

b. Because fetal organ systems develop at different times, specific teratogenic effects depend mainly on the point of gestation when the drug was ingested.

c. The Food and Drug Administration has developed a **classification system** that groups drugs according to the degree of their potential risk during pregnancy [*Federal Register* 44(124) 37434–37467, June 26, 1979].

(1) Category A. Controlled studies that were performed in women who took these drugs during pregnancy did not demonstrate a risk to the fetus.

(2) Category B. Either no well-controlled human studies exist or animal reproduction studies with these drugs did not demonstrate any risk to the fetus. Or, the animal reproduction studies demonstrated an adverse effect on animal fetuses, but well-controlled human studies did not demonstrate similar results.

(3) Category C. The human fetal risk associated with drugs in this category is unknown. Either adverse effects in animal studies were demonstrated, and similar human studies were not performed, or studies in animals and humans are not available.

(4) Category D. Drugs in this category demonstrated evidence of human fetal risk. However, pregnant women may benefit from treatment of a serious disease or a life-threatening situation with these drugs, which may be acceptable despite the risk to the fetus.

(5) **Category X.** Drugs in this category caused fetal abnormalities in human or animal studies, or there is evidence of fetal risk based on human experience, or both. The risk to the fetus from using these drugs clearly outweighs any possible benefit to the pregnant woman. Also, drugs in this category should not be used in women who are planning to conceive.

d. **Examples** of teratogenic and potentially toxic drugs include the following.

(1) **Vitamin A derivatives.** The drugs in this group–which includes vitamin A, isotretinoin, and etretinate–are potent animal teratogens. Using these agents shortly before or during pregnancy may result in severe human deformities.

(2) **ACE inhibitors.** It remains unclear if this class of antihypertensive drugs produces structural abnormalities in the developing human fetus. These drugs may, however, compromise the fetal renal system and result in severe renal failure and possibly fetal death.

(3) **Warfarin and warfarin derivatives.** The use of warfarin during the first trimester has been associated with a pattern of defects that commonly include nasal hypoplasia and a depressed nasal bridge. The characteristic defects are collectively referred to as fetal warfarin syndrome (FWS). Warfarin use during the second and third trimesters is associated with increased risk of fetal central nervous system (CNS) malformations. Heparin, which is poorly transferred across the placenta, may be substituted for warfarin when anticoagulant therapy is necessary.

(4) **Estrogen and androgens.** These category X drugs may cause serious genital tract malformations.

(5) **Other hormonal agents.** Drugs such as thyroid preparations and cortisone may affect the development of fetal endocrine glands. Methimazole and carbimazole have been associated with malformations in newborns exposed in utero. Propylthiouracil (PTU) is the drug of choice in pregnancy and lactation for antithyroid therapy.

(6) **Ethanol.** Alcohol consumed in large amounts or for prolonged periods during pregnancy has been associated with a pattern of defects collectively referred to as fetal alcohol syndrome (FAS). Features of FAS include abnormalities in growth and in cardiac, skeletal, craniofacial, muscular, genitourinary, cutaneous, and CNS development.

(7) **Antibiotics**

(a) Mottling of the teeth may occur when **tetracycline** is taken by the mother after week 18 of pregnancy. This teratogenic effect does not become evident until later in childhood when the teeth erupt.

(b) **Metronidazole** is mutagenic in animals and is contraindicated for treating trichomoniasis during the first trimester. Use for other indications must be carefully evaluated, especially in the first trimester.

(c) **Quinolone** antibiotics are not recommended for use during pregnancy because of arthropathies observed in immature animals.

(8) **Anticonvulsants** such as phenytoin, trimethadione, valproic acid, and sodium valproate have been associated with malformations when used during the first trimester.

(9) **Lithium.** Congenital malformations, primarily in the cardiovascular system, have been associated with first trimester administration of lithium. Ebstein's anomaly (i.e., tricuspid valve malformation) has been reported in a significant number of fetuses exposed to the drug during this period. Exposure to the drug near term has resulted in neonatal lithium toxicity, which is generally reversible.

(10) **Antineoplastics.** Many agents belonging to this class of drugs have been associated with fetal malformations following first trimester exposures. Examples include busulfan, chlorambucil, cyclophosphamide, and methotrexate.

(11) **Finazteride** may cause abnormal development of the genitalia of male fetuses exposed to the drug in utero. Pregnant women should avoid handling crushed tablets of the drug and should avoid contact with the semen of men who are taking this medication.

6. **Fetotoxic drug effects** are the result of pharmacologic activity of a drug that may physiologically affect the developing fetus.

a. During the **fetal period,** these effects are more likely to occur than are teratogenic effects.

b. **Clinically significant** fetotoxic effects include the following:

(1) **CNS depression** may occur with barbiturates, tranquilizers, antidepressants, and narcotics. Also, analgesics and anesthetics commonly given during labor may cause significant CNS and respiratory depression in newborns.

(2) **Neonatal bleeding.** Maternal ingestion of agents such as nonsteroidal anti-inflammatory drugs (NSAIDs) and anticoagulants at therapeutic doses near term may cause bleeding problems in the newborn. NSAIDs may prolong gestation and interfere with the progress of labor. Acetaminophen is a safe and effective analgesic for use in pregnancy.

(3) **Drug withdrawal.** Habitual maternal use of barbiturates, narcotics, benzodiazepines, alcohol, and other substances of abuse may lead to withdrawal symptoms in newborns.

(4) **Reduced birth weight.** Pregnant women who smoke cigarettes, consume large amounts of alcohol, or abuse drugs have an increased risk of delivering a low–birth-weight infant.

(5) **Constriction of the ductus arteriosus.** Maternal use of NSAIDs in the third trimester may cause the ductus arteriosus to close prematurely and may result in pulmonary hypertension in the newborn.

C. Drug excretion in breast milk. Recent appreciation of the benefits of breast feeding for the infant and mother has become evident. Today more than 60% of women choose to breast feed their infants. Of these women, 90%–95% receive a medication during the first postpartum week. It is important to understand the principles of drug excretion in breast milk and specific information on the various medications in order to minimize risks from drug effects in the nursing infant.

1. **Transfer of drugs from plasma to breast milk** is governed by many of the same principles that influence human membrane drug transfer.
   a. Many drugs cross the mammary epithelium via **passive diffusion** along a concentration gradient formed by the un-ionized drug content on each side of the membrane.
   b. This membrane is a **semipermeable lipid barrier** like other human membranes.
   c. The membrane also consists of **small pores** that allow for direct passage of low molecular weight substances (i.e., less than 200 d).
      (1) **Larger drug molecules,** which are unable to pass through the pores, must dissolve in the lipid part of the membrane in order to pass through to the breast milk.
      (2) **Active transport mechanisms** are described for some substances; however, there are no drugs known to use this process.

2. **Physiochemical characteristics of the drug** and its environment that **influence the rate and extent** of drug passage into the breast milk include:
   a. **Molecular weight of the drug** (see II C 1 c)
   b. The **pit gradient between the breast milk and plasma.** Human milk tends to be more acidic than plasma.
      (1) Therefore, weak acids may diffuse across the membrane and remain un-ionized, allowing for passage back into the plasma.
      (2) Weak bases may diffuse into the breast milk and ionize, which causes drug trapping (i.e., a clinically significant increase in the concentration of weak bases in the breast milk).
   c. **Degree of drug ionization.** Only the ionized form of a drug is able to pass through the lipid membrane. Drugs that exist unionized in large concentrations in the plasma would not be available to diffuse across the lipid membrane.
   d. **Plasma protein binding.** Only the unbound portion of a drug is available to pass into the breast milk. In general, drugs with high plasma protein binding properties tend to remain in the plasma and pass into the breast milk in low concentrations. While milk proteins exist and drug binding to these proteins may occur, the clinical relevance is limited.
   e. **Lipid solubility of the drug.** Lipid solubility is necessary for a drug to pass into the breast milk. Highly lipid-soluble drugs (e.g., diazepam) may pass into the breast milk in relatively high amounts and therefore may present a significant dose of drug to the nursing infant.

3. **After a drug is administered to a nursing mother,** the drug may be partially activated or inactivated in the maternal liver. The drug may be metabolized to active or inactive metabolites.

a. **Maternal pharmacology** plays a significant role in the rate and extent of drug passage into breast milk. The extent of plasma protein binding as well as changes in the mother's ability to metabolize or eliminate the drug influence the amount of drug in the plasma that is available to pass into the breast milk.
b. Equally important in affecting drug concentrations in breast milk are the **maternal dose of the drug,** the **dosing schedule or frequency,** and the **route of administration.**

4. **Drugs affecting hormonal influence of breast milk production.** The primary hormone responsible for controlling breast milk production is **prolactin.**
   a. **Following delivery,** serum prolactin levels increase to promote the production and secretion of breast milk. Prolactin continues to be released in response to infant feeding.
   b. However, infant feeding is not the only influence on serum prolactin levels. There are frequently prescribed **medications that may alter serum prolactin levels** and therefore the amount of breast milk produced.
      (1) A decrease in milk production may result in diminished weight gain in the nursing infant, the need for supplementation, or premature cessation of breast feeding.
      (2) **Drugs that decrease serum prolactin levels.** Drugs such as **bromocriptine** have been used to suppress lactation in women who choose not to breast feed. Other drugs include:
         (a) Ergot alkaloids
         (b) L-dopa
      (3) **Drugs that increase serum prolactin levels. Metoclopramide and sulpiride** have been useful therapeutically to enhance milk production. The following drugs are known to increase serum prolactin levels, but they have not been used therapeutically.
         (a) Methyldopa
         (b) Amphetamines
         (c) Haloperidol
         (d) Phenothiazines
         (e) Theophylline

5. **Factors to assess the risk of toxicity to the infant** include:
   a. Inherent toxicity of the drug
   b. Amount of drug ingested
   c. Degree of prematurity
   d. Nursing pattern of the infant

6. **Factors to minimize drug exposure to the infant.** One of the goals when using medications in the breast-feeding mother is to maintain a natural, uninterrupted pattern of nursing. In many instances, it may be possible to withhold a drug when it is not essential or delay therapy until after weaning. Other factors include:
   a. **Product selection.** When a specific product is being selected from a class of drugs, it is important to choose the product that is distributed into the milk the least.
      (1) Other desirable characteristics include a short half-life, inactive metabolites, and no accumulation in breast milk.
      (2) Additionally, it is desirable to select a particular route of administration associated with a lower concentration of the drug in breast milk.
   b. **Maternal dose relative to infant feeding.** One of the goals of drug dosing in lactating women is minimal infant exposure to the drug. In drugs taken on a scheduled basis, it is desirable to adjust the dosing and nursing schedules so that a drug dose is administered immediately before the infant's feeding.

7. **Examples of drugs that readily enter breast milk** and should be used with caution in nursing mothers include the following.
   a. **Narcotics, barbiturates, and benzodiazepines,** such as diazepam, may have a hypnotic effect on the nursing infant. These effects are related to the maternal dose. Alcohol consumption may have a similar effect.
   b. **Antidepressants and antipsychotics.** These classes of drugs appear to pass into the breast milk; however no serious adverse effects are reported. The long-term behavioral effects of chronic exposure to these drugs on developing newborns are unknown.
   c. **Metoclopramide.** This antiemetic passes readily into the breast milk and may accumulate as a result of ion trapping. There are no published reports involving serious effects associated with using this drug in lactating women. Its use may be of concern because of its potential strong CNS effects.

d. **Anticholinergic compounds.** These drugs may result in adverse CNS effects in the infant and may reduce lactation in the mother. Dicyclomine is contraindicated in nursing mothers because it may result in neonatal apnea.

III. DRUG USE IN GERIATRIC PATIENTS

A. General considerations

1. The elderly currently represent approximately 12% of the population, and they consume 25% of all prescription medications. If the amount of nonprescription medications is added to this number, estimates increase the drug usage of those over age 65 to 50% of all drugs used in the United States.

2. Drug response in elderly patients is affected by age-related changes in physiology and pharmacokinetics.

3. Numerous reasons help explain why the elderly are more susceptible than younger patients to adverse drug reactions.
   a. Many geriatric patients have multiple diseases that directly affect the body's ability to handle various medications.
   b. As the number of diseases increase in any given patient, the number of medications that the patient is likely to take also increases. Recent studies reveal that most people over age 65 take five or six different medications per day.
   c. As the number of medications in any given patient increases, so does the likelihood of an adverse drug reaction.
   d. In many cases, more than one physician may be prescribing medications for a single patient without knowledge of other agents being prescribed by another physician.
   e. Studies reveal that on average, geriatric patients self-medicate more frequently than their younger counterparts, who self-medicate as much as 1.5 times every 2 weeks.
   f. Studies reveal that as many as 40% of elderly patients stop taking their medications prematurely.
   g. The methods of administration, frequency of dosing, and combinations of drug products add to noncompliance of dose regimens.
   h. Changes in body composition, renal elimination, metabolism, and distribution can make it difficult to predict geriatric responses to many medications.

B. Pharmacokinetics in geriatric patients

1. **Drug absorption**
   a. **Age-related changes** in the stomach and small intestine, such as increased gastric pH and delayed gastric emptying time, do not create significant variations in the parameters of absorption in the elderly.
   b. Drugs such as antacids, which increase gastric pH, and anticholinergics, which further delay gastric emptying, may lead to significant decreases in bioavailability of various products such as digoxin, chlorpromazine, cimetidine, and tetracycline.

2. **Volume of distribution**
   a. **Body composition.** As a group, the elderly tend to be smaller than the young, with a greater composition of fat (approximately 35%), less muscle, and less body water.
   b. **Lipophilic and hydrophilic drugs.** Drugs that are lipid soluble (i.e., lipophilic) show increased volumes of distribution in the elderly, while those that are water soluble (i.e., hydrophilic) show decreased volumes of distribution. This becomes significant because many drugs are dosed based on lean body weight.
   c. **Serum albumin** tends to be reduced in the elderly, resulting in an increased amount of unbound (free) drug for those agents that are highly bound to albumin (e.g., warfarin).
   d. **Other factors** that affect the volume of distribution include obesity, drug interactions, malnutrition, and bed rest. Several of these factors are common in the geriatric population.

3. **Metabolism.** It is difficult to quantify metabolizing capabilities for numerous drugs in special patient populations.
   a. The **size of the liver** and its capacity for metabolism result in a reduction in the rate of active drug metabolism in the elderly.

b. **Reduced hepatic artery flow,** as well as a consistent reduction in various microsomal enzyme reactions, may lead to prolonged serum half-lives of drugs and potential toxicity.

4. **Renal elimination.** Unlike metabolism, the effect of aging on renal clearance can be quantified.
   a. **Serum creatinine levels** may be considered to be normal, when, in reality, the elderly do have a reduction in creatinine clearance.
   b. The **Cockcroft-Gault formula** has been used with several other nomograms to depict the relationship that exists between serum creatinine and creatinine clearance.
   c. Drugs that are excreted unchanged in the urine (e.g., digoxin, aminoglycosides, and penicillins) may remain in the body for longer periods of time, and may result in a higher incidence of toxicity.

C. Pharmacologic considerations in the geriatric population

1. The **site of action** of a given drug plays a major role in the response elicited by an elderly patient.

2. **Reductions in the cell population of organs,** oxygen consumption, tissue blood flow, and overall organ efficiency create a significant degree of scatter in the physiologic responses of elderly patients receiving numerous drugs. This typically results in either a heightened or diminished response to a drug.

3. **Drugs that act on the CNS** occasionally result in bizarre responses in elderly patients (e.g., increased excitement, mania). Barbiturates, benzodiazepines, antidepressants, and antiparkinsonian agents must be monitored closely for the development of such effects.

4. **Cardiotonics,** such as digitalis, tend to accumulate in the elderly because of decreased excretion, and they pose a significant risk for toxicity. Additionally, hypokalemia, hypothyroidism, and hypercalcemia also increase such toxicity.

5. **Anticoagulants,** because of the numerous reported drug–drug interactions encountered clinically, pose a significant threat to the elderly and should be monitored closely.

6. The elderly seem to have a higher incidence of fluid and electrolyte disturbances as compared with younger people, and this may pose a potential problem in those patients receiving diuretics.

7. The elderly are predisposed to a higher than normal rate of falls as compared with the younger population. Consequently, medications with **hypotensive** properties (e.g., calcium channel blockers, beta-adrenergic blockers, ACE inhibitors, centrally acting sympatholytics, and peripherally acting vasodilators) pose a major threat in causing falls among the elderly.

8. Frequently, the elderly suffer adverse side effects from drug substances owing to the failure of health professionals to recognize many of the traditionally accepted complaints of aging. Nausea, vomiting, fatigue, and upset stomach are not insignificant and may need further investigation.

9. When it comes to initiating drug therapy in the elderly, start low, and go slow.

D. Principles of drug therapy in the elderly. Before preparing any pharmaceutical for the elderly, the following should help the practitioner decide on specific therapeutic options.

1. The practitioner must be convinced that the drug therapy is required and that the diagnosed illness is amenable to drug therapy.

2. Elderly patients present with various obstacles when taking medications. In many situations, it is the dosage form of a drug and the frequency of administration that best determine the chances for a successful outcome, based on the establishment of maximal patient compliance.

3. Elderly patients cannot be expected to respond to all drugs in the same way that younger patients do. Efficacy of a product in the young does not always translate to the elderly.

4. Ensure that the patient is given appropriate medication instructions and stress the importance of taking the medication as directed.

5. Provide the elderly with an added amount of empathy and be prepared to discuss their concerns. Listen extra carefully for messages that others may ignore.

STUDY QUESTIONS

Directions: Each of the numbered items or incomplete statements in this section is followed by answers or by completions of the statement. Select the **one lettered answer** or completion that is **best** in each case.

1. All of the following medications should not be used routinely in pregnant patients during the third trimester EXCEPT

(A) acetaminophen
(B) nonsteroidal anti-inflammatory drugs
(C) warfarin
(D) lithium
(E) aspirin

2. Factors that affect the absorption of drugs in the elderly include all of the following EXCEPT

(A) lengthened gastric emptying time
(B) decreased plasma albumin
(C) elevated gastric pH
(D) decreased intestinal blood flow
(E) decreased gastrointestinal motility

3. Placental transfer of a drug is affected by all of the following characteristics EXCEPT

(A) molecular weight
(B) fetal gender
(C) gestational age
(D) lipid solubility of the drug
(E) plasma protein binding

4. All of the following are taken into account when calculating dosage for children EXCEPT

(A) height
(B) weight
(C) hepatic and renal function
(D) age
(E) body surface area

5. When selecting a benzodiazepine product for a woman who has chronic panic disorder, all of the following drug properties are desirable for breast-feeding her 8-month-old infant who was born at term EXCEPT

(A) hepatic metabolism to inactive metabolites
(B) a short half-life
(C) a rapid onset of action
(D) a tendency to bind to milk proteins

6. All of the following drugs may enhance breast milk production by increasing prolactin levels EXCEPT

(A) haloperidol
(B) methyldopa
(C) metoclopramide
(D) bromocriptine
(E) theophylline

Directions: The question below contains three suggested answers of which **one or more** is correct. Choose the answer

A if **I only** is correct
B if **III only** is correct
C if **I and II** are correct
D if **II and III** are correct
E if **I, II, and III** are correct

7. According to the principles of drug excretion into the breast milk, which combination of the following properties would result in the *highest* drug concentration in breast milk?

I. Low molecular weight, moderately lipophilic
II. Low plasma protein bound, weakly basic
III. Highly plasma protein bound, weakly acidic

ANSWERS AND EXPLANATIONS

1. The answer is A *[II B 5 d (3), (9), 6 b (2)].*
Acetaminophen is a safe and effective analgesic that can be used in therapeutic doses during pregnancy. Nonsteroidal anti-inflammatory drugs (NSAIDs) may interfere with the onset or progress of labor when used in the third trimester. NSAIDs and warfarin, when used near delivery, may cause bleeding problems in the newborn infant. Additionally, warfarin use in the third trimester may be associated with fetal central nervous system (CNS) abnormalities. Lithium use in the third trimester may cause neonatal lithium toxicity.

2. The answer is B *[III B 1, 2].*
Lengthened gastric emptying time, elevated gastric pH, decreased intestinal blood flow, and decreased gastrointestinal motility all may affect drug absorption. Decreases in plasma albumin may alter a drug's distribution but would not affect its absorption.

3. The answer is B *[II B 3].*
Fetal gender does not affect placental transfer of a drug. The molecular weight and the lipid solubility of a drug greatly influence its ability to cross the placental membranes. Plasma protein binding affects the amount of free drug available to cross the placenta. Gestational age influences the volume of distribution of the drug as well as the thickness of the placental membranes.

4. The answer is D *[I E].*
When calculating dosage for children, the child's height, weight, body surface area, and renal and hepatic function must be taken into account. Age, although sometimes used, may result in improper dosing because of the variations in body size and level of development found in children of the same age.

5. The answer is D *[II C 6 a (1)].*
When any drug is used by a nursing mother, it is desirable to have the least amount of active drug available in the maternal circulation to diffuse into the breast milk. A rapidly acting (for maternal onset of action), rapidly eliminated (i.e., short half-life) drug with inactive metabolites is optimal. If the drug binds in high quantities to milk proteins, it may tend to remain or accumulate in the breast milk.

6. The answer is D *[II C 4 b (2) (3)].*
Bromocriptine effectively decreases serum prolactin levels and has been used therapeutically to suppress lactation. Haloperidol, methyldopa, metoclopramide, and theophylline may increase serum prolactin levels. Of these drugs, only metoclopramide (as well as sulpiride) has been useful therapeutically to enhance milk production.

7. The answer is C (I, II) *[II C 1–3].*
High molecular weight substances are less likely to pass into breast milk because of their size. Drugs that are highly plasma protein bound may only reach the breast milk in small amounts, because a large portion of the drug is bound to the maternal plasma proteins, and therefore only a small amount is free to diffuse into breast milk. A low molecular weight, moderately lipophilic drug passes easily into breast milk. A drug that has a low degree of plasma protein binding has a significant amount of drug free to diffuse into breast milk. A weakly basic drug may ionize after reaching the breast milk and therefore remain trapped in the milk.

38 Common Clinical Laboratory Tests

Larry N. Swanson
D. Byron May

I. GENERAL PRINCIPLES

A. Monitoring drug therapy

1. **Laboratory test results** are monitored by pharmacists to:
   a. **Assess the therapeutic and adverse effects of a drug** (e.g., monitoring the serum uric acid level after allopurinol is administered or checking for increased liver function test values after administration of isoniazid)
   b. **Determine the proper drug dose** (e.g., assessment of the serum creatinine or creatinine clearance value before use of a renally excreted drug)
   c. **Assess the need for additional or alternate drug therapy** [e.g., assessment of white blood cell (WBC) count after an antibiotic is administered]
   d. **Prevent test misinterpretation resulting from drug interference** (e.g., determination of a false positive for a urine glucose test after cephalosporin administration)

2. These tests can be **very expensive** and requests for them must be balanced against potential benefits for patients.

B. Definition of normal values

1. **Normal laboratory test results** fall within a predetermined range of values, and **abnormal values** fall outside that range.
   a. **Normal limits may be defined somewhat arbitrarily;** thus, values outside the normal range may not necessarily indicate disease or the need for treatment (e.g., asymptomatic hyperuricemia).
   b. Many factors (e.g., age, sex, time since last meal) must be taken into account when evaluating test results.
   c. **Normal values also vary among institutions** and may depend on the method used to perform the test.
   d. Attempts have been made in recent years to standardize the presentation of laboratory data by using the International System of Units (SI units). Controversy surrounds this issue in the United States, and resistance to adopt this system continues. The SI unit of measure is a method of reporting clinical laboratory data in a standard metric format. The basic unit of mass for the SI is the mole. The mole is not influenced by the addition of excess weight of salt or ester formulations. Technically and pharmacologically, the mole is more meaningful than the gram because each physiological reaction occurs on a molecular level.

      Efforts to implement the SI system began in the 1970s resulting in the adoption of full SI-transition policies by a few major medical and pharmaceutical journals in the 1980s. Reluctance to use this system by many clinicians in the United States has forced changes in the policies by some journals to report both conventional and SI units or to report the conversion factor between the two systems. It is still controversial which method should be used to report clinical laboratory values. There are arguments for and against the universal conversion to the SI system. Readers should be aware that some journals report SI and/or conventional units in their text. Particular attention should be paid to the units associated with a reported laboratory value and access to a conversion table may be necessary to avoid confusion in the interpretation of the data. When appropriate, both conventional and SI units will be reported in this chapter.

2. **Laboratory error** must always be considered when **test results do not correlate with expected results for a given patient.** If necessary, the test should be repeated. Common sources of laboratory error include spoiled specimens, incomplete specimens, specimens taken at the wrong time, faulty reagents, technical errors, incorrect procedures, and failure to take diet or medication into account.

3. During hospital admission or routine physical examination, a **battery of tests** is usually given to augment the history and physical examination. Basic tests may include an electrocardiogram (ECG), a chest x-ray, a sequential multiple analyzer **(SMA) profile, electrolyte tests,** a **hemogram,** and **urinalysis**.

II. HEMATOLOGICAL TESTS.

Blood contains three types of formed elements; RBCs, WBCs, and platelets (Figure 38-1). A complete blood count (CBC) includes Hb, hematocrit (Hct), total WBCs, total RBCs, mean cell volume (MCV), and platelet count.

A. RBCs (erythrocytes)

1. The **RBC count,** which reports the number of RBCs found in a cubic millimeter (mm^3) of whole blood, provides an indirect estimate of the blood's Hb content. **Normal values** are:
   a. 4.3–5.9 million/mm^3 of blood for men ($\times 10^{12}$/L)
   b. 3.5–5.0 million/mm^3 of blood for women ($\times 10^{12}$/L)

2. The **Hct or packed cell volume (PCV)** measures the percentage by volume of packed RBCs in a whole blood sample after centrifugation. The Hct value is usually three times the Hb value (see II A 3) and is given as a percent or fraction of 1 (39%–40% for men; 33%–43% for women).
   a. Low Hct values indicate such conditions as anemia, overhydration or blood loss.
   b. High Hct values indicate such conditions as polycythemia vera or dehydration.

3. The **Hb test** measures the grams of Hb contained in 1 dl of whole blood and provides an estimate of the oxygen-carrying capacity of the RBCs. The Hb value depends on the **number of RBCs** and the **amount of Hb in each RBC.**
   a. Normal values are 14–18 g/dl for men and 12–16 g/dl for women.
   b. Low Hb values indicate anemia.

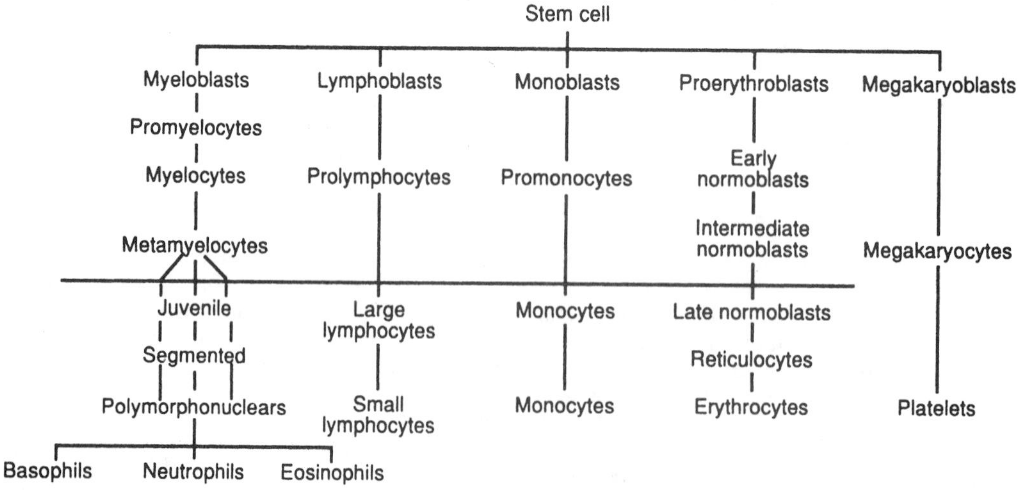

Figure 38-1. Derivation of blood elements from stem cells. Cells located below the *horizontal line* are found in normal peripheral blood with the exception of the late normoblasts.

4. **RBC indices** (also known as **Wintrobe indices**) provide important information regarding RBC size, Hb concentration, and Hb weight. They are used primarily to categorize anemias, although they may be affected by average cell measurements. A peripheral blood smear can provide most of the information obtained through RBC indices. Observations of a smear may show variation in RBC shape (**poikilocytosis**), as might occur in sickle-cell anemia, or it may show a variation in RBC size (**anisocytosis**), as might occur in a mixed anemia (folic acid and iron deficiency).
   a. **Mean cell volume (MCV)** is the ratio of the Hct to the RBC count. It essentially assesses average RBC size and reflects any anisocytosis.

$$\frac{\text{Hct (\%)} \times 10}{\text{RBC count (in millions)}} = \text{MCV}$$

      (1) **Low MCV** indicates **microcytic** (undersized) **RBCs,** as occurs in iron deficiency.
      (2) **High MCV** indicates **macrocytic** (oversized) **RBCs,** as occurs in a vitamin B_{12} or folic acid deficiency.
      3) Normal range for MCV is 90 ± 10.
   b. **Mean cell Hb (MCH)** assesses the amount of Hb in an average RBC.
      (1) MCH is defined as:

$$\frac{\text{Hb} \times 10}{\text{RBC count (in millions)}} = \text{MCH}$$

      (2) **Normal range for MCH** is 30 ± 4.
   c. **Mean cell Hb concentration (MCHC)** represents the average concentration of Hb in an average RBC, defined as:

$$\frac{\text{Hb} \times 100}{\text{Hct}} = \text{MCHC}$$

      (1) **Normal range for MCHC** is 34 ± 3.
      (2) **Low MCHC** indicates **hypochromia** (pale RBCs resulting from decreased Hb content), as occurs in iron deficiency.
   d. **RBC distribution width (RDW)** is a relatively new index of RBCs. Normally, most RBCs are approximately equal in size, so that only one bell-shaped histogram peak is generated. Disease may change the size of some RBCs—for example, the gradual change in size of newly produced RBCs in folic acid or iron deficiency. The difference in size between the abnormal and less abnormal RBCs produces either more than one histogram peak or a broadening of the normal peak.
      (1) **An increased RDW** is found in factor deficiency anemia (e.g., iron, folate, vitamin B_{12}).
      (2) **A normal RDW** is found in such conditions as anemia of chronic disease.
      (3) The **RDW index** is never decreased.

5. The **reticulocyte count** provides a measure of immature RBCs (reticulocytes), which contain remnants of nuclear material (reticulum). Normal RBCs circulate in the blood for about 1–2 days in this form. Hence, this test provides an index of bone marrow production of mature RBCs.
   a. Reticulocytes normally comprise 0.1%–2.4% of the total RBC count.
   b. **Increased reticulocyte count** occurs with such conditions as hemolytic anemia, acute blood loss, and response to the treatment of a factor deficiency (e.g., an iron, vitamin B_{12}, or folate deficiency). **Polychromasia** (the tendency to stain with acidic or basic dyes) noted on a peripheral smear laboratory report, usually indicates increased reticulocytes.
   c. **Decreased reticulocyte count** occurs with such conditions as drug-induced aplastic anemia.

6. The **erythrocyte sedimentation rate (ESR)** measures the rate of RBC settling of whole, uncoagulated blood over time, and it primarily reflects plasma composition. Most of the sedimentation effect results from alterations in plasma proteins.
   a. **Normal ESR rates** range from 0 mm/hr to 20 mm/hr for males and from 0 mm/hr to 30 mm/hr for females.
   b. **ESR values increase** with acute or chronic infection, tissue necrosis or infarction, well-established malignancy, and rheumatoid collagen diseases.

Table 38-1. Normal Percentage Values for White Blood Cell (WBC) Differential

Cell Type	Normal Percentage Value
Polymorphonuclear leukocytes	50%–70%
Bands	3%–5%
Lymphocytes	20%–40%
Monocytes	0%–7%
Eosinophils	0%–5%
Basophils	0%–1%

c. **ESR values** are used to:
   (1) Follow the clinical course of a disease
   (2) Demonstrate the presence of occult organic disease
   (3) Differentiate conditions with similar symptomatology [e.g., angina pectoris (no change in ESR value) as opposed to a myocardial infarction (increase in ESR value)]

B. WBCs (leukocytes)

1. The **WBC count** reports the number of WBCs in a cubic millimeter of whole blood.
   a. **Normal values** range from 4,000 WBC/mm^3 to 11,000 WBC/mm^3
   b. **Increased WBC count (leukocytosis)** usually signals infection; it may also result from leukemia or from tissue necrosis. It is most often found with **bacterial infection.**
   c. **Decreased WBC count (leukopenia)** indicates bone marrow depression, which may result from metastatic carcinoma, lymphoma, or toxic reactions to substances such as antineoplastic agents.

2. The **WBC differential** evaluates the distribution and morphology of the five major types of WBCs—the **granulocytes** (i.e., **neutrophils, basophils, eosinophils**) and the **nongranulocytes** (i.e., **lymphocytes, monocytes**). A certain percentage of each type comprises the total WBC count (Table 38-1).
   a. **Neutrophils** may be mature (**polymorphonuclear leukocytes,** also known as PMNs, "polys," segmented neutrophils, or "segs") or immature ("**bands**" or "stabs").
      (1) **Chemotaxis.** Neutrophils that **phagocytize and degrade many types of particles** serve as the body's first line of defense when tissue is damaged or foreign material gains entry. They congregate at sites in response to a specific stimulus, through a process known as chemotaxis.
      (2) **Neutrophilic leukocytosis.** This describes a response to an appropriate stimulus in which the total neutrophil count increases, often with an increase in the percentage of immature cells (**a shift to the left**). This may represent a systemic bacterial infection, such as pneumonia (Table 38-2).
         (a) **Certain viruses** (e.g., chicken pox, herpes zoster); some **rickettsial diseases** (e.g., Rocky Mountain spotted fever); some **fungi;** and **stress** (e.g., physical ex-

Table 38-2. Examples of Changes in Total White Blood Cell (WBC) Count and WBC Differential in Response to Bacterial Infection

	WBC Count	
Cell Type	Normal	With Bacterial Infection
Total WBCs	8000 (100%)	15,500 (100%)
Neutrophils		
Polymorphonuclear leukocytes	60%	82%
Bands	3%	6%
Lymphocytes	30%	10%
Monocytes	4%	1%
Eosinophils	2%	1%
Basophils	1%	0%

ercise, acute hemorrhage or hemolysis, acute emotional stress) may also cause this response.

(b) Other causes include **inflammatory diseases** (e.g., acute rheumatic fever, rheumatoid arthritis, acute gout); **hypersensitivity reactions to drugs; tissue necrosis** (e.g., from myocardial infarction, burns, certain cancers); **metabolic disorders** (e.g., uremia, diabetic ketoacidosis); **myelogenous leukemia;** and **use of certain drugs** (e.g., epinephrine, lithium).

(3) **Neutropenia.** This is a decreased number of neutrophils. It may occur with an **overwhelming infection of any type** (bone marrow is unable to keep up with the demand). It may also occur with **certain viral infections** (e.g., mumps, measles), with **idiosyncratic drug reactions,** and as a result of chemotherapy.

b. Basophils stain deeply with blue basic dye. Their function in the circulation is not clearly understood; in the tissues they are referred to as **mast cells.**

(1) **Basophilia,** an increased number of basophils, may occur with chronic myelogenous leukemia (CML) as well as other conditions.

(2) A decrease in basophils is generally not apparent because of the small numbers of these cells in the blood.

c. Eosinophils stain deep red with acid dye and are classically associated with immune reactions. **Eosinophilia,** an increased number of eosinophils, may occur with such conditions as **acute allergic reactions** (e.g., **asthma, hay fever, drug allergy)** and **parasitic infestations** (e.g., trichinosis, amebiasis).

d. Lymphocytes play a dominant role in immunological activity and appear to produce antibodies. They are classified as B lymphocytes or T lymphocytes; T lymphocytes are further divided into helper-inducer cells (T_4 cells) and suppressor cells (T_8 cells).

(1) **Lymphocytosis,** an increased number of lymphocytes, usually accompanies a normal or decreased total WBC count and is most commonly caused by **viral infection.**

(2) **Lymphopenia,** a decreased number of lymphocytes, may result from **severe debilitating illness, immunodeficiency,** or from **acquired immune deficiency syndrome (AIDS),** which has a propensity to attack T_4 cells.

(3) **Atypical lymphocytes** (i.e., T lymphocytes in a state of immune activation) are classically associated with **infectious mononucleosis.**

e. Monocytes are phagocytic cells. **Monocytosis,** an increased number of monocytes, may occur with **tuberculosis (TB), subacute bacterial endocarditis,** and during the recovery phase of some **acute infections.**

C. Platelets (thrombocytes). These are the smallest formed elements in the blood, and they are involved in **blood clotting** and vital to the formation of a hemostatic plug after vascular injury.

1. **Normal values for a platelet count** are $150{,}000/mm^3$—$300{,}000/mm^3$ (1.5–$3.0 \times 10^{11}/L$)

2. **Thrombocytopenia,** a decreased platelet count, can occur with a variety of conditions, such as idiopathic thrombocytopenic purpura or, occasionally, from such drugs as quinidine and sulfonamides.

   a. Thrombocytopenia is **moderate** when the platelet count is less than $100{,}000/mm^3$.

   b. Thrombocytopenia is **severe** when the platelet count is less than $50{,}000/mm^3$.

III. COMMON SERUM ENZYME TESTS.

Small amounts of enzymes (catalysts) circulate in the blood at all times and are released into the blood in larger quantities when tissue damage occurs. Thus, serum enzyme levels can be used to **aid in the diagnosis of certain diseases.**

A. Creatine kinase

1. Creatine kinase (CK), known formerly as creatine phosphokinase (CPK), is found primarily in heart muscle, skeletal muscle, and brain tissue.

2. CK levels are used primarily to **aid in the diagnosis of acute myocardial** (Figure 38-2) **or skeletal muscle damage.** However, vigorous exercise, a fall, or deep intramuscular injections can cause significant increases in CK levels.

3. The **isoenzymes** of CK—**CK-MM,** found in skeletal muscle; **CK-BB,** found in brain tissue; and **CK-MB,** found in heart muscle—can be used to differentiate the source of damage.

   a. Normally, serum CK levels are virtually all the **CK-MM isoenzyme.**

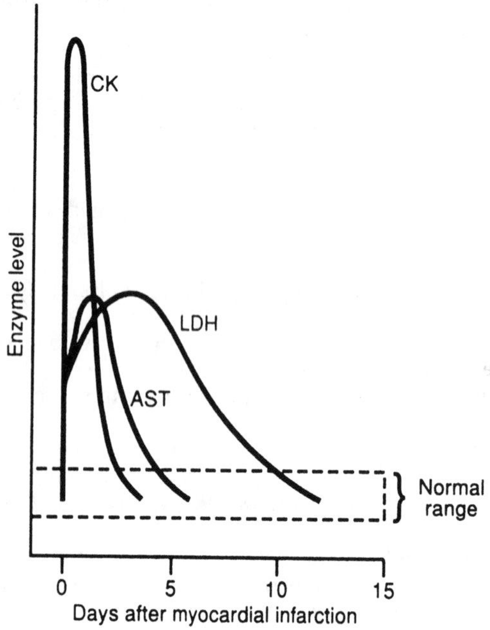

Figure 38-2. The graph shows the increase of serum creatine kinase (CK), lactate dehydrogenase (LDH), and aspartate aminotransferase (AST) levels after a myocardial infarction.

b. Increase in **CK-MB** levels provides a sensitive indicator of myocardial necrosis.

B. Lactate dehydrogenase

1. Lactate dehydrogenase (LDH) catalyzes the interconversion of lactate and pyruvate and represents a group of enzymes present in almost all metabolizing cells.
2. Five individual **isoenzymes** make up the total LDH serum level.
   a. **LDH_1** and **LDH_2** appear primarily in the heart.
   b. **LDH_3** appears primarily in the lungs.
   c. **LDH_4** and **LDH_5** appear primarily in the liver and in skeletal muscles.
3. The distribution pattern of LDH isoenzymes may aid in diagnosing myocardial infraction, hepatic disease, and lung disease.

C. Alkaline phosphatase

1. Alkaline phosphatase (ALP) is produced primarily in the **liver** and in the **bones.**
2. Serum ALP levels are **particularly sensitive to partial or mild biliary obstruction**—either extrahepatic (e.g., caused by a stone in the bile duct) or intrahepatic, both of which cause levels to increase.
3. **Increased osteoblastic activity,** as occurs in Paget's disease, hyperparathyroidism, osteomalacia, and others, also increases serum ALP levels.

D. Aspartate aminotransferase

1. Aspartate aminotransferase **(AST)**, formerly known as **serum glutamic-oxaloacetic transaminase (SGOT),** is found in a number of organs, primarily in heart and liver tissues and, to lesser extent, in skeletal muscle, kidney tissue, and pancreatic tissue.
2. **Damage to the heart** (e.g., from **myocardial infarction;** see Figure 38-2) results in increased AST levels about 8 hours after injury.
   a. Levels are **increased markedly** with **acute hepatitis;** they are **increased mildly** with **cirrhosis** and a **fatty liver.**
   b. Levels are also **increased** with **passive congestion of the liver** [as occurs in congestive heart failure (CHF)].

E. Alanine aminotransferase

1. Alanine aminotransferase (ALT), formerly known as **serum glutamic-pyruvic transaminase (SGPT),** is found in the liver with lesser amounts in the heart, skeletal muscles, and kidney.

2. Although ALT values are **relatively specific for liver cell damage,** ALT is **less sensitive than AST,** and extensive or severe liver damage is necessary before abnormally increased levels are produced.

3. ALT also **increases less consistently and less markedly than AST** after an **acute myocardial infarction.**

IV. LIVER FUNCTION TESTS

A. Liver enzymes

1. **Levels of certain enzymes** (e.g., LDH, ALP, AST, ALT) **increase with liver dysfunction,** as discussed in III.

2. These **enzyme tests indicate only that the liver has been damaged.** They do not assess the liver's ability to function. Other tests provide indications of liver dysfunction.

B. Serum bilirubin

1. Bilirubin, a breakdown product of Hb, is the **predominant pigment in bile.** Effective bilirubin conjugation and excretion depend on **hepatobiliary function** and on the **rate of RBC turnover.**

2. Serum bilirubin levels are reported as **total bilirubin** (conjugated and unconjugated) and as **direct bilirubin** (conjugated only).
   a. Bilirubin is released by Hb breakdown and is bound to albumin as water-insoluble **indirect bilirubin** (unconjugated bilirubin), which is not filtered by the glomerulus.
   b. **Unconjugated bilirubin** travels to the liver, where it is separated from albumin, conjugated with diglucuronide, and then actively secreted into the bile as **conjugated bilirubin** (direct bilirubin), which is filtered by the glomerulus (Figure 38-3).

3. **Normal values of total serum bilirubin** are 0.1–1.0 mg/dl (2–18 μmol/L); of **direct bilirubin,** 0.0 mg/dl–0.2 mg/dl (0–4 μmol/L).

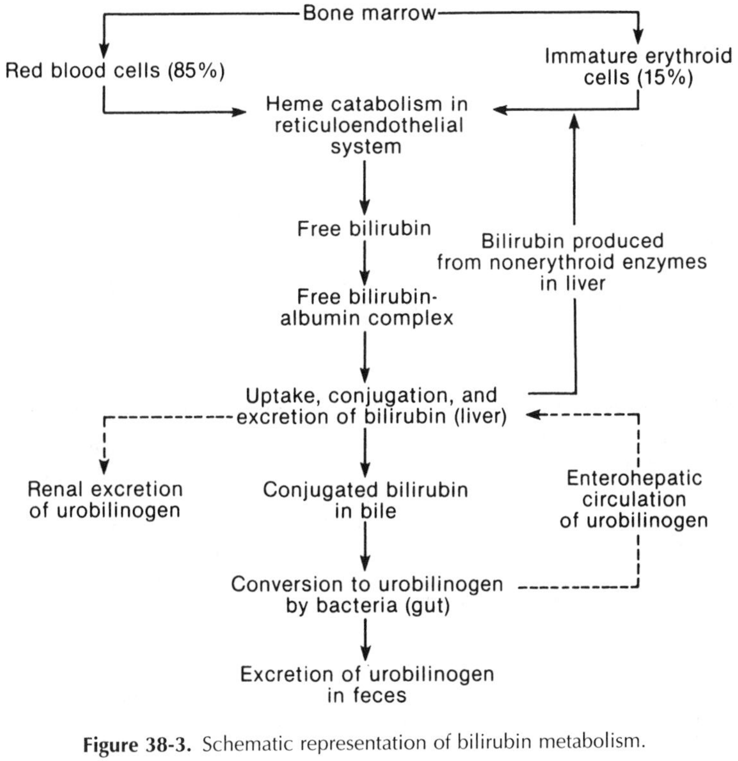

Figure 38-3. Schematic representation of bilirubin metabolism.

4. **Increase in serum bilirubin** results in **jaundice** from bilirubin deposition in the tissues. There are three major causes of increased serum bilirubin.
   a. **Hemolysis** increases total bilirubin; direct bilirubin (conjugated) is usually normal or slightly increased. Urine color is normal, and no bilirubin is found in the urine.
   b. **Biliary obstruction,** which may be intrahepatic (as with a chlorpromazine reaction) or extrahepatic (as with a biliary stone) increases total bilirubin and direct bilirubin; intrahepatic cholestasis (e.g., from chlorpromazine) may increase direct bilirubin as well. Urine color is dark, and bilirubin is present in the urine.
   c. **Liver cell necrosis,** as occurs in viral hepatitis, may cause an increase in both direct bilirubin (because inflammation causes some bile sinusoid blockage) and indirect bilirubin (because the liver's ability to conjugate is altered). Urine color is dark, and bilirubin is present in the urine.

C. Serum proteins

1. **Primary serum proteins** measured are **albumin** and the **globulins** (i.e., alpha, beta, gamma).
   a. **Albumin** (4.0–6.0 g/dl) maintains serum oncotic pressure and serves as a transport agent. Because it is primarily manufactured by the liver, liver disease can decrease albumin levels.
   b. **Globulins** (23–35 g/L) function as transport agents and play a role in certain immunological mechanisms. A decrease in albumin levels usually results in a compensatory increase in globulin production.
2. **Normal values** for total serum protein levels are 6.0–8.0 g/dl (60–80 g/L).

V. URINALYSIS. Standard urinalysis provides basic information regarding renal function, urinary tract disease, and the presence of certain systemic diseases. Components of a standard urinalysis include appearance, pH, specific gravity, protein level, glucose level, ketone level, and microscopic examination.

A. Appearance. Normal urine is **clear** and ranges in color from **pale yellow to deep gold. Changes in color** can result from drugs, diet, or disease.

1. A **red color** may indicate, among other things, the presence of blood or phenolphthalein (a laxative).
2. A **brownish-yellow color** may indicate the presence of conjugated bilirubin.
3. **Other shades of red, orange, or brown** may be caused by ingestion of various drugs.

B. pH

1. **Normal pH** ranges from 4.5 to 9 but is typically **acid** (around 6).
2. **Alkaline pH** may indicate such conditions as alkalosis, a *Proteus* infection, or acetazolamide use. It may also reflect changes caused by leaving the urine sample at room temperature.

C. Specific gravity

1. **Normal range** for specific gravity is 1.003–1.035; it is usually between 1.010 and 1.025.
2. Specific gravity is influenced by the number and nature of solute particles in the urine.
   a. **Increased specific gravity** may occur with such conditions as diabetes mellitus (DM; excess glucose in the urine) or nephrosis (excess protein in the urine).
   b. **Decreased specific gravity** may occur with diabetes insipidus, which decreases urine concentration.
   c. **Specific gravity, fixed at 1.010** (the same as plasma), occurs when the kidneys lose their power to concentrate or dilute.

D. Protein

1. **Normal values** for urine protein are 50–80 mg/24 hr, as the glomerular membrane prevents most protein molecules in the blood from entering the urine.

2. **Proteinuria** occurs with many conditions (e.g., renal disease, bladder infection, venous congestion, fever).
   a. The presence of a **specific protein** can help to identify a specific disease state (e.g., Bence Jones protein may indicate multiple myeloma).
   b. Most often, the protein in urine is **albumin.** Albuminuria may indicate abnormal glomerular permeability.

E. Glucose

1. The normal **renal threshold** for glucose is a blood glucose level of about 180 mg/dl; **glucose does not normally appear in urine** as detected by popular testing methods.
2. **Glycosuria** usually indicates diabetes mellitus. There are certain less common causes (e.g., a lowered renal threshold for glucose).

F. Ketones

1. Ketones **do not normally appear in urine.** They are excreted when the body has used available glucose stores and begins to metabolize fat stores.
2. The **three ketone bodies** are **betahydroxybutyric acid** (80%), **acetoacetic acid** (about 20%), and acetone (a small percentage). Some commercial tests (e.g., Ames products) measure only acetoacetic acid, but usually all three are excreted in parallel proportions.
3. **Ketonuria** usually indicates uncontrolled diabetes mellitus, but it may also occur with starvation and with zero- or low-carbohydrate diets.

G. Evaluation. Microscopic examination of centrifuged urine sediment normally reveals 0–1 RBC, 0–4 WBCs, and only an occasional cast per high-power field (HPF).

1. **Hematuria** (i.e., the presence of RBCs) may indicate such conditions as trauma, a tumor, or a systemic bleeding disorder. In women, a significant number of **squamous cells** suggests vaginal contamination (menstruation).
2. **Casts** (i.e., protein conglomerations outlining the shape of the renal tubules in which they were formed) may or may not be significant. Excessive numbers of certain types of casts indicate renal disease.
3. **Crystals,** which are pH-dependent, may occur normally in acid or alkaline urine. **Uric acid crystals** may form in acid urine; **phosphate crystals** may form in alkaline urine.
4. **Bacteria** do not normally appear in urine. The finding of 20 or more bacteria per HPF may indicate a urinary tract infection (UTI); smaller values may indicate urethral contamination.

VI. COMMON RENAL FUNCTION TESTS

A. Introduction

1. Renal function may be assessed by measuring **blood urea nitrogen (BUN)** and **serum creatinine.** Renal function decreases with age, which must be taken into account when interpreting test values.
   a. These tests primarily evaluate glomerular function by assessing the **glomerular filtration rate (GFR).**
   b. In many **renal diseases,** urea and creatinine accumulate in the blood because they are not excreted properly.
   c. These tests also aid in determining **drug dosage** for drugs excreted through the kidneys.
2. **Azotemia** describes excessive retention of nitrogenous waste products (BUN and creatinine) in the blood. The clinical syndrome resulting from decreased renal function and azotemia is called **uremia.**
   a. **Renal azotemia** results from renal disease, such as glomerulonephritis and chronic pyelonephritis.
   b. **Prerenal azotemia** results from such conditions as severe dehydration, hemorrhagic shock, and excessive protein intake.

c. **Postrenal azotemia** results from such conditions as ureteral or urethral stones or tumors and prostatic obstructions.

3. **Clearance**—a theoretical concept defined as the volume of plasma from which a measured amount of substance can be completely eliminated, or cleared, into the urine per unit time—can be used to estimate glomerular function.

B. Blood urea nitrogen (BUN)

1. **Urea,** an end product of protein metabolism, is produced in the liver. From there, it travels through the blood and is excreted by the kidneys. Urea is **filtered at the glomerulus,** where the tubules reabsorb approximately 40%. Thus, under normal conditions, **urea clearance** is about 60% of the true GFR.

2. **Normal values for BUN** range from 8 mg/dl to 18 mg/dl (3–6.5 mmol/L).
   a. **Decreased BUN levels** occur with **significant liver disease.**
   b. **Increased BUN levels** may indicate **renal disease.** However, factors other than glomerular function [e.g., protein intake, reduced renal blood flow, blood in the gastrointestinal (GI) tract] readily affect BUN levels, making interpretation of results sometimes difficult.

C. Serum creatinine

1. Creatinine, the metabolic breakdown product of muscle creatine phosphate, has a relatively constant level of daily production. Blood levels vary little in a given individual.

2. Creatinine is **excreted** by glomerular filtration and tubular secretion. **Creatinine clearance** parallels the GFR within a range of ± 10% and is a **more sensitive indicator of renal damage than BUN levels** because renal impairment is almost the only cause of an increase in the serum creatinine level.

3. **Normal values for serum creatinine** range from 0.6 mg/dl to 1.2 mg/dl (50–110 μmol/L)
   a. Values vary with the **amount of muscle mass**—a value of 1.2 mg/dl in a muscular athlete may represent normal renal function, whereas the same value in a small, sedentary person with little muscle mass may indicate significant renal impairment.
   b. Generally, the **serum creatinine value doubles with each 50% decrease in GFR.** For example, if a patient's normal serum creatinine is 1 mg/dl, 1 mg/dl represents 100% renal function, 2 mg/dl represents 50% function, and 4 mg/dl represents 25% function.

D. Creatinine clearance

1. Creatinine clearance, which represents the **rate at which creatinine is removed from the blood by the kidneys,** roughly approximates the GFR.
   a. The value is given in units of milliliters per minute, representing the volume of blood cleared of creatinine by the kidney per minute.
   b. **Normal values** for men range from 75 ml/min to 125 ml/min.

2. Calculation requires knowledge of **urinary creatinine excretion** (usually over 24 hours) and concurrent **serum creatinine levels. Creatinine clearance is calculated** as follows:

$$Cl_{CR} = \frac{C_U V}{C_{CR}}$$

   Here, Cl_{CR} is the creatinine clearance in milliliters per minute, C_u is the concentration of creatinine in the urine, V is the urine volume (in milliliters per minute of urine formed over the collection period), and C_{CR} is the serum creatinine concentration.

3. Suppose the serum creatinine concentration is 1 mg/dl, and 1440 ml of urine were collected in 24 hours (1440 min) for a urine volume of 1 ml/min. The urine contains 100 mg/dl of creatinine. Creatinine clearance is calculated as:

$$\frac{100 \text{ mg/dl} \times 1 \text{ ml/min}}{1 \text{ mg/dl}} = 100 \text{ ml/min.}$$

4. Incomplete bladder emptying and other problems may interfere with obtaining an accurate timed urine specimen. Thus, **estimations of creatinine clearance** may be necessary. These

estimations require only a serum creatinine value. One estimation uses the method of **Cockroft and Gault,** which is based on body weight, age, and gender.

a. This formula provides an **estimated value,** calculated for **males** as:

$$Cl_{CR} = \frac{(140 - \text{age in years})\ (\text{body weight in kg})}{72\ (C_{CR}\ \text{in mg/dl})}$$

Again, Cl_{CR} is the creatinine clearance in milliliters per minute, and C_{CR} is the serum creatinine concentration.

b. For **females,** use 0.85 of the value calculated for males.

c. **Example:** A 20-year-old man weighing 72 kg has a Cl_{CR} = 1.0 mg/dl; thus,

$$Cl_{CR} = \frac{(140 - 20)\ (72)}{72(1)}$$

$$Cl_{CR} = 120 \text{ ml/min.}$$

VII. ELECTROLYTES

A. Sodium

1. Sodium (Na) is the major cation of the **extracellular** fluid. Na along with chloride (Cl), potassium (K) and water is important in the regulation of osmotic pressure and water balance between intracellular and extracellular fluids. **Normal values** are 135–147 mEq/L or mmol/L.

2. The Na concentration is defined as the ratio of Na to water, not the absolute amounts of either. Laboratory tests for Na are used mainly to detect disturbances in water balance and body osmolality. The kidneys are major organs of Na and water balance.

3. An increase in Na concentration **(hypernatremia)** may indicate impaired Na excretion or dehydration. A decrease in Na concentration (hyponatremia) may reflect overhydration, abnormal Na loss, or decreased Na intake.

4. Patients with kidney, heart, or pulmonary disease may have difficulty with Na and water balance. In adults, changes in Na concentrations most often reflect changes in water balance not salt imbalances. Therefore Na concentration is often used as an indicator of fluid status rather than salt imbalance.

5. Control of Na by the body is accomplished mainly through the hormones antidiuretic hormone (ADH) and aldosterone. ADH is released from the pituitary in response to signals from the hypothalamus. ADH's presence in the distal tubules and collecting ducts of the kidney causes them to become more permeable to the reabsorption of water, therefore concentrating urine. Aldosterone affects the distal tubular reabsorption of Na as opposed to water. Aldosterone is released from the adrenal cortex in response to low Na, high K, low blood volume, and angiotensin II. Aldosterone causes the spilling of K from the distal tubules in to the urine in exchange for Na reabsorption.

6. **Hyponatremia** is usually related to total body depletion of Na (mineralocorticoid deficiencies, Na-wasting renal disease, replacement of fluid loss with nonsaline solutions, GI losses, renal losses, or loss of Na through the skin), or dilution of serum Na [cirrhosis, CHF, nephrosis, renal failure, excess water intake or syndrome of inappropriate diuretic hormone (SIADH) release].

7. **Hypernatremia** usually results from a loss of free water, or hypotonic fluid or through excessive Na intake. Free water loss is most often associated with diabetes insipidus, but fluid loss can be via the GI tract, renal, skin, or respiratory systems. Excess Na intake can occur through the administration of hypertonic intravenous (IV) solutions, mineralocorticoid excess, excessive Na ingestion, or after administration of drugs high in Na content [e.g., ticarcillin, Na bicarbonate (HCO_3^-)].

B. Potassium

1. Potassium (K) is the most abundant **intracellular** cation (intracellular fluid K averages 141 mEq/L). Approximately 3500 mEq of K are contained in the body of a 70-kg adult. Only 10% of the body's K is extracellular. Normal values are 3.5–5.0 mEq/L or mmol/L.

2. The serum K concentration is not an adequate measure of the total body K because most of the body's K is intracellular. Fortunately the clinical signs/symptoms of K deficiency [malaise, confusion, dizziness, electrocardiogram (ECG) changes, muscle weakness, and pain] correlate well with serum concentrations. The serum K concentration is buffered by the body and may be "normal" despite total body K loss. K depletion causes a shift of intracellular K to the extracellular fluid to maintain K concentrations. There is approximately a 100 mEq total body K deficit when the serum K concentration decreases by 0.3 mEq/L. This may result in misinterpretation of serum K concentrations as they relate to total body K.

3. The role/function of K is in the maintenance of proper electrical conduction in cardiac and skeletal muscles (muscle and nerve excitability), it exerts an influence on the body's water balance (intracellular volume) and plays a role in acid-base equilibrium.

4. K is regulated by:
   a. Kidneys (renal function)
   b. Aldosterone
   c. Arterial pH
   d. Insulin
   e. K intake
   f. Na delivery to distal tubule

5. **Hypokalemia** can occur. The kidneys are responsible for approximately 90% of the daily K loss. Other losses occur mainly through the GI system. Even in states of no K intake, the kidneys still excrete up to 20 mEq of K daily. Therefore, prolonged periods of K deprivation can result in hypokalemia. Hypokalemia can also result from K loss through vomiting or diarrhea, nasogastric suction, laxative abuse, and by diuretic use (mannitol, thiazides or loop diuretics). Excessive mineralocorticoid activity and glucosuria can also result in hypokalemia. K can be shifted into cells with alkalemia and after administration of glucose and insulin.

6. **Hyperkalemia** most commonly results from decreased renal elimination, excessive intake, or from cellular breakdown (tissue damage, hemolysis, burns, infections). Metabolic acidosis may also result in a shift of K extracellularly as hydrogen ions move into cells and are exchanged for K and Na ions. As a general guideline, for every 0.1 unit pH change from 7.4, the K concentration will change by about 0.6 mEq/L. If a patient has a pH of 7.1 and a measured K of 4.5 mEq/L, the actual K concentration would be [(0.3 units less than 7.4) x 0.6 = 1.8; 4.5 − 1.8 = 2.7 mEq/L K concentration]. Correction of the acidosis in this situation will result in a dramatic decrease in K unless supplementation is instituted.

C. Chloride

1. Chloride is the major anion of the extracellular fluid and is important in the maintenance of acid-base balance. Alterations in the serum Cl concentration are rarely a primary indicator of major medical problems. Cl itself is not of primary diagnostic significance. It is usually measured to confirm the serum Na concentration. The relationship among Na, Cl, and bicarbonate (HCO_3^-) is described by the following: $Cl^- + HCO_3^- + R = Na^+$, where R is the anion gap. The **normal value** for Cl is 95–105 mEq/L or mmol/L.

2. **Hypochloremia** is a decreased Cl concentration, and it is often accompanied by metabolic alkalosis or acidosis caused by organic or other acids. Other causes include chronic renal failure, adrenal insufficiency, fasting, prolonged diarrhea, severe vomiting, and diuretic therapy.

3. **Hyperchloremia** is an increased Cl concentration that may be indicative of hyperchloremic metabolic acidosis. Hyperchloremia in the absence of metabolic acidosis is unusual because Cl retention is often accompanied by Na and water retention. Other causes include acute renal failure, dehydration, and excess Cl administration.

D. Bicarbonate/carbon dioxide content

1. The carbon dioxide (CO_2) content represents the sum of the bicarbonate (HCO_3^-) concentration and the concentration of CO_2 dissolved in the serum. The HCO_3^-/CO_2 system is the most important buffering system to maintain pH within physiological limits. Most disturbances of acid-base balance can be considered in terms of this system. Normal values are 22–28 mEq/L or mmol/L.

2. The relationship among this system is defined as follows: $HCO_3^- + H^+ \leftrightarrows H_2CO_3 \leftrightarrows H_2O + CO_2$, bicarbonate ions bind hydrogen ions to form carbonic acid. Clinically, the serum HCO_3^- concentration is measured because acid-base balance can be inferred if the patient has normal pulmonary function.

3. **Hypobicarbonatemia** is usually caused by metabolic acidosis, renal failure, hyperventilation, severe diarrhea, drainage of intestinal fluid, and by drugs such as acetazolamide. Toxicity caused by salicylates, methanol, and ethylene glycol can also decrease the HCO_3^- level.

4. **Hyperbicarbonatemia** is usually caused by alkalosis, hypoventilation, pulmonary disease, persistent vomiting, excess HCO_3^- intake with poor renal function, and diuretics.

VIII. MINERALS

A. Calcium

1. Calcium plays an important role in nerve impulse transmission, muscle contraction, pancreatic insulin release, hydrogen ion release from the stomach, as a cofactor for some enzyme reactions and blood coagulation, and most importantly bone and tooth structural integrity. Normal values are: total Ca 8.8–10.3 mg/dl or 2.20–2.56 mmol/L

2. The total Ca content of normal adults is 20 to 25 g/kg of fat-free tissue, and about 44% of this Ca is in the body skeleton. Approximately 1% of skeletal Ca is freely exchangeable with that of the extracellular fluid. The reservoir of Ca in bones maintains the concentration of Ca in the plasma constant. About 40% of the Ca in the extracellular fluid is bound to plasma proteins (especially albumin), 5% to 15% is complexed with phosphate and citrate, and about 45% to 55% is in the unbound, ionized form. Most laboratories measure the total Ca concentration; however, it is the free, ionized Ca that is important physiologically. Ionized Ca levels may be obtained from the laboratory. Clinically the most important determinant of ionized Ca is the amount of serum protein (albumin) available for binding. The normal serum Ca range is for a serum albumin of 4 g/dl. A good approximation is that for every 1 gm/dl decrease in albumin, 0.8 g/dl should be added to the Ca lab result. Doing this corrects the total plasma concentration to reflect the additional amount of free (active) Ca.

3. **Hypocalcemia** usually implies a deficiency in either the production or response to parathyroid hormone (PTH) or vitamin D. PTH abnormalities include hypoparathyroidism, pseudohypoparathyroidism, or hypomagnesemia. Vitamin D abnormalities can be caused by decreased nutritional intake, decreased absorption of vitamin D, a decrease in production or an increase in metabolism. Administration of loop diuretics causing diuresis can also decrease serum Ca.

4. **Hypercalcemia** is an increased Ca concentration, and it is usually associated with malignancy or metastatic diseases. Other causes include hyperparathyroidism, Paget's disease, milk-alkali syndrome, granulomatous disorders, thiazide diuretics, excessive Ca intake, or vitamin D intoxication.

B. Phosphate

1. **Phosphate** (PO_4) is a major intracellular anion and is the source of phosphate for adenosine triphosphate (ATP) and phospholipid synthesis. Serum Ca and PO_4 are influenced by many of the same factors. It is useful to consider Ca and PO_4 together when interpreting lab results. Normal PO_4 values are 2.5–5.0 mg/dl or 0.80–1.60 mmol/L.

2. **Hyperphosphatemia** and **hypophosphatemia** can occur. The extracellular fluid concentration of phosphate is influenced by PTH, intestinal absorption, renal function, nutrition, and bone metabolism. Hyperphosphatemia is usually caused by renal insufficiency, although increased vitamin D or phosphate intake, hypoparathyroidism, and hyperthyroidism are also causes. Hypophosphatemia can occur in malnutrition, especially when anabolism is induced, after administration of aluminum-containing antacids or Ca acetate, in chronic alcoholics, and in septic patients. Hyperparathyroidism and insufficient vitamin D intake can also induce hypophosphatemia.

C. Magnesium

1. Magnesium (Mg) is the second most abundant intracellular and extracellular cation. It is an activator of numerous enzyme systems that control carbohydrate, fat and electrolyte metabolism, protein synthesis, nerve conduction, muscular contractility, as well as membrane transport and integrity. Normal values are 1.6–2.4 mEq/L or 0.80–1.20 mmol/L.

2. **Hypomagnesemia** and **hypermagnesemia** can occur. **Hypomagnesemia** is found more often than hypermagnesemia. Depletion of Mg usually results from excessive loss from the GI tract or the kidneys. Depletion can occur from either poor intestinal absorption or excessive GI fluid loss. Signs and symptoms include weakness, muscle fasciculations with tremor, tetany, and increased reflexes. Decreased intracardiac Mg may manifest as an increased QT interval with an increased risk of arrhythmia. **Hypermagnesemia** is most commonly caused by increased Mg intake in the setting of renal insufficiency. Other causes include excess Mg intake, hepatitis, and Addison's disease. Signs and symptoms of hypermagnesemia include bradycardia, flushing, sweating, nausea and vomiting, decreased Ca level, decreased deep-tendon reflexes, flaccid paralysis, increased pulse rate and QRS intervals, respiratory distress, and asystole.

STUDY QUESTIONS

Directions: Each of the numbered items or incomplete statements in this section is followed by answers or by completions of the statement. Select the **one** lettered answer or completion that is **best** in each case.

1. Hematological testing of a patient with acquired immune deficiency syndrome (AIDS) is most likely to show which of the following abnormalities?

(A) Basophilia
(B) Eosinophilia
(C) Lymphopenia
(D) Reticulocytosis
(E) Agranulocytosis

2. Hematological studies are most likely to show a low reticulocyte count in a patient who has which one of the following abnormalities?

(A) Aplastic anemia secondary to cancer chemotherapy
(B) Acute hemolytic anemia secondary to quinidine treatment
(C) Severe bleeding secondary to an automobile accident
(D) Iron deficiency anemia 1 week after treatment with ferrous sulfate
(E) Megaloblastic anemia due to folate deficiency 1 week after treatment with folic acid

3. All of the following findings on a routine urinalysis would be considered normal EXCEPT

(A) pH: 6.5
(B) glucose: negative
(C) ketones: negative
(D) WBC: 3 per high-power field (HPF), no casts
(E) RBC: 5 per HPF

4. A 12-year-old boy is treated for otitis media with cefaclor (Ceclor). On the seventh day of therapy, he "spikes" a fever and develops an urticarial rash on his trunk. Which of the following laboratory tests could best confirm the physician's suspicion of a hypersensitivity (allergic) reaction?

(A) Complete blood count (CBC) and differential
(B) Serum hemoglobin (Hb) and reticulocyte count
(C) Liver function test profile
(D) Lactate dehydrogenase (LDH) isoenzyme profile
(E) Red blood cell (RBC) count and serum bilirubin

5. An increased hematocrit (Hct) is a likely finding in all of the following individuals EXCEPT

(A) a man who has just returned from a 3-week skiing trip in the Colorado Rockies
(B) a woman who has polycythemia vera
(C) a hospitalized patient who mistakenly received 5 L of intravenous (IV) dextrose 5% in water (D_5W) over the last 24 hours
(D) a man who has been rescued from the Arizona desert after spending 4 days without water
(E) a woman who has chronic obstructive pulmonary disease

6. A 29-year-old white man is seen in the emergency room. His white blood cell (WBC) count is 14,200 with 80% "polys." All of the following conditions could normally produce these laboratory findings EXCEPT

(A) a localized bacterial infection on the tip of the index finger
(B) acute bacterial pneumonia caused by *Streptococcus pneumoniae*
(C) a heart attack
(D) a gunshot wound to the abdomen with a loss of 2 pints of blood
(E) an attack of gout

7. A 52-year-old male construction worker who drinks "fairly heavily" when he gets off work is seen in the emergency room with, among other abnormal laboratory results, an increased creatine kinase (CK) level. All of the following circumstances could explain this increase EXCEPT

(A) he fell against the bumper of his car in a drunken stupor and bruised his right side
(B) he is showing evidence of some liver damage due to the heavy alcohol intake
(C) he has experienced a heart attack
(D) he received an intramuscular (IM) injection a few hours before the blood sample was drawn
(E) he pulled a muscle that day in lifting a heavy concrete slab

8. A 45-year-old man with jaundice has spillage of bilirubin into his urine. All of the following statements could apply to this patient EXCEPT

(A) his total bilirubin is increased
(B) his direct bilirubin is increased
(C) he may have viral hepatitis
(D) he may have hemolytic anemia
(E) he may have cholestatic hepatitis

Directions: Each item below contains three suggested answers of which **one or more** is correct. Choose the answer

A if **I only** is correct
B if **III only** is correct
C if **I and II** are correct
D if **II and III** are correct
E if **I, II, and III** are correct

9. Factors likely to cause an increase in the blood urea nitrogen (BUN) level include

I. intramuscular (IM) injection of diazepam (Valium)
II. severe liver disease
III. chronic kidney disease

10. A patient who undergoes serum enzyme testing is found to have an increased aspartate aminotransferase (AST) level. Possible underlying causes of this abnormality include

I. methyldopa-induced hepatitis
II. congestive heart failure (CHF)
III. pneumonia

11. Serum enzyme tests that may aid in the diagnosis of myocardial infarction include

I. alkaline phosphatase
II. creatine kinase (CK)
III. lactate dehydrogenase (LDH)

Directions: The group of items in this section consists of lettered options followed by a set of numbered items. For each item, select the **one** lettered option that is most closely associated with it. Each lettered option may be selected once, more than once, or not at all.

Questions 12-14

A 70-year-old black man weighing 154 lb complains of chronic fatigue. Several laboratory tests were performed with the following results:

Blood urea nitrogen (BUN): 15 mg/dl
Aspartate aminotransferase (AST): within normal limits
White blood cell (WBC) count: 7500/mm_3
Red blood cell (RBC) count: 4.0 million/mm_3
Hematocrit (Hct): 29%
Hemoglobin (Hb): 9.0 g/dl

12. This patient's mean cell hemoglobin (Hb) concentration (MCHC) is

(A) 27.5
(B) 28.9
(C) 31.0
(D) 33.5
(E) 35.4

13. His mean cell volume (MCV) is

(A) 61.3
(B) 72.5
(C) 77.5
(D) 90.2
(E) 93.5

14. From the data provided above and from the calculations in questions 12 and 13, this patient is best described as

(A) normal except for a slightly increased blood urea nitrogen (BUN)
(B) having normochromic, microcytic anemia
(C) having sickle-cell anemia
(D) having hypochromic, normocytic anemia
(E) having folic acid deficiency

15. All of the following statements about sodium (Na) are true EXCEPT

(A) The normal range for sodium (Na) is 135–147 mEq/L.
(B) Na is the major cation of the extracellular fluid and the laboratory test is used mainly to detect disturbances in water balance.
(C) Hyponatremia usually results from the total body depletion of Na or through a dilutional effect.
(D) Control of the Na concentration is mainly through regulation of arterial pH.

16. A 53-year-old woman with diabetes mellitus is seen in the emergency room. Her blood glucose is 673 mg/dl and ketones are present in her blood. A diagnosis of diabetic ketoacidosis (DKA) is made. Other important laboratory values are: potassium (K) 4.8 mEq/L, 4+ glucose in urine, and an arterial pH of 7.1. All of the following statements apply to this patient EXCEPT

(A) Her potassium (K) value is normal, therefore no K supplementation is likely to be necessary.
(B) Her K value should be corrected due to her acidosis; a corrected K would be 3.0 mEq/L.
(C) K supplementation should be instituted because her total body K is depleted.
(D) Factors affecting K in this patient include glycosuria and arterial pH.

17. A 50-year-old man presents with bicarbonate of 18 mEq/L. All of the following could be a cause of his low bicarbonate level EXCEPT

(A) metabolic acidosis
(B) salicylate toxicity
(C) diuretic therapy
(D) diarrhea

18. All of the following statements about calcium (Ca) and phosphorus (PO_4) are true EXCEPT

(A) An alcoholic with a serum albumin of 2 g/dl, and a serum total calcium (Ca) of 8.0 mg/dl has a corrected total Ca of 9.6 mg/dl.
(B) Ca and phosphorus (PO_4) levels should be interpreted together because many of the same factors influence both minerals.
(C) Metastatic cancer often induces a decrease in serum Ca levels.
(D) A patient with renal failure may present with hypocalcemia and hyperphosphatemia.

19. All of the following are important functions of magnesium (Mg) EXCEPT

(A) nerve conduction
(B) phospholipid synthesis
(C) muscle contractility
(D) carbohydrate, fat and electrolyte metabolism

ANSWERS AND EXPLANATIONS

1. The answer is C *[II B 2 d (2)].*
Valuable diagnostic information can be obtained through quantitative and qualitative testing of the cells of the blood. A finding of lymphopenia (i.e., decreased number of lymphocytes) suggests an attack on the immune system or some underlying immunodeficiency. Acquired immune deficiency syndrome (AIDS) attacks the T_4 population of lymphocytes and thus may result in lymphopenia.

2. The answer is A *[II A 5].*
The reticulocyte count measures the amount of circulating immature red blood cells (RBCs), which provides information about bone marrow function. A low reticulocyte count is a likely finding in a patient with aplastic anemia—a disorder characterized by a deficiency of all cellular elements of the blood due to a lack of hematopoietic stem cells in bone marrow. A variety of drugs (e.g., those used in anticancer therapy) and other agents produce marrow aplasia. A high reticulocyte count would likely be found in a patient with hemolytic anemia or acute blood loss or in a patient who has been treated for an iron, vitamin B_{12}, or folate deficiency.

3. The answer is E *[V B, E–G].*
Microscopic examination of the urine sediment normally shows fewer than 1 red blood cell (RBC) and from 0–4 white blood cells (WBCs) per high-power field (HPF). Other normal findings on urinalysis include an acid pH (i.e., around 6) and an absence of glucose and ketones.

4. The answer is A *[II B 2 c].*
An allergic drug reaction will usually produce an increase in the eosinophil count (eosinophilia). This could be determined by ordering a white blood cell (WBC) differential.

5. The answer is C *[II A 2].*
Overhydration with an excess infusion of dextrose 5% in water (D_5W) produces a low hematocrit (Hct). The other situations described in the question result in increases of the Hct.

6. The answer is A *[II B 2 a].*
The patient has leukocytosis with an increased neutrophil count (neutrophilia). A localized infection does not normally result in an increase in the total leukocyte count or neutrophil count. The other situations given in the question can produce a neutrophilic leukocytosis.

7. The answer is B *[III A].*
Because creatine kinase (CK) is not present in the liver, alcoholic liver damage would not result in an increase in the level of this enzyme. CK is present primarily in cardiac and skeletal muscle. The other situations described in the question could all result in the release of increased amounts of CK into the bloodstream.

8. The answer is D *[IV B].*
The patient with jaundice (deposition of bilirubin in the skin) usually has an increase in the total bilirubin serum level. Spillage of bilirubin into the urine requires an increased level of direct bilirubin, which is likely with viral hepatitis or cholestatic hepatitis. In hemolytic anemia, direct bilirubin is not usually increased, and therefore, there would be no spillage of bilirubin into the urine.

9. The answer is B (III) *[VI B 2].*
Chronic kidney disease can cause an increase in the blood urea nitrogen (BUN) level; a heavy protein diet and bleeding into the gastrointestinal (GI) tract are other factors that can produce this finding. Severe liver disease can prevent the formation of urea and, therefore, is likely to cause a decrease in the blood urea nitrogen (BUN) level. Although an intramuscular (IM) injection of diazepam (Valium) may cause an increase in the serum creatine kinase (CK) or aspartate aminotransferase (AST) level, it would have no effect on the BUN.

10. The answer is C (I, II) *[III D].*
A lung infection, such as pneumonia, normally would not cause an increase in the release of aspartate aminotransferase (AST), an enzyme primarily found in the liver and heart. In acute hepatitis, a marked increase of AST is a likely finding. AST levels also can be increased with passive congestion of the liver, as occurs in congestive heart failure (CHF).

11. The answer is D (II, III) *[III A–C].*
Usually, the creatine kinase (CK), alanine aminotransferase (ALT), aspartate aminotransferase (AST), and lactate dehydrogenase (LDH) enzyme levels are increased after a myocardial infarction. Alkaline phosphatase is not present in cardiac tissue and, therefore, would not be useful in the diagnosis of a myocardial infarction.

12–14. The answers are: 12-C *[II A 4 c],* **13-B** *[II A 4 a],* **14-B** *[II A 4; VI B 2].*
The mean cell hemoglobin (Hb) concentration (MCHC) is calculated as follows:

$$\text{MCHC} = \frac{\text{Hemoglobin (Hb)} \times 100}{\text{Hematocrit (Hct)}} = \frac{9 \times 100}{29} = 31.0$$

The mean cell volume (MCV) is calculated as follows:

$$\text{MCV} = \frac{\text{Hct (\%)} \times 10}{\text{RBC count (in millions)}} = \frac{29 \times 10}{4} = 72.5$$

The patient described in the question is anemic because his Hb is 9 (normal: 14–18). The anemia is normochromic because the patient's MCHC of 31 is normal (normal range: 31–37), but the anemia is microcytic because the patient's MCV is 72.5 (normal: 80–100). The patient's blood urea nitrogen (BUN), 15 mg/dl, is within the normal range of 10–20 mg/dl.

15. The answer is D. *[VII A 1, 5, 6, 7]*
Sodium (Na), the major extracellular cation, is measured mainly to assist in the determination of fluid status/water balance. Regulation of Na is mainly through the kidneys via antidiuretic hormone (ADH) and aldosterone.

16. The answer is A. *[VII B 2,4,6]*
A "normal" potassium (K) level in the setting of metabolic acidosis, especially in a patient with diabetic ketoacidosis (DKA) should be treated appropriately. If the serum K level is corrected for the patient's acidosis, the corrected level is 3.0 mEq/L. This corresponds to a depletion in total body K stores. Once the acidosis and hyperglycemia begin to correct with appropriate treatment, K levels will decrease precipitously unless supplementation is begun. It is important to recognize that a laboratory value in the "normal" range may not actually be normal, especially when K is involved.

17. The answer is C *[VII D 3, 4]*
Low bicarbonate (HCO_3^-) is usually found in patients with acidosis or renal failure and after hyperventilation or severe diarrhea. In general, disturbances in acid-base balance cause alteration in the serum HCO_3^- or carbon dioxide (CO_2) content. Diuretic therapy can cause an alkalosis and an increase in HCO_3^-.

18. The answer is C *[VIII A 2–4; B 2]*
Malignancy or other metastatic diseases are most often associated with hypercalcemia not hypocalcemia. Ionized calcium (Ca) is the free active form and this level is increased in the setting of a low albumin. Therefore the total Ca level must be adjusted to account for an increased ionized Ca in this setting. Both minerals are influenced by many of the same factors and thus are often interpreted together. Renal function is one such factor whereby a decrease in renal function (i.e., renal failure) can result in a low level of Ca and a high level of phosphorus (PO_4).

19. The answer is B *[VIII C 1]*
Magnesium (Mg) is the second most abundant intracellular and extracellular cation. It is an activator of numerous enzyme systems that control carbohydrate, fat and electrolyte metabolism, protein synthesis, nerve conduction, muscular contractility, as well as membrane transport and integrity. Phosphorus (PO_4) on the other hand is important for adenosine triphosphate (ATP) and phospholipid synthesis.

39
Ischemic Heart Disease

Barbara Szymusiak-Mutnick

I. INTRODUCTION

A. Definition. Ischemic heart disease (IHD) is a condition in which there is an insufficient supply of oxygen to the myocardium (cardiac tissue) so that oxygen demand exceeds oxygen supply.

B. Manifestations

1. **Angina pectoris,** an episodic, reversible oxygen insufficiency, is the most common form of IHD (see II).
2. **Acute myocardial infarction** (MI) occurs with a severe, prolonged deprivation of oxygen to a portion of the myocardium, resulting in irreversible myocardial tissue necrosis (see III).
3. **Sudden death.** Myocardial ischemia or infarction can trigger the abrupt onset of ventricular fibrillation (the most disorganized arrhythmia), which can stop cardiac output. Without immediate intervention—such as precordial thump, cardiopulmonary resuscitation, or defibrillation countershock—the result is death. Episodic recurrences of ventricular fibrillation, sudden death, and resuscitation are known as the **sudden death syndrome.**

C. Etiology. The processes, singly or in combination, that produce IHD include decreased blood flow to the myocardium, increased oxygen demand, and decreased oxygenation of the blood.

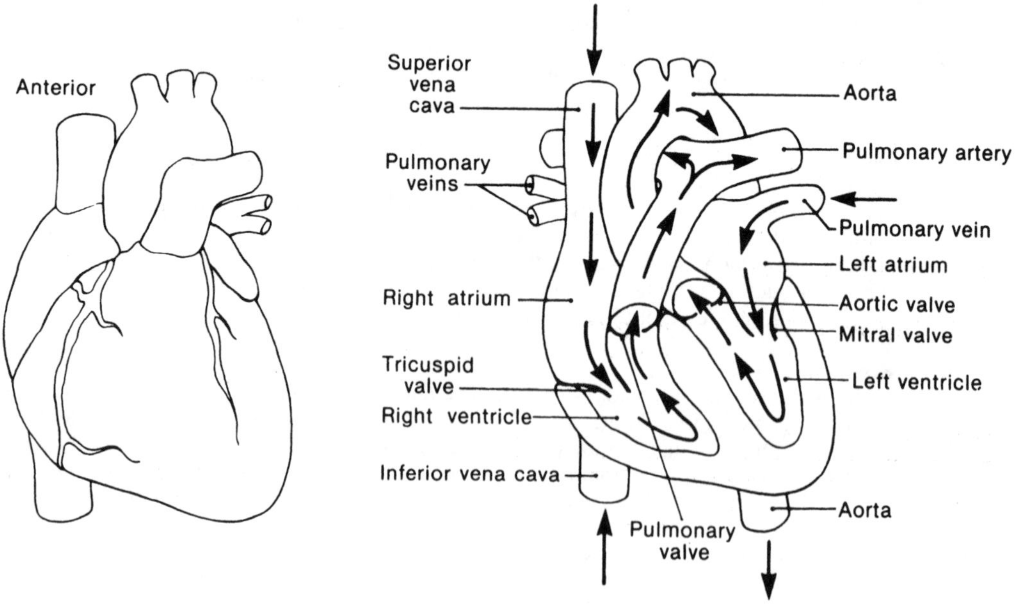

Figure 39-1. Oxygen and other nutrients are borne to the myocardium through the two major coronary arteries (the left and right) and their tributaries. The hemodynamic consequences of ischemic heart disease (IHD) depend on which of the coronary vessels is involved and what part of the myocardium that vessel supplies.

1. **Decreased blood flow.** (Coronary blood flow is illustrated in Figure 39-1.)
   a. **Atherosclerosis,** with or without coronary thrombosis, is the most common cause of IHD. In this condition, the coronary arteries are progressively narrowed by smooth muscle cell proliferation and the accumulation of lipid deposits (plaque) along the inner lining (intima) of the arteries.
   b. **Coronary artery spasm,** a sustained contraction of one or more coronary arteries, can occur spontaneously or be induced by irritation (e.g., by coronary catheter or intimal hemorrhage), exposure to the cold, or ergot-derivative drugs. These spasms can cause Prinzmetal's angina and even MI.
   c. **Traumatic injury,** whether blunt or penetrating, can interfere with myocardial blood supply (e.g., the impact of a steering wheel on the chest causing a myocardial contusion in which the capillaries hemorrhage).
   d. **Embolic events,** even in otherwise normal coronary vessels, can abruptly restrict the oxygen supply to the myocardium.

2. **Increased oxygen demand** can occur with exertion (e.g., exercise, shoveling snow) and emotional stress, which increases sympathetic stimulation and, thus, the heart rate. Some factors affecting cardiac workload, and therefore myocardial oxygen supply and demand, are listed in Table 39-1.
   a. **Diastole.** Under normal circumstances, almost all of the oxygen is removed (during diastole) from the arterial blood as it passes through the heart. Thus, little remains to be extracted if oxygen demand increases. To increase the coronary oxygen supply, blood flow has to increase. The normal response mechanism is for the blood vessels, particularly the coronary arteries, to dilate, thereby increasing blood flow.
   b. **Systole.** The two phases of systole—contraction and ejection—strongly influence oxygen demand.
      (1) The **contractile (inotropic) state of the heart** influences the amount of oxygen it requires to perform.
      (2) **Increases in systolic wall tension,** influenced by left ventricular volume and systolic pressure, increase oxygen demand.
      (3) **Lengthening of ejection time** (i.e., the duration of systolic wall tension per cardiac cycle) also increases oxygen demand.
      (4) **Changes in heart rate** influence oxygen consumption by changing the ejection time.

3. **Reduced blood oxygenation.** The oxygen-carrying capacity of the blood may be reduced, as occurs in various anemias.

D. **Risk factors** for IHD appear in Table 39-2.

E. **Therapeutic considerations.** Because most IHD occurs secondary to atherosclerosis, which is a long-term, cumulative process, medical efforts focus on reducing risk factors through individual patient education and media campaigns. Once manifestations occur, treatment addresses their variables.

II. ANGINA PECTORIS

A. **Definition.** The term **angina pectoris** is applied to varying forms of transient chest discomfort that are attributable to insufficient myocardial oxygen.

Table 39-1. Factors Affecting Cardiac Parameters That Control Myocardial Oxygen Demand

Factors	Heart Rate	Blood Pressure	Ejection Time	Ventricular Volume	Inotropic Effect
Exercise	Increase	Increase	Decrease	Increase or decrease	Increase
Cold	Increase	Increase	. . .	. . .	. . .
Smoking	Increase	Increase	Increase	. . .	Increase
Nitroglycerin	Increase	Decrease	Decrease	Decrease	Increase
β-Blockers	Decrease	Decrease	Increase	Increase	Decrease

Table 39-2. Risk Factors for Ischemic Heart Disease

Hyperlipidemia
Excess serum cholesterol
Increased ratio of low-density lipoproteins (LDLs) to high-density lipoproteins (HDLs)
Excess triglycerides
Hypertension
Smoking
Diabetes mellitus
Obesity
Family history of ischemic heart disease (IHD)
Sedentary life-style
Chronic stress or type A personality (i.e., aggressive, ambitious, chronically impatient, competitive)
Age and gender (i.e., prevalence is higher among men than among premenopausal women and increases for both genders with age)
Oral contraceptive use
Gout

B. Common etiologies. Atherosclerotic lesions that produce a narrowing of the coronary arteries are the major cause of angina. However, tachycardia, anemia, hyperthyroidism, hypotension, and arterial hypoxemia can all cause an oxygen imbalance.

C. Types

1. Stable (classic) angina

a. In this most common form, exertion, emotional stress, or a heavy meal usually precipitates chest discomfort, which is relieved by rest, nitroglycerin, or both.

b. Characteristically, the discomfort builds to a peak, radiating to the jaw, neck, shoulder, and arms, and then subsides without residual sensation. If the angina is related to physical exertion, the discomfort usually subsides quickly (i.e., in 3–5 minutes) with rest; if precipitated by emotional stress, the episode tends to last longer (i.e., about 10 minutes).

c. Stable angina is characteristically due to a fixed obstruction in a coronary artery.

2. Unstable angina

a. Angina is considered unstable and requires further evaluation if patients experience:

(1) New-onset angina

(2) Pattern changes (i.e., an increase in intensity, duration, frequency)

(3) Occurrences at rest for the first time

(4) Decreased response to rest or nitroglycerin

b. Progressive, unstable angina may signal incipient MI and should be reported promptly to a physician.

3. Angina decubitus (nocturnal angina)

a. This angina occurs in the recumbent position and is not specifically related to either rest or exertion.

b. Increased ventricular volume increases oxygen needs and produces angina decubitus, which may indicate cardiac decompensation.

c. Diuretics alone or in combination effectively reduce left ventricular volume and may aid the patient.

d. Nitrates such as nitroglycerin may relieve the paroxysmal nocturnal dyspnea associated with angina decubitus by reducing preload and improving left ventricular dysfunction.

4. Prinzmetal's angina (vasospastic or variant angina)

a. Coronary artery spasm that reduces blood flow precipitates this angina. The spasm may be superimposed on a coronary artery that already has a fixed obstruction due to thrombi or plaque formation.

b. It usually occurs at rest (i.e., pain may disrupt sleep) rather than with exertion or emotional stress.

c. Characteristically, an electrocardiogram (ECG) taken during an attack reveals a transient ST-segment elevation.

d. Calcium-channel blockers, rather than β-blockers, are most effective for this form of angina. Nitroglycerin may not provide relief, depending on the cause of vasospasm.

D. Characteristic patient complaints. Patients' descriptions of angina include squeezing pressure, sharp pain, burning, aching, bursting, and indigestion-like discomfort, sensations that commonly radiate or move to the arms, legs, neck, shoulders, and back.

E. Physical examination is usually not revealing, especially between attacks. However, the patient's history, risk factors, and full description of attacks—precipitation pattern, intensity, duration, relieving factors—usually prove diagnostic.

F. Diagnostic test results

1. The **ECG** is normal in 50%–70% of patients at rest and who are asymptomatic. During chest pain, the ST segment is usually depressed, except in Prinzmetal's angina (see II C 4 c).
2. **Stress testing (exercise ECG)** aids the diagnosis in patients who have normal resting ECGs. ST-segment depression of more than 1 mm is fairly indicative of a vascular abnormality, but the degree of positivity is most indicative of the degree of abnormality.
3. **Pharmacologic stress testing** is useful in patients with suspected coronary artery disease (CAD) who are unable to exercise. Intravenous dipyridamole, adenosine, and high-dose dobutamine induce detectable cardiac ischemia in conjunction with ECG testing.
4. **Coronary arteriography and cardiac catheterization** are very specific and sensitive but are also invasive, expensive, and risky (the mortality rate is about 1%–2%); therefore, they must be used judiciously when trying to confirm suspected angina and to differentiate its etiology.

G. Treatment goals

1. To reduce the risk of sudden death
2. To prevent MI
3. To increase myocardial oxygen supply or reduce oxygen demand
4. To reduce discomfort and anxiety associated with an angina attack
5. To remove or reduce **risk factors.** The management of angina pectoris includes therapies aimed at reversing cardiac risk factors.
   a. **Hyperlipidemia** should be treated. Reducing cholesterol and low-density lipoproteins (LDL-C) is associated with a reduced risk of cardiovascular disease and incidence of ischemic cardiac events, as demonstrated by several recent studies using HMG-CoA reductase inhibitors (see section II G 5 a (2)). A desirable serum cholesterol is less than 200 mg/dl. If serum cholesterol levels are above this mark, management depends on the presence of CAD and risk factors present in the patient, and further fractionation of high-density lipoproteins (HDL-C) and LDL-C should be carried out. If LDL-C is less than 100 mg/dl, patients with CAD should be given instructions on diet and exercise and have levels monitored annually. If LDL-C is 100 mg/dl or higher in patients with CAD, patients should begin therapy. Dietary therapy is the first step, with the goal of reducing serum LDL-C levels. Drug therapy is added after 2–3 months if dietary therapy fails.
      (1) Bile acid sequestrant resins (cholestyramine is dosed at 8–16 g per day in a single dose or two doses a day and colestipol is dosed at 2–16 g per day in a single dose or two doses a day).
         (a) **Mechanism of action.** These insoluble, nonabsorbable, anion-exchange resins bind bile acids within the intestines. Bile acids are synthesized from cholesterol.
         (b) **Indications.** These agents have been shown to be safe and effective in lowering LDL-C.
         (c) **Precautions and monitoring effects**
            (i) These resins are taken just before meals and present palatability problems in patients.
            (ii) Gastrointestinal (GI) intolerance, especially constipation, is frequent.
            (iii) Absorption of many other drugs can be affected.
      (2) **HMG-CoA reductase inhibitors** (lovastatin is dosed at 20–80 mg per day in a single dose or two doses a day, simvastatin is dosed at 5–40 mg in a single daily dose, pravastatin is dosed at 10–40 mg in a single daily dose, and fluvastatin is dosed at 20–40 mg in a single daily dose).

(a) **Mechanism of action.** These agents inhibit enzyme activity. Decrease in the enzyme results in the limitation of cholesterol production and reduction of LDL-C levels.
(b) **Indications.** These agents are effective in lowering LDL-C levels up to 40%.
(c) **Precautions and monitoring effects**
(i) GI adverse effects are less frequently seen than with other classes of agents. Headache and rash frequently occur.
(ii) These agents can elevate liver function tests; routine monitoring should be carried out.
(iii) Routine monitoring of creatine phosphokinase (CPK) may be necessary in patients with skeletal muscle complaints or risk factors that may predispose them to myositis, which is a rare effect of these agents.

(3) **Fibric acid derivatives** (gemfibrozil is dosed at 1200 mg per day in two divided doses and clofibrate is dosed at 2 g per day in divided doses).
(a) **Mechanism of action.** These agents are presumed to inhibit cholesterol synthesis and lower LDL-C.
(b) **Precautions and monitoring effects**
(i) GI effects are the most commonly experienced adverse effect.
(ii) These agents can elevate liver function tests; routine monitoring should be carried out.
(iii) Myositis has occurred with these agents.

b. **Hypertension** controlled (see Chapter 41).

c. **Smoking** should be stopped unless increased anxiety offsets the benefits. Quitting is associated with a 50% decline in cardiovascular mortality within 2 years up until the age of 65.
(1) Transdermal use of nicotine-containing patches has become one strategy for aiding the cessation of smoking. Products such as Nicotrol, Habitrol, Nicoderm, and others are available in varying strengths to wean patients off the use of cigarettes over an 8–12 week period, using descending doses.
(2) Nicotine gum (oral nicotine polacrilex chewing pieces) is available in 2 mg or 4 mg pieces. Nicorette is usually used for 3 months to aid in cessation of smoking.

d. **Obesity** should be reduced through diet and an appropriate exercise program.

H. Therapeutic agents

1. Nitrates (e.g., nitroglycerin)

a. Mechanism of action
(1) The primary value of nitrates is venous dilation, which reduces left ventricular volume (preload) and myocardial wall tension, decreasing oxygen requirements (demand).
(2) Nitrates may also reduce arteriolar resistance, helping to reduce afterload, which decreases myocardial oxygen demand.
(3) By reducing pressure in cardiac tissues, nitrates also facilitate collateral circulation, which increases blood distribution to ischemic areas.

b. Indications
(1) Acute attacks of angina pectoris can be managed with sublingual, transmucosal (spray or buccal tablets), or intravenous delivery.
(2) Indications include the prevention of anticipated attacks, using tablets (oral or buccal) or transdermal paste or patches. Sublingual nitrates can be used before eating, sexual activity, or a known stressful event.

c. **Choice of preparation** should be based on onset of action, duration of action, and patient compliance and preference because all nitrates have the same mechanism of action.
(1) Sublingual nitroglycerin is dosed at 0.3–0.6 mg as required (up to 3 tablets).
(2) Oral nitroglycerin capsules are dosed at 2.5–6.5 mg two to four times a day.
(3) Topical nitroglycerin ointment is 1′ to 2′ every 4 hours for 12–14 hours a day. Patches are used 12–14 hours a day.
(4) Various isosorbide dinitrate preparations vary from 2.5–10 mg every 2–3 hours to 60–120 mg once daily for extended-release product. A once-a-day product is also available in the mononitrate salt.

d. Precautions and monitoring effects

(1) To maximize the therapeutic effect, patients should thoroughly understand the use of their specific dosage forms (e.g., sublingual tablets, transdermal patches or pastes, tablets, capsules).
(2) Blood pressure and heart rate should be monitored because all nitrates can increase heart rate while lowering blood pressure.
(3) Preload reduction can be assessed through reduction of pulmonary symptoms such as shortness of breath, paroxysmal nocturnal dyspnea, or dyspnea.
(4) Nitrate-induced headaches are the most common side effect.
(a) Patients should be warned of the nature, suddenness, and potential strength of these headaches to minimize the anxiety that might otherwise occur.
(b) Compliance can be enhanced if the patient understands that the effect is transient and that the headaches usually disappear with continued therapy.
(c) Acetaminophen ingested 15–30 minutes before nitrate administration may prevent the headache.

e. **Effective therapy** should result in fewer anginal attacks without inducing significant adverse effects (e.g., postural hypotension, hypoxia). If maximal doses are reached and the patient still experiences attacks, additional agents should be administered.

2. β-Adrenergic blockers

a. **Mechanism of action.** β-Blockers reduce oxygen demand, both at rest and during exertion, by decreasing the heart rate and myocardial contractility, which also decreases arterial blood pressure.

b. **Indications.** These agents reduce the frequency and severity of exertional angina that is not controlled by nitrates.

c. **Precautions and monitoring effects**
(1) Doses should be increased until the anginal episodes have been reduced or until unacceptable side effects occur.
(2) β-Blockers should be avoided in Prinzmetal's angina (caused by coronary vasospasm) because they increase coronary resistance.
(3) Asthma is a relative contraindication because all β-blockers increase airway resistance and have the potential to induce bronchospasm in susceptible patients.
(4) Patients with diabetes and others predisposed to hypoglycemia should be warned that β-blockers mask tachycardia, which is a key sign of developing hypoglycemia.
(5) Patients should be monitored for excessive negative inotropic effects. Findings such as fatigue, shortness of breath, edema, and paroxysmal nocturnal dyspnea may signal developing cardiac decompensation, which also increases the metabolic demands of the heart.
(6) Sudden cessation of β-blocker therapy may trigger a withdrawal syndrome that can exacerbate anginal attacks (especially in patients with CAD) or cause MI.

d. **Choice of preparations.** All β-blockers are likely to be equally effective for stable (exertional) angina. For further review of β-adrenergic blockers, see Chapter 41.

3. Calcium-channel blockers

a. **Mechanism of action.** Two actions are most pertinent in the treatment of angina.
(1) These agents prevent and reverse coronary spasm by inhibiting calcium influx into vascular smooth muscle and myocardial muscle. This results in increased blood flow, which enhances myocardial oxygen supply.
(2) Calcium-channel blockers decrease total peripheral vascular resistance by dilating peripheral arterioles and reduce myocardial contractility, resulting in decreased oxygen demand.

b. **Indications**
(1) Calcium-channel blockers are used in stable (exertional) angina that is not controlled by nitrates and β-blockers and in patients for whom β-blocker therapy is inadvisable. Combination therapy—with nitrates, β-blockers, or both—may be most effective.
(2) These agents, alone or with a nitrate, are particularly valuable in the treatment of Prinzmetal's angina.

c. **Individual agents**
(1) Diltiazem, verapamil, and bepridil
(a) These drugs produce negative inotropic effects, and patients must be monitored closely for signs of developing cardiac decompensation (i.e., fatigue, shortness of breath, edema, paroxysmal nocturnal dyspnea). When coadministered with

β-blockers or other agents that produce negative inotropic effects (e.g., disopyramide, quinidine, procainamide, flecainide), the negative effects are additive.
- **(b)** Patients should be monitored for signs of developing bradyarrhythmias and heart block because these agents have negative chronotropic effects.
- **(c)** Verapamil frequently causes constipation, which must be treated as needed to prevent straining at stool, which could cause an increased oxygen demand (Valsalva maneuver). Verapamil is not recommended in patients with sick sinus syndromes, A-V nodal disease, or congestive heart failure (CHF).
- **(d)** Doses of diltiazem for the treatment of angina are 30–60 mg every 6–8 hours initially, up to 360 mg/day or 180–300 mg once a day using diltiazem hydrochloride (HCl) (Cardizem).
- **(e)** Doses of verapamil are 80–120 mg three times a day initially, up to a maximum of 480 mg/day. Twice daily doses of 120–240 mg may be accomplished with sustained-release products.

(2) Nifedipine
- **(a)** This calcium-channel blocker does not seem to have a strongly negative inotropic effect; therefore, it is preferred for combination therapy with agents that do. Nifedipine 10 mg (chewed or swallowed) has been used to treat Prinzmetal's angina or refractory spasm in patients who are not hypotensive.
- **(b)** Because nifedipine increases the heart rate somewhat, it can produce tachycardia, which would increase oxygen demand. Coadministration of a β-blocker should prevent reflex tachycardia.
- **(c)** Its potent peripheral dilatory effects can decrease coronary perfusion and produce excessive hypotension, which can aggravate myocardial ischemia.
- **(d)** Dizziness, light-headedness, and lower extremity edema are the most common adverse effects, but these tend to disappear with time or dose adjustment.
- **(e)** Doses of nifedipine are 10–20 mg three times a day (up to a maximum dose of 20–30 mg three to four times a day or 30–130 mg once a day).

(3) Nicardipine (Cardene) doses are 20–40 mg three times a day or 30–60 mg every 12 hours.

(4) Bepridil (Vascor), amlodipine (Norvasc), felodipine (Plendil), and isradipine (DynaCirc) are second-generation calcium-channel blockers. They have been used effectively as once or twice a day agents due to their long activity. These agents are not recommended in patients with CHF.
- **(a)** Bepridil doses are 200–400 mg/day.
- **(b)** Amlodipine doses are 2.5–10 mg/day.
- **(c)** Felodipine doses are 5–10 mg twice a day.
- **(d)** Isradipine doses are 2.5–10 mg twice a day.

III. MYOCARDIAL INFARCTION (MI)

A. Definition. In MI, a portion of the cardiac muscle suffers a severe and prolonged restriction of oxygenated coronary blood. In the majority of patients, the cause of MI is an occlusive or near occlusive thrombus overlying or adjacent to a ruptured atherosclerotic plaque. This results in cellular ischemia, tissue injury, and tissue necrosis.

1. Recently, the introduction of thrombolytic agents for the acute management of MI has removed thrombus formation in coronary vessels.
2. However, the damage on myocardial tissue is not reversible as it is in angina pectoris, because the myocardial tissue dies.

B. Signs and symptoms

1. The foremost characteristic of an MI is persistent, severe chest pain or pressure, commonly described as crushing, squeezing, or heavy (likened to having an elephant sitting on the chest). The pain generally begins in the chest and, like angina, may radiate to the left arm, the abdomen, back, neck, jaw, or teeth. The onset of pain generally occurs at rest or with normal daily activities; it is not commonly associated with exertion.
2. Unlike an angina attack, sensations associated with an MI usually persist—longer than 30 minutes—and are unrelieved by nitroglycerin. However, it has been estimated that 20%–30% of heart attacks are associated with no pain (silent MI).

3. Other common complaints include a sense of impending doom, sweating, nausea, vomiting, and difficulty breathing. In some patients, fainting and sudden death may be the initial presentation of an acute MI.

4. Observable findings include extreme anxiety, restless, agitated behavior, and ashen pallor.

5. Some patients, particularly those with diabetes or the elderly, may experience only mild or indigestion-like pain or a clinically silent MI, which may only manifest in worsening CHF, loss of consciousness, acute confusion, dyspnea, a sudden drop in blood pressure, or a lethal arrhythmia.

C. **Diagnostic test results.** Because an MI is a life-threatening emergency, diagnosis is presumed—and treatment is instituted—based on the patient's complaints and the results of an immediate 12-lead ECG. Laboratory tests and further diagnostic tests can rule out or provide confirmation of an MI and help to identify the locale and extent of myocardial damage.

1. **Serial 12-lead ECG.** Abnormalities may be absent or inconclusive during the first few hours after an MI and may not aid the diagnosis in about 15% of the cases. When present, characteristic findings show progressive changes.
   a. First, ST-segment elevation (injury current) appears in the leads, reflecting the injured area.
   b. Then T waves invert (reflecting ischemia), and Q waves develop (indicating necrosis) in those leads where the ST segment was elevated.
   c. Unequivocal diagnosis can only be made in the presence of all three abnormalities. However, the manifestations depend on the area of injury. For example, in the non–Q-wave infarction only ST-segment depression may appear.
   d. The most serious arrhythmic complication of an acute MI is ventricular fibrillation, which may occur without warning.
   e. Ventricular premature beats (VPBs) are the most commonly encountered arrhythmias and may require treatment.

2. **Chest radiograph** findings are commonly normal unless CHF is developing, indicated by cardiomegaly, pulmonary vascular congestion, or pleural effusion.

3. **Myocardial scanning** with technetium 99m (^{99m}Tc) pyrophosphate, for example, is useful in confirming or localizing damage; a "hot spot" on the film indicates the area of uptake by damaged tissue. This is usually positive between 1 day and 1 week after the MI.

4. **Cardiac enzyme studies.** Changes in some of the laboratory values do not appear until 6–24 hours after the MI (Table 39-3). Cardiac troponin-I may have higher specificity than creatine kinase of the muscle and brain [CK_2 (MB)]. Myoglobin or isotoms of CK_2 (MB) now prove to be useful in cardiac detection of MI.

Table 39-3. Serum Cardiac Enzyme Values in Myocardial Infarction

Test	Approximate Post-Myocardial Infarction Appearance (Time)	Comments
CK (creatine kinase) or CPK (creatine phosphokinase)	4–8 hours	CK_2 (MB) isoenzyme elevation is particularly telling because it derives almost exclusively in the myocardium; peaks at 12–20 hours and returns to baseline in 30–48 hours
AST (aspartate aminotransferase) or SGOT (serum glutamic-oxaloacetic transaminase)	8–12 hours	Activity peaks in 24–48 hours; returns to normal in 3–5 days
LDH (lactate dehydrogenase)	Detectable in 12 hours	LDH_1 exceeds LDH_2; peaks at 24–48 hours and returns to baseline in 10–14 days
WBC (white blood cells)	24 hours	A count of 12,000–15,000/μl indicates necrosis

D. Treatment goals

1. To relieve chest pain and anxiety
2. To reduce cardiac workload and stabilize cardiac rhythm
3. To reduce MI by limiting the area affected and preserving pump function
4. To prevent or arrest complications, such as lethal arrhythmias, CHF, or sudden death
5. To reopen (or reperfuse) closed coronary vessels with thrombolytic drugs

E. Therapeutic agents. Intramuscular drug administration in MI therapy can invalidate the results of cardiac enzyme studies; therefore, this route should be avoided if possible.

1. **Nitrates (e.g., nitroglycerin)**
   a. **Mechanism of action.** The nitrates decrease oxygen demand and facilitate coronary blood flow, as detailed in II H 1 a.
   b. **Indications.** These agents help to relieve chest pain. Controlling pain is crucial to relieve anxiety and to prevent the release of catecholamines, which may be triggered when pain persists. Catecholamines can produce coronary spasm and increased oxygen demand.
2. **Morphine**
   a. **Mechanism of action.** Morphine causes venous pooling and reduces preload, cardiac workload, and oxygen consumption. Morphine should be administered intravenously, starting with 2 mg and titrating at 5–15-minute intervals until the pain is relieved or toxicity becomes evident.
   b. **Indications.** Morphine is the drug of choice for MI pain and anxiety.
   c. **Precautions and monitoring effects**
      (1) Because morphine increases peripheral vasodilation and decreases peripheral resistance, it can produce orthostatic hypotension and fainting.
      (2) Patients should be monitored for hypotension and signs of respiratory depression.
      (3) Morphine has a vagomimetic effect that can produce bradyarrhythmias. If ECG monitoring reveals excess bradycardia, it should be reversed by administering atropine (0.5–1 mg).
      (4) Nausea and vomiting may occur, especially with initial doses, and patients must be protected against aspiration of stomach contents.
      (5) Severe constipation is a potential problem with ongoing morphine administration. The patient may use a Valsalva maneuver while straining at the stool, which can produce a bradycardia or can overload the cardiac system and trigger cardiac arrest. Docusate (100 mg twice daily) is a useful prophylactic.
3. **Oxygen.** Current **advanced cardiac life support recommendations** require the institution of oxygen therapy at 2–4 liters/minute via nasal cannula in any patient who has chest pain and who may be ischemic. Increasing the oxygen content of the blood, thus improving oxygenation of the myocardium, is a top priority as continuing hypoxia rapidly increases myocardial damage.
4. **Lidocaine**
   a. **Mechanism of action.** This antiarrhythmic agent has a rapid effect and is highly controllable because its effects diminish rapidly once infusion is withdrawn. Usual doses begin with a 100-mg loading dose intravenously, followed by a continuous infusion at 2.0–4.0 mg/min.
   b. **Precautions and monitoring effects**
      (1) Only lidocaine preparations without sympathomimetic amines or other vasoconstrictors should be used in MI. Other forms can cause lethal arrhythmias and are, therefore, contraindicated.
      (2) The risk of lidocaine toxicity increases with an increased rate of infusion.
      (3) Doses should be adjusted downward by as much as 50% in patients with heart failure, liver disease, hypotension, and advanced age.
   c. **Significant interactions.** Coadministration of a β-**blocker** diminishes the metabolism of lidocaine and may result in lidocaine toxicity. At the first signs of toxicity (e.g., dizziness, somnolence, confusion, paresthesias, convulsions), the lidocaine should be withdrawn.
5. **Thrombolytic agents**
   a. **Mechanism of action**. Administration of thrombolytic agents causes the thrombus clot to be lysed in 60%–90% of patients, restoring blood flow.

b. Indications

(1) Thrombolytic agents were used in patients with suspected MI with chest pain for hours. Successful early reperfusion has been shown to reduce infarct size, improve ventricular function, and improve mortality. However, recent studies suggest that benefits may be seen in patients using thrombolytic therapy as late as 12 hours after pain starts.

(2) Intravenous administration of streptokinase (SK), recombinant tissue-type plasminogen activator (t-PA), or anisoylated plasminogen streptokinase activator complex (APSAC) may restore blood flow in an occluded artery if administered within 12 hours of an acute MI, although less than 6 hours is optimal.

(a) t-PA is relatively fibrin-specific and is able to lyse clots without depleting fibrinogen. SK activates the fibrinolytic system and has a greater likelihood of causing systemic effects than t-PA. This effect may result in a greater degree of systemic bleeding as compared with t-PA.

(b) Though which agent—t-PA or SK—is best is still controversial, most studies have shown that both drugs, when used early, can reopen (reperfuse) occluded coronary arteries and reduce mortality from MI.

c. Individual agents

(1) Streptokinase (SK)

(a) Absolute contraindications to SK include active internal bleeding, recent cerebrovascular accident (CVA), intracranial or intraspinal surgery, intracranial neoplasm, pregnancy, arteriovenous malformation, aneurysm, bleeding diathesis, and severe uncontrolled hypertension or hemorrhagic ophthalmic conditions.

(b) Precautions and monitoring effects

(i) Patients who have received SK within the previous 6 months have an added predisposition to allergic reactions as well as a refractory response to SK due to systemic antibody formation.

(ii) Patients must be monitored for bleeding, arrhythmias, anaphylactoid reactions, and hypotension. Many patients develop arrhythmias, which do not require treatment, within 30–45 minutes of SK administration; these arrhythmias are called **reperfusion arrhythmias,** referring to a clot that has been removed and resulted in coronary reperfusion.

(c) Dosage. An intravenous dose of 1.5 million IU is infused over 60 minutes. Other treatments are currently being used, including bolus doses followed by continuous infusions, as well as combination therapy with t-PA.

(2) Recombinant tissue-type plasminogen activator (t-PA)

(a) Absolute contraindications to t-PA include active internal bleeding; recent CVA; intracranial neoplasm; aneurysm; pregnancy; arteriovenous malformations; recent (within 2 months) intracranial surgery, spinal surgery, or trauma; and severe uncontrolled hypertension, bleeding diathesis, or hemorrhagic ophthalmic conditions.

(b) Dosage for patients over 65 kg. A total of 100 mg of t-PA is generally administered to all patients who weigh over 65 kg over a 3-hour period. Though many regimens have been used, generally speaking, 6–10 mg of t-PA is given as an intravenous bolus dose over 1–2 minutes, followed by the remaining infusion rates over the next 3 hours:

(i) A 54–60-mg intravenous infusion over the first hour

(ii) A 20-mg intravenous infusion over the second hour

(iii) A 20-mg intravenous infusion over the third hour

(c) Dosage for patients under 65 kg. For patients who weigh less than 65 kg, a dose of 1.25 mg/kg is given over a 3-hour period with 10% of the total dose given initially as a bolus dose over 1–2 minutes.

(d) Recent studies suggest a "front-loaded" regimen of a total dose of 100 mg or less that is dosed over 1 $\frac{1}{2}$ hours may be more beneficial. The initial dose of 15 mg is bolused, intravenously, 1–2 minutes, while an infusion is begun to:

(i) infuse t-PA at the rate of 0.75 mg/kg over 30 minutes (not to exceed 50 mg)

(ii) followed by t-PA infused at 0.5 mg/kg over 60 minutes (not to exceed 35 mg).

(3) Anisoylated plasminogen streptokinase activator complex (APSAC)

(a) APSAC is the newest thrombolytic agent to be approved in the United States. It is effective for treating acute MI and has many properties similar to those of SK.

(b) The **major advantage** of APSAC over the other agents is its ease of administration as a rapid intravenous bolus dose of 30 units over a short time (less than 5 minutes).

(c) Further evaluation is needed to identify its place in the treatment of acute MI.

d. **Adjunctive therapy**

(1) **Aspirin** administered (160–325 mg) during acute thrombolytic therapy has been shown to affect thrombolysis positively by preventing platelet aggregation. Though the data are not totally conclusive at this time, most cardiologists favor the early use of aspirin after an MI and continue doses of 160–325 mg daily indefinitely

(2) **Heparin** has been administered along with the thrombolytics to prevent re-occlusion once a coronary artery has been opened. It also appears to decrease mortality in patients with an MI even if they have not received thrombolytic therapy. In the United States, heparin has been given intravenously as a 5000-unit bolus, followed by a continuous infusion of 1000 units/hour; the goal is to maintain the activated partial thromboplastin time (APTT) between one and a half to two and a half times normal. Heparin has also been administered subcutaneously in some centers but that seems to be the exception rather than the rule at this time.

(3) **Warfarin** therapy should be used for 3–6 months in patients with mural thrombus or extensive anterior MI. It may be as useful as aspirin in secondary prevention.

6. **β-Adrenergic blockers**

a. If administered early in the acute phase, β-blockers (e.g., propranolol, metoprolol, atenolol, timolol) have been shown to reduce the potential zone of infarction, decrease oxygen demands, and decrease cardiac workload.

b. β-Blocker therapy has also been shown to reduce significantly postmyocardial infarction (PMI) mortality due to sudden death.

c. **Precautions and monitoring effects** (see II H 2 c).

7. Calcium-channel blocking agents are not used in acute phases of MI and may be harmful to patients with impaired left ventricular function.

a. Verapamil, when started in the first week after an MI, appears to reduce the incidence of reinfarction in patients without heart failure who are not receiving β-adrenergic blocking therapy. Its use may decrease mortality.

b. In patients with non–Q-wave MI and good left ventricular function, diltiazem appears to decrease reinfarction rates.

8. The use of angiotensin-converting enzyme (ACE) inhibitors has benefited patients with depressed left ventricular function secondary to an MI. The patients showing most benefit were groups with CHF, anterior MI, and previous MI.

F. **Complications.** MI potentiates many complications; the most common of these include:

1. **Lethal arrhythmias.** Arrhythmias refractory to lidocaine may respond to procainamide, and bretylium.

2. **Congestive heart failure.** (See Chapter 42 for a more detailed discussion.)

a. Left ventricular failure causes pulmonary congestion. Diuretics, especially furosemide, help reduce the congestion.

b. Digitalis glycosides have a positive inotropic effect, which improves myocardial contractility, helping to compensate for myocardial damage.

3. **Cardiogenic shock**

a. In this life-threatening complication, cardiac output is decreased and pulmonary artery and pulmonary capillary wedge pressures are increased. This typically occurs when the area of infarction exceeds 40% of muscle mass and compensatory mechanisms only strain the already compromised myocardium.

b. Vasopressors [e.g., norepinephrine, epinephrine, dopamine (high doses)] enhance blood pressure through α-receptor stimulation and may be indicated.

c. Inotropic drugs [e.g., epinephrine, dopamine (middle doses), dobutamine, isoproterenol, digitalis) are rapidly acting agents used to increase myocardial contractility and improve cardiac output.

d. Vasodilators (e.g., nitroprusside) reduce preload; they lower pulmonary capillary wedge pressure by dilating veins and reduce afterload by decreasing resistance to left ventricular ejection.

e. Additional treatment may include invasive procedures such as intra-aortic balloon pumping.

G. Recent advances in adjunctive therapy

1. The role of warfarin is currently being explored for its beneficial effects post myocardial infarction. Initial effects seem promising.

2. In preliminary trials, magnesium sulfate has been shown to protect the myocardium against ischemia-induced reperfusion injury, to limit CHF, and to reduce early mortality.

3. ACE inhibitors have been used in clinical trials after MIs and have been shown to be effective in preventing and treating CHF. Further studies are ongoing.

STUDY QUESTIONS

Directions: Each of the numbered items or incomplete statements in this section is followed by answers or by completions of the statement. Select the **one** lettered answer or completion that is **best** in each case.

1. Exertion-induced angina, which is relieved by rest, nitroglycerin, or both, is referred to as

(A) Prinzmetal's angina
(B) unstable angina
(C) classic angina
(D) variant angina
(E) preinfarction angina

2. Myocardial oxygen demand is increased by all of the following factors EXCEPT

(A) exercise
(B) smoking
(C) cold temperatures
(D) isoproterenol
(E) propranolol

3. Which of the following agents used in Prinzmetal's angina has spasmolytic actions, which increase coronary blood supply?

(A) Nitroglycerin
(B) Nifedipine
(C) Timolol
(D) Isosorbide mononitrate
(E) Propranolol

4. Patients with angina pectoris receiving propranolol plus diltiazem must be monitored for what adverse drug effect?

(A) Decreased cardiac output
(B) Decreased heart rate
(C) Increased heart rate
(D) Decreased cardiac output and decreased heart rate
(E) Decreased cardiac output and increased heart rate

5. Maximal medical therapy for treating angina pectoris is represented by which of the following choices?

(A) Diltiazem, verapamil, nitroglycerin
(B) Atenolol, isoproterenol, diltiazem
(C) Verapamil, nifedipine, propranolol
(D) Isosorbide, atenolol, diltiazem
(E) Nitroglycerin, isosorbide, atenolol

6. The term ischemic heart disease (IHD) is used to designate all of the following conditions EXCEPT

(A) angina pectoris
(B) sudden cardiac death
(C) congestive heart failure (CHF)
(D) arrhythmias
(E) myocardial infarction (MI)

7. The development of ischemic pain occurs when the demands for oxygen exceed the supply. Determinants of oxygen demand include all of the following choices EXCEPT

(A) contractile state of the heart
(B) myocardial ejection time
(C) left ventricular volume
(D) right atrial pressure
(E) systolic pressure

8. The use of morphine in the patient who has had an MI centers around three distinct pharmacologic properties. Which of the following choices includes these properties?

(A) Relief of pain, relief of anxiety, and increased oxygen supply
(B) Relief of anxiety, afterload reduction, increased preload
(C) Relief of anxiety, preload reduction, and relief of pain
(D) Vagomimetic effect, relief of anxiety, respiratory depression
(E) Bradycardia, preload reduction, and increased afterload

9. Myositis is an adverse effect of all the following agents EXCEPT

(A) lovastatin
(B) simvastatin
(C) pravastatin
(D) gemfibrozil
(E) colestipol

Directions: Each item below contains three suggested answers of which **one or more** is correct. Choose the answer

A if **I only** is correct
B if **III only** is correct
C if **I and II** are correct
D if **II and III** are correct
E if **I, II, and III** are correct

Questions 10–11

A 55-year-old white man is seen in the emergency room of a local hospital with the signs and symptoms of an acute MI. This is the second such attack within the last 4 months, and the patient has not altered his life-style to eliminate important risk factors. Previous therapy included a thrombolytic agent (name unknown), a blood thinner, and daily aspirin.

10. Which of the following thrombolytic agents would be appropriate at this time?

I. Anisoylated plasminogen streptokinase activator complex (APSAC)
II. Streptokinase (SK)
III. Recombinant tissue-type plasminogen activator (t-PA)

11. Which of the following agents should be recommended during the acute MI to help prevent sudden death?

I. Atenolol
II. Metoprolol
III. Propranolol

ANSWERS AND EXPLANATIONS

1. The answer is C *[II C 1 a].*
Classic, or stable, angina refers to the syndrome in which physical activity or emotional excess causes chest discomfort, which may spread to the arms, legs, neck, and so forth. This type of angina is relieved promptly (within 1–10 minutes) with rest, nitroglycerin, or both.

2. The answer is E *[I C 2].*
Due to the β-adrenergic blocking effects of propranolol (e.g., decreased heart rate, decreased blood pressure, decreased inotropic effect), there is a net decrease in myocardial oxygen demand. This is the direct opposite of the effects seen with the β-agonist isoproterenol. Exercise, cigarette smoking, and exposure to cold temperatures have all been shown to increase myocardial oxygen demand.

3. The answer is B *[II C 4 d]*
Due to the calcium-channel blocking properties of nifedipine, primarily coronary dilation and spasmolytic effects, there is proven benefit from this agent in the treatment of Prinzmetal's angina, a syndrome believed due more to a spastic event than to a fixed coronary occlusion.

4. The answer is D *[II H 2, 3].*
Because propranolol (a β-adrenergic blocker) and diltiazem (a calcium-channel blocker) both reduce heart rate (a negative chronotropic effect) and reduce cardiac contractility (negative inotropic effect), patients receiving both drugs must be monitored for signs of decompensation (reduced cardiac output) and bradyarrhythmias.

5. The answer is D *[II H 1 a, 3 b (1)].*
The use of a nitrate (isosorbide) in conjunction with a β-adrenergic blocker (atenolol) and a calcium-channel blocker (diltiazem) represents the maximal medical regimen that presently could be used in a nonresponsive angina patient. Venous dilation and coronary dilation due to nitrates reduce oxygen demand while increasing oxygen supply, respectively. The addition of diltiazem further reduces oxygen demand by decreasing the heart rate and cardiac contractility. The use of a β-blocker such as atenolol reduces oxygen demand even more, resulting in a total net reduction in myocardial oxygen demand.

6. The answer is C *[I B].*
Ischemic heart disease (IHD) is a clinical condition that exists when there is a lack of oxygen to the heart. This may be due to increased demands of or decreased supplies to the heart. Angina pectoris, sudden cardiac death due to toxic ventricular arrhythmias, and MI represent the various conditions associated with IHD.

7. The answer is D *[I C 2].*
As with most muscles in the body, the contractile force of the heart dictates the amount of oxygen that the heart needs to perform. Consequently, as contractility decreases, the oxygen needs of the heart increase. As contractility continues to decrease, the volume of fluid in the left ventricle increases due to poor muscle performance and increasing tension within the ventricle, resulting in additional oxygen requirements. As the amount of tension within the ventricle increases per cardiac cycle, there is again an added requirement for oxygen by the heart muscle.

8. The answer is C *[III E 2].*
Venous dilation (preload reduction) along with relief of pain and anxiety make morphine a very helpful agent in the patient who has had an MI. In the clinical situation, the patient's pain and anxiety represent an added stress, which only increases myocardial oxygen demands further, thus adding potential insult to the already compromised myocardium. Venous dilation would help reduce venous return to the heart and, therefore, reduce oxygen demands placed on the myocardium. Both of these physiologic responses aid in reestablishing the balance between myocardial oxygen supply and demand.

9. The answer is E *[II G 5 a (1)–(3)]*
Myositis is an adverse effect of all the HMG CoA reductase inhibitors (lovastatin, simvastatin, pravastatin, and fluvastatin) and has been seen with use of fibric acid derivatives (gemfibrozil and clofibrate).

10. and 11. The answers are: 10-B (III) *[III E 5 b]*, **II-E (all)** *[III E 6 a, b].*
Streptokinase (SK) and anisoylated plasminogen streptokinase activator complex (APSAC) are derived from exogenous substances, which initiate antibody formation after initial exposure. A patient receiv-

ing either agent within 6 months of previous exposure may have a refractory response to them due to excess antibody production. It has also been speculated that such patients may have an increased likelihood of developing an allergic reaction. Recombinant tissue-type plasminogen activator (t-PA) represents recombinant DNA technology where exogenous substances are not introduced into the body. The likelihood for antibody formation is nil, and therefore, this agent, barring any absolute contraindications, would be the agent of choice.

Recent studies have made it relatively clear that when atenolol, metoprolol, and propranolol are given during the acute phases of an MI, there is a significant reduction in sudden death and overall mortality in the patients treated. Each of these β-adrenergic blockers is given intravenously, followed by oral therapy, in an attempt to eliminate sudden death as a consequence of MI. Because of the negative inotropic, chronotropic effects, it is still imperative to monitor the patient closely for signs of cardiac decompensation and bradyarrhythmias.

40
Cardiac Arrhythmias

Alan H. Mutnick

I. INTRODUCTION

A. Definition. Cardiac arrhythmias are deviations from the normal heartbeat pattern. They include **abnormalities of impulse formation,** such as heart rate, rhythm, or site of impulse origin, and **conduction disturbances,** which disrupt the normal sequence of atrial and ventricular activation.

B. Electrophysiology

1. Conduction system

a. Two electrical sequences that cause the heart chambers to fill with blood and contract are initiated by the conduction system of the heart.

(1) Impulse formation, the first sequence, takes place when an electrical impulse is generated automatically.

(2) Impulse transmission, the second sequence, occurs once the impulse has been generated, signaling the heart to contract.

b. Four main structures composed of tissue that can generate or conduct electrical impulses comprise the conduction system of the heart.

(1) The **sinoatrial (SA) node,** in the wall of the right atrium, contains cells that spontaneously initiate an action potential. Serving as the main pacemaker of the heart, the SA node initiates 60–100 beats/min.

(a) Impulses generated by the SA node trigger atrial contraction.

(b) Impulses travel through internodal tracts—the anterior tract, middle tract (Wenckebach's bundle), posterior tract (Thorel's bundle), and anterior interatrial tract (Bachmann's bundle) [Figure 40-1].

(2) At the **atrioventricular (AV) node,** situated in the lower interatrial septum, the impulses are delayed briefly to permit completion of atrial contraction before ventricular contraction begins.

(3) At the **bundle of His**—muscle fibers arising from the AV junction—impulses travel along the left and right bundle branches, located on either side of the intraventricular septum.

(4) The impulses reach the **Purkinje fibers,** a diffuse network extending from the bundle branches and ending in the ventricular endocardial surfaces. Ventricular contraction then occurs.

c. Latent pacemakers. The AV junction, bundle of His, and Purkinje fibers are latent pacemakers; they contain cells capable of generating impulses. However, these regions have a slower firing rate than the SA node. Consequently, the SA node predominates except when it is depressed or injured, which is known as **overdrive suppression.**

2. Myocardial action potential. Before cardiac contraction can take place, cardiac cells must depolarize and repolarize.

a. Depolarization and **repolarization** result from changes in the electrical potential across the cell membrane, caused by the exchange of sodium and potassium ions.

b. Action potential, which reflects this electrical activity, has five phases (Figure 40-2).

(1) Phase 0 (rapid depolarization) takes place as sodium ions enter the cell through fast channels; the cell membrane's electrical charge changes from negative to positive.

(2) Phase 1 (early rapid repolarization). As fast sodium channels close and potassium ions leave the cell, the cell rapidly repolarizes (i.e., returns to resting potential).

(3) Phase 2 (plateau). Calcium ions enter the cell through slow channels while potassium ions exit. As the cell membrane's electrical activity temporarily stabilizes, the

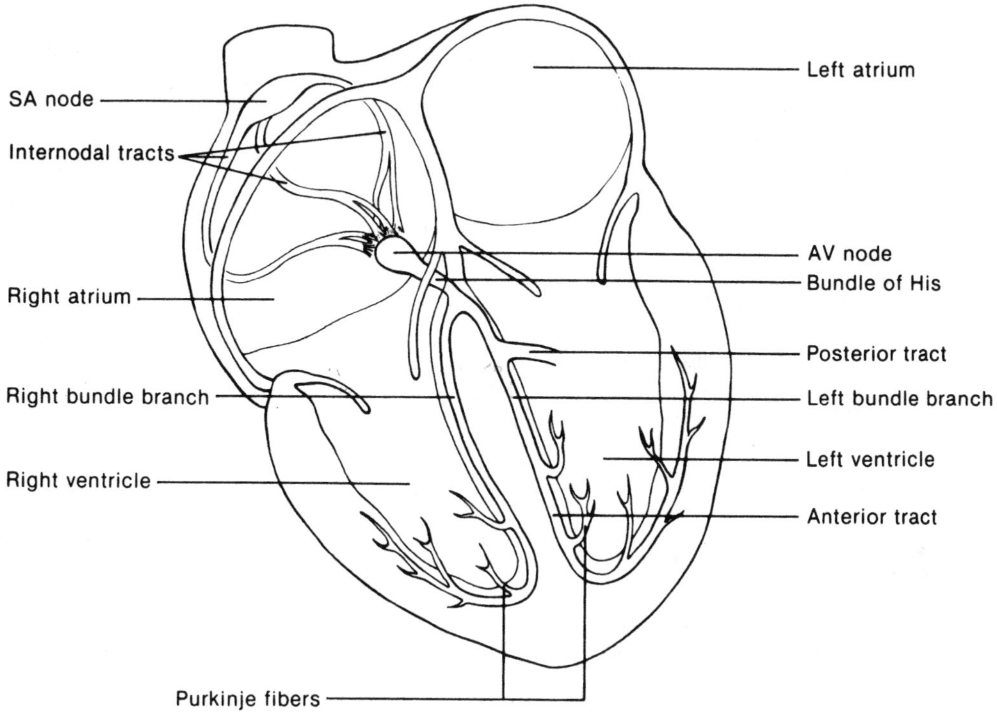

Figure 40-1. Electrical pathways of the heart. *SA* = sinoatrial; *AV* = atrioventricular.

action potential reaches a plateau (represented by the notch at the beginning of this phase in Figure 40-2).

(4) Phase 3 (final rapid repolarization). Potassium ions are pumped out of the cell as the cell rapidly completes repolarization and resumes its initial negativity.

(5) Phase 4 (slow depolarization). The cell returns to its resting state with potassium ions inside the cell and sodium and calcium ions outside.

c. During both depolarization and repolarization, a cell's ability to initiate an action potential varies.

(1) The cell cannot respond to any stimulus during the **absolute refractory period** (beginning during phase 1 and ending at the start of phase 3).

(2) A cell's ability to respond to stimuli increases as repolarization continues. During the **relative refractory period,** which occurs during phase 3, the cell can respond to a strong stimulus.

(3) When the cell has been completely repolarized, it can again respond fully to stimuli.

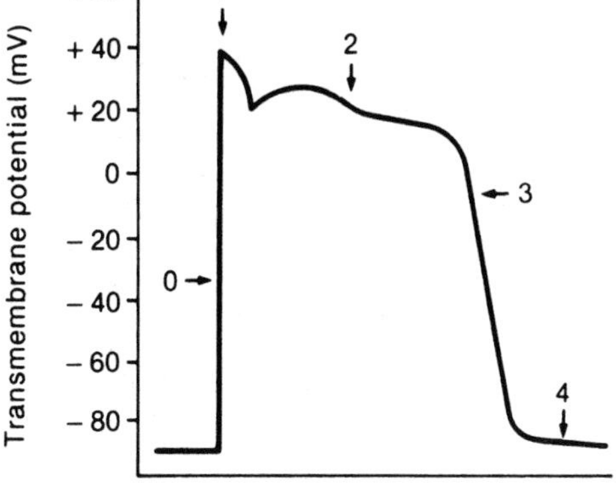

Figure 40-2. Myocardial action potential curve. This curve represents ventricular depolarization/repolarization. *0* = phase 0 (rapid depolarization); *1* = phase 1 (early rapid repolarization); *2* = phase 2 (plateau); *3* = phase 3 (final rapid repolarization); *4* = phase 4 (slow depolarization).

d. Cells in different cardiac regions depolarize at various speeds, depending on whether fast or slow channels predominate.

(1) Sodium flows through fast channels; calcium flows through slow channels.

(2) Where fast channels dominate (e.g., in cardiac muscle cells), depolarization occurs quickly. Where slow channels dominate (e.g., in the electrical cells of the SA node and AV junction), depolarization occurs slowly.

3. Electrocardiography. The electrical activity occurring during depolarization–repolarization can be transmitted through electrodes attached to the body and transformed by an **electrocardiograph (ECG) machine** into a series of waveforms (ECG waveform). Figure 40-3 shows a normal ECG waveform.

a. The **P wave** reflects atrial depolarization.

b. The **PR interval** represents the spread of the impulse from the atria through the Purkinje fibers.

c. The **QRS complex** reflects ventricular depolarization.

d. The **ST segment** represents phase 2 of the action potential—the absolute refractory period (part of ventricular repolarization).

e. The **T wave** shows phase 3 of the action potential—ventricular repolarization.

C. Classification. Arrhythmias generally are classified by origin (i.e., supraventricular or ventricular).

1. Supraventricular arrhythmias stem from enhanced automaticity of the SA node (or another pacemaker region) or from re-entry conduction.

2. Ventricular arrhythmias occur when an ectopic (abnormal) pacemaker triggers a ventricular contraction before the SA node fires (e.g., from a conduction disturbance or ventricular irritability).

D. Etiology

1. Precipitating causes. Arrhythmias result from various conditions, including:

a. Heart disease (e.g., infection, coronary artery disease (CAD), valvular heart disease, rheumatic heart disease, ischemic heart disease)

b. Myocardial infarction (MI)

c. Toxic doses of cardioactive drugs (e.g., digitalis preparations)

d. Increased sympathetic tone

e. Decreased parasympathetic tone

f. Vagal stimulation (e.g., straining at stool)

g. Increased oxygen demand (e.g., from stress, exercise, fever)

h. Metabolic disturbances

i. Cor pulmonale

j. Systemic hypertension

k. Hyperkalemia

l. Chronic obstructive pulmonary disease (COPD) [e.g., chronic bronchitis, emphysema]

m. Thyroid disorders

2. Mechanisms of arrhythmias. Abnormal impulse formation, abnormal impulse conduction, or a combination of both may give rise to arrhythmias.

a. Abnormal impulse formation may stem from:

(1) Depressed automaticity, as in escape beats and bradycardia

(2) Increased automaticity, as in premature beats, tachycardia, and extrasystole

(3) Depolarization and triggered activity, leading to sustained ectopic firing

b. Abnormal impulse conduction results from:

(1) A conduction block or delay

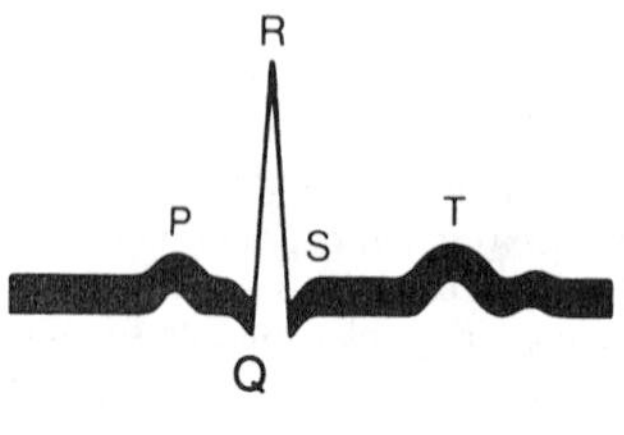

Figure 40-3. Normal ECG waveform.

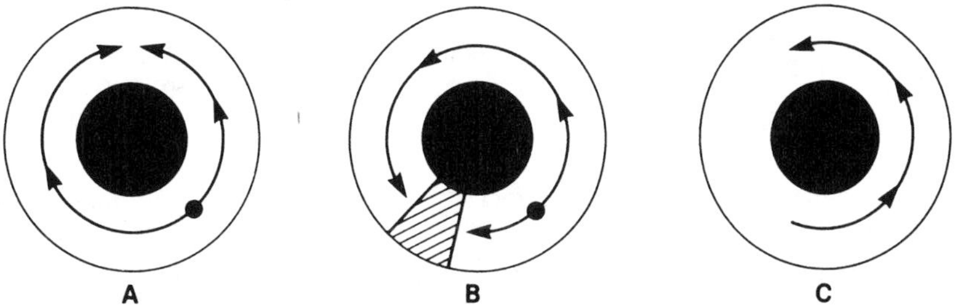

Figure 40-4. Re-entry arrhythmias. *A* shows two waves of excitation going in opposite directions; *B* represents a unidirectional wave of excitation; *C* shows re-excitation of tissue in a slow conduction area.

(2) Re-entry, which occurs when an impulse is re-routed through certain regions in which it has already traveled. The impulse, thus, depolarizes the same tissue more than once, producing an additional impulse (Figures 40-4 and 40-5). Re-entry sites include the SA and AV nodes as well as various accessory pathways in the atria and ventricles (Figure 40-6). For re-entry to occur, the following conditions must exist:

(a) Markedly shortened refractoriness or a slow conduction area that allows an adequate delay so that depolarization recurs

(b) Unidirectional conduction

E. Pathophysiology. Arrhythmias may decrease cardiac output, reduce blood pressure, and disrupt perfusion of vital organs. Specific pathophysiologic consequences depend on the arrhythmia present (see III).

F. Clinical evaluation

1. Physical findings. Although some arrhythmias are silent, most produce signs and symptoms. Only an ECG can definitively identify an arrhythmia. However, physical findings may suggest which arrhythmia is present; they also yield information about the patient's clinical status and may help to identify associated complications. **Signs and symptoms** that typically accompany arrhythmias include:

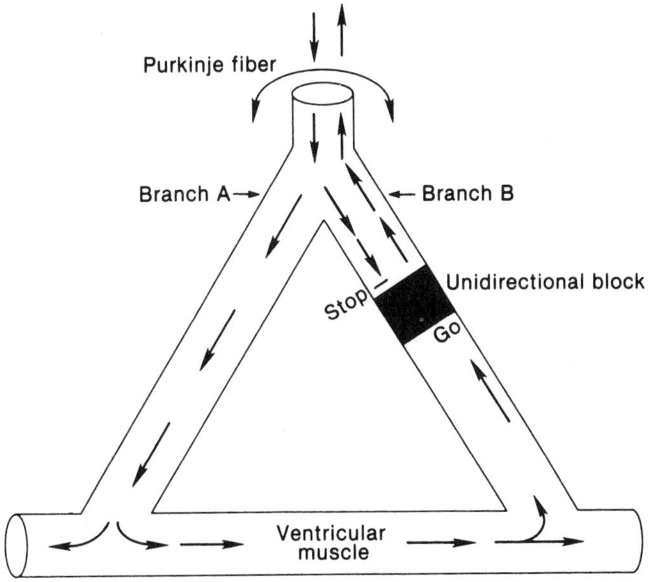

Figure 40-5. Ventricular reentry. This diagram shows a branched Purkinje fiber joining ventricular muscle. The *dark-ended area* represents the site of a unidirectional block; in this depolarization region, the impulse heading toward the AV node continues upward whereas the impulse traveling toward the muscle is blocked. Because retrograde conduction in *branch B* is slow, cells in *branch A* have time to recover and respond to the re-entrant impulse.

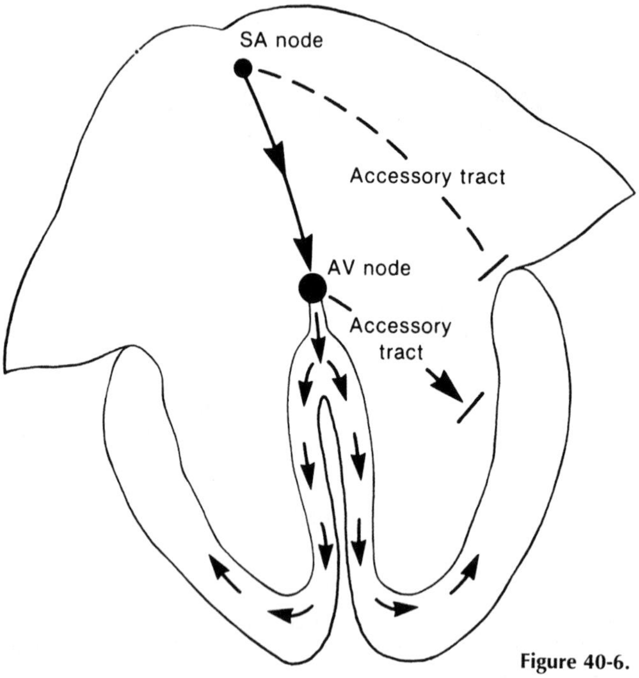

Figure 40-6. Re-entry sites.

a. Chest pain
b. Anxiety and confusion (from reduced brain perfusion)
c. Dyspnea
d. Skin pallor or cyanosis
e. Abnormal pulse rate, rhythm, or amplitude
f. Reduced blood pressure
g. Palpitations
h. Syncope
i. Weakness
j. Convulsions
k. Hypotension
l. Decreased urinary output

2. Diagnostic test results

a. An **ECG** can identify a specific arrhythmia; usually, a 12-lead ECG is used. (For ECG findings in specific arrhythmias, see III.)

b. Electrophysiologic (EP) testing. This intracardiac procedure determines the location of ectopic foci and bypass tracts and may help assess therapeutic response to antiarrhythmic drug therapy. It also can determine the need for a pacemaker or surgical intervention.

(1) Intracardiac catheters and pacing wires are placed transvenously or transarterially.

(2) The heart is divided into imaginary sections, and each section is stimulated until an arrhythmia is induced. The section in which the arrhythmia occurs is identified as the origin of the ectopic foci.

c. His bundle study, a type of EP testing, can locate the origin of a heart block or re-entry pattern.

d. Laboratory findings. Some arrhythmias result from electrolyte abnormalities—most commonly, hyperkalemia and hypocalcemia.

(1) A serum potassium level above 5 mEq/L reflects hyperkalemia; a serum calcium level below 4.5 mEq/L signifies hypocalcemia.

(2) An ECG tracing may suggest an electrolyte abnormality. For example, prolonged QRS complexes, tented T waves, and lengthened PR intervals may signal hyperkalemia; prolonged QT intervals and flattened, or inverted, T waves suggest hypocalcemia.

G. Treatment objectives

1. **Terminate** or **suppress the arrhythmia,** if it causes hemodynamic compromise or disturbing symptoms.
2. **Maintain adequate cardiac output and tissue perfusion.**
3. **Correct or maintain fluid balance** (some arrhythmias cause hypervolemia).

II. THERAPY.

Antiarrhythmic agents directly or indirectly alter the duration of the myocardial action potential. Most antiarrhythmics fall into one of four classes, depending on their specific effects on the heart's electrical activity (Table 40-1). Class I drugs are further subdivided into three groups.

A. Class I antiarrhythmics

1. **Indications**
   a. **Class IA drugs**
      (1) **Quinidine** is used to treat and prevent acute and chronic ventricular and supraventricular arrhythmias, especially paroxysmal supraventricular tachycardias (PSVTs), premature ventricular contractions (PVCs), premature atrial contractions (PACs), and ventricular tachycardia.
      (2) **Procainamide** is therapeutic for the same arrhythmias for which quinidine is given. It is used more frequently than quinidine because it can be administered intravenously and in sustained-release oral preparations. Quinidine poses added concern when used intravenously because of increased cardiovascular effects (i.e., hypotension, syncope, myocardial depression).
      (3) **Disopyramide** may be used as an alternative to quinidine or procainamide for treating ventricular arrhythmias (e.g., PVCs, moderate ventricular tachycardia).
   b. **Class IB drugs**
      (1) **Lidocaine** is used therapeutically for ventricular arrhythmias (especially PVCs and ventricular tachycardia) that result from digitalis therapy, acute MI, and open-heart surgery. Controversy still exists as to the benefits of lidocaine when used prophylactically in patients with acute MI to prevent ventricular fibrillation.
      (2) **Tocainide,** closely related to lidocaine, is used to treat and prevent ventricular arrhythmias, including frequent PVCs and ventricular tachycardia. It may be given after an acute MI.
      (3) **Phenytoin** most commonly is used to treat digitalis-induced ventricular and supraventricular arrhythmias. It is also given to suppress ventricular arrhythmias associated with acute MI, open-heart surgery, or ventricular arrhythmias that are refractory to lidocaine or procainamide, but its efficacy is less significant for these indications than it is for digitalis-induced arrhythmias.

Table 40-1. Currently Available Antiarrhythmic Agents

Class	Agents
IA	Quinidine, procainamide, disopyramide
IB	Lidocaine, phenytoin, tocainide, mexiletine
IC	Flecainide, propafenone, moricizine
II*	Propranolol, esmolol, metoprolol, nadolol, atenolol, timolol, pindolol, labetalol, acebutolol, betaxolol, carteolol, penbutolol, bisoprolol, carredilol
III†	Amiodarone, bretylium, sotalol
IV‡	Verapamil, diltiazem, nifedipine, bepridil, nicardipine, isradipine, felodipine, amlodipine

*Only propranolol, esmolol, and acebutolol are currently approved for use as antiarrhythmics.

†Sotalol is a β-adrenergic blocker, which is available and has been classified as a type III antifibrillatory agent.

‡Nifedipine, bepridil, nicardipine, isradipine, amlodipine, and felodipine, though currently available, are not considered agents for arrhythmias.

(4) **Mexiletine,** another drug that closely resembles lidocaine, is used to suppress ventricular arrhythmias, including those following an acute MI. It is effective against ventricular tachycardia that has not responded to other antiarrhythmics.

c. **Class IC drugs**

(1) **Flecainide** suppresses PVCs and ventricular tachycardia; it may be used to treat some arrhythmias that are refractory to other agents. Flecainide is reserved for patients with refractory life-threatening ventricular arrhythmias who do not have CAD.

(2) **Propafenone** also suppresses PVCs and ventricular tachycardia and has been used successfully for treating sustained ventricular tachycardia when the arrhythmia is life-threatening.

(3) **Moricizine** is a difficult antiarrhythmic to classify based on the fact that it has properties of all three class I antiarrhythmic groups. Because it prolongs the QRS interval like other class IC agents, it has been classified as a class IC agent throughout this discussion. Moricizine is effective for suppressing PVCs, and may offer some benefits over other agents because of a lower incidence of proarrhythmia effects.

2. **Mechanism of action.** Class I antiarrhythmics slow impulse conduction through the AV node by depressing the flow of sodium ions into cells during phase 0 of the action potential. Class I subgroups (i.e., IA, IB, IC) differ in the degree and onset of their myocardial depressant actions and in their effects on the duration of the action potential and repolarization phase.

a. **Class IA drugs** moderately reduce the depolarization rate and prolong repolarization (refractory period).

b. **Class IB drugs** shorten repolarization (refractory period); they also weakly affect the repolarization rate.

c. **Class IC drugs** strongly depress depolarization but have a negligible effect on the duration of repolarization or refractoriness.

3. **Administration and dosage**

a. **Quinidine** is administered orally, usually in three or four daily doses of 200–300 mg. Sustained-release products may be given every 8–12 hours, depending on the salt form. (In special circumstances, it can be given intravenously or intramuscularly with caution.) To achieve an effective plasma concentration rapidly, a loading dose of 600–1000 mg may be administered in doses of 200 mg every 2 hours to a maximum of 1000 mg.

b. **Procainamide** is available for oral, intravenous, or intramuscular use.

(1) For **acute therapy,** intravenous administration is preferred.

(a) Intermittent intravenous administration calls for infusion of 100 mg over 2–4 minutes, repeated every 5 minutes until the arrhythmia is abolished, side effects occur, or 1 g has been given. The usual effective dose is 500–1000 mg.

(b) Rapid intravenous administration calls for infusion of 1–1.5 g at a rate of 20–50 mg/min.

(c) Once the arrhythmia is terminated, 2–6 mg/min is given as a continuous infusion.

(2) For **long-term therapy,** oral administration is used. The usual daily dosage is 3–6 g, given at intervals of 4–6 hours or less frequently with the sustained-release form of the drug (every 6–8 hours).

c. Disopyramide is available in oral form. Usually, 400–800 mg/day is administered in divided doses or less frequently with the controlled-release product. (A loading dose of 300–400 mg may be given to attain an effective plasma level rapidly.)

d. Lidocaine may be administered intravenously or intramuscularly.

(1) An intravenous loading dose rapidly achieves a therapeutic plasma level.

(a) Initially, 1–1.5 mg/kg is administered.

(b) A second injection of half the initial dose may be required 5 minutes later.

(2) Continuous intravenous infusion of 1–4 mg/min produces an effective plasma level in 7–10 hours.

(3) In an emergency, an intramuscular injection rapidly achieves an effective plasma level. The usual dosage is 300–400 mg injected into the deltoid muscle.

e. **Tocainide** is administered orally. Initially, 400 mg is given every 8 hours; then, 1200–1800 mg/day is given in two or three divided doses.

f. **Phenytoin** is given orally or in intermittent intravenous doses.

(1) For oral administration, a loading dose of 1 g is divided over the first 24 hours; for the next 2 days, 300–500 mg/day is administered. The maintenance dosage is 300–400 mg/day.

(2) For intermittent intravenous administration, 100 mg is given every 5 minutes at a rate not exceeding 25–50 mg/min, until the arrhythmia disappears, adverse effects develop, or 1 g has been given. The usual effective dosage is 700 mg.

g. **Mexiletine** is given orally in an initial dosage of 200–400 mg, followed by 200 mg every 8 hours. If this fails to control the arrhythmia, the dosage may be increased to 400 mg every 8 hours. (Alternatively, doses may be given every 12 hours.)

h. **Flecainide** is administered orally in a dosage of 50–100 mg every 12 hours. To obtain satisfactory arrhythmia control, the dosage may be increased in twice-daily increments of 50 mg every 4 days to a maximum of 400-600 mg/day.

i. **Propafenone** is administered orally in an initial dose of 150 mg every 8 hours. This dose may be slowly increased at 3- to 4-day intervals to a maximum dose of 300 mg every 8 hours.

j. **Moricizine** is administered orally in doses ranging from 600–900 mg divided into three equal doses throughout the day.

4. Precautions and monitoring effects

a. Quinidine

(1) This drug is contraindicated in patients with:

(a) Complete AV block unless a ventricular pacemaker is in place

(b) Marked prolongation of the QT interval or prolonged QT syndrome because ventricular tachyarrhythmia (torsades de pointes) may arise, resulting in quinidine syncope (i.e., syncope or sudden death)

(2) An increase of 50% or more in the duration of the QRS complex necessitates dosage reduction.

(3) Quinidine has a narrow therapeutic index. Toxicity may cause acute cardiac effects, such as pronounced slowing of conduction in all heart regions; this, in turn, may lead to SA block or arrest, ventricular tachycardia, or asystole.

(4) The ECG should be monitored during quinidine therapy to detect signs of cardiotoxicity. To counteract quinidine-induced ventricular tachyarrhythmias, catecholamines, glucagon, or sodium lactate may be given.

(5) In patients receiving quinidine for atrial tachyarrhythmias, vagolytic effects may increase impulse conduction at the AV node, resulting in an accelerated ventricular response. To prevent this, agents that slow AV nodal conduction (e.g., verapamil, digoxin) may be administered.

(6) The dosage should be reduced in elderly patients (over 60 years old) and in patients with hepatic dysfunction or congestive heart failure (CHF).

(7) Embolism may occur upon restoration of normal sinus rhythm after prolonged atrial fibrillation. To prevent or minimize this complication, anticoagulants may be administered before quinidine therapy begins.

(8) Quinidine may cause cinchonism at high serum concentrations, manifested by tinnitus, hearing loss, blurred vision, and GI disturbances. In severe cases, nausea, vomiting, diarrhea, headache, confusion, delirium, photophobia, diplopia, and psychosis may occur.

(9) Gastrointestinal (GI) reactions are the most common adverse reactions to quinidine. About 30% of patients experience diarrhea; nausea and vomiting may also occur. Arising almost immediately after the first dose, these symptoms sometimes warrant discontinuing the drug. However, aluminum hydroxide or use of the polygalacturonate salt may reverse this.

(10) Hypersensitivity reactions include anaphylaxis, thrombocytopenia, respiratory distress, and vascular collapse.

(11) Plasma quinidine levels of 2–6 μg/ml are therapeutic.

b. Procainamide

(1) This drug is contraindicated in patients with hypersensitivity to procaine and related drugs, myasthenia gravis, second- or third-degree AV block with no pacemaker, a history of procainamide-induced systemic lupus erythematosus (SLE), prolonged QT syndrome, or torsades de pointes.

(2) An increase of 50% or more in the duration of the QRS complex necessitates dosage reduction.

(3) Procainamide has a narrow therapeutic index. Toxicity may cause acute cardiac effects (e.g., pronounced slowing of conduction in all heart regions), which, in turn, may lead to SA block or arrest, ventricular tachycardia, or asystole.

(4) High serum procainamide levels may induce ventricular arrhythmias (e.g., PVCs, ventricular tachycardia or fibrillation). The ECG should be monitored continuously to detect these problems. Catecholamines, glucagon, or sodium lactate may be administered to counteract these arrhythmias.
(5) Hypotension may occur with rapid intravenous administration.
(6) GI effects are less common than with quinidine therapy.
(7) Hypersensitivity reactions are the most severe adverse effects of procainamide. These reactions include drug fever, agranulocytosis, and an SLE-like syndrome.
   (a) An SLE-like syndrome is manifested by fatigue, arthralgia, myalgia, and low-grade fever.
   (b) Antinuclear antibody titer is positive in 50%–80% of patients receiving procainamide. However, only 20%–30% of these patients develop symptoms of the SLE-like syndrome.
   (c) Drug discontinuation usually is necessary when symptomatic SLE-like syndrome occurs.
(8) N-Acetylprocainamide (NAPA), an active procainamide metabolite, may accumulate in patients with renal dysfunction, increasing the risk of drug toxicity.
(9) The dosage should be reduced and given over 6 hours to patients with renal or hepatic impairment, as the drug half-life is increased in these patients.
(10) Lower doses may be needed in patients with CHF to adjust for the lower volume of distribution.
(11) Embolism may occur upon restoration of normal sinus rhythm after prolonged atrial fibrillation. An anticoagulant is frequently administered before procainamide therapy begins to prevent this complication.
(12) Plasma levels of both procainamide and NAPA should be monitored. Generally, a procainamide level of 4–8 μg/ml and a NAPA level of 15–25 μg/ml are considered therapeutic. Controversy still exists as to the routine monitoring of both of these levels.

c. Disopyramide

(1) This drug may cause marked hemodynamic compromise and ventricular dysfunction. It is contraindicated in patients with cardiogenic shock or second- or third-degree AV block with no pacemaker.
(2) Disopyramide should be avoided or used with extreme caution in patients with CHF. It should also be used cautiously in patients with urinary tract disorders, myasthenia gravis, and renal or hepatic dysfunction.
(3) In patients receiving this drug for atrial tachyarrhythmias, vagolytic effects may increase impulse conduction at the AV node, resulting in an accelerated ventricular response. To prevent this, agents that slow AV nodal conduction (e.g., verapamil, digoxin) may be given.
(4) Anticholinergic effects of this drug include dry mouth, constipation, urinary hesitancy or retention, and blurred vision.
(5) Therapeutic plasma levels range from 2–4 μg/ml.

d. Lidocaine

(1) This drug may cause hemodynamic compromise in patients with severe cardiac dysfunction. Generally, however, it has few untoward cardiovascular effects.
(2) Lidocaine should be used cautiously and in reduced dosage in patients with CHF or renal or hepatic impairment.
(3) Central nervous system (CNS) reactions are the most pronounced adverse effects of lidocaine. These reactions may range from light-headedness and restlessness to confusion, tremors, stupor, and convulsions.
(4) Tinnitus, blurred vision, and anaphylaxis have been reported.
(5) Plasma lidocaine levels of 1.5–6.5 μg/ml are therapeutic.
(6) Lidocaine's metabolites—glycinexylidide and monoethylglycinexylidide—may have neurotoxic as well as antiarrhythmic effects.

e. Tocainide

(1) This drug is contraindicated in patients with hypersensitivity to lidocaine and related agents.
(2) Tocainide must be used cautiously in patients with CHF or reduced cardiac reserve.
(3) Neurologic effects, including light-headedness, paresthesias, restlessness, confusion, and tremors, are encountered in 30%–50% of patients.
(4) Nausea, vomiting, epigastric pain, and diarrhea occur frequently.

(5) Other adverse effects of tocainide include hypotension, blurred vision, aplastic anemia, hepatitis, skin rash, and pulmonary fibrosis.
(6) Dosage reduction may be necessary in patients with renal or hepatic impairment.
(7) Plasma tocainide levels of 3–10 μg/ml are therapeutic.

f. Phenytoin

(1) This drug is contraindicated in patients with sinus bradycardia or heart block.
(2) Phenytoin must be used cautiously in patients with CHF, renal or hepatic impairment, myocardial insufficiency, respiratory depression, or hypotension.
(3) During acute therapy, this drug may cause CNS reactions (e.g., drowsiness, vertigo, nystagmus, ataxia, nausea). Cardiotoxicity also may occur, especially with fast intravenous infusion rates.
(4) Chronic phenytoin may lead to vestibular and cerebellar effects, behavioral changes, GI distress, gingival hyperplasia, megaloblastic anemia, and osteomalacia.
(5) Hypersensitivity reactions may be manifested by liver, skin, and hematologic problems.
  (a) Toxic hepatitis may occur.
  (b) Skin reactions include exfoliative dermatitis, Stevens-Johnson syndrome, scarlatiniform or morbilliform rash, SLE, toxic epidermal necrolysis, eosinophilia, and erythema multiforme.
  (c) Hematologic reactions include agranulocytosis, megaloblastic anemia, leukopenia, thrombocytopenia, and pancytopenia.
(6) Therapeutic plasma phenytoin levels range from 10–20 μg/ml.

g. Mexiletine

(1) This drug is contraindicated in patients with cardiogenic shock or second- or third-degree AV block with no pacemaker.
(2) Tremor is an early sign of mexiletine toxicity. Dizziness, ataxia, and nystagmus indicate an increasing plasma drug concentration.
(3) Hypotension, bradycardia, and widened QRS complexes may develop during mexiletine therapy.
(4) Adverse GI effects include nausea and vomiting.
(5) Therapeutic serum levels range from 0.50–2.0 μg/ml.

h. Flecainide

(1) This drug is contraindicated in patients with cardiogenic shock or second- or third-degree AV block with no pacemaker.
(2) The ECG should be monitored during flecainide therapy because this drug may exacerbate existing arrhythmias or precipitate new ones.
(3) This drug has a significant negative inotropic effect and may bring on or worsen CHF and cardiomyopathy.
(4) Adverse CNS effects (e.g., dizziness, headache, tremor) and GI effects (e.g., nausea, abdominal pain) may occur.
(5) Blurred vision and dyspnea have been reported.

i. Propafenone

(1) This drug, like other antiarrhythmic agents, may cause new or worsened arrhythmias. Such proarrhythmic properties range from an increased frequency of PVCs to the development of severe ventricular tachycardia, ventricular fibrillation, and torsades de pointes. This proarrhythmic effect has been under discussion for the class IC agents, and, thus, this agent should be monitored closely. Most recently, encainide was taken off the market in the United States due to significant arrhythmogenic properties in the completed Cardiac Arrhythmia Suppression Trial (CAST). The findings from this trial must be weighed against the benefits of using these agents for treating significant ventricular arrhythmias.
(2) Dizziness is a side effect that has been reported in as many as 10%–15% of patients taking the drug.
(3) Other associated side effects include vomiting; a metallic, bitter taste in the mouth; constipation; headache; and new or worsening CHF and asthma.

j. Moricizine

(1) This drug has been reported to have proarrhythmic properties. However, it has been reported that the incidence of this effect may be less than with other antiarrhythmics. Patients predisposed to the development of such proarrhythmic effects include those with a history of coronary artery bypass surgery, pacemakers, CAD, CHF, and conduction abnormalities. As most patients receiving this agent have at least one of the

previously mentioned risk factors, this agent must be used cautiously. The benefits of using this agent must be weighed against its associated risks.
(2) Dizziness is the most commonly reported adverse effect associated with the drug and has been reported in up to 15% of all patients.
(3) Other associated side effects include nausea, intraventricular conduction delays, headache, fatigue, palpitations, and shortness of breath.

5. **Significant interactions**
a. **Quinidine**
(1) Quinidine may increase serum levels of **digoxin** and increase the effects of **digitalis** on the heart, with a resultant increase in toxicity.
(2) Severe orthostatic hypotension may occur with concomitant administration of **vasodilators** (e.g., **nitroglycerin**).
(3) **Phenytoin, rifampin,** and **barbiturates** may antagonize quinidine activity and reduce its therapeutic efficacy.
(4) **Nifedipine** may reduce plasma quinidine levels.
(5) **Antacids, sodium bicarbonate,** and **sodium acetazolamide** may increase plasma quinidine levels, possibly resulting in toxicity.
(6) Quinidine may produce additive hypoprothrombinemic effects with **coumarin** anticoagulants.
b. **Amiodarone** and **cimetidine** may increase plasma procainamide levels, possibly leading to drug toxicity.
c. **Phenytoin** accelerates disopyramide metabolism, possibly reducing its therapeutic efficacy.
d. **Lidocaine**
(1) **Phenytoin** may increase the cardiodepressant effects of lidocaine.
(2) **β-Blockers** (class II antiarrhythmics) may reduce lidocaine metabolism, possibly leading to drug toxicity.
e. **Phenytoin**
(1) The risk of phenytoin toxicity increases with concomitant administration of **diazepam, antihistamines, isoniazid, chloramphenicol, dicumarol, cimetidine, salicylates, sulfisoxazole, phenylbutazone, amiodarone,** and **valproate.**
(2) **Carbamazepine** may enhance phenytoin metabolism and thus reduce plasma phenytoin levels and therapeutic efficacy. (Phenytoin has the same effect on carbamazepine.)
f. **Mexiletine. Phenobarbital, rifampin,** and **phenytoin** reduce plasma mexiletine levels and may decrease therapeutic efficacy.

B. Class II antiarrhythmics

1. **Indications.** These drugs—**β-adrenergic blockers**—are used mainly to treat systemic hypertension. Among the drugs in this class, propranolol and esmolol are approved for antiarrhythmic use. (The use of class II drugs in the treatment of hypertension is discussed in Chapter 41.)
a. **Propranolol** may be given to:
(1) Control supraventricular arrhythmias (e.g., atrial fibrillation or flutter, PSVTs)
(2) Treat tachyarrhythmias caused by catecholamine stimulation (e.g., in hypothyroidism, during anesthesia)
(3) Suppress severe ventricular arrhythmias in **prolonged QT syndrome**
(4) Treat digitalis-induced ventricular arrhythmias
(5) Terminate certain ventricular arrhythmias (e.g., PVCs in patients without structural heart disease)
b. **Esmolol** is used to treat supraventricular tachycardias; it possesses a very short (9-minute) half-life and has been used to control the ventricular response to atrial fibrillation or flutter during or after surgery.

2. **Mechanism of action.** Class II antiarrhythmics reduce sympathetic stimulation of the heart, decreasing impulse conduction through the AV node and lengthening the refractory period. As a result, the heart rate slows, decreasing myocardial oxygen demand.

3. **Administration and dosage**
a. **Propranolol** may be given intravenously or orally when used as an antiarrhythmic.

(1) Emergency therapy calls for slow intravenous administration of 1–3 mg diluted in 50 ml dextrose 5% in water or normal saline solution. This dose is infused slowly (no faster than 1 mg/min). A second dose of 1–3 mg may be given 2 minutes later.

(2) For oral therapy, 10–80 mg/day is given in three or four doses. (However, 1000 mg or more may be required for resistant ventricular arrhythmias.)

b. Esmolol is given intravenously. A loading dose of 500 μg/kg/min is infused over 1 minute, followed by a 4-minute maintenance infusion of 50 μg/kg/min. If a satisfactory response is not achieved within 5 minutes, the loading dose is repeated and followed by a maintenance infusion of 100 μg/kg/min.

4. Precautions and monitoring effects

a. Propranolol

(1) This drug is contraindicated in patients with sinus bradycardia, second- or third-degree AV block, cardiogenic shock, severe CHF, or asthma.

(2) The β-blocking effects of this drug may lead to marked hypotension, exacerbation of CHF and left ventricular failure, or cardiac arrest.

(3) Blood pressure, heart rate, and the ECG should be monitored during intravenous infusion.

(4) Embolism may occur upon restoration of normal sinus rhythm after sustained atrial fibrillation. An anticoagulant may be given before propranolol therapy begins to prevent this complication.

(5) Propranolol may depress AV node conduction and ventricular pacemaker activity, resulting in AV block or asystole.

(6) This drug may mask the signs and symptoms of hypoglycemia. It also may mask signs of shock.

(7) Fatigue, lethargy, increased airway resistance, and skin rash have been reported.

(8) Nausea, vomiting, and diarrhea may occur.

(9) Sudden withdrawal of propranolol may lead to acute MI, arrhythmias, or angina in cardiac patients. Drug therapy is discontinued by tapering the dose over 4–7 days.

b. Esmolol

(1) This drug is contraindicated in patients with severe CHF or sinus bradycardia.

(2) Hypotension occurs in approximately 30% of patients receiving esmolol. This effect can be reversed by reducing the dosage or stopping the infusion.

(3) This drug is for short-term use only and should be replaced by a long-acting antiarrhythmic once the patient's heart stabilizes.

(4) Dizziness, headache, fatigue, and agitation may occur.

(5) Other adverse effects include nausea, vomiting, and bronchospasm.

5. Significant interactions

a. Propranolol

(1) Severe vasoconstriction may occur with concomitant **epinephrine** administration.

(2) **Digitalis** preparations can cause excessive bradycardia.

(3) **Calcium-channel blockers** (e.g., **diltiazem, verapamil**) and other negative **inotropic** and **chronotropic drugs** (e.g., **disopyramide, quinidine**) add to the myocardial depressant effects of propranolol.

b. Esmolol. Morphine may raise plasma esmolol levels.

C. Class III antiarrhythmics

1. Indications

a. Amiodarone is given to control refractory ventricular arrhythmias and may be used prophylactically against ventricular tachycardia and fibrillation. It usually is reserved as a last-line agent for arrhythmias that are unresponsive to first- and second-line agents.

b. Bretylium is used solely to treat life-threatening ventricular arrhythmias, including ventricular tachycardia and ventricular fibrillation, that have not responded to other agents. It should be given only in intensive care facilities.

c. Sotalol is used to treat supraventricular and ventricular tachyarrhythmias. It does not have nonselective β-blocking activity and works by delaying atrial and ventricular repolarization. This property is its main distinguishing factor and is the reason why it is classified as a type III antiarrhythmic drug rather than a type II agent (β-blocker).

2. Mechanism of action. Class III antiarrhythmic drugs prolong the refractory period and action potential; they have no effect on myocardial contractility or conduction time.

3. Administration and dosage

a. Amiodarone—Oral/Intravenous Use

(1) Available for oral use where 800–1600 mg is given daily for 1–3 weeks until a satisfactory response occurs. A maintenance dose of 200–600 mg/day is then given.

(2) Oral treatment is used to suppress ventricular and supraventricular arrhythmias but can take days or weeks to take effect.

(3) Intravenous formulation has been recently approved for treatment and prophylaxis of recurrent ventricular fibrillation or hemodynamically unstable ventricular tachycardia in refractory patients.

(4) Intravenous form is rapidly distributed throughout the body. Recommended doses include a rapid loading infusion of 150 mg over 10 minutes followed by a slow infusion of 1 mg/min for 6 hours (360 mg) and then a maintenance infusion of 0.5 mg/min for the remainder of the 24-hour period. Patients usually receive 2–4 days of infusions before conversion to oral form. However, a maintenance infusion can be continued for 2–3 weeks.

b. Bretylium is used for short-term intravenous or intramuscular therapy.

(1) For ventricular fibrillation, 5 mg/kg is given by rapid intravenous injection. As needed, the dosage may be increased to 10 mg/kg and repeated every 15–30 minutes up to a total of 30 mg/kg.

(2) For other ventricular arrhythmias, 500 mg are diluted to 50 ml with dextrose 5% or normal saline solution and infused intravenously at 5–10 mg/kg over more than 8 minutes. The dose may be repeated in 1–2 hours, then given every 6–8 hours.

(3) Bretylium has also been used successfully as a continuous infusion at a rate of 1–2 mg/min, after diluting 500 mg in 50 ml dextrose 5% in water or normal saline solution.

(4) Intramuscular therapy calls for administration of 5–10 mg/kg undiluted. As needed, the dose may be repeated in 1–2 hours, then given every 6–8 hours.

c. Sotalol

(1) Sotalol is available commercially as an oral tablet in two divided doses of 160–480 mg/day.

(2) An intravenous preparation has been used in the acute treatment of arrhythmias with doses of 0.2–1.0 mg/kg.

4. Precautions and monitoring effects

a. Amiodarone

(1) Life-threatening pulmonary toxicity may occur during amiodarone therapy, especially in patients receiving more than 400 mg/day. Baseline as well as routine pulmonary function tests reveal relevant pulmonary changes.

(2) Most patients develop corneal microdeposits 1–4 months after amiodarone therapy begins. However, this reaction rarely causes visual disturbance, but the patient should be monitored with routine ophthalmologic examinations.

(3) Blood pressure and heart rate and rhythm should be monitored for hypotension and bradyarrhythmias.

(4) Patients should be monitored routinely for the possible development of hepatic dysfunction, thyroid disorders (e.g., hyperthyroidism, hypothyroidism), and photosensitivity.

(5) CNS reactions include fatigue, malaise, peripheral neuropathy, and extrapyramidal effects.

(6) Nausea and vomiting have been reported.

(7) This drug has an extremely long half-life (up to 50 days). Therapeutic response may be delayed for weeks after oral therapy begins; adverse reactions may persist up to 4 months after therapy ends.

b. Bretylium

(1) This drug is contraindicated in digitalis-induced arrhythmias.

(2) Severe hypotension, especially orthostatic hypotension, may develop when bretylium is administered intravenously for the treatment of acute arrhythmias.

(3) Rapid intravenous injection may cause severe nausea and vomiting.

(4) Patients with renal impairment may require dosage reduction.

c. Sotalol

(1) Side effects of this drug are directly related to β-blockade and prolongation of repolarization.

(2) Transient hypotension, bradycardia, myocardial depression, and bronchospasm have all been associated with this drug.

(3) This drug carries all the contraindications associated with other β-blockers along with those due to its electrophysiologic properties.

5. **Significant interactions**

   a. **Amiodarone**

      (1) Amiodarone may increase the plasma levels of **quinidine, procainamide, diltiazem, digitalis,** and **flecainide.**

      (2) It may increase the pharmacologic effect of **β-blockers, calcium-channel blockers,** and **warfarin.**

   b. **Bretylium. Antihypertensives** may potentiate bretylium-induced hypotension.

   c. **Sotalol**

      (1) Sotalol must be used cautiously in those patients receiving agents with cardiac depressant properties.

      (2) Agents such as sotalol, which prolong the QT interval, may induce malignant arrhythmias when used in combination with other type IA antiarrhythmics, especially in the presence of low potassium levels.

D. Class IV antiarrhythmics

1. **Indications**

   a. **Calcium-channel blockers** (e.g., verapamil, diltiazem) are used mainly to treat and prevent supraventricular arrhythmias.

      (1) They are first-line agents for the suppression of PSVTs stemming from AV nodal reentry.

      (2) They can rapidly control the ventricular response to atrial flutter and fibrillation.

   b. Other calcium-channel blockers available include nicardipine, nifedipine, bepridil, amlodipine, and felodipine, but these agents have primarily been used in the treatment of angina pectoris and hypertension. For information on these agents see Chapters 39 and 41.

2. **Mechanism of action.** Class IV antiarrhythmics are calcium-channel blockers. They inhibit AV node conduction by depressing the SA and AV nodes, where calcium channels predominate.

3. **Administration and dosage**

   a. To control atrial arrhythmias, verapamil usually is administered intravenously. A dose of 5–10 mg is given over at least 2 minutes and may be repeated in 30 minutes, if necessary. A 5–10 mg/hr continuous intravenous infusion has also been used in treating arrhythmias.

   b. To prevent PSVTs, verapamil may be given orally in four daily doses of 80–120 mg each.

   c. To control atrial arrhythmias, diltiazem usually is administered intravenously. A dose of 20 mg (0.25 mg/kg) is given over 2 minutes. If an adequate response is not obtained, a second dose of 25 mg (0.35 mg/kg) is administered after 15 minutes. A 5–15 mg/hr intravenous continuous infusion has also been used in treating arrhythmias.

4. **Precautions and monitoring effects**

   a. Verapamil and diltiazem are contraindicated in patients with AV block, left ventricular dysfunction, severe hypotension, concomitant intravenous, β-blocking, and atrial fibrillation with an accessory AV pathway.

   b. These drugs must be used cautiously in patients with CHF, sick sinus syndrome, MI, and hepatic or renal impairment.

   c. Because of the negative chronotropic effect, verapamil and diltiazem must be used cautiously in patients who have slow heart rates or who are receiving digitalis glycosides.

   d. The ECG (especially the RR interval) should be monitored during therapy.

   e. Patients over 60 years old should receive reduced dosages and slower injection rates.

   f. Constipation and nausea have been reported with verapamil.

5. **Significant interactions**

   a. Concomitant administration of **β-blockers** or **disopyramide** may precipitate heart failure.

   b. **Quinidine** may increase the risk of calcium-channel blocker–induced hypotension.

   c. Verapamil may increase serum **digoxin** concentrations, and diltiazem may do the same to a lesser extent.

d. **Rifampin** may enhance the metabolism of calcium-channel blockers with a resultant decrease in pharmacologic effect.
e. Verapamil and diltiazem may inhibit **theophylline** metabolism and may require reductions in theophylline dosage.
f. Diltiazem and verapamil inhibit the metabolism of **cyclosporine** and may require reductions in cyclosporine dosages.

E. Unclassified antiarrhythmics

1. **Atropine**
   a. **Indications.** Atropine is therapeutic for symptomatic sinus bradycardia and junctional rhythm.
   b. **Mechanism of action.** An anticholinergic, atropine blocks vagal effects on the SA node, promoting conduction through the AV node and increasing the heart rate.
   c. **Administration and dosage.** For antiarrhythmic use, atropine is administered in a dose of 0.4–1 mg by intravenous push; the dose is given every 5 minutes to a maximum of 2 mg.
   d. **Precautions and monitoring effects**
      (1) Thirst and dry mouth are the most common adverse effects of atropine.
      (2) CNS reactions (e.g., restlessness, headache, disorientation, dizziness) may occur with doses over 5 mg.
      (3) Tachycardia and ophthalmic disturbances (e.g., mydriasis, blurred vision, photophobia) may occur with doses of 1 mg or more.
      (4) Initial doses may induce a reflex bradycardia due to incomplete suppression of vagal impulses.

2. **Adenosine**
   a. **Indications.** Adenosine is indicated for the conversion of acute supraventricular tachycardia to normal sinus rhythm.
   b. **Mechanism of action.** Adenosine is a naturally occurring nucleoside, which is normally present in all cells of the body. It has been shown to:
      (1) Slow conduction through the AV node.
      (2) Interrupt re-entry pathways through the AV node.
      (3) Restore normal sinus rhythm in patients with PSVTs.
   c. **Administration and dosage.** For antiarrhythmic effects, adenosine is given as a rapid bolus intravenous injection in a 6-mg dose over 1–2 seconds. If the first dose does not eliminate the arrhythmia within 1–2 minutes, the dose should be increased to 12 mg and again given as a rapid intravenous dose. An additional 12-mg dose may be repeated if necessary.
   d. **Precautions and monitoring effects**
      (1) The effects of adenosine are antagonized by methylxanthines, such as caffeine and theophylline. Theophylline has been successfully used for treating adenosine-induced side effects, such as hypotension, sweating, and palpitations. If side effects are encountered, aggressive therapy is not required because of the ultra-short half-life of the drug (10 seconds or less).
      (2) The main side effect associated with adenosine use in up to 18% of patients is facial flushing, but this effect is normally very short-lived.
      (3) Other side effects associated with adenosine use include shortness of breath, chest pressure, nausea, headache, and a metallic taste.
   e. **Additional use.** Adenosine has recently been used as an adjunctive agent in patients undergoing various types of pharmacologic stress testing (e.g., with thallium). In this situation, adenosine is given as a continuous infusion over a period of about 4–6 minutes and is able to provide a form of exercise tolerance test in patients not able to exert themselves due to age, fatigue, and various other physical handicaps.

III. MAJOR ARRHYTHMIAS

A. Supraventricular arrhythmias

1. **Sinus bradycardia**
   a. **Description.** This arrhythmia occurs when the heart rate is fewer than 60 beats/min and impulses originate in the SA node. Signs and symptoms include light-headedness, palpitations, fatigue, hypotension, and ventricular ectopy.

b. **Causes** include hyperkalemia, drugs, vagal stimulation, severe pain, and MI. (In well-conditioned athletes, sinus bradycardia is considered normal.)

c. **Therapy**

(1) Asymptomatic sinus bradycardia usually requires no treatment.

(2) When this arrhythmia leads to hemodynamic compromise, atropine may be administered intravenously in a dose of 0.4–1.0 mg every 5–10 minutes until the desired heart rate is attained.

(3) Artificial pacing may be indicated in some cases.

2. **Sinus tachycardia**

a. **Description.** This arrhythmia occurs when the heart rate ranges from 100–160 beats/min; impulses originate from the SA node. Sinus tachycardia commonly causes palpitations but is usually benign.

b. **Causes** include decreased vagal tone, increased sympathetic tone, digitalis toxicity, and increased myocardial oxygen demand as well as fever, stress, and inflammation. Nonpathologic causes include caffeine and alcohol consumption.

c. **Therapy.** A class II antiarrhythmic (e.g., propranolol) may be given if treatment is required and if heart failure is not present. Digitalis may be helpful in the patient with heart failure.

3. **Sinus arrest**

a. **Description.** This arrhythmia occurs when the SA node fails to initiate an electrical impulse. On ECG, the P wave is dropped or absent, and the PP interval is not a multiple of the sinus rhythm.

b. **Causes** include MI, digitalis toxicity, increased vagal tone, and degenerative heart disease.

c. **Therapy.** The underlying cause should be treated if symptomatic bradycardia develops. Drug therapy has not shown long-term benefits, and a permanent pacemaker may be indicated in the symptomatic patient.

4. **Sick sinus syndrome**

a. **Description.** In this conduction disturbance (also known as Stokes-Adams syndrome), tachycardia and bradycardia alternate; these arrhythmias are interrupted by a long sinus pause. Symptoms include dizziness and syncope.

b. **Causes** include cardiomyopathy, atherosclerosis, MI, neuromuscular disorders, and drug therapy.

c. **Therapy.** Chronic sick sinus syndrome may warrant drugs (digitalis or propranolol), permanent pacing, or both.

5. **Premature atrial contractions (PACs)**

a. **Description.** PACs occur when an ectopic pacemaker generates premature beats before the SA node fires again. On the ECG, the P wave is premature and abnormal (possibly buried in the preceding T wave); PR intervals are abnormally short or long. Nonconducted PACs, which occur when the impulse reaches the ventricles during the absolute refractory period, cause absent QRS complexes. PACs typically produce an irregular pulse and palpitations.

b. **Causes** include coronary heart disease, valvular heart disease, drug therapy (e.g., procainamide, digitalis), infection, and inflammation. Nonpathologic causes include fatigue, stress, caffeine or alcohol consumption, and nicotine.

c. **Therapy.** Usually, PACs are clinically insignificant and do not require treatment. However, when they occur frequently or lead to prolonged tachycardia, therapy with digitalis, propranolol, or another drug that prolongs the atrial refractory period (e.g., quinidine or procainamide) may be given.

6. **Paroxysmal supraventricular tachycardias (PSVTs)**

a. **Description.** This category includes two tachyarrhythmias originating above the bundle of His bifurcation: paroxysmal atrial tachycardia (PAT) and paroxysmal junctional tachycardia (PJT). These arrhythmias result from AV nodal re-entry mechanism.

(1) The heart rate is from 140–240 beats/min; the rhythm is regular.

(2) On the ECG, PSVTs are manifested by aberrant QRS complexes and a P wave contour that deviates from that of sinus beats.

(3) PSVTs may cause no symptoms or may produce mild chest pain, palpitations, nausea, and dyspnea.

b. **Causes** include digitalis toxicity, primary cardiac disease (e.g., MI, congenital heart disease), hyperthyroidism, and cor pulmonale.

c. **Therapy.** Most PSVTs subside spontaneously.

(1) If patients have underlying cardiac disease or if PSVTs cause hemodynamic compromise, an emergency mechanical measure (e.g., Valsalva maneuver, carotid sinus massage, synchronized cardioversion) or drug therapy (e.g., adenosine, digitalis, diltiazem, verapamil) may be needed.

(2) Chronic PSVTs may warrant maintenance therapy with digitalis, propranolol, verapamil, diltiazem, quinidine, or procainamide.

7. **Atrial flutter**

a. **Description.** This arrhythmia occurs when ectopic impulses are at a rate of 220–350 beats/min. However, a protective mechanism of the AV node allows only some of these impulses to reach the ventricles. The ventricular rate determines how much danger this arrhythmia poses. On the ECG, sawtoothed F (flutter) waves appear; the ratio of atrial to ventricular contractions may be constant or variable.

b. **Causes** include MI, valvular heart disease, cor pulmonale, CAD, cardiac infection, CHF, COPD, thyrotoxicosis, and quinidine therapy.

c. **Therapy**

(1) Atrial flutter, causing a rapid ventricular rate and decreased cardiac output, calls for emergency measures, such as:

(a) Synchronized cardioversion, if hypotension, severe heart failure, and angina are present with a rapid ventricular rate

(b) A class IV antiarrhythmic (e.g., verapamil, diltiazem)

(2) Digoxin (used for chronic atrial flutter) possibly can be given in combination with verapamil or a β-blocker.

8. **Atrial fibrillation**

a. **Description.** In this arrhythmia, many ectopic loci fire at different times. However, the AV node blocks many impulses from reaching the ventricles.

(1) The atrial rate is 400–600 beats/min.

(2) The atrial rhythm is chaotic.

b. **Causes** include valvular, ischemic, or rheumatic heart disease; CAD; systemic hypertension; cardiomyopathy; thyrotoxicosis; COPD; CHF; and MI.

c. **Therapy.** The goal of treatment is to control the ventricular response.

(1) Immediate synchronized cardioversion is necessary in hemodynamically unstable patients.

(2) Verapamil or diltiazem (administered intravenously) is the drug of choice in acute atrial fibrillation.

(3) Digoxin frequently is used in chronic atrial fibrillation. It may be administered in combination with a calcium-channel blocker or a β-blocker.

(4) Type I antiarrhythmics may be useful in converting atrial fibrillation to sinus rhythm or preventing recurrence.

B. **Pre-excitation syndromes.** This arrhythmia category includes **Wolff-Parkinson-White (WPW)** syndrome and **Lown-Ganong-Levine (LGL)** syndrome.

1. **Description.** In these arrhythmias, early ventricular depolarization occurs.

a. In **WPW syndrome,** the ECG shows a PR interval of less than 0.12 second and a QRS complex greater than 0.12 second.

(1) The ventricular rate may be as high as 300 beats/min. At rates of 180 beats/min or more, atrial fibrillation may develop.

(2) Delta waves, the hallmark of WPW, appear as a slurring of the initial portion of the QRS complex.

b. In **LGL syndrome,** the ECG shows short but constant PR intervals and normal P waves and QRS complexes.

2. **Cause.** Pre-excitation syndromes result from abnormal conduction of impulses from the atria to the ventricles. Impulses travel along accessory pathways, which connect the atria and ventricles at abnormal locations and provide a re-entry route for impulses.

3. **Therapy**

a. In an emergency, vagotonic maneuvers or drugs (e.g., propranolol, procainamide, verapamil, diltiazem, lidocaine) may be necessary. If no response occurs, cardioversion may be used.

b. Long-term management may involve administration of a class IA antiarrhythmic (to increase refractoriness in the bypass tract), a class II or IV antiarrhythmic, or digoxin.

c. In resistant cases, electrophysiologic testing, surgical ablation of the bypass tract, or therapy with amiodarone, flecainide, or propafenone may be necessary.

C. Ventricular arrhythmias

1. Premature ventricular contractions (PVCs)

a. Description. These common arrhythmias, when associated with frequent or complex ventricular ectopy in patients with heart disease, may be associated with an increased risk of sudden death.

(1) A premature heart beat occurs, followed by a compensatory pause (as evidenced on heart auscultation or radial pulse palpation).

(2) On the ECG, PVCs appear as wide, bizarre QRS complexes; absent P waves; and large, wide T waves pointing in the direction opposite the QRS complexes.

(3) PVCs occur in the following patterns:

(a) **Couplet,** consisting of two consecutive PVCs

(b) **Salvo** (run of ventricular tachycardia), consisting of three or more consecutive PVCs

(c) **Ventricular bigeminy,** consisting of a PVC following each normal beat

(d) **Ventricular trigeminy,** consisting of two normal beats followed by a PVC

(4) PVCs may be **unifocal** or **multifocal.**

(a) In **unifocal PVCs,** QRS complexes are identical in configuration, reflecting a single ectopic ventricular pacemaker.

(b) In **multifocal PVCs,** QRS complexes have varying configurations, reflecting two ectopic ventricular pacemakers.

(5) The **R-on-T phenomenon** occurs when the PVC falls on the T wave of the preceding beat.

b. Causes include cardiomyopathy, CAD, and mitral valve prolapse. In people with normal hearts, PVCs may arise from caffeine or alcohol consumption or tobacco use. The mechanism underlying this arrhythmia is unknown.

c. Therapy

(1) Treatment is always required for the following types of PVCs:

(a) Multifocal PVCs

(b) Frequent (more than 6 beats/min) PVCs

(c) Couplets or salvos

(d) R-on-T phenomenon

(2) Treatment may involve a class IA, IB, or IC antiarrhythmic agent (lidocaine is commonly given).

(3) Asymptomatic patients with benign PVC types and no underlying heart disease do not require treatment.

(4) Benefits of treatment need to be weighed against the risks associated with antiarrhythmic agents (e.g., flecainide), which may increase mortality.

2. Ventricular tachycardia

a. Description. This dangerous arrhythmia, which may be brief or sustained, is defined as three or more consecutive PVCs.

(1) Uncoordinated atrial and ventricular activity may lead to a drastic reduction in cardiac output; ventricular fibrillation may occur.

(2) The ventricular rate is 150-240 beats/min; the rhythm is fairly regular.

(3) On the ECG, QRS complexes are wide and bizarre, P waves are absent, T waves appear in the direction opposite the QRS complexes, and RR intervals are regular or slightly irregular.

b. Causes. Ventricular tachycardia results from myocardial irritability or ischemia (e.g., from MI, valvular heart defects, cardiomyopathy, or heart failure).

c. Therapy

(1) Immediate intervention is necessary to prevent acute ventricular tachycardia from evolving into ventricular fibrillation.

(a) In unconscious patients, cardiopulmonary resuscitation (CPR) and defibrillation are warranted.

(b) In less acute cases, lidocaine is given.

(2) Long-term drug therapy may include quinidine, procainamide, disopyramide, tocainide, mexiletine, flecainide, propafenone, moricizine, and finally amiodarone.

3. **Ventricular fibrillation**
   a. **Description.** This deadly arrhythmia is the most common cause of cardiac arrest after an acute MI. The ventricles quiver rather than contract; as a result, cardiac output is interrupted, and death may ensue.
      (1) Typically, the patient does not register a pulse, is apneic, and may have seizures. Acidosis and hypoxemia develop.
      (2) The ECG shows a rapid, chaotic ventricular rhythm and an undulating baseline; P waves, T waves, and QRS complexes cannot be discerned.
   b. **Causes.** PVCs and ventricular tachycardia most commonly cause this arrhythmia. Rarely, it arises spontaneously.
   c. **Therapy.** Ventricular fibrillation calls for immediate emergency measures, such as CPR and defibrillation. Emergency intravenous-drug therapy may include epinephrine, lidocaine, bretylium, procainamide, or propranolol.

D. **AV blocks.** These arrhythmias reflect disturbances in impulse conduction from the atria to the ventricles. AV block occurs in three major variations—first degree, second degree, and third degree.

1. **Description**
   a. **First-degree AV block.** All supraventricular impulses are delayed. On the ECG, the PR interval is prolonged (greater than 0.20 second) but constant, QRS complexes are normal, and the rhythm is regular.
   b. **Second-degree AV block.** Some impulses are blocked at the AV node. Second-degree AV block occurs in two types.
      (1) **Type I** (also called **Mobitz I** or **Wenckebach**). Each successive impulse is conducted at an earlier stage of the refractory period, until one impulse arrives during the absolute refractory period and cannot be conducted. The next impulse, arriving during the relative refractory period, is conducted normally. The dropped ventricular beats have a predictable pattern. ECG evidence of this arrhythmia includes grouped beating, an irregular rhythm, progressively lengthening PR intervals, progressively shortening RR intervals, and constant PP intervals.
      (2) Type II (also called **Mobitz II**). Abnormal conduction in the bundle of His and the bundle branches causes dropped ventricular beats at unpredictable times. ECG manifestations include a sudden dropped beat with normal PR intervals and QRS complexes.
   c. **Third-degree AV block** (also known as **complete heart block**). All supraventricular impulses are blocked at the AV junction. As a result, the atria and ventricles beat independently of one another.
      (1) An ectopic pacemaker in the AV junction or the ventricles stimulates ventricular contractions.
      (2) On the ECG, QRS complexes may be wide or narrow depending on the location of the secondary pacemaker, PP intervals are constant, and P waves have no relationship to QRS complexes.
      (3) Usually, the ventricular rate exceeds 45 beats/min.

2. **Causes.** AV heart block typically results from drug toxicity (e.g., digitalis, quinidine), degenerative disease of myocardial conductive tissue, acute MI, rheumatic fever, or severe CAD. In some cases, this arrhythmia is congenital.

3. **Therapy**
   a. First- and second-degree AV blocks usually do not require treatment. If the underlying cause is drug toxicity, the offending drug is withdrawn. If the arrhythmia reduces cardiac output, atropine may be given.
   b. Type II second-degree AV block may warrant drug therapy to maintain cardiac output if the patient is hypotensive. Long-term management may involve artificial pacing to prevent ventricular standstill.
   c. Third-degree AV block may warrant drug therapy (e.g., atropine, isoproterenol) if the arrhythmia has compromised cardiac output. Artificial pacing frequently is necessary.

STUDY QUESTIONS

Directions: Each of the numbered items or incomplete statements in this section is followed by answers or by completions of the statement. Select the **one** lettered answer or completion that is **best** in each case.

1. Strong anticholinergic effects limit the antiarrhythmic use of

(A) quinidine
(B) procainamide
(C) tocainide
(D) flecainide
(E) disopyramide

2. A pronounced slowing of phase 0 of the myocardial action potential would be reflected on the electrocardiogram (ECG) as a

(A) shortened QRS complex
(B) shortened P wave
(C) prolonged QRS complex
(D) flipped T wave
(E) ST segment depression

3. Which of the following class I antiarrhythmics would be most capable of inducing the torsades de pointes type of ventricular tachycardia?

(A) Lidocaine
(B) Amiodarone
(C) Quinidine
(D) Flecainide
(E) Diltiazem

4. A patient receiving a class I antiarrhythmic agent on a chronic basis complains of fatigue, low-grade fever, and joint pain suggestive of systemic lupus erythematosus (SLE). The patient is most likely receiving

(A) lidocaine
(B) procainamide
(C) quinidine
(D) flecainide
(E) propranolol

5. Class IA antiarrhythmics do all of the following to the cardiac cell's action potential EXCEPT

(A) slow the rate of rise for phase 0 of depolarization
(B) delay the fast-channel conductance of sodium ions
(C) prolong phases 2 and 3 of repolarization
(D) inhibit the slow-channel conductance of calcium ions
(E) prolong the refractory period of the action potential

6. Which of the following drugs is a class IV antiarrhythmic that is primarily indicated for the treatment of supraventricular tachyarrhythmias?

(A) Nifedipine
(B) Mexiletine
(C) Diltiazem
(D) Quinidine
(E) Propranolol

7. Sinus tachycardia is characterized by a heart rate

(A) in excess of 100 with impulses initiated by the AV node
(B) in excess of 60 with impulses initiated by the SA node
(C) less than 60 with impulses initiated by the AV node
(D) less than 60 with impulses initiated by the SA node
(E) in excess of 100 with impulses initiated by the SA node

8. Which of the following agents has a direct effect on the AV node, delaying calcium-channel depolarization?

(A) Lidocaine
(B) Verapamil
(C) Bretylium
(D) Quinidine
(E) Nifedipine

9. Which of the following drugs is a class III antiarrhythmic agent that is effective in the acute management of ventricular tachycardia, including ventricular fibrillation?

(A) Bretylium
(B) Lidocaine
(C) Metoprolol
(D) Disopyramide
(E) Diltiazem

10. All of the following problems represent concerns when patients are started on amiodarone EXCEPT

(A) extremely long elimination half-life
(B) need for multiple daily doses
(C) development of hyper- or hypothyroidism
(D) development of pulmonary fibrosis
(E) interactions with other antiarrhythmic drugs

Directions: The group of items in this section consists of lettered options followed by a set of numbered items. For each item, select the **one** lettered option that is most closely associated with it. Each lettered option may be selected once, more than once, or not at all.

Questions 11–15

For each description of a phase of an action potential in Purkinje fibers, choose the corresponding letter in the accompanying diagram.

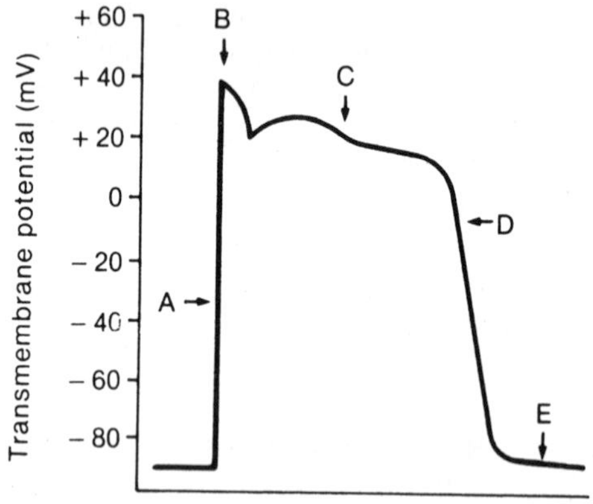

11. Slow-channel depolarization—calcium influx

12. Resting phase—diastole

13. Rapid repolarization

14. Fast-channel depolarization—sodium influx

15. Early repolarization

ANSWERS AND EXPLANATIONS

1. The answer is E *[II A 4 c (4)].*
Disopyramide has anticholinergic actions about one-tenth the potency of atropine. Effects include dry mouth, constipation, urinary retention, and blurred vision. Therefore, it cannot be used in patients with glaucoma or with conditions causing urinary retention. Moreover, disopyramide has a negative inotropic effect and must, therefore, be used with great caution, if at all, in patients with preexisting ventricular failure.

2. The answer is C *[I B 2 b, 3].*
A slowing in phase 0 of the myocardial action potential corresponds to a slowing down of depolarization within the myocardium. This results in a prolongation of either atrial depolarization [causing a prolonged P wave on the electrocardiogram (ECG) or ventricular depolarization (causing a prolonged QRS complex)].

3. The answer is C *[II A 4 a (1)].*
Torsades de pointes is a form of ventricular tachyarrhythmia characterized by electrocardiographic (ECG) changes, which include a markedly prolonged QT interval. This potentially fatal reaction to quinidine causes syncopal episodes (quinidine syncope) or sudden death. Therefore, quinidine should not be used in patients whose QT interval is long or shows a marked prolongation in response to quinidine administration.

4. The answer is B *[II A 4 b (7)].*
The patient's complaints are typical of a systemic lupus erythematosus (SLE)-like hypersensitivity reaction to procainamide. Symptoms of an SLE-like syndrome include fatigue, arthralgia, myalgia, a low-grade fever, and a positive antinuclear antibody titer. The patient's symptoms should subside if procainamide therapy is stopped and an alternative antiarrhythmic agent is given instead.

5. The answer is D *[II A 2].*
Class IA antiarrhythmic agents delay phase 0 of depolarization. Fast-channel conduction of sodium and phases 2 and 3 of repolarization are also slowed. The net effect is to extend the refractory period of myocardial tissue. Class IA antiarrhythmic agents do not inhibit the slow-channel conductance of calcium ions; that is an action of class IV agents such as verapamil.

6. The answer is C *[II D 1 a].*
Of the agents listed, diltiazem and nifedipine are calcium-channel blockers and, along with verapamil, represent the class IV antiarrhythmics. Diltiazem, but not nifedipine, has been used for its direct-acting effects on impulse conduction throughout the heart. Thus, diltiazem is used to treat and prevent supraventricular arrhythmias, whereas nifedipine is used mainly to control angina pectoris. Mexiletine is a class IB drug that closely resembles lidocaine. Quinidine is a class IA drug, and propranolol, a β-adrenergic blocker, is class II. Mexiletine, quinidine, and propranolol are all also effective for supraventricular arrhythmias.

7. The answer is E *[III A 2].*
The term sinus tachycardia denotes a rapid heart rate with impulses originating in the sinoatrial (SA) node. In sinus tachycardia, the heart rate ranges from 100–160 beats/min. Though a sinus tachycardia commonly causes palpitations, it is usually a benign condition.

8. The answer is B *[II D 2].*
Verapamil, a calcium-channel blocker, inhibits calcium influx through slow channels into myocardial cells. Verapamil's direct actions on the slow–channel-dependent SA node and AV node; along with its availability in injection form, make it an ideal agent for the acute intravenous treatment of such re-entry arrhythmias as paroxysmal supraventricular tachyarrhythmias.

9. The answer is A *[II C I b].*
Bretylium, amiodarone, and sotalol are class III antiarrhythmic agents. Class III agents prolong the refractory period and myocardial action potential; they are used to treat ventricular arrhythmias. Bretylium is considered a second-line drug for controlling ventricular fibrillation. When used intravenously, bretylium requires close monitoring for hypotension, especially orthostatic hypotension, and may cause severe nausea and vomiting.

10. The answer is B *[II C 3 a, 4 a, 5 a].*
Amiodarone, like bretylium and sotalol, is a class III antiarrhythmic agent and acts by prolonging repolarization of cardiac cells. Amiodarone is given orally, often in once-a-day or twice-a-day maintenance dosage. Because of its very long elimination half-life, therapeutic response may be delayed for weeks. Therefore, an initial loading phase is often advisable. This requires hospitalization with close monitoring for desired effects, untoward reactions, and adjustments in dosage. Amiodarone may increase the plasma levels of quinidine, procainamide, diltiazem, and digitalis. During therapy with amiodarone, patients may develop hypo- or hyperthyroidism, pulmonary disorders, hepatic dysfunction, and various other unwanted effects. Because of amiodarone's extremely long half-life, adverse reactions may persist for months after therapy ends.

11–15. The answers are: 11-C, 12-E, 13-D, 14-A, 15-B *[I B 2 b].*

The action potential of cardiac Purkinje fibers reflects the depolarization and repolarization of the cardiac cells. This electrical activity involves the transport of sodium, calcium, and potassium ions across the cell membrane. The action potential has five phases. Phase 0 (rapid depolarization) is primarily dependent on the conduction of sodium ions into the cell through fast channels. Phase 0 is followed by phase 1 (early repolarization), which precedes phase 2, a slight notch that represents the inward flow of calcium ions into the cardiac cell via slow channels. Phase 3 (rapid repolarization) represents the inward flow of potassium ions. Phase 4 (slow repolarization), ending the action potential, represents electrical diastole.

41
Systemic Hypertension

Alan H. Mutnick

I. GENERAL CONSIDERATIONS

A. Definition. Hypertension is blood pressure elevated enough to perfuse tissues and organs. Elevated systemic blood pressure is usually defined as a systolic reading greater than or equal to 140 mm Hg and a diastolic reading greater than or equal to 90 mm Hg (≥ 140/90).

B. Classification of hypertension is shown in Table 41-1. This table reflects the latest recommendations of the Fifth Report of the Joint National Committee on Detection, Evaluation, and Treatment of High Blood Pressure (JNC-V).

C. Incidence. Hypertension is the most common cardiovascular disorder. Approximately 50 million Americans have blood pressure measurements > 140/90. Incidence increases with age—that is, 54%–65% of people over age 60 have hypertension.

1. **Primary (or essential) hypertension,** in which no specific cause can be identified, constitutes approximately 95% of all cases of systemic hypertension. The average age of onset is about 35 years.

2. **Secondary hypertension,** resulting from an identifiable cause, such as renal disease and adrenal hyperfunction, accounts for the remaining 5% of cases of systemic hypertension. This type usually develops between the ages of 30 and 50.

D. Physiology

Blood pressure = (stroke volume × heart rate) × systemic vascular resistance.

Altering any of the factors on the right side of the blood pressure equation results in a change in blood pressure, as shown in Figure 41-1.

1. **Sympathetic nervous system. Baroreceptors** (pressure receptors) in the carotids and aortic arch respond to changes in blood pressure and influence vasodilation or vasoconstriction. When stimulated to vasoconstriction, the contractile force strengthens, increasing the heart rate and augmenting peripheral resistance, thus increasing cardiac output. If pressure remains elevated, the baroreceptors reset at the higher levels and so sustain the hypertension.

2. **Renin-angiotensin-aldosterone system.** Decreased renal perfusion pressure in afferent arterioles stimulates the release of renin from juxtaglomerular cells. The renin reacts with circulating angiotensinogen to produce angiotensin I (a weak vasoconstrictor). This, in turn, is hydrolyzed to form angiotensin II (a very potent natural vasoconstrictor). This vasopressor

Table 41-1. Classification of Hypertension Based on the Fifth Report of the Joint National Committee on Detection, Evaluation, and Treatment of High Blood Pressure (JNC-V)

Category	Systolic Blood Pressure (mm Hg)	Diastolic Blood Pressure (mm Hg)
High normal	130–139	85–89
Stage 1 (mild)	140–159	90–99
Stage 2 (moderate)	160–179	100–109
Stage 3 (severe)	180–209	110–119
Stage 4 (very severe)	> 210	> 120

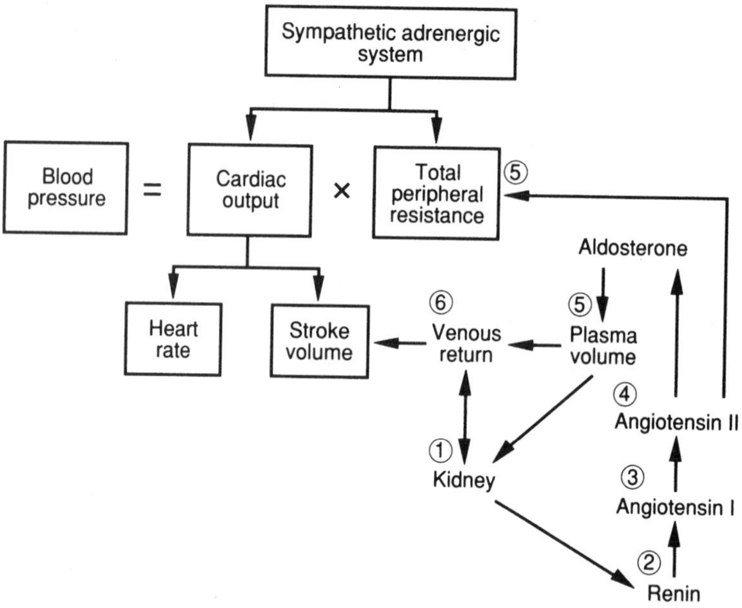

Figure 41-1. Blood pressure regulation. This figure depicts the various determinants of blood pressure as they relate to cardiac output and total peripheral resistance. Angiotensin II, a potent vasopressor, not only increases total peripheral resistance but, by stimulating aldosterone release, leads to an increase in plasma volume, venous return, stroke volume, and ultimately an increase in cardiac output.

stimulates aldosterone release, which results in increased sodium reabsorption and fluid volume.

3. **Fluid volume regulation. Increased fluid volume** increases venous system distention and venous return, affecting cardiac output and tissue perfusion. These changes **alter vascular resistance,** increasing the blood pressure.

E. **Complications.** Untreated systemic hypertension, regardless of cause, results in inflammation and necrosis of the arterioles, narrowing of the blood vessels, and restriction of the blood flow to major body organs (Table 41-2). When blood flow is severely compromised, target organ damage ensues.

1. **Cardiac effects**
   a. Left ventricular hypertrophy compensates for the increased cardiac workload. Signs and symptoms of heart failure occur, and the increased oxygen requirements of the enlarged heart may produce angina pectoris.
   b. Hypertension can be caused by accelerated atherosclerosis. Atheromatous lesions in the coronary arteries lead to decreased blood flow, resulting in angina pectoris. Myocardial infarction (MI) and sudden death may ensue.

2. **Renal effects**
   a. Decreased blood flow leads to an increase in renin-aldosterone secretion, which heightens the reabsorption of sodium and water and increases blood volume.
   b. Accelerated atherosclerosis decreases the oxygen supply, leading to renal parenchymal damage with decreased filtration capability and to azotemia. The atherosclerosis also decreases blood flow to the renal arterioles, leading to nephrosclerosis and, ultimately, renal failure (acute as well as chronic).

3. **Cerebral effects.** Decreased blood flow, decreased oxygen supply, and weakened blood vessel walls lead to transient ischemic attacks, cerebral thromboses, and the development of aneurysms with hemorrhage. There are alterations in mobility, weakness and paralysis, and memory deficits.

4. **Retinal effects.** Decreased blood flow with retinal vascular sclerosis and increased arteriolar pressure with the appearance of exudates and hemorrhage result in visual defects (e.g., blurred vision, spots, blindness).

Table 41-2. Findings in Hypertension

Findings	Basis of Findings
Cardiovascular	
Blood pressure persistently ≥ 140 mm Hg systolic and/or 90 mm Hg diastolic	Constricted arterioles, causing abnormal resistance to blood flow
Angina pain	Insufficient blood flow to coronary vasculature
Dyspnea on exertion	Left-sided heart failure
Edema of extremities	Right-sided heart failure
	Decrease in blood supply
Neurologic	
Severe occipital headaches with nausea and vomiting; drowsiness; giddiness; anxiety; mental impairment	Vessel damage within the brain characteristic of severe hypertension, resulting in transient ischemic attacks or strokes
Renal	
Polyuria, nocturia, and diminished ability to concentrate urine; protein and red blood cells in urine; elevated serum creatinine	Arteriolar nephrosclerosis (hardening of arterioles within the kidney)
Ocular	
Retinal hemorrhage and exudates	Damage to arterioles that supply the retina
Peripheral vascular	Absence of pulses in extremities with or without intermittent claudication; development of an aneurysm

II. SECONDARY HYPERTENSION

A. Clinical evaluation. Because most patients presenting with high blood pressure have primary rather than secondary hypertension, extensive screening is unwarranted. A thorough history and physical examination followed by an evaluation of common laboratory tests should rule out most causes of secondary hypertension. If a secondary cause is not found, the patient is considered to have essential hypertension.

1. A patient's **history** and **other physical findings** suggest an underlying cause of hypertension. These include the following:
   - **a.** Weight gain, moon face, truncal obesity, hirsutism, hypokalemia, diabetes, and increased plasma cortisol may signal Cushing syndrome.
   - **b.** Weight loss, episodic flushing, diaphoresis, increased urinary catecholamines, headaches, intermittent hypertension, tremors, and palpitations suggest pheochromocytoma.
   - **c.** Steroid or estrogen intake, including oral contraceptives, nonsteroidal anti-inflammatory drugs (NSAIDs), nasal decongestants, tricyclic antidepressants, appetite suppressants, cyclosporine, erythropoietin, and monoamine oxidase (MAO) inhibitors, suggests drug-induced hypertension.
   - **d.** Repeated urinary tract infections, nocturia, hematuria, and pain on urinating may signal renal involvement.
   - **e.** Abdominal bruits, recent onset, and accelerated hypertension indicate renal artery stenosis.
   - **f.** Muscle cramps, weakness, excess urination, and hypokalemia may suggest primary aldosteronism.

2. **Laboratory findings**
   - **a.** Blood urea nitrogen (BUN) and creatinine elevations suggest renal disease.
   - **b.** Increased urinary excretion of catecholamine or its metabolites (e.g., vanillylmandelic acid, metanephrine) confirms pheochromocytoma.
   - **c.** Serum potassium evaluation revealing hypokalemia suggests primary aldosteronism or Cushing syndrome.

3. **Diagnostic tests**
   - **a.** Renal arteriography or renal venography may show evidence of renal artery stenosis.

b. Electrocardiography (ECG) may reveal left ventricular hypertrophy or ischemia.

B. Etiology

1. **Primary aldosteronism.** Hypersecretion of aldosterone by the adrenal cortex increases distal tubular sodium retention, expanding the blood volume, which increases total peripheral resistance.

2. **Pheochromocytoma.** A tumor of the adrenal medulla stimulates hypersecretion of epinephrine and norepinephrine, which results in increased total peripheral resistance.

3. **Renal artery stenosis.** Decreased renal tissue perfusion activates the renin-angiotensin-aldosterone system (see I D 2).

C. Treatment. Secondary hypertension requires treatment of the underlying cause (e.g., surgical intervention accompanied by supplementary control of hypertensive effects) [see III B].

III. ESSENTIAL (PRIMARY) HYPERTENSION

A. Clinical evaluation requires a thorough history and physical examination followed by a careful analysis of common laboratory test results.

1. **Objectives**
   - a. To rule out uncommon secondary causes of hypertension
   - b. To determine the presence and extent of target organ damage
   - c. To determine the presence of other cardiovascular risk factors in addition to high blood pressure
   - d. To lower blood pressure, with minimal side effects

2. **Predisposing factors**
   - a. **Family history** of essential hypertension, stroke, and premature cardiac disease
   - b. **Patient history** of intermittent elevations in blood pressure
   - c. **Racial predisposition.** Hypertension is more common among blacks than whites.
   - d. **Obesity.** Weight reduction has been shown to reduce blood pressure in a large proportion of hypertensive patients who are more than 10% above ideal body weight.
   - e. **Smoking,** resulting in vasoconstriction and activation of the sympathetic nervous system. Smoking is a major risk factor for cardiovascular disease.
   - f. Stress
   - g. High dietary intake of saturated fats or sodium
   - h. Sedentary life style
   - i. Diabetes mellitus
   - j. Hyperlipidemia

3. **Physical findings**
   - a. Serial blood pressure readings greater than or equal to 140/90 should be obtained on at least two occasions before specific therapy is begun, unless the initial blood pressure levels are markedly elevated (i.e., $\geq$ 210 mm Hg systolic, $\geq$ 120 mm Hg diastolic, or both) or are associated with target organ damage. A single elevated reading is an insufficient basis for a diagnosis.
   - b. Essential hypertension usually does not become clinically evident—other than through serial blood pressure elevations—until vascular changes affect the heart, brain, kidneys, or ocular fundi.
   - c. Examination of the ocular fundi is valuable; their condition can indicate the duration and severity of the hypertension.
     - (1) **Early stages.** Hard shiny deposits, tiny hemorrhages, and elevated arterial blood pressure occur.
     - (2) **Late stages.** Cotton-wool patches, exudates, retinal edema, papilledema caused by ischemia and capillary insufficiency, hemorrhages, and microaneurysms become evident.

B. Treatment (Tables 41-3 and 41-4; Figure 41-2).

1. **General principles.** Treatment primarily aims to lower blood pressure toward "normal" with minimal side effects and to prevent or reverse organ damage.

Table 41-3. Common Antihypertensive Drugs

I. Diuretics
- **A.** Thiazide diuretics
  - Bendroflumethiazide
  - Benzthiazide
  - Chlorothiazide
  - Chlorthalidone
  - Hydrochlorothiazide
  - Hydroflumethiazide
  - Indapamide
  - Methyclothiazide
  - Metolazone
  - Polythiazide
  - Trichlormethiazide
- **B.** Loop diuretics
  - Bumetanide
  - Ethacrynic acid
  - Furosemide
  - Torsemide
- **C.** Potassium-sparing diuretics
  - Amiloride
  - Spironolactone
  - Triamterene

II. Vasodilators (direct acting)
- Diazoxide
- Hydralazine
- Minoxidil
- Nitroprusside

III. Angiotensin-converting enzyme (ACE) inhibitors
- Benazepril
- Captopril
- Enalapril
- Enalaprilat (IV)
- Fosinopril
- Lisinopril
- Moexipril
- Quinapril
- Ramipril

II. Angiotensin II receptor antagonist
- Losartan

V. Sympatholytics
- **A.** β-Adrenergic blocking agents
  - Acebutolol
  - Atenolol
  - Betaxolol
  - Bisoprolol
  - Carteolol
  - Carvedilol
  - Esmolol
  - Labetalol
  - Metoprolol
  - Nadolol
  - Penbutolol
  - Pindolol
  - Propranolol
  - Timolol
- **B.** Centrally acting α-agonists
  - Clonidine
  - Guanabenz
  - Guanfacine
  - Methyldopa
- **C.** Postganglionic adrenergic neuron blockers
  - Guanadrel
  - Guanethidine
  - Reserpine
- **D.** α-Adrenergic blocking agents
  - Doxazosin
  - Prazosin
  - Terazosin
- **E.** Calcium-channel blockers
  - Amlodipine
  - Diltiazem
  - Felodipine
  - Isradipine
  - Nicardipine
  - Nifedipine
  - Verapamil

a. Candidates for treatment

(1) All patients with a diastolic pressure of ≥ 90 mm Hg, a systolic pressure of ≥ 140 mm Hg, or a combination of both should receive antihypertensive drug therapy.

(2) For those patients with a diastolic pressure of 85–90 mm Hg or a systolic pressure of 130–139 mm Hg (high normal), treatment should be individualized with risk factors considered.*

b. Nonspecific measures. Before initiating antihypertensive drug therapy, patients are encouraged to eliminate or minimize controllable risk factors (see III A 2).

c. Pharmacologic treatment

(1) The recent recommendations of the JNC-V reveal that:

(a) Diuretics and β-adrenergic blocking agents are the only drugs that have been shown to lower morbidity and mortality rates.

---

*The risks associated with certain antihypertensive agents (e.g., β-blockers, diuretics) may outweigh or partially cancel the treatment benefits. However, treatment to reduce risk factors through nonpharmacologic intervention should be initiated.

Table 41-4. Common Combination Products for Hypertension

I.	**Diuretics**
	Hydrochlorothiazide—spironolactone (Aldactazide)
	Hydrochlorothiazide—triamterene (Dyazide, Maxzide)
	Hydrochlorothiazide—amiloride (Moduretic)
II.	**Diuretics—Adrenergic Blockers**
	Bendroflumethiazide—nadolol (Corzide)
	Hydrochlorothiazide—propranolol (Inderide)
	Hydrochlorothiazide—metoprolol (Lopressor HCT)
	Chlorthalidone—atenolol (Tenoretic)
	Hydrochlorothiazide—timolol (Timolide)
	Hydrochlorothiazide—bisoprolol (Ziac)
III.	**Diuretics—ACE Inhibitors**
	Hydrochlorothiazide—captopril (Capozide)
	Hydrochlorothiazide—benazepril (Lotensin HCT)
	Hydrochlorothiazide—lisinopril (Prinzide, Zestoretic)
	Hydrochlorothiazide—enalapril (Vaseretic)
IV.	**Diuretic—Angiotensin II receptor antagonist**
	Hydrochlorothiazide—losartan (Hyzaar)
V.	**Calcium-channel blocker—Adrenergic blocker**
	Amlodipine—benazepril (Lotrel)
VI.	**Other**
	Hydrochlorothiazide—methyldopa (Aldoril)
	Hydrochlorothiazide—hydralazine (Apresazide)
	Hydrochlorothiazide—guanethidine (Esimil)
	Hydrochlorothiazide—reserpine (Hydropres)

(b) β-Blockers and diuretics should be considered initial agents for treatment unless a contraindication exists for a given patient.

(c) Agents such as angiotensin-converting enzyme (ACE) inhibitors, α-blockers, α–β-blockers, and calcium-channel blockers have all been recommended for patients that cannot receive a diuretic or a β-blocker as initial therapy.

(2) Unlike previous reports describing a "stepped-care approach" for treating hypertension, the term is not actively used by the JNC-V but can be used to show the systematic approach needed.

d. Monitoring guidelines. Specific monitoring guidelines for the various drug categories are covered in III B 2–6.

(1) Blood pressure should be monitored routinely to determine the therapeutic response and to encourage patient compliance.

(2) Clinicians must be alert to indications of adverse drug effects. Many patients do not link side effects to drug therapy or are embarrassed to discuss them, especially effects related to sexual function or effects that appear late in therapy.

e. Patient compliance

(1) Because hypertension is usually a symptomless disease, "how the patient feels" does not reflect the blood pressure level. In fact, the patient may actually report "feeling normal" with an elevated blood pressure and "abnormal" during a hypotensive episode because of the light-headedness associated with a sudden drop in blood pressure. Because essential hypertension requires a lifelong drug regimen, it is difficult to impress on patients the need for compliance.

(2) Recognizing the seriousness of the consequences of noncompliance is key. Patients should be told that prolonged, untreated hypertension, known as the "silent killer," can affect the heart, brain, kidneys, and ocular fundi.

2. Diuretics

a. Thiazide diuretics and their derivatives are currently recommended as initial therapy for hypertension.

(1) Actions. Antihypertensive effects are produced by directly dilating the arterioles and reducing the total fluid volume. Thiazide diuretics increase:

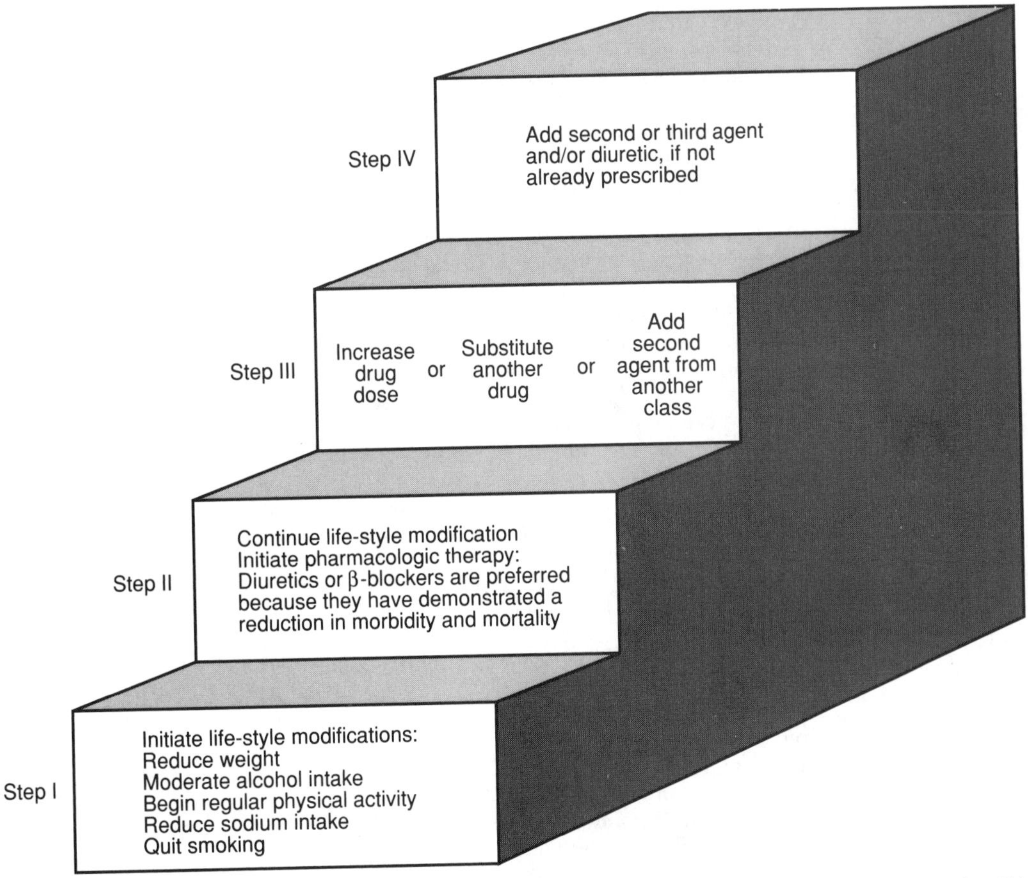

Figure 41-2. Algorithm for the treatment of hypertension. Based on the most recent recommendations from the Fifth Report of the Joint National Committee on Detection, Evaluation, and Treatment of High Blood Pressure (JNC-V).

- **(a)** Urinary excretion of sodium and water by inhibiting sodium and chloride reabsorption in the distal renal tubules
- **(b)** Urinary excretion of potassium and, to a lesser extent, bicarbonate
- **(c)** The effectiveness of other antihypertensive agents by preventing reexpansion of extracellular and plasma volumes

(2) **Significant interactions. NSAIDs,** such as the now common over-the-counter forms of ibuprofen, interact to diminish the antihypertensive effects of the thiazide diuretics.

(3) **Usual effective doses**
- **(a)** **Bendroflumethiazide** 2.5–5.0 mg daily
- **(b)** **Benzthiazide** 12.5–50 mg daily
- **(c)** **Chlorothiazide,** 125–500 mg daily
- **(d)** **Chlorthalidone,** 12.5–50 mg daily
- **(e)** **Hydrochlorothiazide,** 12.5–50 mg daily
- **(f)** **Hydriflurathiazide** 12.5–50 mg daily
- **(g)** **Methyclothiazide,** 2.5–5.0 mg daily
- **(h)** **Polythiazide** 1–4 mg daily
- **(i)** **Trichlormethiazide** 1–4 mg daily
- **(j)** **Metolazone,** 0.5–5.0 mg daily
- **(k)** **Indapamide,** 2.5–5.0 mg daily

(4) **Precautions and monitoring effects**
- **(a)** Potassium ion (K^+) depletion may require supplementation, increased dietary intake, or the use of a potassium-sparing diuretic.
- **(b)** Uric acid retention may occur; this is potentially significant in patients who are predisposed to gout and related disorders.

(c) Blood glucose levels may increase, which may be significant in the patient with diabetes.
(d) Calcium levels may increase because of the potential for retaining calcium ions.
(e) Patients with known allergies to sulfa-type drugs should be questioned to determine the significance of the allergy.
(f) Other common effects include fatigue, headache, palpitations, rash, vertigo, and transitory impotence.
(g) Hyperlipidemia, including **hypertriglyceridemia,** hypercholesterolemia, increased low-density lipoprotein (LDL) cholesterol, and decreased high-density lipoprotein (HDL) cholesterol must be evaluated routinely to prevent an added risk for coronary artery disease.
(h) Fluid losses must be evaluated and monitored to prevent dehydration, postural hypotension, and even hypovolemic shock.
(i) Alterations in fluid and electrolytes (e.g., hypokalemia, hypomagnesemia, hypercalcemia) may predispose patients to cardiac irritability, with a resultant increase in cardiac arrhythmias. ECGs are performed routinely to prevent the development of life-threatening arrhythmias.

b. JNC-V selected diuretics and β-adrenergic blockers as first-line therapy because they have shown long-term reductions in mortality rates in hypertensive patients.

c. Loop (high-ceiling) diuretics

(1) **Indications.** These agents are indicated when patients are unable to tolerate thiazides, experience a loss of thiazide effectiveness, or have impaired renal function (clearance < 30 ml/min).

(2) **Actions. Furosemide, ethacrynic acid, bumetanide,** and **torsemide** act primarily in the loop of Henle; hence, they are called "loop" diuretics. Their action is more intense but of shorter duration (1–4 hours) than that of the thiazides; they may also be more expensive.

(3) **Significant interactions.** As with the thiazides, the antihypertensive effect of loop diuretics may be diminished by **NSAIDs.**

(4) **Precautions and monitoring effects.** Loop diuretics have the same effects as thiazides (see III B 2 a) in addition to the following:
(a) Loop diuretics have a complex influence on renal hemodynamics; thus, patients must be monitored closely for signs of hypovolemia.
(b) Because these agents should be used cautiously in patients with episodic or chronic renal impairment, BUN and serum creatinine levels should be checked routinely.
(c) Transient deafness has been reported. If the patient is taking a potentially ototoxic drug (e.g., an aminoglycoside antibiotic), another class of diuretic (e.g., a thiazide diuretic) should be substituted.

(5) **Usual effective doses**
(a) **Bumetanide,** 0.5–5.0 mg daily
(b) **Ethacrynic acid,** 25–100 mg daily
(c) **Furosemide,** 20–320 mg daily
(d) **Torsemide,** 5–20 mg in one or two doses

d. Potassium-sparing diuretics

(1) **Indications.** The diuretics in this group—**spironolactone, amiloride, and triamterene**—are indicated for patients in whom potassium loss is significant and supplementation is not feasible. These agents are often used in combination with a thiazide diuretic because they potentiate the effects of the thiazide while minimizing potassium loss. **Spironolactone** is particularly useful in patients with hyperaldosteronism as it has direct antagonistic effects on aldosterone.

(2) **Actions.** Potassium-sparing diuretics achieve their diuretic effects differently and less potently than the thiazides and loop diuretics. Their most pertinent shared feature is that they promote potassium retention.

(3) **Significant interactions.** Coadministration with **ACE inhibitors** or **potassium supplements** significantly increases the risk of hyperkalemia.

(4) **Precautions and monitoring effects**
(a) Potassium-sparing diuretics should be avoided in patients with acute renal failure and used with caution in patients with impaired renal function because they can retain potassium.

(b) **Triamterene** should not be used in patients with a history of kidney stones or hepatic disease.

(c) **Hyperkalemia** is a major risk, requiring routine monitoring of serum electrolytes. BUN and serum creatinine levels should be checked routinely to signal incipient excess potassium retention and impaired renal function.

(5) **Usual effective doses**

(a) **Amiloride,** 5–10 mg in one or two doses

(b) **Spironolactone,** 25–100 mg daily and 100–400 mg daily to treat hyperaldosteronism

(c) **Triamterene,** 50–150 mg in one or two doses

e. **Combination products.** Four agents combine a thiazide and a potassium-sparing diuretic.

(1) **Aldactazide,** 25 mg spironolactone/25 mg hydrochlorothiazide (2–4 tablets daily)

(2) **Moduretic,** 5 mg amiloride/50 mg hydrochlorothiazide (1–2 tablets daily)

(3) **Dyazide,** 50 mg triamterene/25 mg hydrochlorothiazide (1–2 capsules daily)

(4) **Maxzide,** 75 mg triamterene/50 mg hydrochlorothiazide (½–1 tablet daily)

3. **Sympatholytics**

a. **β-Adrenergic blockers**

(1) **Indications.** These agents are used for the initial treatment of hypertension. β-Blockers are particularly effective in patients with rapid resting heart rates or concomitant ischemic heart disease.

(2) **Actions.** Proposed mechanisms of action include the following:

(a) Stimulation of renin secretion is blocked.

(b) Cardiac contractility is decreased, thus diminishing cardiac output.

(c) Sympathetic output is decreased centrally.

(d) Reduction in heart rate decreases cardiac output.

(e) β-Blocker action may combine all of the above mechanisms.

(3) **Epidemiology.** Young (< 45 years) whites with high cardiac output and heart rate and normal vascular resistance respond best to β-blocker therapy.

(4) **Precautions and monitoring effects**

(a) Patients must be monitored for signs and symptoms of **cardiac decompensation** (i.e., increasingly reduced cardiac output) because decreased contractility can trigger compensatory mechanisms, leading to congestive heart failure (CHF).

(b) ECGs should be monitored routinely because all β-blockers can decrease electrical conduction within the heart.

(c) Relative cardioselectivity is dose-dependent and is lost as dosages are increased. Therefore, **no β-blocker is totally safe in patients with bronchospastic disease** [e.g., asthma, chronic obstructive pulmonary disease (COPD)].

(d) Suddenly stopping β-blocker therapy puts the patient at risk for a **withdrawal syndrome** that may produce:

(i) Exacerbated anginal attacks, particularly in patients with coronary artery disease

(ii) MI

(iii) A life-threatening rebound of blood pressure to levels exceeding pretreatment readings

(e) β-Blocker therapy should be used with caution in patients with the following conditions:

(i) **Diabetes.** β-Blockers can mask hypoglycemic symptoms, such as tachycardia.

(ii) **Raynaud's phenomenon or peripheral vascular disease.** Vasoconstriction can occur.

(iii) **Neurologic disorders.** Several β-blockers enter the central nervous system (CNS), potentiating related side effects (e.g., fatigue, lethargy, poor memory, weakness, or mental depression).

(f) Hypertriglyceridemia, reduced HDL cholesterol, or increased LDL cholesterol have been reported as major consequences of β-blockers, which require routine lipid evaluations with chronic therapy.

(g) Impotence and decreased libido may result in reduced patient compliance.

(5) **Significant interactions.** β-Adrenergic blockers interact with numerous agents, requiring cautious selection, administration, and monitoring.

(6) **β-Blocker terms**

(a) **Relative cardioselective activity.** Relative to propranolol, β-blockers have a greater tendency to occupy the β_1-receptor in the heart, rather than the β_2-receptors in the lungs.

(b) **Intrinsic sympathomimetic activity.** These agents have the ability to release catecholamines and to maintain a satisfactory heart rate. Intrinsic sympathomimetic activity may also prevent bronchoconstriction and other direct β-blocking actions.

(7) **Specific agents**

(a) **Propranolol** was the first β-blocking agent shown to block both β_1- and β_2-receptors. The **average daily dose** is 80–240 mg.

(b) **Metoprolol** was the first β-blocking agent with relative cardioselective blocking activity. The **average daily dose** is 50–200 mg.

(c) **Nadolol** was the first β-blocking agent that allowed once-daily dosing. It blocks both β_1- and β_2-receptors. The **average daily dose** is 20–240 mg.

(d) **Atenolol** was the first β-blocking agent to combine once-daily dosing with relative cardioselective, blocking activity. The **average daily dose** is 25–100 mg.

(e) **Timolol** was the first β-blocking agent shown to be effective after an acute MI to prevent sudden death. It blocks both β_1- and β_2-receptors. The **average daily dose** is 10–40 mg.

(f) **Pindolol** was the first β-blocking agent shown to have high intrinsic sympathomimetic activity. The **average daily dose** is 10–60 mg.

(g) **Labetalol** was the first β-blocking agent shown to possess both α- and β-blocking activity. The **average daily dose** is 200–1200 mg. Labetalol is also effective for treating hypertensive crisis (Table 41-5).

(h) **Acebutolol** was the first β-blocking agent that combined efficacy with once-daily dosing, possessing intrinsic sympathomimetic activity and having relative cardioselective blocking activity. The **average daily dose** is 200–1200 mg.

(i) **Esmolol** was the first β-blocking agent to have an ultrashort duration of action. This agent is not used routinely in treating hypertension owing to its duration of action and the need for intravenous administration.

(j) **Betaxolol** is a new β-blocker, which possesses relative cardioselective blocking activity similar to metoprolol but has a half-life that allows for once-daily dosing. The **average daily dose** is 5–40 mg.

(k) **Carteolol** is a new β-blocking agent, which has low lipid solubility so less drug penetrates the CNS, has moderate intrinsic sympathomimetic activity like pindolol, and allows for once-daily dosing. The **average daily dose** is 2.5–10.0 mg.

(l) **Penbutolol** is a new β-blocking agent that has weak intrinsic sympathomimetic activity like pindolol and allows for once-daily dosing. The **average daily dose** is 20–80 mg.

(m) **Bisoprolol** is a new β-blocking agent that is cardioselective and has no intrisic sympathomimetic activity. It allows for once-a-day dosing, and the **average daily dose** is 5–20 mg.

(n) **Carvedilol** is a new β-blocking agent that has β-blocking properties as well as vasodilating properties. The drug is administered twice daily with a starting dose of 6.25 mg titralet at 7–14 day intervals to a dose of 25 mg twice daily. **Maximum daily doses** are 50 mg twice daily.

b. **Peripheral α_1-adrenergic blockers** (e.g., prazosin, terazosin, doxazosin)

(1) **Actions.** The α_1-blockers (indirect vasodilators) block the peripheral postsynaptic α_1-adrenergic receptor, causing vasodilation of both arteries and veins. Also, the incidence of reflex tachycardia is lower with these agents than with the vasodilator hydralazine. These hemodynamic changes reverse the abnormalities in hypertension and preserve organ perfusion. Recent studies have also shown that these agents have no adverse effect on serum lipids and other cardiac risk factors.

(2) **Indications.** This group of drugs has been added to the current recommendations for initial therapy in hypertensive patients as alternatives for those who cannot take diuretics or β-blockers.

(3) **Precautions and monitoring effects**

(a) **First-dose phenomenon.** A syncopal episode may occur within 30–90 minutes of the first dose; similarly associated are postural hypotension, nausea, dizziness, headache, palpitations, and sweating. To minimize these effects, the first dose should be limited to 1.0 mg of each agent and administered just before bedtime.

Table 41-5. Rapid-Acting Parenteral Antihypertensive Agents for Hypertensive Crisis

Drug	Mode of Administration	Dose	Onset of Action	Duration of Action	Precautions	Side Effects
Diazoxide	IV bolus (usually 10–30 seconds)	50–150 mg or 15–30 mg/min as infusion	1–2 minutes	6–12 hours	Use with care in cerebral vascular disease, coronary artery disease, aortic dissections; blood glucose monitoring is necessary	Hyperglycemia; hyperuricemia; hypotension, tachycardia; chest pain; nausea; vomiting; sodium retention
Enalaprilat	IV	0.625-1.25 mg every 6 hours	15–60 minutes	12–24 hours		Hypotension; declining renal function; potential renal failure
Esmolol	IV	500 μg/kg load then 50 μg/kg/min × 4 minutes then 50–200 μg/kg/min as maintenance	2–10 minutes	10–30 minutes	Use with care in bronchiospastic patients	Hypotension, bradycardia, dizziness, peripheral ischemia
Hydralazine	IM or IV	IV 10–20 mg or IM 10–40 mg	10 minutes 20–30 minutes	2–6 hours	Relatively contraindicated in patients with angina pectoris; aortic dissections	Flushing; headache; tachycardia; nausea; vomiting; possible aggravation of angina
Labetalol	IV	20–80 mg every 10 minutes or 2 mg/min as infusion	5–10 minutes	2–4 hours		Dizziness; fatigue; nausea; dyspnea; congestive heart failure (CHF); bradycardia; bronchoconstriction
Methyldopate	IV	250–500 mg every 6 hours as infusion	30–60 minutes	12–24 hours		Drowsiness; headache; nasal stuffiness; weight gain
Nitroglycerin	IV drip	5–200 μg/min infusion	2–5 minutes	3–5 minutes		Bradycardia, tachycardia, headache, flushing
Sodium nitroprusside	IV drip	Titration 0.25–10 μg/kg/min	Instantaneous	2–3 minutes after cessation of drip	Use fresh solution every 4–8 hours; shield solution from light; constant monitoring is needed	Nausea; vomiting; hypotension; thiocyanate intoxication; sodium retention
Trimethaphan camsylate	IV drip	1–4 mg/min as infusion	2–5 minutes	5 minutes after cessation of drip	Requires constant monitoring; resistance develops in 24–48 hours; not advised for postoperative patients or those with a history of allergies	Paresis of the bowel, bladder; hypotension; visual blurring; dry mouth; sodium retention

(b) Additional adverse effects include diarrhea, weight gain, peripheral edema, dry mouth, urinary urgency, constipation, and priapism.

(4) **The average daily doses** are:

(a) Prazosin, 1–20 mg in two doses

(b) Terazosin, 1–20 mg in one dose

(c) Doxazosin, 1–16 mg in one dose

c. **Centrally active α-agonists** have been used in the past as alternatives to initial antihypertensives, but they are currently recommended as "supplemental" agents in patients that do not respond to initial antihypertensive agents. They act primarily within the CNS on α_2-receptors to decrease sympathetic outflow to the cardiovascular system.

(1) **Methyldopa**

(a) **Actions.** Methyldopa decreases total peripheral resistance through the above mechanism while having little effect on cardiac output or heart rate (except in older patients).

(b) **Precautions and monitoring effects**

(i) Common untoward effects include orthostatic hypotension, fluid accumulation (in the absence of a diuretic), and rebound hypertension upon abrupt withdrawal. Sedation is a common finding upon initiating therapy and when increasing doses; however, the sedative effect usually decreases with continued therapy.

(ii) Fever and other flulike symptoms occasionally occur and may represent hepatic dysfunction, which should be monitored by liver function tests.

(iii) A positive Coombs' test develops in 25% of patients with chronic use (longer than 6 months). Fewer than 1% of these patients develop a hemolytic anemia. (Red blood cells, hemoglobin, and blood count indices should be checked.) The anemia is reversible by discontinuing the drug.

(iv) Other effects include dry mouth, subtly decreased mental activity, sleep disturbances, depression, impotence, and lactation in either gender.

(c) The **average daily dose** is 250 mg–2.0 g in two doses.

(2) **Clonidine**

(a) **Indications.** Clonidine is effective in patients with renal impairment, although they may require a reduced dose or a longer dosing interval.

(b) **Actions.** Clonidine stimulates α_2-receptors centrally, decreasing vasomotor tone and heart rate.

(c) **Precautions and monitoring effects**

(i) Intravenous administration causes an initial paradoxical increase in pressure (diastolic and systolic), which is followed by a prolonged drop. As with methyldopa, abrupt withdrawal can cause rebound hypertension.

(ii) Sedation and dry mouth are common but usually disappear with continued therapy.

(iii) Clonidine has a tendency to cause or worsen depression and it heightens the depressant effects of alcohol and other sedating substances.

(d) The **average daily dose** is 0.1–0.6 mg in two doses.

(e) Patient compliance is a major issue for most hypertensive patients. The recently released once-weekly patch, which provides 0.1–0.3 mg/24-hr, may improve compliance.

(3) **Guanabenz and guanfacine**

(a) **Actions.** Guanabenz and guanfacine are centrally active α_2-agonists that have actions similar to clonidine.

(b) **Indications.** These agents are recommended as adjunctive therapy with other antihypertensives for additive effects when initial therapy has failed.

(c) **Precautions and monitoring effects.** These agents should be used cautiously with other sedating medications and in patients with severe coronary insufficiency, recent MI, cerebrovascular accident (CVA), and hepatic or renal disease. Side effects include sedation, dry mouth, dizziness, and reduced heart rate.

(d) The **average daily doses** are 4–64 mg in two doses for guanabenz and 1–3 mg in one dose for guanfacine.

d. **Postganglionic adrenergic neuron blockers.** This class of antihypertensive drugs is best avoided unless it is necessary to treat severe refractory hypertension that is unresponsive to all other medications, because agents in this class are poorly tolerated by most patients.

(1) **Reserpine**

(a) **General considerations.** Because of the high incidence of adverse effects, other agents are usually chosen first. When used, reserpine is given in low doses and in conjunction with other antihypertensive agents. Reserpine in very low doses (0.05 mg) combined with a diuretic such as chlorothiazide (50–100 mg) may be an alternative to traditional doses of 0.1–0.25 mg/day.

(b) **Actions.** Reserpine acts centrally as well as peripherally by depleting catecholamine stores in the brain and in the peripheral adrenergic system.

(c) **Precautions and monitoring effects**

(i) A history of depression is a contraindication for reserpine. Even low doses, such as 0.25 mg/day, can trigger a range of psychic responses, from nightmares to suicide attempts. Drug-induced depression may linger for months after the last dose.

(ii) Peptic ulcer is also a contraindication for using reserpine. Even a single dose tends to increase gastric acid secretion.

(iii) Common adverse effects include drowsiness, dizziness, weakness, lethargy, memory impairment, sleep disturbances, and weight gain. Nasal congestion is also common but may decrease with continued therapy.

(d) The **average daily dose** is 0.05–0.1 mg in one dose.

(2) **Guanethidine**

(a) **Actions.** Guanethidine acts in peripheral neurons, where it first produces a sympathetic blockade. Administered chronically, its cumulative effect reduces tissue concentrations of norepinephrine. This lasts several days after discontinuing the drug.

(b) **Significant interactions**

(i) Patients should avoid **over-the-counter preparations** that contain sympathomimetic substances (e.g., cold medicines) because the combination may potentiate an acute hypertensive effect.

(ii) **Tricyclic antidepressants** and **chlorpromazine** antagonize the therapeutic effect of guanethidine.

(c) **Precautions and monitoring effects**

(i) Pheochromocytoma is a contraindication for guanethidine use because of the risk of a severe hypertensive reaction.

(ii) Postural and exercise hypotension are common side effects, which may be heightened by heat (e.g., hot weather, hot showers) and ingesting alcohol. The patient should be warned of these effects with changes in body position, particularly upon standing.

(iii) Fluid retention can occur, diminishing the antihypertensive effect and usually requiring a diuretic.

(iv) Sexual dysfunction (primarily inhibited ejaculation) can occur and should be considered before initiating therapy.

(v) Bradycardia, CHF, and exacerbated angina are possible side effects for which the patient should be monitored.

(d) The **average daily dose** is 10–100 mg in one dose.

(3) **Guanadrel**

(a) **Actions.** Guanadrel decreases adrenergic neuronal activity like guanethidine and does not cross into the CNS.

(b) **Significant interactions** are similar to those of guanethidine.

(c) **Precautions and monitoring effects.** Guanadrel should be avoided in patients with CHF, angina, and cerebrovascular disease. Side effects include faintness, orthostatic hypotension, diarrhea, and severe volume depletion.

(d) The **average daily dose** is 10–75 mg in two doses.

4. **Vasodilators.** These drugs are used as second-line agents in patients refractory to initial therapy with diuretics, β-blockers, or supplemental agents such as ACE inhibitors or calcium-channel blockers. Vasodilators directly relax peripheral vascular smooth muscle—arterial, venous, or both. The direct vasodilators should not be used alone owing to increases in plasma renin activity, cardiac output, and heart rate.

a. **Hydralazine**

(1) **Actions.** Hydralazine directly relaxes arterioles, decreasing systemic vascular resistance. It is also used intravenously or intramuscularly in managing hypertensive crisis.

(2) **Precautions and monitoring effects**

(a) Because hydralazine triggers compensatory reactions that counteract its antihypertensive effects, it is most useful when combined with a β-blocker, central α-agonist, or diuretic as a latter-step agent.

(b) Reflex tachycardia is common and should be considered before initiating therapy.

(c) Hydralazine may induce angina, especially in patients with coronary artery disease and those not receiving a β-blocker.

(d) Drug-induced systemic lupus erythematosus (SLE) may occur.

(i) Baseline and serial complete blood counts (CBCs) with antinuclear antibody titers should be followed routinely to detect SLE.

(ii) Slow acetylators of this drug have an increased incidence of SLE; their risk may be reduced by administering doses of less than 200 mg/day.

(iii) Fatigue, malaise, low-grade fever, and joint aches may signal SLE.

(e) Other adverse effects may include headache, peripheral neuropathy, nausea, vomiting, fluid retention, and postural hypotension.

(3) The **average daily dose** is 40–200 mg in two to four doses.

b. Minoxidil

(1) **Actions.** A more potent vasodilator than hydralazine, minoxidil relaxes arteriolar smooth muscle directly, decreasing peripheral resistance. It also decreases renal vascular resistance while preserving renal blood flow. Effective in most patients, minoxidil is commonly used to treat patients with severe hypotension that has been refractory to conventional drug regimens.

(2) **Precautions and monitoring effects**

(a) Peripheral dilation results in a reflex activation of the sympathetic nervous system and an increase in heart rate, cardiac output, and renin secretion.

(b) Because this agent promotes sodium and water retention, particularly in the presence of renal impairment, patients should be monitored for fluid accumulation and signs of cardiac decompensation. Administering minoxidil along with a sympatholytic agent and a potent diuretic (e.g., furosemide) minimizes increased sympathetic stimulation and fluid retention.

(c) Hypertrichosis (i.e., excessive hair growth) is a common side effect, particularly if the drug is continued for more than 4 weeks.

(3) The **average daily dose** is 2.5–80 mg in one or two doses.

c. Nitroprusside

(1) **Actions.** A direct-acting peripheral dilator, this agent has potent effects on both the arterial and venous systems. It is usually used only in short-term emergency treatment of acute hypertensive crisis, when a rapid effect is required. Onset of action is almost instantaneous and is maximal in 1–2 minutes. Nitroprusside is administered intravenously with continuous blood pressure monitoring.

(2) **Precautions and monitoring effects.** To prevent acute hypotensive episodes, initial doses should be very low, followed by slow titration upward until the desired effect is achieved.

(a) Once the solution is prepared, it should be protected from light. Color changes are a signal that replacement is needed.

(b) Thiocyanate toxicity may develop with long-term treatment—particularly in patients with reduced renal activity—but can be treated with hemodialysis. Symptoms may include fatigue, anorexia, disorientation, nausea, psychotic behavior, or muscle spasms.

(c) Cyanide toxicity can occur (rarely) with long-term, high-dose administration. It may present as altered consciousness, convulsions, tachypnea, or even coma.

(3) The **average daily dose** is 0.25–10 μg/kg/min as a continuous intravenous infusion.

d. Diazoxide

(1) **Indications.** Diazoxide exerts a direct action on the arterioles but has little effect on venous capacity. It is used intravenously in the emergency treatment of acute hypertensive crisis.

(2) **Administration**

(a) Because the antihypertensive effect of diazoxide increases with the speed of infusion, recent recommendations suggest that a slow infusion spread over 15–30 minutes may achieve more predictable, controllable, hypotensive effects than rapid, high-dose administration.

(b) Alternatively, maximal reductions in mean arterial pressure may be obtained after 2 minutes through bolus injections of 50–150 mg for 5–10 seconds, repeated every 5–10 minutes, if needed. Additionally, the drug may be administered as a continuous infusion of 15–30 mg/min.

(3) **Precautions and monitoring effects**

(a) Diazoxide is closely related to the thiazides chemically; therefore, patients with thiazide sensitivity cross-react to diazoxide. In patients with impaired cerebral or cardiac function, the risks may outweigh the benefits of diazoxide administration.

(b) Diazoxide also produces transient hyperglycemia, requiring caution if administered to patients with diabetes.

(c) Hypotensive reactions may be severe.

(d) Unlike the thiazides, this agent promotes sodium and water retention, potentiating edema.

5. **ACE inhibitors**

a. **General considerations.** The ACE inhibitors (e.g., benazepril, captopril, enalapril, fosinopril, lisinopril, moexipril, quinapril, ramipril) are a rapidly growing group of drugs, which most recently have been recommended for the initial treatment of hypertension in those patients who cannot take diuretics or β-blockers. Eight agents are currently available for use, but as the number of agents continues to grow, the differences among them must be considered.

b. **Indications.** Although the use of ACE inhibitors was initially restricted to patients with refractory hypertension, they currently are indicated as first-line alternatives for treating hypertension. This has been primarily because of studies documenting their clinical efficacy as well as minimal impact on patients' abilities to maintain normal function. However, as reported by the JNC-V, ACE inhibitors have not been tested and shown to reduce morbidity and mortality.

c. **Actions**

(1) These agents inhibit the conversion of angiotensin I (a weak vasoconstrictor), to angiotensin II (a potent vasoconstrictor), which decreases the availability of angiotensin II.

(2) ACE inhibitors indirectly inhibit fluid volume increases when interfering with angiotensin II by inhibiting angiotensin II–stimulated release of aldosterone, which promotes sodium and water retention. The net effect appears to be a decrease in fluid volume, along with peripheral vasodilation.

d. **Significant interactions**

(1) The antihypertensive effect of ACE inhibitors may be diminished by **NSAIDs** (e.g., over-the-counter forms of ibuprofen).

(2) **Potassium-sparing diuretics** increase serum potassium levels when used with ACE inhibitors, and potassium levels need to be very closely monitored in these patients.

e. **Precautions and monitoring effects**

(1) Neutropenia is rare (especially with **enalapril**) but serious; there is an increased incidence in patients with renal insufficiency or autoimmune disease.

(2) Proteinuria occurs, particularly in patients with a history of renal disease. Urinary proteins should be monitored regularly.

(3) Serum potassium levels should be monitored regularly for hyperkalemia. The mechanism of action tends to increase potassium levels somewhat. Patients with renal impairment are at increased risk.

(4) Renal insufficiency can occur in patients with predisposing factors, such as renal stenosis, and when ACE inhibitors are administered with thiazide diuretics. Renal function should be monitored (e.g., through monitoring levels of serum creatinine and BUN).

(5) A dry cough may occur but disappears within a few days after the ACE inhibitor is discontinued. All ACE inhibitors have the potential to cause this side effect, but switching to an alternative agent may improve the symptoms.

(6) Other untoward effects include rashes, an altered sense of taste (dysgeusia), vertigo, headache, fatigue, first-dose hypotension, and minor gastrointestinal disturbances.

f. **Specific agents**

(1) **Captopril.** The original ACE inhibitor is given initially as a 6.25-mg dose three times daily and is increased to an **average daily dose** of 12.5–150 mg in two or three doses.

(2) **Enalapril** is a prodrug, which is rapidly converted to its active metabolite enalaprilat. Initial doses are 5.0 mg daily, with an **average daily dose** of 2.5–40 mg. Additionally, the enalaprilat form of the drug has been used effectively for treating acute hypertensive crisis (see Table 41-5).

(3) **Lisinopril** is a long-acting analog of enalapril, given initially as a 5–10 mg daily dose and adjusted to **an average daily dose** of 5–40 mg in one dose.

(4) **Benazepril, fosinopril, moexipril, quinapril, and ramipril are five recently released ACE inhibitors** whose major benefit appears to be once-daily dosing. **Average daily doses** for these agents are:

Benazepril: 10–40 mg
Fosinopril: 10–40 mg
Moexipril: 7.5–30 mg
Quinapril: 5–80 mg
Ramipril: 1.25–20 mg

Further study for each of these agents is currently underway to determine specific benefits of each agent in hypertensive patients as well as in patients with CHF.

6. Calcium-channel blockers

a. Indications. Similar to the ACE inhibitors, the calcium-channel blockers have rapidly become alternative drugs for the initial treatment of hypertensive patients who cannot take diuretics or β-blockers. Currently, seven agents (e.g., amlodipine, diltiazem, felodipine, isradipine, nicardipine, nifedipine, verapamil) are available, but as the number of agents continues to grow, the differences among them must be considered.

b. Actions

(1) Calcium-channel blockers inhibit the influx of calcium through slow channels in vascular smooth muscle and cause relaxation. Low-renin hypertensive, black, and elderly patients respond well to these agents.

(2) Although the calcium-channel blockers share a similar mechanism of action, each agent produces different degrees of systemic and coronary arterial vasodilation, sinoatrial (SA) and atrioventricular (AV) nodal depression, and a decrease in myocardial contractility.

c. Significant interactions. β-Adrenergic blockers, when used with calcium-channel blockers, may have an additive effect on inducing CHF and bradycardia. Electrical conduction to the AV node may be further depressed when patients are given agents such as verapamil and diltiazem along with β-blockers.

d. Precautions and monitoring effects

(1) Diltiazem and verapamil must be used with extreme caution or not at all in patients with conductive disturbances involving the SA or AV node, such as second- or third-degree AV block, sick sinus syndrome, and digitalis toxicity.

(2) Nifedipine use has been associated with flushing, headache, and peripheral edema; the patient may find these very troublesome, thus jeopardizing compliance. Using the sustained-release product once daily has been shown to effectively reduce these effects.

(3) Verapamil use has been associated with a significant degree of constipation, which must be treated to prevent stool straining and noncompliance.

e. Specific agents

(1) **Diltiazem.** The release of the extended-release product, Dilacor XR (Cardizem CO), has greatly increased this agent's role in the treatment of hypertension. Daily doses of 90–360 mg are effective for treating mild to moderate hypertension. Diltiazem already has proven efficacy as an antiarrhythmic and an antianginal agent. This product contrasts with a previously released sustained-release product (Cardizem SR), which required two daily doses for maximal effect.

(2) **Nifedipine.** The release of once-daily sustained-release preparations (Procardia XL, Adalat CC) has made this agent very effective for long-term treatment of hypertension. A previously reported long list of side effects has been reduced with the sustained-release product at a daily dose of 30–120 mg.

(3) **Verapamil.** This drug is similar to diltiazem in its actions (though with more potent effects on electrical conduction depression). Sustained-release products (Calan SR, Isoptin S) at doses of 120–480 mg daily have been shown to be efficacious for long-term management of mild to moderate hypertension, while side effects such as

dizziness, constipation, and hypotension are reduced. An additional form of verapamil (Verelan) has recently been released with the hope of providing 24-hour blood pressure control.

(4) **Amlodipine, isradipine, felodipine,** and **nicardipine** are second-generation calcium-channel blockers. These agents have been developed to produce more selective effects on specific target tissues than the first-generation agents diltiazem, nifedipine, and verapamil. These agents are chemically similar to nifedipine and are referred to as dihydropyridine derivatives. The daily dose ranges are:

(a) **Amlodipine,** 2.5–10.0 mg in one dose
(b) **Isradipine,** 5–10 mg in one or two doses
(c) **Felodipine,** 5.0–20 mg in one dose
(d) **Nicardipine,** 60–120 mg in three doses or an extended-release product, Cardene SR, can be given in doses of 60–120 mg in two doses.

7. **Angiotensin II type I receptor antagonists**

a. **Losartan** is the first drug released in this new class of drugs to treat mild to moderate hypertension.

b. **Actions.** Losartan works by blocking the binding of angiotensin II to the angiotensin II receptors. By blocking the receptor site, losartan inhibits the reconstrictor effects of angiotensin II as well as prevents the release of aldosterone due to angiotensin II. These two properties of angiotensin II have been shown to be important causes for developing hypertension.

c. **Precautions and monitoring effects**

(1) Similar to ACE inhibitors, increases in serum potassium levels can occur, especially in patients receiving potassium-sparing diuretics. When used alone, hyperkalemia has not been reported to be severe enough to require stopping its use. However, as in patients receiving ACE inhibitors, potassium levels need to be monitored closely in those with compromised renal function.

(2) Cough associated with ACE inhibitors does not appear to occur with losartan because of its specificity for the angiotensin II receptor rather than direct effects on the losartan or prostaglandin system.

d. **Dosage**

(1) Usual starting dose is 50 mg daily; however, patients receiving diuretics or those with an impaired liver should start with 25 mg daily.

(2) Most patients require daily maintenance doses of 25–100 mg taken in one or two doses.

(3) A combination product containing losartan 50 mg with 12.5 mg of hydrochlorothiazide (see Table 41-4) has been released for those patients who are candidates for combination therapy.

e. **Current studies**

(1) Losartan is currently being investigated for treating diabetic nephropathy. As of this publication, there are unknown long-term benefits/harm in this condition.

(2) Currently there is no evidence that losartan, like ACE inhibitors, prolongs survival in patients with heart failure or after an MI.

IV. HYPERTENSIVE EMERGENCIES

A. Definition. A hypertensive emergency is a severe elevation of blood pressure (i.e., > 200 mm Hg systolic or > 140 mm Hg diastolic) that demands reduction—either immediate (within minutes) or prompt (within hours).

1. Conditions requiring immediate reduction include hypertensive encephalopathy, acute left ventricular failure with pulmonary edema, dissecting aortic aneurysm, acute MI, and intracranial hemorrhage.

2. Conditions requiring prompt reduction include malignant or accelerated hypertension.

B. Treatment

1. The **reduction in blood pressure must be gradual** (e.g., a 15-mm Hg decrease in mean arterial pressure over the first hour) rather than precipitous to avoid compromising perfusion of critical organs, particularly cerebral perfusion.

2. **Diuretics should be avoided initially,** because they may exacerbate hypovolemia and induce severe vasoconstriction, unless intravascular fluid overload has been demonstrated. They may be introduced later to treat sodium and fluid retention resulting from drug therapy with agents such as diazoxide or sodium nitroprusside.

3. **Specific agents** used in hypertensive crisis are shown in Table 41-5; for further information on vasodilators, see III B 4.

STUDY QUESTIONS

Directions: Each of the numbered items or incomplete statements in this section is followed by answers or by completions of the statement. Select the **one** lettered answer or completion that is **best** in each case.

1. Which of the following agents represents a new class of drugs used in treating hypertension?

(A) Propranolol
(B) Atenolol
(C) Nadolol
(D) Losartan
(E) Metoprolol

2. Reflex tachycardia, headache, and postural hypotension are adverse effects that limit the use of which of the following antihypertensive agents?

(A) Prazosin
(B) Captopril
(C) Methyldopa
(D) Guanethidine
(E) Hydralazine

3. A 60-year-old man presents with moderate hypertension that is refractory to diuretics, β-blockers, and methyldopa. He has renovascular hypertension with elevated renin levels confirmed on laboratory evaluation. This patient's antihypertensive regimen would be enhanced best by adding which of the following agents?

(A) Prazosin
(B) Hydralazine
(C) Fosinopril
(D) Nitroprusside
(E) Clonidine

4. A hypertensive patient who is asthmatic and very noncompliant would be best treated with which of the following β-blocking agents?

(A) Timolol
(B) Penbutolol
(C) Esmolol
(D) Acebutolol
(E) Propranolol

5. Long-standing hypertension leads to tissue damage in all of the following organs EXCEPT the

(A) heart
(B) lungs
(C) kidneys
(D) brain
(E) eyes

6. According to the Fifth Report of the Joint National Committee on Detection, Evaluation, and Treatment of High Blood Pressure (JNC-V), all of the following agents are suitable as initial therapy for treating hypertension EXCEPT

(A) hydrochlorothiazide
(B) fosinopril
(C) atenolol
(D) guanadrel
(E) nifedipine

Directions: Each question below contains three suggested answers, of which **one or more** is correct. Choose the answer

A if **I only** is correct
B if **III only** is correct
C if **I and II** are correct
D if **II and III** are correct
E if **I, II, and III** are correct

7. A patient treated with a thiazide diuretic should be monitored regularly for altered plasma levels of

I. potassium
II. glucose
III. uric acid

8. Before antihypertensive therapy begins, secondary causes of hypertension should be ruled out. Laboratory findings that suggest an underlying cause of hypertension include

I. a decreased serum potassium level
II. an increased urinary catecholamine level
III. an increased blood cortisol level

9. In an otherwise healthy adult with mild hypertension, appropriate initial antihypertensive therapy would be

I. hydrochlorothiazide
II. metoprolol
III. bisoprolol

Directions: Each group of items in this section consists of lettered options followed by a set of numbered items. For each item, select the **one** lettered option that is most closely associated with it. Each lettered option may be selected once, more than once, or not at all.

Questions 10–14

Match the adverse effects with the antihypertensive agent that is most likely to cause them.

(A) Ramipril
(B) Methyldopa
(C) Nitroprusside
(D) Terazosin
(E) Penbutolol

10. Thiocyanate intoxication, hypotension, and convulsions

11. Bradycardia, bronchospasm, and cardiac decompensation

12. Cough, skin rash, and proteinuria

13. Postural hypotension, fever, and a positive Coombs' test

14. First-dose syncope, postural hypotension, and palpitations

Questions 15–19

Match each description of a β-blocker with the most appropriate β-adrenergic blocking agent.

(A) Esmolol
(B) Labetalol
(C) Bisoprolol
(D) Nadolol
(E) Pindolol

15. A β-blocker with intrinsic sympathomimetic activity

16. A β-blocker that also blocks α-adrenergic receptors

17. A β-blocker with an ultrashort duration of action

18. A β-blocker with a long duration of action and nonselective blocking activity

19. A β-blocker with relative cardioselective blocking activity

ANSWERS AND EXPLANATIONS

1. The answer is D *[III B 7 a].*
Losartan is the first angiotensin II, type 1 receptor antagonist that blocks the production of angiotensin II and consequently its effects as a powerful vasoconstrictor and stimulant for aldosterone release.

2. The answer is E *[III B 4 a].*
Hydralazine is a vasodilator that works by directly relaxing arterioles, thereby reducing peripheral vascular resistance. Its effectiveness as an antihypertensive agent is compromised, however, by the compensatory reactions it triggers (e.g., reflex tachycardia) and by its other adverse effects (e.g., headache, postural hypotension, nausea, palpitations). Fortunately, the unwanted effects of hydralazine are minimized when it is used in combination with a diuretic agent and a β-blocker. Thus, hydralazine is most effective as a supplemental antihypertensive drug in combination with first-line therapy.

3. The answer is C *[III B 5 f].*
Fosinopril, an angiotensin-converting enzyme (ACE) inhibitor, acts by inhibiting the conversion of angiotensin I (a weak vasoconstrictor) to angiotensin II (a potent vasoconstrictor). Because this patient has renovascular hypertension, a response would be expected from an ACE inhibitor such as fosinopril; fosinopril works directly on the renin-angiotensin system, which is activated by renal artery stenosis. ACE inhibitors are indicated as initial therapy for hypertension if the patient is unable to take diuretics or β-blockers.

4. The answer is D *[III B 3 a (7) h].*
The β-adrenergic blocking agents are used as initial agents in treating hypertension. A major feature of some of these agents is their relative selectivity for β_1-receptors (in the heart) rather than for β_2-receptors (in the lung), which provides advantages in the treatment of certain (e.g., asthmatic) patients. Of the β-blockers listed in the question, acebutolol is less likely than the rest to block β_2-receptors because of its relative cardioselective blocking activity. Acebutolol also has a long duration of action, which could be helpful in the noncompliant patient by requiring fewer doses per day. Penbutolol is a new β-blocker that has weak intrinsic sympathomimetic activity like pindolol but lacks relative cardioselectivity despite its long duration of action.

5. The answer is B *[I E; Table 41-2].*
Left untreated, hypertension can be lethal because of its progressively destructive effects on major organs, such as the heart, kidneys, and brain. The eyes also suffer damage; the lungs, however, do not. End-organ damage caused by hypertension includes left ventricular hypertrophy, congestive heart failure (CHF), angina pectoris, myocardial infarction, renal insufficiency caused by atherosclerotic lesions, nephrosclerosis, cerebral aneurysm and hemorrhage, retinal hemorrhage, and papilledema.

6. The answer is D *[III B 6; Figure 41-2].*
Calcium-channel blockers such as nifedipine, β-adrenergic blockers such as atenolol, angiotensin-converting enzyme (ACE) inhibitors such as fosinopril, and diuretics such as hydrochlorothiazide are considered initial agents for treating mild to moderate hypertension. Because of adverse drug reactions, guanadrel, a postganglionic adrenergic neuronal blocker, like reserpine and guanethidine, should be reserved for those patients who do not respond to all other antihypertensive drugs. Strictly speaking, diuretics and β-blockers are initial agents for treating hypertension because they have been shown to reduce mortality and morbidity rates, whereas ACE inhibitors, calcium-channel blockers, and α_1-blockers are considered supplemental therapy whereas only if the patient cannot take diuretics or β-blockers.

7. The answer is E (all) *[III B 2 a].*
Thiazide diuretics act directly on the kidneys by increasing the excretion of sodium and water and, to a lesser extent, the excretion of potassium. Patients who are treated with thiazides should be monitored for hypokalemia, which may require potassium supplementation or addition of a potassium-sparing diuretic to the antihypertensive regimen. Thiazide diuretics have the opposite effect on uric acid and glucose excretion. Thus, patients receiving these drugs also should be monitored for increased plasma levels of uric acid (especially if they are predisposed to gout) and glucose (especially if they are predisposed to diabetes).

8. The answer is E (all) *[II A 1].*
Low serum potassium levels in a hypertensive patient suggest primary aldosteronism. Elevated urinary catecholamines suggest a pheochromocytoma; other signs and symptoms of this tumor include weight

loss, episodic flushing, and sweating. Elevated serum cortisol levels suggest Cushing syndrome; the patient is also likely to have a round face and truncal obesity. Secondary hypertension requires treatment of the underlying cause; supplementary antihypertensive drug therapy may also be needed.

9. The answer is E (I) *[III B 2 a, c; Figure 41-2].*
Thiazide diuretics, such as hydrochlorothiazide, and β-adrenergic blockers, such as metoprolol and bisoprolol, are indicated as initial antihypertensive agents for treating hypertension.

10–14. The answers are: 10-C *[III B 4 c (2)],* **11-E** *[III B 3 a (7) (l)],* **12-A** *[III B 5 f (4)],* **13-B** *[III B 3 c (1) (b)],* **14-D** *[III B 3 b (4)].*
The goal of treatment in hypertension is to lower blood pressure toward "normal" with minimal side effects. All antihypertensive drugs can cause adverse effects. Therefore, the stepped-care approach has evolved on the principle that combination therapy allows for lower doses of each drug and, thus, reduces the risk of adverse effects while providing optimal therapeutic benefits.

15–19. The answers are: 15-E, 16-B, 17-A, 18-D, 19-C *[III B 3 a (7)].*
The β-adrenergic blocking agents are valuable for managing hypertension and are used as initial antihypertensives. The β-blockers are sympathetic antagonists: They act by blocking various receptors of the sympathetic nervous system. They differ in their selectivity for these sympathetic receptors. For example, β_1-blockers have relative cardioselective activity; that is, they block β_1-receptors (in the heart) rather than β_2-receptors (in bronchial smooth muscle) and, therefore, are highly useful antihypertensive agents. Intrinsic sympathomimetic activity also appears to reduce the problem of bronchoconstriction; moreover, drugs with this property can also maintain a satisfactory heart rate.

42 Congestive Heart Failure

Alan H. Mutnick

I. INTRODUCTION

A. Definition. Congestive heart failure (CHF) is a clinical syndrome with multiple etiologies in which an abnormality in myocardial function results in the inability of the ventricles to deliver adequate quantities of blood to the metabolizing tissues during normal activity or at rest. The condition is termed **congestive** because of the **edematous state** commonly produced by the fluid backup resulting from poor pump function.

B. Mortality rate. According to the Framingham Heart Disease Epidemiology Study, of those who were diagnosed as having CHF, less than 50% of the men and less than 60% of the women survived 5 years after the initial diagnosis.

C. Etiology

1. Although the disease occurs most commonly among the elderly, it may appear at any age as a consequence of underlying cardiovascular disease (Table 42-1).
2. CHF should not be considered an independent diagnosis, as it is superimposed on an underlying cause.
   a. Hypertension and coronary artery disease are the two major underlying causes of CHF development.
   b. Myocardial stress may be caused by trauma, disease, or other abnormal state (e.g., pulmonary embolism, infection, anemia, pregnancy, drug use or abuse, fluid overload, arrhythmia, valvular heart disease, cardiomyopathies, and congenital heart disease).

D. Forms of heart failure

1. **Low-output versus high-output failure**
   a. If metabolic demands are within normal limits but the heart is unable to meet them, the failure is designated **low output** (the most common type).
   b. If metabolic demands increase (e.g., hyperthyroidism, anemia), and the heart is unable to meet them, the failure is designated **high output.**
2. **Left-sided versus right-sided failure**
   a. **General symptomatology**
      (1) The signs and symptoms of heart failure usually result from the effects of blood backing up behind the failing ventricle (except in heart failure due to increased body demands).
      (2) Initially, the signs and symptoms tend to be specific to failure of one side of the heart, but eventually bilateral involvement is evidenced.

Table 42-1. Cardiac Diseases Commonly Underlying Congestive Heart Failure

Age Range (Years)	Common Underlying Causes
20–40	Rheumatic fever, rheumatic heart disease
40–50	Myocardial infarction, hypertension, pulmonary disease
Over 50	Calcific aortic stenosis

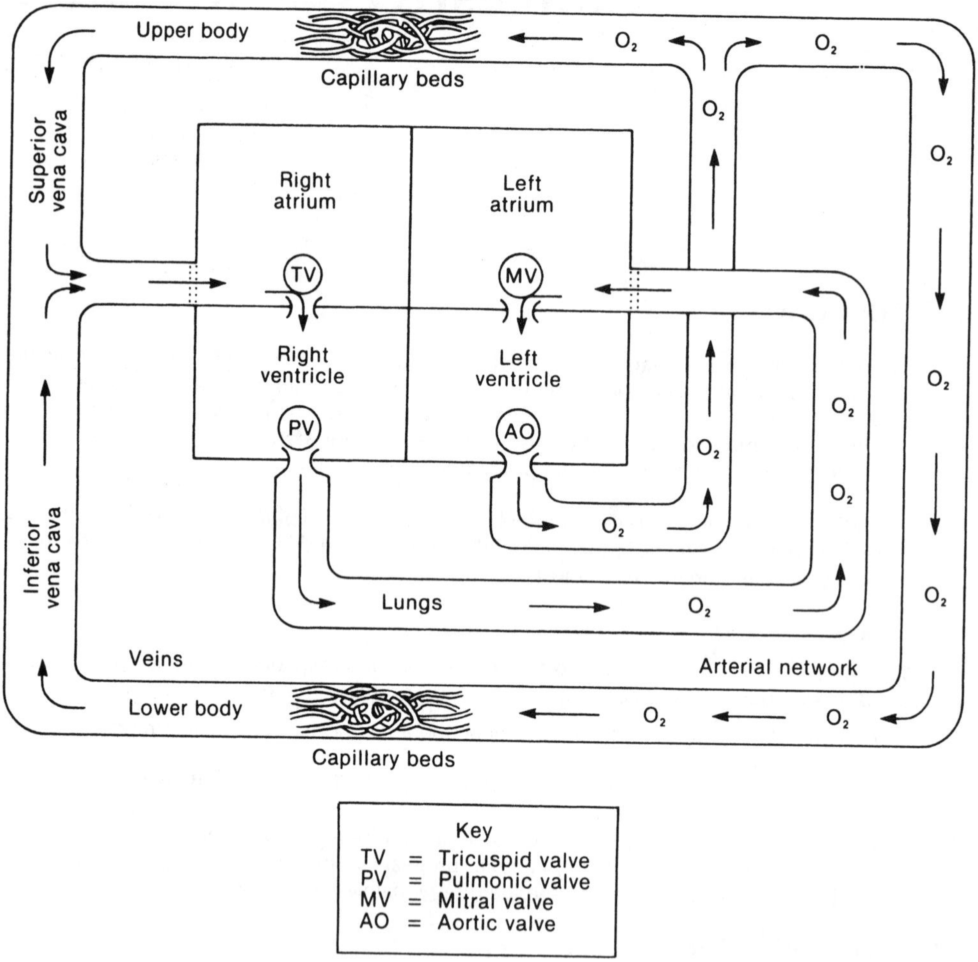

Figure 42-1. An overview of blood flow through the cardiovascular system.

(3) This progression occurs because the cardiovascular system is a closed system (Figure 42-1); thus, over time, right-sided failure causes left-sided failure and vice versa.

b. Left-sided failure

(1) If blood cannot be adequately pumped from the left ventricle to the peripheral circulation and it accumulates within the left ventricle, the failure is designated **left-sided.**

(2) Given this accumulation, the left ventricle is unable to accept blood from the left atrium and lung; therefore, the fluid portion of the blood backs up into the pulmonary alveoli, producing pulmonary edema.

c. Right-sided failure

(1) When blood cannot be pumped from the right ventricle into the lungs and it accumulates within the right ventricle, the failure is designated **right-sided.**

(2) When blood is not pumped from the right ventricle, the fluid portion of the blood backs up throughout the body (e.g., in the veins, liver, legs, bowels), producing systemic edema.

E. Treatment goals. CHF requires a two-pronged therapeutic approach, the overall goals of which are:

1. To remove or mitigate the underlying cause; for example, by eliminating ingestion of certain drugs or other substances (Table 42-2) that can produce or exacerbate CHF or by correcting an anemic syndrome, which can increase cardiac demands

Table 42-2. Substances that May Exacerbate Congestive Heart Failure

Promote Sodium Retention	Produce Osmotic Effect	Decrease Contractility
Androgens	Albumin	Antiarrhythmic agents (e.g., quinidine, disopyramide, procainamide, flecainide)
Corticosteroids	Glucose	β-Adrenergic blocking agents
Diazoxide	Mannitol	Calcium-channel blockers (e.g., verapamil, diltiazem)
Estrogens	Saline	Doxorubicin hydrochloride
Guanethidine	Urea	
Licorice		
Lithium carbonate		
Methyldopa		
NSAIDs		
Salicylates		

2. **To relieve the symptoms and improve pump function by:**
   a. Reducing metabolic demands through rest, relaxation, and pharmaceutical controls
   b. Reducing fluid volume excess through dietary and pharmaceutical controls
   c. Administering digitalis and other inotropic substances
   d. Promoting patient compliance and self-regulation through education
   e. Selecting appropriate patients for cardiac transplantation

II. PATHOPHYSIOLOGY.

Heart failure and decreased cardiac output trigger a complex scheme of compensatory mechanisms designed to normalize cardiac output (cardiac output = stroke volume × heart rate).

A. Compensation. These mechanisms are represented schematically in Figure 42-2.

1. **Sympathetic responses.** Inadequate cardiac output stimulates reflex (norepinephrine and epinephrine) activation of the sympathetic nervous system and an increase in circulating catecholamines. The heart rate increases, and blood flow is redistributed to ensure perfusion of the most vital organs (the brain and the heart).
2. **Hormonal stimulation.** The redistribution of blood flow results in reduced renal perfusion, which decreases the glomerular filtration rate (GFR). Reduction in GFR results in:
   a. Sodium and water retention
   b. Activation of the renin-angiotensin-aldosterone system, which further enhances sodium retention and, thus, volume expansion
3. **Concentric cardiac hypertrophy** describes a mechanism that thickens cardiac walls, providing larger contractile cells and diminishing the capacity of the cavity in an attempt to precipitate expulsion at lower volumes.
4. **Frank-Starling mechanism.** The premise of this response is that increased fiber dilation heightens the contractile force, which then increases the energy released.
   a. Within physiologic limits, the heart pumps all the blood it receives without allowing excessive accumulation within the veins or cardiac chambers.
   b. As blood volume increases, the various cardiac chambers dilate (stretch) and enlarge in an attempt to accommodate the excess fluid.
   c. As these stretched muscles contract, the contractile force increases in proportion to their distention. Then the extended fibers "snap back" (as a rubber band would), expelling the extra fluid into the arteries.

B. Decompensation. Over time, the compensatory mechanisms become exhausted and increasingly ineffective, entering a vicious spiral of decompensation in which the mechanisms surpass their limits and become self-defeating—as they work harder, they only exhaust the system's capacity to respond.

1. As the strain continues, total peripheral resistance and afterload increase, thereby decreasing the percentage of blood ejected per unit of time. Afterload is determined by the amount of contractile force needed to overcome intraventricular pressure and eject the blood.

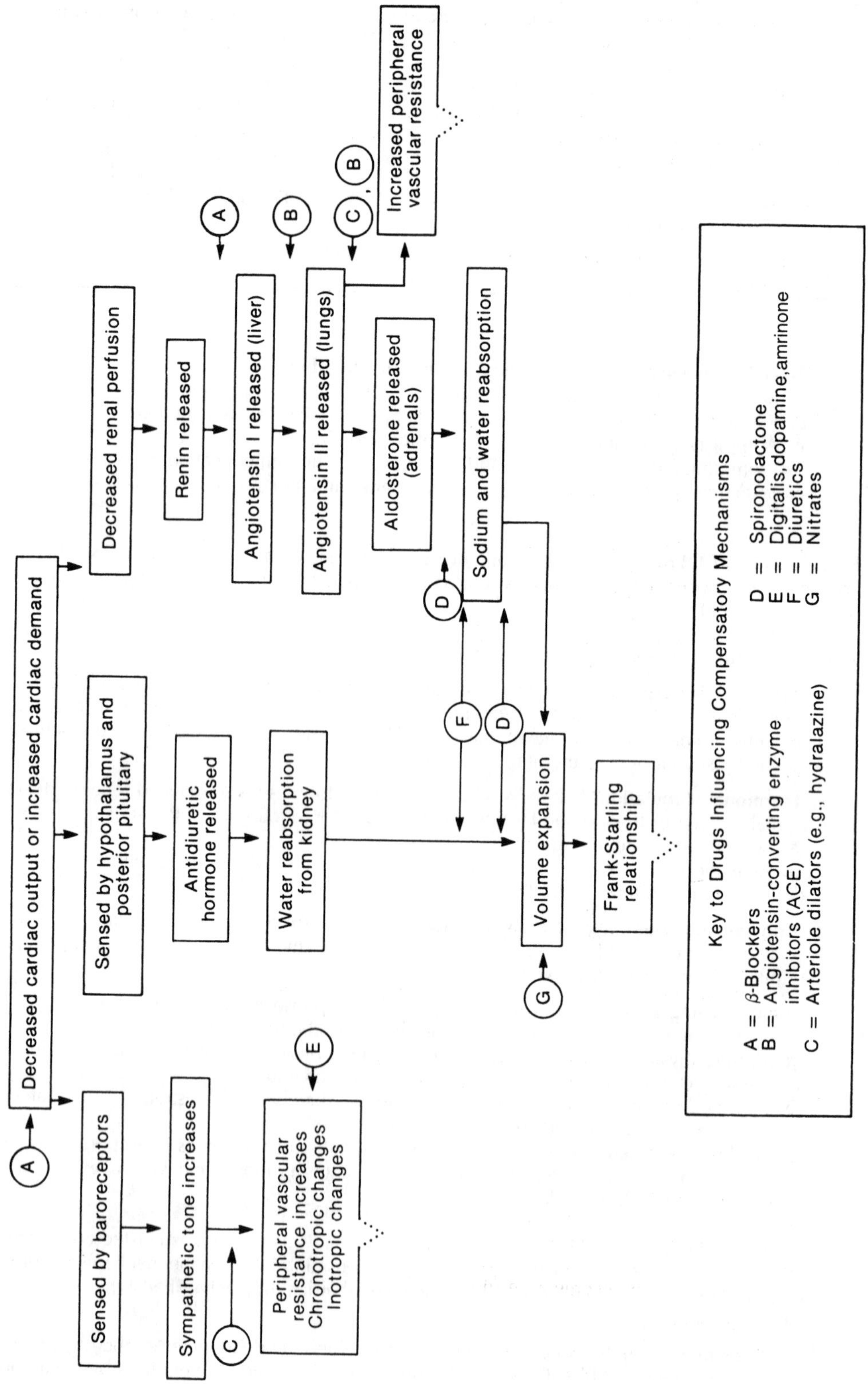

Figure 42-2. Compensatory mechanisms in congestive heart failure (CHF).

a. **Afterload** is the tension in ventricular muscles during contraction. In the left ventricle, this tension is determined by the amount of force needed to overcome pressure in the aorta. Afterload (also known as intraventricular systolic pressure) is sometimes used to describe the amount of force needed in the right ventricle to overcome pressure in the pulmonary artery.

b. **Preload** is the force exerted on the ventricular muscle at the end of diastole that determines the degree of muscle fiber stretch. This concept is also known as ventricular end-diastolic pressure. Preload is a key factor in contractility because the more these muscles are stretched in diastole, the more powerfully they contract in systole.

2. As the fluid volume expands, so do the demands on an already exhausted pump, allowing increased volume to remain in the ventricle.

3. The resulting fluid backup (from the left ventricle into the lungs; from the right ventricle into peripheral circulation) produces the signs and symptoms of CHF.

III. CLINICAL EVALUATION

A. Left-sided heart failure

1. Signs and symptoms

a. Dyspnea

(1) As CHF progresses, the amount of effort required to trigger **exertional dyspnea** lessens.

(2) **Both paroxysmal nocturnal dyspnea** and **orthopnea** result from volume pooling in the recumbent position and can be relieved by propping with pillows or sitting upright. (Orthopnea is often gauged by the number of pillows the patient needs to sleep comfortably.)

b. Dry, wheezing cough

c. Exertional fatigue and weakness

d. Nocturia. Edematous fluids that accumulate during the day migrate from dependent areas when the patient is in a recumbent position and renal perfusion increases.

2. Physical findings

a. Rales (or crackles) indicate the movement of air through fluid-filled passages.

b. Tachycardia is an early compensatory response detected through an increased pulse rate.

c. S_3 ventricular gallop is a vibration produced by rapid filling of the left ventricle early in diastole.

d. S_4 atrial gallop is a vibration produced by increased resistance to sudden, forceful ejection of atrial blood in late diastole; it does not vary with inspiration in left-sided failure and is more common in diastolic dysfunction.

3. Diagnostic test results

a. Cardiomegaly (heart enlargement), left ventricular hypertrophy, and pulmonary congestion may be evidenced by chest radiograph, electrocardiogram (ECG), and echocardiography.

b. Arm-to-tongue circulation time is prolonged.

c. Transudative pleural effusion may be suggested by radiograph and confirmed by analysis of aspirated pleural fluid.

B. Right-sided heart failure

1. Signs and symptoms

a. Complaints by the patient of tightness and swelling (e.g., "My ring is too tight," "My skin feels too tight") suggest edema.

b. Nausea, vomiting, anorexia, bloating, or abdominal pain on exertion may reflect hepatic and visceral engorgement, resulting from venous pressure elevation.

2. Physical findings

a. Jugular vein distention reflects increased venous pressure and is a cardinal sign of CHF.

b. S_3 ventricular gallop is described in III A 2 c.

c. S_4 atrial gallop intensifies on inspiration in right-sided failure.

d. Hepatomegaly (a tender, enlarged liver) is revealed when pushing on the edge of the liver results in a fluid reflux into the jugular veins, causing bulging (positive hepatojugular reflux).
e. Bilateral leg edema is an early sign of right-sided heart failure; pitting ankle edema signals more advanced heart failure. However, edema is common to many disorders, and a pattern of associated findings, such as concurrent neck vein distention, is required for differential diagnosis.

3. **Laboratory findings. Elevated levels of hepatic enzymes** [e.g., alanine aminotransferase (ALT)] reflect hepatic congestion.

IV. THERAPY

A. Bed rest

1. **Advantages**
   a. Bed rest decreases metabolic needs, which reduces cardiac workload.
   b. Reduced workload, in turn, reduces pulse rate and dyspnea.
   c. Bed rest also helps decrease excess fluid volume by promoting diuresis.

2. **Disadvantages.** The risk of venous stasis increases with bed rest and can result in thromboembolism. Antiembolism stockings help minimize this risk, as do passive or active leg exercises, when the patient's condition permits.

3. **Progressive ambulation** should follow adequate bed rest.

B. Dietary controls

1. **Consuming small, but frequent meals** (4–6 daily) that are low in calories and residue provide nourishment without unduly increasing metabolic demands.

2. **Sodium restriction** is a primary tool in reducing central volume in CHF.
   a. Renal function should be evaluated to assess sodium conservation if severe sodium restriction is contemplated.
   b. Moderate sodium restriction (2–4 g of dietary sodium/day) can be achieved with relative ease by limiting the addition of salt during cooking and at the table.
   c. The patient should be advised about medications and common products that contain sodium and cautioned about their use (e.g., antacids, sodium bicarbonate or baking soda, commercial diet food products, water softeners). Table 42-2 lists other substances that promote sodium retention.

C. Digitalis glycosides.

Digitalis usually is considered a mainstay of CHF treatment, but its use, particularly in chronic CHF, has become somewhat controversial. Some authorities feel that digitalis use should be reserved for cases refractory to therapy combining rest, dietary controls, diuretics, and vasodilators.

1. **Therapeutic effects**
   a. **Positive inotropic effects** provide most of the benefits:
      (1) Increased cardiac output
      (2) Decreased cardiac filling pressure
      (3) Decreased venous and capillary pressure
      (4) Decreased heart size
      (5) Increased renal blood flow
      (6) Deactivation of renin-angiotensin-aldosterone compensation, promoting diuresis
      (7) Decreased fluid volume
      (8) Diminished edema
   b. **Negative chronotropic effects** accrue from the effect of digitalis on the sinoatrial (SA) node when given in doses that produce high total body stores (e.g., 15–18 μg/kg).

2. **Choice of agent.** All of the digitalis glycosides have similar properties; thus, selection is based on absorption, elimination kinetics, speed of onset, and duration of effect. Overall, digoxin is the most versatile and widely used and is, therefore, used as the therapeutic prototype.
   a. Digoxin is available in tablet, injection, elixir, and capsule forms.

b. Calculation of doses must factor in the differences in systemic availability among these forms. For example, digoxin solution in capsules is more bioavailable than digoxin tablets; therefore, 0.125-mg tablets are equivalent to 0.1-mg capsules.

3. **Dosage and administration.** The range between therapeutic and toxic doses is extremely narrow. There is no "magic threshold" level for digitalis therapy, but serum concentrations of 0.8–2.0 ng/ml for digoxin (10–35 ng/ml for digitoxin) have been associated with therapeutic response and minimal toxicity.
   a. **Rapid digitalization**
      (1) In this method, the effects (and steady-state levels) are achieved within 24 hours, but the actual administration rate is usually slow and delivered in divided doses.
      (2) In the presence of an acute need for an immediate effect, intravenous digitalization with digoxin may be required—if the patient has not received any digitalis in the previous 2 weeks. Intravenous digitoxin is not usually used in acute situations because it has a long latency period.
   b. **Slow digitalization.** When urgency is not the driving force, oral administration of maintenance doses should achieve steady-state levels in 7–8 days for the average patient (3–4 weeks in a patient with renal dysfunction).

4. **Precautions and monitoring effects**
   a. **Potassium** seems to antagonize digitalis preparations.
      (1) Decreased potassium levels favor digoxin binding to cardiac cells and increase its effect, thus increasing the likelihood of digitalis toxicity. This antagonism is particularly significant for the CHF patient who is receiving a diuretic (many of which decrease potassium levels).
      (2) Conversely, increased potassium levels seem to decrease digoxin binding and decrease its effect. This is likely in patients taking potassium or a captopril-like agent (which increases potassium reabsorption).
   b. **Calcium** ions act synergistically with digoxin and increased levels increase the force of myocardial contraction. At excessive levels, arrhythmias and systolic standstill can develop.
   c. **Magnesium** levels are inversely related to digoxin activity. As magnesium levels decrease, the predisposition to toxicity increases and, within reason, vice versa.
   d. **Serum digoxin levels**
      (1) In cardiac glycoside therapy, the patient's clinical state is the most practical barometer of a successful regimen. However, should questions arise as to compliance, absorption, or a drug–drug interaction, serum digoxin levels may be helpful.
      (2) After oral ingestion of digoxin, serum levels rise rapidly, then drop sharply as the drug enters the myocardium and other tissues. Therefore, a meaningful evaluation requires a determination of the relationship between serum digoxin levels and myocardial tissue levels.
      (3) The most meaningful results are obtained if serum samples are taken after steady state has been reached and 6–8 hours after an oral dose (3–4 hours after an intravenous dose).
   e. **Renal function studies.** Because the kidney is the primary metabolic route for **digoxin,** renal function studies such as serum creatinine levels aid the evaluation of elimination kinetics for digoxin. (For **digitoxin,** which is eliminated primarily through the liver, evaluation of metabolizing capabilities is more difficult.)

5. Digitalis toxicity is a fairly common occurrence because of the narrow therapeutic range and can be fatal in a significant percentage of patients experiencing a toxic reaction.
   a. **Risk of toxicity** increases with co-administration of quinidine, verapamil, and amiodarone and is influenced by the electrolyte effects described in IV C 4 a–c.
   b. **Signs of toxicity** include:
      (1) Anorexia, a common and early sign
      (2) Fatigue, headache, malaise
      (3) Nausea and vomiting
      (4) Mental confusion and disorientation
      (5) Alterations in visual perception (e.g., blurring, yellowing, or a halo effect)
      (6) Cardiac effects, which include:
         (a) Premature ventricular contractions; ventricular tachycardia and fibrillation
         (b) SA and atrioventricular (AV) block

(c) Atrial tachycardia with AV block

c. **Treatment of toxicity**

(1) Digitalis is discontinued immediately, as is any potassium-depleting diuretic.

(2) If the patient is hypokalemic, potassium supplements are administered and serum levels are monitored to avoid hyperkalemia through overcompensation. However, potassium supplements are contraindicated in a patient with severe AV block.

(3) Arrhythmias are treated with lidocaine (usually a 100-mg bolus, followed by infusion at 2–4 mg/min) or phenytoin (as a slow intravenous infusion of 25–50 mg/min, to a maximum of 1.0 g).

(4) Cholestyramine, which binds to digitalis glycosides, may help prevent absorption and reabsorption of digitalis in the bile.

(5) Patients with very high serum digoxin levels (such as those resulting from a suicidal overdose) may benefit from the use of purified digoxin-specific Fab fragment antibodies. One vial (40 mg) will bind 0.6 mg of digitalis. The dosage is calculated based on the estimated total body store of digitalis.

D. **Diuretics** (see Chapter 18). All diuretics reduce excess sodium and water. Thus, they reduce preload by decreasing venous return, which is essential in managing CHF.

1. **Thiazide diuretics** are effective and commonly used, but they deplete potassium stores in the process.

2. The **loop** diuretics furosemide and bumetanide are frequently used diuretics that have this effect plus the added advantage of reducing venous return independent of diuresis. Also, because furosemide's action is more intense, it is useful as a rapid-acting intravenous agent in reversing acute pulmonary edema, due to its direct dilating effects on pulmonary vasculature.

3. **Potassium-sparing diuretics** may help avoid the exacerbating effects of hypokalemia, but they have a weaker diuretic effect than the other diuretics. As the number of CHF patients receiving angiotensin-converting enzyme (ACE) inhibitor therapy continues to increase, fewer patients may require supplemental potassium therapy.

E. **Vasodilators**

1. These agents reduce pulmonary congestion and increase cardiac output by reducing preload and afterload.

2. Because of the complexity of vasodilator actions in patients with CHF, their use requires close hemodynamic monitoring and individualized adjustments to avoid excessive vasodilation and its adverse effects.

3. Some vasodilators exert their action primarily on the veins (preload reduction) or on the arteries (afterload reduction); others act on venous and arterial beds almost equally, providing a balanced effect (preload–afterload reduction).

4. **Individual agents**

a. **Nitroprusside** is administered intravenously in doses of 0.5–10 μg/kg/min to provide potent dilation of both arteries and veins.

b. **Hydralazine**

(1) This arteriole dilator decreases afterload and increases cardiac output in patients with CHF.

(2) Effective long-term therapy has been achieved with doses of 50–75 mg taken orally up to four times daily.

c. **Prazosin**

(1) This α-adrenergic blocker acts as a balanced arteriovenous dilator.

(2) It has been shown to be effective in long-term therapy in doses of 2–10 mg taken up to four times daily.

d. **Nitrates**

(1) Venous dilation by nitrates increases venous pooling, which decreases preload.

(2) Their arterial effects seem to result in decreased afterload with continued therapy.

(3) Nitrates are available in many forms and doses. Because individual reactions vary widely, dosages have to be adjusted, but, in general, they are higher for CHF than for angina. Table 42-3 provides examples of nitrate doses used in CHF patients.

Table 42-3. Examples of Nitrates Used in Congestive Heart Failure

Form	Typical Dose	Interval
Intravenous nitroglycerin	5–20 μg/min	Continuous infusion
Nitroglycerin buccal tablets	1–3 mg	4–6 hours
Nitroglycerin capsules (sustained-release)	6.5–19.5 mg	4–6 hours
Nitroglycerin ointment	1–3 inches	4–6 hours
Sublingual nitroglycerin	0.4 mg	1–2 hours
Oral isosorbide dinitrate	10–60 mg	4–6 hours
Sublingual isosorbide dinitrate	5–10 mg	4 hours

e. Combination therapy. Hydralazine has been used with isosorbide dinitrate to reduce afterload (or with nitroglycerin to reduce preload) for treating chronic CHF. A recently completed multicenter study within the Veterans Administration Hospitals has shown that combination therapy with hydralazine and isosorbide dinitrate significantly reduced mortality in patients unresponsive to digitalis and diuretics.

f. Angiotensin-converting enzyme (ACE) inhibitors

(1) Inhibit the conversion of angiotensin I to angiotensin II (a potent vasoconstrictor). This action significantly decreases total peripheral resistance, which aids in reducing afterload.

(2) Inhibiting the production of angiotensin II interferes with stimulation of aldosterone release, thus indirectly reducing retention of sodium and water, which decreases venous return and preload.

(3) Recently, a new class of drugs, "angiotensin II receptor antagonists," has been approved for use in the treatment of mild to moderate hypertension. Losartan is the first agent available, and currently studies are underway to assess its potential use for treating heart failure.

(4) See Table 42-4 for a comparative review of those ACE inhibitors currently used in CHF.

F. Inotropic agents have been used in the emergency treatment of patients with CHF and in patients refractory to, or unable to take, digitalis.

1. Dopamine (intravenous)

a. Low doses of 2–5 μg/kg/min stimulate specific dopamine receptors within the kidney to increase renal blood flow, and thus increase urine output.

b. Moderate doses of 5–10 μg/kg/min increase cardiac output in CHF patients.

c. High doses

(1) As doses are raised above 10 μg/kg/min, alpha peripheral activity increases, resulting in increased total peripheral resistance and pulmonary pressures.

(2) When the infusion exceeds 8–9 μg/kg/min, the patient should be monitored for tachycardia. If the infusion is slowed or interrupted, the adverse effect should disappear, as dopamine has a very short half-life in plasma.

2. Dobutamine (intravenous)

Table 42-4. Comparative Doses of ACE-Inhibitor Therapy Doses for the Treatment of CHF

Drug	Initial Dose	Target Dose
Benazepril	Not currently indicated in CHF	
Captopril	6.25 mg TID	50 mg TID
Enalapril	2.5 mg BID	10 mg BID
Fosinopril	10 mg QD	20 mg QD
Lisinopril	5 mg QD	20 mg QD
Moexipril	Not currently indicated in CHF	
Quinapril	5 mg BID	20 mg BID
Ramipril	2.5 mg BID	5 mg BID

ACE = angiotensin-converting enzyme
CHF = congestive heart failure

a. Patients who are unresponsive to, or adversely affected by, dopamine may benefit from dobutamine in doses of 5–20 μg/kg/min.

b. Although dobutamine resembles dopamine chemically, its actions differ somewhat. For example, dobutamine does not directly affect renal receptors and, therefore, does not act as a renal vasodilator. It increases urinary output only through increased cardiac output.

c. Serious arrhythmias are a potential occurrence, although less likely to occur than with dopamine. Slowing or interrupting the infusion usually reverses this effect, as it does for dopamine.

d. Dobutamine and dopamine have been used together to treat cardiogenic shock, but similar use in CHF has yet to be accepted.

3. Amrinone (intravenous) is the first of a class of drugs referred to as nonglycoside, nonsympathomimetic inotropic agents.

a. A derivative of bipyridine, amrinone has both a positive inotropic effect and a vasodilating effect.

b. By inhibiting phosphodiesterase located specifically in the cardiac cells, it increases the amount of cyclic adenosine monophosphate (cAMP).

c. Amrinone has been used in patients with heart failure that has been refractory to treatment with other inotropic agents.

d. Effective regimens have used loading intravenous infusions of 0.75 mg/kg over 3–4 minutes followed by maintenance infusions of 5–10 μg/kg/min.

e. Precautions and monitoring effects

(1) Amrinone is unstable in dextrose solutions and should be added to saline solutions instead. Because of fluid balance concerns, this can be a potential problem in patients with CHF.

(2) Because of the peripheral dilating properties, patients should be monitored for hypotension.

(3) Thrombocytopenia has occurred and is dose-dependent and asymptomatic.

(4) Ventricular rates may increase in patients with atrial flutter or fibrillation.

4. Milrinone (intravenous) is the newest inotropic agent released and is similar to amrinone. It possesses both inotropic and vasodilatory properties.

a. This agent has been used as short-term management to treat patients with heart failure.

b. Most milrinone patients in clinical trials have also been receiving digoxin and diuretics.

c. Effective dosing regimens have used a loading dose of 50 μg/kg, administered slowly over 10 minutes intravenously, followed by maintenance doses of 0.59–1.13 mg/kg/day by continuous infusion, based on the clinical status of the patient.

d. Precautions and monitoring effects

(1) Renal impairment significantly prolongs the elimination rate of milrinone, and infusions need to be reduced accordingly.

(2) Monitoring is necessary for the potential arrhythmias occurring in CHF, which may be increased by drugs such as milrinone and other inotropic agents.

(3) Blood pressure and heart rate should be monitored when administering milrinone, due to its vasodilatory effects and its potential to induce arrhythmias.

(4) Additional side effects include mild-to-moderate headache, tremor, and thrombocytopenia.

G. Patient education

1. The patient should be made aware of the importance of taking the digitalis glycoside (and any other medications) exactly as prescribed and should be advised to watch for signs of toxicity (see IV C 5 b).

2. Dietary sodium restrictions should be emphasized.

3. The patient should understand the need for regular checkups and be able to recognize symptoms that require immediate physician notification; for example, an unusually irregular pulse rate, palpitations, shortness of breath, swollen ankles, visual disturbances, or weight gain exceeding 3–5 lb in 1 week.

4. The patient needs to be educated about drugs such as calcium-channel blockers; NSAIDs (nonsteroidal anti-inflammatory drugs), which may cause a problem in CHF by retaining fluid; and sodium.

STUDY QUESTIONS

Directions: Each of the numbered items or incomplete statements in this section is followed by answers or by completions of the statement. Select the **one** lettered answer or completion that is **best** in each case.

1. Which of the following groups of symptoms is most often associated with a patient who has right-sided heart failure?

(A) Nocturia, rales, paroxysmal nocturnal dyspnea
(B) Paroxysmal nocturnal dyspnea, pedal edema, jugular venous distention, hepatojugular reflux
(C) Jugular venous distention, hepatojugular reflux, pedal edema, shortness of breath
(D) Hepatojugular reflux, jugular venous distention, pedal edema, abdominal distention
(E) Paroxysmal nocturnal dyspnea, jugular venous distention, abdominal distention, shortness of breath

2. Which of the following combinations of drugs, when used together, reduce both preload and afterload?

(A) Nitroglycerin and isosorbide dinitrate
(B) Hydralazine and isosorbide dinitrate
(C) Captopril and methyldopa
(D) Prazosin and angiotensin II
(E) Hydralazine and methyldopa

3. When digitalis glycosides are used in the patient with congestive heart failure (CHF), they work by exerting a positive effect on

(A) stroke volume
(B) total peripheral resistance
(C) heart rate
(D) blood pressure
(E) venous return

Questions 4–5

A 60-year-old hypertensive woman is currently being treated with atenolol, nitroglycerin, nifedipine, aspirin, and dipyridamole. She is admitted with a diagnosis of congestive heart failure (CHF).

4. Which agent is most likely to be discontinued in this patient?

(A) Nifedipine
(B) Atenolol
(C) Aspirin
(D) Nitroglycerin
(E) Dipyridamole

5. It is later found that the patient has developed CHF as a result of a serious anemia due to aspirin-induced bleeding. What type of heart failure does the patient have?

(A) High-output
(B) Low-output
(C) Left-sided
(D) Right-sided
(E) Low-output, left-sided

6. Because of direct dilating effects on the lung, certain agents aid in the treatment of congestive heart failure (CHF) patients suffering from pulmonary congestion. Which of the following agents is in this category?

(A) Hydrochlorothiazide
(B) Triamterene
(C) Furosemide
(D) Metolazone
(E) Spironolactone

7. Which of the following vasodilators is an orally effective preload–afterload reducer in the patient with congestive heart failure (CHF)?

(A) Hydralazine
(B) Felodipine
(C) Isosorbide dinitrate
(D) Prazosin
(E) Nitroprusside

8. For treating the patient with congestive heart failure (CHF), which of the following dosages of dopamine is selected for its positive inotropic effects?

(A) 2.0 μg/kg/min
(B) 5–10 μg/kg/min
(C) 10–20 μg/kg/min
(D) 40 μg/kg/min
(E) > 40 μg/kg/min

9. The use of angiotensin-converting enzyme (ACE) inhibitors in congestive heart failure (CHF) centers around their ability to cause

(A) direct reduction in renin levels with a resultant decrease in angiotensin II and aldosterone levels
(B) indirect reduction in angiotensin II and aldosterone levels due to inhibition of ACE
(C) direct reduction in aldosterone secretion and angiotensin I production by inhibiting ACE
(D) increase in afterload due to an indirect decrease in angiotensin II as well as a decrease in preload due to an indirect reduction in aldosterone secretion
(E) inhibition of the angiotensin II receptor, which results in reduced angiotensin II levels and reduced secretion of aldosterone.

Directions: Each item below contains three suggested answers, of which **one or more** is correct. Choose the answer

A if **I only** is correct
B if **III only** is correct
C if **I and II** are correct
D if **II and III** are correct
E if **I, II, and III** are correct

10. Which of the following have been shown to be effective in the acute management of digitalis toxicity?

I. Cholestyramine resin
II. Lidocaine or phenytoin
III. Potassium administration

11. Situations that predispose a digitalis-treated patient to toxicity include

I. hypercalcemia
II. hyperkalemia
III. hypermagnesemia

12. Guidelines necessary for monitoring the patient with congestive heart failure (CHF) include which of the following questions?

I. Does the patient have therapeutic blood levels of digoxin in the range of 0.8–2.0 ng/ml?
II. Is the patient taking a product that may decrease the effectiveness of therapy (e.g., antacids, baking soda)?
III. Does the patient have signs of digitalis toxicity or a digoxin-drug interaction?

13. Correct statements about dobutamine include which of the following?

I. Doses of 5–20 μg/kg/min have been associated with a positive inotropic effect in treating the patient with congestive heart failure (CHF)
II. Patients receiving dobutamine should be monitored for increases in peripheral vascular resistance
III. Dobutamine is considered a nonglycoside, nonsympathomimetic positive inotropic agent

ANSWERS AND EXPLANATIONS

1. The answer is D *[III B 2].*
A patient with right-sided heart failure would present with symptoms and signs of peripheral edema, due to the backup of fluid behind the failing right ventricle. The patient's symptoms and signs result from the peripheral accumulation of fluid within the liver, the legs, the abdomen, and the venous system in general. Pulmonary signs (e.g., rales, shortness of breath, paroxysmal nocturnal dyspnea) are more the consequence of the backup of fluid behind the failing left ventricle, characteristically seen in left-sided heart failure.

2. The answer is B *[IV E 4 d–e].*
The venous dilating properties of isosorbide dinitrate (preload) in conjunction with the arteriolar dilating effects of hydralazine (afterload) make this combination of agents effective in reducing both preload and afterload. The Veterans Administration Cooperative Vasodilator-Heart Failure Trial demonstrated that, as compared to placebo, the combination of the vasodilators hydralazine and isosorbide dinitrate reduced mortality in patients with mild-to-moderate heart failure previously treated with digoxin and diuretics.

3. The answer is A *[IV C 1 a].*
Digitalis glycosides are used in congestive heart failure (CHF) as positive inotropic agents to increase stroke volume. By increasing stroke volume, digitalis glycosides increase the cardiac output by increasing the right side of the following equation:

$$\text{Cardiac output} = \text{stroke volume} \times \text{heart rate.}$$

4-5. The answers are: 4-B *[I E 1, 2; Table 42-2];* **5-A** *[I D 1 b].*
Because they produce negative inotropic effects, β-adrenergic receptor blockers such as atenolol must be used very cautiously in patients who develop congestive heart failure (CHF). All β-blockers have the potential to reduce cardiac output. The physician must determine whether the benefit of such therapy for a patient with angina, hypertension, arrhythmia, and so forth is worth the risk of inducing heart failure. In many situations, the risk is worth taking; in other situations, it may not be if alternative therapy is available.

In anemia, the lack of oxygen-carrying capacity by the red blood cells puts an added stress on the heart, which must work harder to provide better oxygenation to the metabolizing tissues. Initially, the heart may be able to compensate, either by increasing the heart rate or by increasing stroke volume through cardiac dilation and hypertrophy. However, if the anemia is allowed to continue, the heart is unable to meet the metabolic demands placed on it, resulting in the signs and symptoms of heart failure.

6. The answer is C *[IV D 2].*
Furosemide has been shown to possess direct pulmonary dilating effects, which are independent of a diuretic effect and which occur prior to the diuretic effect.

7. The answer is D *[IV E 4 c].*
Prazosin acts as an α-adrenergic blocking agent. The physiologic response seen includes both arteriolar and venous dilation. Prazosin has been shown to produce a balanced dilating effect, making it a useful agent in the ambulatory setting. Unlike hydralazine (which produces afterload reduction), isosorbide dinitrate (producing preload reduction), and nitroprusside (a parenteral agent), prazosin is effective orally in reducing both preload and afterload when used alone. Felodipine is a calcium-channel blocker, which has not yet shown beneficial effects in reducing preload and afterload in CHF.

8. The answer is B *[IV F 1].*
Dopamine has shown great versatility in its effects. At doses of 2–5 μg/kg/min, it increases renal blood flow through its dopaminergic effects. At doses of 5–10 μg/kg/min, it increases cardiac output through its β-adrenergic stimulating effect. At doses of 10–20 μg/kg/min, it increases peripheral vascular resistance through its α-adrenergic stimulating effects. There is no specific cutoff for any of these effects, so close titration is required to provide for individual response.

9. The answer is B *[IV E 4 f (2); Figure 42-2].*
By directly inhibiting the angiotensin-converting enzyme (ACE), production of angiotensin II is reduced, as is angiotensin II-mediated secretion of aldosterone from the adrenal gland. Losartan is a

newly released angiotensin II receptor blocker which decreases angiotensin II product and reduces subsequent secretion of aldosterone. It is currently not used to treat CHF.

10. The answer is E (all) *[IV C 5 c].*
Cholestyramine resin has been used in the acute situation to decrease the absorption of digoxin within the gastrointestinal tract. This results in lower digoxin levels if the resin is administered before all the digoxin has been absorbed. Potassium administration has been shown to be effective in protecting the myocardium from the toxic effects of digoxin while toxic levels return to normal. Both lidocaine and phenytoin have been shown to be useful in preventing and treating toxic arrhythmias associated with digitalis toxicity.

11. The answer is A (I) *[IV C 4 a–c].*
Calcium ions act synergistically with digitalis. Therefore, when hypercalcemia occurs, digitalis exerts an added pharmacologic effect on the heart. This may present itself as toxic arrhythmias, cardiac standstill, and even death. Elevated potassium levels or elevated magnesium levels seem to aid in the prevention of digitalis-induced toxicity. There is building evidence that digitalis preparations need calcium ions to work, and consequently low calcium levels may negate the pharmacologic potential of digitalis.

12. The answer is E (all) *[IV B 2 c; C 3, 5 a–b; G 1–4].*
Digitalis has a narrow therapeutic range; serum levels of 0.8–2.0 ng/ml provide a therapeutic response with minimal toxicity. Monitoring serum digoxin levels is especially helpful during initial dosage titrations and when questions arise as to compliance, absorption, or a drug–drug interaction. Patients with congestive heart failure (CHF) must be informed of the need to take their medication appropriately and accurately so that blood levels for all drugs will be within the therapeutic range. Patients must also be told to inform their pharmacist of any additional drugs they are taking since these could aggravate the disease or interact with digoxin or with other drugs. Patients should also be monitored for those symptoms related to CHF that effective therapy should prevent. Reporting symptoms such as swollen legs or shortness of breath enables the physician to add different drugs or increase the dosage of current medications.

13. The answer is A (I) *[IV F 2 a].*
Dobutamine in doses of 5–20 μg/kg/min is an inotropic agent that is useful in the treatment of congestive heart failure (CHF). Dobutamine does not have the versatility that dopamine offers, lacking comparable effects on renal blood flow or peripheral vascular resistance. Rather, dobutamine has a peripheral dilating effect that offers a benefit to patients who have reduced cardiac output due to elevated peripheral resistance.

43
Infectious Diseases

Paul F. Souney
Cheryl A. Stoukides

I. PRINCIPLES OF ANTI-INFECTIVE THERAPY

A. Definition. Anti-infective agents treat infection by suppressing or destroying the causative microorganisms—bacteria, mycobacteria, fungi, protozoa, or viruses. Anti-infective agents derived from natural substances are called **antibiotics;** those produced from synthetic substances are called **antimicrobials.** These two terms now are used interchangeably.

B. Indications. Anti-infective agents should be used only when:

1. A significant infection has been diagnosed or is strongly suspected
2. An established indication for prophylactic therapy exists

C. Gram stain, microbiologic culturing, and susceptibility tests. These tests should be performed before anti-infective therapy is initiated. Test materials must be obtained by a method that avoids contamination of the specimen by the patient's own flora.

1. **Gram stain.** Performed on all specimens except blood cultures, the Gram stain helps to identify the cause of infection immediately. By determining if the causative agent is gram-positive or gram-negative, the test allows a better choice of drug therapy, particularly when an anti-infective regimen must begin without delay.
   a. **Gram-positive** microorganisms stain **blue** or **purple.**
   b. **Gram-negative** microorganisms stain **red** or **rose-pink.**
   c. **Fungi** may also be identified by Gram stain.

2. **Microbiologic cultures.** To identify the specific causative agent, specimens of body fluids or infected tissue are collected for analysis.

3. **Susceptibility tests.** Different strains of the same pathogenic species may have widely varying susceptibility to a particular anti-infective agent. Susceptibility tests determine microbial susceptibility to a given drug and, thus, can be used to predict whether the drug will combat the infection effectively.
   a. **Microdilution method.** The drug is diluted serially in various media containing the test microorganism.
      (1) The lowest drug concentration that prevents microbial growth after 18–24 hours of incubation is called the **minimum inhibitory concentration (MIC).**
      (2) The lowest drug concentration that reduces bacterial density by 99.9% is called the **minimum bactericidal concentration (MBC).**
      (3) **Breakpoint** concentrations of antibiotics are used to characterize antibiotic activity: the interpretive categories are **susceptible, moderately susceptible (intermediate),** and **resistant.** These concentrations are determined by considering pharmacokinetics, serum and tissue concentrations following normal doses, and the **population distribution** of MICs of a group of bacteria for a given drug.
   b. **Kirby-Bauer disk diffusion technique.** This test is less expensive but less reliable than the microdilution method; however, it provides qualitative susceptibility information.
      (1) Filter paper disks impregnated with specific drug quantities are placed on the surface of agar plates streaked with a microorganism culture. After 18 hours, the size of a clear inhibition zone is determined; drug activity against the test strain is then correlated to zone size.
      (2) The Kirby-Bauer technique does not reliably predict therapeutic effectiveness against certain microorganisms (e.g., *Staphylococcus aureus, Shigella*).

D. Choice of agent. An anti-infective agent should be chosen on the basis of its pharmacologic properties and spectrum of activity as well as on various host (patient) factors.

1. **Pharmacologic properties** include the drug's ability to reach the infection site and to attain a desired level in the target tissue.

2. **Spectrum of activity.** To treat an infectious disease effectively, an anti-infective drug must be active against the causative pathogen. Susceptibility testing or clinical experience in treating a given syndrome may suggest the effectiveness of a particular drug.

3. **Patient factors.** Selection of an anti-infective drug regimen must take various patient factors into account to determine which type of drug should be administered, the correct drug dosage and administration route, and the potential for adverse drug effects.
   a. **Immunologic status.** A patient with impaired immune mechanisms may require a drug that rapidly destroys pathogens (i.e., **bactericidal agent**) rather than one that merely suppresses a pathogen's growth or reproduction (i.e., **bacteriostatic agent**).
   b. **Presence of a foreign body.** The effectiveness of anti-infective therapy is reduced in patients who have prosthetic joints or valves, cardiac pacemakers, and various internal shunts.
   c. **Age.** A drug's pharmacokinetic properties may vary widely in patients of different ages. In very young and very old patients, drug metabolism and excretion commonly decrease. Elderly patients also have an increased risk of suffering ototoxicity when receiving certain antibiotics.
   d. **Underlying disease**
      (1) Preexisting **kidney** or **liver disease** increases the risk of nephrotoxicity or hepatotoxicity during the administration of some antibacterial drugs.
      (2) Patients with **central nervous system (CNS) disorders** may suffer neurotoxicity (motor seizures) during penicillin therapy.
      (3) Patients with **neuromuscular disorders** (e.g., myasthenia gravis) are at increased risk for developing neuromuscular blockade during aminoglycoside or polymyxin B therapy.
   e. **History of drug allergy or adverse drug reactions.** Patients who have had previous allergic or other untoward reactions to a particular antibiotic have a higher risk of experiencing the same reaction during subsequent administration of that drug. Except in life-threatening situations, patients who have had serious allergic reactions to penicillin, for example, should not receive the drug again.
   f. **Pregnancy and lactation.** Because drug therapy during pregnancy and lactation can cause unwanted effects, the mother's need for the antibiotic must be weighed against the drug's potential harm.
      (1) Pregnancy can increase the risk of adverse drug effects for both mother and fetus. Also, plasma drug concentrations tend to decrease in pregnant women, reducing a drug's therapeutic effectiveness.
      (2) Most drugs, including antibiotics, appear in the breast milk of nursing mothers and may cause adverse effects in infants. For example, sulfonamides may lead to toxic bilirubin accumulation in a newborn's brain.
   g. **Genetic traits**
      (1) Sulfonamides may cause hemolytic anemia in patients with glucose-6-phosphate dehydrogenase (G6PD) deficiency.
      (2) Patients who rapidly metabolize drugs (i.e., rapid acetylators) may develop hepatitis when receiving the antitubercular drug isoniazid.

E. Empiric therapy. In serious or life-threatening disease, anti-infective therapy must begin before the infecting organism has been identified. In this case, the choice of drug (or drugs) is based on clinical experience, suggesting that a particular agent is effective in a given setting.

1. A **broad-spectrum antibiotic** usually is the most appropriate choice until the specific organism has been determined.

2. In all cases, **culture specimens must be obtained** before therapy begins.

F. Multiple antibiotic therapy. A combination of drugs should be given only when clinical experience has shown such therapy to be more effective than single-agent therapy in a particular setting. A multiple-agent regimen can increase the risk of toxic drug effects and, in a few cases, may result in drug antagonism and subsequent therapeutic ineffectiveness. Indications for multiple-agent therapy include:

1. **Need for increased antibiotic effectiveness.** The **synergistic** (intensified) effect of two or more agents may allow a dosage reduction or a faster or enhanced drug effect.
2. **Treatment of an infection caused by multiple pathogens** (e.g., intra-abdominal infection)
3. **Prevention of proliferation of drug-resistant organisms** (e.g., during treatment of tuberculosis)

G. Duration of anti-infective therapy. To achieve the therapeutic goal, anti-infective therapy must continue for a sufficient duration.

1. **Acute uncomplicated infection.** Treatment generally should continue until the patient has been afebrile and asymptomatic for at least 72 hours.
2. **Chronic infection** (e.g., endocarditis, osteomyelitis). Treatment may require a longer duration (4–6 weeks) with follow-up culture analyses to assess therapeutic effectiveness.

H. Monitoring therapeutic effectiveness. To assess the patient's response to anti-infective therapy, appropriate specimens should be cultured and the following parameters monitored:

1. **Fever curve.** An important assessment tool, the fever curve may be a reliable indication of response to therapy. Defervescence usually indicates favorable response.
2. **White blood cell (WBC) count.** In the initial stage of infection, the neutrophil count from a peripheral blood smear may rise above normal (neutrophilia) and immature neutrophil forms ("bands") may appear ("left shift"). In patients who are elderly, debilitated, or suffering overwhelming infection, the WBC count may be normal or subnormal.
3. **Radiographic findings.** Small effusions, abscesses, or cavities that appear on radiographs indicate the focus of infection.
4. **Pain** and **inflammation** (as evidenced by swelling, erythema, and tenderness) may occur when the infection is superficial or within a joint or bone, also indicating a possible focus of infection.
5. **Erythrocyte sedimentation rate (ESR or "sed rate").** Large elevations in ESR are associated with acute or chronic infection, particularly endocarditis, chronic osteomyelitis, and intra-abdominal infections. A normal ESR does not exclude infection; more often ESR is elevated due to noninfectious causes such as collagen vascular disease.
6. **Serum complement concentrations,** particularly C3 component, are often reduced in serious infections because of consumption during the host defense process.

I. Lack of therapeutic effectiveness. When an antibiotic drug regimen fails, other drugs should not be added indiscriminately or the regimen otherwise changed. Instead, the situation should be reassessed and diagnostic efforts intensified. Causes of therapeutic ineffectiveness include:

1. **Misdiagnosis.** The isolated organism may have been misidentified by the laboratory or may not be the causative agent for infection (e.g., the patient may have an unsuspected infection).
2. **Improper drug regimen.** The drug dosage, administration route, dosing frequency, or duration of therapy may be inadequate or inappropriate.
3. **Inappropriate choice of antibiotic agent.** As discussed in I D, patient factors and the pharmacologic properties and spectrum of activity of a given drug must be considered when planning anti-infective drug therapy.
4. **Microbial resistance.** By acquiring resistance to a specific antibiotic, microorganisms can survive in the drug's presence. Many gonococcal strains, for instance, now resist penicillin. Drug resistance is particularly common in geographic areas where a specific drug has been used excessively (and perhaps improperly).
5. **Unrealistic expectations.** Antibiotics are ineffective in certain circumstances.
   a. Patients with conditions that require **surgical drainage** frequently cannot be cured by anti-infective drugs until the drain has been removed. For example, the presence of

necrotic tissue or pus in patients with pneumonia, empyema, or renal calculi is a common cause of antibiotic failure.

b. Fever should not be treated with anti-infective drugs unless infection has been identified as the cause. Although fever frequently signifies infection, it sometimes stems from noninfectious conditions (e.g., drug reactions, phlebitis, neoplasms, metabolic disorders, arthritis). These conditions do not respond to antibiotics. One exception to this position is neutropenic cancer patients; such patients with no signs or symptoms of infection other than fever are widely treated with antimicrobial agents.

6. Infection by two or more types of microorganisms. If not detected initially, an additional cause of infection may lead to therapeutic failure.

J. Perioperative antibiotic prophylaxis

1. Definition. Perioperative antibiotic prophylaxis is a short course of antibiotic administered before there is clinical evidence of infection.

2. General considerations

a. Timing. The antibiotic should be administered at the site of contamination before the incision. Initiation of prophylaxis is often at induction of anesthesia, just before the surgical incision. This ensures peak serum and tissue antibiotic levels.

b. Duration. Prophylaxis should be maintained for the duration of surgery. Long surgical procedures (e.g., more than 3 hours) may require additional doses. There is little evidence to support continuation of prophylaxis beyond 24 hours.

c. Antibiotic spectrum should be appropriate for the usual pathogens.

(1) In general, **first-generation cephalosporins** (e.g., cefazolin) are the drugs of choice for most procedures and patients. These agents have an appropriate spectrum, a low frequency of side effects, a favorable half-life, and a low cost.

(2) **Vancomycin** is a suitable alternative in penicillin-sensitive patients and in situations where methicillin-resistant *S. aureus* is a concern.

d. Route of administration. Intravenous (IV) or intramuscular routes are preferred to guarantee good serum and tissue levels at the time of incision.

II. ANTIBACTERIAL AGENTS

A. Definition and classification. Used to treat infections caused by **bacteria,** antibacterial agents fall into several major categories: **aminoglycosides, cephalosporins, erythromycins, penicillins** (including various subgroups), **sulfonamides, tetracyclines, fluoroquinolones, urinary tract antiseptics,** and **miscellaneous antibacterials** (Table 43-1).

B. Aminoglycosides. These drugs, containing amino sugars, are used primarily in infections caused by gram-negative enterobacteria and in suspected sepsis. They have little activity against anaerobic and facultative organisms. The toxic potential of these drugs limits their use. Major aminoglycosides include **amikacin, kanamycin, gentamicin, neomycin, netilmicin, streptomycin,** and **tobramycin.**

1. Mechanism of action. Aminoglycosides are **bactericidal;** they inhibit bacterial protein synthesis by binding to and impeding the function of the 30S ribosomal subunit. (Some aminoglycosides also bind to the 50S ribosomal subunit.) Their mechanism of action is not fully known.

2. Spectrum of activity

a. Streptomycin is active against both gram-positive and gram-negative bacteria. However, widespread resistance to this drug has restricted its use to the organisms that cause plague and tularemia; gram-positive streptococci (given in combination with penicillin); and *Mycobacterium tuberculosis* (given in combination with other antitubercular agents, as described in V C 3).

b. Amikacin, kanamycin, gentamicin, tobramycin, neomycin, and **netilmicin** are active against many gram-negative bacteria (e.g., *Proteus, Serratia,* and *Pseudomonas* organisms).

(1) **Gentamicin** is active against some *Staphylococcus* strains; it is more active than tobramycin against *Serratia* organisms.

Table 43-1. Some Important Parameters of Anti-Infective Drugs

Agent	Elimination Route	Half-Life	Administration Route	Common Dosage Range (Adults)
Aminoglycosides				
Amikacin	Renal	2–3 hours	IV, IM	15 mg/kg/day
Gentamicin	Renal	2 hours	IV, IM	3 mg/kg/day
Kanamycin	Renal	2–4 hours	Oral, IV	15 mg/kg q 8–12 hours
Neomycin	Renal	2–3 hours	Oral, topical	50–100 mg/kg/day (oral); 10–15 mg/day (topical)
Netilmicin	Renal	2–7 hours	IV, IM	3–6 mg/kg/day
Streptomycin	Renal	2–3 hours	IM	15 mg/kg/day†
Tobramycin	Renal	2–5 hours	IV, IM	3–5 mg/kg/day
Cephalosporins				
First-generation				
Cefadroxil	Renal	1.5 hours	Oral	1–2 g/day
Cefazolin	Renal	1.4–2.2 hours	IV	250 mg–1 g q 8 hours
Cephalexin	Renal	0.9–1.3 hours	Oral	250–500 mg q 6 hours
Cephalothin	Renal (H)	0.5–0.9 hour	IV, IM	500 mg–2 g q 4–6 hours
Cephapirin	Renal (H)	0.6–0.8 hour	IV, IM	500 mg–2 g q 4–6 hours
Cephradine	Renal	1.3 hours	Oral, IV	250–500 mg q 6 hours
Second-generation				
Cefaclor	Renal (H)	0.8 hour	Oral	250–500 mg q 8 hours
Cefamandole	Renal	1 hour	IV	500 mg–1 g q 4–8 hours
Cefmetazole	Renal	72 minutes	IV	2 g q 6–12 hours
Cefonicid	Renal	4 hours	IV	1–2 g/day
Ceforanide	Renal	2.2–3 hours	IV	0.5 mg–1 g q 12 hours
Cefotetan	Renal	2.8–4.6 hours	IV, IM	1–2 g q 12 hours
Cefoxitin	Renal	0.8 hour	IV	1–2 g q 6–8 hours
Cefpodoxime	Renal	2.5 hours	Oral	100–400 mg q 12 hours
Cefprozil	Renal	78 minutes	Oral	250–500 mg q 12–24 hours
Cefuroxime	Renal	1.5–2.2 hours	IV, IM	750 mg–1.5 g q 8 hours
Loracarbef	Renal	1 hour	Oral	200 mg q 12 hours or 400 mg/day
Third-generation				
Cefixime	Renal	3–4 hours	Oral	400 mg/day
Cefoperazone	Hepatic	1.6–2.4 hours	IV	2–4 g q 12 hours
Cefotaxime	Renal (H)	1.5 hours	IV	1–2 g q 6–8 hours
Cefotetan	Renal	4.2 hours	IV, IM	1–2 g q 12 hours
Ceftazidime	Renal	1.8 hours	IV, IM	1–2 g q 8–12 hours
Ceftibuten	Renal	2.5 hours	Oral	400 mg/day
Ceftizoxime	Renal	1.7 hours	IV	1–2 g q 8–12 hours
Ceftriaxone	Renal	8 hours	IV, IM	1–2 g/day
Moxalactam	Renal	2.2 hours	IV, IM	2–4 g q 8–12 hours
Fourth-generation				
Cefepime	Renal	2 hours	IV, IM	1–2 g q 12 hours
Erythromycins and other macrolides				
Azithromicin	Hepatic	68 hours	Oral	250 mg/day
Clarithromycin	Renal	3–7 hours	Oral	250–500 mg q 12 hours
Dirithromycin	Hepatic	8 hours	Oral	500 mg daily
Erythromycin base, estolate, ethylsuccinate, and stearate	Hepatic	1.2–2.6 hours	Oral	250–500 mg q 6 hours
Erythromycin gluceptate and lactobionate			IV	0.5–2 g q 6 hours
Troleandomycin	Hepatic (R)	1.05 hours	Oral	250–500 mg q 12 hours

(continued on next page)

Table 43-1. (continued) Some Important Parameters of Anti-Infective Drugs

Agent	Elimination Route	Half-Life	Administration Route	Common Dosage Range (Adults)
Natural penicillins				
Penicillin G	Renal (H)	0.5 hour	Oral, IV, IM	200,000–500,000 units q 6–8 hours
Penicillin V	Renal	1 hour	Oral	500 mg–2 g/day
Penicillin G procaine	Renal	24–60 hours	IM	300,000–600,000 units/day
Penicillin G benzathine	Renal	24–60 hours	IM	300,000–600,000 units/day
Penicillinase-resistant penicillins				
Cloxacillin	Renal (H)	0.5 hour	Oral	250–500 mg q 6 hours
Dicloxacillin	Renal (H)	0.5–0.9 hour	Oral	500 mg–1 g/day
Methicillin	Renal (H)	0.5–1 hour	IV, IM	1–2 g q 4–6 hours
Nafcillin	Hepatic (R)	0.5 hour	Oral, IV, IM	0.25–2 g q 6 hours
Oxacillin	Renal (H)	0.5 hour	Oral, IV, IM	500 mg–2 g q 4–6 hours
Aminopenicillins				
Amoxicillin	Renal (H)	0.9–2.3 hours	Oral	250–500 mg q 8 hours
Amoxicillin/ clavulanic acid	Renal	1 hour	Oral	250–500 mg q 8 hours
Ampicillin	Renal (H)	0.8–1.5 hours	Oral, IV, IM	250 mg–2 g q 4–6 hours
Ampicillin/sulbactam	Renal	1–1.8 hours	IV, IM	1.5–3 g q 6 hours
Bacampicillin	Renal	1 hour	Oral	400–800 mg q 12 hours
Cyclacillin	Renal (H)	0.5 hour	Oral	250–500 mg q 6 hours
Extended-spectrum penicillins				
Azlocillin	Renal (H)	0.8–1.5 hours	IV	100–300 mg/kg/day
Carbenicillin	Renal (H)	1.5 hours	IM, IV	1–5 g q 4–6 hours
Carbenicillin indanyl	Renal (H)	1.5 hours	Oral	382–764 mg qid
Mezlocillin	Renal (H)	0.6–1.2 hours	IV, IM	1–3 g q 4–6 hours
Piperacillin	Renal (H)	0.8–1.4 hours	IV, IM	1–1.5 mg/kg q 6–12 hours
Piperacillin/tazobactam	Renal	0.7–1.2 hours	IV	3.375 g q 6 hours
Ticarcillin	Renal	0.9–1.5 hours	IV, IM	1–3 g q 4–6 hours
Ticarcillin/ clavulanic acid	Renal	1–1.5 hours	IV	3.1 g q 4–6 hours
Sulfonamides				
Sulfacytine	Renal	4–4.5 hours	Oral	250 mg q 6 hours
Sulfadiazine	Renal (H)	6 hours	Oral, IV	2–4 g/day
Sulfamethoxazole	Hepatic (R)	9–11 hours	Oral	1–3 g/day
Sulfisoxazole	Renal (H)	3–7 hours	Oral, IV	2–8 g/day
Tetracyclines				
Demeclocycline	Renal	10–17 hours	Oral	300 mg–1 g/day
Doxycycline	Hepatic	14–25 hours	Oral, IV	100–200 mg q 12 hours
Methacycline	Renal	16 hours	Oral	150 mg q 6 hours to 300 mg q 12 hours
Minocycline	Hepatic	12–15 hours	Oral, IV	100–200 mg q 12 hours
Oxytetracycline	Renal	6–12 hours	Oral, IM	250–500 mg q 6 hours
				250–500 mg qid or 300 mg/day in one or two divided doses
Tetracycline‡	Renal	6–12 hours	Oral, IV, IM	1–2 g/day
Fluoroquinolones				
Ciprofloxacin	Renal (H)	5–6 hours	IV	200–600 mg q 12 hours
		3–5 hours	Oral	250–750 mg q 12 hours
Enoxacin	Renal (H)	6.2 hours	Oral	200 mg/day–600 mg q 12 hours

Table 43-1. (continued) Some Important Parameters of Anti-Infective Drugs

Agent	Elimination Route	Half-Life	Administration Route	Common Dosage Range (Adults)
Lomefloxacin	Renal	6.35–7.77 hours	Oral	400 mg/day
Ofloxacin	Renal	5–7.5 hours 5–10 hours	Oral IV	100 mg/day–400 mg q 12 hours (IV and Oral)
Urinary tract antiseptics				
Cinoxacin	Renal	1–1.5 hours	Oral	250 mg q 6 hours or 500 mg q 12 hours
Methenamine hippurate and mandelate	Renal	1–3 hours	Oral	0.5–2 g qid
Nalidixic acid	Renal	8 hours	Oral	4 g/day
Nitrofurantoin	Renal	0.3–1 hour	Oral	5–7 mg/kg/day
Norfloxacin	Hepatic	3–4 hours	Oral	400 bid
Miscellaneous antiinfectives				
Atovaquone	Renal		Oral	750 mg TID × 21 days
Aztreonam	Renal	1.7 hours	IV, IM	500 mg–2 g q 8–12 hours
Chloramphenicol	Hepatic	1.5–4.1 hours	Oral, IV	50–100 mg/kg/day
Ciprofloxacin	Hepatic (R)	3–5 hours	Oral	250–750 mg q 12 hours
Clindamycin	Hepatic	2–4 hours	Oral, IM, IV	300–900 mg q 6–8 hours
Clofazimine	Hepatic	70 days	Oral	100 mg/day
Dapsone	Hepatic (R)	28 hours	Oral	50–100 mg/day
Imipenem	Renal	1 hour	IV	250 mg–1 g q 6 hours
Lincomycin	Hepatic (R)	4.4–6.4 hours	IV, IM	600 mg–1 g q 8–12 hours
Meropenem	Renal	1.5 hours	IV,IM	0.5–2 g q 8 hours
Mupirocin	Renal	19–35 minutes	Topical	Apply q 8–12 hours
Spectinomycin	Renal	1.2–2.8 hours	IM	2–4 g (single dose)
Trimethoprim	Renal (H)	8–15 hours	Oral	100–200 mg/day
Vancomycin	Renal	6–8 hours	Oral, IV	500 mg q 6 hours
Antifungal agents				
Amphotericin B	Unknown	24 hours	IV	1–1.5 mg/kg/day
Fluconazole	Renal	30 hours	IV, Oral	100–200 mg/day
Flucytosine	Renal	3–6 hours	Oral	50–150 mg/kg/day
Griseofulvin	Hepatic (R)	9–24 hours	Oral	300–375 mg/day
Intraconazole	Hepatic	34–42 hours	Oral	200–400 mg/day
Ketoconazole	Hepatic	1.5–3.3 hours	Oral	200–400 mg/day
Miconazole	Hepatic	20–24 hours	IV	600 mg–3 g/day
Nystatin	Fecal	. . .	Oral	500,000–1,000,000 units tid
Antiprotozoal agents				
Atovaquone	Hepatic	2.9 days	Oral	750 mg/day for 21 days
Chloroquine hydrochloride phosphate	Renal	3 days	IM, Oral	160–200 mg/day§ 500 mg–1 g/day
Diloxanide furoate	Renal	. . .	Oral	500 mg tid
Eflornithine	Renal	3 hours	IV	100 mg/kg/dose q 6 hours
Emetine	Renal	4–7 days	SC, IM	1 mg/kg/day to 60 mg/day maximum
Fansidar	Hepatic (R)	150 hours	Oral	3 tablets for one dose
Iodoquinol	Fecal	. . .	Oral	650 mg tid for 20 days
Mefloquine	Hepatic	15–33 days	Oral	5 tablets for one dose
Metronidazole	Hepatic (R)	6–14 hours	Oral	250–500 mg q 6–8 hours
Paramomycin	Fecal	. . .	Oral	25–35 mg/kg/day
Pentamidine	Renal	6–9 hours	IV	4 mg/kg qid for 14 days (treatment IV) 300 mg q 4 weeks (prophylaxis INH)

(continued on next page)

Table 43-1. (continued) Some Important Parameters of Anti-Infective Drugs

Agent	Elimination Route	Half-Life	Administration Route	Common Dosage Range (Adults)
Primaquine phosphate	Renal	3–6 hours	Oral	15 mg (base)/day
Pyrimethamine	Renal	4 days	Oral	25 mg/week
Quinacrine	. . .	5 days	Oral	100 mg/day
Quinine sulfate	Renal	12 hours	Oral	650 q 8 hours‖
Antitubercular agents				
Aminosalicylic acid	Renal	1 hour	Oral	10–12 g/day
Capreomycin	Renal	4–6 hours	IM	15 mg/kg/day to 1 g/day maximum
Cycloserine	Renal	10 hours	Oral	500 mg/day to 1 g/day maximum
Ethambutol	Hepatic	3.3 hours	Oral	15 mg/kg/day
Ethionamide	Hepatic	3 hours	Oral	500 mg–1 g/day
Isoniazid	Hepatic	1–4 hours	Oral, IM	5 mg/kg/day to 300 mg/day maximum
Pyrazinamide	Hepatic	9–10 hours	Oral	20–35 mg/kg/day to 3 g/day maximum
Rifampin	Hepatic	3 hours	Oral	600 mg/day
Rifabutin	Renal	4–5 hours	Oral	300 mg/day
Antiviral agents				
Acyclovir	Renal	2.1–3.8 hours	Oral, IV, topical	200 mg q 4 hours (oral); 5 mg/kg q 8 hours (IV)
Amantadine	Renal	12 hours	Oral	100–200 mg/day
Cidofovir	Renal	6.5 hours	IV	5 mg/kg once weekly for 2 weeks, then 5 mg/kg q 2 weeks (administer with probenecid)
Didanosine	Hepatic (R)	1.6 hours	Oral	125–300 mg q 12 hours
Foscarnet	Renal	2–8 hours	IV	60 mg/kg q 8 hours
Ganciclovir	Renal	2.9 hours	IV	5 mg/kg q 12 hours
		4.8 hours	Oral	1000 mg induction 500 mg 6 × day every 30 maintenance
Indinavir	Hepatic	NA	Oral	800 mg TID
Ribavirin	Renal	9.5 hours	Aerosol	6 g q 24 hours
Rotinavir	Hepatic	3–5 hours	Oral	600 mg BID
Saquinavir	Hepatic	NA	Oral	600 mg BID
Vidarabine	Renal (H)	1.5 hours	IV, topical	15 mg/kg/day
Zalcitabine	Renal	1–3 hours	Oral	0.75 mg q 8 hours
Zidovudine	Renal (H)	1 hour	Oral	200 mg q 4 hours
Famciclovir	Renal	2–2.5 hours	IV, Oral	500 mg q 8 hours for 7 days
Stavudine (D4T) hours	Renal	1.5 hours	Oral	≥ 60 kg = 40 mg q 12 < 60 kg = 30 mg q 6 hours
Rimantadine	Renal	25 hours	Oral	100 mg twice daily
Lamivudine	Renal	5–7 hours	Oral	150 mg BID with zidovudine
Valacyclovir	Renal	2.5–3.3 hours	Oral	1 g TID for 7 days
Anthelmintics				
Diethylcarbamazine	Renal	30 hours	Oral	25 mg/day for 3 days, then 50 mg/day for 5 days, then 100 mg/day for 3 days, then 150 mg/day for 12 days

Table 43-1. (continued) Some Important Parameters of Anti-Infective Drugs

Agent	Elimination Route	Half-Life	Administration Route	Common Dosage Range (Adults)
Mebendazole	Hepatic	0.83–11.5 hours	Oral	100 mg q 12 hours
Niclosamide	Fecal	. . .	Oral	2 g/day
Praziquantel	Renal	0.8–1.5 hours	Oral	20 mg/kg for 3 doses
Pyrantel	Hepatic	. . .	Oral	11 mg/kg for 1 dose (maximum, 1 g)
Oxamniquine	Renal	1–2.5 hours	Oral	12–15 mg/kg for 1 dose
Thiabendazole	Renal	. . .	Oral	< 70 kg, 25 mg/kg > 70 kg, 1.5 g

(H) = secondary hepatic elimination; IM = intramuscular; IV = intravenous; (R) = secondary renal elimination; and SC = subcutaneous.

†Dosage applies to infections other than tuberculosis; for tuberculosis, dosage is 1 g/day.

‡Intravenous agent withdrawn from U.S. market.

§For short-term therapy.

||For initial therapy.

(2) **Amikacin** is the broadest spectrum aminoglycoside with activity against most aerobic gram-negative bacilli as well as many anaerobic gram-negative bacterial strains that resist gentamicin and tobramycin. It is also active against *M. tuberculosis.*

(3) **Tobramycin,** as compared to gentamicin, may be more active against *Pseudomonas aeruginosa.*

(4) **Netilmicin** may be active against gentamicin-resistant organisms; it appears to be less ototoxic than other aminoglycosides.

(5) **Neomycin,** in addition to its activity against such gram-negative organisms as *Escherichia coli* and *Klebsiella pneumoniae,* is active against several gram-positive organisms (e.g., *S. aureus, M. tuberculosis*). *P. aeruginosa* and most streptococci are now neomycin-resistant.

3. **Therapeutic uses**

a. **Streptomycin** is used to treat plague, tularemia, acute brucellosis (given in combination with tetracycline), bacterial endocarditis caused by *Streptococcus viridans* (given in combination with penicillin), and tuberculosis (given in combination with other antitubercular agents, as described in V C 2).

b. **Gentamicin, tobramycin, amikacin,** and **netilmicin** are therapeutic for serious gram-negative bacillary infections (e.g., those caused by *Enterobacter, Serratia, Klebsiella, P. aeruginosa*), pneumonia (given in combination with a cephalosporin or penicillin), meningitis, complicated urinary tract infections, osteomyelitis, bacteremia, and peritonitis.

c. **Neomycin** is used for preoperative bowel sterilization; hepatic coma (as adjunctive therapy); and, in topical form, for skin and mucous membrane infections (e.g., burns).

4. **Precautions and monitoring effects.** Aminoglycosides can cause serious adverse effects. To prevent or minimize such problems, blood drug concentrations and blood urea nitrogen (BUN) and serum creatinine levels should be monitored during therapy.

a. **Ototoxicity.** Aminoglycosides can cause vestibular or auditory damage.

(1) Gentamicin and streptomycin cause primarily **vestibular** damage (manifested by tinnitus, vertigo, and ataxia). Such damage may be bilateral and irreversible.

(2) Amikacin, kanamycin, and neomycin cause mainly **auditory** damage (hearing loss).

(3) Tobramycin can result in both vestibular and auditory damage.

b. **Nephrotoxicity.** Because aminoglycosides accumulate in the proximal tubule, mild renal dysfunction develops in up to 25% of patients receiving these drugs for several days or more. Usually, this adverse effect is reversible.

(1) Neomycin is the most nephrotoxic aminoglycoside; streptomycin, the least nephrotoxic. Gentamicin and tobramycin are nephrotoxic to approximately the same degree.

(2) **Risk factors** for increased nephrotoxic effects include:

(a) Preexisting renal disease

(b) Previous or prolonged aminoglycoside therapy
(c) Concurrent administration of another nephrotoxic drug
(d) Impaired renal flow unrelated to renal disease (e.g., from hypotension, severe hepatic disease)

(3) Trough levels above 2 μg/ml for gentamicin and tobramycin and above 10 μg/ml for amikacin are associated with nephrotoxicity.

c. **Neuromuscular blockade.** This problem may arise in patients receiving high-dose aminoglycoside therapy.

(1) **Risk factors** for neuromuscular blockade include:
(a) Concurrent administration of a neuromuscular blocking agent or an anesthetic
(b) Preexisting hypocalcemia or myasthenia gravis
(c) Intraperitoneal or rapid IV drug administration

(2) Apnea and respiratory depression may be reversed with administration of calcium or an anticholinesterase.

d. **Hypersensitivity** and **local reactions** are rare adverse effects of aminoglycosides.

e. **Therapeutic levels**

(1) Gentamicin and tobramycin peak at 6–10 μg/ml. Their trough level is 0.5–1.5 μg/ml.
(2) Amikacin peaks at 25–30 μg/ml. The trough level is 5–8 μg/ml.

5. **Significant interactions**

a. **IV loop diuretics** can result in increased ototoxicity.
b. **Other aminoglycosides, cephalothin, cisplatin, amphotericin B,** and **methoxyflurane** can cause increased nephrotoxicity when given concurrently with streptomycin.

C. **Cephalosporins.** These agents are known as **β-lactam antibiotics** because their chemical structure consists of a β-lactam ring adjoined to a thiazolidine ring. Cephalosporins generally are classified in three major groups based mainly on their spectrum of activity (Table 43-2).

1. **Mechanism of action.** Cephalosporins are **bactericidal;** they inhibit bacterial cell wall synthesis, reducing cell wall stability, thus causing membrane lysis.

Table 43-2. Classification of Cephalosporins

First-Generation	Second-Generation	Third-Generation	Fourth-Generation
Cefadroxil* (Duricef, Ultracef)	Cefaclor* (Ceclor)	Cefixime* (Suprax)	Cefepime (Maxpime)
Cefazolin (Ancef, Kefzol)	Cefamandole (Mandol)	Cefoperazone (Cefobid)	
Cephalexin* (Keflex)	Cefmetazole (Zefazone)	Cefotaxime (Claforan)	
Cephalothin (Keflin)	Cefonicid (Monocid)	Ceftazidime (Fortax, Taxicef, Tazidime)	
Cephapirin (Cefadyl)	Ceforanide (Precef)	Ceftibuten* (Cedax)	
Cephradine* (Anspor, Velosef)	Cefotetan (Cefotan)	Ceftizoxime (Cefizox)	
	Cefoxitin (Mefoxin)	Ceftriaxone (Rocephin)	
	Cefuroxime (Zinacef)	Moxalactam (Moxam)	
	Cefuroxime axetil* (Ceftin)		
	Cefpodoxime* (Vantin)		
	Cefprozil* (Cefzil)		
	Loracarbef* (Lorabid)		

*Oral agents

2. Spectrum of activity

a. First-generation cephalosporins are active against most gram-positive cocci (except enterococci) as well as enteric aerobic gram-negative bacilli (e.g., *E. coli, K. pneumoniae, Proteus mirabilis*).

b. Second-generation cephalosporins are active against the organisms covered by first-generation cephalosporins and have extended gram-negative coverage, including β-lactamase–producing strains of *Haemophilus influenzae*.

c. Third-generation cephalosporins have wider activity against most gram-negative bacteria; for example, *Enterobacter, Citrobacter, Serratia, Providencia, Neisseria,* and *Haemophilus* organisms, including β-lactamase–producing strains.

d. Fourth-generation cephalosporins. Cefepime is the first member of this group to be marketed. Cefepime is highly resistant to β-lactamases and has a low propensity for selection of β-lactam–resistant mutant strains. Its clinical value continues to be defined.

e. Each generation of cephalosporin has shifted toward increased gram-negative activity but has lost activity toward gram-positive organisms.

3. Therapeutic uses

a. First-generation cephalosporins commonly are administered to treat serious *Klebsiella* infections and gram-positive and some gram-negative infections in patients with mild penicillin allergy. These agents also are used widely in perioperative prophylaxis. For most other indications, they are not the preferred drugs.

b. Second-generation cephalosporins are valuable in the treatment of urinary tract infections resulting from *E. coli* organisms and gonococcal disease caused by organisms that resist other agents.

(1) Cefaclor is useful in otitis media and sinusitis in patients who are allergic to ampicillin and amoxicillin.

(2) Cefoxitin is therapeutic for mixed aerobic–anaerobic infections, such as intra-abdominal infection. **Cefprozil, cefotetan, cefpodoxime,** and **loracarbef** are second-generation cephalosporins that can be administered twice daily but offer no important spectrum differences.

(3) Cefamandole and **cefuroxime** commonly are administered for community-acquired pneumonia.

c. Third-generation cephalosporins penetrate the cerebrospinal fluid (CSF) and, thus, are valuable in the treatment of meningitis caused by such organisms as meningococci, pneumococci, *H. influenzae,* and enteric gram-negative bacilli.

(1) These agents also are used to treat sepsis of unknown origin in immunosuppressed patients and to treat fever in neutropenic immunosuppressed patients (given in combination with an aminoglycoside).

(2) Third-generation cephalosporins are useful in infections caused by many organisms resistant to older cephalosporins.

(3) These agents frequently are administered as empiric therapy for life-threatening infection in which resistant organisms are the most likely cause.

(4) Initial therapy of mixed bacterial infections (e.g., sepsis) commonly involves third-generation cephalosporins.

4. Precautions and monitoring effects

a. Because all cephalosporins (except cefoperazone) are eliminated renally, doses must be adjusted for patients with renal impairment.

b. Cross-sensitivity with penicillin has been reported in up to 10% of patients receiving cephalosporins. More recent information indicates that true cross-reactivity is rare.

c. Cephalosporins can cause hypersensitivity reactions similar to those resulting from penicillin [see II E 1 e (1)]. Manifestations include fever, maculopapular rash, anaphylaxis, and hemolytic anemia.

d. Other adverse effects include nausea, vomiting, diarrhea, superinfection, and nephrotoxicity; *Clostridium difficile*-induced colitis; with cefoperazone, moxalactam, and cefamandole, bleeding diatheses may occur. Bleeding can be reversed by vitamin K administration.

e. Cephalosporins may cause false-positive glycosuria results on tests using the copper reduction method.

5. Significant interactions

a. **Probenecid** may impair the excretion of cephalosporins (except ceftazidime and moxalactam), causing increased cephalosporin levels and possible toxicity.
b. **Alcohol consumption** may result in a disulfiram-type reaction in patients receiving moxalactam, cefoperazone, and cefamandole.
c. **Aminoglycosides** may cause additive toxicity when administered with cephalothin.

D. **Erythromycins.** The chemical structure of these macrolide antibiotics is characterized by a lactone ring to which sugars are attached. Erythromycin base and the estolate, ethylsuccinate, and stearate salts are given orally; erythromycin lactobionate and gluceptate are given parenterally.

1. **Mechanism of action.** Erythromycins may be **bactericidal** or **bacteriostatic;** they bind to the 50S ribosomal subunit, inhibiting bacterial protein synthesis.

2. **Spectrum of activity.** Erythromycins are active against many gram-positive organisms, including streptococci (e.g., *Streptococcus pneumoniae*), and *Corynebacterium* and *Neisseria* species as well as some strains of *Mycoplasma, Legionella, Treponema,* and *Bordetella.* Some *S. aureus* strains that resist penicillin G are susceptible to erythromycins.

3. **Therapeutic uses**
   a. Erythromycins are the preferred drugs for the treatment of *Mycoplasma pneumoniae* and *Campylobacter* infections, legionnaires' disease, chlamydial infections, diphtheria, and pertussis.
   b. In patients with penicillin allergy, erythromycins are important alternatives in the treatment of pneumococcal pneumonia, *S. aureus* infections, syphilis, and gonorrhea.
   c. Erythromycins may be given prophylactically before dental procedures to prevent bacterial endocarditis.

4. **Precautions and monitoring parameters**
   a. Serious adverse effects from erythromycins are rare.
   b. Gastrointestinal (GI) distress (nausea, vomiting, diarrhea, epigastric discomfort) may occur with all erythromycin forms.
   c. Allergic reactions (rare) may present as skin eruptions, fever, and eosinophilia.
   d. Cholestatic hepatitis may arise in patients treated for 1 week or longer with erythromycin estolate; symptoms usually disappear within a few days after drug therapy ends. There have been infrequent reports of hepatotoxicity with other salts of erythromycin.
   e. Intramuscular injections of over 100 mg produce severe pain persisting for hours.
   f. Transient hearing impairment may develop with high-dose erythromycin therapy.

5. **Significant interactions**
   a. Erythromycin inhibits the hepatic metabolism of **theophylline,** resulting in toxic accumulation.
   b. Erythromycin interferes with the metabolism of **digoxin, corticosteroids, carbamazepine, cyclosporin,** and **lovastatin,** possibly potentiating the effect and toxicity of these drugs.
   c. Clarithromycin and erythromycin increase terfenadine concentrations. Cardiac arrhythmia may result. Azithromycin and dirithromycin do not appear to interfere with terfenadine metabolism; however, if used concomitantly, patients should be closely monitored.

6. **Alternatives to erythromycin**
   a. **Clarithromycin, azithromycin,** and **dirithromycin** are semisynthetic macrolide antibiotics. These expensive but well-tolerated alternatives to erythromycin are administered once daily.
      (1) **Clarithromycin**
         (a) **Therapeutic uses.** This agent is indicated for the prevention of *Mycobacterium avium* complex infection and is useful in otitis media, sinusitis, mycoplasmal pneumonia, and pharyngitis. Clarithromycin is also used with omeprazole for *Helicobacter pylori* eradication.
         (b) **Spectrum of activity. Clarithromycin** is more active than erythromycin against staphylococci and streptococci. In addition to activity against other organisms covered by erythromycin, it is also active in vitro against *Mycobacterium avium-intracellulare* (MAI), *Toxoplasma gondii,* and *Cryptosporidium* species.
      (2) **Azithromycin**
         (a) **Therapeutic uses.** This agent is useful in nongonococcal urethritis caused by chlamydia, lower respiratory tract infections, *Mycobacterium avium* complex

infection and prophylaxis, pharyngitis, and legionnaires' disease. Azithromycin is also indicated for pediatric use.

(b) Spectrum of activity. Azithromycin is less active than erythromycin against gram-positive cocci but more active against *H. influenzae* and other gram-negative organisms. Azithromycin concentrates within cells, and tissue levels are higher than serum levels.

(3) Dirithromycin is indicated for the treatment of acute exacerbations of chronic bronchitis, pharyngitis and tonsillitis caused by *Streptococcus pyogenes,* and uncomplicated skin and skin structure infections caused by *S. aureus.*

b. Troleandomycin is similar to erythromycin in most respects, but generally is less active against susceptible organisms.

E. Penicillins

1. Natural penicillins. As with cephalosporins and all other penicillins, natural penicillins are β-lactam antibiotics. Among the most important antibiotics, natural penicillins are the preferred drugs in the treatment of many infectious diseases.

a. Available agents

(1) Penicillin G sodium and potassium salts can be administered orally, intravenously, or intramuscularly.

(2) Penicillin V, a soluble drug form, is administered orally.

(3) Penicillin G procaine and **penicillin G benzathine** are repository drug forms. Administered intramuscularly, these insoluble salts allow slow drug absorption from the injection site and, thus, have a longer duration of action (12–24 hours).

b. Mechanism of action. Penicillins are bactericidal; they inhibit bacterial cell wall synthesis in a manner similar to that of the cephalosporins.

c. Spectrum of activity

(1) Natural penicillins are highly active against gram-positive cocci and against some gram-negative cocci.

(2) Penicillin G is five to ten times more active than penicillin V against gram-negative organisms and some anaerobic organisms.

(3) Because natural penicillins are readily hydrolyzed by penicillinases (β-lactamases), they are ineffective against *S. aureus* and other organisms that resist penicillin.

d. Therapeutic uses

(1) Penicillin G is the preferred agent for all infections caused by *S. pneumoniae* organisms, including:

(a) Pneumonia
(b) Arthritis
(c) Meningitis
(d) Peritonitis
(e) Pericarditis
(f) Osteomyelitis
(g) Mastoiditis

(2) Penicillins G and V are highly effective against other streptococcal infections, such as pharyngitis, otitis media, sinusitis, and bacteremia.

(3) Penicillin G is the preferred agent in gonococcal infections, syphilis, anthrax, actinomycosis, gas gangrene, and *Listeria* infections.

(4) Administered when an oral penicillin is needed, penicillin V is most useful in skin, soft-tissue, and mild respiratory infections.

(5) Penicillin G procaine is effective against syphilis and uncomplicated gonorrhea.

(6) Used to treat syphilis infections outside the CNS, penicillin G benzathine also is effective against group A β-hemolytic streptococcal infections.

(7) Penicillins G and V may be used prophylactically to prevent streptococcal infection, rheumatic fever, and neonatal gonorrhea ophthalmia. Patients with valvular heart disease may receive these drugs preoperatively.

(8) There is emerging resistance to penicillin G by *S. pneumoniae* in some areas of the country. The alternative therapy is vancomycin.

e. Precautions and monitoring effects

(1) Hypersensitivity reactions. These occur in up to 10% of patients receiving penicillin. Manifestations range from mild rash to anaphylaxis.

(a) The rash may be urticarial, vesicular, bullous, scarlatiniform, or maculopapular. Rarely, thrombopenic purpura develops.

(b) Anaphylaxis is a life-threatening reaction that most commonly occurs with parenteral administration. Signs and symptoms include severe hypotension, bronchoconstriction, nausea, vomiting, abdominal pain, and extreme weakness.
(c) Other manifestations of hypersensitivity reactions include fever, eosinophilia, angioedema, and serum sickness.
(d) Before penicillin therapy begins, the patient's history should be evaluated for reactions to penicillin. A positive history places the patient at heightened risk for a subsequent reaction. In most cases, such patients should receive a substitute antibiotic. (However, hypersensitivity reactions may occur even in patients with a negative history.)

(2) **Other adverse effects** of natural penicillins include GI distress (e.g., nausea, diarrhea); bone marrow suppression (e.g., impaired platelet aggregation, agranulocytosis); and superinfection. With high-dose therapy, seizures may occur, particularly in patients with renal impairment.

f. Significant interactions

(1) **Probenecid** increases blood levels of natural penicillins and may be given concurrently for this purpose.
(2) Antibiotic antagonism occurs when **erythromycins, tetracyclines,** or **chloramphenicol** is given within 1 hour of the administration of penicillin. The clinical significance of such antagonism is not clear.
(3) With penicillin G procaine and benzathine, precaution must be used in patients with a history of hypersensitivity reactions to penicillins because prolonged reactions may occur. Intravascular injection should be avoided. Procaine hypersensitivity is a contraindication to the use of procaine penicillin G.
(4) Parenteral products contain either potassium (1.7 mEq/million units) or sodium (2 mEq/million units).

2. **Penicillinase-resistant penicillins.** These penicillins are not hydrolyzed by staphylococcal penicillinases (β-lactamases). These agents include **methicillin, nafcillin,** and the **isoxazolyl penicillins—cloxacillin, dicloxacillin,** and **oxacillin.**

a. Mechanism of action (see II E 1 b)

b. Spectrum of activity. Because these penicillins resist penicillinases, they are active against staphylococci that produce these enzymes.

c. Therapeutic uses

(1) Penicillinase-resistant penicillins are used solely in staphylococcal infections resulting from organisms that resist natural penicillins.
(2) These agents are less potent than natural penicillins against organisms susceptible to natural penicillins and, thus, make poor substitutes in the treatment of infections caused by these organisms.
(3) **Nafcillin** is excreted by the liver and, thus, may be useful in treating staphylococcal infections in patients with renal impairment.
(4) **Oxacillin, cloxacillin,** and **dicloxacillin** are most valuable in long-term therapy of serious staphylococcal infections (e.g., endocarditis, osteomyelitis) and in the treatment of minor staphylococcal infections of the skin and soft tissues.

d. Precautions and monitoring effects

(1) As with all penicillins, the penicillinase-resistant group can cause hypersensitivity reactions [see II E 1 e (1)].
(2) Methicillin may cause nephrotoxicity and interstitial nephritis.
(3) Oxacillin may be hepatotoxic.
(4) Complete cross-resistance exists among the penicillinase-resistant penicillins.

e. Significant interactions. Probenecid increases blood levels of these penicillins and may be given concurrently for that purpose.

3. **Aminopenicillins.** This penicillin group includes the semisynthetic agents **ampicillin** and **amoxicillin** and their derivatives, **bacampicillin** and **cyclacillin.** Because of their wider antibacterial spectrum, these drugs are also known as **broad-spectrum penicillins.**

a. Mechanism of action (see II E 1 b)

b. Spectrum of activity. Aminopenicillins have a spectrum that is similar to but broader than that of the natural and penicillinase-resistant penicillins. Easily destroyed by staphylococcal penicillinases, aminopenicillins are ineffective against most staphylococcal organisms. Against most bacteria sensitive to penicillin G, aminopenicillins are slightly less effective than this agent.

c. **Therapeutic uses.** Aminopenicillins are used to treat gonococcal infections, upper respiratory infections, uncomplicated urinary tract infections, and otitis media caused by susceptible organisms.
   (1) For infections resulting from penicillin-resistant organisms, **ampicillin** may be given in combination with sulbactam.
   (2) **Amoxicillin** is less effective than ampicillin in shigellosis.
   (3) **Amoxicillin** is more effective against *S. aureus, Klebsiella,* and *Bacteroides fragilis* infections when administered in combination with clavulanic acid (amoxicillin/potassium clavulanate) because clavulanic acid inactivates penicillinases.

d. **Precautions and monitoring effects**
   (1) Hypersensitivity reactions may occur [see II E 1 e (1)].
   (2) Diarrhea is most common with ampicillin.
   (3) In addition to the urticarial hypersensitivity rash seen with all penicillins, ampicillin and amoxicillin frequently cause a generalized erythematous, maculopapular rash. (This occurs in 5%–10% of patients receiving ampicillin.)

e. **Significant interactions** (see II E 2 e)

4. **Extended-spectrum penicillins.** These agents have the widest antibacterial spectrum of all penicillins. Also called **antipseudomonal penicillins,** this group includes the **carboxypenicillins** (e.g., **carbenicillin, carbenicillin indanyl, ticarcillin**) and the **ureidopenicillins** (e.g., **azlocillin, mezlocillin, piperacillin**).
   a. **Mechanism of action** (see II E 1 b)
   b. **Spectrum of activity.** These drugs have a spectrum similar to that of the aminopenicillins but also are effective against *Klebsiella* and *Enterobacter* species, some *B. fragilis* organisms, and indole-positive *Proteus* and *Pseudomonas* organisms.
      (1) **Carbenicillin** frequently is active against ampicillin-resistant *Proteus* strains and some other gram-negative organisms.
      (2) **Ticarcillin** is two to four times as active as carbenicillin against *P. aeruginosa.* Combined with clavulanic acid, ticarcillin has enhanced activity against organisms that resist ticarcillin alone.
      (3) **Azlocillin** and **piperacillin** are 10 times as active as carbenicillin against *Pseudomonas* organisms and are more active than carbenicillin against streptococcal organisms.
      (4) **Piperacillin and tazobactam**. Tazobactam is a β-lactamase inhibitor that expands the spectrum of activity to include some organisms not sensitive to piperacillin alone (if resistance is due to β-lactamase production), including strains of staphylococci, *Haemophilus, Bacteroides,* and *Enterobacteriaceae.* Generally, tazobactam does not enhance activity versus *Pseudomonas.*
      (5) **Mezlocillin** and **piperacillin** are more active than carbenicillin against *Klebsiella* organisms.
   c. **Therapeutic uses.** Extended-spectrum penicillins are used mainly to treat serious infections caused by gram-negative organisms (e.g., sepsis; pneumonia; infections of the abdomen, bone, and soft tissues).
   d. **Precautions and monitoring effects**
      (1) Hypersensitivity reactions may occur [see II E 1 e (1)].
      (2) Carbenicillin and ticarcillin may cause hypokalemia.
      (3) The high sodium content of carbenicillin and ticarcillin may pose a danger to patients with congestive heart failure (CHF).
      (4) All inhibit platelet aggregation, which may result in bleeding.
   e. **Significant interactions** (see II E 2 e)

F. **Sulfonamides.** Derivatives of sulfanilamide, these agents were the first drugs to prevent and cure human bacterial infection successfully. Although their current usefulness is limited by the introduction of more effective antibiotics and the emergence of resistant bacterial strains, sulfonamides remain the drugs of choice for certain infections. The major sulfonamides are **sulfadiazine, sulfamethoxazole, sulfisoxazole, sulfacytine,** and **sulfamethizole.**

1. **Mechanism of action.** Sulfonamides are **bacteriostatic;** they suppress bacterial growth by triggering a mechanism that blocks folic acid synthesis, thereby forcing bacteria to synthesize their own folic acid.

2. **Spectrum of activity.** Sulfonamides are broad-spectrum agents with activity against many gram-positive organisms (e.g., *Streptococcus pyrogenes, S. pneumoniae)* and certain gram-

negative organisms (e.g., *H. influenzae, E. coli, P. mirabilis*). They also are effective against certain strains of *Chlamydia trachomatis, Nocardia, Actinomyces,* and *Bacillus anthracis.*

3. **Therapeutic uses**
   a. Sulfonamides most often are used to treat urinary tract infections caused by *E. coli,* including acute and chronic cystitis, and chronic upper urinary tract infections.
   b. These agents have value in the treatment of nocardiosis, trachoma and inclusion conjunctivitis, and dermatitis herpetiformis.
   c. **Sulfadiazine** may be administered in combination with pyrimethamine to treat toxoplasmosis.
   d. **Sulfamethoxazole** may be given in combination with trimethoprim to treat such infections as *Pneumocystis carinii* pneumonia, *Shigella* enteritis, *Serratia* sepsis, urinary tract infections, respiratory infections, and gonococcal urethritis (see II J 7 c).
   e. **Sulfisoxazole** is sometimes used in combination with erythromycin ethylsuccinate to treat acute otitis media caused by *H. influenzae* organisms. For the initial treatment of uncomplicated urinary tract infections, sulfisoxazole may be given in combination with phenazopyridine for relief of symptoms of pain, burning, or urgency.
   f. Prophylactic sulfonamide therapy has been used successfully to prevent streptococcal infections and rheumatic fever recurrences.

4. **Precautions and monitoring effects**
   a. Sulfonamides may cause blood dyscrasias (e.g., hemolytic anemia—particularly in patients with G6PD deficiency, aplastic anemia, thrombocytopenia, agranulocytosis, eosinophilia).
   b. Hypersensitivity reactions to sulfonamides probably result from sensitization and most commonly involve the skin and mucous membranes. Manifestations include various types of skin rash, exfoliative dermatitis, and photosensitivity. Drug fever and serum sickness also may develop.
   c. Crystalluria and hematuria may occur, possibly leading to urinary tract obstruction. (Adequate fluid intake and urine alkalinization can prevent or minimize this risk.) Sulfonamides should be used cautiously in patients with renal impairment.
   d. Life-threatening hepatitis caused by drug toxicity or sensitization is a rare adverse effect. Signs and symptoms include headache, nausea, vomiting, and jaundice.
   e. AIDS patients have increased frequency of cutaneous hypersensitivity reactions to sulfamethoxazole.

5. **Significant interactions.** Sulfonamides may potentiate the effects of **phenytoin, oral anticoagulants,** and **sulfonylureas.**

G. **Tetracyclines.** These broad-spectrum agents are effective against certain bacterial strains that resist other antibiotics. Nonetheless, they are the preferred drugs in only a few situations. The major tetracyclines include **demeclocycline, doxycycline, methacycline, minocycline,** and **chlortetracycline.**

1. **Mechanism of action.** Tetracyclines are **bacteriostatic;** they inhibit bacterial protein synthesis by binding to the 30S ribosomal subunit.

2. **Spectrum of activity.** Tetracyclines are active against gram-negative and gram-positive organisms, spirochetes, *Mycoplasma* and *Chlamydia* organisms, rickettsial species, and certain protozoa.
   a. *Pseudomonas* and *Proteus* organisms are now resistant to tetracyclines. Many coliform bacteria, pneumococci, staphylococci, streptococci, and *Shigella* strains are increasingly resistant.
   b. Cross-resistance within the tetracycline group is extensive.

3. **Therapeutic uses**
   a. Tetracyclines are the agents of choice in rickettsial (Rocky Mountain spotted fever), chlamydial, and mycoplasmal infections; amebiasis; and bacillary infections (e.g., cholera, brucellosis, tularemia, some *Salmonella* and *Shigella* infections).
   b. Tetracyclines are useful alternatives to penicillin in the treatment of anthrax, syphilis, gonorrhea, Lyme disease, nocardiosis, and *H. influenzae* respiratory infections.
   c. Oral or topical tetracycline may be administered as a treatment for acne.
   d. **Doxycycline** is highly effective in the prophylaxis of "traveler's diarrhea" (commonly caused by *E. coli*). Because the drug is excreted mainly in the feces, it is the safest tetracycline for the treatment of extrarenal infections in patients with renal impairment.

e. **Demeclocycline** is used commonly as an adjunctive agent to treat the **syndrome of inappropriate antidiuretic hormone (SIADH)** secretion.

4. **Precautions and monitoring effects**
   a. GI distress (e.g., diarrhea, abdominal discomfort, nausea, anorexia) is a common adverse effect of tetracyclines. This problem can be minimized by administering the drug with food or temporarily decreasing the dosage.
   b. Skin rash, urticaria, and generalized exfoliative dermatitis signify a hypersensitivity reaction. Rarely, angioedema and anaphylaxis occur.
   c. Cross-sensitivity within the tetracycline group is common.
   d. Phototoxic reactions (severe skin lesions) can develop with exposure to sunlight. This reaction is most common with demeclocycline and doxycycline.
   e. Tetracyclines may cause hepatotoxicity, particularly in pregnant women. Manifestations include jaundice, acidosis, and fatty liver infiltration.
   f. Renally impaired patients may experience a significant increase in BUN secondary to catabolic effects of tetracyclines.
   g. Tetracyclines may induce permanent tooth discoloration, tooth enamel defects, and retarded bone growth in infants and children.
   h. Use of outdated and degraded tetracyclines can lead to renal tubular dysfunction, possibly resulting in renal failure.
   i. Minocycline can cause vestibular toxicity (e.g., ataxia, dizziness, nausea, vomiting).
   j. IV tetracyclines are irritating and may cause phlebitis.

5. **Significant interactions**
   a. **Dairy products** and other foods, **iron preparations,** and **antacids** and **laxatives** containing aluminum, calcium, or magnesium can cause reduced tetracycline absorption. Absorption of doxycycline is not inhibited by these factors.
   b. **Methoxyflurane** may exacerbate the tetracyclines' nephrotoxic effects.
   c. **Barbiturates** and **phenytoin** decrease the antibiotic effectiveness of tetracyclines.
   d. Demeclocycline antagonizes the action of **antidiuretic hormone (ADH)** and may be given as a diuretic in patients with SIADH.

H. **Fluoroquinolones** are agents related to nalidixic acid [see II I 1 c, 2 c (1), 4 c (1)] and include **ciprofloxacin, enoxacin, lomefloxacin, norfloxacin,** and **ofloxacin.** They are bactericidal for growing bacteria.

1. **Mechanism of action.** Fluoroquinolones inhibit DNA gyrase.

2. **Spectrum of activity.** Fluoroquinolones are highly active against enteric gram-negative bacilli, *Salmonella, Shigella, Campylobacter, Haemophilus,* and *Neisseria.*
   a. **Ciprofloxacin** has good activity against *P. aeruginosa,* but the fluoroquinolones as a group have variable activity against non–*P. aeruginosa.* Ciprofloxacin is active against many anaerobes; it has moderate activity against *M. tuberculosis.*
   b. Gram-positive organisms are less susceptible than gram-negative organisms but usually are sensitive except for *Enterococcus faecalis* and methicillin-resistant staphylococci.
   c. **Ofloxacin** has the greatest activity against *Chlamydia.*

3. **Therapeutic uses**
   a. Norfloxacin is indicated for the oral treatment of urinary tract infections, uncomplicated gonococcal infections, and prostatitis.
   b. Ciprofloxacin and ofloxacin are available orally and intravenously. Ciprofloxacin is approved for use in urinary tract infections; lower respiratory infections; bone, joint, and skin structure infections; typhoid fever; urethral and cervical gonococcal infections; and infectious diarrhea. Ofloxacin is approved for use in lower respiratory infections, uncomplicated gonococcal and chlamydial cervicitis and urethritis, skin and skin structure infections, prostatitis, and urinary tract infections.
   c. Lomefloxacin and enoxacin are approved for the treatment of urinary tract infections. Lomefloxacin is also used in lower respiratory infections and enoxacin in uncomplicated gonococcal infections. These agents offer no improvement in the spectrum of activity as compared to other fluoroquinolones.

4. **Precautions and monitoring effects**
   a. Occasional adverse effects include nausea, dyspepsia, headache, dizziness, and insomnia.

b. Infrequent adverse effects include rash, urticaria, leukopenia, and elevated liver enzymes.
c. Crystalluria occurs with high doses at alkaline pH.
d. Cartilage erosion has been observed in young animals; thus, fluoroquinolones should not be used in children or in women who are pregnant or nursing.

5. **Significant interactions**
   a. Ciprofloxacin has been shown to increase **theophylline** levels. Variable effects on theophylline levels have been reported from other members of the group. In patients requiring fluoroquinolones, theophylline levels should be monitored.
   b. **Antacids** and **sucralfate** may significantly decrease the absorption of fluoroquinolones.
   c. Fluoroquinolones may increase prothrombin times in patients receiving **warfarin.**
   d. Concurrent use with **nonsteroidal anti-inflammatory drugs** (NSAIDs) may increase the risk of CNS stimulation (seizures).

I. **Urinary tract antiseptics.** Concentrating in the renal tubules and bladder, these agents exert local antibacterial effects; most do not achieve blood levels high enough to treat systemic infections. [However, some new quinolone derivatives, such as ciprofloxacin and ofloxacin, are valuable in the treatment of certain infections outside the urinary tract (see II H 3 b).]

1. **Mechanism of action**
   a. **Methenamine** is hydrolyzed to ammonia and formaldehyde in acidic urine; formaldehyde is antibacterial against gram-positive and gram-negative organisms. Mandelic and hippuric acids, with which methenamine is combined, provide supplementary antibacterial action.
   b. **Nitrofurantoin** is **bacteriostatic;** in high concentrations, it may be **bactericidal.** Presumably, it disrupts bacterial enzyme systems.
   c. **Quinolones. Nalidixic acid** and its analogues and derivatives—**oxolinic acid, norfloxacin, cinoxacin, ciprofloxacin, pefloxacin,** and others—interfere with DNA gyrase and inhibit DNA synthesis during bacterial replication.

2. **Spectrum of activity**
   a. **Methenamine** is active against both gram-positive and gram-negative organisms (e.g., *Enterobacter, Klebsiella, Proteus, P. aeruginosa, S. aureus).*
   b. **Nitrofurantoin** is active against many gram-positive and gram-negative organisms, including some strains of *E. coli, S. aureus, Proteus, Enterobacter,* and *Klebsiella.*
   c. **Quinolones** (see II H)
      (1) **Nalidixic acid** and **oxolinic acid** are active against most gram-negative organisms that cause urinary tract infections, including *P. mirabilis, E. coli, Klebsiella,* and *Enterobacter* organisms. These drugs are not effective against *Pseudomonas* organisms.
      (2) **Norfloxacin** is active against *E. coli, Enterobacter, Klebsiella, Proteus, P. aeruginosa, S. aureus, Citrobacter,* and some *Streptococcus* organisms.
      (3) **Cinoxacin** is active against *E. coli, Klebsiella, P. mirabilis, Proteus vulgaris, Proteus morganii, Serratia,* and *Citrobacter* organisms.

3. **Therapeutic uses**
   a. **Methenamine** and **nitrofurantoin** are used to prevent and treat urinary tract infections.
   b. **Quinolones** are administered to treat urinary tract infections; some also are used in such diseases as osteomyelitis and respiratory tract infections.

4. **Precautions and monitoring effects**
   a. **Methenamine** may cause nausea, vomiting, and diarrhea; in high doses, it may lead to urinary tract irritation (e.g., dysuria, frequency, hematuria, albuminuria). Skin rash also may develop.
   b. **Nitrofurantoin** may cause various adverse effects.
      (1) GI distress (e.g., nausea, vomiting, diarrhea) is relatively common.
      (2) Hypersensitivity reactions to nitrofurantoin may involve the skin, lungs, blood, or liver; manifestations include fever, chills, hepatitis, jaundice, leukopenia, hemolytic anemia, granulocytopenia, and pneumonitis.
      (3) Adverse CNS effects include headache, vertigo, and dizziness. Polyneuropathy may develop with high doses or in patients with renal impairment.
   c. **Quinolones**
      (1) **Nalidixic acid** and **oxolinic acid** may cause nausea, vomiting, abdominal pain, urticaria, pruritus, skin rash, fever, eosinophilia, and CNS effects, such as headache, dizziness, confusion, vertigo, drowsiness, and weakness.

(2) **Cinoxacin** may induce nausea, vomiting, diarrhea, headache, insomnia, skin rash, pruritus, and urticaria.

5. **Significant interactions**
   a. The effects of methenamine are inhibited by **alkalinizing agents** and are antagonized by **acetazolamide.**
   b. Nitrofurantoin absorption is decreased by **magnesium-containing antacids.** Nitrofurantoin blood levels are increased and urine levels decreased by **sulfinpyrazone** and **probenecid,** leading to increased toxicity and reduced therapeutic effectiveness.
   c. **Quinolones**
      (1) Cinoxacin urine levels are decreased by **probenecid,** reducing therapeutic effectiveness.
      (2) Norfloxacin is rendered less effective by **antacids.**

J. Miscellaneous antibacterial agents

1. **Aztreonam.** This agent was the first commercially available monobactam (monocyclic β-lactam compound). It resembles the aminoglycosides in its efficacy against many gram-negative organisms but does not cause nephrotoxicity or ototoxicity. Other advantages of this drug include its ability to preserve the body's normal gram-positive and anaerobic flora, activity against many gentamicin-resistant organisms, and lack of cross-allergenicity with penicillin.
   a. **Mechanism of action.** Aztreonam is **bactericidal;** it inhibits bacterial cell wall synthesis.
   b. **Spectrum of activity.** This drug is active against many gram-negative organisms, including *Enterobacter* and *P. aeruginosa.*
   c. **Therapeutic uses.** Aztreonam is therapeutic for urinary tract infections, septicemia, skin infections, lower respiratory tract infections, and intra-abdominal infections resulting from gram-negative organisms.
   d. **Precautions and monitoring effects**
      (1) Aztreonam sometimes causes nausea, vomiting, and diarrhea.
      (2) Liver enzymes may increase transiently during aztreonam therapy.
      (3) This drug may induce skin rash.

2. **Chloramphenicol.** A nitrobenzene derivative, this drug has broad activity against rickettsia as well as many gram-positive and gram-negative organisms. It also is effective against many ampicillin-resistant strains of *H. influenzae.*
   a. **Mechanism of action.** Chloramphenicol is primarily **bacteriostatic,** although it may be bactericidal against a few bacterial strains.
   b. **Spectrum of activity.** This agent is active against rickettsia and a wide range of bacteria, including *H. influenzae, Salmonella typhi, Neisseria meningitidis, Bordetella pertussis, Clostridium, B. fragilis, S. pyogenes,* and *S. pneumoniae.*
   c. **Therapeutic uses.** Because of its toxic side effects, chloramphenicol is used only to suppress infections that cannot be treated effectively with other antibiotics. Such infections typically include:
      (1) Typhoid fever
      (2) Meningococcal infections in cephalosporin-allergic patients
      (3) Serious *H. influenzae* infections, particularly in cephalosporin-allergic patients
      (4) Anaerobic infections (e.g., those originating in the pelvis or intestines)
      (5) Anaerobic or mixed infections of the CNS
      (6) Rickettsial infections in pregnant patients, tetracycline-allergic patients, and renally impaired patients
   d. **Precautions and monitoring effects**
      (1) Chloramphenicol can cause bone marrow suppression (dose-related) with resulting pancytopenia; rarely, the drug leads to aplastic anemia (non–dose-related).
      (2) Hypersensitivity reactions may include skin rash and, in extremely rare cases, angioedema or anaphylaxis.
      (3) Chloramphenicol therapy may lead to gray baby syndrome in neonates (especially premature infants). This dangerous reaction, which stems partly from inadequate liver detoxification of the drug, is manifested by vomiting, gray cyanosis, rapid and irregular respirations, vasomotor collapse, and, in some cases, death.
   e. **Significant interactions**

(1) Chloramphenicol inhibits the metabolism of **phenytoin, tolbutamide, chlorpropamide,** and **dicumarol,** leading to prolonged action and intensified effect of these drugs.
(2) **Phenobarbital** shortens chloramphenicol's half-life, thereby reducing its therapeutic effectiveness.
(3) **Penicillins** can cause antibiotic antagonism.
(4) **Acetaminophen** elevates chloramphenicol levels and may cause toxicity.

3. **Clindamycin.** This agent has essentially replaced lincomycin, the drug from which it is derived. It is used to treat skin, respiratory tract, and soft-tissue infections caused by staphylococci, pneumococci, and streptococci.
   a. **Mechanism of action.** Clindamycin is **bacteriostatic;** it binds to the 50S ribosomal subunit, thereby suppressing bacterial protein synthesis.
   b. **Spectrum of activity.** This agent is active against most gram-positive and many anaerobic organisms, including *B. fragilis.*
   c. **Therapeutic uses.** Because of its marked toxicity, clindamycin is used only against infections for which it has proven to be the most effective drug. Typically, such infections include abdominal and female genitourinary tract infections caused by *B. fragilis.*
   d. **Precautions and monitoring effects**
      (1) Clindamycin may cause rash, nausea, vomiting, diarrhea, and pseudomembranous colitis as evidenced by fever, abdominal pain, and bloody stools.
      (2) Blood dyscrasias (e.g., eosinophilia, thrombocytopenia, leukopenia) may occur.
   e. **Significant interactions.** Clindamycin may potentiate the effects of **neuromuscular blocking agents.**

4. **Dapsone.** A member of the sulfone class, this drug is the primary agent in the treatment of all forms of leprosy.
   a. **Mechanism of action.** Dapsone is **bacteriostatic** for *Mycobacterium leprae;* its mechanism of action probably resembles that of the sulfonamides.
   b. **Spectrum of activity.** This drug is active against *M. leprae;* however, drug resistance develops in up to 40% of patients. Dapsone also has some activity against *P. carinii* organisms and the malarial parasite *Plasmodium.*
   c. **Therapeutic uses**
      (1) Dapsone is the drug of choice for treating leprosy.
      (2) This agent may be used to treat dermatitis herpetiformis, a skin disorder.
      (3) Maloprim, a dapsone-pyrimethamine product, is valuable in the prophylaxis and treatment of malaria.
      (4) Dapsone, with or without trimethoprim, is used for prophylaxis of *P. carinii* pneumonia in patients with AIDS.
   d. **Precautions and monitoring effects**
      (1) Hemolytic anemia can occur with daily doses above 200 mg. Other adverse hematologic effects include methemoglobinemia and leukopenia.
      (2) Nausea, vomiting, and anorexia may develop.
      (3) Adverse CNS effects include headache, dizziness, nervousness, lethargy, paresthesias, and psychosis.
      (4) Dapsone occasionally results in a potentially lethal mononucleosis-like syndrome.
      (5) Paradoxically, this drug sometimes exacerbates leprosy.
      (6) Other adverse effects include skin rash, peripheral neuropathy, blurred vision, tinnitus, hepatitis, and cholestatic jaundice.
   e. **Significant interactions. Probenecid** elevates blood levels of dapsone, possibly resulting in toxicity.

5. **Imipenem.** Formerly known as thienamycin, imipenem is the first carbapenem compound introduced in the United States. A β-lactam antibiotic, it resists destruction by most β-lactamases. Because it is inhibited by renal dipeptidases, imipenem must be combined with cilastatin sodium, a dipeptidase inhibitor.
   a. **Mechanism of action.** Imipenem is **bactericidal;** it inhibits bacterial cell wall synthesis.
   b. **Spectrum of activity.** This drug has the broadest spectrum of all β-lactam antibiotics. It is active against most gram-positive cocci (including many enterococci), gram-negative rods (including many *P. aeruginosa* strains), and anaerobes. It has good activity against many bacterial strains that resist other antibiotics.

c. **Therapeutic uses.** Imipenem has most value in the treatment of severe infections caused by drug-resistant organisms susceptible only to imipenem.

d. **Precautions and monitoring effects**
   (1) Imipenem may cause nausea, vomiting, diarrhea, and pseudomembranous colitis.
   (2) Seizures, dizziness, and hypotension may develop.
   (3) Patients who are allergic to penicillin or cephalosporins may suffer cross-allergy during imipenem therapy.

e. **Meropenem,** recently introduced, has a similar antimicrobial spectrum. It appears less likely to cause seizures, which may make this drug more useful than imipenem to treat meningitis. It does not require the addition of cilastatin because it is not metabolized by the same enzyme as imipenem.

6. **Spectinomycin.** An aminocyclitol agent related to the aminoglycosides, this antibiotic is useful against penicillin-resistant strains of gonorrhea.
   a. **Mechanism of action.** Spectinomycin is **bacteriostatic;** it selectively inhibits protein synthesis by binding to the 30S ribosomal subunit.
   b. **Spectrum of activity.** This agent is active against various gram-negative organisms.
   c. **Therapeutic uses.** Spectinomycin is used only to treat gonococcal infections in patients with penicillin allergy or when such infection stems from penicillinase-producing gonococci (PPNG).
   d. **Precautions and monitoring effects.** Because spectinomycin is given only as a single-dose intramuscular injection, it causes few adverse effects. Nausea, vomiting, urticaria, chills, dizziness, and insomnia occur rarely.

7. **Trimethoprim.** A substituted pyrimidine, trimethoprim is most commonly combined with sulfamethoxazole (a sulfonamide discussed in II F) in a preparation called co-trimoxazole. However, it may be used alone for certain urinary tract infections.
   a. **Mechanism of action.** Trimethoprim inhibits dihydrofolate reductase, thus blocking bacterial synthesis of folic acid.
   b. **Spectrum of activity.** This agent is active against various gram-negative organisms.
      (1) Trimethoprim is active against most gram-negative and gram-positive organisms. However, drug resistance may develop when this drug is used alone.
      (2) Trimethoprim–sulfamethoxazole is active against a variety of organisms, including *S. pneumoniae, N. meningitidis,* and *Corynebacterium diphtheriae* and some strains of *S. aureus, Staphylococcus epidermidis, P. mirabilis, Enterobacter, Salmonella, Shigella, Serratia,* and *Klebsiella* species, and *E. coli.*
      (3) The trimethoprim–sulfamethoxazole combination is synergistic; many organisms resistant to one component are susceptible to the combination.
   c. **Therapeutic uses**
      (1) Trimethoprim may be used alone or in combination with sulfamethoxazole to treat uncomplicated urinary tract infections caused by *E. coli, P. mirabilis,* and *Klebsiella* and *Enterobacter* organisms.
      (2) Trimethoprim–sulfamethoxazole is therapeutic for acute gonococcal urethritis, acute exacerbation of chronic bronchitis, shigellosis, and *Salmonella* infections.
      (3) Trimethoprim–sulfamethoxazole may be given as prophylactic or suppressive therapy in *P. carinii* pneumonia.
   d. **Precautions and monitoring effects**
      (1) Most adverse effects involve the skin (possibly from sensitization). These include rash, pruritus, and exfoliative dermatitis.
      (2) Rarely, trimethoprim–sulfamethoxazole causes blood dyscrasias (e.g., acute hemolytic anemia, leukopenia, thrombocytopenia, methemoglobinemia, agranulocytosis, aplastic anemia).
      (3) Adverse GI effects including nausea, vomiting, and epigastric distress glossitis may occur.
      (4) Neonates may develop kernicterus.
      (5) Patients with AIDS sometimes suffer fever, rash, malaise, and pancytopenia during trimethoprim therapy.

8. **Vancomycin.** This glycopeptide destroys most gram-positive organisms.
   a. **Mechanism of action.** Vancomycin is **bactericidal;** it inhibits bacterial cell wall synthesis.
   b. **Spectrum of activity.** This drug is active against most gram-positive organisms, including methicillin-resistant strains of *S. aureus.*

c. **Therapeutic uses.** Vancomycin usually is reserved for serious infections, especially those caused by methicillin-resistant staphylococci. It is particularly useful in patients who are allergic to penicillin or cephalosporins. Typical uses include endocarditis, osteomyelitis, and staphylococcal pneumonia.

(1) Oral vancomycin is valuable in the treatment of antibiotic-induced pseudomembranous colitis caused by *Clostridium difficile* or *S. aureus* enterocolitis. Because vancomycin is not absorbed after oral administration, it is not useful for systemic infections. Because of resistance, the Centers for Disease Control recommend vancomycin as the second choice to metronidazole for *C. difficile* infections.

(2) Because 1 g provides adequate blood levels for 7–10 days, IV vancomycin is particularly useful in the treatment of anephric patients with gram-positive bacterial infections.

d. **Precautions and monitoring effects**

(1) Ototoxicity may arise; nephrotoxicity is rare but can occur with high doses.

(2) Vancomycin may cause hypersensitivity reactions, manifested by such symptoms as anaphylaxis or skin rash.

(3) Therapeutic levels peak at 20–40 μg/ml. The trough is less than 10 μg/ml.

(4) "Red man's syndrome" may occur. This is facial flushing and hypotension due to too rapid infusion of the drug. Infusion should be over a minimum of 60 minutes for a 1-g dose.

(5) IV solutions are very irritating to the vein.

e. **Vancomycin-resistant enterococci.** A few strains of vancomycin-resistant enterococci are susceptible to teicoplanin (investigational by Marion Merrel Dow) and Quinupristin/dalfopristin (Synercid) by Rhone Poulenac Rorer. These agents may be useful for multiple drug-resistant *Enterococcus faecium.*

9. **Clofazimine** is Phenazine dye with antimycobacterial and anti-inflammatory activity.

a. **Mechanism of action.** Clofazimine appears to bind preferentially to mycobacterial DNA, inhibiting replication and growth. It is **bactericidal** against *M. leprae,* and it appears to be **bacteriostatic** against *M. avium-intracellulare.*

b. **Spectrum of activity.** Clofazimine is active against various *Mycobacterium,* including *M. leprae, M. tuberculosis,* and *M. avium-intracellulare.*

c. **Therapeutic uses.** Clofazimine is used to treat leprosy and a variety of atypical *Mycobacterium* infections.

d. **Precautions and monitoring effects**

(1) Pigmentation (pink to brownish) occurs in 75%–100% of patients within a few weeks. This skin discoloration has led to severe depression (and suicide).

(2) Urine, sweat, and other body fluids may be discolored.

(3) Other effects include ichthyosis and dryness of skin (8%–28%), rash and pruritus (1%–5%), and GI intolerance (e.g, abdominal/epigastric pain, diarrhea, nausea, vomiting) in 40%–50% of patients. Clofazimine should be taken with food.

III. ANTIFUNGAL AGENTS

A. **Definition.** These agents treat systemic and local fungal (mycotic) infections—diseases that resist treatment with antibacterial drugs.

B. **Amphotericin B.** This polyene antibiotic is therapeutic for various fungal infections that frequently proved fatal before the drug became available. It is used increasingly in the empiric treatment of severely immunocompromised patients in certain clinical situations.

1. **Mechanism of action.** Amphotericin B is both fungicidal and fungistatic; it binds to sterols in the fungal cell membrane, thereby increasing membrane permeability and permitting leakage of intracellular contents. Other mechanisms may be involved as well.

2. **Spectrum of activity.** Amphotericin B is a broad-spectrum antifungal agent with activity against *Histoplasma capsulatum, Cryptococcus neoformans, Coccidioides immitis,* and *Candida* species. Many strains of *Aspergillus* and *Sporothrix schenckii* also are susceptible.

3. **Therapeutic uses.** Amphotericin B is the most effective antifungal agent in the treatment of systemic fungal infections, especially in immunocompromised patients.

a. It is therapeutic for meningitis, histoplasmosis, coccidioidomycosis, blastomycosis, cryptococcosis, disseminated moniliasis, aspergillosis, and phycomycosis.
b. This agent may be used to treat coccidioidal arthritis.
c. Topical preparations are given to eradicate cutaneous and mucocutaneous candidiasis.

4. **Precautions and monitoring effects.** Because amphotericin B can cause many serious adverse effects, it should be administered in a hospital setting—at least during the initial therapeutic stage.
   a. Nephrotoxicity occurs in most patients; those with serious preexisting renal impairment may require dosage reduction or temporary drug discontinuation.
   b. Adverse CNS effects include headache, peripheral neuropathy, convulsions, and seizures.
   c. Adverse GI effects include nausea, vomiting, diarrhea, anorexia, and cramps.
   d. Fever, malaise, and chills may be minimized by pretreatment with aspirin, acetaminophen, diphenhydramine, or by the addition of hydrocortisone to the IV infusion.
   e. Parenteral administration may cause local pain, thrombophlebitis, burning, stinging, irritation, and tissue damage with extravasation. Addition of heparin (100 units/infusion) helps minimize these effects.

5. **Significant interactions.** Other nephrotoxic drugs may cause additive nephrotoxicity.

6. Amphotericin B lipid complex (Abelcet) injection offers an alternative formulation of amphotericin B indicated for the treatment of aspergillosis in patients who are intolerant of or whose disease is refractory to conventional treatment.

C. **Flucytosine.** This fluorinated pyrimidine usually is given in combination with amphotericin B.

1. **Mechanism of action.** Flucytosine penetrates fungal cells and is converted to fluorouracil, a metabolic antagonist. Incorporated into the RNA of the fungal cell, flucytosine causes defective protein synthesis.

2. **Spectrum of activity.** This drug is active against some strains of *Cryptococcus, Candida, Aspergillus, Torulopsis,* and certain other fungal species. In combination with amphotericin B, flucytosine results in synergistic activity against *C. neoformans* and some strains of *Candida tropicalis* and *Candida albicans.*

3. **Therapeutic uses.** Flucytosine is therapeutic for systemic infections (e.g., septicemia, endocarditis, pulmonary and urinary tract infections, meningitis). In most cases, it is given with amphotericin B.

4. **Precautions and monitoring effects**
   a. Although flucytosine is less toxic than amphotericin B, it may cause serious adverse effects, including bone marrow suppression, severe enterocolitis, and hepatomegaly.
   b. Nausea, vomiting, diarrhea, dizziness, drowsiness, and skin rash also may occur.
   c. Flucytosine may increase serum creatinine values on tests using the EKTACHEM method.

D. **Griseofulvin.** Produced from *Penicillium griseofulvum dierckx,* this drug is deposited in the skin, bound to keratin.

1. **Mechanism of action.** This agent is **fungistatic;** it inhibits fungal cell activity by interfering with mitotic spindle structure.

2. **Spectrum of activity.** Griseofulvin is active against various strains of *Microsporum, Epidermophyton,* and *Trichophyton.*

3. **Therapeutic uses.** Griseofulvin is effective in tinea infections of the skin, hair, and nails (including athlete's foot) caused by *Microsporum, Epidermophyton,* and *Trichophyton.*
   a. Generally, this agent is given only for infections that do not respond to topical antifungal agents.
   b. Griseofulvin is available only in oral form.

4. **Precautions and monitoring effects**
   a. Griseofulvin rarely results in serious adverse effects. However, the following problems have been reported:
      (1) Headache, fatigue, confusion, impaired performance, syncope, and lethargy
      (2) Leukopenia, neutropenia, and granulocytopenia

(3) Serum sickness, angioedema, urticaria, erythema, and hepatotoxicity

b. The dosage is dependent on the particle size of the product: 250 mg of ultramicrosize is equivalent in therapeutic effects to 500 mg of microsize.

5. **Significant interactions**

a. Griseofulvin may increase the metabolism of **warfarin,** leading to decreased prothrombin time.

b. **Barbiturates** may reduce griseofulvin absorption.

c. **Alcohol consumption** may cause tachycardia and flushing.

E. **Imidazoles.** The substituted imidazole derivatives **ketoconazole, miconazole, fluconazole,** and **itraconazole** are valuable in the treatment of a wide range of systemic fungal infections.

1. **Mechanism of action.** Imidazoles inhibit sterol synthesis in fungal cell membranes and increase cell wall permeability; this, in turn, makes the cell more vulnerable to osmotic pressure. These agents are **fungistatic.**

2. **Spectrum of activity.** These agents are active against many fungi, including yeasts, dermatophytes, actinomycetes, and some *Phycomycetes.*

3. **Therapeutic uses**

a. **Ketoconazole,** an oral agent, successfully treats many fungal infections that previously yielded only to parenteral agents.

(1) It is therapeutic for systemic and vaginal candidiasis, mucocandidiasis, candiduria, oral thrush, histoplasmosis, coccidioidomycosis, chromomycosis, and paracoccidioidomycosis.

(2) Because ketoconazole is slow-acting and requires a long duration of therapy (up to 6 months for some chronic infections), it is less effective than other antifungal agents for the treatment of severe and acute systemic infections.

b. **Miconazole,** primarily administered as a topical agent, also is available in parenteral form.

(1) Topical miconazole is highly effective in vulvovaginal candidiasis, ringworm, and other skin infections.

(2) Parenteral miconazole serves as a second-line agent in severe systemic fungal infections only when other antifungal drugs are ineffective or cannot be tolerated.

c. **Fluconazole.** Available in oral and parenteral forms, fluconazole can be used against systemic and CNS infections involving *Cryptococcus* and *Candida. Candida* oropharyngeal infection and esophagitis may also be treated with fluconazole. *Aspergillus, coccidioides,* and *Histoplasma* have demonstrated in vitro sensitivity.

d. **Itraconazole** is available as an oral agent with activity against systemic and invasive pulmonary aspergillosis without the hematologic toxicity of amphotericin B. Other deep mycotic infections susceptible to itraconazole include blastomycosis, coccidioidomycosis, cryptococcosis, and histoplasmosis.

4. **Precautions and monitoring effects**

a. **Ketoconazole** may cause nausea, vomiting, diarrhea, abdominal pain, and constipation. Rarely, it leads to headache, dizziness, gynecomastia, and fatal hepatotoxicity.

b. **Parenteral miconazole therapy** frequently induces nausea, vomiting, diarrhea, phlebitis, pruritic rash, anaphylactoid reaction, CNS toxicity, and hyponatremia. Dose-related anemia and thrombocytosis may also occur.

c. **Fluconazole** commonly causes GI disturbances (e.g., nausea, vomiting, epigastric pain, diarrhea). Reversible elevations in serum aminotransferase, exfoliative skin reactions, and headaches have been reported.

d. **Itraconazole** may cause nausea, vomiting, hypertriglyceridemia, hypokalemia, rash, and elevations in liver enzymes.

5. **Significant interactions**

a. Both **ketoconazole** and **miconazole** may enhance the anticoagulant effect of **warfarin.**

b. **Ketoconazole** may antagonize the antibiotic effects of **amphotericin B.**

c. **Fluconazole** has been shown to elevate serum levels of **phenytoin, cyclosporine, warfarin,** and **sulfonylureas.** Concurrent hepatic enzyme inducers, such as **rifampin,** have resulted in increased elimination of both fluconazole and itraconazole.

d. Coadministration of **itraconazole** or **ketoconazole** with **astemizole** or **terfenadine** may result in increased astemizole or terfenadine levels, possibly leading to life-threatening dysrhythmias and death.

F. Nystatin. A polyene antibiotic, nystatin has a chemical structure similar to that of amphotericin B.

1. **Mechanism of action.** Nystatin is **fungicidal** and **fungistatic;** binding to sterols in the fungal cell membrane, it increases membrane permeability and permits leakage of intracellular contents.

2. **Spectrum of activity.** Nystatin is active against *Candida, Cryptococcus, Histoplasma,* and *Blastomyces* organisms.

3. **Therapeutic uses**
   a. This drug is used primarily as a topical agent in vaginal and oral *Candida* infections.
   b. Oral nystatin is therapeutic for *Candida* infections of the GI tract, especially oral and esophageal infections.

4. **Precautions and monitoring effects.** Oral nystatin occasionally causes GI distress (e.g., nausea, vomiting, diarrhea). Rarely, hypersensitivity reactions occur.

IV. ANTIPROTOZOAL AGENTS

A. Classification. These drugs fall into two main categories: **antimalarial agents,** used to treat malaria infection; and **amebicides** and **trichomonacides,** used to treat amebic and trichomonal infections.

B. Antimalarial agents. Still a leading cause of illness and death in tropical and subtropical countries, malaria results from infection by any of four species of the protozoal genus *Plasmodium.* Antimalarial agents are selectively active during different phases of the protozoan life cycle. Major antimalarial drugs include **chloroquine, primaquine, pyrimethamine, quinine, fansidar,** and **mefloquine.**

1. **Mechanism of action**
   a. **Chloroquine** binds to and alters the properties of microbial and mammalian DNA.
   b. The mechanism of action of **primaquine, quinine, fansidar,** and **mefloquine** is unknown.
   c. **Pyrimethamine** impedes folic acid reduction by inhibiting the enzyme dihydrofolate reductase.

2. **Spectrum of activity**
   a. **Chloroquine,** a suppressive agent, is active against the asexual erythrocyte forms of *Plasmodium vivax* and *Plasmodium falciparum* and gametocytes of *P. vivax, Plasmodium malariae,* and *Plasmodium ovale.*
   b. **Primaquine,** a curative agent, is active against liver forms of *P. vivax* and *P. ovale* and the primary exoerythrocyte forms of *P. falciparum.*
   c. **Pyrimethamine** is active against chloroquine-resistant strains of *P. falciparum* and some strains of *P. vivax.*
   d. **Quinine,** a generalized protoplasmic poison, is toxic to a wide range of organisms. In malaria, this drug has both suppressive and curative action against chloroquine-resistant strains.
   e. **Fansidar** is a blood **schizonticidal** agent that is active against the erythrocytic forms of susceptible plasmodia. It is also active against *T. gondii.*
   f. **Mefloquine** is a blood schizonticidal agent that is active against *P. falciparum* (both chloroquine-susceptible and resistant strains) and *P. vivax.*

3. **Therapeutic uses**
   a. **Chloroquine** is used to suppress malaria symptoms and to terminate acute malaria attacks resulting from *P. falciparum* and *P. malariae* infections.
      (1) It is more potent and less toxic than quinine.
      (2) Except where drug-resistant *P. falciparum* strains are prevalent, chloroquine is the most useful antimalarial agent.
   b. **Primaquine** is used to cure relapses of *P. vivax* and *P. ovale* malaria and to prevent malaria in exposed persons returning from regions where malaria is endemic.
   c. **Pyrimethamine** is effective in the prevention and treatment of chloroquine-resistant strains of *P. falciparum.* It is now used almost exclusively in combination with a sulfonamide or sulfone.

d. Quinine

(1) Quinine sulfate, an oral form, is therapeutic for acute malaria caused by chloroquine-resistant strains.

(2) Quinine dihydrochloride, a parenteral form, is used in severe cases of chloroquine-resistant malaria. (It is available only from the Centers for Disease Control in Atlanta.)

(3) Quinine is almost always given in combination with another antimalarial agent.

e. Fansidar

(1) Fansidar is used for the suppression or prophylaxis of chloroquine-resistant *P. falciparum* malaria.

(2) It has been used for the prophylaxis of *P. carinii* infections in AIDS patients unable to tolerate co-trimoxazole (trimethoprim–sulfamethoxazole).

f. Mefloquine is indicated for the treatment of acute malaria and the prevention of *P. falciparum* and *P. vivax* infections.

4. Precautions and monitoring effects

a. Chloroquine

(1) Because this drug concentrates in the liver, it should be used cautiously in patients with hepatic disease.

(2) Chloroquine must be administered with extreme caution in patients with neurologic, hematologic, or severe GI disorders.

(3) Visual disturbances, headache, skin rash, and GI distress have been reported.

b. Primaquine

(1) This agent is contraindicated in patients with rheumatoid arthritis and lupus erythematosus and in those receiving other potentially hemolytic drugs or bone marrow suppressants.

(2) Primaquine may cause agranulocytosis, granulocytopenia, and mild anemia; in patients with G6PD deficiency, it may cause hemolytic anemia.

(3) Abdominal cramps, nausea, vomiting, and epigastric distress sometimes occur.

c. Pyrimethamine

(1) In high doses, this drug may cause agranulocytosis, megaloblastic anemia, aplastic anemia, and thrombocytopenia.

(2) Erythema multiforme (Stevens-Johnson syndrome), nausea, vomiting, and anorexia may develop during pyrimethamine therapy.

d. Quinine

(1) Quinine is contraindicated in patients with G6PD deficiency, tinnitus, and optic neuritis.

(2) Quinine overdose or hypersensitivity reactions may be fatal. Manifestations of quinine poisoning include visual and hearing disturbances; GI symptoms (e.g., nausea, vomiting); hot, flushed skin; headache; fever; syncope; confusion; shallow, then depressed, respirations; and cardiovascular collapse.

(3) Quinine must be used cautiously in patients with atrial fibrillation.

(4) Renal damage and anuria have been reported.

e. Fansidar

(1) Severe, sometimes fatal, hypersensitivity reactions have occurred. In most cases, death resulted from severe cutaneous reactions, including erythema multiforme, Stevens-Johnson syndrome, and toxic epidermal necrolysis.

(2) Adverse hematologic and hepatic effects as seen with sulfonamides have been reported.

f. Mefloquine

(1) Concomitant use of mefloquine with quinine, quinidine, or β-adrenergic blockade may produce electrocardiographic (ECG) abnormalities or cardiac arrest.

(2) Concomitant use of mefloquine and quinine or chloroquine may increase the risk of convulsions.

C. Amebicides and trichomonacides. These agents are crucial in the treatment of amebiasis, giardiasis, and trichomoniases—the most common protozoal infections in the United States. The major amebicides include **diloxanide, emetine, iodoquinol, metronidazole, paromomycin,** and **quinacrine.**

1. Mechanism of action

a. **Diloxanide,** a dichloroacetamide derivative, is **amebicidal;** its mechanism of action is unknown. (It is available only from the Centers for Disease Control in Atlanta.)
b. **Emetine,** an alkaloid obtained from ipecac, is **amebicidal;** it kills amebae by inhibiting amebic protein synthesis.
c. **Metronidazole** is a synthetic compound with direct **amebicidal** and **trichomonacidal** action; it works at both intestinal and extraintestinal sites. Its mechanism of action involves disruption of the helical structure of DNA.
d. **Quinacrine** is an acridine derivative that inhibits DNA metabolism.
e. **Iodoquinol** is a luminal or contact amebicide that is effective against the trophozoites of *Entamoeba histolytica* located in the lumen of the large intestines.
f. **Paromomycin** is a poorly absorbed amebicidal aminoglycoside whose mechanism of action parallels other aminoglycosides (i.e., protein synthesis inhibitor). It is also effective against enteric bacteria *Salmonella* and *Shigella.*

2. **Spectrum of activity and therapeutic uses**
   a. **Diloxanide**
      (1) This drug is used to treat asymptomatic carriers of amebic and giardiac cysts.
      (2) Diloxanide is therapeutic for invasive and extraintestinal amebiasis (given in combination with a systemic or mixed amebicide).
      (3) Diloxanide is not effective as single-agent therapy for extraintestinal amebiasis.
   b. **Emetine**
      (1) This drug is widely used to treat severe invasive intestinal amebiasis, amebic abscess, and amebic hepatitis.
      (2) Because of its toxicity, emetine generally is used only when other drugs are contraindicated or have proven to be ineffective.
      (3) Usually, emetine is administered in combination with another amebicidal agent.
   c. **Metronidazole**
      (1) This agent is the preferred drug in amebic dysentery, giardiasis, and trichomoniasis.
      (2) Metronidazole also is active against all anaerobic cocci and gram-negative anaerobic bacilli.
      (3) This agent is the treatment of choice by the Centers for Disease Control for the treatment of *Clostridium difficile* colitis infections due to emerging vancomycin-resistant enterococci. This therapy is cost effective.
   d. **Quinacrine** is useful in the treatment of giardiasis and tapeworms (see VII G).
   e. **Iodoquinol** is indicated for treatment of intestinal amebiasis. It is active against the protozoa *Entamoeba histolytica.*
   f. **Paromomycin** is indicated for acute and chronic intestinal amebiasis; it is not useful for extraintestinal amebiasis because it is not absorbed. Paromomycin has been used for *Dientamoeba fragilis, Taenia saginata, Dipylidium caninum,* and *Hymenolepis nana.*

3. **Precautions and monitoring effects**
   a. **Diloxanide** rarely causes serious adverse effects. Vomiting, flatulence, and pruritus have been reported.
   b. **Emetine**
      (1) This drug may induce potentially lethal systemic toxicity. Manifestations may be cardiovascular (e.g., ECG abnormalities, tachycardia, hypotension, CHF), GI (e.g., nausea, vomiting, diarrhea), or neurologic (e.g., dizziness, headache, changes in central or peripheral nerve function).
      (2) Emetine usually is contraindicated in patients with cardiac disease, renal impairment, muscle disease, and polyneuropathy; in children; and in patients who have taken the drug in the past 6–8 weeks.
      (3) IV injection is contraindicated.
      (4) Deep subcutaneous administration (preferred over the intramuscular route) may cause muscle weakness at the injection site.
   c. **Metronidazole**
      (1) The most common adverse effects of this drug are nausea, epigastric distress, and diarrhea.
      (2) Metronidazole is carcinogenic in mice and should not be used unnecessarily.
      (3) Headache, vomiting, metallic taste, and stomatitis have been reported.
      (4) Occasionally, neurologic reactions (e.g., ataxia, peripheral neuropathy, seizures) develop.

(5) A disulfiram-type reaction may occur with concurrent ethanol use.

d. **Quinacrine** (see VII G 4)

(1) This drug frequently causes dizziness, headache, nausea, and vomiting. Nervousness and seizures also have been reported.

(2) Quinacrine should not be taken in combination with primaquine because this may increase primaquine toxicity.

(3) Quinacrine should be administered with extreme caution in patients with psoriasis because it may cause marked exacerbation of this disease.

e. **Iodoquinol** may produce optic neuritis or atrophy or peripheral neuropathy with high-dose, long-term use. Protein-bound iodine levels may be increased during treatment and may interfere with the results of thyroid tests for 6 months after treatment. Iodoquinol should not be used in patients who are hypersensitive to 8-hydroxyquinolone (e.g., iodoquinol, iodochlorhydroxyquin) or iodine-containing agents or in patients with hepatic disorders.

f. **Paromomycin** may cause nausea, cramping, and diarrhea at high doses (more than 3 g/day). Inadvertent absorption through ulcerative bowel lesions may result in ototoxicity or renal damage.

D. **Pentamidine isethionate** is an aromatic diamide antiprotozoal agent. It can be administered intramuscularly, intravenously, and by inhalation.

1. **Mechanism of action** is not fully understood, but in vitro studies indicate interference with nuclear metabolism and inhibition of DNA, RNA, phospholipid, and protein synthesis.

2. **Therapeutic uses**

a. Pentamidine is indicated for the prevention and treatment of infections due to *P. carinii.*

b. Unlabeled uses include treatment of trypanosomiasis and visceral leishmaniasis.

3. **Precautions and monitoring effects**

a. This agent must be used cautiously in patients with hypertension, hypotension, hypoglycemia, hyperglycemia, hypocalcemia, leukopenia, thrombocytopenia, anemia, hepatic or renal dysfunction, ventricular tachycardia, or pancreatitis.

b. Inhalation of pentamidine may produce bronchospasm.

c. Laboratory tests before and during therapy include BUN, serum creatinine, complete blood count (CBC) and platelets, liver function tests (LFTs), serum calcium, blood glucose, and ECG.

E. **Atovaquone** is a hydroxynaphthoquinone initially synthesized as an antimalarial drug.

1. **Mechanism of action.** Atovaquone blocks mitochondrial electron transport at complex III of the respiratory chain of protozoa, resulting in inhibition of pyrimidine species.

2. **Spectrum of activity.** It is active against *P. carinii, T. gondii, Cryptosporidium parvum,* and *Plasmodium falciparum.*

3. **Therapeutic uses.** Atovaquone is used for second-line treatment of mild-to-moderate *P. carinii* pneumonia in patients intolerant to co-trimoxazole or other sulfonamides, or non-responsive to co-trimoxazole.

4. **Precautions and monitoring effects**

a. Oral absorption significantly increases when administered with food.

b. Rash, nausea, diarrhea, headache, fever, abdominal pain, dizziness, and elevated liver function tests commonly are reported.

5. **Significant interactions.** Atovaquone is highly bound to plasma protein. It should be used with caution when administered with other highly protein-bound drugs with a narrow therapeutic range.

F. **Eflornithine HCl** is an IV antiprotozoal agent. Its activity has been attributed to the inhibition of the enzyme ornithine decarboxylase.

1. **Mechanism of action** is a specific, enzyme-activated, irreversible inhibitor of ornithine decarboxylase.

2. **Spectrum of activity and therapeutic uses.** Eflornithine is active in the treatment of the meningoencephalitic stage of *Trypanosoma brucei gambiense* (sleeping sickness).

3. **Precautions and monitoring effects**
   a. Myelosuppression is the most frequent serious side effect.
   b. Seizures occur in about 8% of treated patients.
   c. Cases of hearing impairment have been reported.

V. ANTITUBERCULAR AGENTS

A. Definition and classification. Drugs used to treat tuberculosis suppress or kill the slow-growing mycobacteria that cause this disease. Antitubercular agents fall into two main categories: **primary** and **retreatment** agents. Because the causative organisms tend to develop resistance to any single drug, combination drug therapy has become standard in the treatment of tuberculosis.

1. The **incidence** of tuberculosis in the United States is increasing due to shifts in populations considered to be endemic for tuberculosis, the rise in HIV-positive patients, and drug resistance.
2. Agents chosen for **therapy** must eradicate mycobacterium. Agents available include isoniazid, streptomycin, quinolones, ethambutol, pyrazinamide, rifampin, and rifabutin. **Combination chemotherapy** is essential. Agents showing the lowest incidence of resistance (isoniazid, rifampin, streptomycin) are usually used in combination with pyrazinamide or ethambutol.
3. Choice of therapy is dependent upon many patient and disease factors (e.g., duration of therapy needed, likelihood of drug resistance, and HIV status).
4. Most patients are started on isoniazid, rifampin, and pyrazinamide. A fourth drug (ethambutol, streptomycin) is added with suspected resistance (i.e., if patients were previously treated or if resistance is expected). Patients failing this therapy must be treated with five drugs (isoniazid, rifampin, pyrazinamide, ethambutol, and streptomycin). If one or more of these agents cannot be used, ethionamide, para-aminosalicylic acid, cycloserine, or capreomycin (older, more toxic agents) can be used.
5. **Treatment choices based on Centers for Disease Control recommendations**
   a. The first choice is isoniazid, rifampin, and pyrazinamide for 8 weeks, then isoniazid for 16 weeks with rifampin daily. In cases of suspected isoniazid resistance, add ethambutol or streptomycin. Administer for at least 6 months.
   b. The second choice includes isoniazid, rifampin, pyrazinamide, and either streptomycin or ethambutol daily for 2 weeks, then two times a week for 6 weeks, followed by isoniazid and rifampin two times a week for 16 weeks.
   c. The third choice is isoniazid, rifampin, pyrazinamide, plus either streptomycin or ethambutol three times a week for 6 months.
   d. For HIV-positive patients, use any of the previous recommendations, but continue therapy for at least 9 months.

B. Primary agents. These drugs, isoniazid, ethambutol, rifampin, pyrazinamide, and streptomycin, usually offer the greatest effectiveness with the least toxicity; they are successful in most tuberculosis patients. Frequently, two or three are administered together; in most cases, the combination of isoniazid, rifampin, and pyrazinamide is most effective.

1. **Ethambutol** is a synthetic water-based compound.
   a. **Mechanism of action.** This drug is **bacteriostatic;** its precise mechanism of action is unknown.
   b. **Spectrum of activity and therapeutic uses.** Ethambutol is active against many *M. tuberculosis* strains. However, drug resistance develops fairly rapidly when it is used alone. In most cases, ethambutol is given adjunctively in combination with isoniazid or rifampin.
   c. **Precautions and monitoring effects.** Rarely, ethambutol causes such adverse effects as reversible dose-related ($\geq$ 15 mg/kg/day) optic neuritis, drug fever, abdominal pain, headache, dizziness, and confusion.
2. **Isoniazid** is a hydrazide of isonicotinic acid. The mainstay of antitubercular therapy, this drug should be included (if tolerated) in all therapeutic regimens.
   a. **Mechanism of action.** Isoniazid is **bacteriostatic** for resting bacilli and **bactericidal** for rapidly dividing organisms. Its mechanism of action is not fully known; the drug probably disrupts bacterial cell wall synthesis by inhibiting mycolic acid synthesis.

b. **Spectrum of activity.** Isoniazid is active against most tubercle bacilli; some atypical mycobacteria are resistant.

c. **Therapeutic uses**

(1) The most widely used antitubercular agent, isoniazid should be given in combination with another antitubercular drug (such as rifampin or ethambutol) to prevent drug resistance.

(2) For uncomplicated pulmonary tuberculosis, isoniazid therapy may last 6 months to 2 years.

(3) Prophylactic isoniazid may be administered alone for 1 year in children who have a positive tuberculin test result but lack active lesions.

d. **Precautions and monitoring effects**

(1) The most common adverse effects of isoniazid are skin rash, fever, jaundice, and peripheral neuritis.

(2) Hepatitis, an occasional reaction, can be severe and, in some cases, fatal. The risk of hepatitis increases with the patient's age and rises with alcohol abuse.

(3) Blood dyscrasias (e.g., agranulocytosis, aplastic or hemolytic anemia, thrombocytopenia) may occur.

(4) Adverse GI effects include nausea, vomiting, and epigastric distress.

(5) CNS toxicity may result from pyridoxine deficiency. Signs and symptoms include insomnia, restlessness, hyperreflexia, and convulsions.

e. **Significant interactions**

(1) With concurrent **phenytoin** therapy, blood levels of both phenytoin and isoniazid may increase, possibly causing toxicity.

(2) **Aluminum-containing antacids** may reduce isoniazid absorption.

(3) Concurrent **carbamazepine** therapy may increase the risk of hepatitis.

3. **Rifampin** is a complex macrocyclic agent.

a. **Mechanism of action.** This drug is **bactericidal;** it impairs bacterial RNA synthesis by binding to DNA-dependent RNA polymerase.

b. **Spectrum of activity.** Rifampin is active against most gram-negative and many gram-positive organisms.

c. **Therapeutic uses**

(1) The combination of rifampin and isoniazid is the most effective therapy for tuberculosis. Rifampin should not be administered alone because this can lead to the emergence of highly drug-resistant organisms.

(2) Prophylactic rifampin is effective when administered to carriers of meningococcal disease caused by *H. influenzae* organisms.

d. **Precautions and monitoring effects**

(1) Serious hepatotoxicity may result from rifampin therapy.

(2) In rare cases, this drug induces an influenza-like syndrome.

(3) Other adverse effects include skin rash, drowsiness, headache, fatigue, confusion, nausea, vomiting, and abdominal pain.

(4) Rifampin colors urine, sweat, tears, saliva, and feces orange-red.

e. **Significant interactions**

(1) Rifampin induces hepatic microspinal enzymes and, thus, may decrease the therapeutic effectiveness of **corticosteroids, warfarin, oral contraceptives, quinidine, digitoxin,** and **barbiturates.**

(2) **Probenecid** may increase blood levels of rifampin.

4. **Streptomycin** (see II B 3)

5. **Pyrazinamide** is a pyrazine analog of nicotinamide.

a. **Mechanism of action** is bactericidal and/or bacteriostatic, depending on cell concentration achieved.

b. **Spectrum of activity and therapeutic uses.** Pyrazinamide is used as a primary agent with isoniazid and rifampin for at least 2 months, followed by isoniazid and rifampin.

c. **Precautions and monitoring effects.** This agent may result in hepatotoxicity and, rarely, hepatic necrosis resulting in death. Anorexia, nausea, vomiting, malaise, and fever have been reported. Hyperuricemia may result in gouty exacerbations.

C. **Retreatment agents.** These agents include aminosalicylic acid, capreomycin, cycloserine, ethionamide and kanamycin. Retreatment agents are less effective, more toxic, and are used in combination with primary agents.

1. **Mechanism of action**
   a. **Aminosalicylic acid** is **bacteriostatic;** it probably inhibits the enzymes responsible for folic acid synthesis.
   b. **Cycloserine** can be **bacteriostatic** or **bactericidal,** depending on its concentration at the infection site; it impairs amino acid utilization, thereby inhibiting bacterial cell wall synthesis.
   c. The mechanism of action of capreomycin (**bacteriostatic**), ethionamide (**bactericidal**), and pyrazinamide (**bactericidal**) is unknown.

2. **Spectrum of activity and therapeutic uses.** Second-line antitubercular agents are active against various microorganisms, including *M. tuberculosis.* These agents generally are reserved for patients with extensive extrapulmonary or drug-resistant disease or for patients who need retreatment. These drugs are almost always administered in combination.

3. **Precautions and monitoring effects**
   a. Adverse effects of **aminosalicylic acid** include leukopenia, agranulocytopenia, thrombocytopenia, hemolytic anemia, mononucleosis-like syndrome, malaise, joint pain, fever, and skin rash.
   b. **Capreomycin** and **streptomycin** are ototoxic and nephrotoxic; they should not be administered together.
   c. **Cycloserine** may cause adverse CNS effects, including headache, suicidal and psychotic tendencies, hyperirritability, confusion, paranoia, and nervousness.
   d. **Ethionamide** may induce nausea, vomiting, orthostatic hypotension, metallic taste, epigastric distress, and peripheral neuropathy.

D. Alternative agents

1. **Rifater.** A combination of rifampin 120 mg, isoniazid 50 mg, and pyrazinamide 300 mg in one tablet is used in patients expected to have low compliance with tuberculosis drug therapy. One **disadvantage** is that many patients are required to take as many as 5–6 tablets daily, which may reduce compliance.

2. **Quinolones.** Ciprofloxacin and ofloxacin are used in tuberculosis therapy. Ofloxacin is preferred due to increased serum concentrations. Ofloxacin is usually used in combination with other tuberculosis agents for active treatment. For prophylaxis, ofloxacin is combined with pyrazinamide.

3. **Macrolides.** Clarithromycin and azithromycin have shown limited activity against *M. tuberculosis.*

4. **Rifabutin** is an antimycobacterial agent that is similar to rifampin, with activity against both tubercular and nontubercular mycobacterium, and offers no clear advantage over rifampin.
   a. **Mechanism of action.** In addition to its antimycobacterial activity against tubercular and nontubercular mycobacterium, rifabutin has been reported to inhibit reverse transcriptase and block the in vitro infectivity and replication of HIV.
   b. **Therapeutic uses.** Rifabutin is indicated for the prevention of disseminated *M. avium-intracellulare* complex disease in patients with advanced HIV infections.
   c. **Precautions and monitoring effects.** The use of rifabutin has resulted in mild elevation of liver enzymes and thrombocytopenia.
   d. **Significant interactions**
      (1) Rifabutin antagonizes and potentially negates the immune response mediated by the bacillus Calmette-Guérin (BCG) vaccine.
      (2) Rifabutin may increase the clearance of **cyclosporine.** Serum cyclosporine levels should be monitored in patients receiving both agents.

VI. ANTIVIRAL AGENTS

A. Definition.
These drugs alleviate viral disease by influencing viral replication. Because viruses lack independent metabolic activity and can replicate only within living host cells, antiviral agents tend to injure host as well as viral cells. Consequently, few antiviral drugs have been introduced; most are active against only one virus.

1. **DNA viruses.** Currently approved antiviral therapy against the *Herpesviridae* family of DNA viruses [herpes simplex virus (HSV) 1 and 2, varicella-zoster virus (VZV), cytomegalovirus (CMV)] are virustatic and arrest DNA synthesis by inhibiting viral DNA polymerase. With the exception of the broad-spectrum antiviral drug **foscarnet,** these agents are prodrugs and require viral and host cellular enzymes (e.g., thymidine, deoxyguanosine kinase) to phosphorylate them into the active triphosphate form before being incorporated. Hence, a common mechanism of resistance is a deficiency or structural alteration in viral thymidine kinase (Table 43-3).

2. **RNA viruses.** Currently approved antiretroviral agents active against HIV-1 include the reverse transcriptase inhibitors **zidovudine, didanosine, zalcitabine, stavudine, lamivudine,** and **nevirapine,** as well as the recently approved protease inhibitors **saquinavir, ritonavir,** and **indinavir.** These agents are virustatic and involve life-long therapy.

B. **Acyclovir** is a synthetic purine nucleoside analogue that is therapeutic for various herpes infections. It is the least toxic antiviral agent.

1. **Mechanism of action.** Acyclovir becomes incorporated into viral DNA and inhibits viral replication.

2. **Spectrum of activity.** This agent is active against herpes viruses, particularly HSV-1.
   a. Acyclovir is used to treat mucocutaneous HSV infections in immunocompromised patients and to reduce pain and speed healing of herpes zoster, genital herpes, and neonatal herpes.
   b. This agent is available in topical, oral, and IV forms. Topical acyclovir is applied directly on herpes lesions in primary herpes infection and in non–life-threatening mucocutaneous HSV infection in immunocompromised patients.
   c. Acyclovir may be administered intravenously in the treatment of initial and recurrent mucocutaneous HSV infection in immunocompromised patients and in the treatment of severe initial herpes infection in patients with normal immunity.

3. **Precautions and monitoring effects**
   a. Oral acyclovir may induce nausea, vomiting, diarrhea, and headache.
   b. IV administration may cause nephrotoxicity, neurologic effects (e.g., lethargy, confusion, tremors, agitation, seizures, coma, obtundation), hypotension, rash, itching, and inflammation and phlebitis at the injection site.
   c. Local discomfort and pruritus may result from topical administration.
   d. Acyclovir is removed in hemodialysis. Doses should be adjusted in renal impairment and hemodialysis.

4. **Significant interactions. Probenecid** may increase blood concentrations of acyclovir, possibly causing toxicity.

C. **Amantadine,** a synthetic tricyclic amine with a unique chemical structure, serves as a valuable agent against influenza A viral infection.

1. **Mechanism of action.** Amantadine inhibits replication of the influenza A virus by interfering with viral attachment and uncoating.

2. **Spectrum of activity and therapeutic uses**

Table 43-3. Activity of Anti-DNA Viral Agents

Agent	HSV-1	HSV-2	VZV	CMV	Influenza A
Ribavirin	+	+	. . .	. . .	. . .
Vidarabine*	+	+	+	. . .	. . .
Acyclovir*	+	+	+	. . .	. . .
Ganciclovir*	. . .	. . .	. . .	+	. . .
Amantadine	. . .	. . .	. . .	. . .	+
Foscarnet	+	+	+	+	. . .
Famciclovir	+	+	+	. . .	. . .
Valacyclovir*	+	+	+	. . .	. . .
Cidofovir	. . .	. . .	. . .	+	. . .

*Requires activation into triphosphate form.

a. Amantadine is effective in the prophylaxis and treatment of influenza A virus.
b. Clinicians recommend that all nonimmunized high-risk patients receive this drug at the first sign of community influenza A activity.
c. Suppressive therapy should continue for 24–48 hours after influenza symptoms disappear or, if necessary, up to 90 days for repeated exposure to the virus.
d. This drug may be used to treat some patients with parkinsonism.

3. **Precautions and monitoring effects**
   a. The most pronounced adverse effects of amantadine are ataxia, nightmares, and insomnia. Other CNS effects include depression, confusion, dizziness, fatigue, anxiety, and headache. Patients with a history of epilepsy and psychiatric disorders should be monitored closely during therapy.
   b. Anticholinergic reactions (e.g., dry mouth, blurred vision, tachycardia) have been reported.

D. **Ribavirin** is a synthetic nucleoside analogue that plays a key role in the treatment of respiratory syncytial virus.

1. **Mechanism of action.** Ribavirin may inhibit RNA and DNA synthesis by depleting intracellular nucleotide reserves.

2. **Spectrum of activity.** This agent is active in vitro against RNA and DNA viruses, such as influenza A and B, respiratory syncytial virus, and herpes simplex.

3. **Therapeutic uses.** Administered in aerosol form, ribavirin is used to relieve symptoms and speed recovery in young adults with influenza A and B and in children with respiratory syncytial virus.

4. **Precautions and monitoring effects**
   a. Ribavirin must be administered only with a specific small-particle aerosol generator (Viratek SPAG-2).
   b. This agent is contraindicated in patients using respirators because it may precipitate on respirator valves and tubing, causing lethal malfunction. (However, use of a prefilter may permit ribavirin therapy in such patients.)
   c. Serious adverse effects include cardiac arrest, deterioration of pulmonary function, bacterial pneumonia, and apnea.
   d. Rash, conjunctivitis, and reticulocytosis have been reported.

E. **Vidarabine,** an adenosine analogue, is useful in the treatment of serious herpes infections.

1. **Mechanism of action.** Vidarabine inhibits viral multiplication by becoming incorporated into viral DNA.

2. **Spectrum of activity and therapeutic uses.** Vidarabine is effective against herpes simplex encephalitis (administered intravenously) and herpes simplex keratoconjunctivitis (administered as a topical ophthalmic agent). In immunocompromised patients, vidarabine is given intravenously to treat herpes zoster infection.

3. **Precautions and monitoring effects**
   a. The most common adverse effects of vidarabine are nausea, diarrhea, and rash.
   b. Dose-related CNS toxicity (manifested by tremors, dizziness, confusion, and ataxia) may develop.
   c. IV administration requires dilution in a large volume of fluid, posing a danger to patients with cardiac or renal disease.
   d. Vidarabine may be carcinogenic and mutagenic.

4. **Significant interactions. Allopurinol** increases the risk of CNS toxicity.

F. **Ganciclovir** is a synthetic purine nucleoside analogue that is used for CMV infections.

1. **Mechanism of action.** Ganciclovir triphosphate is incorporated into viral DNA, inhibits viral DNA polymerase, and thus terminates viral replication.

2. **Spectrum of activity.** Ganciclovir has in vitro activity against HSV-1 and -2, VZV, and Epstein-Barr viruses, but due to its enhanced ability to penetrate host cells, it is indicated for

CMV infections, such as colitis, pneumonia, and retinitis. However, ganciclovir use in CMV infections of the CNS has not been successful even though it is capable of CNS penetration.

a. Conversion into the triphosphate form is greater in infected host cells, even though drug penetration occurs in both uninfected and infected cells.
b. Inhibitory concentrations for the viral DNA polymerase are lower than those of the host cellular polymerase.
c. In cases of CMV pneumonia or bone marrow transplant patients, CMV immune globulin is added to the regimen.
d. Maintenance therapy for 75 days after the initial 14 days of therapy is required to prevent relapse.

3. **Precautions and monitoring effects**
   a. The main side effects of IV ganciclovir are neutropenia and thrombocytopenia. Phlebitis and pain may occur at the site of infusion.
   b. Because ganciclovir is cleared by glomerular filtration and tubular secretion, renal function and adequate hydration should be monitored. The drug is removed in hemodialysis. Doses should be adjusted in cases of renal impairment and hemodialysis.

4. **Significant interactions**
   a. **Probenecid** may increase ganciclovir levels and possibly toxicity.
   b. **Zidovudine** and **cytotoxic agents** in combination with ganciclovir may result in neutropenia; careful monitoring of granulocyte levels is required when they are taken concurrently with ganciclovir.
   c. **Imipenem–cilastatin** in combination with ganciclovir may induce generalized seizures.

G. **Foscarnet** (trisodium phosphonoformate hexahydrate, PFA) is a synthetic pyrophosphate analogue, which directly inhibits enzymes involved in viral DNA synthesis without incorporation into viral DNA. It is a broad-spectrum antiviral agent and is the drug of choice in cases of acyclovir or ganciclovir resistance.

1. **Mechanisms of action**
   a. Viral DNA replication requires the addition of deoxynucleoside triphosphates at the end of the DNA strand by DNA polymerase and the subsequent cleavage of pyrophosphate from the newly attached nucleotide. Foscarnet competitively binds directly to DNA polymerase to form an inactive complex and prevents pyrophosphate cleavage. Viral DNA chain elongation is thus terminated.
   b. Foscarnet is also active against HIV-1, an RNA retrovirus. It is a noncompetitive, reversible inhibitor of HIV reverse transcriptase, the enzyme responsible for converting viral RNA to viral DNA.

2. **Spectrum of activity and therapeutic uses.** Foscarnet has in vitro activity against HSV-1 and -2, CMV, VZV, and Epstein-Barr DNA polymerases, influenza polymerase, and HIV reverse transcriptase. Therapeutically, the drug may be used in HSV-1 and -2, VZV, CMV, and HIV-1 infections.
   a. The most experience with foscarnet is in the treatment of CMV retinitis in immunocompromised patients. An initial induction therapy lasts 2–4 weeks. Maintenance therapy within 1 month after induction may be needed to prevent relapse.
   b. Foscarnet may be used with zidovudine either synergistically in HIV therapy or concurrently in CMV infections in AIDS patients where neutropenia contraindicates ganciclovir therapy.
   c. Foscarnet is able to cross the blood–brain barrier.

3. **Precautions and monitoring effects**
   a. IV foscarnet is highly nephrotoxic, causing acute tubular necrosis. Renal failure can be prevented if adequate hydration is maintained throughout therapy and with daily renal function monitoring.
   b. Other common adverse effects include hypercalcemia, hypocalcemia, hypomagnesemia, and hyperphosphatemia.
   c. Foscarnet is removed by hemodialysis.

4. **Significant interactions**
   a. Intravenous **pentamidine** increases the risk of renal toxicity and severe hypocalcemia.
   b. Foscarnet is exclusively eliminated by glomerular filtration and tubular secretion. **Probenecid** may prolong elimination and possibly cause toxicity.

c. Other concurrent nephrotoxic agents should be avoided whenever possible.

H. Zidovudine is a synthetic thymidine analogue. Formerly called azidothymidine (AZT), this agent is the first available drug for the treatment of HIV infection in patients with AIDS and AIDS-related complex (ARC).

1. Mechanism of action. Zidovudine is phosphorylated by human cellular kinases to a triphosphate and then incorporated into viral DNA, where it can terminate viral DNA synthesis by inhibiting the viral enzyme reverse transcriptase or terminating DNA strand elongation. HIV replication is thus prevented.

2. Spectrum of activity and therapeutic uses

a. Zidovudine has been shown to slow HIV-1 production, alleviate symptoms, and prolong life in some patients with AIDS.

b. More recent clinical trials have revealed that maintenance doses of 500–600 mg/day are as effective as the higher and potentially more toxic dose of 800 mg/day.

c. There is evidence that treating HIV-1–positive patients with $CD4^+$ lymphocyte counts of less than 500 cells/mm^3 (early in the natural history of the disease before the definitive AIDS diagnosis of $CD4^+$ count < 200), using maintenance doses, prolongs survival. Further testing on the use of zidovudine early in the disease is likely.

d. Zidovudine can cross the blood–brain barrier.

3. Precautions and monitoring effects

a. Zidovudine can cause severe bone marrow suppression leading to anemia, granulocytopenia, and thrombocytopenia. Patients may require blood transfusions to reverse anemia.

b. The use of erythropoietin or granulocyte colony-stimulating factor (G-CSF) is an alternative adjunctive therapy in zidovudine-induced anemia. There is a theoretical but yet unproven risk of activating latent HIV-1 in monocyte/macrophages when granulocyte/macrophage CSF (GM-CSF) is used. Studies using GM-CSF have not observed increased viremia.

c. Other adverse effects include headache, agitation, confusion, anxiety, insomnia, rash, and itching.

4. Significant interactions

a. Co-trimoxazole may impair zidovudine metabolism, causing increased zidovudine toxicity.

b. Other **cytotoxic drugs** can cause additive bone marrow suppression.

c. Fatigue and lethargy may develop with concurrent **acyclovir** therapy.

I. Dideoxyinosine (Didanosine DDI), a synthetic purine analogue, inhibits HIV-1 replication and is unique in having a long intracellular half-life (> 12 hours versus 3 hours for zidovudine) and rare hematologic toxicities. This agent is approved for patients who have failed or are intolerant of zidovudine therapy.

1. Mechanism of action. DDI is phosphorylated in human cells by the enzyme 5′-nucleotidase and other cellular kinases before it competitively inhibits the viral enzyme reverse transcriptase. This results in viral DNA synthesis termination and prevention of HIV-1 replication.

2. Spectrum of activity. DDI has demonstrated a dose-dependent activity against HIV-1, resulting in lower virus production (p24 antigens); increases in peripheral blood $CD4^+$ cell counts; and increases in appetite, weight, and energy without significant neutropenia.

a. Clinical trials are assessing synergy, alternating therapy, or equivalent efficacy with zidovudine.

b. DDI is well absorbed orally but is acid unstable, requiring administration with buffers or antacids.

c. DDI is able to cross the blood–brain barrier.

3. Precautions and monitoring effects

a. DDI can cause reversible peripheral neuropathy and acute, potentially lethal pancreatitis. Serum triglycerides should be monitored, and DDI should be withheld when potential pancreatitis-inducing agents (e.g., IV pentamidine, sulfonamides) are given. Transiently elevated serum amylase may not reflect pancreatitis.

b. Other adverse effects include headaches, insomnia, hepatitis, and hyperuricemia (because DDI is catalyzed to uric acid).

4. **Significant interactions.** Pancreatitis-inducing drugs, such as **cimetidine, ranitidine, sulfonamides, pentamidine,** and **alcohol,** should not be used with DDI.

J. **Zalcitabine** is a synthetic pyrimidine nucleoside analogue that is active against HIV.

1. **Mechanism of action.** Within cells, zalcitabine is converted to the active metabolite dideoxycytidine-5′-triphosphate (ddCTP) by cellular enzymes. ddCPT serves as an alternate substrate to deoxycytidine triphosphate (dCTP) for HIV reverse transcriptase and inhibits in vitro replication of HIV-1 by inhibition of viral DNA synthesis.

2. **Spectrum of activity and therapeutic uses.** Zalcitabine is indicated for combination therapy with zidovudine in advanced HIV infection; that is, for the treatment of adult patients with advanced infection ($CD4^+$ cell count $< 300/mm^3$) who have demonstrated significant clinical or immunologic deterioration.

3. **Precautions and monitoring effects**
   a. The major clinical toxicity of zalcitabine is peripheral neuropathy, which occurs in up to 31% of patients.
   b. Documented pancreatitis has occurred alone or in combination with zidovudine. Serum amylase must be monitored.
   c. Other adverse effects include esophageal ulcers, cardiomyopathy/CHF, anaphylactoid reactions, and impaired renal or hepatic function.

4. **Significant interactions**
   a. Drugs that have the potential to cause peripheral neuropathy should be avoided. These include **chloramphenicol, cisplatin, dapsone, disulfiram, ethionamide, glutethimide, gold, hydralazine, iodoquinol, isoniazid, metronidazole, nitrofurantoin, phenytoin, ribavirin,** and **vincristine.**
   b. Zalcitabine treatment should be interrupted when a drug with the potential to cause pancreatitis is needed (i.e., **pentamidine**).

K. **Rimantadine** is a synthetic antiviral agent and an α-methyl derivative of amantadine that blocks the early step in the replication of the influenza A virus.

1. **Mechanism of action.** Rimantadine inhibits the early viral replication cycle, possibly inhibiting the uncoating of the virus.

2. **Spectrum of activity and therapeutic uses**
   a. Rimantidine plays a role in the inhibition of the influenza virus. Rimantidine has been shown to be safe and effective in preventing signs and symptoms of infection caused by various strains of influenza A virus.
   b. The method of choice for prophylaxis against influenza is vaccination; however, in some cases vaccine is contraindicated or not available.
   c. Rimantidine therapy should be considered in people who develop flu-like symptoms during influenza A season. Therapy should be initiated within 48 hours of symptoms' onset.

3. **Precautions and monitoring effects**
   a. Use with caution in patients with a history of seizure because rimantidine may increase the incidence of seizure.
   b. The most frequent adverse reactions include GI disturbance (nausea, vomiting, anorexia) and CNS toxicity (insomnia, dizziness, headache).

4. **Significant interactions**
   a. Cimetidine may reduce the clearance of rimantidine therapy and increase levels of rimantidine.
   b. Aspirin and acetaminophen may cause small reductions in rimantidine serum levels.

L. **Stavudine (d4T)** is a synthetic thymidine nucleoside analog that is active against HIV infection.

1. **Mechanism of action.** Stavudine is phosphorylated by cellular kinase to stavudine triphosphate. Stavudine triphosphate inhibits HIV replication by inhibiting HIV reverse transcriptase and inhibiting viral DNA synthesis by causing DNA chain termination.

2. Spectrum of activity and therapeutic uses

a. Stavudine is active against the HIV virus by inhibiting replication of HIV in human cells in vitro.

b. Stavudine is indicated only in patients with advanced HIV infections who are intolerant to other antiviral therapies or who have experienced significant deterioration while on those agents.

3. Precautions and monitoring effects

a. The major toxicity with stavudine is a dose-related peripheral neuropathy.

b. Initial HIV therapy should be with zidovudine; stavudine should be held in reserve.

c. Fatal episodes of pancreatitis have been reported; monitor patients closely.

M. Famciclovir is a prodrug of the antiviral agent penciclovir. It acts against HSV-1, HSV-2, and VZV.

1. Mechanism of action. Famciclovir is rapidly phosphorylated in virus-infected cells by viral thymidine kinase to penciclovir monophosphate. Penciclovir is a competitive inhibitor of viral DNA polymerase and prevents viral replication by inhibition of herpes virus DNA synthesis.

2. Spectrum of activity

a. Famciclovir has activity against HSV-1, HSV-2, and VZV. Therapeutically the drug is indicated for management of acute herpes zoster (also known as shingles).

b. The most experience with famciclovir is in herpes zoster. Therapy must be promptly initiated as soon as herpes zoster is diagnosed (within 48–72 hrs), at a dose of 500 mg every 8 hours for 7 days.

3. Precautions and monitoring effects. Common adverse events include fatigue, GI complaints such as nausea, diarrhea, vomiting, constipation, and anorexia. Headache is also commonly reported.

4. Significant interactions

a. Use of probenecid and other drugs requiring elimination by use of active renal tubular secretion may result in increased plasma concentration of penciclovir.

b. Famciclovir may increase digoxin levels.

N. Lamivudine (3TC) is a synthetic nucleoside analog that has activity against HIV infection.

1. Mechanism of action. Lamivudine inhibits HIV reverse transcription by viral DNA chain termination and inhibition of the RNA- and DNA-dependent DNA polymerase activity of the reverse transcriptase.

2. Spectrum of activity and therapeutic uses

a. Lamivudine is active against HIV.

b. Lamivudine is indicated for use only in combination with zidovudine for the treatment of HIV infection with disease progression. Currently there are no controlled clinical trials evaluating progression of HIV disease as measured by opportunistic infection or long-term survival.

3. Precautions and monitoring effects

a. Reported adverse reactions include headache, fatigue, GI reactions such as nausea, vomiting, and diarrhea. CNS toxicity includes neuropathy, dizziness, and insomnia. Lab test abnormalities such as neutropenia and elevations in liver enzymes are also reported.

b. As with other antiviral therapies used for the treatment of HIV infection, lamivudine is not a cure for HIV infection, and patients may continue to acquire illnesses associated with HIV infection.

c. Long-term effects of lamivudine are currently unknown.

d. Lamivudine has not been shown to reduce the risk of transmission of HIV through sexual contact.

O. Valacyclovir

1. Mechanism of action. Valacyclovir is rapidly converted to acyclovir. Acyclovir is selective for the thymidine kinase enzyme, beginning the conversion of acyclovir to acyclovir triphosphate, stopping the replication of herpes viral DNA.

2. **Spectrum of activity and therapeutic uses**
   a. Valacyclovir is active against HSV-1, HSV-2 and VZV.
   b. This agent is used for the therapy of herpes zoster (shingles) in immunocompetent adults.

3. **Precautions and monitoring effects**
   a. Valacyclovir is not indicated in immunocompromised individuals (e.g., advanced HIV disease, bone marrow transplant) due to the occurrence of thrombotic thrombocytopenic purpura/hemolytic uremic syndrome.
   b. Begin therapy within 72 hours of herpes zoster diagnosis (or rash onset).
   c. Most commonly reported adverse reactions are nausea, headache, and vomiting.

P. **Protease inhibitors** include **saquinavir, rotinavir,** and **indinavir.** In some patients with HIV infection, the introduction of a protease inhibitor into their regimen has led to marked clinical improvement.

1. **Mechanism of action.** These agents block the enzyme protease. When used in combination with nucleoside analogues, two of the enzymes needed to replicate HIV may be blocked.

2. **Spectrum of activity.** These agents are active against HIV.

3. **Therapeutic use.** Saquinavir is indicated for use in combination with nucleoside analogues (zidovudine, zalcitabine) for the treatment of advanced HIV infection in selected patients. Currently, there are no controlled studies evaluating the effects of saquinavir on clinical progression of HIV infection or on survival. Treatment with saquinavir (in combination with zidovudine) has been shown to increase CD4 counts in zidovudine-naive patients more than zidovudine monotherapy. When added to a regimen of prolonged prior zidovudine, studies have shown little benefit.
   a. Saquinavir- and zidovudine-resistant HIV isolates are generally susceptible to rotinavir.
   b. Studies show combination therapy, including ritonivar or indinavir alone, may decrease HIV levels in some patients.

4. **Precautions and monitoring effects**
   a. The **most common adverse events** in clinical trials were diarrhea, nausea, and abdominal discomfort.
   b. Saquinavir should be administered with caution to patients with hepatic insufficiency, because patients with baseline LFTs higher than five times normal were not included in clinical studies.
   c. Other adverse effects with rotinavir include asthenia, circumoral and peripheral parasthesias, altered taste, and elevated triglycerides, cholesterol, and liver enzymes.
   d. Indinavir causes mild elevation of indirect bilirubin in approximately 10% of patients, which usually resolves without intervention; kidney stones are reported in 2%–3% of patients. Patients should drink at least 48 ounces of water daily.

5. **Significant interactions.** Rifampin reduces saquinavir concentrations by 80%. Rifabutin, phenobarbital, phenytoin, dexamethasone, and carbamazepine also lower saquinavir plasma concentrations.
   a. Saquinavir may interfere with metabolism by CYP3A4 of various drugs, including terfenadine and astemizole, which in high concentrations can cause fatal cardiac arrhythmias.
   b. Ritinovir should be taken with food; indinavir should be taken 1 hour before or 2 hours after meals.
   c. Indinavir may interfere with absorption of didanosine.
   d. Check product information for the most current interaction information; these drugs have high potential to interact with many drugs.

Q. **Cidofovir** is a recently approved antiviral with limited indications.

1. **Mechanism of action.** Cidofovir suppresses CMV replication by selective inhibition of DNA synthesis.

2. **Spectrum of activity. In vitro** activity has been demonstrated against CMV, VZV, EBV, and HHV-6. Controlled clinical studies are limited to patints with AIDS and CMV retinitis.

3. **Therapeutic use** includes the treatment of CMV retinitis in patients with AIDS.

4. **Precautions and monitoring effects**
   a. Avoid using this drug in patients with serum creatinine > 1.5 mg/dl or creatinine clearance < 55ml/min.
   b. Cidofovir is contraindicated in patients with a history of severe hypersensitivity to probenecid or other sulfa-containing medications.
   c. The dose-limiting toxicity of cidofovir is nephrotoxicity; granulocytopenia also has been reported.
   d. Probenecid must be administered with each cidofovir dose.

VII. ANTHELMINTICS

A. **Definition.** These drugs are used to rid the body of worms **(helminths)**. These agents may act locally to rid the GI tract of worms or work systemically to eradicate worms that are invading organs or tissues.

B. **Mebendazole** is a synthetic benzimidazole-derivative anthelmintic.

1. **Mechanism of action.** Mebendazole interferes with reproduction and survival of helminths by inhibiting the formation of microtubules and irreversibly blocking glucose uptake, thereby depleting glycogen stores in the helminth.

2. **Spectrum of activity.** Mebendazole is active against *Trichuris trichiura* (whipworm), *Enterobius vermicularis* (pinworm), *Ascaris lumbricoides* (roundworm), *Ancylostoma duodenale* (common hookworm), and *Necator americanus* (American hookworm).

3. **Therapeutic uses.** Mebendazole is used for the treatment of single or mixed infections. Immobilization and subsequent death of helminths are slow, with complete GI clearance up to 3 days after therapy.

4. **Precautions and monitoring effects**
   a. In cases of massive infection, abdominal pain and nausea may result.
   b. If the patient is not cured in 3 weeks, retreatment is necessary.

5. **Significant interactions.** Agents that may reduce the blood levels and subsequent efficacy of mebendazole include carbamazepine and hydantoins.

C. **Diethylcarbamazine citrate**

1. **Mechanism of action.** Diethylcarbamazine citrate is a synthetic organic compound highly specific for several common parasites.

2. **Spectrum of activity.** This agent is active against *Wuchereria bancrofti, Onchocerca volvulus, Loa loa,* and *Ascaris lumbricoides.*

3. **Therapeutic uses.** Diethylcarbamazine citrate is a used for the treatment of Bancroft's filariasis, onchocerciasis, ascariasis, tropical eosinophilia, and loiasis.

4. **Precautions and monitoring effects**
   a. Patients treated for *W. bancrofti* infection often present with headache and general malaise. Severe allergic phenomena in conjunction with a skin rash have been reported.
   b. Patients treated for onchocerciasis present with pruritus and facial edema. Severe reaction may be noted after a single dose.
   c. Children who are undernourished or are suffering from debilitating ascariasis infection may experience giddiness, malaise, nausea, and vomiting after treatment.

D. **Pyrantel** is a pyrimidine derivative anthelmintic.

1. **Mechanism of action.** Pyrantel is a depolarizing neuromuscular blocking agent that causes a spastic paralysis of the helminth.

2. **Spectrum of activity.** Pyrantel is active against *A. lumbricoides* (roundworm) and *E. vermicularis* (pinworm).

3. **Therapeutic uses.** Pyrantel is used for the treatment of ascariasis (roundworm) and enterobiasis (pinworm).

4. **Precautions and monitoring effects**
   a. Most commonly reported reactions include anorexia, nausea, vomiting, diarrhea, headache, and rash.
   b. A single dose may be taken with food, milk, juice, or on an empty stomach.

5. **Significant interactions**
   a. When **piperazine** is used with pyrantel, the agents are antagonistic.
   b. **Theophylline** serum levels may increase with concomitant pyrantel administration.

E. **Thiabendazole,** a pyrazinoisoquinolone derivative, is a synthetic heterocyclic anthelmintic.

1. **Mechanism of action.** Thiabendazole has both **vermicidal** and **vermifugal** activity.

2. **Spectrum of activity.** It is active against *A. lumbricoides* (roundworm), *E. vermicularis* (pinworm), *Strongyloides stercoralis* (threadworm), *N. americanus* (American hookworm), *A. duodenale* (common hookworm), T. *trichiura* (whipworm), *Ancylostoma braziliense* (dog and cat hookworm), *Toxocara canis,* and *Toxocara cati* (ascarides).

3. **Therapeutic uses.** Thiabendazole is used for the treatment of strongyloidiasis (threadworm), cutaneous larva migrans (creeping eruption), and visceral larva migrans. It is used for the treatment of uncinariasis (hookworm), *N. americanus, A. duodenale,* trichuriasis (whipworm), and ascariasis (large roundworm) when more specific therapy is unavailable or further treatment is required with a second agent.

4. **Precautions and monitoring effects**
   a. If hypersensitivity develops, the drug should be discontinued. Erythema multiforme (including Stevens-Johnson syndrome) has been reported.
   b. **CNS effects** related to therapy have been reported. Activities requiring mental alertness should be avoided.

5. **Significant interactions**
   a. Serum **xanthine** levels may increase.
   b. Serum theophylline levels may increase.

F. **Piperazine**

1. **Mechanism of action.** Piperazine causes flaccid paralysis of the helminth by blocking the response of ascaris muscle to acetylcholine.

2. **Spectrum of activity.** It is active against *A. lumbricoides* (roundworm) and *E. vermicularis* (pinworm).

3. **Therapeutic uses.** Piperazine is used for the treatment of enterobiasis (pinworm) and ascariasis (roundworm).

4. **Precautions and monitoring effects**
   a. The most commonly reported reactions include GI and CNS effects. If these effects become significant, therapy should be discontinued.
   b. Piperazine should be taken on an empty stomach.
   c. Prolonged, repeated, and excessive therapy (particularly in children) should be avoided due to potential neurotoxicity.

G. **Quinacrine** (see also IV)

1. **Mechanism of action.** Quinacrine eradicates intestinal cestodes.

2. **Spectrum of activity.** Quinacrine is active against *Taenia saginata* (beef tapeworm), *Taenia solium* (pork tapeworm), *Hymenolepis nana* (dwarf tapeworm), *Diphyllobothrium latum* (fish tapeworm), and the protozoa, *Giardia lamblia.*

3. **Therapeutic uses.** Quinacrine is used for the treatment of *giardiasis* and *cestodiasis.*

4. **Precautions and monitoring effects**
   a. This agent should be used with caution in patients with hepatic disease.
   b. It may cause a transitory psychosis and should, therefore, be used with caution in those individuals over 60 years of age or with a history of psychosis.

H. Niclosamide

1. **Mechanism of action.** Niclosamide inhibits the oxidative phosphorylation in the mitochondria of cestodes.

2. **Therapeutic uses.** Niclosamide is used against *T. saginata* (beef tapeworm), *D. latum* (fish tapeworm), and *H. nana* (dwarf tapeworm).

3. **Precautions and monitoring effects**
   - **a.** This agent may cause nausea, vomiting, dizziness, and drowsiness.
   - **b.** It is not active against cysticercosis as it affects the cestodes of the intestine only.

I. Oxamniquine

1. **Mechanism of action.** Oxamniquine eradicates male and female schistosomes. Although it is less effective against female schistosomes, the residual females cease to lay eggs and lose the parasitologic activity.

2. **Therapeutic uses.** This agent is active against *Schistosoma mansoni* infection, including the acute and chronic phases with hepatosplenic involvement.

3. **Precautions and monitoring effects**
   - **a.** Convulsions may occur within a few hours of the first dose in patients with a previous seizure history.
   - **b.** Transitory dizziness, drowsiness, nausea, vomiting, and urticaria may occur.
   - **c.** Oxamniquine should be taken with food to increase GI tolerance.

J. Praziquantel

1. **Mechanism of action.** Praziquantel increases cell membrane permeability in susceptible helminths with loss of intracellular calcium and paralysis of their musculature. Vacuolization and disintegration of the schistosome tegument result, followed by attachment of phagocytes to the parasite and death.

2. **Therapeutic uses.** Praziquantel is active against *Schistosoma mekongi, S. japonicum, S. haematobium,* and infections due to liver flukes *(Clonorchis sinensis/Opisthorchis viverrini).*

3. **Precautions and monitoring effects**
   - **a.** Treatment of ocular cysticercosis should be avoided because parasite destruction within the eyes may cause irreparable lesions.
   - **b.** CNS effects are related to therapy, and activities requiring mental alertness should be avoided.
   - **c.** Side effects are transient and may include malaise, headache, dizziness, and abdominal discomfort.

STUDY QUESTIONS

Directions: Each of the numbered items or incomplete statements in this section is followed by answers or by completions of the statement. Select the **one** lettered answer or completion that is **best** in each case.

1. Isoniazid is a primary antitubercular agent that

(A) requires pyridoxine supplementation
(B) may discolor the tears, saliva, urine, or feces orange-red
(C) causes ocular complications that are reversible if the drug is discontinued
(D) may be ototoxic and nephrotoxic
(E) should never be used due to hepatotoxic potential

2. All of the following factors may increase the risk of nephrotoxicity from gentamicin therapy EXCEPT

(A) age over 70 years
(B) prolonged courses of gentamicin therapy
(C) concurrent amphotericin B therapy
(D) trough gentamicin levels below 2 μg/ml
(E) concurrent cisplatin therapy

3. In which of the following groups do all four drugs warrant careful monitoring for drug-related seizures in high-risk patients?

(A) Penicillin G, imipenem, amphotericin B, metronidazole
(B) Penicillin G, chloramphenicol, tetracycline, vancomycin
(C) Imipenem, tetracycline, vancomycin, sulfadiazine
(D) Cycloserine, metronidazole, vancomycin, sulfadiazine
(E) Metronidazole, imipenem, doxycycline, erythromycin

4. Spectinomycin is an aminoglycoside-like antibiotic indicated for the treatment of

(A) gram-negative bacillary septicemia
(B) tuberculosis
(C) penicillin-resistant gonococcal infections
(D) syphilis
(E) gram-negative meningitis due to susceptible organisms

5. A man has an *Escherichia coli* bacteremia with a low-grade fever (101.6°F). Appropriate management of his fever would be to

(A) give acetaminophen 650 mg orally every 4 hours
(B) give aspirin 650 mg orally every 4 hours
(C) give alternating doses of aspirin and acetaminophen every 4 hours
(D) withhold antipyretics, and use the fever curve to monitor his response to antibiotic therapy
(E) use tepid water baths to reduce the fever

6. A woman has an upper respiratory infection. Six years ago she experienced an episode of bronchospasm following penicillin V therapy. The cultures now reveal a strain of *Streptococcus pneumoniae* that is sensitive to all of the following drugs. Which of these drugs would be the best choice for this patient?

(A) Amoxicillin/clavulanate
(B) Erythromycin
(C) Ampicillin
(D) Cefaclor
(E) Cyclacillin

7. All of the following drugs are suitable oral therapy for a lower urinary tract infection due to *Pseudomonas aeruginosa* EXCEPT

(A) norfloxacin
(B) trimethoprim–sulfamethoxazole
(C) ciprofloxacin
(D) carbenicillin
(E) methenamine mandelate

8. A woman's neglected hangnail has developed into a mild staphylococcal cellulitis. Which of the following regimens would be appropriate oral therapy?

(A) Dicloxacillin 125 mg q 6h
(B) Vancomycin 250 mg q 6h
(C) Methicillin 500 mg q 6h
(D) Cefazolin 1 g q 8h
(E) Penicillin V 500 mg q 6h

9. Which of the following drugs has demonstrated in vitro activity against *Mycobacterium avium-intracellulare* (MAI)?

(A) Azithromycin
(B) Clarithromycin
(C) Erythromycin base
(D) Troleandomycin
(E) Erythromycin estolate

10. All of the following statements regarding pentamidine isethionate are true EXCEPT

(A) it is indicated for treatment or prophylaxis of infection due to *Pneumocystis carinii*
(B) it may be administered intramuscularly, intravenously, or by inhalation
(C) it has no clinically significant effect on serum glucose
(D) it is effective in the treatment of leishmaniasis

Directions: Each item below contains three suggested answers of which **one or more** is correct. Choose the answer

A if **I only** is correct
B if **III only** is correct
C if **I and II** are correct
D if **II and III** are correct
E if **I, II, and III** are correct

11. Drugs usually active against penicillinase-producing *Staphylococcus aureus* include which of the following?

I. Timentin (ticarcillin–clavulanate)
II. Augmentin (amoxicillin–clavulanate)
III. Oxacillin

12. Antiviral agents that are active against cytomegalovirus (CMV) include which of the following?

I. Ganciclovir
II. Foscarnet
III. Acyclovir

Directions: The group of items in this section consists of lettered options followed by a set of numbered items. For each item, select the **one** lettered option that is most closely associated with it. Each lettered option may be selected once, more than once, or not at all.

Questions 13–15

Match the following statements about effects or dosages with the appropriate drug.

(A) Clofazimine
(B) Itraconazole
(C) Lomefloxacin
(D) Neomycin

13. It may be administered once per day for the treatment of urinary tract infections

14. It may cause pink-to-brownish skin pigmentation within a few weeks of the initiation of therapy

15. Coadministration with astemizole or terfenadine may lead to life-threatening cardiac dysrhythmias

ANSWERS AND EXPLANATIONS

1. The answer is A *[V B 2 d (5)].*
Isoniazid increases the excretion of pyridoxine, which can lead to peripheral neuritis, particularly in poorly nourished patients. Pyridoxine (a form of vitamin B_6) deficiency may cause convulsions as well as the neuritis, involving synovial tenderness and swelling. Treatment with the vitamin can reverse the neuritis and prevent or cure the seizures.

2. The answer is D *[II B 4 b].*
Trough serum levels below 2 μg/ml are considered appropriate for gentamicin and are recommended to minimize the risk of toxicity from this aminoglycoside. Because aminoglycosides accumulate in the proximal tubule of the kidney, nephrotoxicity can occur.

3. The answer is A *[II E 1 e (2), J 5 d (2); III B 4 b; IV C 3 c].*
Seizures have been attributed to the use of penicillin G, imipenem, amphotericin B, and metronidazole. Seizures are especially likely with high doses in patients with a history of seizures and in patients with impaired drug elimination.

4. The answer is C *[II J 6].*
Although active against various gram-negative organisms, spectinomycin is approved only for the treatment of gonorrhea and is particularly recommended for treatment of uncomplicated forms of the disease.

5. The answer is D *[I H 1].*
The fever curve is very useful for monitoring a patient's response to antimicrobial therapy. Antipyretics can be used to reduce high fever in patients at risk for complications (e.g., seizures) or, in some cases, to make the patient more comfortable.

6. The answer is B *[II D 3 b].*
Amoxicillin, ampicillin, and cyclacillin are all penicillins and should be avoided in patients with histories of hypersensitivity to other penicillin compounds. Although the risk of cross-reactivity with cephalosporins (e.g., cefaclor) is now considered very low, most clinicians avoid the use of these agents in patients with histories of type I hypersensitivity reactions (anaphylaxis, bronchospasm, giant hives).

7. The answer is B *[II E 4, H 3 a, b, I 2 a, 3 a, J 7].*
Norfloxacin, ciprofloxacin, carbenicillin, and methenamine mandelate achieve urine concentrations high enough to treat urinary tract infection due to *Pseudomonas aeruginosa.* Trimethoprim–sulfamethoxazole is not useful for infection due to this organism, although the combination is useful for certain other urinary tract infections.

8. The answer is A *[II C, E 1 c (3), 2 b, J 8].*
Although vancomycin, methicillin, and cefazolin have excellent activity against staphylococci, they are not effective orally for systemic infections. Vancomycin is prescribed orally for infections limited to the gastrointestinal tract, but because it is poorly absorbed orally, it is not effective for systemic infections. Most hospital- and community-acquired staphylococci are currently resistant to penicillin V. Thus, of the drugs listed in the question, the most appropriate drug for oral therapy of staphylococcal cellulitis is dicloxacillin.

9. The answer is B *[II D 6 a, b].*
Clarithromycin, an alternative to erythromycin, has demonstrated in vitro activity against *Mycobacterium avium-intracellulare* (MAI). Clarithromycin is also used against *Toxoplasma gondii* and *Cryptosporidium* species, and it is more active than erythromycin against staphylococci and streptococci. Azithromycin is also an alternative to erythromycin, but it is more active against gram-negative organisms. Troleandomycin is similar to erythromycin but is generally less active against these organisms.

10. The answer is C *[IV D].*
Pentamidine isethionate is indicated for both treatment and prophylaxis of infection due to *Pneumocystis carinii.* It can be administered intramuscularly, intravenously, or by inhalation. Inhalation may produce bronchospasm. Blood glucose should be carefully monitored because pentamidine may produce either hyperglycemia or hypoglycemia.

11. The answer is E (all) *[II E 2–4].*
Timentin and Augmentin each include a β-lactamase inhibitor, combined with ticarcillin and amoxicillin, respectively. These combinations offer activity against *Staphylococcus aureus* similar to that of the penicillinase-resistant penicillins, such as oxacillin.

12. The answer is C (I and II) *[VI B, F, G].*
Only ganciclovir and foscarnet are active against cytomegalovirus (CMV) infections. These agents are virustatic and arrest DNA synthesis by inhibiting viral DNA polymerase. Although ganciclovir can penetrate the central nervous system (CNS), the use of ganciclovir in the treatment of CMV infections in the CNS has not been successful. Foscarnet is a broad-spectrum antiviral agent and is used in patients with ganciclovir resistance. Acyclovir is not clinically useful for the treatment of CMV infections because CMV is relatively resistant to acyclovir in vitro.

13–15. The answers are: 13-C *[II H 3 c],* **14-A** *[II J 9],* **15-B** *[III E 5 d].*
Lomefloxacin may be administered daily for treating urinary tract infections. Enoxacin is another fluoroquinolone used to treat urinary tract infections. Compared to other fluoroquinolones, neither lomefloxacin nor enoxacin improves the spectrum of activity.

Because clofazimine contains phenazine dye, it can cause pink-to-brown skin pigmentation. This change in pigmentation occurs in 75%–100% of patients taking clofazimine, and it occurs within a few weeks of the initiation of therapy. The discoloration of skin has reportedly led to severe depression and even suicide in some patients. Clofazimine is used in the treatment of leprosy and several atypical *Mycobacterium* infections.

Administration of itraconazole or ketoconazole with astemizole or terfenadine may increase the level of astemizole or terfenadine, which can lead to life-threatening dysrhythmias and death. Itraconazole, which is an imidazole, is a fungistatic agent. Specifically, itraconazole can be taken orally to treat aspergillosis infections and other deep fungal infections, such as blastomycosis, coccidioidomycosis, cryptococcosis, and histoplasmosis.

44
Seizure Disorders

Azita Razzaghi

I. INTRODUCTION

A. Definitions

1. **Seizures** are characterized by an excessive, hypersynchronous discharge of cortical neuron activity, which can be measured by the electroencephalogram (EEG). In addition, there may be disturbances in consciousness, sensory motor systems, subjective well-being, and objective behavior; seizures are usually brief, with a beginning and an end, and may produce postseizure impairment.
2. **Epilepsy** is defined as a chronic disorder, or group of disorders, characterized by seizures that usually recur unpredictably in the absence of a consistent provoking factor. The term epilepsy is derived from the Greek word meaning "to seize upon" or "taking hold of." It was first described by Hughlings Jackson in the 19th century as an intermittent derangement of the nervous system due to a sudden, excessive, disorderly discharge of cerebral neurons.
3. **Convulsions** are violent, involuntary contractions of the voluntary muscles. A patient may have epilepsy or a seizure disorder without convulsions.

B. Classification. There are two systems of classification: The first system is based on the seizure type and the characteristics of the seizures (Table 44-1), and the second system is based on the characteristics of the epilepsy, including age at onset, etiologic factors, and frequency, as well as the characteristics of the seizures as in the first classification system (Table 44-2).

1. **Partial seizures** are the most common seizure type, occurring in approximately 80% of epileptic patients.
   a. **Clinical and EEG changes** indicate initial activation of a system of neurons limited to part of one cerebral hemisphere that may extend to other or all brain areas. Manifestations of the seizures depend on the site of the epileptogenic focus in the brain.
   b. Partial seizures are subclassified as **simple** (usually unilateral involvement) and **complex** (usually bilateral involvement). Loss of consciousness is found in complex seizures. Consciousness is defined as the degree of awareness and responsiveness of the patient to externally applied stimuli.
      (1) **Simple partial seizures** generally do not cause loss of consciousness. **Signs and symptoms** of simple partial seizures may be primarily motor, sensory, somatosensory, autonomic, or psychic. These signs and symptoms may help pinpoint the site of the abnormal brain discharge; for example, localized numbness or tingling reflects a dysfunction in the sensory cortex, located in the parietal lobe.
         (a) **Motor signs** include convulsive jerking, chewing motions, and lip smacking.
         (b) **Sensory and somatosensory manifestations** include paresthesias and auras.
         (c) **Autonomic signs** include sweating, flushing, and pupil dilation.
         (d) **Psychic manifestations,** which are sometimes accompanied by impaired consciousness, include déjà vu experiences, structured hallucinations, and dysphasia.
      (2) **Complex partial seizures** are accompanied by impaired consciousness; however, in some cases, the impairment precedes or follows the seizure. These seizures have variable manifestations.
         (a) Purposeless behavior is common.
         (b) The affected person may have a glassy stare, may wander about aimlessly, and may speak unintelligibly.

Table 44-1. International Classification of Epileptic Seizures

I. Partial seizures (seizures beginning locally)
- **A. Simple partial seizures** (consciousness not impaired)
  - **1.** With motor symptoms
  - **2.** With somatosensory or special sensory symptoms
  - **3.** With autonomic symptoms
  - **4.** With psychic symptoms
- **B. Complex partial seizures** (with impairment of consciousness)
  - **1.** Beginning as simple partial seizures and progressing to impairment of consciousness
    - **a.** Without automatisms
    - **b.** With automatisms
  - **2.** With impairment of consciousness at onset
    - **a.** With no other features
    - **b.** With features of simple partial seizures
    - **c.** With automatisms
- **C. Partial seizures** (simple or complex), secondarily generalized

II. Generalized seizures (bilaterally symmetric, without localized onset)
- **A. Absence seizures**
  - **1. True absence seizures (petit mal)**
  - **2. Atypical absence seizures**
- **B. Myoclonic seizures**
- **C. Clonic seizures**
- **D. Tonic seizures**
- **E. Tonic–clonic seizures** (grand mal)
- **F. Atonic seizures**

III. Unclassified seizures

Reprinted from Commission on Classification and Terminology of the International League Against Epilepsy: Proposal for classification of epilepsies and epileptic syndromes. *Epilepsia* 26(3):268-278, 1985.

(c) Psychomotor (temporal lobe) epilepsy may lead to aggressive behavior (e.g., outbursts of rage or violence).

(d) Postictal confusion usually persists for 1–2 minutes after the seizure ends.

(e) Automatism (e.g., picking at clothes) is common and may follow visual, auditory, or olfactory hallucinations.

2. Generalized seizures are diffuse, affecting both cerebral hemispheres.

a. Clinical and EEG changes indicate initial involvement of both hemispheres.

(1) Consciousness may be impaired, and this impairment may be the initial manifestation.

(2) Motor manifestations are bilateral.

(3) The ictal EEG patterns initially are bilateral and presumably reflect neuronal discharge, which is widespread in both hemispheres.

b. There are three **types** of generalized seizures.

(1) Idiopathic epilepsies have an age-related onset, typical clinical and EEG characteristics, and a presumed genetic etiology.

(2) Symptomatic epilepsies are considered the consequence of a known or suspected disorder of the central nervous system (CNS).

(3) Cryptogenic epilepsy refers to a disorder whose cause is hidden or occult; it is presumed to be symptomatic, but the etiologic factors are unknown. It is age-related, but often does not have well-defined clinical and EEG characteristics.

c. Signs and symptoms of generalized seizures may be minor or major.

(1) Absence (petit mal) seizures present as alterations of consciousness (absences) lasting 10–30 seconds.

(a) Staring (with occasional eye blinking) and loss or reduction in postural tone are typical. If the seizure takes place during conversation, the individual may break off in midsentence.

(b) Enuresis and other autonomic components may occur during absence seizures.

(c) Some patients experience 100 or more absences daily.

Table 44-2. Proposed International Classification of Epilepsies and Epileptic Syndromes

- **I. Localized-related (focal, local, partial) epilepsies** and **syndromes**
  - **A. Idiopathic** (with age-related onset)
    - **1.** Benign childhood epilepsy with centrotemporal spikes (rolandic epilepsy)
    - **2.** Childhood epilepsy with occipital paroxysms
  - **B. Symptomatic**
    - **1.** Chronic progressive epilepsia partialis continua of childhood
    - **2.** Syndromes characterized by specific modes of precipitation
    - **3.** Temporal lobe epilepsies
    - **4.** Frontal lobe epilepsies
    - **5.** Parietal lobe epilepsies
    - **6.** Occipital lobe epilepsies
  - **C. Cryptogenic**
- **II. Generalized epilepsies and syndromes**
  - **A. Idiopathic** (with age-related onset)
    - **1.** Benign neonatal familial convulsions
    - **2.** Benign neonatal convulsions
    - **3.** Benign myoclonic epilepsy in infancy
    - **4.** Childhood absence epilepsy (pyknolepsy)
    - **5.** Juvenile absence epilepsy
    - **6.** Juvenile myoclonic epilepsy
    - **7.** Epilepsy with generalized tonic–clonic seizures on awakening
    - **8.** Other generalized idiopathic epilepsies not defined above
    - **9.** Epilepsies with seizures precipitated by specific modes of activation
  - **B. Cryptogenic or symptomatic** (in order of age)
    - **1.** West syndrome (infantile spasms)
    - **2.** Lennox-Gastaut syndrome
    - **3.** Epilepsy with myoclonic–astatic seizures
    - **4.** Epilepsy with myoclonic absences
  - **C. Symptomatic**
    - **1. Nonspecific etiology**
      - **a.** Early myoclonic encephalopathy
      - **b.** Early infantile epileptic encephalopathy with suppression burst
      - **c.** Other symptomatic generalized epilepsies not defined above
    - **2. Specific syndromes** and generalized seizures complicating other disease states
- **III. Epilepsies and syndromes undetermined whether focal or generalized**
  - **A. With both focal and generalized seizures**
    - **1.** Neonatal seizures
    - **2.** Severe myoclonic epilepsy in infancy
    - **3.** Epilepsy with continuous spike-waves during slow-wave sleep
    - **4.** Acquired epileptic aphasia (Landau-Kleffner syndrome)*
    - **5.** Other undetermined epilepsies not defined above
  - **B. Without unequivocal generalized or focal features**
- **IV. Special situations**
  - **A.** Febrile convulsions
  - **B.** Isolated seizures or isolated status epilepticus
  - **C.** Seizures occurring only when there is an acute metabolic or toxic event due to such factors as alcohol, drugs, eclampsia, and nonketotic hyperglycemia

*Believed to be a localized-related epilepsy.

Reprinted from Bleck TP: Convulsive disorders: the use of anticonvulsant drugs. *Clin Neuropharmacol* 13(3):198–209, 1990.

(d) Onset of this seizure type occurs from ages 3–16 years; in most patients, absence seizures disappear by age 40.

(2) Myoclonic (bilateral massive epileptic myoclonus) seizures present as involuntary jerking of the facial, limb, or trunk muscles, possibly in a rhythmic manner.

(3) Clonic seizures are characterized by sustained muscle contractions alternating with relaxation.

(4) Tonic seizures involve sustained tonic muscle extension (stiffening).

(5) **Generalized (grand mal) tonic–clonic seizures** cause sudden loss of consciousness.
  (a) The individual becomes rigid and falls to the ground. Respirations are interrupted. The legs extend, and the back arches; contraction of the diaphragm may induce grunting. This tonic phase lasts for about 1 minute.
  (b) A clonic phase follows, marked by rapid bilateral muscle jerking, muscle flaccidity, and hyperventilation. Incontinence, tongue biting, tachycardia, and heavy salivation sometimes occur.
  (c) During the postictal phase, the individual may experience headache, confusion, disorientation, nausea, drowsiness, and muscle soreness. This phase may last for hours.
  (d) Some epileptics have serial grand mal seizures, regaining consciousness briefly between attacks. In some cases, grand mal seizures occur repeatedly with no recovery of consciousness between attacks (**status epilepticus**); this disorder is discussed in III A.

(6) **Atonic seizures (drop attacks)** are characterized by a sudden loss of postural tone so that the individual falls to the ground. They occur primarily in children.

C. Epidemiology

1. Epilepsy has a prevalence of approximately 1% (i.e., 500,000 cases per 50 million persons worldwide).
2. In the United States, the prevalence of epilepsy is 6.42 cases per 1000 population.
3. The onset of seizures is greatest during the first year of life; this probability decreases each decade after the first year until age 60.
4. Approximately 70% of epileptics have only one seizure type; the remainder have two or more seizure types.

D. Etiology.

Some seizures arise secondary to other conditions. However, in most cases, the cause of the seizure is unknown.

1. **Primary (idiopathic) seizures** have no identifiable cause.
   a. This type of seizure affects about 75% of epileptics.
   b. The onset of primary seizures typically occurs before age 20.
   c. Birth trauma, hereditary factors, and unexplained metabolic disturbances have been proposed as possible causes.
2. **Secondary seizures** (**symptomatic** or **acquired seizures**) occur secondary to an identifiable cause.
   a. Disorders that may lead to secondary seizures include:
      (1) Intracranial neoplasms
      (2) Infectious diseases, such as meningitis, influenza, toxoplasmosis, mumps, measles, and syphilis
      (3) High fever (in children)
      (4) Head trauma
      (5) Congenital diseases
      (6) Metabolic disorders, such as hypoglycemia and hypocalcemia
      (7) Alcohol or drug withdrawal
      (8) Lipid storage disorders
      (9) Developmental abnormalities
   b. Age at seizure onset suggests the precipitating cause (Table 44-3).

E. Pathophysiology.

Seizures reflect a sudden, abnormal, excessive neuronal discharge in the cerebral cortex. Any abnormal neuronal discharge could precipitate a seizure (Figure 44-1).

1. **Normal firing of neurons,** which usually originate from the gray matter of one or more cortical or subcortical areas, requires the following elements.
   a. **Voltage-dependent ion channels** are involved in action potential propagation or burst generation.
   b. **Neurotransmitters** control neuronal firing, including excitatory neurotransmitters, acetylcholine, norepinephrine, histamine, corticotropin-releasing factors (CRF), inhibitory neurotransmitters, γ-aminobutyric acid (GABA), and dopamine; therefore, for normal neu-

Table 44-3. Probable Causes of Recurrent Seizures by Age-Group

Age at Seizure Onset	Probable Cause of Seizure
Birth–1 month	Birth injury or anoxia, congenital or hereditary diseases, and metabolic disorders
1–6 Months	As above, plus infantile spasms
6 Months–2 years	Infantile spasms, febrile convulsions, birth injury or anoxia, meningitis, and head trauma
3–10 Years	Birth injury or anoxia, meningitis, cerebral vessel thrombosis, and idiopathic epilepsy
10–18 Years	Idiopathic epilepsy and head trauma
18–25 Years	Idiopathic epilepsy, trauma, neoplasm, and withdrawal from alcohol or drugs
35–60 Years	Trauma, neoplasm, vascular disease, and withdrawal from alcohol or drugs
Over 60 years	Vascular disease, neoplasm, degenerative disease, and trauma

ronal activity, there is a need for adequate ions (e.g., sodium, potassium, calcium); excitatory and inhibitory neurotransmitters; and glucose, oxygen, amino acids, and adequate systemic pH.

c. Epileptics may be **genetically** predisposed to a **lower seizure threshold.**

d. A **diencephalic nerve group** that normally suppresses excessive brain discharge may be deafferentated, hypersensitive, and vulnerable to activation by various stimuli in epileptics.

e. During seizures, there is an increased use of energy, oxygen, and, consequently, an increased production of carbon dioxide. Because of the limited capacity to increase the blood flow to the brain, the blood supply may be **oxygen deficient.** The ratio of supply and demand decreases when the seizure episode is prolonged, leading to increased ischemia and neuronal destruction. Thus, it is crucial to diagnose seizures and treat them as soon as possible.

2. **Abnormal electrical brain activity** occurring during a seizure usually produces **characteristic changes on the EEG.** Each part of the cortical area has its own function, and the clinical

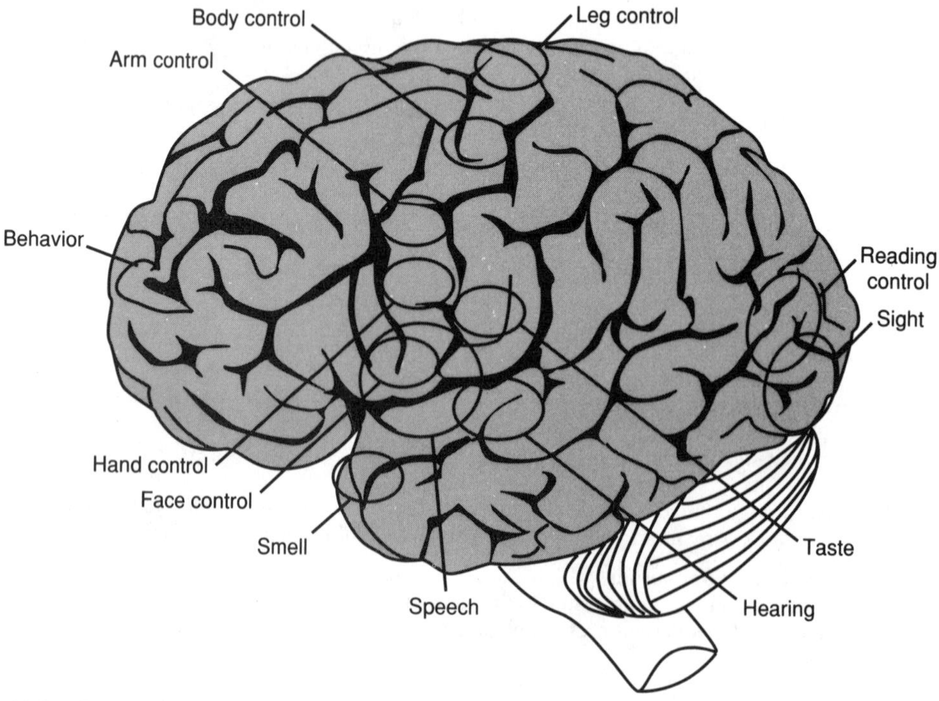

Figure 44-1. Gross anatomy of the brain. Clinical presentation of seizures depends on the area of the cortex that is affected and its function, the degree of irritability, and the identity of the impulse.

presentation of a seizure depends on the site, the degree of irritability of the area, and the intensity of the impulse.

3. Seizure activity may include three major **phases**.
   a. A **prodrome** may precede the seizure by hours or days.
      (1) Changes in behavior or mood typically occur during the prodrome.
      (2) This phase may include an aura—a subjective sensation, such as an unusual smell or flashing light.
   b. The **ictal phase** is the seizure itself. In some cases, its onset is heralded by a scream or cry.
   c. The **postictal phase** takes place immediately after the seizure.
      (1) Extensor plantar reflexes may appear.
      (2) The patient typically exhibits lethargy, confusion, and behavioral changes.

F. Clinical evaluation

1. **History** includes an evaluation of the seizure, including interviews of the patient's family and eyewitness accounts to establish:
   a. The frequency and duration of the episodes
   b. Precipitating factors
   c. The times at which episodes occur
   d. The presence or absence of an aura
   e. Ictal activity
   f. Postictal state
2. **Physical and neurological examinations** are the tools with which to identify an underlying etiology to rule out diseases that manifest as seizures (Table 44-4).
3. **Laboratory tests** may also identify an underlying etiology.
   a. Liver and kidney function tests, complete blood count (CBC), urinalysis, and serum drug levels (e.g., antidepressants and amphetamines may precipitate seizures) are necessary.
   b. Lumbar puncture may be required for evidence of cerebrospinal fluid (CSF) infection for the patient with a fever who has seizures.
4. **Neurological imaging studies,** including magnetic resonance imaging (MRI) or computed tomography (CT)–complement electrophysiological studies, can identify structural brain disorders (anatomic abnormalities).
   a. An MRI can detect cerebral lesions related to epilepsy.
   b. Positron-emission tomography (PET), single-photoemission CT (SPECT), and stable xenon-enhanced x-ray CT offer functional views of the brain to detect hypometabolism or relative hypoperfusion. PET and SPECT scans are not available in all institutions.
   c. EEG studies measure the electrical activity of the brain.
      (1) An EEG is useful for classifying the seizure, but the EEG by itself cannot rule seizures in or out, as there are patients with normal EEGs who have seizure disorders.
      (2) The best time to obtain an EEG is *during* a seizure episode. The EEG may be performed during a sleep-induced state under normal conditions or in a sleep-deprived state.

G. Treatment objectives

Table 44-4. Disorders That Mimic Epilepsy

Gastroesophageal reflux	Movement disorders
Breath-holding spells	Shuddering attacks
Migraine	Paroxysmal choreoathetosis
Confusional	Nonepileptic myoclonus
Basilar	Tics and habit spasms
With recurrent abdominal pain and cyclic vomiting	Psychological disorders
Sleep disorders (especially parasomnias)	Panic disorder
Cardiovascular events	Hyperventilation attacks
Pallid infantile syncope	Pseudoseizures
Vasovagal attacks	Rage attacks
Vasomotor syncope	
Cardiac arrhythmias	

Reprinted from Scheurer ML, Pedley TA: The evaluation and treatment of seizures. *N Eng J Med* 323:1469, 1990.

1. To prevent or suppress seizures or reduce their frequency through drug therapy
2. To control or eliminate the factors that cause or precipitate seizures
3. To prevent serious consequences of seizures, such as anoxia, airway occlusion, or injury, by protecting the tongue and placing a pillow under the victim's head
4. To encourage a normal lifestyle and prevent an invalid attitude

II. THERAPY

A. Principles of drug therapy

1. **Seizure control.** Approximately 50% of epileptics achieve complete seizure control through drug therapy. In another 25%, drugs reduce the frequency of seizures. Epileptics generally require continuous drug therapy for at least 4 seizure-free years before the drug can be discontinued.

2. **Initial treatment**
   a. Before any drug treatment is instituted, remedial causes of the seizure activity should be excluded.
   b. A single primary drug that is most appropriate for the seizure type must be selected. If there is more than one appropriate primary drug, age, sex, and compliance of the patient must be considered.
   c. Approximately one-fourth–one-third of the maintenance dose of a single medication is used to begin therapy; it is then increased over 3–4 weeks, except phenytoin or phenobarbital, which can be started with the loading or maintenance dose. The dose should be titrated until seizure control or intolerable side effects occur.
   d. With the initiation of therapy, blood concentrations of medications should be measured:
      (1) To establish therapeutic ranges and dosage regimens based on symptomatic toxicity or seizure frequency
      (2) To assess the patient's compliance with therapy
      (3) To control the correlation among the dose, blood levels, and clinical therapeutic levels or toxicity
         (a) Phenytoin follows nonlinear kinetics as drug levels increase dramatically (more than one-fold) with only a small increase in the dose; however, before this dose increase, there is a predictable linear increase with dose increases. Thus, the maximum rate of hepatic enzyme clearance is reached, and the body can no longer clear the drug as fast as it is introduced into the body.
         (b) If physical examination reveals a new onset of nystagmus (except with phenytoin in which nystagmus develops before clinical intoxication), ataxia, and unsteady, wide gait, the next dose increase should be minimal.
         (c) Carbamazepine has an autoinduction metabolism property, which means that if the dose is increased twofold, blood levels increase less than twofold because of increased metabolism.
      (4) To determine the free drug level, which is helpful in patients who are in the therapeutic range but have side effects or no response. The plasma protein binding may be altered in these patients by some other disease state or medication. Because of this alteration, there is more free drug available in the system than the total level shows, especially with phenytoin, valproic acid, and carbamazepine.

3. **Additional therapy.** If seizures recur after the maximal tolerated dose is reached, a second drug is added at a low dose.
   a. The dose of the second drug is increased until a therapeutic level is reached.
   b. The first drug is maintained until the optimal dose of the second drug is determined; then the first drug is discontinued gradually to avoid triggering seizure activity.

4. **Diseases and conditions that alter antiepileptic drug–protein bindings**
   a. Liver disease
   b. Hypoalbuminemia
   c. Burns
   d. Pregnancy

Table 44-5. Uses of Antiepileptic Medications Based on Seizure Type

	Choices of Drug Therapy			
Seizure Type	**1**	**2**	**3**	**4**
Simple partial	Carbamazepine	Phenytoin	Primidone	Gabapentin (alone or combination)
Complex partial	Carbamazepine	Phenytoin	Phenobarbital	Valproic acid (primidone)
Primary generalized tonic–clonic	Valproic acid	Carbamazepine	Phenytoin (valproic acid)	Phenobarbital
Absence	Ethosuximide	Valproic acid		
Myoclonic	Valproic acid	Clonazepam		Felbamate (alone or combination)
Atonic	Valproic acid	Clonazepam		

e. High protein-binding drugs or antiepileptic agents. (Most important interactions are discussed under individual agents.)

5. Medications. There are medications that decrease levels of phenytoin, carbamazepine, phenobarbital, and primidone by enhancing their metabolism. These drugs also cause false decreases in thyroid function tests.

a. Oral contraceptives
b. Oral hypoglycemics
c. Glucocorticoids
d. Tricyclic antidepressants
e. Azathioprine
f. Cyclosporine
g. Quinidine
h. Theophylline
i. Warfarin
j. Doxycycline
k. Levodopa

B. Specific antiseizure agents. Table 44-5 lists the uses of antiepileptic medications based on seizure type. Table 44-6 lists classifications of anticonvulsive drugs.

1. Carbamazepine

a. Mechanisms of action. Carbamazepine is chemically related to the tricyclic antidepressants. It was originally used to control the pain of trigeminal neuralgia. Its mechanism of action is unknown in the treatment of seizure disorders, but it is thought to act by reducing polysynaptic responses and blocking the post-tetanic potentiation. Carbamazepine is the drug of choice for simple partial and complex partial seizures.

b. Administration and dosage (Table 44-7)

(1) Adults and children older than 12 years receive an initial oral dose of 200 mg twice daily. This may be increased gradually to 800–2000 mg daily (usually given in divided doses).

(2) Children under age 12 usually receive 10–20 mg/kg daily in two or three divided doses.

c. Precautions and monitoring effects

Table 44-6. Anticonvulsive Drug Classification

Barbiturates	Hydantoins	Succinimides	Oxazolidinediones	Benzodiazepin	Miscellaneous
Phenobarbital	Phenytoin	Ethosuximide	Paramethadione	Clonazepam	Lamotrigine
Primidone	Mephenytoin	Methsuximide	Trimethadione		Felbamate
Mephobarbital	Ethotoin	Phensuximide			Gabapentin
	Phenacemide				Carbamazepine
					Valproic acid

Table 44-7. Dosages Characteristic of Antiepileptic Medications

Drug	Loading Dose	Usual Adult Dose (mg/day)	Half-life (hours)	Therapeutic Range of Total Plasma Concentration (μg/ml)	Major Mode of Elimination	Protein Binding Level
Carbamazepine	No	800–2000	11*–22	8–12	Hepatic	40%–90%
Phenytoin	Yes	300–700	22–72	10–20 1–2(free)	Hepatic	90%
Phenobarbital	Yes	90–300	100	15–40	Hepatic > renal	50%
Primidone	No	750–3000	15*†	5–12	Hepatic	80%
Valproic acid	No	1000–3000	15–20	50–120	Hepatic	90%–95%
Ethosuximide	No	750–1000	50	40–100	Hepatic > renal	0%
Felbamate	No	2400	20–23	30–100	Hepatic > renal	22%–25%
Gabapentin	No	900–1000	5–7	2–6	Renal > hepatic	0%
Lamotrigine	No	200–400	25 12.6a 70b	2–6	Hepatic > renal	55%

a = receiving other enzyme-inducing drugs
b = Valproic acid slows the metabolism
*The half-life decreases autometabolism after chronic use.
†Metabolized in part to phenobarbital.
Adapted from Commission on Classification and Terminology of the International League Against Epilepsy: Proposal for classification of epilepsies and epileptic syndromes. *Epilepsia* 26(3):268–278, 1985.

(1) Carbamazepine should be used with caution in patients with bone marrow depression. A CBC should be obtained and platelets measured to determine baseline levels before therapy and levels should be monitored during therapy.

(2) Tricyclic antidepressants should be avoided if there is a history of hypersensitivity to tricyclics. Monoamine oxidase (MAO) inhibitors should be discontinued 2 weeks before carbamazepine therapy.

(3) Carbamazepine should be used cautiously in patients with glaucoma because of its mild anticholinergic effects.

(4) Carbamazepine is an enzyme inducer; therefore, the half-life decreases over 3–4 weeks ($t_{1/2}$ = 18–54 hours; $t_{1/2}$ = 10–25 hours); for maximal enzyme induction, levels should be rechecked to avoid breakthrough seizures.

(5) **Adverse effects.** The physician should be notified if any of the following adverse effects occur: jaundice, abdominal pain, pale stool, darkened urine, unusual bruising and bleeding, fever, sore throat, or an ulcer in the mouth.

- **(a)** **CNS effects.** These include dizziness, ataxia, and diplopia. If diplopia and ataxia are common and occur after a dose, the schedule could be adjusted to include more frequent administration or a larger proportion of the dose at night. CNS side effects may decrease with chronic administration.
- **(b)** **Gastrointestinal (GI) effects.** These most commonly include nausea, vomiting, and anorexia.
- **(c)** **Metabolic effects.** Hyponatremia occurs after several weeks to months of therapy, and the incidence increases with age. The antidiuretic hormone (ADH) level may be low. Levels of 125–135 mEq/L without symptoms should be monitored. Fluid restriction should be instituted when levels decrease to less than 125 mEq/L with or without symptoms. Another agent should be used if fluid dose reduction does not help or the seizures recur.
- **(d)** **Hematopoietic effects.** Aplastic anemia is rare. Thrombocytopenia and anemia have a 5% incidence and they respond to a cessation of drug therapy. Leukopenia is the most common hematopoietic side effect: 10% of cases are transient, and about 2% of patients have persistent leukopenia but do not seem to have increased infections even with white blood cell (WBC) counts of 3000/ml.
- **(e)** **Dermatologic effects.** Pruritic and erythematous rashes, the Stevens-Johnson syndrome, and lupus erythematosus have been reported.

d. Significant interactions

(1) **Antiepileptic drugs,** such as **phenytoin, primidone,** and **phenobarbital,** decrease the level of carbamazepine (increase metabolism). **Valproic acid** increases the level of carbamazepine (decreases metabolism).

(2) **Other medications,** such as **erythromycin, isoniazid, cimetidine, propoxyphene, diltiazem,** and **verapamil** increase the level of carbamazepine (decrease metabolism).

2. Phenytoin

a. Mechanism of action

(1) Phenytoin inhibits the spread of seizures at the motor cortex and blocks post-tetanic potentiation by influencing synaptic transmission. There is an alternation of ion fluxes in depolarization, repolarization, and membrane stability phase and alternating calcium uptake in presynaptic terminals.

(2) Phenytoin is effective for the treatment of generalized tonic–clonic (grand mal) seizures and for partial seizures, both simple and complex. It is not effective for absence seizures.

b. Administration and dosage (see Table 44-7)

(1) The usual daily dose for **adults** is 300–700 mg, with adjustments made as needed.

(a) Regular daily doses above 500 mg are poorly tolerated.

(b) A loading dose of 900 mg to 1.5 g may be given intravenously (IV). The infusion rate should not exceed 50 mg/min. (Alternatively, an oral loading dose may be given.)

(2) The usual daily dose for **children** is 4–7 mg/kg divided every 12 hours. An IV loading dose of 15 mg/kg may be given.

(3) Phenytoin sodium is available as capsules and parenteral solution. Phenytoin is available as tablets and oral suspension.

c. Precautions and monitoring effects

(1) IV phenytoin should not be used in patients with sinus bradycardia, sinoatrial block, second- and third-degree atrioventricular (AV) block, or Adams-Stokes syndrome.

(2) Phenytoin should be used cautiously in patients with myocardial insufficiency and hypotension.

(3) Elimination of phenytoin converts from first-order elimination (proportional to its concentration) to zero-order elimination (a fixed amount per unit time), usually at high therapeutic levels. The daily dose of phenytoin can be increased 100 mg daily until therapeutic blood levels are attained after which increases of 30–50 mg will avoid two- to threefold increases in blood levels.

(4) It is necessary to measure free drug levels or correct the total level when aluminum levels are abnormal or the patient has renal failure.

(5) **Adverse effects.** The physician should be notified if any of the following adverse effects occur: swollen or tender gums, skin rash, nausea and vomiting, swollen glands, bleeding, jaundice, fever, or sore throat (i.e., signs of infection or bleeding).

(a) **CNS effects** include, ataxia (limiting side effect), dysarthria, and insomnia. Transient hyperkinesia may follow IV phenytoin infusion. Alcoholic beverages should be avoided while on this medication.

(b) **GI effects** most commonly include nausea and vomiting. Phenytoin should be taken with food to enhance absorption and decrease GI upset.

(c) **Dermatologic effects** include maculopapular rashes sometimes with fever, Stevens-Johnson syndrome, and lupus erythematosus. Gingival hyperplasia may be reduced by frequent brushing and appropriate oral care.

(d) **Connective tissue disorders** include a coarsening of the facial features.

(e) **Hematopoietic effects** include thrombocytopenia, leukopenia, and granulocytopenia.

(f) **Miscellaneous effects** include hyperglycemia and increased body hair.

d. Significant interactions

(1) **Antiepileptic drugs,** such as **carbamazepine, valproic acid, clonazepam,** and **phenobarbital** decrease the level of phenytoin (increase metabolism). **Phenytoin** increases the conversion of primidone to phenobarbital (increases metabolism).

(2) **Other medications** such as **disulfiram, isoniazid, chloramphenicol,** and **propoxyphene** increase the level of phenytoin (decrease metabolism). Drugs whose efficacy is impaired by phenytoin include **corticosteroids, digitoxin, doxycycline estrogens,**

furosemide, oral contraceptives, quinidine, rifampin, theophylline, vitamin D, and enteral nutritional therapy. Coumarin anticoagulants increase the serum phenytoin levels and prolong the serum half-life of phenytoin by inhibiting its metabolism.

3. Valproic acid

a. Mechanism of action

(1) Increases levels of GABA

(2) Potentiates a postsynaptic GABA response by inhibiting the enzymatic response for the catabolism of GABA

(3) Affects the potassium channel, creating a direct membrane-stabilizing effect

b. Administration and dosage (see Table 44-7)

(1) For **adults**, valproic acid is administered orally in a usual dose of 1000–3000 mg daily in divided doses.

(2) For **children**, valproic acid is administered orally in a dose of 15–60 mg/kg daily, divided into two or three doses.

(3) Medication should be taken with food to reduce GI upset.

(4) Tablets or capsules should be swallowed, not chewed, to avoid irritation of the mouth and throat.

c. Precautions and monitoring effects. There are some reports of hepatotoxicity and increased liver function tests, which are mostly reversible. The severity and incidence of hepatotoxicity increase when the patient is younger than 2 years old.

d. Adverse effects

(1) **CNS effects** include tremor, ataxia, diplopia, lethargy, drowsiness, behavioral changes, and depression.

(2) **GI effects** include nausea and increased appetite. Enteric-coated divalproex sodium may reduce these side effects.

(3) **Dermatologic effects** include alopecia and petechiae.

(4) **Hematopoietic effects** include thrombocytopenia, bruising, hematoma, and bleeding.

(5) **Hepatic effects** include minor elevations of aspartate aminotransferase (AST), alanine aminotransferase (ALT), and lactate dehydrogenase (LDH).

(6) **Endocrine effects** include decreased levels of prolactin, resulting in irregular menses, and secondary amenorrhea.

(7) **Pancreatic effects** include acute pancreatitis.

(8) **Metabolic effects** include hyperammonemia due to renal origin. Discontinuation may be considered if lethargy develops.

e. Significant interactions

(1) Antiepileptic drugs

(a) **Primidone** decreases valproic acid clearance (increases metabolism).

(b) **Phenobarbital** and **phenytoin** displace protein binding, resulting in an increased total phenytoin level and an increase or no change of free phenytoin.

(c) **Clonazepam** increases CNS toxicity in patients on valproic acid.

(2) Other medications

(a) **Aspirin** increases the level of valproic acid.

(b) **Warfarin** inhibits the secondary phase of platelet aggregation.

(c) **Antacids** increase the level of valproic acid.

(3) Laboratory tests

(a) False-positive urine ketone tests may result in patients taking valproic acid; thus, diabetic patients must use caution when using urine tests.

(b) Thyroid function tests may be altered by antiepileptic drugs.

4. Phenobarbital

a. Mechanism of action. Phenobarbital increases the seizure threshold by decreasing postsynaptic excitation by stimulating postsynaptic GABA-A receptor inhibitor responses as a CNS depressant.

b. Administration and dosage (see Table 44-7)

(1) For **adults**, phenobarbital is administered orally at 90–300 mg daily (in three divided doses or as a single dose at bedtime).

(2) **Children** typically receive 3–6 mg/kg daily in two divided doses. Adjustment is made as needed.

c. Precautions and monitoring effects

(1) Phenobarbital produces respiratory depression, especially with parenteral administration.

(2) Phenobarbital should be used with caution in patients with hepatic disease who may need dose adjustments.

(3) Phenobarbital has sedative effects in adults and produces hyperactivity in children.

(4) Abrupt discontinuation of phenobarbital produces withdrawal convulsions. If the drug must be discontinued, another GABA-A agonist (e.g., benzodiazepine, paraldehyde) should be substituted.

(5) **Adverse effects.** The physician should be notified if any of the following adverse effects occur: sore throat, mouth sores, easy bruising or bleeding, and any signs of infection.

(a) **CNS effects** include agitation, confusion, lethargy, and drowsiness. Patients should avoid alcohol and other CNS depressants.

(b) **Respiratory effects** include hypoventilation and apnea.

(c) **Cardiovascular effects** include bradycardia and hypotension.

(d) **GI effects** include nausea, diarrhea, and constipation. If GI upset is experienced, phenobarbital should be taken with food.

(e) **Hematologic effects** include megaloblastic anemia after chronic use (a rare side effect).

(f) **Miscellaneous effects** include osteomalacia and Stevens-Johnson syndrome, both of which are rare.

d. Significant interactions

(1) **Antiepileptic drugs,** such as **valproic acid** and **phenytoin,** increase the level of phenobarbital (decrease metabolism).

(2) **Other drugs,** such as **acetazolamide, chloramphenicol, cimetidine,** and **furosemide** increase the level of phenobarbital (decrease metabolism). **Rifampin, pyridoxine,** and **ethanol** decrease the level of phenobarbital (increase metabolism).

5. Primidone

a. Mechanism of action. Primidone is a metabolite of phenobarbital and phenylethylmalonamide (PEMA), which has some anticonvulsive effects. It has drug characteristics similar to phenobarbital with some differences in dose and half-life.

b. Administration and dosage

(1) Primidone has a short half-life of 7 hours, which may require three times daily dosing.

(2) Primidone is tolerated better if started at 50 mg at night for 3 days until the target daily dose is reached.

6. Ethosuximide

a. Mechanism of action

(1) Ethosuximide may inhibit the sodium–potassium adenosine triphosphatase (Na^+–K^+ ATPase) system and the reduced form of nicotinamide-adenine dinucleotide phosphate (NADPH)–linked aldehyde reductase (which is necessary for the formation of γ-hydroxybutyrate, which is associated with the induction of absence seizures).

(2) Ethosuximide reduces or eliminates the EEG abnormality; however, absence seizures are the only seizures in which the normal EEG has clinical value (i.e., when the EEG abnormality is corrected, the seizures are also controlled).

(3) Ethosuximide is a relatively benign anticonvulsant with minimum protein binding.

b. Administration and dosage (see Table 44-7). Ethosuximide is usually given orally in an initial dose of 500 mg daily in adults and older children and 250 mg daily in children ages 3–6 years. The dose may be raised by 250 mg every week to a maximum of 1.5 g daily in adults.

c. Precautions and monitoring effects

(1) Blood dyscrasias have been reported, making periodic blood counts necessary.

(2) There have been reports of hepatic and renal toxicity; thus periodic renal and liver function monitoring is necessary.

(3) Cases of systemic lupus erythematosus have been reported.

(4) **Adverse effects**

(a) **GI effects** include nausea and vomiting. Small doses may lessen these effects. Ethosuximide should be taken with food if GI upset occurs.

(b) **CNS effects** include drowsiness, blurred vision, fatigue, lethargy, hiccups, and headaches. Alcoholic beverages should be avoided with this medication.

(c) **Miscellaneous effects** include skin rashes, lupus, and blood dyscrasias (all rare).

d. **Significant interactions. Antiepileptic drugs,** such as **carbamazepine,** decrease the level of ethosuximide (increase metabolism), and **valproic acid** increases the level of ethosuximide (decreases metabolism).

7. **Clonazepam**

a. **Mechanism of action.** Clonazepam is a potent GABA-A agonist, but its efficacy decreases over several months of treatment.

b. **Administration and dosage**

(1) For **adults**, clonazepam is an oral agent that may be given in an initial dose of 1.5 mg daily divided two or three times. The dose may be increased to a maximum of 20 mg daily.

(2) **Children** should receive 0.01–0.03 mg daily in two or three doses. The dosage may be increased to a maximum of 0.2 mg/kg daily.

c. **Precautions and monitoring effects**

(1) Patients with psychoses, acute narrow-angle glaucoma, and significant liver disease should use this medicine cautiously.

(2) **Adverse effects**

(a) **CNS effects** include drowsiness, ataxia, and behavior disturbances in children; these may be corrected by dose reduction.

(b) **Respiratory effects** include hypersalivation and bronchial hypersecretion.

(c) **Miscellaneous effects** include anemia, leukopenia, thrombocytopenia, and respiratory depression.

d. **Significant interactions**

(1) **Antiepileptic drugs,** such as **phenytoin,** increase the level of clonazepam (decrease metabolism).

(2) **Other drugs.** Clonazepam decreases the efficacy of **levodopa** and increases the serum level of **digoxin.**

8. **Felbamate**

a. **Mechanism of action.** A proposed mechanism of action is that the drug interacts with glycine modulatory site on *N*-methyl-D-aspartate (NMDA) receptors. Blockade of NMDA may contribute to neuroprotective effects of felbamate. Felbamate is used as monotherapy or adjunctive or without secondary generalization in adults and generalized seizures associated with Lennox-Gastaut syndrome in children. The United States Food and Drug Administration (FDA) recommended that use of felbamate be restricted to use in only those patients who are refractory to other medications and in whom the risk–benefit relationship warrants its use.

b. **Administration and dosage**

(1) Adults and children older than 14 years

(2) Monotherapy, initially 1.2 g in three to four doses daily. The dosage may be increased in 600-mg increments every 2 weeks to 2.4 g daily based on clinical response and thereafter 3.6 g daily if necessary.

(3) Adjunctive, 1.2 g in three to four doses daily, with reduction of the dosage of other antiepileptic drugs by 20%–33%. The dosage of felbamate may be increased in increments of 1.2 g at weekly intervals to a maximum of 3.6 g daily.

(4) Conversion to monotherapy initially 1.2 g daily in three to four doses, with reduction of the dosage of other antiepileptic drugs by 33% at week 3. The felbamate dosage may be increased to 3.6 g daily and other antiepileptic drugs discontinued or dosage further reduced in stepwise fashion.

(5) Children 2 to 14 years with Lennox-Gastaut syndrome, as adjunctive therapy, initially 15 mg/kg daily in three to four doses. The dosage of other antiepileptic drugs is reduced by 20%. The amount of felbamate may be increased in increments of 15 mg/kg at weekly intervals to 45 mg/kg daily. Further reduction in the dosage of other antiepileptic drugs may be necessary.

c. **Precaution and monitoring effects.** There are two very serious toxic effects, aplastic anemia and liver failure, which lead to death for some patients.

(1) For aplastic anemia, the onset ranged from 5–30 weeks of initiation of therapy. Weekly or biweekly CBCs are recommended initially.

(2) For liver, toxicity time between initiation of treatment and diagnosis of these cases ranged from 14–257 days. It is recommended that liver function tests be performed before initiation of therapy to recognize patients who have evidence of preexisting

liver damage. Liver function tests should also be performed weekly or biweekly. The FDA recommends this drug be used only in patients who are refractory to other medications and in whom the risk–benefit relationship warrants its use.

(3) Photoallergy or phototoxicity may occur; patients should take protective measures against exposure to ultraviolet light or sunlight.

(4) Instruct patients to store medication in its own tightly closed container at room temperature away from excessive heat, direct sunlight, or moisture.

(5) Adverse effects

(a) This drug has potential aplastic anemia (bone marrow).

(b) The patient should be monitored for these toxicities by CBCs and liver function tests weekly or biweekly until discontinuation of any sign of these toxicities occurs.

(c) CNS effects are insomnia, headache, and fatigue.

(d) GI side effects are anorexia, weight decrease, and nausea.

(e) Hematological effects may include lymphadenopathy, leukopenia, and thrombocytopenia.

(f) Metabolic/nutrition effects may include hypokalemia and hyponatremia.

d. Significant interactions

(1) Felbamate and phenytoin. Felbamate causes an increase in phenytoin plasma concentration. Phenytoin doubles felbamate clearance, resulting in 45% decrease in felbamate levels.

(2) Felbamate and carbamazepine. Felbamate causes a decrease in carbamazepine levels and an increase in carbamazepine metabolites. In addition, carbamazepine causes a 50% increase in felbamate clearance, resulting in a 40% decrease in steady-state trough levels.

(3) Felbamate and valproic acid. Felbamate causes an increase in valproic acid levels, but valproic acid does not affect felbamate levels.

(4) Adverse effects. Signs and symptoms associated with increased plasma level and toxicity are anorexia, nausea, vomiting, insomnia, and headache.

9. Gabapentin

a. Mechanism of action. It is an analogue of GABA. It increases GABA turnover, but it does not bind to GABA or any other established neurotransmitter receptor. Its mechanism of action is currently unknown, although it binds to a specific receptor in the brain and inhibits voltage-dependent sodium currents. It has been shown to be effective as an add-on drug in patients with partial seizure without or with secondary generalization.

b. Administration and dosage

(1) Patients older than 12 years receive 900 mg to 1.8 g daily administered as adjunctive therapy in three divided doses. Titrate to an effective dose normally can be achieved within 3 days by initiating therapy with 300 mg and then increasing the dose in 300-mg increments over the next 2 days to establish a dosage of 900 mg daily in three doses. If necessary, the dosage may be increased to 1.8 g daily. To minimize potential side effects, especially somnolence, dizziness, or fatigue, the first dose on day 1 may be administered at bedtime.

(2) The drug is primarily excreted renally; therefore, the dosage should be adjusted for patients who have compromised renal function.

(3) The drug does not bind to plasma protein. There are no significant pharmacokinetic interactions with other commonly used antiepileptic drugs.

(4) If gabapentin is discontinued or an alternate anticonvulsant medication is added, it should be done gradually over a minimum of 1 week.

c. Precautions and monitoring effects

(1) The value of monitoring blood concentration has not been established and would not alter blood concentration of other antiepileptic drugs when used together.

(2) It has a low level of toxic side effects, which include somnolence, dizziness, ataxia, and minimal interaction with other drugs.

(3) Gabapentin is useful in patients who are taking other medications for epilepsy or other chronic diseases. It may be especially useful for elderly patients.

(4) Gabapentin is well absorbed orally; it can be taken with or without food. However, patients who have GI problems might have problems with absorption.

(5) Adverse effects

(a) CNS effects are somnolence, dizziness, ataxia, and fatigue.

(b) GI effects include dyspepsia, dryness of mouth, constipation, increased appetite.

(c) Vision effects are diplopia, blurred vision, and nystagmus.

d. **Significant interactions**

(1) **Antacids and gabapentin.** Antacids reduce the bioavailability of gabapentin by 20% and could be taken 2 hours after antacid use.

(2) **Cimetidine and gabapentin.** Cimetidine decreases the renal excretion of gabapentin by 14% and consequently increases gabapentin plasma levels (this amount is not clinically significant).

(3) **Oral contraceptives and gabapentin.** Oral contraceptives increase the level of norethindrone by 13%; this amount may not be clinically significant.

10. **Lamotrigine**

a. **Mechanism of action.** Its antiepileptic effect is similar to that of phenytoin. Its effect may be due to inhibition of voltage-dependent sodium currents and reduction of sustained repetitive neuronal activity. It is indicated for the treatment of partial seizures and secondary generalized tonic–clonic seizures that are not controlled with other drugs.

b. **Administration and dosage**

(1) Adults (older than 16 years), initially receive 50 mg twice daily for the first 2 weeks followed by maintenance doses of 200–400 mg daily in two doses.

(2) For patients taking valproic acid, the initial dose is 50 mg daily for the next 2 weeks, followed by maintenance doses of 100–200 mg daily in two doses.

(3) Reduced clearance in the elderly necessitates dosage reduction.

(4) Patients with hepatic impairment may require dosage reduction because of reduction in metabolism.

c. **Precautions and monitoring effects**

(1) The value of monitoring plasma concentration has not been established.

(2) Caution should be used for patients taking this drug. It may adversely affect the patient's metabolism or complicate the elimination of the drug because of renal, hepatic, or cardiac impairment.

(3) Lamotrigine binds to melanin and can accumulate in melanin-rich tissue over time. Periodic ophthalmological monitoring is recommended.

(4) Photosensitization (photoallergy and phototoxicity) patients should take protective measures against exposure to ultraviolet or sunlight.

(5) **Adverse effects**

(a) CNS side effects are headache, dizziness, and ataxia.

(b) GI effects are nausea, vomiting, diarrhea, and dyspepsia.

(c) Vision effects are diplopia, blurred vision, and vision abnormality.

(d) Dermatological effects are pruritus, and a rash may form similar to that found when using phenytoin and carbamazepine. In many cases, the rash disappears during continued therapy, and 1%–2% of patients with the rash represent more serious allergic reaction. Occasionally patients have developed the Stevens-Johnson syndrome. Concomitant use with valproic acid may increase the likelihood of serious rash.

d. **Significant interactions**

(1) Carbamazepine decreases lamotrigine concentration by 70% and increases carbamazepine levels.

(2) Phenobarbital or primidone decreases lamotrigine concentration by 40%.

(3) Valproic acid increases lamotrigine concentration twofold and valproic acid concentration by 25%.

11. **Less common drugs** (Table 44-8)

C. **Surgery.** If seizures do not respond to drug therapy, surgery may be performed to remove the epileptogenic brain region.

1. **Indications** for surgery are intractable or disabling seizures recurring for 6–12 months.

2. In **stereotaxic surgery,** the surgeon uses three-dimensional coordinates to guide a needle through a hole drilled in the skull, then destroys abnormal pathways via small intracerebral incisions.

Table 44-8. Less Common Drugs Used in Practice

Drug	Labeled Indication	Half-Life (Hours)	Therapeutic Range of Total Plasma Concentration (mg/ml)	Usual Adult Dose (mg/day)	Major Mode of Elimination	Protein-Binding Level
Mephobarbital	• Grand mal • Petit mal • Gets converted to phenobarbital • Indicated when phenobarbital must be d/c because of excessive drowsiness • Hyperexcitability • Mood disturbances	11–67	NA	400–600	Liver	40–60
Mephenytoin	• Tonic–clonic • Psychomotor • Status epilepticus • Used with phenytoin; together more sedative compared to phenytoin alone	95 (Active metabolite)	NA	200–600	Liver > > renal	90
Ethotoin	• Tonic–clonic • Psychomotor • Used as second-line therapy; less toxic than phenytoin and less effective (alone or combined)	3–9a	15–50	2000–3000	Liver	NA
Phenacemide	• Severe mixed psychomotor • Toxic drug (hydantoin toxicity) • Second-line therapy	NA	NA	2000–3000	Liver	NA
Methsuximide	• Absence • Does not precipitate tonic–clonic (compared to other succinimides)	2–40b	NA	1200	Liver	NA
Phensuximide	• Absence • Less toxic, less effective compared to other succinimides	8b	NA	1000–3000	Urine, bile	NA
Paramethadione	• Absence • Useful when other seizures exist with absence seizure • Note: Do not use with mephenytoin or phenacemide because of high toxicity	NA	NA	900–2400	Liver > renal	NA
Trimethadione	• Same as paramethadione	6–13 **days**	NA	900–2400	Liver	0

a = At high doses non-liner kinetic like phenytoin
b = Active metabolite

3. **Other surgical approaches** include temporal lobe resection, removal of the temporal lobe tip, and cerebral hemispherectomy.

III. COMPLICATIONS

A. Convulsive status epilepticus. This disorder is characterized by rapid repetition of generalized tonic–clonic seizures with no recovery of consciousness between seizures. This life-threatening condition may persist for hours or even days; if it lasts longer than 1 hour, severe permanent brain damage may result.

1. **Causes** of status epilepticus include poor therapeutic compliance, intracranial infection or neoplasm, alcohol withdrawal, drug overdose, and metabolic imbalance.
2. **Management**
   - **a.** A patent airway must be maintained.
   - **b.** If the cause of the condition is unknown, 50% dextrose in water (25–30 ml) is given via IV in case hypoglycemia is the cause.
   - **c.** If the seizures persist, **diazepam** (10 mg) is administered via IV at a rate not exceeding 2 mg/min until the seizures stop or 20 mg have been given.
   - **d. Phenytoin** is then administered via IV no faster than 50 mg/min to a maximum dose of 11–18 mg/kg. Blood pressure is monitored to detect hypotension.
   - **e.** If these measures do not stop the seizures, one of the following drugs is given.
     - **(1) Diazepam** is given as an IV drip of 50–100 mg diluted in 500 ml dextrose 5% in water, infused at 40 ml/hr until the seizures stop.
     - **(2) Phenobarbital** is given as an IV infusion of 8–20 mg/kg no faster than 100 mg/min.
   - **f.** If seizures continue despite these measures, one of the following steps is then taken.
     - **(1) Paraldehyde** is given via IV in a dosage of 0.10–0.15 ml/kg diluted to a 4% solution in normal saline solution.
     - **(2) Lidocaine** is given in an IV loading dose of 50–100 mg, followed by an infusion of 1–2 mg/min.
     - **(3) General anesthesia** is induced with ventilatory assistance and neuromuscular junction blockade.

B. Nonconvulsive status epilepticus. This condition presents as repeated absence seizures or complex partial seizures. The patient's mental state fluctuates; confusion, impaired responses, and automatisms are prominent. **Initial management** typically involves intravenous diazepam. Complex partial status epilepticus may also necessitate administration of such drugs as phenytoin or phenobarbital.

STUDY QUESTIONS

Directions: Each of the numbered items or incomplete statements in this section is followed by answers or by completions of the statement. Select the **one** lettered answer or completion that is **best** in each case.

1. Phenytoin is effective for the treatment of all of the following types of seizures EXCEPT

(A) generalized tonic–clonic
(B) simple partial
(C) complex partial
(D) absence
(E) grand mal

2. Which of the following anticonvulsants is contraindicated in patients with a history of hypersensitivity to tricyclic antidepressants?

(A) Phenytoin
(B) Ethosuximide
(C) Acetazolamide
(D) Carbamazepine
(E) Phenobarbital

3. Which anticonvulsant drug requires therapeutic monitoring of phenobarbital serum levels as well as its own serum levels?

(A) Phenytoin
(B) Primidone
(C) Clonazepam
(D) Ethotoin
(E) Carbamazepine

4. A 23-year-old patient is diagnosed with simple partial seizures. What would the drug of choice be in this patient?

(A) Carbamazepine
(B) Phenytoin
(C) Primidone
(D) Clonazepam
(E) Ethosuximide

ANSWERS AND EXPLANATIONS

1. The answer is D *[I B 2 c (1); II B 2].*
Phenytoin (diphenylhydantoin) is the most commonly prescribed hydantoin for seizure disorders. It is one of the preferred drugs for generalized tonic–clonic (grand mal) seizures and for partial seizures, both simple and complex. However, phenytoin is not effective for absence (petit mal) seizures.

2. The answer is D *[II B 1 c (2)].*
Carbamazepine is structurally related to the tricyclic antidepressants (e.g., amitriptyline, desipramine, imipramine, nortriptyline, protriptyline) and should not be administered to patients with hypersensitivity to any of the tricyclic antidepressants.

3. The answer is B *[II B 5].*
Primidone's antiseizure activity may be partly attributable to phenobarbital. In patients receiving primidone, serum levels of both primidone and phenobarbital should be measured.

4. The answer is A *[I B 1 b (1); II B 1 a].*
For simple partial seizures, the drug of choice is carbamazepine, especially in young individuals, because it has fewer side effects. The patient should begin with a low dose; if the patient continues to have seizures without limiting side effects, the dose is increased until therapeutic effects are seen or the patient develops side effects. In the case of limiting side effects or a lack of response, a second drug (phenytoin) should be added. Optimally, the carbamazepine dose may be tapered as the patient responds to the second therapy.

45
Parkinson's Disease

Azita Razzaghi

I. DISEASE STATE AND PATHOLOGY

A. Definition. Parkinson's disease is a slowly progressive degenerative neurologic disease characterized by tremor, rigidity, bradykinesia (sluggish neuromuscular responsiveness), and postural instability. Parkinson's disease was first described by Dr. James Parkinson in 1817 as "shaking palsy."

B. Incidence

1. It is one of the most common neurologic disorders that occur after age 50 (with an incidence of 100–150/100,000 population).
2. Onset generally occurs between age 50 and 65; usually in the 60s.

C. Pathogenesis. Parkinson's disease is a neurodegenerative disease associated with **depigmentation of the substantia nigra** and the **loss of dopaminergic input to the basal ganglia** (extrapyramidal system); it is characterized by distinctive **motor disability** (Figure 45-1).

D. Etiology. Several forms of Parkinson's disease have been recognized.

1. **Primary (idiopathic) Parkinson's disease**
   a. This is also called classic Parkinson's disease or **paralysis agitans.**
   b. The cause is unknown, and while treatment may be palliative, the disease is incurable.
   c. Most patients suffer from this type of parkinsonism.
   d. **Hypotheses of neuronal loss** in idiopathic Parkinson's disease are:
      (1) **Absorption of highly potent neurotoxins,** such as carbon monoxide, manganese, solvents, and *N*-methyl-4-phenyl-1,2,3,6-tetrahydropyridine (MPTP), which is a product of improper synthesis of a synthetic heroin-like compound. Exposure to these agents, alone or in combination with the neuronal loss of age, may be the cause of Parkinson's disease.
      (2) **Exposure to the free radicals.** Normally, dopamine is catabolized by monoamine oxidase (MAO). Hydrogen peroxide and production of free radicals—both toxic to cells—are products of catabolism. Protective mechanisms, enzymes, and free radical scavengers, such as vitamins E and C, protect cells from damage. It is proposed that either a decrease in these protective mechanisms or an increase in the production of dopamine causes a destruction of the neurons by free radicals.
2. **Secondary parkinsonism—from a known cause**
   a. Only a small percentage of cases are secondary, and many of these are curable.
   b. Secondary parkinsonism may be caused by drugs, including dopamine antagonists, such as:
      (1) Phenothiazines (e.g., chlorpromazine, perphenazine)
      (2) Butyrophenones (e.g., haloperidol)
      (3) Reserpine
   c. Poisoning by chemicals or toxins may be the cause, including:
      (1) Carbon monoxide poisoning
      (2) Heavy metal poisoning, such as that by manganese or mercury
      (3) MPTP, a commercial compound used in organic synthesis and found (as a side product) in an illegal meperidine analogue
   d. Infectious causes include:
      (1) Encephalitis (viral)

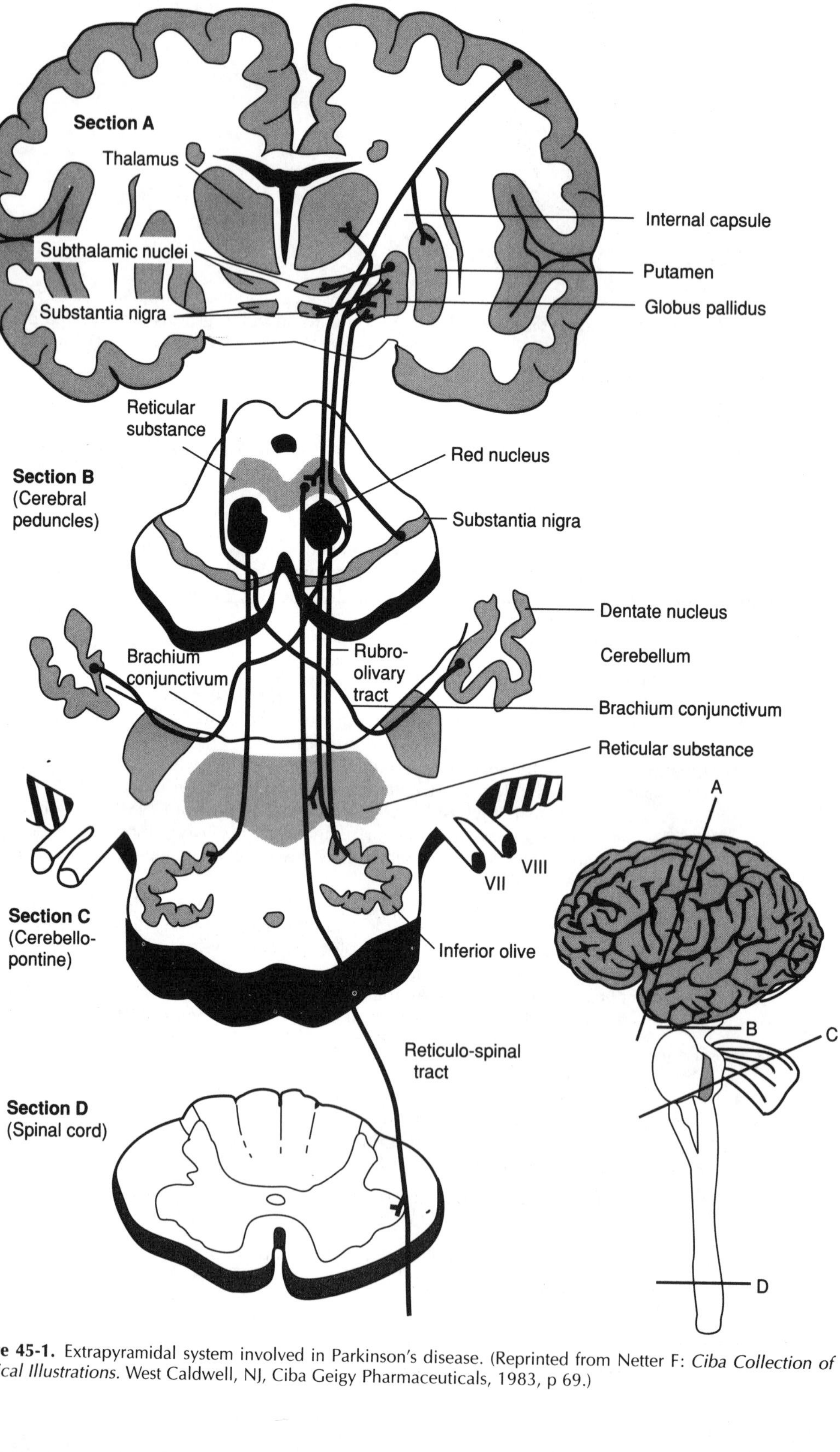

Figure 45-1. Extrapyramidal system involved in Parkinson's disease. (Reprinted from Netter F: *Ciba Collection of Medical Illustrations.* West Caldwell, NJ, Ciba Geigy Pharmaceuticals, 1983, p 69.)

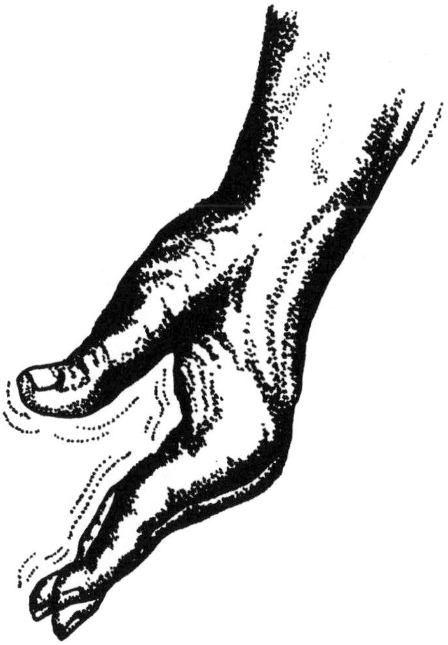

Figure 45-2. Resting (or static) tremors. (Adapted from Bates B: *A Guide to Physical Examination and History Taking,* 5th ed. Philadelphia, JB Lippincott, 1991, p 554.)

(2) Syphilis

e. Other causes include:
   (1) Arteriosclerosis
   (2) Degenerative diseases of the central nervous system (CNS), such as progressive supranuclear palsy
   (3) Metabolic disorders, such as Wilson's disease

E. Signs and symptoms

1. **Tremor**
   a. Tremor may be the initial complaint in some patients. It is most evident at rest **(resting tremor)** and with low-frequency movement. When the thumb and forefinger are involved, it is known as the **pill-rolling tremor.** Before pills were made by machine, pharmacists made tablets (pills) by hand, hence the name (Figure 45-2).
   b. Some patients experience **action tremor** (most evident during activity), which can exist with or before the resting tremor develops.

2. **Limb rigidity** is present in almost all patients. It is detected clinically when the arm responds with a ratchet-like (i.e., cogwheeling) movement when the limb is moved passively. This is owing to a tremor that is superimposed on the rigidity.

3. **Akinesia or bradykinesia.** Akinesia is characterized by difficulty in initiating movements, and bradykinesia is a slowness in performing common voluntary movements, including standing, walking, eating, writing, and talking. The lines of the patient's face are smooth, and the expression is fixed **(masked face)** with little evidence of spontaneous emotional responses (Figure 45-3).

4. **Gait and postural difficulties.** Characteristically, patients walk with a stooped, flexed posture; a small shuffling stride; and a diminished arm swing in rhythm with the legs. There may be a tendency to accelerate or festinate (Figure 45-4).

5. **Changes in mental status.** Mental status changes, including depression (50%), dementia (25%), and psychosis, are associated with the disease and may be precipitated or worsened by drugs.

F. Stages of Parkinson's disease (Table 45-1)

G. Diagnosis

1. Diagnosis depends on clinical findings.

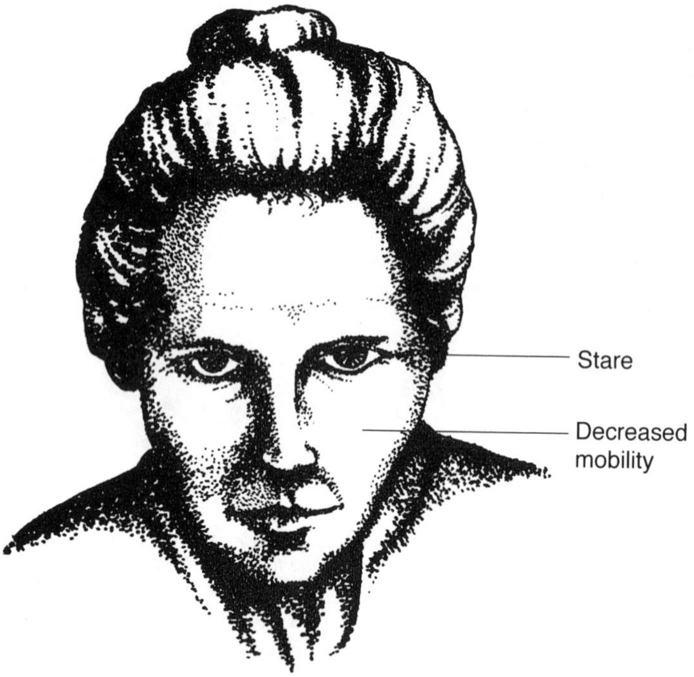

Figure 45-3. Masked face of Parkinson's disease. (Adapted from Bates B: *A Guide to Physical Examination and History Taking,* 5th ed. Philadelphia, JB Lippincott, 1991, p 197.)

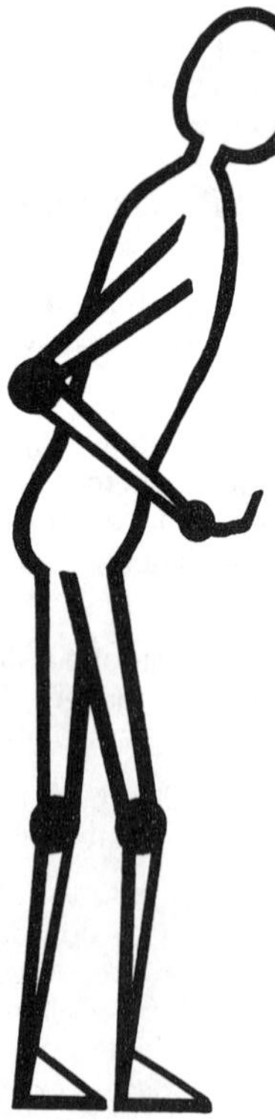

Figure 45-4. Characteristic walk of patients with Parkinson's disease. (Adapted from Bates B: *A Guide to Physical Examination and History Taking,* 5th ed. Philadelphia, JB Lippincott, 1991, p 553.)

Table 45-1. Stages of Parkinson's Disease

Stage I	Unilateral involvement
Stage II	Bilateral involvement but no postural abnormalities
Stage III	Bilateral involvement with mild postural imbalance; patient leads independent life
Stage IV	Bilateral involvement with postural instability; patient requires substantial help
Stage V	Severe, fully developed disease; patient restricted to bed or chair

Reprinted from Hoehn MM, Yahr MD: Parkinsonism: onset, progression, and mortality. *Neurology* 17:427, 1967.

2. Tests (including imaging) are mostly used to rule out an etiology of secondary Parkinson's disease.
3. New technologies [e.g., positron emission tomography (PET scan)] are used to visualize dopamine uptake in the substantia nigra and basal ganglia. The PET scan measures the extent of neuronal loss in these areas, but it is not yet widely available.

H. Treatment

1. **Drug therapy for symptomatic relief.** Four classes of drugs are available.
   a. Anticholinergics (for resting tremor)
   b. Precursor of dopamine (e.g., carbidopa/levodopa)
   c. Direct-acting dopamine agonists (e.g., bromocriptine, pergolide)
   d. Indirect-acting dopamine agonists
      (1) Decrease re-uptake (e.g., amantadine)
      (2) Decrease metabolism (e.g., selegiline)
2. **Drug therapy for treating associated symptoms**
   a. **Tricyclic antidepressants** are used to treat **depression.** They exhibit some dopaminergic and anticholinergic effects.
   b. **β-Blockers,** especially **propranolol** with its high lipophilicity, **benzodiazepines,** and **primidone** are medications used for **action tremor.** Usually patients show a clinical response in low doses.
   c. **Antihistamine.** Diphenhydramine hydrochloride has some mild anticholinergic effects and is used for symptomatic release of mild tremor and because of its adverse reaction in the CNS, is used with caution in the elderly
3. **General principles of drug therapy**
   a. If a patient does not respond to an agent in one class, another class should be tried. The two dopamine agonists, bromocriptine and pergolide, are two exceptions. Studies show that some patients respond to one agent when they fail to respond to another. This could be because of their different potencies or the limited information available on pergolide.
   b. Therapy should be started with a low dose and titrated up. Response usually is seen within a few days after starting therapy.
   c. If a second agent is added to the drug therapy, the dose of the first medication should be decreased to minimize side effects.
   d. Drug therapy should never be discontinued suddenly because withdrawal may exacerbate the symptoms.
4. **Definitions concerning drug therapy**
   a. **Dyskinesias** are typically oral–facial movements, grimacing, or jerky and writhing movements of the trunk and extremities. They are always reversible with antiparkinsonian medications, and they decrease or diminish with dose reduction. Symptoms of Parkinson's disease may reappear by reducing the dose, and it is the clinical judgment of the physician or the preference of the patient whether to continue with the drug regimen or tolerate the side effects.
   b. **On–off effect** describes oscillations in response (at the receptor site) and sudden changes in mobility from no symptoms to full parkinsonian symptoms in a matter of minutes. No direct relationship between the on–off effect and drug levels has been found. Usually, a second drug is added to the therapy regimen to correct the effect. Reducing the dose of one drug and adding a second drug may also be useful.
   c. **End-dose effect,** known also as the **wearing-off effect,** occurs at a latter part of the dosing interval; it may improve by shortening the dosing interval.

d. **Drug holiday.** Long-term levodopa use results in down-regulation of dopamine receptors. A drug holiday allows striatal nigra dopamine receptors to be re-sensitized, although controversy exists regarding the consequences and the outcome of this "holiday."

5. **Physical rehabilitation** restores patients' physical function and independence by physical and occupational therapy. These will help patients with managing big and small muscle groups by focusing on maintaining coordination, dexterity, flexibility, and range of motions.

6. **Psychological rehabilitation** provides support for patients and their families. Keep in mind that patients with Parkinson's disease have a high incidence of depression, and in later stages of the disease they develop dementia (Table 45-2).

II. INDIVIDUAL DRUGS

A. **Anticholinergic agents** are used for mild symptoms, predominantly tremors.

1. **Mechanism of action.** This class of drugs blocks the excitatory neurotransmitter cholinergic influence in the basal ganglia. These drugs are more effective for tremor and rigidity than for bradykinesia and less effective for postural imbalance.
2. **Administration and dosage** (Table 45-3)
3. **Precautions and monitoring effects**
   a. Anticholinergics should be used with caution in patients with obstructed gastrointestinal (GI) or genitourinary (GU) tracts, narrow-angle glaucoma, or severe cardiac disease. Physicians should be notified if a rapid heartbeat or eye pain are experienced. (Frequent ophthalmologic visits are recommended.)
   b. The sedative side effects of antihistamines may be beneficial in some patients.
   c. Alcohol and other CNS depressants should be used with caution.
   d. **Adverse effects** of anticholinergic therapy include the following:
      (1) **Peripheral anticholinergic effects** include dry mouth (hard candies may be helpful); decreased sweating, resulting in decreased tolerance to heat; urinary retention; constipation (stool softeners may be helpful); increased intraocular tension;

Table 45-2. Overview of Parkinson's Disease Management

		Treatment Considerations	
Stage	**Characteristics**	**Physical**	**Psychosocial**
Early	Fully functional May have unilateral tremor, rigidity	Preventative exercise program	Education Information
Early middle	Symptoms bilateral, bradykinesia, rigidity Mild speech impairment Axial rigidity, stooped posture, stiffness Gait impairment begins	Corrective exercise program	Counseling Support group Monitor for depression
Late middle	All symptoms worse but independent in ADLs[a] May need minor assistance Balance problems	Compensatory and corrective exercise Speech therapy Occupational therapy	Caregiver issues (medications, mobility) Monitor for dementia
Late	Severely disabled, impaired Dependent with ADLs	Compensatory exercise Dietary concerns Skin care Hygiene Pulmonary function	Dementia Depression

[a]ADLS = activities of daily living.

Reprinted from Custin TM: Overview of Parkinson's disease management, *Physical Therapy* 75:363–373, 1995.

Table 45-3. Dosage Range and Characteristics of Drug Treatment

Drugs	Time to Peak Concentration (hours)	Half-Life (hours)	Daily Dosage Range (mg/day)
Anticholinergic agents			
Benztropine	Not available	Not available	1–6
Biperiden	1–1.5	18.4–24.3	2–8
Procyclidine	1.1–2	11.5–12.6	6–20
Trihexyphenidyl	1–1.3	5.6–10.2	2–15
Amantadine	4–8	9.7–14.5	100–400
Levodopa/carbidopa	1	1–1.75	10/100–25/100 tid q 3 hours
Sustained release	2	> standard treatment	10/400–25/1000 in 2–3 divided doses
Dopaminergic agents			
Bromocriptine	1–3	48	2.50–25
Pergolide	2	8	0.1–5
Selegiline	0.5–2	2–20.5	5–10

and nausea. Because of patients' decreased tolerance to heat, these agents should be used with caution in hot weather. They should also be taken with food to minimize GI upset.

(2) **CNS effects** include dizziness, delirium, disorientation, anxiety, agitation, hallucinations, and impaired memory. The incidence of CNS effects increases in elderly individuals.

(3) **Cardiovascular effects** include hypotension and orthostatic hypotension.

4. Significant interactions

a. Side effects may be potentiated by other drugs with anticholinergic activity such as **antihistamines, antidepressants,** and **phenothiazines.**

b. Anticholinergic agents increase **digoxin** levels.

c. When anticholinergic agents are taken with **haloperidol,** the following occurs:

(1) Schizophrenic symptoms may increase.

(2) Haloperidol levels may decrease.

(3) The severity of (not the risk of) tardive dyskinesia may increase.

d. When **phenothiazines** are taken with anticholinergic drugs, the effects of the phenothiazines decrease and the anticholinergic symptoms increase.

e. Patients on high doses of anticholinergics combined with **levodopa** should be watched for decreased levodopa activity because of a delayed gastric emptying time.

B. Dopamine precursor. Levodopa/carbidopa is the most effective drug for managing Parkinson's disease; however, prolonged use decreases its therapeutic effects (there is a decline in efficacy after 3–5 years) and increases adverse drug reactions. Dopamine does not cross the blood–brain barrier; therefore a precursor is used. Peripheral conversion of levodopa to dopamine causes adverse reactions like nausea, vomiting, cardiac arrhythmias, and postural hypotension. To decrease the peripheral conversion and peripheral adverse effects, a peripheral dopa decarboxylase inhibitor (carbidopa) is added to levodopa (Sinemet).

1. Mechanism of action

a. Levodopa is converted to dopamine by the enzyme dopa decarboxylase, which elevates CNS levels of dopamine.

b. The sustained-release formulation is designed to release the drug over 4–6 hours, thereby inhibiting variation in plasma concentration and decreasing motor fluctuation "off" time, or to improve overall dose response in patients with advanced disease.

2. Administration and dosage (see Table 45-3)

a. It is necessary to give at least 100 mg daily of carbidopa to decrease the incidence of the peripheral conversion of levodopa and GI side effects (e.g., nausea) and increase the bioavailability of levodopa for the CNS.

b. If carbidopa is given in a separate dosage form, the dose of levodopa can be decreased by 75%.

c. If patients still complain of GI side effects after combination levodopa/carbidopa, plain carbidopa (supplied by Merck & Co., Inc.) can be given.
d. Sustained-release preparations are approximately 30% less bioavailable as compared with levodopa/carbidopa. Because of this lower bioavailability, the daily dosage should be higher. If a patient is receiving a standard preparation and needs to be converted to the sustained-release dose, approximately 10% more levodopa should initially be added to daily dosage and at least 3 days should pass between increased dosages; then gradually increase the levodopa dose up to 30% of standard preparation.
e. With the sustained-release preparation the peak plasma concentration is lower and the trough plasma concentration is higher.
f. The sustained-release preparation could be divided in half at the scored point only. The tablet should not be chewed or crushed.

3. **Precautions and monitoring effects**
   a. Levodopa must be used with caution in patients with narrow-angle glaucoma.
   b. Levodopa may activate a malignant melanoma in patients with suspicious undiagnosed skin lesions or a history of melanoma.
   c. The efficacy of levodopa declines with long-term therapy by desensitizing the receptors or because of the decreased number of receptors, resulting from the progression of the disease.
   d. **Adverse drug reactions**
      (1) **GI effects** include anorexia, nausea and vomiting, and abdominal distress. Levodopa should be taken with food to minimize stomach upset.
      (2) **Cardiovascular effects** include postural hypotension and tachycardia.
      (3) **Musculoskeletal effects** include dystonia or choreiform muscle movement.
      (4) **CNS effects** include confusion, memory changes, depression, hallucinations, and psychosis. Physicians should be notified if any of these symptoms occur.
      (5) **Hematologic effects** include hemolytic anemia, leukopenia, and agranulocytosis (rare).

4. **Significant interactions**
   a. **Antacids** cause rapid and complete intestinal levodopa absorption (by decreasing gastric emptying time).
   b. **Hydantoin** decreases the effectiveness of levodopa.
   c. **Methionine** increases the clinical signs of Parkinson's disease.
   d. **Metoclopramide** increases the bioavailability of levodopa, which decreases the effects of metoclopramide on gastric emptying and on lower esophageal pressure. As a dopamine blocker, it may also precipitate parkinsonian symptoms.
   e. False-positive results are seen with the Coombs' test.
   f. The uric acid test increases with the calorimetric method but not with the uricase method.
   g. Hypertensive reactions may occur if levodopa is administered to patients receiving **MAO inhibitors** and **furazolidone.** MAO inhibitors must be discontinued 2 weeks before starting levodopa.
   h. Administering **papaverine** may decrease the effect of levodopa.
   i. **Tricyclic antidepressants** decrease the rate and extent of absorption of levodopa; hypertensive episodes have been reported when levodopa is combined with tricyclic antidepressants.
   j. **Food** decreases the rate and extent of absorption and transport to the CNS across the blood–brain barrier. A **protein-restricted diet** may also help to minimize the "fluctuations" (i.e., the decreased response to levodopa) at the end of each day or at various times of the day.

C. Direct-acting dopamine agonists

1. **Bromocriptine**
   a. **Mechanism of action.** Bromocriptine is responsible for directly stimulating postsynaptic dopamine receptors; it is most commonly used as an adjunct to levodopa therapy in patients:
      (1) With a deteriorating response to levodopa
      (2) With a limited clinical response to levodopa secondary to an inability to tolerate higher doses
      (3) Who are experiencing fluctuations in response to levodopa

b. Administration and dosage (see Table 45-3)
  (1) Initially, patients are given 1/2 tablet twice daily, which is then increased to one tablet twice daily every 2–3 days.
  (2) Patients' responses are extremely variable. Many patients show a dopamine antagonist response at both low and high doses, with the desirable agonist response in the midrange.
  (3) Because postural hypotension may result from the first few doses of bromocriptine, the first dose should be administered with the patient lying down, and sudden changes in posture should be avoided.

c. Precautions and monitoring effects
  (1) Bromocriptine may cause a first-dose phenomenon that can trigger sudden cardiovascular collapse. It should be used with caution in patients with a history of myocardial infarction or arrhythmias.
  (2) Early in therapy, dizziness, drowsiness, and fainting may occur, so patients should be cautious about driving or operating machinery. A physician should be notified if these symptoms appear.
  (3) **Cardiac dysrhythmias.** Patients on bromocriptine were found to have significantly more episodes of atrial premature contractions and sinus tachycardia.
  (4) **Other adverse effects**
    (a) **GI effects,** including anorexia, nausea, vomiting, and abdominal distress, may be decreased by taking bromocriptine with food.
    (b) **Cardiovascular effects** include postural hypotension (to which tolerance develops) and tachycardia. Blood pressure must be monitored, particularly for patients taking antihypertensive medication.
    (c) **Pulmonary effects,** including reversible infiltrations, pleural effusions, and pleural thickening, may develop after long-term treatment, so pulmonary function should be monitored in patients treated longer than 6 months.
    (d) **CNS effects,** including confusion, memory changes, depression, and hallucinations, and psychosis, may be exacerbated by bromocriptine; thus, patients with psychiatric illnesses must be monitored.

d. Significant interactions
  (1) A combination of **antihypertensive drugs** and bromocriptine could decrease blood pressure.
  (2) **Dopamine antagonists** increase the effect of bromocriptine.

2. Pergolide

a. Mechanism of action. Pergolide is a semisynthetic ergosine derivative. In Parkinson's disease, it exerts its effect by directly stimulating postsynaptic dopamine receptors in the nigrostriatal system, with D_1-agonist properties.
  (1) It is 10 times more potent than bromocriptine on a milligram basis.
  (2) It inhibits the secretion of prolactin, increases the serum concentration of growth hormone, and decreases the serum concentration of luteinizing hormone.
  (3) It is most commonly used as adjunctive treatment to levodopa/carbidopa.

b. Administration and dosage (see Table 45-3)

c. Precautions and monitoring effects
  (1) Hypersensitivity reactions to pergolide and other ergot derivatives can occur.
  (2) Caution must be used with patients who are at high risk for ventricular arrhythmia, especially when doses higher than 3 mg/day are used.
  (3) **Cardiac dysrhthmias.** Adverse effects are similar to those experienced with bromocriptine [see II C 1 c (3)].
  (4) **CNS effects** include dyskinesia, hallucinations, somnolence, and insomnia.
  (5) **GI effects** include nausea, constipation, diarrhea, and dyspepsia.
  (6) **Cardiovascular effects** include premature atrial contractions and sinus tachycardia (alone or in combination with levodopa).
  (7) **Miscellaneous effects** include transient elevations of aspartate aminotransferase, alanine aminotransferase, and alkaline phosphatase, and pleural thickening.

d. Significant interactions
  (1) Because pergolide is 90% protein bound, it must be used with caution with other highly **protein-bound drugs.**
  (2) **Antipsychotic agents** (e.g., phenothiazines, haloperidol, metoclopramide) combined with dopamine agonists decrease the dopamine action and decrease the therapeutic action of the antipsychotic agent.

D. Indirect-acting dopamine agonists

1. Selegiline

a. Mechanism of action

(1) MAO catabolizes various catecholamines (e.g., dopamine, norepinephrine, epinephrine), serotonin, and various exogenous amines (e.g., tyramines) found in foods (e.g., aged cheese, beer, wine, smoked meat) and drugs. Lack of MAO in the intestinal tract causes absorption of these amines, creating a hypertensive crisis. MAO type A is predominantly found in the intestinal tract, and MAO type B in the brain. They differ in their substrate specificity and tissue distribution. This specificity decreases with selegiline as the dose increases. Most patients experience side effects at doses of selegiline higher than 30–40 mg/day.

(2) Selegiline is a selective inhibitor of MAO type B, which prevents the breakdown of dopamine selectively in the brain at recommended doses.

(3) Selegiline is most commonly used as an adjunct with levodopa/carbidopa when patients experience a "wearing-off" phenomenon; it decreases the amount of "off" time and decreases the dose needed of levodopa/carbidopa by 10%–30%.

(4) Results of some studies show that selegiline delays the time before a treatment with a more potent dopaminergic drug like levodopa is needed; the proposed mechanism of action is that an oxidation mechanism contributes to the emergence and progression of Parkinson's disease.

b. Administration and dosage (see Table 45-3). Exceeding the recommended dose of 10 mg/day increases the risk of losing MAO selectivity. The precise selectivity dose is unknown but seems to be above 30–40 mg/day.

c. Precautions and monitoring effects

(1) Hypertensive crisis [see II D 1 a (1)]

(2) Levodopa-associated side effects may be increased because the increased amounts of dopamine react with supersensitive postsynaptic receptors. Reducing the dose of levodopa/carbidopa by 10%–30% may decrease levodopa side effects.

(3) Patients should be educated about foods and drugs containing tyramine and the signs and symptoms of hypertensive reactions.

(4) CNS effects include dizziness, confusion, headache, hallucinations, vivid dreams, dyskinesias, behavioral and mood changes, and depression. Patients who experience insomnia should avoid taking the drug late in the day.

(5) Cardiovascular effects include orthostatic hypotension, hypertension, arrhythmia, palpitation, sinus bradycardia, and syncope.

(6) GI effects includes nausea, abdominal pain, and **lead to GI bleed,** weight loss, poor appetite, and dysphagia.

(7) GU effects include slow urination, transient nocturia, and prostatic hypertrophy.

(8) Dermatologic effects include increased sweating, diaphoresis, and photosensitivity.

(9) Hepatic effects include mild and transient elevations in liver function tests.

d. Significant interactions. MAO inhibitors are contraindicated with **meperidine** and other opioids. Because the mechanism of action is unknown, administration with opioids should be avoided. When used with fluoxetine, at least 5 weeks should elapse between discontinuing fluoxetine and starting selegiline and at least 14 days between discontinuing selegiline and starting fluoxetine. This is based on one death report; no cause and effect has been established but the manufacturer recommends that these two drugs not be given together.

2. Amantadine

a. Mechanism of action. Amantadine is an antiviral agent (used to prevent influenza).

(1) Amantadine increases dopamine levels at postsynaptic receptor sites by decreasing presynaptic re-uptake and enhancing dopamine synthesis and release.

(2) It may also have some anticholinergic effects. It decreases tremor, rigidity, and bradykinesia.

(3) It can be given in combination with levodopa as Parkinson's disease progresses.

(4) Clinical effects of amantadine can be seen within the first few weeks of therapy, unlike the other antiparkinsonian medications (e.g., carbidopa/levodopa), which need weeks to months to show their full clinical effect.

b. Administration and dosage (see Table 45-3)

(1) Amantadine should be started at 100 mg/day. This may be increased to 200–300 mg/day as a maintenance dose.

(2) Patients experiencing a decline in response may benefit from the following:
 (a) Discontinuing the drug for a few weeks, then restarting it
 (b) Using the drug episodically, only when the patient's condition most needs a therapeutic boost

(3) Amantadine is also available in liquid form for patients with dysphagia.

c. Precautions and monitoring effects

(1) Amantadine should be used with caution in patients with renal disease, congestive heart failure (CHF), peripheral edema, history of seizures, and mental status changes. It may be necessary to modify dosages in patients with renal failure.

(2) Tolerance usually develops within 6–12 months. If tolerance occurs, another drug from a different class can be added, or the dose may be increased.

(3) Patients should be informed about the side-effect profile.
 (a) **Peripheral anticholinergic effects** include those mentioned in II A 3 d (1).
 (b) **CNS effects** include seizures as well as those mentioned in II A 3 d (2).
 (c) **Cardiovascular effects.** Patients may develop CHF. Periodic blood pressure monitoring and electrocardiograms (ECGs) are necessary in patients with myocardial infarction or arrhythmias.
 (d) **Dermatologic effects** include **livedo reticularis,** a diffuse rose color mottling of the skin, which is reversible upon discontinuing the drug.
 (e) **Hematologic effects.** Periodic complete blood counts (CBCs) should be done for patients with long-term therapy.

d. Significant interactions

(1) Amantadine increases the anticholinergic effects of **anticholinergic drugs,** requiring a decrease in the dosage of the anticholinergic drug.

(2) **Hydrochlorothiazide** plus **triamterene** decrease the urinary excretion of amantadine and increase its plasma concentration.

III. SURGICAL TREATMENT includes autologous adrenal medulla or fetal substantia nigra transplants, but the validity, applicability, and long-term benefits of surgery are unknown at present.

STUDY QUESTIONS

Directions: Each of the numbered items or incomplete statements in this section is followed by answers or by completions of the statement. Select the **one** lettered answer or completion that is **best** in each case.

1. The maximum recommended daily dose of levodopa is

(A) 500 mg
(B) 1 g
(C) 2 g
(D) 4 g
(E) 8 g

2. When administered with carbidopa, the dosage of levodopa is usually decreased by

(A) 75%
(B) 50%
(C) 40%
(D) 20%
(E) 10%

3. Which of the following agents should NOT be used concurrently with levodopa?

(A) Diphenhydramine
(B) Benztropine
(C) Amantadine
(D) Monoamine oxidase (MAO) inhibitors
(E) Carbidopa

Directions: Each item below contains three suggested answers of which **one or more** is correct. Choose the answer

A if **I only** is correct
B if **III only** is correct
C if **I and II** are correct
D if **II and III** are correct
E if **I, II, and III** are correct

4. Levodopa is associated with which of the following problems?

I. Gastrointestinal side effects
II. Involuntary movements
III. A decline in efficacy after 3–5 years

5. Amantadine has which of the following advantages over levodopa?

I. More rapid relief of symptoms
II. Higher success rate
III. Better long-term effects

ANSWERS AND EXPLANATIONS

1. The answer is E *[II B 2; Table 45-3].*
The maximum total daily dose of levodopa should be 8 g, administered in divided doses at least three times a day. Levodopa is used in treating Parkinson's disease to replenish the brain's supply of dopamine, the neurotransmitter that is deficient in this disorder. Dopamine itself does not cross the blood–brain barrier, and therefore its precursor, levodopa, is administered. Levodopa is metabolized to dopamine in the body by dopa decarboxylase. Dosage of levodopa must be carefully titrated for each patient to produce the maximum improvement with the least side effects.

2. The answer is A *[II B 2 b].*
Administering carbidopa in combination with levodopa reduces the required dose of levodopa by about 75%. When levodopa is given alone, much of the dose is metabolized before the drug reaches the brain. Therefore, large doses are required and these are apt to cause unwanted side effects. Carbidopa inhibits the peripheral decarboxylation of levodopa. This action simultaneously reduces the likelihood of peripheral side effects and allows more levodopa to reach the brain. Because carbidopa does not cross the blood–brain barrier, the levodopa in the brain is converted there to dopamine. Thus, coadministering carbidopa plus levodopa allows the levodopa dosage to be significantly reduced without reducing the desired effects.

3. The answer is D *[II B 4 g].*
Levodopa causes a significant rise in blood pressure as well as flushing and palpitations when given to patients receiving monoamine oxidase (MAO) inhibitors. Levodopa can be used in combination with any of the other agents listed in the question without adverse interactions. Amantadine increases the body's dopamine supply and carbidopa prevents decarboxylation of levodopa. Diphenhydramine (an antihistamine) and benztropine have anticholinergic effects; they are used to treat Parkinson's disease because they decrease the body's acetylcholine supply.

4. The answer is E (all) *[II B 3 c, d].*
Levodopa can cause gastrointestinal side effects such as nausea and vomiting, particularly when starting treatment. Bowel irregularity and gastrointestinal bleeding can also occur. With long-term levodopa therapy, involuntary choreiform movements can develop, and the efficacy of the drug declines. Other unwanted effects of levodopa include tachycardia and cardiac arrhythmias, postural hypotension, and psychiatric disturbances such as confusion or depression.

5. The answer is A (I) *[II D 2 a (4), c (2)].*
Amantadine is most efficacious within the first few weeks, whereas benefits from levodopa may not be seen for weeks to months. Amantadine is more beneficial than the anticholinergics, but is less effective than levodopa. Unfortunately, the efficacy of amantadine declines after 6–12 months of therapy. The efficacy of levodopa declines after 3–5 years of therapy.

46
Schizophrenia

Helen L. Figge

I. INTRODUCTION

A. Definition. Schizophrenia is a group of disorders involving disruption of thought and disintegration of personality. Symptoms involve alterations in behavior, thought, affect, and perception. Schizophrenia is characterized by all of the following disturbances in the content and form of thought:

1. Hallucinations
2. Delusions
3. Flat or grossly inappropriate affect
4. Catatonic behavior
5. Incoherence or marked loosening of associations

B. Incidence. Schizophrenia occurs in about 0.5%–1% of the general population. Onset is usually between the ages of 15 and 45 years with an equal distribution between men and women.

C. Etiology. Although the actual cause of schizophrenia is unproven, theorized etiologies can be categorized broadly as genetic, neurophysiologic, and psychosocial.

1. **Genetic studies** have provided significant data supporting a genetic basis for schizophrenia. The risk factor in the general population is 0.5%–1% but increases to 5%–10% if one parent has a history of schizophrenia. It may be as high as 46% if both parents are affected.

2. **Neurophysiologic theories** focus on a possible imbalance of brain neurotransmitter physiology. The predominant theory, the **dopamine hypothesis,** suggests that overactivity of dopamine in the brain is responsible. However, the recent introduction of clozapine, an antipsychotic agent with little effect on the dopamine system but marked efficacy, seriously challenges the dopamine hypothesis. Additional theories in this category focus on other neurotransmitters.

3. **Psychosocial theories,** though largely unproven, do exist. Among the proposed causes are stress, lack of interpersonal skills, conflicting and contradictory family communication, and socioeconomic influences. Each theory has its supporters, but none is definitive.

D. Clinical presentation. Characterization of the disorder has not been standardized.

1. **Four A's.** Swiss psychiatrist Eugen Bleuler (1857–1939) described the four A's of schizophrenia; however, these have been criticized as nonspecific symptoms because they are also seen in nonschizophrenics.
   a. **Association defect** entails impaired thinking as evidenced by illogical or idiosyncratic thought processes. One idea is not obviously connected with the next, and verbalization ranges from subtly confusing to grossly disorganized.
   b. **Affect.** The patient experiences an alteration of mood or feelings; the affect may be flat with no emotional responsiveness or inappropriate.
   c. **Ambivalence.** Opposing attitudes may exist simultaneously, or there may be rapid fluctuations among contradictory emotions.
   d. **Autism.** The patient may withdraw into a private world, absorbed in inner thoughts.

2. **Additional features** of importance include the following:

a. **Hallucinations.** Sensory perceptions may be abnormal, occurring without external stimuli. Any sense may be affected, but **auditory** hallucinations are the **most common.**
b. **Delusions.** Firmly held but false beliefs are expressed that have absolutely no basis in fact. These may be simple or multiple, poorly or well organized, and bizarre or seemingly realistic. Often they feature persecutory content. Patients may complain that their thoughts are being read by others or are being broadcast to others, that people are spying on them or talking about them, or that they are being controlled.

E. Diagnostic criteria. The current approach to diagnostic criteria is based on the *Diagnostic and Statistical Manual of Mental Disorders,* 3rd ed. (revised) *[DSM-III-R],** as summarized following.

1. During a phase of the illness, at least one of the following symptoms must be present for at least 1 week.
   a. Two of the following:
      (1) Delusions
      (2) Prominent hallucinations
      (3) Incoherence or marked loosening of associations
      (4) Catatonic behavior
      (5) Flat or grossly inappropriate affect
   b. Bizarre delusions
   c. Prominent hallucinations of a voice with content having no apparent relation to depression or elation, or a voice keeping up a running commentary on the person's behavior or thoughts
2. During the course of the disturbance, functioning in areas such as work, social relations, and self-care is markedly impaired.
3. Other disorders, such as schizoaffective disorders and mood disorders with psychotic features, must be ruled out.
4. Continuous signs of the disturbance must be present for at least 6 months.
5. An organic factor that initiates or maintains the disturbance cannot be established.
6. If there is a history of autistic disorder, prominent delusions or hallucinations must be present.

F. Classification of schizophrenia is based on the symptoms predominating at the time of evaluation, but these symptoms may change over time.

1. **Disorganized (hebephrenic)** schizophrenia is characterized by marked incoherence with inappropriate responses or unresponsiveness. Delusions or hallucinations are disorganized and fragmented. The patient may giggle, grimace, and act in an incongruous or silly manner. Hypochondriacal behavior may be present.
2. **Catatonic** schizophrenia is distinguished by marked psychomotor disturbances. The patient may demonstrate rigidity, immobility, or posturing and may also be withdrawn and silent. At the other extreme is characteristic excitement, such as pacing and shouting. Fluctuations between these behavioral extremes may occur.
3. **Paranoid** schizophrenia is identified by its most prominent characteristics: delusions of grandeur or persecution, during which the patient may be extremely aggressive, argumentative, and even violent. Many of these patients are intensely concerned with homosexual impulses in themselves or others.
4. **Undifferentiated** schizophrenia may incorporate prominent delusions, hallucinations, incoherence, or grossly disorganized behavior, but the overall picture either does not meet the criteria for one of the specific types or meets the criteria for more than one type.
5. **Residual** schizophrenia designates a patient who, while not currently acutely psychotic, has a history of at least one prior episode of prominent psychotic symptoms. Residual symptoms such as loose or vague associations, illogical thinking, withdrawal, or inappropriate affect may be present, and daily living skills may be impaired.

---

*American Psychiatric Association: *Diagnostic and Statistical Manual of Mental Disorders,* 3rd ed. (revised). Washington, DC, 1987.

G. Treatment objectives. Because there is no known cure for schizophrenia, treatment is primarily aimed at relieving symptoms. The **two major therapeutic approaches**—psychotherapy and pharmacotherapy with antipsychotic (neuroleptic) agents—share the following goals:

1. Bring the patient's thoughts and behavior under control
2. Prevent self-inflicted harm
3. Restore contact with reality
4. Return the patient to society
5. Prevent a relapse

II. THERAPY: ANTIPSYCHOTIC AGENTS

A. Choice of agent. With the exception of clozapine, all antipsychotic agents are therapeutically equivalent when administered in appropriate doses, but responses vary from patient to patient and drug to drug. Consideration should be given before medical experience, if applicable. A patient who has failed to respond to a particular drug in the past is not likely to respond to that drug at any time. The **major difference** among these agents is their **adverse effects** (see II F).

B. Mechanism of action is not understood. It has been thought that the drugs work by antagonizing dopamine action; however, this view has been challenged by the introduction of clozapine, which appears to be more therapeutically effective than other agents; yet, it has only weak antidopaminergic effects. The dopamine theory has rested on the premise that most neuroleptics have antidopaminergic activity.

C. Specific agents (Table 46-1)

D. Administration and dosage

1. **General guidelines**
   a. A drug-response history should be obtained, and potential side effects should be considered.
   b. Therapy should be initiated, using a single drug administered in divided doses.
   c. The first symptoms to respond are usually aggressiveness, paranoia, and irritability; later symptoms to be reduced are hallucinations and changes in social skills.

Table 46-1. Currently Available Antipsychotic Agents

Agent	Nonproprietary Name	Approximate Equivalent Dose (mg)	Daily Dose Range
Phenothiazines	–	–	–
Aliphatics	Chlorpromazine	100	30–800
	Promazine	200	40–1200
	Triflupromazine	25	60–150
Piperidines	Thioridazine	100	150–800
	Mesoridazine	50	30–400
Piperazines	Acetophenazine	20	60–120
	Perphenazine	10	12–64
	Prochlorperazine	15	15–150
	Fluphenazine	2	0.5–40
	Trifluoperazine	5	2–40
Thioxanthenes	Chlorprothixene	100	75–600
	Thiothixene	4	8–30
Butyrophenone	Haloperidol	2	1–15
Dihydroindolone	Molindone	10	15–225
Dibenzoxazepine	Loxapine	15	20–250
Dibenzodiazepine	Clozapine	50	300–900
Benzisoxazole	Risperidone	ND	4–16
Diphenylbutylpiperidine	Pimozide	0.3–0.5	1–10

d. When the patient has been stabilized, attempts should be made to lower the dose. The lowest possible dose should be used for maintenance.

e. When discontinuing therapy, withdrawal should be tapered.

2. Gradual control method. This is the standard therapeutic method.

a. Initial doses should be at the lower end of the usual daily dose schedule (see Table 46-1), such as 300–400 mg of chlorpromazine daily. Doses should be divided initially to allow for observation of effect and toxicity.

b. If no improvement is noted after 1 week, doses may be increased by 25%–33% weekly, if necessary. Increases should be smaller in the elderly and in other individuals known to be at particular risk for adverse effects. For patients who are acutely psychotic and agitated, increases may be larger.

c. Maximal improvement may take 6–8 weeks or longer if this is not initial therapy.

d. When a patient's response and tolerance have been determined, the drug may be administered in one or two daily doses.

3. Rapid control method. This approach usually is reserved for patients who are acutely psychotic with agitation.

a. High-potency agents, such as fluphenazine or haloperidol, usually are injected intramuscularly; for example, haloperidol may be initiated at a dose of 5–10 mg every hour until the acute symptoms are controlled, adverse effects occur, or the patient falls asleep.

b. When control has been established, therapy should be converted to oral administration. The physician may elect to administer the same agent, but in oral form, at a dose appropriate for initial therapy. Dosage may then be adjusted in accordance with the patient's response.

4. Maintenance therapy to prevent relapse has less clear guidelines.

a. Some practitioners suggest that therapy be continued for 6 months after an acute episode before drug withdrawal is considered. Signs favoring discontinuation of therapy include the following:

(1) Continued control of symptoms during maintenance therapy

(2) No history of relapse ensuing from drug withdrawal

(3) Willingness of the patient to discontinue therapy

b. Other practitioners suggest that therapy be continued for 6 months in a patient who has had one episode, for 1 year after a second episode, and indefinitely after a third episode.

c. Long-acting (depot) preparations are primarily for maintenance therapy and are administered intramuscularly. Depot preparations may improve compliance and help to prevent relapse.

(1) Although the three preparations currently available are therapeutically equivalent, they differ in duration of action and in therapeutic dose.

(a) **Fluphenazine decanoate** has a longer duration of action than fluphenazine enanthate and may produce fewer extrapyramidal effects. A dose may last 3–4 weeks.

(b) **Fluphenazine enanthate** may require administration every 2 weeks.

(c) **Haloperidol decanoate** may be administered every 4 weeks.

(2) Therapy should be initiated at low doses to minimize adverse effects.

(3) If the patient has been receiving oral therapy, continuing the oral medication for the first few weeks of depot therapy may be beneficial while the blood levels of the depot preparation accumulate to steady-state levels.

(4) Before converting to long-acting preparations, it would be helpful if the patient were first converted to oral fluphenazine or haloperidol. Several formulas are available to guide the conversion, but they are only rough guidelines for initiation of therapy.

(5) When depot therapy has begun, the patient must be monitored carefully to facilitate dosage adjustments.

E. Evaluation of patient response should focus on target symptoms to determine therapeutic effectiveness.

1. Positive symptoms, such as hallucinations, delusions, hostility, and hyperactivity, are most likely to respond to antipsychotic agents.

2. Negative symptoms, such as poor judgment, apathy, social incompetence, and withdrawal, are less likely to respond.

F. Precautions and monitoring effects. Table 46-2 lists the association of major side effects with specific antipsychotic agents.

1. **Sedative effects** are common, particularly with the **phenothiazines.**

2. **Extrapyramidal effects**

   a. **Dystonic reactions** involve sudden muscle spasms of the neck, face, or trunk. These reactions include torticollis (neck twisting), trismus (clenched jaw), and oculogyric crisis (fixed upward gaze). The risk of dystonias is highest during the first 24–48 hours of therapy and when the dose is increased; they are most likely to occur in young patients, in men, and in patients receiving high doses. Dystonias can be managed initially through intramuscular or intravenous administration of anticholinergic agents, such as diphenhydramine or benztropine mesylate. Further reactions may be prevented by a short course of oral anticholinergic therapy.

   b. **Akathisia** is associated with an inner tension or agitation that is relieved by activity. Patients usually manifest this restlessness in an inability to keep their legs and feet still. This side effect most commonly appears within the first few weeks of therapy and may respond to anticholinergic agents or diazepam. If not, a change in neuroleptic agent or discontinuation of therapy may be necessary.

   c. **Drug-induced parkinsonism** includes parkinsonian symptoms such as akinesia, rigidity, resting tremor, shuffling gait, mask-like facial expression, and slowed speech. The onset of symptoms may occur within weeks or months. A related but less common effect, known as the **rabbit syndrome,** compels the patient to movements resembling the chewing motions typical of rabbits. Anticholinergic agents should manage these effects.

   d. **Tardive dyskinesia**

      (1) This disorder is characterized by abnormal facial movements with chewing, tongue protrusion, and puckering of the mouth. The reaction may progress to the extremities and trunk, producing involuntary movements, disturbance of the gag reflex, or respiratory distress.

      (2) A late-onset effect, tardive dyskinesia usually does not appear for months or years. It is thought to be caused by prolonged dopamine receptor blockade, which leads to increased receptor sensitivity, so that dopamine stimulation tends to produce movement disorders. The syndrome may begin when drugs are discontinued; in fact, a short drug holiday may reveal symptoms, allowing early detection.

      (3) **Treatment. Anticholinergics do not alleviate the syndrome** and may even worsen it. Treatment attempts have been aimed at increasing cholinergic activity, using such compounds as physostigmine, lecithin, and choline, or decreasing dopamine activity. Agents that increase γ-aminobutyric acid (GABA) activity have had some success. No definitive treatment has been identified; the emphasis is on prevention.

Table 46-2. Likelihood of Adverse Effects with Antipsychotic Agents

Agent	Sedative	Extrapyramidal	Anticholinergic	Cardiovascular (Alpha Blockade)
Acetophenazine	Medium	High	Low	Low
Chlorpromazine	High	Medium	Medium	High
Chlorprothixene	High	Medium	Medium	Medium
Clozapine	High	Very low	High	High
Fluphenazine	Low	High	Low	Low
Haloperidol	Very low	Very high	Very low	Very low
Loxapine	Low	Medium	Low	Low
Mesoridazine	High	Low	High	Medium
Molindone	Very low	Medium	Low	Low
Perphenazine	Low	High	Low	Low
Pimozide	Medium	High	Medium	Low
Prochlorperazine	Medium	High	Low	Low
Promazine	Medium	Medium	High	Medium
Risperidone	Low	Very low	Low	Low
Thioridazine	High	Low	High	High
Thiothixene	Low	High	Low	Low
Trifluoperazine	Low	High	Low	Low
Triflupromazine	High	Medium	High	Medium

(a) **Antipsychotics** and **anticholinergics** should be used only when needed and in the lowest possible doses.
(b) Patients should be examined for early signs of **dyskinesia** (e.g., fine worm-like movements when the tongue is at rest, facial tics, increased frequency of blinking). If any are discovered, antipsychotics should be discontinued gradually, if feasible. Nevertheless, symptoms may persist for months to years and may be irreversible.
(c) If the patient's condition necessitates continuing the medication, the lowest therapeutic dosage should be used.

3. **Anticholinergic effects** include dry mouth, blurred vision, constipation, and urinary retention. Administering the dose at night or reducing the dosage may reduce significant or persistent effects.

4. Cardiovascular effects include orthostatic hypotension resulting from α-blockade. Other potential effects include reflex tachycardia and electrocardiogram abnormalities, specifically S-T depression, flattened T waves, Q-T prolongation, and the appearance of U waves.

5. **Ocular effects**
   a. **Degenerative pigmentary retinopathy** may occur with high doses of **thioridazine** (the maximum daily dose should be 800 mg).
   b. **Corneal lens opacities** have been associated with antipsychotic therapy, especially with **chlorpromazine.** Slit-lamp examination helps detect deposits in the cornea or lens. These deposits usually do not affect vision and may resolve within months after discontinuation of the drug.

6. Decreased seizure threshold may occur with neuroleptics, and they should be used cautiously in a patient with a seizure disorder. Anticonvulsant dose increases may be necessary.

7. **Neuroleptic malignant syndrome** is an uncommon but serious and potentially life-threatening complication of therapy. It is a complex of extrapyramidal effects, hyperthermia, altered consciousness, and autonomic changes (e.g., tachycardia, unstable blood pressure, diaphoresis, incontinence). The onset is sudden, and recovery may take 5–10 days after discontinuation of therapy. Specific management includes discontinuation of the drug; supportive measures, such as temperature control; and drug therapy with dantrolene or bromocriptine.

8. **Additional effects**
   a. **Temperature regulation** may be impaired, causing the patient to assume the environmental temperature. This can result in hyperthermia or hypothermia.
   b. **Sexual dysfunction** may include impotence, inability to ejaculate, retrograde ejaculation, diminished libido, amenorrhea, galactorrhea, and gynecomastia. These effects are seen most commonly with **thioridazine.**
   c. **Photosensitivity** in the form of gray to purple pigmentation has been reported with chlorpromazine, thioridazine, and the thiothixenes. A correlation has been noted between skin and ocular pigmentation; patients with a photosensitive reaction should have an ocular examination.

G. Clozapine therapy

1. **Overview.** Clozapine is one of the first **effective antipsychotic agents** to have few of the extrapyramidal side effects that are typical of nearly all of the neuroleptic agents in clinical use today.
   a. It can be effective in treating some patients who are unresponsive to standard neuroleptic drugs.
   b. It has only weak dopaminergic activity.
   c. In 14 double-blind studies, clozapine produced superior clinical results in 79% of subjects as compared with a standard neuroleptic agent.

2. **Precautions and monitoring effects**
   a. The **major side effect** is **agranulocytosis,** which may be fatal. Thus, patients taking clozapine must be routinely monitored by blood counts at intervals established by the physician but usually as often as once a week. This has contributed to the relatively **high annual cost** for providing this drug to individual patients.
   b. Other possible **side effects** are seizures, hypotension, fatigue, sedation, nausea, and vomiting.

STUDY QUESTIONS

Directions: Each of the numbered items or incomplete statements in this section is followed by answers or by completions of the statement. Select the **one** lettered answer or completion that is **best** in each case.

1. All of the following statements concerning antipsychotic agents are true EXCEPT

(A) studies have proven chlorpromazine to be the most effective antipsychotic agent
(B) patients who have responded to a particular drug in the past are likely to respond to retreatment with that same drug
(C) the major differences among antipsychotic drugs are their side effects
(D) any given patient may or may not respond to any given antipsychotic drug
(E) newly diagnosed, young patients tend to respond to drugs better than older chronic schizophrenic patients

2. The four A's that Bleuler used to characterize schizophrenia include all of the following EXCEPT

(A) anxiety
(B) ambivalence
(C) association defect
(D) autism
(E) alteration of affect

3. Which of the following is an example of delusion?

(A) Hearing strange voices
(B) Seeing someone who is not really there
(C) The feeling that ants are crawling all over the body
(D) The lack of any emotional response to any situation
(E) The belief that an advertisement on television is directed to the individual and contains a secret message

4. Most antipsychotic agents except clozapine are potent blockers of which neurotransmitters?

(A) Acetylcholine
(B) Dopamine
(C) Calcium
(D) Zinc
(E) Norepinephrine

5. The earliest movement disorder to appear during neuroleptic therapy is

(A) pseudoparkinsonism
(B) dystonia
(C) tardive dyskinesia
(D) akathisia
(E) resting tumor

6. Specific therapy for an acute extrapyramidal reaction to chlorpromazine is

(A) physostigmine
(B) diphenhydramine
(C) bethanechol
(D) propranolol
(E) metoclopramide

Questions 7–10

A 35-year-old man was brought to the emergency room because he was swinging at passersby in a shopping mall. He required four-point restraints for acute agitation. No history could be obtained except for the patient declaring that multiple voices were telling him to knock down the people in the mall who were chasing him.

On physical examination, the patient was extremely agitated and uncooperative. Blood pressure was 120/85, pulse 94, and respirations 16. General examination was superficially unremarkable; neurological examination was grossly nonfocal except for the mental status examination, which revealed elements of hallucinations, delusions of persecution, and multiple loose associations. Local authorities reported that the patient had escaped from a local psychiatric facility and had been missing for 3 days. His previous treatment regimen was chlorpromazine (800 mg daily in divided doses). When compliant with the medication, the patient's symptoms were well controlled.

7. What therapeutic agent could be given to control the patient's present symptoms?

(A) Haloperidol
(B) Clozapine
(C) Lithium
(D) Fluoxetine

8. Which subtype of schizophrenia is the patient likely to have?

(A) Hebephrenic
(B) Catatonic
(C) Paranoid
(D) Residual

9. After initial therapy, the patient develops trismus associated with torticollis. Which of the following agents should be administered to control these reactions?

(A) Haloperidol
(B) Clozapine
(C) Diphenhydramine
(D) Diazepam

10. What is the usual dose of the appropriate agent from question number 7?

(A) 5–10 mg every hour intramuscularly until control of symptoms is achieved
(B) 50–100 mg every hour intramuscularly until control of symptoms is achieved
(C) 5–10 mg orally for a single dose
(D) 50–100 mg for a single dose

Directions: The group of items in this section consists of lettered options followed by a set of numbered items. For each item, select the **one** lettered option that is most closely associated with it. Each lettered option may be selected once, more than once, or not at all.

Questions 11–15

Match the drug with the phrase that most accurately describes it.

(A) Used in depot preparations
(B) Used in the management of neuroleptic malignant syndrome
(C) High doses may cause degenerative pigmentary retinopathy
(D) Counteracts dystonias
(E) Produces minimal sedative effects

11. Thioridazine

12. Benztropine mesylate

13. Dantrolene

14. Molindone

15. Haloperidol

ANSWERS AND EXPLANATIONS

1. The answer is A *[II A, G].*
Those individuals most likely to respond to antipsychotic drugs are young patients. Current evidence suggests that clozapine may be more effective than chlorpromazine. Any given patient may respond to any given antipsychotic drug; however, when selecting a drug to treat a patient with schizophrenia, a past history of success with a particular drug indicates that the patient will probably respond to that drug again. The major differences among antipsychotic drugs are their side effects.

2. The answer is A *[I D 1].*
Bleuler described the four A's of schizophrenia by using the symptoms of association defect, abnormal affect, ambivalence, and autism. Anxiety disorders are a different class of psychologic disorders.

3. The answer is E *[I D 2 b].*
A hallucination is an abnormal sensory perception, such as hearing or seeing something that is not there. The lack of an emotional response to any situation is due to an abnormal affect. A delusion is a firmly held but false belief, such as having one's thoughts read or the belief that an advertisement is speaking directly to you with a secret message.

4. The answer is B *[II B].*
The classic neuroleptics block dopamine receptors, but clozapine has only weak dopaminergic action. Clozapine has potent antimuscarinic receptor activity.

5. The answer is B *[II F 2 a].*
In patients given antipsychotic drugs, dystonic reactions have the earliest onset—that is, the risk is highest during the first 24–48 hours of therapy and when the dose is increased. Pseudoparkinsonism, which is characterized in part by a resting tremor, may not begin for weeks to months after initiation of antipsychotic therapy; and tardive dyskinesia is usually not seen for months to years. Akathisia begins within the first few weeks of therapy.

6. The answer is B *[II F 2 a–c].*
Acute extrapyramidal reactions are due to excess cholinergic activity resulting from the blockade of dopamine receptors by the neuroleptic agent. Specific treatment is the administration of an agent with anticholinergic activity, such as diphenhydramine.

7–10. The answers are: 7-A *[II D 3 a],* **8-C** *[I F 3],* **9-C** *[II F 2 a],* **10-A** *[II D 3 a].*
Haloperidol can be used effectively for the acute treatment of psychosis. Clozapine is reserved for recalcitrant cases. Lithium is used to treat bipolar disorder, which this patient does not have. Fluoxetine is used to treat depression.

The patient described in the question exhibits the classic features of paranoid schizophrenia, including delusions of grandeur or persecution, during which the patient may become extremely aggressive and violent. Some paranoid schizophrenics become obsessed with homosexual impulses.

The patient is experiencing a dystonic reaction from the haloperidol; this should be treated with the intravenous administration of an anticholinergic agent such as diphenhydramine. Clozapine would not be an appropriate choice for this acute intervention.

Standard dosing of haloperidol for an acute situation is 5–10 mg intramuscularly every hour until the acute symptoms are controlled, adverse effects occur, or the patient falls asleep.

11-15. The answers are: 11-C *[II F 5 a],* **12-D** *[II F 2 a],* **13-B** *[II F 7],* **14-E** *[Table 46-2],* **15-A** *[II D 4 c].*
Pigmentary retinopathy may be caused by thioridazine when administered in doses over 800 mg/day. Benztropine mesylate has anticholinergic activity and may be used to manage the extrapyramidal side effects associated with antipsychotic therapy. Dantrolene, through its effects on muscles, may be able to control the signs of neuroleptic malignant syndrome. Although sedation is common to all antipsychotic agents, molindone, thiothixene, and most piperazine phenothiazines are associated with a lower incidence of this effect. Two antipsychotic agents are currently available in depot (long-acting) formulations: fluphenazine (as the decanoate or the enanthate) and haloperidol decanoate.

47
Affective Disorders

Helen L. Figge

I. INTRODUCTION

A. Definition. Affective disorders are characterized by disturbances of mood, such as low and depressed states or periods of exhilaration to the point of mania. Affective disorders are considered in two major classifications.

1. **Unipolar disorder.** The patient experiences depressive episodes.

2. **Bipolar disorder.** The patient experiences depressive and manic episodes or, less commonly, manic episodes alone.

B. Incidence. Affective disorders rank as the **most common psychiatric disorders.**

1. **Unipolar disorder.** Estimates indicate that 18%–23% of adult women and 8%–11% of adult men experience at least one major depressive episode. Onset of a major depressive illness may occur at any age but is most common in the late twenties.

2. **Bipolar disorder.** This form of affective disorder is much less common than the unipolar type. Its incidence ranges between 0.4% and 1.2% of the adult population with approximately equal distribution among men and women. Onset generally occurs before age 30.

C. Etiology. Although no consensus has been achieved on precise causes for affective disorders, theorists focus on genetic, biologic, and psychological factors.

1. **Genetic factors**
   a. Research indicates an increased frequency of occurrence in families of patients with affective disorders as compared with the general population.
   b. Studies of monozygotic and dizygotic twins support theories of genetic influence on the development of major affective disorders. However, they also indicate that other factors are involved.

2. **Neurochemical factors**
   a. The **biogenic amine hypothesis** proposes that depression is due to a deficiency of either norepinephrine or serotonin and that mania results from an excess of norepinephrine.
   b. The **permissive hypothesis** states the following:
      (1) Serotonin deficiencies may create a predisposition to a major affective disorder.
      (2) Deficiencies of both serotonin and norepinephrine result in depression.
      (3) A serotonin deficiency accompanied by a norepinephrine excess results in mania.
   c. The **receptor sensitivity theory** proposes that there is an alteration of receptor sensitivity to neurotransmitters; consequently, antidepressants exert their effects by altering receptor sensitivity.

3. **Psychological factors.** Theories proposing a psychological basis for the origin of major depressive episodes abound. For example, one hypothesis suggests that stress or loss may result in an episode of clinical depression, especially if coupled with the patient's inability to cope with the event.

D. Treatment goals

1. To shorten the episode

2. To prevent recurrence

II. CLINICAL EVALUATION

A. General. Diagnosis of an affective disorder requires the following determinations.

1. The mood disturbance (unipolar or bipolar) should be evident.
2. The symptoms should not be superimposed on a schizophrenic disorder.
3. The mood disturbance must not be due to an organic mental disorder or simple bereavement.

B. Unipolar disorders

1. Major depressive illness is characterized by mood depression or loss of interest or pleasure in all or almost all usual activities.
2. The mood disturbance must be prominent and relatively persistent.
3. Differential diagnosis requires that four or more of the following associated signs accompany the mood disturbance for 2 weeks:
   a. Appetite loss or increase with a correlative weight change
   b. Insomnia or hypersomnia
   c. Psychomotor retardation, agitation, or both
   d. Loss of interest in or gratification from family, sexual activity, work, hobbies, clubs, and other social activities
   e. Feelings of worthlessness or guilt
   f. Loss of energy; feeling of chronic fatigue or lack of pep
   g. Decreased ability to think clearly or concentrate; impaired memory
   h. Suicidal thoughts, plans, or attempts; thoughts focusing on death

C. Bipolar disorders

1. A diagnosis of bipolar disorder requires one or more periods in which the predominant mood is elated, expansive, or irritable. The mood must predominate for a distinct period, although it may alternate with depressive periods.
2. The diagnosis of the manic phase also requires that at least three of the following associated symptoms have been significant and persistent during the period (four if the mood is solely irritable):
   a. Increase in activity or restlessness
   b. Unusual verbosity or rapid or pressured speech
   c. Flight of ideas, characterized by rapid changes in subject; racing thoughts, which can compromise coherence
   d. Ease of distractibility, in which almost anything can disrupt concentration
   e. Inflation of self-esteem, which can reach delusional proportions
   f. Decreased need for sleep
   g. Impairment of judgment, which may lead to involvement in highly consequential activities such as buying sprees; reckless driving; sexual indiscretions; and flamboyant, intrusive socializing (such as making late-night phone calls or visits)
3. The disorder must be severe enough to interfere with work, relationships, or social activities, or require hospitalization to prevent harmful activities.

III. CLINICAL COURSE

A. Depressive episodes

1. These episodes are usually self-limiting, lasting 6 months or less.
2. With proper and timely therapy, up to 85% of patients who experience depressive episodes may achieve a complete response.
3. The clinical course may be:
   a. **Limited**—to a single episode
   b. **Recurrent**—with two or more episodes separated by intervals of varying lengths (episodes may also occur in clusters)

c. **Chronic**—in which some symptoms may persist for up to 2 years with asymptomatic periods of less than 2 months

4. The major risk for these patients is suicide.

B. Manic episodes

1. If untreated, manic episodes may last from days to months.
2. Recurrence intervals are unpredictable, but it is not unusual for episodes to occur at 1- to 2-year intervals.
3. The sequence of episodes in bipolar disorder is also unpredictable. Manic episodes are not necessarily followed by depressive periods.

IV. TREATMENT OF UNIPOLAR (DEPRESSIVE) DISORDERS. Depressive episodes may be managed with pharmacotherapy, psychotherapy, electroconvulsive therapy, or a combination of modalities. This discussion will be limited to pharmacotherapy; specifically, antidepressants and monoamine oxidase (MAO) inhibitors.

A. Antidepressants

1. **Types available in the United States***
   a. Aminoketone. Bupropion (Wellbutrin)
   b. Tricyclics
      (1) Amitriptyline (Elavil)
      (2) Doxepin (Adapin)
      (3) Imipramine (Tofranil)
      (4) Trimipramine (Surmontil)
      (5) Desipramine (Norpramin)
      (6) Nortriptyline (Pamelor)
      (7) Protriptyline (Vivactil)
      (8) Amoxapine (Asendin)
   c. Tetracyclic. Maprotiline (Ludiomil)
   d. Triazolopyridine. Trazodone (Desyrel)
   e. Selective serotonin reuptake inhibitors
      (1) Fluoxetine (Prozac)
      (2) Paroxetine (Paxil)
      (3) Sertraline (Zoloft)
   f. Phenethylamine. Venlafaxine (Effexor)
   g. Other. Nefazodone (Serzone)

2. **Pharmacologic properties**
   a. **Blockade of 5-hydroxytryptamine 1A (5-HT1A) [serotonin] receptors**
      (1) **Highest affinities** shown by trazodone, amitriptyline, amoxapine, doxepin, and nortriptyline
      (2) **Possible clinical consequences.** Ejaculatory disturbances
   b. **Blockade of 5-HT2 (serotonin) receptors**
      (1) **Highest affinities** shown by amoxapine, trazodone, doxepin, amitriptyline, and trimipramine
      (2) **Possible clinical consequences.** Hypotension and alleviation of migraine headaches
   c. **Blockade of norepinephrine uptake**
      (1) **Highest potency** shown by desipramine, protriptyline, nortriptyline, amoxapine, maprotiline, and venlafaxine
      (2) **Possible clinical consequences.** Tremors, tachycardia, insomnia, erectile dysfunction, blockade of antihypertensive effects of guanethidine and guanadrel, and augmentation of pressor effects of sympathomimetic amines
   d. **Blockade of serotonin uptake**
      (1) **Highest potency** shown by fluoxetine, paroxetine, sertraline, imipramine, amitriptyline, trazodone, nortriptyline, and venlafaxine

*Clomipramine is not marketed in the United States as an antidepressant and, therefore, is not discussed further.

(2) **Possible clinical consequences.** Gastrointestinal disturbances, dose-dependent increase or decrease in anxiety, sexual dysfunction, extrapyramidal side effects, interactions with L-tryptophan and MAO inhibitors

e. **Blockade of histamine H_1-receptors**

(1) **Highest affinities** shown by doxepin, trimipramine, amitriptyline, maprotiline, and nortriptyline

(2) **Possible clinical consequences.** Potentiation of central depressant drugs, sedation, weight gain, and hypotension

f. **Blockade of muscarinic receptors**

(1) **Highest affinities** shown by amitriptyline, protriptyline, trimipramine, doxepin, and imipramine

(2) **Possible clinical consequences.** Blurred vision, dry mouth, sinus tachycardia, constipation, urinary retention, and memory dysfunction

g. **Blockade of α_1-adrenergic receptors**

(1) **Highest affinities** shown by doxepin, trimipramine, amitriptyline, trazodone, and amoxapine

(2) **Possible clinical consequences.** Potentiation of the antihypertensive effects of prazosin and terazosin, postural hypotension, dizziness, and reflex tachycardia

h. **Blockade of α_2-adrenergic receptors**

(1) **Highest affinities** shown by trazodone, trimipramine, amitriptyline, doxepin, and nortriptyline

(2) **Possible clinical consequences.** Blockade of the antihypertensive effects of clonidine, guanabenz, methyldopa, and guanfacine; and priapism

i. **Blockade of dopamine D_2-receptors**

(1) **Highest potency** shown by amoxapine but basically shows weak activity

(2) **Possible clinical consequences.** Extrapyramidal movement disorders, endocrine changes, and sexual dysfunction

j. **Blockade of dopamine uptake**

(1) **Highest potency** shown by bupropion but basically shows weak activity

(2) **Possible clinical consequences.** Improvement of parkinsonism and aggravation of psychosis

3. **Mechanism of action** of cyclic antidepressants remains poorly understood. It may result from a supersensitivity of catecholamine receptors in the presence of low levels of serotonin or possibly neurotransmitter receptor downregulation.

4. **Choice of agent.** All antidepressants are equally effective with similar periods of time for onset of action. The choice of an agent depends on the medical status of the patient (the type of depression), the side effect profile of the drug, and the history of a previous response of the patient or a family member to a particular antidepressant. Recommended agents for specific situations include the following:

a. **Cardiovascular effects**

(1) Congestive heart failure (CHF) or coronary disease: nortriptyline

(2) Conduction defect: maprotiline

(3) Untreated mild hypertension: imipramine

(4) Postural hypotension: bupropion, fluoxetine, and maprotiline

b. **Neurologic effects**

(1) Seizure disorder: MAO inhibitor

(2) Chronic pain syndrome: amitriptyline and doxepin

(3) Migraine headaches: trazodone, doxepin, trimipramine, and amitriptyline

c. **Gastrointestinal effects**

(1) Chronic diarrhea: doxepin, trimipramine, amitriptyline, imipramine, and protriptyline

(2) Chronic constipation: trazodone, bupropion, fluoxetine, amoxapine, maprotiline, and desipramine

(3) Peptic ulcer disease: doxepin, trimipramine, amitriptyline, and imipramine

5. **Administration and dosage**

a. **Initiation of treatment**

(1) The recommended daily dosage ranges for antidepressants are presented in Table 47-1. The high end of these dosage ranges is usually reserved for the severely ill hospitalized patient.

Table 47-1. Daily Antidepressant Doses in Adults*

Agents	Starting Dosage (mg/day)	Usual Daily Dose (mg)	Usual Dosage Range (mg/day)	Therapeutic Serum Levels (ng/ml)
Tricyclics				
Amitriptyline	50	150–200	50–300	80–250†
Nortriptyline	20	75–100	30–125	50–150
Imipramine	50	75–150	50–300	150–250†
Desipramine	50	100–200	50–300	125–300
Protriptyline	10	15–40	10–60	70–260
Doxepin	50	75–150	50–300	150–250†
Trimipramine	50	100–200	50–300	150–250
Others				
Maprotiline	50	100–150	50–225	200–600
Amoxapine	50	200–300	50–400	200–600†
Bupropion	100 b.i.d.	300‡	100–450	Unidentified
Trazodone	50	150–400	50–600	800–1600
Fluoxetine	20	20–80	20–80	Unidentified
Paroxetine	20	20–50	20–50	Unidentified
Sertraline	50	50–200	50–200	Unidentified
Venlafaxine	75	75–225	75–375	Unidentified
Nefazodone	200	300–600	300–600	Unidentified

*Dosages should be divided initially for all listed drugs, and elderly individuals should be treated with about half of the usual dosage for adults.

†Active metabolites included.

‡Divided dose (100 mg t.i.d.) should be given starting on the fourth day of treatment. No single dose should exceed 150 mg, and the total dose should not exceed 450 mg/day because of the risk of seizures.

(2) Therapy should be initiated with one fourth of the target dose. For example, 50 mg of amitriptyline should be administered in divided doses to minimize adverse effects.

(3) The dose may be increased once or twice a week until a response is obtained.

(4) Further increases of 50 mg weekly may be necessary until improvement, toxicity, or the upper end of the dosing range is reached.

(5) After a gradual transition, most of these drugs may be administered in a single daily dose, usually at bedtime.

(6) The elderly and patients with cardiovascular disease require lower initial doses and a slower rate of increase.

(7) Response rate

(a) Physiologic symptoms (e.g., sleep disturbances, anorexia, psychomotor disturbance) usually respond within 1 week.

(b) Psychosocial symptoms usually respond after 2–4 weeks.

(c) Full response may require about 4 weeks. If there is no response after 4 weeks, serum drug levels should be checked, as discussed in IV A 6 b.

b. Maintenance therapy

(1) Therapy is usually maintained for 6 months after recovery to prevent a relapse.

(2) The maintenance dose is one third to one half of the dose needed to achieve remission.

(3) After the 6 months, the drug is tapered off over 4–8 weeks.

c. Prophylaxis. A patient with a history of frequent or severe episodes may require prophylactic therapy to prevent future episodes.

6. Precautions and monitoring effects

a. Contraindications

(1) Cyclic antidepressants should be avoided in patients with severely impaired liver function or with cardiac conduction defects.

(2) Coadministration of MAO inhibitors and cyclic antidepressants can result in serious reactions, including hyperpyrexia, seizures, excitation, and death. Such combination therapy is rarely warranted and should be initiated with great caution.

(3) Caution is required with administering these agents to patients with cardiovascular disease, glaucoma, benign prostatic hypertrophy, or a history of seizures or urinary retention.

b. Serum level monitoring

(1) Although therapeutic serum levels have been identified for most antidepressants (see Table 47-1), the correlation between levels and activity is unclear. Therapeutic levels do not guarantee either the desired response or a lack of adverse effects. Patients should, therefore, be evaluated by their response to therapy. Therapeutic plasma concentrations have been firmly established for only imipramine, nortriptyline, and desipramine.

(2) Orders for serum levels should account for active metabolites, as applicable.

(3) Assessment of serum levels provides several major benefits, such as helping in the detection and management of antidepressant overdose [see IV A 6 c (6)].

(4) Serum level monitoring is particularly useful in the **nonresponsive patient.**

(a) A **subtherapeutic or low-end serum level** indicates the need for incremental dosage increases.

(b) A **lower than expected serum level** despite a reasonable dose may reveal patient noncompliance.

(c) An **upper-end serum level** suggests the need to change to a different drug.

(d) **Achieving therapeutic serum levels** without obtaining patient response after 4 weeks suggests the need for re-evaluation of the diagnosis. If the physician is confident of the diagnosis, a change in medications is recommended.

c. Adverse effects (Table 47-2)

(1) **Sedative effects,** which may be desirable in a patient with insomnia, are usually undesirable in a patient with psychomotor retardation.

(2) **Anticholinergic effects** include dry mouth, constipation, blurred vision, and urinary retention.

(3) **Cardiac effects**

(a) Orthostatic hypotension is the most common cardiac effect (with an incidence as high as 20%).

(b) Tachycardia of the mild sinus type is common.

(c) Arrhythmias and electrocardiogram (ECG) disturbances

(i) ECG changes may include T-wave flattening or prolongation of the P-R, QRS, or Q-T intervals.

Table 47-2. Incidence of Adverse Effects with Cyclic Antidepressant Use

Agents	Sedation	Anticholinergic Effects	Orthostatic Hypotension	Delay in Conduction or Arrhythmias	Lowered Seizure Threshold
Tricyclics					
Amitriptyline	High	High	High	Yes	Moderate
Nortriptyline	Moderate	Low	Low	Yes	Low
Imipramine	Moderate	Moderate	High	Yes	Moderate
Desipramine	Low	Low	Low	Yes	Low
Protriptyline	Low	Moderate	Low	Yes	Low
Doxepin	High	Moderate	High	Yes	Moderate
Trimipramine	High	High	Moderate	Yes	Moderate
Others					
Maprotiline	Moderate	Low	Moderate	Low	High
Amoxapine	Moderate	Low	Moderate	Low	Moderate
Bupropion	Very low	Very low	Very low	Low	High
Trazodone	High	Very low	Moderate	Low	Low
Fluoxetine	Very low	Very low	Very low	Low	Low
Paroxetine	Very low	Very low	Very low	Low	Low
Sertraline	Very low	Very low	Very low	Low	Low
Venlafaxine	Very low	Very low	Very low	Low	Low
Nefazodone	Low	Very low	Low	Low	Low

(ii) Tricyclic compounds may interfere with atrioventricular conduction, similar to the effect of quinidine. In the presence of bundle-branch block or atrioventricular block, these effects can be life-threatening. Therefore, these agents should be avoided in patients with conduction defects.

(4) Neurologic effects

(a) Most cyclic antidepressants tend to lower the seizure threshold.

(i) Cautious administration is required in patients with a history of seizures.

(ii) Anticonvulsant doses may need to be increased.

(iii) Maprotiline has been associated with an increased risk of seizures at doses exceeding 225 mg/day, even in patients without a history of seizures. To minimize this risk, dosage increases should be gradual.

(iv) Bupropion is also associated with increased seizure risk. Careful dosage administration is required (see Table 47-1).

(b) Neuroleptic effects, most common with amoxapine, may include:

(i) Severe restlessness and agitation (akathisia)

(ii) Tardive dyskinesia

(iii) Dystonias

(iv) Drug-induced parkinsonism

(v) Neuroleptic malignant syndrome (e.g., extrapyramidal signs, changes in blood pressure, altered consciousness, hyperpyrexia), a rare but serious complication

(5) Dermatologic effects. Exanthematous rash may erupt in 4%–5% of patients taking maprotiline.

(6) Overdosage

(a) Signs and symptoms may reflect cardiac, central nervous system (CNS), and anticholinergic effects, including arrhythmias, seizures, coma, confusion, respiratory depression, hyperpyrexia, and bladder or bowel dysfunction.

(b) Treatment may initially include emesis or gastric lavage and administration of activated charcoal. Additional measures may include phenytoin or diazepam for seizure control and lidocaine or phenytoin for arrhythmias. Physostigmine may be helpful in certain cases.

(7) Withdrawal symptoms, such as nausea, headache, and malaise, can be avoided by withdrawing the drug gradually.

B. Monoamine oxidase (MAO) inhibitors

1. Mechanism of action. MAO inhibitors block the usual destruction of neurotransmitters by MAO, thus creating a buildup of biogenic amine levels in the brain. This increase probably underlies the antidepressant effect.

2. Indications. MAO inhibitors are reserved for patients who have not responded to cyclic antidepressants (first-line agents) or who cannot tolerate their side effects.

3. Administration and dosage (Table 47-3)

a. When changing from a cyclic antidepressant or another MAO inhibitor to a new MAO inhibitor, the first drug should be discontinued for 10 days before starting the new MAO inhibitor.

b. MAO inhibitors should be initiated at a low dose, and dosage increments should be made slowly and cautiously.

Table 47-3. Recommended Daily Doses for Monoamine Oxidase (MAO) Inhibitors

Agents	Brand Name	Usual Daily Dose (mg)
Hydrazides		
Phenelzine	Nardil	60–90
Isocarboxazid	Marplan	10–50
Nonhydrazide		
Tranylcypromine	Parnate	10–60

c. When changing from an MAO inhibitor to a cyclic antidepressant, at least 10 days must pass after stopping the MAO inhibitor before beginning therapy with the cyclic agent to avoid a potentially serious interaction.
d. Therapeutic effects may not occur for 2–3 weeks or longer.

4. **Precautions and monitoring effects**
   a. **Contraindications**
      (1) MAO inhibitors should not be administered to patients who are debilitated or who have a history of hepatic or renal impairment or cardiovascular or cerebrovascular disease.
      (2) Administration is also contraindicated within 7–10 days of surgery that requires general anesthesia or a local anesthetic containing cocaine or sympathomimetic vasoconstrictors.
   b. **Adverse effects**
      (1) Orthostatic hypotension is common but may be minimized by using smaller incremental dosage increases.
      (2) MAO inhibitors derived from hydrazide may cause hepatocellular damage. Although of low incidence, this toxic effect can have serious consequences; therefore, liver function should be monitored after a baseline is established. Administration should be avoided if the patient has a history of hepatic impairment.
      (3) Weight gain, sexual dysfunction, and edema may occur.
   c. **Overdosage** may be signaled by palpitations, agitation, frequent headaches, hypertension, or severe orthostatic hypotension.
   d. **Significant interactions**
      (1) **Hypertensive crisis,** the most serious and most likely interaction, results from ingestion of sympathomimetic drugs and foods with a high tyramine content.
         (a) The patient should be given a list of **foods to avoid,** particularly:
            (i) Beer and most wines (except white wine)
            (ii) Caviar and herring
            (iii) Chicken livers
            (iv) Chocolate
            (v) Most cheeses (especially blue, cheddar, mozzarella, Parmesan)
            (vi) Sausage and other smoked meats
         (b) Patients should also be warned not to take any medications—including over-the-counter cold, hay fever, or diet preparations—without first consulting a physician or pharmacist.
         (c) Patients should not be given MAO inhibitors if they are unwilling or unable to comply with the restrictions.
         (d) **Early signs** of hypertensive crisis may include:
            (i) Stiff neck
            (ii) Occipital headache
            (iii) Nausea and vomiting
            (iv) Sweating and flushing
            (v) Palpitations
      (2) **Coadministration of a cyclic antidepressant and an MAO inhibitor** must be undertaken with extreme caution, if at all [see IV A 6 a (2)].

V. TREATMENT OF BIPOLAR DISORDERS.

Neuroleptic agents, lithium, and psychotherapy may be used to manage bipolar disorders. Antidepressants are administered with lithium to manage the depressive phase of the illness. Use of antidepressants alone is usually avoided because of their tendency to provoke the re-emergence of the manic phase.

A. Neuroleptic agents

1. **Indications.** Neuroleptic agents are used in the acute manic phase to decrease agitation and hyperactivity, the first treatment priority.

2. **Therapeutic effects**
   a. Neuroleptics such as chlorpromazine and haloperidol quickly lower the arousal level while not interfering with intellectual processes.
   b. Emotional or affective displays are reduced; aggressive and impulsive behavior is diminished.

3. Administration and dosage
- **a.** Because lithium efficacy has a delayed onset (see V B 2 a), neuroleptics are used until the lithium can achieve a therapeutic effect.
- **b.** Neuroleptic therapy is usually initiated at the same time as the lithium therapy.
- **c.** Neuroleptics can be tapered off as symptoms improve and serum lithium levels reach therapeutic concentrations [see V B 3 b (3)].
- **d.** The dosage varies with the severity of the patient's symptoms and whether the patient is treated in the hospital or as an outpatient.
  - **(1)** The usual starting dose of **chlorpromazine** for a hospitalized patient in the manic phase is 25 mg intramuscularly. Doses of 25–50 mg intramuscularly may be administered hourly if necessary. The dose is gradually increased over the next few days to as much as 400 mg every 4–6 hours if needed.
  - **(2)** **Haloperidol** may be initiated at a dose of 2–5 mg intramuscularly in an acutely ill patient. Doses may be repeated hourly as needed.
  - **(3)** Oral administration should be used as soon as the patient is calm.

4. Precautions and monitoring effects
- **a. Chlorpromazine**
  - **(1)** This agent should be used with extreme caution or not at all in patients with cardiovascular disease, glaucoma, benign prostatic hypertrophy, or a history of seizures.
  - **(2)** Chlorpromazine has a strong sedative effect while bearing only moderate extrapyramidal effects.
- **b. Haloperidol**
  - **(1)** Extrapyramidal effects may be seen with haloperidol administration. These effects include parkinsonian symptoms, akathisia, and dystonic reactions.
  - **(2)** Coadministration of haloperidol (or a phenothiazine) with lithium may result in an acute encephalopathy. Patients should be carefully monitored while receiving this combination.
  - **(3)** Haloperidol tends to have a high incidence of extrapyramidal effects (especially akathisia and dystonias) while having a moderate sedative effect.
- **c. General.** These agents should not be withdrawn suddenly unless intolerably severe adverse effects arise.

B. Lithium is the drug of choice for control and prophylaxis of manic episodes.

1. Mechanism of action. Although the exact mechanism remains unknown, lithium is thought to:
- **a.** Affect membrane stabilization
- **b.** Inhibit norepinephrine release
- **c.** Accelerate norepinephrine metabolism
- **d.** Increase presynaptic re-uptake of norepinephrine and serotonin
- **e.** Decrease receptor sensitivity

2. Administration and dosage
- **a. General.** Lithium has a very narrow therapeutic index and a significant lag time (3–5 days, longer in some patients) before the initial therapeutic effect is observable. Therefore, monitoring serum lithium levels and evaluating the patient for signs of toxicity provide the keys to determining and adjusting the dosage regimen.
- **b. Oral dosage**
  - **(1)** For acute episodes, 900 mg twice a day or 600 mg three times a day are given.
  - **(2)** For long-term control, 900–1200 mg/day in 2–3 divided doses are given.
- **c. Maintenance therapy**
  - **(1)** Once the symptoms have diminished, the dose should be decreased to achieve maintenance serum levels [see V B 3 b (3) (b)].
  - **(2)** Manic attacks are usually self-limiting. Unless there is an indication for chronic therapy, lithium may be discontinued after 3–6 months. Long-term therapy is indicated for patients with severe or frequent attacks.

3. Precautions and monitoring effects
- **a. Contraindications**
  - **(1)** Renal, cardiovascular, and thyroid disorders may preclude the use of lithium or necessitate extremely cautious monitoring.
  - **(2)** Lithium is contraindicated during the first trimester of pregnancy because it increases the risk of congenital cardiovascular anomalies, particularly valvular malformations.

b. Serum level monitoring. To minimize the likelihood of lithium toxicity while assuring adequate dosage, the patient's blood levels should be monitored closely.

(1) Levels should be checked twice a week during the first few weeks of therapy and at least every 2 months thereafter.

(2) The ideal time to check serum levels is 12 hours after the last dose. Drawing the sample in the morning before the first dose of the day is generally most convenient.

(3) Therapeutic serum level ranges are as follows:

(a) **Initial therapy:** 1.0–1.5 mEq/L

(b) **Maintenance therapy:** 0.6–1.2 mEq/L

c. Laboratory test results can be affected by lithium intake, including:

(1) Elevations in urinary serum glucose tests

(2) Decreases in serum uric acid levels and serum protein-bound iodine studies

(3) Increased thyroid-stimulating hormone

(4) Decreased thyroxine levels

(5) Increased serum sodium levels, which can increase secondary to diabetes insipidus [see V B 3 e (4) (b)]

d. Breast feeding should be avoided by mothers taking lithium because significant concentrations of the drug have been detected in breast milk.

e. Adverse effects are generally related to increasing serum concentration levels.

(1) Below 1.5 mEq/L, the effects are usually tolerable or manageable by dividing or reducing the dose. These effects include:

(a) Gastrointestinal distress, such as anorexia, nausea, vomiting, and diarrhea. These may be minimized by taking the drug with food or dividing the dose.

(b) Polyuria and polydipsia

(c) Fine hand tremor

(d) Slight muscle weakness

(2) Effects associated with lithium serum levels between 1.5 and 2.5 mEq/L should be considered early **warning signs of toxicity.** These effects include:

(a) Persistent or recurring gastrointestinal distress

(b) Coarse hand tremor

(c) Hyperirritability

(d) Slurred speech

(e) Confusion or somnolence

(3) **Lithium toxicity** usually occurs when levels exceed 2.5 mEq/L. This is a potentially fatal medical emergency requiring immediate attention.

(a) **Signs and symptoms** include:

(i) Increased deep tendon reflexes

(ii) Irregular pulse

(iii) Hypotension

(iv) Seizures

(v) Stupor or coma

(b) **Treatment** of acute toxicity should include attempts to empty the stomach by emesis or gastric lavage. Supportive treatment should be administered, and diuresis may increase urinary lithium elimination. Hemodialysis may be necessary if serum lithium levels exceed 3 mEq/L or if the patient's condition does not improve or begins to decline.

(4) Some effects occur with ongoing therapy but are unrelated to serum levels. These include:

(a) White blood cell counts may range from 10,000 mm^3 to 15,000 mm^3 (leukocytosis) and may remain elevated throughout therapy.

(b) Patients may develop an inability to concentrate urine, with increased urine output and increased thirst (nephrogenic diabetes insipidus syndrome).

(i) Dosage reduction or specific therapy may be needed if urine output becomes excessive.

(ii) Thyroid function tests and serum electrolytes should be monitored before initiating therapy and periodically thereafter to monitor for hypothyroidism and hypernatremia secondary to diabetes insipidus, respectively.

(c) Gain of 10 kg (22 lb) or more may occur.

(d) Clinically evident hypothyroidism or goiter may occur in a few cases.

4. Significant interactions. Lithium interacts with many drugs, only a few of which are discussed following. These interactions either increase lithium levels or increase lithium excretion. Lithium is eliminated through the kidneys by glomerular filtration and competes with sodium for reabsorption in the renal tubules.

a. Thiazide diuretics interfere with sodium reabsorption and, thus, may favor lithium reabsorption, which could lead to lithium toxicity. Care should be given to adjust the dosage of the lithium, and serum levels should be monitored closely. Conversely, lithium doses may need to be increased if the diuretic is discontinued. Furosemide therapy does not present this concern because the increased reabsorption of lithium in the proximal tubule is counteracted by decreased absorption in the loop of Henle.

b. Osmotic diuretics, sodium bicarbonate, and **theophylline** increase lithium excretion, thereby diminishing the therapeutic effect.

STUDY QUESTIONS

Directions: Each of the numbered items or incomplete statements in this section is followed by answers or by completions of the statement. Select the **one** lettered answer or completion that is **best** in each case.

1. All of the following patterns are associated with a bipolar major affective disorder EXCEPT

(A) a history of manic episodes only
(B) a history of depressed episodes only
(C) a history of several depressed episodes and only one manic episode
(D) cycling from manic to depressed episodes with periods of normal mood in between
(E) a history of several manic episodes and only one depressed episode

2. Unipolar affective disorder is characterized by which of the following signs?

(A) Flight of ideas
(B) Unusual verbosity
(C) Poor judgment leading to reckless driving
(D) Loss of interest in the job and family
(E) Ease of distractibility

3. As a group, cyclic antidepressants have which of the following characteristics?

(A) They have similar therapeutic efficacy
(B) They have potent anticholinergic activity
(C) They lack histamine H_1-blocking activity
(D) They prevent the synthesis of neurotransmitters
(E) They have nearly identical side effect profiles

4. Therapeutic serum lithium levels during initiation of therapy are defined as

(A) 0.4–0.8 mEq/L
(B) 1.0–1.5 mEq/L
(C) 0.6–1.0 μg/L
(D) 0.8–1.0 mg/L
(E) 1.2–1.6 μg/L

5. Which of the following relatively mild adverse effects is associated with initiation of lithium therapy?

(A) Blurred vision
(B) Dystonic reactions
(C) Fine hand tremor
(D) Pseudoparkinsonism
(E) Tinnitus

6. Foods high in tyramine such as pickled herring and most cheeses (especially blue, cheddar, Parmesan) should be avoided by patients who are taking

(A) doxepin
(B) phenelzine
(C) maprotiline
(D) alprazolam
(E) trazodone

7. Which of the following drugs prescribed for control of a major affective disorder is associated with an almost immediate onset of activity?

(A) Lithium carbonate
(B) Protriptyline
(C) Tranylcypromine
(D) Chlorpromazine
(E) Isocarboxazid

8. Under the biogenic amine hypothesis, mania is thought to be due to

(A) an excess of epinephrine activity
(B) an excess of norepinephrine activity
(C) an excess of dopamine activity
(D) a deficiency of epinephrine activity
(E) a deficiency of dopamine activity

Questions 9–13

A 28-year-old woman presents with complaints of suicidal ideation. She has lost interest in her usual activities and because of poor appetite, she has lost approximately 15 pounds over the last 6 months. She complains of severe insomnia. She has a poorly formulated suicide plan but states that she would not carry out the plan. There is no history of previous suicide attempts. Her past medical history is unremarkable except for a normal pregnancy at age 23 years (full term, viable infant).

On physical examination, she appears mildly agitated. Blood pressure is 110/70 with a pulse of 72 and respirations 12; she is afebrile. The general examination is unremarkable. Heart, lungs, abdomen, and neurologic examinations are normal. Routine laboratory studies including an electrocardiogram are within normal limits. The patient was prescribed amitriptyline.

9. Which feature of amitriptyline makes it a reasonable therapeutic choice for this patient?

(A) The patient has a bipolar disorder, and amitriptyline is effective in this disorder
(B) The sedative properties of amitriptyline might prove beneficial
(C) Amitriptyline lacks significant H_1-blocking activity
(D) Amitriptyline does not cause any cardiac side effects

10. All of the following symptoms are potential anticholinergic side effects of amitriptyline EXCEPT

(A) blurred vision
(B) constipation
(C) sinus bradycardia
(D) urinary retention

11. What is an appropriate starting dose of amitriptyline?

(A) 50 mg/day
(B) 150 mg/day
(C) 200 mg/day
(D) 250 mg/day

12. How long will it take for the amitriptyline to be fully therapeutically effective?

(A) 1 week
(B) 2 weeks
(C) 1 month
(D) 3 months

13. The patient's husband brings her back to the emergency room and states that the patient has taken an overdose of the amitriptyline. All of the following choices are appropriate EXCEPT

(A) obtain an electrocardiogram
(B) obtain a toxic screen with a tricyclic level included
(C) gastric lavage
(D) observe patient only; no laboratory work would be needed because the drug is not toxic

ANSWERS AND EXPLANATIONS

1. The answer is B *[I A 2; II C 1, 2].*
Bipolar depression is characterized by periods of depression and mania, or mania alone. Therefore, someone with a history of depressed episodes only would not fit the definition of a bipolar disorder.

2. The answer is D *[II B 3 d].*
Loss of interest in the job or family is a common sign of a unipolar affective disorder. Flight of ideas, unusual verbosity, poor judgment that could lead to reckless driving, and ease of distractibility are all signs of the manic phase of a bipolar affective disorder.

3. The answer is A *[IV A 2, 4].*
The cyclic antidepressants all have equivalent therapeutic efficacy when given at the appropriate dose. Each drug has its own unique side effect profile. Several of the drugs are potent antihistamines (e.g., doxepin, amitriptyline). While some of the drugs have potent anticholinergic activity, others are nearly devoid of this activity (e.g., bupropion, trazodone, fluoxetine). Cyclic antidepressants block the reuptake of neurotransmitters but do not block neurotransmitter synthesis.

4. The answer is B *[V B 3 b (3) (a)].*
Therapeutic serum lithium levels during initiation of lithium therapy range from 1.0–1.5 mEq/L. During maintenance therapy, the therapeutic serum level range is 0.6–1.2 mEq/L. It is important to monitor serum levels because lithium, like digoxin, has a narrow range between therapeutic and toxic doses. During the first weeks of therapy, serum levels are checked several times a week until the levels have stabilized. During maintenance therapy, serum lithium levels are checked at least once every 2 months.

5. The answer is C *[V B 3 e].*
The relatively mild adverse effects associated with lithium therapy consist of gastrointestinal disturbances, polyuria, and polydipsia, muscle weakness, and fine hand tremor. Pseudoparkinsonism and dystonic reactions do not occur with lithium therapy; tinnitus and blurred vision are not signs of lithium toxicity.

6. The answer is B *[IV B 4 d (1) (a)].*
Foods high in tyramine should be avoided in patients who are taking monoamine oxidase (MAO) inhibitors such as phenelzine. The enzyme MAO takes part in the oxidative deamination of biogenic amines (e.g., dopamine, norepinephrine, serotonin, tyramine). MAO inhibitors prevent this enzymatic degradation. (This is considered to be the mechanism of their antidepressant effects.) When a person taking an MAO inhibitor eats foods high in tyramine, the tyramine is not degraded in the body. The tyramine can induce the release of stored catecholamines (e.g., norepinephrine), and this may precipitate an episode of severe hypertension. Doxepin, maprotiline, alprazolam, and trazodone are not MAO inhibitors.

7. The answer is D *[IV A 5 a (7), B 3 d; V A 2 a, 3 a].*
Protriptyline is a tricyclic antidepressant. Full response may require about 4 weeks. Tranylcypromine and isocarboxazid are monoamine oxidase (MAO) inhibitors. The onset of antidepressant effects may be delayed for 2–3 weeks. Lithium carbonate has a delayed onset and may take up to 2 weeks for maximum effectiveness. Chlorpromazine is the only agent listed in the question that has an immediate onset of activity.

8. The answer is B *[I C 2 a].*
Under the biogenic amine hypothesis, depression is thought to be due to a deficiency of serotonin or norepinephrine activity, and mania is thought to be due to an excess of norepinephrine activity.

9–13. The answers are: 9-B *[IV A 6 c (1)]*, **10-C** *[IV A 6 c (3) (b)]*, **11-A** *[IV A 5 a (2)]*, **12-C** *[IV A 5 a (7)]*, **13-D** *[IV A 6 c (6)].*
The patient described in the question does not have a bipolar disorder. Amitriptyline is a potent H_1-blocker, and its sedating properties might be beneficial for this patient. Amitriptyline can cause cardiac side effects such as arrhythmias.

Blurred vision, constipation, and urinary retention are anticholinergic side effects. Sinus tachycardia, not sinus bradycardia, is an anticholinergic effect.

An appropriate starting dose of amitriptyline is 50 mg/day (in divided doses); this should be titrated up to the target dose.

Physiologic symptoms usually respond in 1 week, and psychosocial symptoms usually respond after 2–4 weeks. However, full therapeutic effectiveness usually requires about 4 weeks.

Tricyclic overdose is potentially fatal. Treatment may initially include emesis and gastric lavage and administration of activated charcoal. An electrocardiogram and a toxic screen are routine emergency room evaluation tools.

48
Asthma and Chronic Obstructive Pulmonary Disease

Laura Wilson
Mary Ann Dzurec

I. ASTHMA

A. Definition. Asthma is a chronic inflammatory disorder of the airways characterized by variable airway obstruction (reversible either spontaneously or as a result of therapy), airway inflammation, and increased airway responsiveness to a variety of stimuli. The major symptoms are shortness of breath, cough, and wheezing.

B. Classification. Asthma is classified by severity of disease as mild, moderate, or severe. These classifications are based on combinations of symptoms, treatment requirements, and objective measurements. Previous classifications for asthma (i.e., intrinsic, extrinsic) are no longer used. It is now recognized that patients respond to a variety of stimuli. An allergic component can be found in 35%–55% of asthmatics.

1. **Mild asthma**
   - a. Intermittent, brief symptoms up to two times weekly
   - b. Asymptomatic between exacerbations
   - c. Brief symptoms with activity
   - d. Infrequent (less than two times per month) nocturnal symptoms
2. **Moderate asthma**
   - a. Symptoms more than one or two times weekly
   - b. Exacerbations affect sleep and activity level
   - c. Exacerbations may last several days
   - d. Occasional emergency care
3. **Severe asthma**
   - a. Continuous symptoms
   - b. Limited activity level
   - c. Frequent exacerbations
   - d. Frequent nocturnal symptoms
   - e. Occasional hospitalization and emergency treatment

C. Incidence. Asthma affects approximately 10 million Americans. It has been estimated that 5% of adults and 7%–10% of children have asthma.

1. In about half of all cases, onset is before age 10.
2. Up to age 15, asthma is more prevalent in males; older asthmatics are more commonly female.
3. By early adulthood, 30%–70% of those with childhood asthma have marked improvement of symptoms or become symptom-free.
4. Although death from asthma remains uncommon, mortality has been increasing in recent years. The most common cause of death is inadequate assessment of the severity of airway obstruction and inadequate therapy. The key to prevention of death is education of patients and clinicians.

D. Etiology

1. **Precipitating factors** of an acute asthma attack include:
   - a. Allergens (e.g., pollen, dust, animal dander)
   - b. Respiratory tract infections (e.g., rhinovirus, influenza)

c. Exercise
d. Emotions (e.g., anxiety, stress, laughter)
e. Irritant exposure
   (1) Occupational exposure to such agents as gasoline fumes and fresh paint
   (2) Environmental exposure to cold air, sulfur dioxide, and cigarette smoke
f. **Drugs.** Two different mechanisms can trigger drug-related asthma:
   (1) **Hypersensitivity reaction** due to drugs (e.g., aspirin, ibuprofen, penicillin, products containing tartrazine)
   (2) **Extension of pharmacological effect** may develop with antiadrenergic and cholinergic drugs (e.g., β-adrenergic blockers, bethanechol).

2. **The mechanism of airway hyperresponsiveness** has not been determined; however, several theories have been suggested:
   a. **Airway inflammation** is now believed to be a principal factor in airway hyperresponsiveness. Increased levels of inflammatory mediators and infiltration by inflammatory cells are thought to be the primary mechanisms responsible for airway hyperresponsiveness.
   b. Alterations in autonomic neural control of airways
      (1) β-Adrenergic defect producing β-blockade. This theory is based on the principle that β-blockers alter respiratory function, but has not been proven in asthma patients.
      (2) Increased cholinergic response. Asthma patients seem to be more responsive to bronchoconstriction from cholinergic agents. This suggests changes in the parasympathomimetic control of the airways.
   c. Abnormalities in bronchial epithelial integrity lead to increased permeability to inhaled allergens, irritants, and inflammatory mediators. Epithelial injury may be a result of inflammation.
   d. Changes in intrinsic bronchial smooth muscle function. Bronchial smooth muscle hypertrophy is often found in histological sections from asthma patients; however, the importance of these changes in the development of airway hyperresponsiveness is not established.
   e. Airflow obstruction can be influenced by factors such as mucus production, edema, smooth muscle contraction, and hypertrophy. Airflow obstruction is not the primary cause of airway hyperresponsiveness, although it may be a contributing factor.

E. Pathophysiology

1. **Allergic stimuli** produce a biphasic response that has been linked to the inflammatory process.
   a. **Early asthmatic response**
      (1) There is an **immediate response to an allergen with a peak effect at 10–30 minutes** and a duration of **1.5–3.0 hours.**
      (2) The allergen reacts with immunoglobulin E (IgE) attached to mast cells, causing release of inflammatory mediators (see I E 4).
      (3) The early response can be inhibited by premedication with β-agonists, cromolyn, nedocromil, theophylline, or glucocorticoids (when given for the proper duration).
      (4) The response can be reversed by the administration of β-agonists.
   b. **Late asthmatic response**
      (1) A late asthmatic response, characterized by persistent airflow obstruction, airway inflammation, and bronchial hyperresponsiveness, is found in about 50% of asthma patients 4–8 hours after an acute response triggered by inhalation of an allergen. The duration of the response may last several days. Bronchial hyperreactivity may last several weeks.
      (2) Mediators involved in the late response may include those released from mast cells, including eosinophil chemotactic factor, neutrophil chemotactic factor, and basophil chemotactic factor. Platelet-activating factor (PAF) and leukotrienes are released from eosinophils.
      (3) Mediators cause an influx of inflammatory cells including eosinophils, macrophages, neutrophils, and lymphocytes, with release of additional mediators.
      (4) This response can be prevented by administration of anti-inflammatory agents, including cromolyn, nedocromil, or corticosteroids. β-agonists have no effect on this response.

2. **Nonallergic stimuli,** such as exercise, methacholine, or cold air, produce acute bronchospasm that lasts about 1 hour and is not followed by a late asthmatic response. These stimuli may cause bronchoconstriction, using some of the inflammatory mediators, but the process is still controversial.

3. **Acute asthma attacks** are characterized by a response that triggers airway obstruction.
   a. In response to a precipitating factor, mediators from mast cells cause bronchial smooth muscle to become spasmodic, leading to bronchoconstriction, which triggers blood vessel engorgement and infiltration of inflammatory cells (neutrophils).
   b. Mucous glands and **goblet cells,** the mucus-secreting cells of the respiratory tract epithelium, become edematous, which leads to increased mucus production, further narrowing the airway.
   c. Airway obstruction reduces ventilation to some lung regions; this, in turn, causes a ventilation/perfusion (V/Q) imbalance that leads to hypoxemia. This is reflected by a reduction in the partial pressure of arterial oxygen (Pao_2) more frequently in a moderate to severe attack.
   d. In the early stages, hyperventilation results in a decrease in the partial pressure of arterial carbon dioxide ($Paco_2$). If the asthma attack progresses and the airways remain narrowed, respiratory muscles suffer fatigue.
   e. **Respiratory acidosis** develops if hypoxemia worsens and the patient's respiratory rate is not maintained; then the $Paco_2$ level begins to increase.
   f. Peak expiratory flow rate (PEFR) and forced expiratory volume (1 second) [FEV_1] may decrease in the early stages of an acute asthma attack. As the attack worsens, FEV_1 decreases, resulting in **air trapping and lung hyperinflation.**

4. **Immunopathologic events affect asthma.** The adrenergic and cholinergic responses in asthma are governed by immunologic, environmental, and physical stimuli.
   a. After exposure to an asthma "trigger," mediators are released from the mast cells, alveolar macrophages, and eosinophils. The mediators that are released [e.g., histamine, heparin, prostaglandin D_2 (PGD_2), leukotrienes, chymotrypsin/trypsin] cause the early asthmatic response.
   b. Additional mediators (e.g., eosinophil chemotactic factor, neutrophil chemotactic factor, basophil chemotactic factor, and platelet-activating factor) are responsible for the late asthmatic response.
      (1) Some of these mediators may be released in response to nonallergic stimuli, but this is still controversial.
      (2) These mediators are responsible for bronchoconstriction, airway edema, and mucus production (Figure 48-1). Bronchial hyperresponsiveness may also be induced by these mediators and may last up to 4 weeks after the initial asthma attack, increasing sensitivity to stimuli.

F. Clinical evaluation

1. **Physical findings**
   a. An acute attack, which may have a sudden or gradual onset, produces respiratory distress and wheezing of a variable degree, depending on the severity of the attack (Table 48-1).
   b. Other common findings include chest tightness, cough, tachypnea, tachycardia, accessory muscle use, and pulsus paradoxus.
   c. Between acute asthma attacks, the patient may be asymptomatic. Physical findings are dependent on the severity of the disease.

2. **Diagnostic test results**
   a. **Blood analysis** typically shows a slightly increased white blood cell (WBC) count during an acute attack; eosinophilia also may be present.
   b. **Sputum analysis** may reveal Curschmann's spirals (mucous casts of the small airways), eosinophils, Charcot-Leyden crystals (products of eosinophil breakdown), Creola bodies (clumps of epithelial cells), and bacteria (if there is an infection).
   c. **Arterial blood gas measurements** help gauge the severity of the asthma attack (see Table 48-1).
   d. **Pulmonary function tests** help determine the degree of airway obstruction and gas exchange impairment. During an acute asthma attack, FEV_1 decreases while residual volume (RV) and functional residual volume (FRV) increase. Total lung capacity (TLC) may

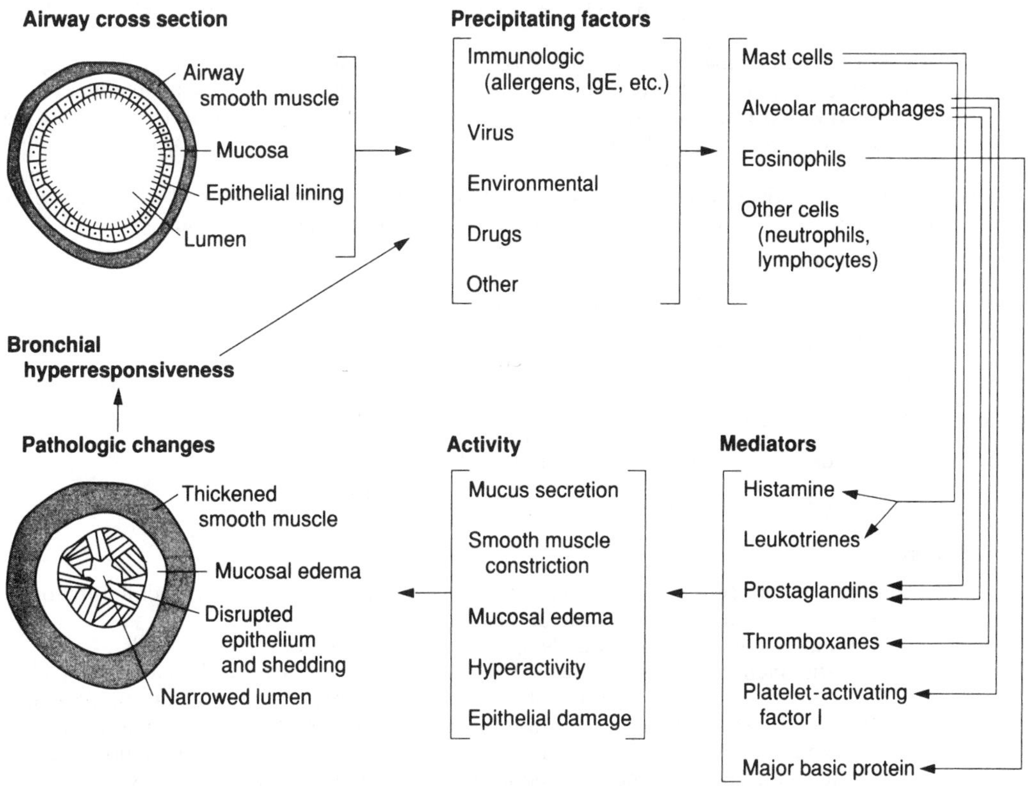

Figure 48-1. Diagrammatic representation of the pathophysiology of asthma.

Table 48-1. Stages of Severity of an Acute Asthmatic Attack

Stage	Symptoms	FEV_1 or FVC	Arterial pH	PaO_2	$PaCO_2$
I: Mild	Mild dyspnea and wheezing	50%–80% of normal	Normal or ↑	Normal or ↓	Normal or ↓
II: Moderate	Respiratory distress at rest and marked wheezing	50% of normal	↑	↓	↓
III: Severe	Marked respiratory distress, loud wheezing, coughing, difficulty speaking, accessory chest muscle use, and chest hyperinflation	< 50% of normal	Normal or ↓	↓	Normal or ↑
IV: Respiratory failure	Severe respiratory distress, confusion, lethargy, cyanosis, disappearance of breath sounds, and pulsus paradoxus > 12 mm Hg	< 25% of normal	↓↓	↓	↑↑

Arrows indicate changes: ↑ = increased; ↓ = decreased; ↑↑ = markedly increased; ↓↓ = markedly decreased. *FEV_1* = forced expiratory volume in 1 second; *FVC* = forced vital capacity; *PaO_2* = partial pressure of arterial oxygen; *$PaCO_2$* = partial pressure of arterial carbon dioxide.

be increased. Changes in the PEFR correlate well with FEV_1 and may be used to evaluate lung function.

e. An **electrocardiogram** (ECG) may show sinus tachycardia.

f. **Chest x-ray** is useful in detecting an accompanying pneumothorax or pneumonia.

g. **Allergy skin tests** may identify allergens that trigger asthma. (Skin tests should not be done during an acute attack.)

G. **Treatment objectives.** The goal of therapy is to provide symptomatic control with normalization of lifestyle and return pulmonary function as close to normal as possible.

1. Maintain control of symptoms
2. Prevent exacerbations and chronic symptoms by reducing inflammation
3. Maintain normal pulmonary function
4. Maintain normal activity levels, including exercise
5. Avoid adverse effects from asthma medications
6. Prevent development of irreversible airway obstruction
7. Prevent asthma mortality

H. **Therapy**

1. **Management of acute asthma.** A stepped approach is used with suggested administration in the order discussed below. The role of theophylline is controversial.

a. **β-Agonists** (e.g., albuterol) usually are given first (Table 48-2).

(1) **Therapeutic effects.** Among their various effects, these agents (also called sympathomimetics) relieve bronchoconstriction and, thus, help reverse an acute asthma attack.

(2) **Mechanism of action.** β-Agonists stimulate β_2-receptors, activating adenyl cyclase, which increases intracellular production of cyclic adenosine monophosphate (cAMP). This produces relaxation of smooth muscle (bronchial relaxation), stabilization of mast cell membranes, and stimulation of skeletal muscles (tremor). Additional effects include gluconeogenesis, insulin secretion, and activation of Na^+, K^+-adenosine triphosphatase (ATPase). β-Agonists differ in their affinity for the β_1- and β_2-receptors. Agents with β_1 effects can cause cardiotoxicity.

(3) **Administration and dosage.** Whenever possible, these agents are given to asthmatics via a nebulizer or a metered dose inhaler (MDI) because of their rapid onset of action, similar duration of action, and fewer side effects when compared with other dosage forms. In an emergency situation, a motorized nebulizer is preferred. This route has been shown to be as effective as parenteral agents in severe acute asthma. Agents can also be administered to patients on mechanical ventilation by insertion of the MDI into the respiratory circuit. For chronic therapy, they are administered orally only to patients who cannot use aerosols with spacer devices properly. For dosage information, see Table 48-2.

(4) **Precautions and monitoring effects**

(a) These drugs should be used cautiously in patients who have a history of arrhythmias, coronary artery disease (CAD), hypertension, or diabetes.

(b) Tremor, nervousness, headache, dizziness, weakness, and insomnia are common central nervous system (CNS) effects of β-agonists.

(c) Palpitations and tachycardia occur. Pulse rate should be monitored closely in patients receiving any of the β-agonists.

(d) The use of nonselective β-agonists can induce myocardial ischemia, myocardial necrosis, and arrhythmias because of excessive cardiac stimulation. Avoidance of these agents (e.g., isoproterenol) and administration of β_2-selective agents (e.g., albuterol, bitolterol, or pirbuterol) is preferred.

(e) The longer-acting β_2-agonist, salmeterol, is indicated for chronic treatment of bronchospasm and should not be used in acute exacerbations due to its slow onset of action.

(f) Drug tolerance or tachyphylaxis can occur with inhaled or oral β-agonists. Suggested mechanisms include:

(i) A decrease in the number of active β-receptors due to movement of receptors from the cell surface into the cell **(downregulation)**

(ii) A decreased sensitivity in the β-receptors to stimuli making them unable to activate adenyl cyclase. The clinical significance of this effect is unclear in patients taking normal doses of β-agonists. Patients may only become tolerant to the extrapulmonary effects and not to the bronchodilation. Tolerance is signaled by an increase in the requirement for β-agonists when they are used on a regular schedule. This effect may potentially be reversed by adding oral or aerosol corticosteroids to the regimen.

(g) Rebound bronchoconstriction found with β-agonists such as isoproterenol and albuterol may occur acutely after administration or after longer periods of treatment (i.e., weeks or months).

(h) Increased bronchial hyperreactivity to irritants such as methacholine and histamine may be observed with chronic β-agonist use.

(i) Although further study on the safety of β-agonists is warranted, limiting the use of these drugs to manufacturer-recommended doses and recognizing that overuse demonstrates a lack of asthma control are essential.

(5) Significant interactions

(a) Concomitant use of systemic β-agonists with **monoamine oxidase (MAO) inhibitors, tricyclic antidepressants, or methyldopa** may lead to severe hypertension. The risk with aerosolized agents may be smaller.

(b) **β-Adrenergic blockers** (e.g., propranolol) block the bronchodilatory and cardiostimulating effects of β-agonists.

(c) **β-Agonists** should not be combined with other **sympathomimetic agents** because of additive cardiovascular effects. Vasoconstrictive and pressor effects of epinephrine are antagonized by **α-adrenergic blocking agents** (e.g., phentolamine).

b. Corticosteroids (e.g., beclomethasone, betamethasone, hydrocortisone, prednisone) may be given if bronchoconstriction fails to respond to β-adrenergics.

(1) Therapeutic effects. When used to treat asthma, corticosteroids suppress the inflammatory response.

(2) Mechanism of action. Mechanisms of action include:

(a) Decreased inflammatory cell activation, recruitment, and infiltration

(b) Decreased production of inflammatory mediators (e.g., prostaglandins, leukotrienes)

(c) Increased synthesis of proteins that enhances the β-adrenergic response

(d) Decreased mucus production

(e) Prevention of increased vascular permeability

(3) Administration and dosage. A lag time may occur with the onset of these agents because they lack direct bronchodilatory effects on smooth muscle. After administration of intravenous (IV), oral, or inhaled agents, some patients may show improvement of pulmonary function tests in 1–3 hours, with a maximum effect in 6–9 hours.

(a) There is no significant difference in the clinical efficacy of the corticosteroid products. The agent should have the following properties: good glucocorticoid activity, minimal mineralocorticoid activity, and short-to-intermediate duration of action. The route of administration is determined by the condition of the patient.

(b) IV corticosteroids are administered when the patient cannot use the oral route during a severe acute asthma attack. The duration of therapy is short but may be continued as oral therapy; the dose is then rapidly tapered. Hydrocortisone and methylprednisolone are most commonly used. An example of dosing is methylprednisolone (or equivalent) 1–2 mg/kg IV, then 0.5–2 mg/kg every 6 hours.

(c) Beclomethasone, dexamethasone, flunisolide, and triamcinolone are available in aerosol form, which is preferred because of the lower incidence of adverse effects. These agents should not be used as primary therapy for a severe acute attack but are useful with other therapies for chronic management (Table 48-3).

(d) Prednisone (1 mg/kg/day), methylprednisolone, and prednisolone are the preferred oral agents. They can be administered in short "bursts" to improve recovery during an acute exacerbation. A typical regimen is 60 mg/day of prednisone or methylprednisolone gradually tapered over several days. If a prolonged course is necessary, side effects may be minimized by a single morning dose given on alternating days.

Table 48-2. β-Adrenergic Agonists Used in the Treatment of Asthma or COPD

Agent	Severe Acute		Chronic		Site of Action	Duration of Action	Comments
	Pediatric	Adult	Pediatric	Adult			
Albuterol							
NEB: 0.5% (5 mg/ml)	0.1 to 0.15 mg/kg/dose q 20 minutes × 3 doses (maximum 5 mg)	2.5 mg q 20 minutes × 3 doses	0.05–0.15 mg/kg q 4–6 hours	2.5 mg q 6–8 hours	β_1-receptors + β_2-receptors ++++	3–8 hours inhalation 4–8 hours oral	Dilute with normal saline or sterile water.
MDI: 0.09 mg/puff	2 puffs q 5 minutes (maximum of 12 puffs)	2 puffs q 20 minutes × 3 doses	1–2 puffs q 4–6 hours	2 puffs q 4–6 hours			
ORAL (various)	NCR	NCR	2 to 4 mg q 6 hours (maximum 24 mg)	2–4 mg q 6 hours or 8 mg SR q 12 hours (maximum 32 mg)			
Bitolterol							
NEB: 0.2% (2 mg/ml)	NCR in children <12 years	1–2.5 mg q 4–8 hours	NCR in children < 12 years	1–2.5 mg q 6–8 hours	β_1-receptors + β_2-receptors ++++	6–8 hours	Dilute with normal saline or sterile water to a total volume of 2–4 ml.
MDI: 0.37 mg/puff	NCR in children <12 years	NCR	NCR in children < 12 years	2–3 puffs q 4–6 hours			
Epinephrine							
SC: 1:1000 (1 mg/ml)	0.01 mg/kg/dose (0.01 ml/kg/dose) q 20 minutes × 3 doses	0.3–0.5 mg/dose (0.3–0.5 ml/dose) q 20 to 30 minutes × 3 doses	NCR	NCR	α-receptors +++ β_1-receptors +++ β_2-receptors +++	1–4 hours subcutaneous 1–3 hours inhalation	Sustained-released product with a longer duration of action than epinephrine solution.
SC: 1:200 (5 mg/ml) sustained release	0.025 mg/kg/dose q 4–6 hours (max single dose for < 30 kg is 0.15 ml)	0.75–1.5 mg q 4–6 hours	NCR	NCR			Dilute with normal saline or sterile water.
NEB (racemic): 2.25% racepinephrine	< 10 kg: 2 ml of 1:8 dilution 10–15 kg: 2 ml of 1:6 dilution 15–20 kg: 2 ml of 1:4 dilution > 20 kg: 2 ml of 1:3 dilution all given over 15 minutes q 1–4 hours	2 ml of 1:2 or 1:3 dilution over 15 minutes q 1–4 hours	NCR	NCR			
MDI (various)	NCR	NCR	NCR	NCR			

Isoetharine							
NEB: 1% (10 mg/ml)	NCR	5 mg q 20 minutes × 3 doses	0.1–0.2 mg/kg/dose q 4 hours	2.5–10 mg q 4 hours	β_1-receptors ++ β_2-receptors +++	1–3 hours	Dilute 1:3 with normal saline or sterile water. Agents with a longer duration of action and greater selectivity may be preferred.
MDI: 0.34 mg/puff	NCR	NCR	1–2 puffs q 3–4 hours	1–2 puffs q 3–4 hours			
Isoproterenol							
NEB: 1:200 (5 mg/ml)	NCR	NCR	NCR	NCR	β_1-receptors +++ β_2-receptors ++++	1–2 hours inhalation	Short duration of action; tolerance and cardiovascular side effects may develop.
MIDI (various)	NCR	NCR	NCR	NCR		1–2 hours intravenous	
Metaproterenol							
NEB: 5% (50 mg/ml)	0.25–0.5 mg/kg/dose q 1 hour	10–15 mg q 1 hour	< 12 yrs: 0.5 mg/kg/dose q 4–6 hours (maximum dose 15 mg)	> 12 yrs: 10–15 mg q 4–6 hours	β_1-receptors ++ β_2-receptors +++	4 hours oral 2–6 hours inhalation	Dilute with normal saline 2.5 ml if used with IPPB. Cardiovascular side effects may develop.
MDI: 0.65 mg/puff	1–3 puffs q 3–4 hours (maximum 12 puffs/day)	2–3 puffs q 3–4 hours (maximum 12 puffs/day)	2 puffs 4–6 hours (maximum 12 puffs/day)	2–3 puffs q 4–6 hours (maximum 12 puffs/day)			
ORAL (various)	NCR	NCR	0.3–0.5 mg/kg/dose q 6–8 hours	20 mg q 6–8 hours			
Pirbuterol							
MDI: 0.2 mg/puff	NCR	NCR	> 12 yrs: 2 puffs q 4–6 hours (maximum 12 puffs/day)	2 puffs q 4–6 hours (maximum 12 puffs/day)	β_1-receptors + β_2-receptors ++++	5 hours	
Salmeterol							
MDI: 0.025 mg/puff	NCR	NCR	> 12 yrs: 1–2 puffs q 12 hours	1–2 puffs q 12 hours	β_1-receptors + β_2-receptors ++++	12 hours	Not indicated for acute exacerbations
Terbutaline							
MDI: 0.2 mg/puff	2 puffs q 5 minutes (maximum 12 puffs)	2 puffs q 4 hours	2 puffs q 4–6 hours	2 puffs q 4–6 hours	β_1-receptors + β_2-receptors ++++	3–6 hours inhalation	Parenteral solution not FDA-approved for nebulization
SC: 0.1% (1 mg/ml)	0.01 mg/kg up to 0.3 mg q 2–6 hours	0.25 mg q 2–6 hours	NCR	NCR		1.5–4 hours parenteral	
ORAL (various)	NCR	NCR	< 12 yrs: 0.05–0.15 mg/kg/dose q 8 hours (maximum 5 mg/24 hrs)	5 mg q 6–8 hours		4–8 hours oral	

FDA = Food and Drug Administration; *MDI* = metered dose inhaler; *NCR* = not currently recommended; *NEB* = solution for nebulizer; *SC* = subcutaneous.

Table 48-3. Aerosol Corticosteroids

Agent	MDI Dose Delivered Per Metered Spray	Recommended Dosage	
		Adults	Pediatric
Dexamethasone sodium phosphate*	84 μg	3 inhalations 3–4 times daily (maximum 12)	2 inhalations 3–4 times daily (maximum 8)
Beclomethasone dipropionate*	42 μg	2 inhalations 3–4 times daily (maximum 20)	1–2 inhalations 3–4 times daily (maximum 10)
Triamcinolone acetonide*	100 μg	2 inhalations 3–4 times daily (maximum 16)	1–2 inhalations 3–4 times daily (maximum 12)
Flunisolide	250 μg	2 inhalations twice daily (maximum 8)	2 inhalations twice daily (maximum 4)

*May be given twice daily in stabilized patients
MDI = metered dose inhaler

(4) Precautions and monitoring effects

(a) Corticosteroids should be used cautiously in elderly and pediatric patients and in those with diabetes mellitus (DM), hypothyroidism, peptic ulcers or other gastrointestinal (GI) diseases, chronic infections, Cushing's syndrome, myasthenia gravis, and psychotic tendencies.

(b) Patients receiving daily or alternate-day oral corticosteroid therapy, using the smallest effective dose, should be monitored closely for adverse systemic effects (Table 48-4).

(c) Inhaled steroids may cause such local effects as dry mouth, hoarseness, and fungal infection of the mouth and throat (spacer devices reduce these adverse effects) and rare systemic side effects.

(d) Significant interactions

(i) Concurrent use of **hepatic microsomal enzyme inducers** (e.g., rifampin, barbiturates, hydantoins) causes enhanced corticosteroid metabolism, reducing therapeutic efficacy.

(ii) Concurrent use of **estrogens, oral contraceptives, ketoconazole, macrolide antibiotics** (e.g., erythromycin, clarithromycin) may decrease corticosteroid metabolism.

(iii) Cyclosporine may decrease plasma clearance of some corticosteroids (i.e., methylprednisone), and these agents may increase the plasma concentration of cyclosporine.

Table 48-4. Systemic Effects of Corticosteroid Therapy

Effect	Clinical Manifestations	Intervention/Prevention
Appetite stimulation	Weight gain	Reduction in caloric intake
Fluid and sodium retention	Edema	Reduction in sodium intake
Hyperacidity	Esophagitis, gastritis	Antacids, histamine$_2$-receptor antagonists (e.g., ranitidine)
Hypertension	Headache, cerebrovascular accident	Blood pressure monitoring
Psychosis	Disruptive behavior	Tranquilizers
Increased intraocular pressure	Glaucoma	Ophthalmologic evaluation
Hypokalemia	Muscle weakness	Potassium replacement therapy
Increased gluconeogenesis	Hyperglycemia	Adjustment of dietary, insulin, or oral hypoglycemic therapy

(iv) Administration of **potassium-depleting diuretics** (e.g., thiazides, furosemide) or other potassium-depleting drugs (e.g., amphotericin) with corticosteroids causes enhanced hypokalemia. Serum potassium should be closely monitored, especially in patients on **digitalis glycosides.**

(v) Corticosteroids can decrease the serum concentrations of **isoniazid** and **salicylates** when the agents are used concurrently.

c. Theophylline compounds (methylxanthines) may be considered if β-agonists and corticosteroids fail to control an acute asthma attack. Whether theophylline should be used in acute asthma is controversial. It has not been consistently shown that any additional beneficial effect is provided in combination with inhaled β-agonists. However, patients on chronic theophylline therapy who present to the emergency department with subtherapeutic levels may benefit from therapy to increase the serum theophylline concentration.

(1) Therapeutic effects. Among their various effects, these drugs relax bronchial smooth muscle, reduce mucus secretions, enhance mucociliary transport, and improve respiratory muscle contractility. There may also be some degree of anti-inflammatory activity, although this is subject to debate.

(2) Mechanism of action. The precise mechanism of action is not known. Inhibition of the enzyme phosphodiesterase, resulting in increased cAMP, occurs in vitro only at concentrations greater than those achieved in vivo. Other suggested mechanisms include alteration of intracellular calcium and increased binding of cAMP to its binding protein. Adenosine antagonism, increasing circulating catecholamines, and inhibition of production of contractile prostaglandins have also been proposed.

(3) Administration and dosage

(a) IV therapy. Theophylline and aminophylline (contains 80% theophylline) are available.

(i) The usual **loading dose** for adults and children not previously receiving a methylxanthine is 5 mg/kg theophylline administered over 20–30 minutes at a rate not exceeding 25 mg/min.

(ii) The usual **maintenance infusion** rate of theophylline is 0.4 mg/kg/hr in nonsmoking adults. This rate should be adjusted for factors that affect the metabolism of theophylline and serum levels obtained after the infusion begins (Table 48-5).

(b) Oral therapy

(i) Oral loading doses of a nonsustained-release theophylline or aminophylline product can be given. The initial dose of theophylline for adults and children older than 1 year of age is the lesser of 400 mg/day or 16 mg/kg/day given in divided doses. The dose can be titrated slowly upward and the serum level monitored until a therapeutic level is obtained. The maximum dose varies with age, from 22 mg/kg/day for children aged 1–9 years to 16 mg/kg/day for adults.

(ii) Other methylxanthine compounds are available (e.g., oxtriphylline, dyphylline); dosing is based on theophylline content.

(iii) Sustained-release forms of theophylline are available to increase the dosing interval and improve compliance. The products can vary in their time to peak concentration (Table 48-6).

Table 48-5. Theophylline Maintenance Doses

Group	Infusion Rate (mg/kg/hr)
Infants (6 weeks to 6 months)	0.5
Infants (6 months to 1 year)	0.6–0.7
Children (1–9 years old)	0.8
Older children (9–12 years old) and adolescent (12–16 years old) smokers	0.7
Adults (over age 16)	0.4
Adult smokers	0.7
Adults with cardiac decompensation, cor pulmonale, liver dysfunction, or a combination of these	0.2

Table 48-6. Selection of Theophylline Products

Salt	Theophylline Content (%)	Equivalent Dose (mg)
Theophylline anhydrous (e.g., most oral solids)	100	100
Theophylline monohydrate (e.g., oral solutions)	91	110
Aminophylline anhydrous	86	116
Aminophylline dihydrate	80	127
Formulation	**Time to Peak**	**Dosing Interval**
Uncoated tablets	1–2 hours	q 6 hours
Oral liquids	1–2 hours	q 6 hours
Sustained-release		
Capsule	3–6 hours	q 8 hours
Tablet	4–10 hours	q 12 hours
Capsule	11–15 hours	q 24 hours

(4) Precautions and monitoring effects

(a) Contraindicated in patients with hypersensitivity to xanthine compounds and in those with a history of arrhythmias.

(b) Cautious use is indicated in patients with peptic ulcer disease, gout, CAD, and DM.

(c) Adverse CNS effects such as dizziness, restlessness, nervousness, insomnia, and seizures may occur.

(d) Palpitations and sinus tachycardia have been reported, even in the therapeutic dosage range.

(e) Adverse GI effects include nausea, vomiting, and anorexia; these effects should be carefully differentiated from theophylline toxicity.

(f) Because individuals metabolize theophylline compounds at different rates, serum drug levels should be monitored to ensure a level in the therapeutic range (10–20 mg/ml). Levels should be monitored at steady-state. During infusion therapy, levels can be measured at 32–40 hours after the start or change in infusion. During oral therapy, a trough level is taken before the dose is given after the first 1½ to 2 days. Peak serum levels should be monitored in patients with rapid theophylline elimination to avoid transient adverse effects.

(g) Cardiac glycosides may be potentiated with increased potential for toxicity.

(h) Drug clearance may be altered by various factors, including significant drug interactions (Table 48-7).

d. Other agents used in the treatment of acute asthma include the following:

(1) Anticholinergics (also called cholinergic blocking agents). These drugs may cause bronchodilation by inhibiting acetylcholine stimulation of efferent vagal pathways, reducing intrinsic vagal tone to bronchial smooth muscle. Bronchoconstriction due to mediator release may be partially mediated through cholinergic stimulation. This effect may vary from patient to patient. During an acute attack, anticholinergics may be synergistic when combined with β-agonists and should be used only as second-line therapy in selected patients.

(a) Aerosolized atropine usage has decreased because of the high incidence of adverse effects and lack of demonstrated efficacy in studies.

(b) Ipratropium bromide can be given to patients with acute and chronic asthma with minimal risk of side effects when poorly controlled by corticosteroids and β-agonists. It is, however, more effective in the chronic obstructive pulmonary disease (COPD) population. The MDI dose is 2–4 inhalations four times daily. The nebulizing solution dose is 500 μg (2.5 ml) four times daily.

(2) Antihistamines. Terfenadine, astemizole, and loratadine compete with histamine for histamine$_1$-receptor sites on effector cells and, thus, help prevent the histamine-mediated responses that influence asthma. However, their use in asthma requires further study. These agents are useful for patients with allergic rhinitis.

Table 48-7. Factors That Alter Theophylline Clearance

Factors that increase clearance (causing a reduced serum drug level)
Age 1–12 years
Fever
Smoking
Concurrent use of carbamazepine, IV isoproterenol, phenobarbital, phenytoin, or rifampin
Low carbohydrate/high protein diet
Charcoal-broiled foods
Factors that decrease clearance (causing an increased serum drug level)
Advanced age
Premature neonates
Term infants < 6 months
Cor pulmonale
Congestive heart failure
Liver failure
Fever/viral illness
Pregnancy
Concurrent use of allopurinol, cimetidine, erythromycin, clarithromycin, oral contraceptives, propranolol, troleandomycin, clindamycin, influenza virus vaccine, amiodarone, ciprofloxacin, ofloxacin, norfloxacin, or enoxacin

(3) **Calcium channel blockers** (e.g., verapamil, nifedipine). Theoretically, these agents may have therapeutic effects in asthma. In vitro, these agents cause relaxation of smooth muscle by inhibition of calcium influx. However, this has not been proved in clinical studies and further investigation is needed.

(4) **Antibiotics.** These are administered if the patient has a known or suspected bacterial infection as suggested by yellow, green, or brown sputum.

(5) **Magnesium sulfate.** This is administered via nebulization and it may be useful because of its modest ability to bronchodilate. Magnesium sulfate improves respiratory (striated) muscle strength in hypomagnesemic patients when administered intravenously. Further study is warranted.

e. Nonpharmacologic treatment may also be used.

(1) Humidified oxygen is administered to all patients with severe, acute asthma to reverse hypoxemia. The fraction of inspired oxygen (FIO_2) administered is based on the patient's arterial blood gas status; generally 1–3 L/min are given via Venturi mask or nasal cannula.

(2) IV fluids and electrolytes may be required if the patient is dehydrated.

2. Management of chronic asthma. A stepped approach to manage chronic asthma based on severity of disease is used.

a. Mild asthma. Pretreatment with an inhaled β-agonist and/or cromolyn or nedocromil is used for exposure to exercise or allergens. Inhaled β-agonists are used as needed for acute symptoms.

b. Moderate asthma. Inhaled β-agonists and anti-inflammatory agents are recommended. Sustained-release theophylline and/or an oral β-agonist can be added if symptoms persist. Short courses of oral corticosteroids followed by inhaled corticosteroids are used for acute exacerbations.

c. Severe asthma. Inhaled β-agonists and anti-inflammatory agents (corticosteroid with or without cromolyn or nedocromil) with or without sustained-release theophylline and/or an oral β-agonist are recommended. Extra inhaled β-agonists and oral corticosteroids are added when exacerbations occur.

d. Chronic asthma. Chronic asthma occurs when the symptoms are frequent and require long-term prophylactic therapy. Medications are added in a stepped approach until symptoms are under control.

(1) β-Agonists by inhalation are used for mild to severe exacerbations. They also can be used chronically in patients with moderate to severe asthma. The proper use of an

MDI with a spacing device increases the efficacy and safety by increasing the pulmonary delivery and reducing the GI delivery of these agents.

- **(a)** Salmeterol may be more suitable for chronic therapy because of its slow onset and longer duration of action.
- **(b)** Inhaled corticosteroids are used for moderate episodes or as chronic prophylaxis. This route is the least likely to cause adverse reactions (see Table 48-3).
- **(c)** Short-course oral therapy ("burst" therapy) is used when the intermittent episodes are severe. Prednisone (or equivalent) is given in high doses (40–80 mg/day in adults; 1–2 mg/kg/day in children) for up to 5–10 days, then rapidly tapered. Improvement in the PEFR is used to monitor therapy.
- **(d)** Chronic oral steroids are used after the failure of other medications to relieve chronic symptoms. Agents should be given in the lowest possible dose to avoid serious complications.

(2) **Cromolyn sodium and nedocromil sodium** are nonsteroidal anti-inflammatory drugs (NSAIDs) used adjunctively to treat mild, moderate, or severe asthma. They sometimes help reduce the amount of corticosteroid needed. They have no value in the treatment of an acute asthma attack. Initial improvement is within 1–2 weeks; the maximum effect may take longer.

- **(a)** **Therapeutic effect.** When used prophylactically, cromolyn and nedocromil prevent both the early and late response as well as asthma induced by exercise, cold air, and sulfur dioxide. When used as maintenance therapy for asthma, they suppress nonspecific airway reactivity.
- **(b)** **Mechanism of action.** Cromolyn and nedocromil are believed to act locally on the lung mucosa by inhibiting the degranulation of sensitized mast cells. There is also evidence for inhibitory effects on inflammatory cells such as macrophages, eosinophils, neutrophils, monocytes, and platelets.
- **(c)** **Administration and dosage.** Cromolyn is available as an MDI, providing 800 μg per inhalation; as a nebulizer solution (20 mg/2 ml); and as 20-mg capsules whose contents are inhaled via a special turboinhaler. Nedocromil is available as an MDI, providing 1.75 mg per inhalation.
  - **(i)** As adjunctive therapy for chronic asthma, two inhalations of the MDI are used four times a day; 20 mg of the nebulized solution is inhaled four times a day; or a 20-mg capsule is given for inhalation four times a day. Nedocromil is dosed as two inhalations four times a day. In some cases, the frequency of cromolyn or nedocromil administration may be reduced to two or three times daily.
  - **(ii)** To prevent asthma attacks, cromolyn or nedocromil is used prior to (e.g., 10–15 minutes) but no more than 1 hour before exposure to the triggering factor (e.g., exercise, allergen).
- **(d)** **Precautions and monitoring effects**
  - **(i)** Cromolyn and nedocromil are not indicated for use during an acute asthma attack or status asthmaticus.
  - **(ii)** Generally, these drugs are well tolerated; occasionally, the inhaled form causes paradoxical bronchospasm, wheezing, and coughing, as well as nasal congestion and irritation or dryness of the throat. There are fewer side effects with the MDI.
  - **(iii)** Hypersensitivity rarely occurs.

(3) **Theophylline** may be added to the regimen when therapy with other inhaled agents has been maximized. Because of the availability of sustained-release products, this agent is most beneficial in patients with early morning symptoms. Monitoring serum levels, adverse reactions, and concomitant drug use is essential for long-term therapy.

(4) **Anticholinergics. Ipratropium bromide** has bronchodilator action in acute exacerbations of asthma and has been shown to increase therapeutic response in combination with β-agonists. However, any benefits in the chronic management of asthma have not been established. The onset of action is more delayed (usually 5–20 minutes) than that of β-agonists.

(5) Investigational agents which may be available for the treatment of chronic asthma include lipo-oxygenase inhibitors and leukotriene receptor antagonists. These drugs inhibit the production or receptor binding of leukotrienes which are responsible for the inflammatory response associated with asthma.

(6) **Spacer devices** are used with MDIs to increase the amount of drug delivered to the lung and decrease oropharyngeal deposition. They are especially beneficial in patients with poor hand-lung coordination. Devices vary in construction and efficacy.
  (a) **Holding chamber** (e.g., Aerochamber, Inhal-Aid, Inspirease)
  (b) **Tube spacer** (e.g., Brethancer)

I. Complications of asthma

1. **Status asthmatics.** This life-threatening condition occurs when a prolonged asthma attack fails to respond to normal treatment.
   a. Findings include altered consciousness, cyanosis (even with oxygen therapy), pulsus paradoxus (greater than 12 mm Hg), peak flow less than 150 L/min in adults or less than 50% of the predicted value, and FEV_1 less than 50%.
   b. Standard therapy for status asthmaticus involves oxygen, fluids, inhaled β-agonists, corticosteroids, and parenteral β-agonists. In some cases, IV aminophylline or oral theophylline is added.
   c. Aggressive therapy is indicated if standard therapy fails. If the patient has respiratory acidosis, tracheal intubation and mechanical ventilation may be indicated.

2. **Pneumothorax.** This condition is characterized by accumulation of air in the pleural space, as sometimes occurs during an acute asthma attack.
   a. **Physical findings** include sudden sharp chest pain, dyspnea, tachypnea, hypotension, diaphoresis, pallor, and anxiety.
   b. **Therapy** includes placing the patient in Fowler's position, oxygen therapy, aspiration or pleural air via a chest tube, and analgesics.

3. **Atelectasis.** This disorder, which inhibits gas exchange during respiration, may occur if bronchiolar obstruction causes collapse of lung tissue. In asthmatics, atelectasis usually involves the right middle lobe but sometimes affects the entire lung.
   a. **Physical findings** include diminished breath sounds, mediastinal shift toward the affected side, worsening dyspnea, anxiety, and cyanosis.
   b. **Therapy** includes incentive spirometry, postural drainage, chest percussion, coughing and deep breathing exercises, and bronchodilators. Bronchoscopy may be necessary to remove secretions.

II. CHRONIC OBSTRUCTIVE PULMONARY DISEASE

A. Definitions. COPD is a general term for conditions characterized by chronic, progressive lower airway destruction, causing reduced pulmonary inspiratory and expiratory capacity. The two major forms of COPD—**chronic bronchitis** and **emphysema**—frequently coexist.

1. **Chronic bronchitis.** In this disorder, excessive mucus production by the tracheobronchial tree results in airway obstruction due to edema and bronchial inflammation. Bronchitis is considered chronic when the patient has a cough producing more than 30 ml of sputum in 24 hours for at least 3 months of the year for 2 consecutive years.

2. **Emphysema.** This condition is marked by permanent alveolar enlargement distal to the terminal bronchioles and destructive changes of the alveolar walls.

B. Incidence. Approximately 10 million Americans have COPD. It is the fourth leading cause of death in the United States. While it is most commonly diagnosed in older men, the incidence is increasing in women because of an increasing population of women smokers.

C. Etiology. Various factors have been implicated in the development of COPD.

1. **Cigarette smoking.** One mechanism suggests that pulmonary hyperreactivity secondary to smoking results in persistent airway obstruction.

2. **Other etiologic factors**. Other etiologic factors include exposure to irritants such as sulfur dioxide (as in polluted air), noxious gases, and organic or inorganic dusts; a history of respiratory infections or bronchial hyperreactivity; and social, economic and hereditary factors (e.g., $alpha_1$-antitrypsin deficiency).

D. Pathophysiology

1. Chronic bronchitis

a. **Respiratory tissue inflammation** (as from smoking) results in vasodilation, congestion, mucosal edema, and goblet cell hypertrophy. These events trigger goblet cells to produce excessive amounts of mucus.

b. **Changes in tissue** include increased smooth muscle, cartilage atrophy, infiltration of neutrophils and other cells, and impairment of cilia.

c. Chronic bronchitis, due to lung impairment, predisposes patients to **lung infections,** both viral and bacterial, which further **destroy small bronchioles.**

d. As the disease progresses:

(1) **Airways are blocked** by thick, tenacious mucus secretions, which trigger a productive cough.

(2) As the **airways degenerate,** overall gas exchange is impaired, causing **exertional dyspnea.**

(3) Hypoxemia results from a V/Q imbalance and is reflected in an increasing arterial CO_2 tension ($Paco_2$).

(4) Sustained hypercapnia (increased $Paco_2$) desensitizes the brain's respiratory control center and central chemoreceptors. As a result, compensatory action to correct hypoxemia and hypercapnia (i.e., a respiratory rate or depth increase) does not occur.

2. Emphysema

a. **Anatomical changes** destroy elasticity.

(1) **Inflammation** and **excessive mucus secretion** (as from long-standing chronic bronchitis) cause **air trapping in the alveoli.** This contributes to breakdown of the bronchioles, alveolar walls, and connective tissue.

(2) As clusters of alveoli merge, the number of alveoli diminishes, leading to increased space available for air trapping.

(3) Destruction of alveolar walls causes collapse of small airways on exhalation and disruption of the pulmonary capillary beds.

(4) These changes result in V/Q abnormalities; blood is shunted away from destroyed areas to maintain a constant V/Q ratio, unlike the case in chronic bronchitis.

(5) Hypercapnia and respiratory acidosis may develop, causing desensitization of brain centers to hypercapnia. When this occurs, hypoxemia serves as the stimulus for breathing.

b. There are **specific lung regions** in which characteristic anatomical changes of emphysema occur.

(1) In **centrilobular** (centriacinar) emphysema, associated with cigarette smoking, the upper lung portions are affected. Typically, bronchioles and alveolar ducts become dilated and merge.

(2) In **panlobular** (panacinar) emphysema, all lung segments are involved. The alveoli enlarge and atrophy, and the pulmonary vascular bed is destroyed. This form of emphysema is associated with alpha$_1$-antitrypsin deficiency.

(3) In **paraseptal** emphysema, the lung periphery adjacent to fibrotic regions is the site of alveolar distention and alveolar wall destruction. This is associated with spontaneous pneumothorax.

E. Clinical evaluation

1. Physical findings

a. **Predominant chronic bronchitis** typically has an insidious onset after age 45.

(1) A **chronic productive cough** is the hallmark of chronic bronchitis. It occurs first in winter, then progresses to year-round. It is usually worse in the morning.

(2) **Exertional dyspnea,** the most common presenting symptom, is progressive. However, the severity of this symptom does not reflect the severity of the disease.

(3) Other common findings include obesity, rhonchi and wheezes on auscultation, cyanosis, prolonged expiration, and a normal respiratory rate. As the disease progresses, right ventricular failure is common which presents as jugular venous distention, peripheral edema, hepatomegaly, and cardiomegaly, hence the term "blue bloater."

b. **Predominant emphysema** has an insidious onset, and symptoms occur after age 55.

(1) The **cough** is chronic but less productive than in chronic bronchitis.

(2) Exertional dyspnea is progressive, constant, severe, and more characteristic of emphysema.
(3) Other common findings include weight loss, tachypnea, pursed-lip breathing, prolonged expiration, accessory chest muscle use, hyperresonance on percussion, diaphragmatic excursion, and diminished breath sounds, hence the term "pink puffer."

c. Patients may have elements and physical findings from each of these diseases simultaneously.

2. Diagnostic test results

a. Chronic bronchitis

(1) Blood analysis usually reveals an increased hematocrit and hemoglobin due to erythropoiesis secondary to hypoxemia. With bacterial infection, the WBC count may be increased.
(2) Sputum inspection reveals thick purulent or mucopurulent sputum tinged yellow, white, green, or gray; the color change is diagnostic of infection. Microscopic analysis may detect neutrophils and microorganisms.
(3) Arterial blood gas studies may show a markedly decreased Pao_2 level (e.g., 45–60 mm Hg) reflecting hypoxemia and a $Paco_2$ level that is normal or elevated (e.g., 50–60 mm Hg), reflecting hypercapnia.
(4) Pulmonary function tests may be normal in the early disease stages. Later, they show an increased RV, a decreased vital capacity (VC), and a decreased FEV. Unlike emphysema, chronic bronchitis patients have normal diffusing capacity, normal static lung compliance, and normal TLC.
(5) Chest x-ray typically identifies lung hyperinflation and increased bronchovascular markings.
(6) An ECG may reveal right ventricular hypertrophy and changes consistent with cor pulmonale.

b. Emphysema

(1) Blood analysis may show a decreased $alpha_1$-antitrypsin level.
(2) Sputum inspection reveals scanty sputum that is clear or mucoid. Infections are less frequent than in chronic bronchitis.
(3) Arterial blood gas studies typically indicate a reduced or normal Pao_2 (e.g., 65–75 mm Hg) level and, in late disease stages, an increased $Paco_2$ level (e.g., 50–60 mm Hg).
(4) Pulmonary function tests show normal or increased static lung compliance, reduced FEV and diffusing capacity, and increased TLC and RV.
(5) Chest x-ray usually reveals bullae, blebs, a flattened diaphragm, lung hyperinflation, vertical heart, enlarged anteroposterior chest diameter, decreased vascular markings in the lung periphery, and a large retrosternal air space.

F. Treatment Objectives

1. Smoking cessation and avoidance of irritants
2. Relieve symptoms and enable the patient to perform normal daily activities
3. Improve pulmonary function
4. Control life-threatening disease exacerbations
5. Prevent complications
6. Teach the patient about the disease and the use of medications and improve therapeutic compliance

G. Therapy

1. **Drug therapy.** β-Agonists and anticholinergic drugs are the most commonly used agents. Methylxanthines are added when the response to other agents is inadequate. Corticosteroids are beneficial when an allergic component has been demonstrated.

a. **Ipratropium bromide and atropine** produce bronchodilation by competitively inhibiting cholinergic responses. Ipratropium also reduces sputum volume without altering viscosity. Some studies have shown an increased response to these agents in COPD when they are combined with β-agonists.

(1) Ipratropium bromide is three to five times more potent and has fewer side effects than atropine. High-dose ipratropium may lead to more prolonged bronchodilation. Initial MDI dosing is two inhalations (40 μg) four times daily but dosing can be increased to six inhalations four times daily without significant risk. Alternatively, ipratropium solution 500 μg/ml 2.5 ml or more may be nebulized four times daily. Ipratropium is more useful when administered regularly because of a slower onset and longer duration of action as compared with β-agonists.

(2) Atropine is administered by diluting 0.025 mg/kg to 0.05 mg/kg in 2–4 ml of normal saline and placing it in a nebulizer for spraying every 6 hours. Because absorption is substantial, side effects are pronounced, including dry mouth, tachycardia, and urinary retention. Use of atropine requires close monitoring.

b. **β-Agonists** (see I H 1 a; Table 48-2) are effective in relieving dyspnea due to airway obstruction. Response is not as significant as in asthmatic patients. These agents may also increase mucociliary clearance by stimulating ciliary activity.

(1) β-Agonists are administered via aerosol (e.g., MDI with or without a spacer, or a nebulizer) unless the patient cannot use the drug properly; then an oral agent is used.

(2) Agents in this class should not be used in combination. An adequate dose of a single agent provides peak bronchodilation.

(3) Prolonged use of high doses of β-agonists may lead to drug intolerance.

c. **Theophylline** compounds (see I H 1 c; Table 48-5) typically are added to the drug regimen after a trial of ipratropium and β-adrenergics.

(1) In COPD, these drugs increase mucociliary clearance, stimulate the respiratory drive, enhance diaphragmatic contractility, improve the ventricular ejection fraction, and stimulate renal diuresis.

(2) A trial of 1–2 months with the serum drug level maintained at 8–12 μg/ml and maximized, if necessary, up to 20 μg/ml is needed to assess therapeutic efficacy. An increase in FEV_1 by more than 15%–20% indicates a positive response. If no change occurs in the patient's condition, theophylline therapy should be discontinued due to the potential for side effects.

(3) Serum drug levels should be closely monitored in patients with congestive heart failure (CHF) or cor pulmonale due to reduced theophylline metabolism.

d. **Corticosteroids** (see I H 1 b; Table 48-3) play a less prominent role in COPD than in asthma.

(1) These agents may be added to the drug regimen after maximal ipratropium, β-agonists, and theophylline therapy.

(2) Candidates for corticosteroid therapy should have a history of submaximal response to the previous drug therapies (i.e., ipratropium, β-agonists, and theophylline). Long-term corticosteroids should be maintained only for patients with documented improvement in airflow and exercise, and at the lowest possible dose.

(3) Corticosteroids may be given via aerosol to minimize adverse effects, but aerosolization may be less effective than oral therapies.

(4) Acute exacerbations can be treated intravenously with methylprednisolone, 0.5-1.0 mg/kg every 6 hours for 72 hours, then tapered off.

(5) For oral use, prednisone is administered in a dosage of 20–40 mg/day for the first 2–4 weeks, then titrated to the lowest effective dosage or discontinued, if possible.

e. **Antibiotics** are used to treat a documented infection as evidenced by an increase in volume or change in color or viscosity of the sputum. Sputum cultures rarely offer additional information as COPD patients are often chronically seeded with the causative organism(s). Prevention of infection with chronic antibiotic therapy is controversial and should be considered only in patients with multiple exacerbations annually (i.e., greater than two per year).

(1) The most common infecting organisms are *Mycoplasma pneumoniae, Streptococcus pneumoniae, Haemophilus influenzae,* and *Moraxella catarrhalis.*

(2) Ambulatory antibiotic treatment of pneumonia in patients with COPD includes either a second-generation cephalosporin (e.g., cefuroxime or ceclor), trimethoprim/sulfamethoxazole, or a β-lactam with or without a β-lactamase inhibitor (e.g., amoxicillin or amoxicillin/clavulanate). If infection with *Mycoplasma pneumoniae* is a concern, a macrolide (e.g., erythromycin or azithromycin) may be added.

(3) Antibiotic treatment of pneumonia in hospitalized patients with COPD includes either a second- or third-generation cephalosporin (e.g., cefuroxime, ceftriaxone, or

cefotaxime) or a β-lactam with or without a β-lactamase inhibitor (e.g., ampicillin or ampicillin/sulbactam). If infection with *Mycoplasma pneumoniae* is a concern, a macrolide (e.g., erythromycin or azithromycin) may be added.

(4) *Streptococcus pneumoniae, Haemophilus influenzae,* and *Moraxella catarrhalis* infections should be treated for approximately 7–10 days. Cases of *Mycoplasma pneumoniae* may need longer therapy ranging from 10 to 14 days. Exceptions to this would be the use of azithromycin whose uniquely long half-life allows 5 days of therapy.

2. Other measures. Depending on individual patient needs, COPD therapy also may include the following:

a. Mucolytics (e.g., acetylcysteine) may improve sputum clearance and disrupt mucus plugs but it does not improve measured pulmonary function and can cause bronchospasm.

b. Expectorants (e.g., guaifenesin) are of limited benefit. Potassium iodide should be avoided because of side effects associated with iodine therapy.

c. Oxygen therapy (administered at a low flow rate) reverses hypoxemia, particularly during exercise or at night. Indications for oxygen include a Pao_2 less than 55 mm Hg or evidence of cor pulmonale, pulmonary hypertension, mental impairment, or polycythemia with a Pao_2 of less than 60 mm Hg.

d. Chest physiotherapy loosens secretions, helps reexpand the lungs, and increases the efficacy of respiratory muscle use. Techniques used include postural drainage, chest percussion and vibration, coughing, and deep breathing.

e. Physical rehabilitation improves the patient's exercise tolerance. A rehabilitation program usually includes exercises that improve diaphragmatic and abdominal muscle tone.

f. Vaccines (e.g., influenza virus, pneumococcal, and *H. influenzae* type b polysaccharide vaccines) are recommended to prevent infection.

g. Avoidance of cigarette smoking or other irritants has been shown to slow the rate of decline of FEV in COPD patients. Nicotine gum or patches, or the use of clonidine may be useful in smoking cessation.

H. Complications of COPD. Patients with COPD have an increased risk for developing several life-threatening complications.

1. Pulmonary hypertension. With decreased pulmonary vascular bed space (due to lung congestion), pulmonary arterial pressure increases. In some cases, pressure increases enough to cause cor pulmonale (right ventricular hypertrophy) with consequent heart failure.

2. Acute respiratory failure. In advanced stages of emphysema, the brain's respiratory center may become seriously compromised, leading to poor cerebral oxygenation and an increased $Paco_2$ level. Hypoxia and respiratory acidosis may ensue. If the condition progresses, respiratory failure occurs.

3. Infection. In chronic bronchitis, trapping of excessive mucus, air, and bacteria in the tracheobronchial tree sets the stage for infection. In addition, impairment of coughing and deep breathing, which normally cleanse the lungs, leads to respiratory cilia destruction. Once an infection sets in, reinfection can easily occur.

STUDY QUESTIONS

Directions: Each of the numbered items or incomplete statements in this section is followed by answers or by completions of the statement. Select the **one** lettered answer or completion that is **best** in each case.

1. The symptoms of allergen-mediated asthma result from

(A) increased release of mediators from mast cells
(B) increased adrenergic responsiveness of the airways
(C) increased vascular permeability of bronchial tissue
(D) decreased calcium influx into the mast cell
(E) decreased prostaglandin production

2. Acute exacerbations of asthma can be triggered by all of the following EXCEPT

(A) bacterial or viral pneumonia
(B) hypersensitivity reaction to penicillin
(C) discontinuation of asthma medication
(D) hot, dry weather
(E) stressful emotional events

3. The selection of an oral theophylline product depends primarily on

(A) the percentage of theophylline content of the product
(B) preexisting disease states (e.g., gout, peptic ulcer disease)
(C) theophylline half-life
(D) concurrent asthma medication
(E) age of the patient

4. In the emergency room, the preferred first-line therapy for asthma is

(A) theophylline
(B) a β-agonist
(C) a corticosteroid
(D) cromolyn sodium
(E) an antihistamine

5. The primary goals of asthma therapy include all of the following EXCEPT

(A) maintain normal activity levels
(B) maintain control of symptoms
(C) avoid adverse effects of asthma medications
(D) prevent acute exacerbations and chronic symptoms
(E) prevent of lung tissue destruction

6. In the treatment of chronic obstructive pulmonary disease (COPD), corticosteroids

(A) are more effective than in the treatment of asthma
(B) are more beneficial when used alone
(C) produce more side effects when used in the aerosol form
(D) should have the dosage titrated upward until side effects are found
(E) should be used for at least 2 weeks before efficacy is assessed

Directions: The item below contains three suggested answers, of which **one or more** is correct. Choose the answer

A if **I only** is correct
B if **III only** is correct
C if **I and II** are correct
D if **II and III** are correct
E if **I, II, and III** are correct

7. The disease process of chronic bronchitis is characterized by

I. the destruction of central and peripheral portions of the acinus
II. an increased number of mucous glands and goblet cells
III. edema and inflammation of the bronchioles

Directions: The item in this section consists of lettered options followed by a set of numbered items. For each item, select the **one** lettered option that is most closely associated with it. Each lettered option may be selected once, more than once, or not at all.

Questions 8–10

Match the description with the appropriate agent.

(A) Cimetidine
(B) Albuterol
(C) Ipratropium bromide
(D) Epinephrine
(E) Atropine

8. Decreases theophylline clearance

9. Has anticholinergic activity with few side effects

10. Has high β_2-adrenergic selectivity

ANSWERS AND EXPLANATIONS

1. The answer is A *[I E 4; Figure 48-1].*
In asthma, airborne antigen binds to the mast cell, activating the immunoglobulin E (IgE)-mediated process. Mediators (e.g., histamine, leukotrienes, prostaglandins) are then released, causing bronchoconstriction and tissue edema.

2. The answer is D *[I D 1; Figure 48-1].*
Exacerbations of asthma can be triggered by allergens, respiratory infections, occupational stimuli (e.g., fumes from gasoline or paint), emotions, and environmental factors. Studies have shown that cold air can cause release of mast cell mediators by an undetermined mechanism. Hot, dry air does not cause this release.

3. The answer is A *[I H 1 c; Table 48-6].*
Theophylline or aminophylline products vary in their percentage of active drug, theophylline content, and the type of preparation. Sustained-release products decrease the absorption rate and do not alter theophylline half-life.

4. The answer is B *[I H 1 a].*
In an emergency situation, the most rapidly acting agent is used first. Selection of the route of administration depends on the severity of the attack. An inhaled β-agonist administered in a nebulizer or administered as a subcutaneous (SC) agent is the most appropriate first-line therapy.

5. The answer is E *[I E, G; II D].*
Asthma is characterized by reversible airway obstruction in response to specific stimuli. Mast cells release mediators, which trigger bronchoconstriction. After an acute attack, in most cases, symptoms are minimal, and pathological changes are not permanent. Unlike asthma, chronic obstructive pulmonary disease (COPD) does cause progressive airway destruction, chronic bronchitis by excessive mucus production and other changes, and emphysema by destruction of the acinus.

6. The answer is E *[II G 1 d].*
In chronic obstructive pulmonary disease (COPD), corticosteroids are used in addition to β-adrenergic agents and theophylline compounds after maximal therapy with these agents. Corticosteroids may be used in aerosol form to minimize side effects. If given orally, dosage is reduced after 2–4 weeks of therapy to the lowest effective dosage. Because the onset of benefit is unknown, an adequate trial of therapy (at least 2–4 weeks) is needed.

7. The answer is D (II, III) *[II D 1, 2].*
Chronic bronchitis is characterized by an increase in the number of mucous and goblet cells due to bronchial irritation. This results in increased mucus production. Other changes include edema and inflammation of the bronchioles and changes in smooth muscle and cartilage. Emphysema is a permanent destruction of the central and peripheral portions of the acinus distal to the bronchioles. In this disease, adequate oxygen reaches the alveolar duct, but there is inadequate blood perfusion.

8-10. The answers are: 8-A *[Table 48-7],* **9-C** *[II G 1 a],* **10-B** *[Table 48-2].*
Cimetidine, a histamine$_2$-receptor antagonist, decreases theophylline clearance by inhibiting hepatic microsomal mixed-function oxidase metabolism. Theophylline clearance can be decreased by 40% during the first 24 hours of concurrent therapy. Anticholinergic agents such as atropine and ipratropium bromide produce bronchodilation by competitively inhibiting cholinergic receptors. The disadvantages of atropine include dry mouth, tachycardia, and urinary retention. Ipratropium bromide is three to five times more potent than atropine and does not have these side effects. Albuterol is one of the most β_2-selective adrenergic agents available. Other such agents include terbutaline, bitolterol, and pirbuterol. Agents with β_2-selectivity dilate bronchioles without causing side effects related to β_1-stimulation (e.g., increased heart rate).

49
Rheumatoid Arthritis

Larry N. Swanson

I. INTRODUCTION

A. Definition. Rheumatoid arthritis (RA) is a chronic, systemic, inflammatory condition that is most apparent in its synovial joint involvement. Inflammation may extend to extra-articular sites such as tendons and organ structures.

B. Classification. Patients are said to have RA if they have satisfied at least four of the following criteria. The first four criteria must be present for at least 6 weeks.

1. **Morning stiffness** must be present in and around the joints lasting at least 1 hour before maximal improvement.
2. **Three joint areas** (at least) must have **soft-tissue swelling** or **fluid** observed by a physician. The possible joint areas are right or left **proximal interphalangeal (PIP) joint, metacarpophalangeal (MCP) joint, wrist, elbow, knee, ankle,** and **metatarsophalangeal (MTP) joint.**
3. **One joint area (at least) in the hand joints** (i.e., a wrist, MCP, PIP) **must be swollen** and observed by a physician.
4. There must be **symmetric arthritis** (i.e., simultaneous involvement of the same joint areas on both sides of the body).
5. **Subcutaneous nodules (rheumatoid nodules)** over bony prominences, over extensor surfaces, or in juxta-articular regions must be observed by a physician.
6. **Abnormal amounts of serum rheumatoid factor** must be demonstrated by any method that has been positive in less than 5% of normal control subjects.
7. **Radiologic changes** typical of RA, including erosions or unequivocal bony decalcification localized to or most marked adjacent to the involved joints, must be present on hand and wrist x-rays.

C. Incidence. RA is more common in women than in men, occurring with a female to male ratio between two and three to one. The condition occurs in approximately 1%–3% of the general adult population and often occurs between the ages of 30 and 40 years, but the incidence is highest between ages 40 and 60 years.

D. Etiology. The cause of this disease remains unknown; however, the following factors may play a role:

1. A specific human leukocyte antigen (HLA-DR4) may be involved. When patients with this antigen are exposed to certain environmental factors, an inappropriate immune response occurs, which results in chronic inflammation. About 73% of white patients with RA have this antigen whereas only 30% of the general population have it.
2. Some infectious agent may be involved in precipitating RA in patients genetically predisposed.
3. Although no specific agent has been identified, for many years investigators have noted the occurrence of polyarthritis in association with microbial organisms, including bacteria (i.e., Lyme disease).

E. Pathogenesis

1. The initial event inciting synovial inflammation (the earliest synovial response) is unknown. Vasodilation, edema, sensation of heat, and loss of function result. Synovial fluid production increases with a resultant accumulation of an effusion. If untreated, the synovitis of RA becomes self-perpetuating and chronic. The synovium becomes thickened and boggy.
2. Inward overgrowth of the enlarged synovium across the surface of the articular cartilage results in the formation of **pannus** (an exuberant synovial thickening). The inflammatory reaction at the cartilage–pannus junction may eventually result in:
   a. Articular cartilage degradation
   b. Loss of adjacent bone
   c. Characteristic marginal erosions, which are observable on x-ray
3. The effect of degradation of cartilage is bone rubbing against bone in the joint, producing bony crepitus and pain.

F. Clinical manifestations

1. Usually, RA presents as **symmetric synovitis** affecting similar joints bilaterally. Occasionally, the disease may present as arthritis in only one joint or in an asymmetric pattern affecting a few joints. Over time, however, the arthritis assumes a symmetric pattern.
2. **Frank joint inflammation in a previously healthy individual** is a common presentation.
3. **A rapidly progressive arthritis affecting many joints,** accompanied by organ system involvement, is an uncommon presentation.
4. **Organ system involvement without clinically evident joint inflammation** is a very uncommon presentation.
5. Extra-articular manifestations of RA are common and may involve almost any organ system in the body. Such manifestations can be severe, and some, including cardiopulmonary complications, diffuse vasculitis, gastrointestinal (GI) complications, and infections, can lead to death. Extra-articular manifestations tend to be more common in patients with high titers of rheumatoid factor, subcutaneous nodules, and severe disease.

G. Clinical course (Figure 49-1)

1. The clinical course of RA is highly variable and often unpredictable.
   a. About 80% of patients have a **polycyclic course** with intermittent partial or complete remissions.

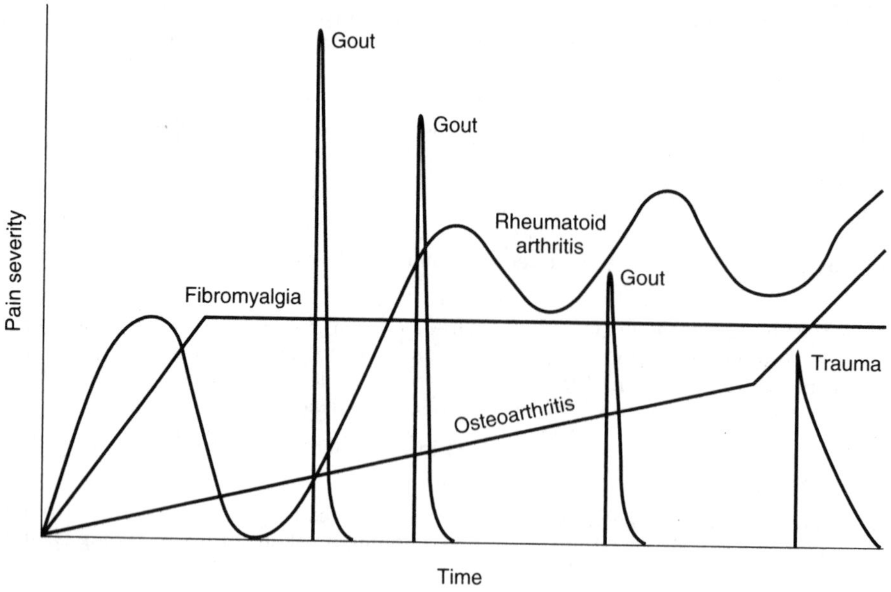

Figure 49-1. Temporal patterns characteristic of various causes of joint pain. (Adapted from *Am Fam Physician,* March 1996.)

b. Most of the remaining patients usually have a **progressive disease** with relentless synovial inflammation that rapidly advances to a destructive and deforming arthritis.
c. A **monocyclic course** with transient arthritis followed by prolonged remission is uncommon.

2. Very early symptoms may be vague and lack evidence of synovial inflammation. The presenting complaints may include variable aching, multiple joint pain, and fatigue. Over months, the synovitis gradually evolves, usually in the feet and hands.
   a. Early involvement occurs most often in the hands, with swelling, warmth, and tenderness affecting mainly the PIP and MCP joints.
   b. Although hand and foot involvement is the most common initial presentation, synovitis can be prominent in the large joints of the knee, ankle, and elbow, as well as in the intervertebral and temporomandibular joints.

3. The **hallmark of RA is maximal pain and stiffness on awakening;** this so-called morning gel typically lasts for more than 30 minutes and may persist for hours.

4. RA is a progressive disease that may result in irreversible joint deformities, such as:
   a. Ulnar deviation of fingers
   b. Swan-neck deformity
   c. Boutonnière deformities of PIP joints

5. Patients typically experience progressive functional decline, work disability, and a decrease in income. The average life expectancy of persons with RA is 4–10 years shorter than that of unaffected persons.

H. Diagnosis and clinical evaluation

1. There is no pathognomonic test for RA. The diagnosis is made primarily on the basis of clinical findings and supported by results of laboratory tests and radiologic studies (see I B, H 4). RA is easily identified in most patients who have well-established disease. Diagnosis is not as simple in early disease, when the manifestations are often atypical.

2. A thorough **joint system evaluation** with documentation of the swelling, synovial thickening, tenderness, pain, and reduced range of motion in peripheral joints is mandatory.

3. **Presence of rheumatoid nodules** (i.e., firm, round, rubbery masses that are pathognomonic for RA) are found in about 20% of patients. These nodules are most commonly located in subcutaneous tissues at sites prone to external pressure (e.g., the elbow), but they may affect other organs.

4. **X-rays** of involved joints may reveal only soft-tissue swelling initially. If inflammation is entrenched, the films may reveal juxta-articular osteoporosis, symmetrical joint space narrowing, and erosions near the joint capsular attachments.

5. **Laboratory findings**
   a. **Rheumatoid factors** (i.e., a heterogeneous group of antibodies produced in most patients with RA) are detectable through various serological techniques and are present in about 80% of patients. The most commonly found rheumatoid factors are **immunoglobulin G (IgG)** and **immunoglobulin M (IgM).** Patients with RA who are seropositive for rheumatoid factors generally follow a more serious disease course than those who are seronegative.
   b. **Erythrocyte sedimentation rate** may be increased, reflecting the inflammatory response.
   c. **Normochromic, normocytic anemia** may be found (anemia of chronic disease).
   d. **Antinuclear antibody test** is positive in 15% of patients, usually in low titer.

I. Treatment objectives

1. To provide pain relief
2. To reduce or suppress inflammation
3. To avoid, minimize, or eliminate adverse effects resulting from therapy
4. To preserve or restore joint function
5. To maintain the patient's lifestyle

J. Monitoring parameters. Selected parameters are used to assess disease activity and drug response to RA. These parameters may include:

1. Duration of morning stiffness
2. Number of painful and tender joints
3. Number of swollen joints
4. Range of joint motion
5. PIP joint circumference
6. Time to onset of fatigue
7. Time to walk 50 feet
8. Erythrocyte sedimentation rate

II. THERAPY.

II. THERAPY. The treatment of RA combines two approaches: mechanical and pharmacologic. Mechanical therapy includes a balanced program of rest and exercise. The pharmacologic component now includes both symptomatic [aspirin and other nonsteroidal anti-inflammatory drugs (NSAIDs)] and disease-modifying therapy (second-line drugs) that usually require a combination of agents.

A. Mechanical therapy. The patient is educated in a balanced daily program of exercise and rest.

1. Initially, the joints are rested.
2. Exercises are then introduced to strengthen muscles and increase the range of motion without undue joint strain.
3. Alignment of the joints in a position of function is ensured during sleep through use of specially designed lightweight splints.
4. Complete immobilization is avoided.
5. When preventive measures fail, surgery to improve function of the hands and knees is sometimes beneficial.

B. Symptomatic pharmacologic therapy. The choice of **aspirin** or **aspirin-like agents** is usually empirical because patients' responses vary widely. Further decisions on the drug regimen should be based on the therapeutic effect after 2–3 weeks. However, an inadequate response to one drug in this group may not reflect a patient's response to another. Furthermore, adverse effects or toxicity may override an adequate therapeutic response.

1. **Aspirin** is the first-line agent, administered initially as an analgesic, then in higher doses as an anti-inflammatory agent. Aspirin is as effective as any other NSAID and is much less expensive.
   a. **Mechanism of action.** In common with other NSAIDs, aspirin appears to work, at least in part, by inhibiting prostaglandin synthesis and release.
   b. **Dosage.** The usual total dose is 3.6–5.4 g daily.
   c. **Precautions and monitoring effects**
      (1) Aspirin interferes with platelet function and can cause serious bleeding; this effect may persist for 4–7 days after the drug has been discontinued.
      (2) Tinnitus and, rarely, hepatitis or renal damage can occur with high-dose aspirin therapy.
      (3) The intolerable GI effects experienced by some patients may be avoided by using an enteric-coated agent.
2. **Other NSAIDs** (e.g., ibuprofen, naproxen, sulindac, piroxicam) [Table 49-1]. Many patients tolerate effective doses of the NSAIDs better than high-dose aspirin therapy. However, the newer drugs are much more expensive. No clinical evidence has proven that any one of these drugs is consistently more effective than another, but research shows that a patient who does not respond to one NSAID may respond to another. By trial and error, patients may need to try three or four of these agents. Generally, a 2- to 3-week trial of an adequate dose is required to identify treatment success or failure.

Table 49-1. Nonsteroidal Anti-inflammatory Drugs

Propionic acids	**Brand name**	**Half-life**	**Maximum dose**
Fenoprofen	Nalfon	2–3 hrs	3200 mg
Flurbiprofen	Ansaid	5.7 hrs	300 mg
Ibuprofen	Motrin	1.8–2.5 hrs	3200 mg
Ketoprofen	Orudis	2–4 hrs	300 mg
Naproxen	Naprosyn	12–15 hrs	1500 mg
Oxaprozin	Daypro	42–50 hrs	1800 mg
Acetic acids			
Diclofenac	Voltaren	1–2 hrs	200 mg
Etodolac	Lodine	7.3 hrs	1200 mg
Indomethacin	Indocin	4.5 hrs	200 mg
Ketorolac	Toradol	2.4–8.6 hrs	PO 40 mg
Nabumetone	Relafen	22.5–30 hrs	2000 mg
Sulindac	Clinoril	7.8 hrs	400 mg
Tolmetin	Tolectin	1–1.5 hrs	2000 mg
Anthranilic acids			
Meclofenamate	Meclomen	2 hrs	400 mg
Mefenamic acid	Ponstel	2–4 hrs	1000 mg
Oxicams			
Piroxicam	Feldene	30–86 hrs	20 mg

a. **Mechanism of action** (see II B I a)

b. **Precautions and monitoring effects.** The NSAIDs differ somewhat in adverse effects and it is not clear whether an equally effective dose of any NSAID is demonstrably safer in all patients. See (8) below for selected points of concern for specific NSAIDS.

(1) NSAIDs should be avoided in asthmatic patients who are sensitive to aspirin because they may trigger bronchospasm and respiratory failure.

(2) All NSAIDs interfere with platelet function and prolong bleeding time. However, unlike the effect with aspirin, this effect is quickly reversible with discontinuation of the drug.

(3) All NSAIDs produce GI effects, including peptic ulceration. The combined effect of GI irritation and platelet interference can yield severe gastric hemorrhage.

(a) **Misoprostol** (Cytotec) is currently the only agent proven effective in preventing gastric and duodenal ulcers in chronic NSAID users. H_2-receptor antagonists appear to decrease the incidence of duodenal lesions, but they have failed to significantly prevent gastric ulcers. Sucralfate and antacids are of unproven benefit as well.

(b) Misoprostol is given in a dose of 100–200 μg four times daily. The 100-μg dose is slightly less effective, but less diarrhea occurs. Patients at particularly high risk for NSAID-induced ulceration (i.e., female patients older than 60 years of age) may benefit from administration of this agent.

(4) Renal blood flow is decreased somewhat by these agents, and renal failure may ensue in some patients. The potential for renal damage increases when NSAIDs are used in patients at risk for decreased intravascular volume, as occurs in such conditions as congestive heart failure (CHF) and diuretic use. (This risk may be lower with sulindac.)

(5) Mild hepatic dysfunction and, rarely, severe hepatitis may occur.

(6) All NSAIDs can cause adverse central nervous system (CNS) effects such as drowsiness, dizziness, anxiety, tinnitus, and confusion initially, but these symptoms usually disappear with continued use. CNS effects, including severe headache, occur more frequently with indomethacin (especially in high doses).

(7) Rarely, these agents may cause blood dyscrasias.

(8) Specific NSAID information

(a) There is some evidence that **ibuprofen** (e.g., Motrin) and **naproxen** (Naprosyn) have a lower risk of serious GI complications than other NSAIDs.

(b) **Nabumetone** (Relafen) may cause less gastric irritation than other NSAIDs.

(c) **Meclofenamate** (Meclomen) may cause a high incidence of diarrhea, which may sometimes be severe.

(d) **Piroxicam** (Feldene), which has a longer half-life, may cause a higher incidence of GI bleeding than other NSAIDs and probably should be avoided in elderly patients.

(e) **Indomethacin** (Indocin) may cause more severe CNS adverse effects than other NSAIDs including severe headache at higher doses.

3. **Nonacetylated salicylates** (e.g., choline salicylate, salsalate) are safer for aspirin-sensitive patients. They do not usually trigger the respiratory effects produced by aspirin and other NSAIDs [see II B 2 b (1)]. Nonacetylated salicylates have less effect on platelet function than aspirin and other NSAIDs, but they may also have fewer anti-inflammatory effects.

C. **Second-line agents.** These are also referred to as **slow-acting antirheumatic drugs** (SAARDs) and **disease-modifying antirheumatic drugs** (DMARDs). Patients with sustained disabling arthritis may require more than an anti-inflammatory agent. Altering the course of the disease is attempted initially through the use of hydroxychloroquine, methotrexate, gold compounds, penicillamine, and sulfasalazine.

1. **General considerations**

a. Although the precise mechanism of action in RA remains undetermined, these agents attempt to modulate the immune response. Progression of erosion may be delayed or prevented in some patients. Alteration of disease progression evolves slowly and gradually, and therapeutic effect—if it occurs—may not be evident for months, with the exception of methotrexate (i.e., gold, penicillamine, and hydroxychloroquine may require 3 or more months before a therapeutic benefit develops).

b. Generally, the agents in this group are tried one at a time in combination with an NSAID. However, many clinicians now advocate using combinations of these agents. If a drug proves ineffective, it is discontinued before another is introduced. No consensus has been formed as to which agent should be tried first; often hydroxychloroquine is used for mild RA and methotrexate if the disease is more severe.

c. All of these agents exhibit potentially severe adverse reactions and, therefore, require careful monitoring of patients.

d. Some clinicians now begin the second-line drugs early (some at the time of diagnosis) in the course of the disease because prolonged prior use of NSAIDs often has not prevented deformity and joint destruction.

2. **Hydroxychloroquine (Plaquenil)**

a. **Administration and dosage.** Hydroxychloroquine should be given in dosages of 400 mg daily (200 mg twice a day maximum) or 6.5 mg/kg daily, whichever is less. It may be reduced to 200 mg daily.

b. **Precautions and monitoring effects**

(1) Nausea and epigastric pain can occur, but serious adverse effects are rare.

(2) Hydroxychloroquine can cause severe and sometimes irreversible adverse effects on the eyes, skin, CNS, and bone marrow, but these are rare with recommended doses.

(3) An ophthalmologist should check for loss of visual acuity every 3–6 months. Toxicity can generally be avoided if the drug is discontinued promptly at the first signs of retinal toxicity.

(4) This retinopathy, the most common side effect of hydroxychloroquine, results from deposition of the drug in a melanin layer of the cones. Symptoms include blurred vision, scotomata, and halos, and early damage may occur without warning. Mild defects in accommodation and convergence or corneal deposits are common and reversible.

3. **Methotrexate (Rheumatrex).** This drug is a folic acid antagonist that has been used as an antineoplastic agent. Some rheumatologists now consider it a first-line drug for RA.

a. **Administration and dosage.** Initially, the weekly regimen should consist of 5–10 mg. (Taking divided doses at 12-hour intervals is not more effective or safer than a single weekly dose.) This can be increased slowly—at 3- to 6-week intervals—to 15–20 mg a week. For patients who experience GI effects or for those who lose benefit over time with **oral** methotrexate, giving the same dose **IM** once weekly may be helpful.

b. **Precautions and monitoring effects**

(1) Aspirin (and possibly other NSAIDs) may increase the toxicity of methotrexate by slowing its rate of excretion.

(2) Adverse effects associated with methotrexate include GI effects (e.g., anorexia, nausea, vomiting, abdominal cramps, GI ulceration, bleeding), bone marrow suppression, hepatic toxicity, and hypersensitivity pneumonitis. Because it is immunosuppressive, infections such as herpes zoster and *Pneumocystis carinii* have been reported to be more common in patients taking it for RA. Because the drug is used in lower doses than those for chemotherapy, the serious side effects are not usually seen.

(3) Monitoring should include baseline and follow-up complete blood counts (CBCs), platelet counts, and monthly renal and liver function profiles.

4. Gold compounds. These may be administered in oral or intramuscular (IM) form. Gold has been used for several years and may be effective in delaying or preventing progression of joint erosion in some patients. Some clinicians have questioned their effectiveness, but one meta-analysis placed them among the more effective second-line drugs.

a. IM agents [e.g., **gold sodium thiomalate** (Myochrysine) and aurothioglucose (Solganal)]. These agents are considered equally effective.

(1) **Administration and dosage.** Initially, a test dose of 10 mg is administered, followed by 25 mg once a week for 2 weeks, and then 50 mg in weekly intervals for up to 20 weeks. Once there is a therapeutic effect, treatment intervals are lengthened to every 2 weeks, then every 3 weeks, and finally to regular monthly administration. Patients who respond (response usually occurs within 3 to 6 months after starting treatment) should remain at least on monthly therapy; if therapy is discontinued, arthritic symptoms may recur and may not be controlled when gold is restarted.

(2) **Precautions and monitoring effects**

(a) The **most common side effects** are proteinuria and rash.

(i) Some clinicians obtain a CBC and urinalysis before each injection or every other injection to detect drug-related decreases in blood counts or the presence of proteinuria.

(ii) Pruritus usually precedes stomatitis and a diffuse rash, which can progress to generalized exfoliation; therefore, the drug should be discontinued when pruritus occurs. Lower-dose therapy may be tried later if pruritus does occur.

(b) Leukopenia, thrombocytopenia, and aplastic anemia have been reported.

(c) Anaphylaxis, angioneurotic edema, glossitis, and interstitial pneumonitis can also occur.

(d) Aurothioglucose (fat-soluble) may be safer than gold sodium thiomalate (water-soluble), which is more likely to cause vasodilation and nitritoid reactions. These reactions are rare and usually mild, but hypotension, syncope, and myocardial infarction have been reported.

b. Oral agents. Auranofin (Ridaura) may be slightly less toxic, but slightly less effective, than other forms of gold.

(1) **Administration and dosage.** The initial regimen for auranofin consists of 3 mg twice a day or 6 mg once a day for 6 months. If there is no response, the dosage is increased to 3 mg three times daily (9 mg daily). If there is still no response after 3 more months, auranofin should be discontinued.

(2) **Precautions and monitoring effects.** Common, reversible side effects include diarrhea, abdominal pain, rash, stomatitis, and proteinuria. Oral gold causes less mucocutaneous, bone marrow, and renal toxicity than injectable gold but more diarrhea and other GI reactions.

5. Sulfasalazine (Azulfidine). Although it is not approved for RA by the United States Food and Drug Administration (FDA), it has become increasingly more popular as a treatment for RA.

a. Indications

(1) A meta-analysis of short-term clinical trials found sulfasalazine to be among the most effective second-line drugs.

(2) Sulfasalazine may slow the progress of joint damage.

b. Administration and dosage. The usual starting close of sulfasalazine is 0.5 g twice daily, increased in increments of 0.5 g weekly to a maintenance dose of 2–3 g daily taken in two or three divided doses.

c. Precautions and monitoring effects. Common side effects include GI disturbances and rash. Serious reactions such as blood dyscrasias and hepatitis are rare, but monitoring liver function tests and CBCs is recommended every 2–3 weeks during the first 3 months of treatment and less frequently thereafter.

6. **Penicillamine (Depen).** The effectiveness of this agent as an anti-inflammatory may result from its effect on the altered immune response. It can be effective in patients with refractory RA and may delay progression of erosions.
   a. **Administration and dosage.** Penicillamine should be given on an empty stomach because food decreases absorption. Initially, 125–250 mg should be administered once daily. Then the dosage should be increased (by the same amount) at 1- to 3-month intervals until an effective daily dose has been achieved (usually, 750 mg daily; rarely, 1000–1500 mg daily). The dosing motto for this drug is "go low—go slow."
   b. **Precautions and monitoring effects.** Penicillamine has a high incidence of toxic effects, which limits its usefulness.
      (1) Adverse effects (usually reversible) include rash, fever, hematuria, proteinuria, dysgeusia, and aphthous ulcers.
      (2) Of more serious consequence are potential hematologic effects such as leukopenia, thrombocytopenia, and aplastic anemia.
      (3) Autoimmune conditions such as systemic lupus erythematosus (SLE), Goodpasture's syndrome, and pemphigus have occurred.

7. **Azathioprine (Imuran).** This drug is a purine analogue immunosuppressive drug. It is generally used after other agents have failed (for refractory RA).
   a. **Administration and dosage.** Initially, 50–100 mg (about 1 mg/kg) should be given once or twice daily. After 6–8 weeks and then every 4 weeks, the doses can be increased by 0.5 mg/kg daily up to a maximum of 2.5 mg/kg daily. A maintenance regimen should use the lowest effective dose. The dosage should be reduced in patients with renal dysfunction.
   b. **Precautions and monitoring effects**
      (1) Adverse effects include nausea, vomiting, abdominal pain, hepatitis, and reversible bone marrow depression.
      (2) Severe toxicity is uncommon with the dosage used for RA, but an increased risk of lymphoma has been reported.
      (3) A CBC and liver function profile should be obtained every 2–4 weeks as the dosage is increased.

8. **Cyclophosphamicle (Cytoxan).** This drug has been used primarily as an antineoplastic agent but may be used in refractory RA. However, cyclophosphamide is significantly more toxic than other immunosuppressive agents.
   a. **Administration and dosage.** The usual initial dose is 1.5–3.0 mg/kg daily.
   b. **Precautions and monitoring effects.** Serious toxic effects include bone marrow depression, hemorrhagic cystitis, sterility, alopecia, and malignant diseases (e.g., bladder cancer).

9. **Chlorambucil and cyclosporine.** These are relatively toxic but may play a role in treating refractory RA. **Minocycline** may have a potential role in RA therapy via its effects against the *Mycoplasma* organism, which might be an etiologic factor in the genesis of RA.

D. Corticosteroids

1. **General considerations.** In severe, progressive RA, **prednisone** may afford some degree of control, but corticosteroids are usually recognized as agents of last resort. They occasionally may be used:
   a. For acute flare-ups of the disease
   b. During the interim before the therapeutic effects of slow-acting drugs are observed
   c. In elderly patients as alternatives to the risks of second-line agents
   d. In patients who cannot tolerate NSAIDs
   e. For patients with significant systemic manifestations of RA

2. **Administration and dosage**
   a. Oral **prednisone** in a dose of 5–10 mg daily may benefit some patients. Because adverse effects are related to dose and duration, an effort must be made to keep the dose as low as possible.
   b. If painful symptoms are restricted to one or a few acutely inflamed joints, intra-articular injections may provide relief.

3. **Precautions and monitoring effects.** Long-term administration may produce GI bleeding, poor wound healing, myopathy, cataracts, hyperglycemia, hypertension, and osteoporosis.

E. Topical therapy

1. Topical **capsaicin** (Zostrix) may be useful in the symptomatic treatment of RA. Capsaicin is the primary pungent ingredient of hot pepper. It is thought to work by depleting and preventing reaccumulation of substance P (believed to be the major chemical mediator in pain transmission from the periphery to the CNS) in peripheral sensory neurons. After topical application, capsaicin produces a sensation of warmth in the skin and many patients experience significant relief from joint pain. Patients must be counseled to apply the agent three or four times a day to experience full therapeutic benefit and that several weeks of treatment are necessary for a complete response.

2. **Counterirritants** (e.g., allyl isothiocyanate, methylsalicylate, menthol) produce a mild inflammatory reaction when applied to the skin. Their therapeutic benefit may be partially explained by the massaging action that accompanies drug application.

III. COMBINATION SECOND-LINE THERAPY

A. Over the past decade, conventional therapeutic approaches for RA have been challenged by the recognition of the need for early and more aggressive treatment. However, controversy exists concerning appropriate therapeutic approaches.

B. The toxicity of the NSAIDs and a greater awareness of the bleak prospects for many patients with RA have led to new therapeutic strategies. Combinations of second-line agents **(combination therapy)** are popular alternatives to sequential monotherapy, the rationale being that they may achieve greater efficacy without a corresponding increase in toxicity because each drug has different anti-inflammatory mechanisms. Theoretically, initiating second-line therapies earlier and using them in combination may improve patient outcomes beyond those obtained by more traditional methods. Early in the disease process, the response potential also may be greater. The use of "remission-inducing" agents, either alone or in combination, early in therapy is advocated based on the premise that the rate of joint damage is greatest in the first 2 years. These approaches include:

1. **Step-down bridge approach**
   - **a.** Prednisone is administered for 1 month. Patients who do not respond adequately then receive a combination of antimalarials, oral gold, parenteral gold, and methotrexate. Other second-line agents may be substituted. After 3 months of multiple-drug therapy, the dosages are tapered in the hope that the antimalarials alone will control the disease.
   - **b.** The step-down bridge approach attempts to control early inflammation before joint damage occurs, to shorten the duration of treatment with potentially toxic drugs, and to achieve a simpler and less expensive program than that provided by the conventional pyramid.

2. **Sawtooth strategy.** This approach advocates the use of second-line agents early in the course of RA and then the serial substitution of new agents throughout the disease course as the drugs that are being used lose their therapeutic benefit.

3. **Graduated-step paradigm.** Goals of this strategy include increasing objectivity of therapeutic decision-making throughout the course of disease treatment and exposing only those patients with sufficiently active disease to the risks of combination second-line therapy. Patients are reevaluated at 3 months and disease activity is scored quantitatively. If disease activity is high and therefore unresponsive, treatment is escalated.

STUDY QUESTIONS

Directions: Each of the numbered items or incomplete statements in this section is followed by answers or by completions of the statement. Select the **one** lettered answer or completion that is **best** in each case.

1. A 50-year-old woman is admitted to the hospital with a chief complaint of bilateral swelling of her knees for 3 days, early morning stiffness, and lethargy. She is not responding to 650 mg of aspirin three times daily. The patient is an obese white woman who states that her ability to move about has slowly regressed due to the stiffness and swelling. She has also noticed a progressive swelling of the hands and wrists. A diagnosis of rheumatoid arthritis is made. Initial suggestion for drug therapy of this patient is

(A) hydroxychloroquine, 200 mg daily
(B) steroid injections into all swollen joints
(C) aspirin, 975 mg four times a day
(D) penicillamine, 250 mg four times a day
(E) gold injections, 50 mg intravenously once weekly

2. Which of the following agents and dosage regimens is the best choice of treatment for a patient with rheumatoid arthritis who is considered sensitive to aspirin?

(A) Ibuprofen, 800 mg three times daily
(B) Acetaminophen, 650 mg every 4 hours
(C) Gold injections, 25 mg intramuscularly once a week
(D) Azathioprine, 75 mg daily
(E) Cyclophosphamide, 100 mg daily

3. Which of the following statements best describes the usual course of rheumatoid arthritis?

(A) It is an acute exacerbation of joint pain treated with short-term anti-inflammatory therapy
(B) It is a chronic disease characterized by acute changes within nonsynovial joints
(C) It is an acute disease that is characterized by rapid synovial changes due to inflammation
(D) It is a chronic disease characterized by acute exacerbations followed by remissions, with consequences associated with chronic inflammatory changes
(E) It is a joint disease characterized by a marked loss of calcium from the bones and a resultant thinning of the bones

Directions: Each group of items in this section consists of lettered options followed by a set of numbered items. For each item, select the **one** lettered option that is most closely associated with it. Each lettered option may be selected once, more than once, or not at all.

Questions 4–8

Match the drug characteristic with the appropriate agent.

(A) Corticosteroids
(B) Ibuprofen
(C) Aspirin
(D) Auranofin
(E) Penicillamine

4. Persistent platelet function effect

5. Oral form of gold

6. Given on an empty stomach

7. May be used intra-articularly

8. May cause drowsiness

Questions 9–13

Match the phrase below with the appropriate agent used to treat rheumatoid arthritis.

(A) Indomethacin
(B) Aspirin
(C) Hydroxychloroquine
(D) Methotrexate
(E) Cyclophosphamide

9. May cause hemorrhagic cystitis

10. May cause more severe central nervous system (CNS) adverse effects than other nonsteroidal anti-inflammatory drugs (NSAIDs)

11. Enteric-coated form may be useful in treating some patients

12. Aspirin may slow this drug's rate of excretion

13. Vision should be monitored every 3–6 months

ANSWERS AND EXPLANATIONS

1. The answer is C *[II B 1].*
Unless there are contraindications to the use of salicylates, aspirin administered in anti-inflammatory doses is the agent of choice for initial treatment of the patient with rheumatoid arthritis. The patient in the question has been taking only analgesic doses of aspirin, that is, 650 mg three times a day (1950 mg daily). Parenteral gold preparations are given by intramuscular injection, not intravenously.

2. The answer is C *[II B 2 b (1), C 4 a (1)].*
Patients with nasal polyps, hay fever, or asthma have an increased incidence of aspirin hypersensitivity. In these patients, aspirin administration may result in rhinorrhea, bronchospasm, or anaphylaxis. Patients who are intolerant of aspirin may also show a cross-sensitivity to ibuprofen and other nonsteroidal anti-inflammatory drugs (NSAIDs). Acetaminophen may provide some analgesic effect but has essentially no anti-inflammatory properties and, therefore, would not be a good choice for a patient with rheumatoid arthritis. If available, a nonacetylated salicylate may be given. Many rheumatologists use gold injections (10 mg as a test dose and 25–50 mg at weekly intervals) as the next most appropriate agent. Azathioprine and cyclophosphamide usually are reserved for later therapy.

3. The answer is D *[I A, G].*
Rheumatoid arthritis is a chronic disease that most often follows a sporadic course of acute exacerbations of synovial inflammation followed by remissions, with eventual joint manifestations of chronic inflammation (see Figure 49-1).

4–8. The answers are: 4-C *[II B 1 c (1)],* **5-D** *[II C 4 b],* **6-E** *[II C 6],* **7-A** *[II D 2 b],* **8-B** *[II B 2 b (6)].*
Both aspirin and other nonsteroidal anti-inflammatory drugs (NSAIDs) interfere with platelet function; with aspirin, the effect may persist for 4–7 days after the drug has been discontinued, whereas platelet function usually returns quickly to normal after stopping other NSAID therapy. Most gold preparations are given by intramuscular injection, but auranofin is given orally. Penicillamine is given on an empty stomach because food decreases its absorption. Intra-articular injection of a corticosteroid is helpful when painful symptoms are restricted to one or a few joints. Ibuprofen, like other NSAIDs, may cause drowsiness and other central nervous system effects, but these usually subside with continued use.

9–13. The answers are: 9-E *[II C 8 b],* **10-A** *[II B 2 b (8) (e)],* **11-B** *[II B 1 c (3)],* **12-D** *[II C 3 b (1)],* **13-C** *[II C 2].*
Cyclophosphamide is significantly more toxic than other immunosuppressive agents; one of its serious side effects is hemorrhagic cystitis. Indomethacin does indeed cause more central nervous system (CNS) adverse effects. There are many other less toxic nonsteroidal anti-inflammatory drugs (NSAIDs) that can be used. Many patients taking high doses of aspirin cannot tolerate regular aspirin but can take the enteric-coated form. Aspirin administration may slow the excretion of methotrexate; this can increase the latter drug's toxicity. Because hydroxychloroquine can cause ophthalmic adverse effects, patients receiving this drug should have their vision checked at least every 6 months.

50
Hyperuricemia and Gout

Larry N. Swanson

I. INTRODUCTION

A. Definitions

1. **Hyperuricemia** refers to a serum uric acid level that is elevated more than two standard deviations above the population mean. In most laboratories, the upper limit of normal is 7 mg/dl (uricase methods). However, the level varies with the laboratory method used; the upper limit of normal is about 1 mg/dl lower for women than for men.

2. **Gout** is a disease that is characterized by recurrent acute attacks of urate crystal-induced arthritis. It may include **tophi**—deposits of monosodium urate—in and around the joints and cartilage and in the kidneys, as well as uric acid nephrolithiasis.

B. Incidence

1. Gout affects approximately 0.2%–1.5% of the population in the United States.

2. Most gout victims are men (approximately 95% of cases); most women with the disease are postmenopausal.

3. The mean age at disease onset is 47 years.

4. The risk of developing gout increases as the serum uric acid level rises. Virtually all gout patients have a serum uric acid level above 7 mg/dl.

5. Research shows that among patients with a serum uric acid level above 9 mg/dl, the cumulative incidence of gout reached 22% after 5 years.

6. Gout has a familial tendency; 10%–60% of cases occur in family members of patients with the disease.

7. Obesity, heavy alcohol consumption, and certain other lifestyle factors increase the chances of developing gout.

C. Uric acid production and excretion

1. Uric acid, an end product of **purine metabolism,** is produced from both dietary and endogenous sources. Its formation results from the conversion of adenine and guanine moieties of nucleoproteins and nucleotides (Figure 50-1).

2. **Xanthine oxidase** catalyzes the reaction that occurs as the final step in the degradation of purines to uric acid.

3. The body ultimately excretes uric acid via the kidneys (300–600 mg/day; two-thirds of total uric acid) and via the gastrointestinal (GI) tract (100–300 mg/day; one-third of the total uric acid).

4. Uric acid has no known biologic function.

5. The body has a total uric acid content of 1.0–1.2 g; the daily turnover rate is approximately 600–800 mg.

6. At a pH of 4.0–5.0 (i.e., in urine), uric acid exists as a poorly soluble free acid; at physiologic pH, it exists primarily as **monosodium urate salt.**

7. Uric acid filtration, reabsorption, and secretion sites are shown in Figure 50-2.

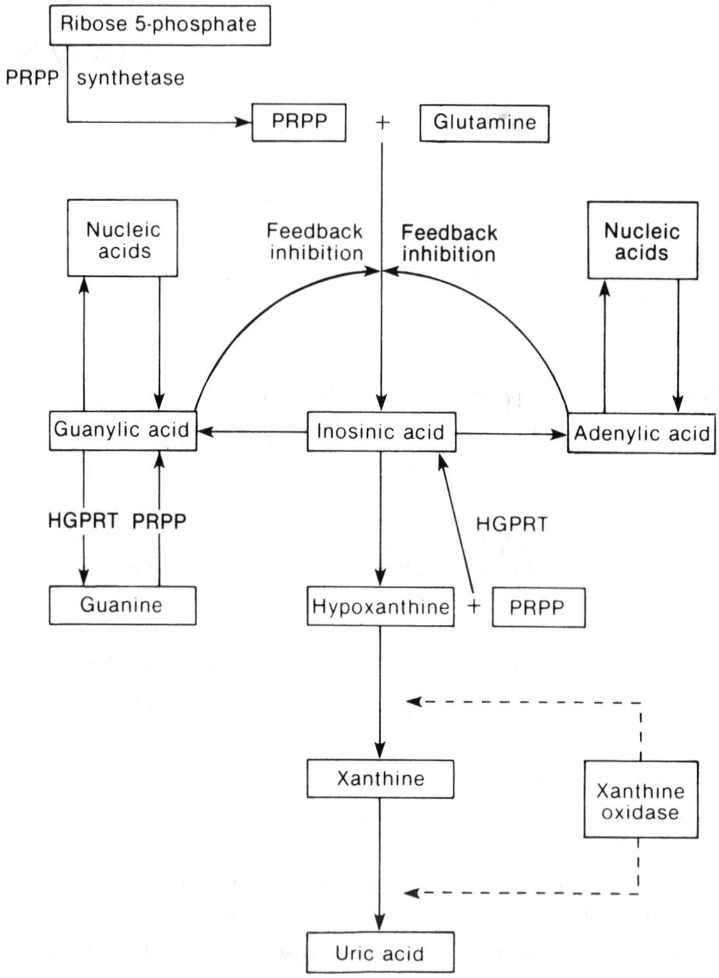

Figure 50-1. Uric acid formation. *PRPP* = phosphoribosyl-1-pyrophosphate; *HGPRT* = hypoxanthine–guanine phosphoribosyltransferase. (Redrawn with permission from DiPiro J, Talbert R, Hayes P, et al: *Pharmacotherapy—A Pathophysiologic Approach.* East Norwalk, CT, Appleton & Lange, 1993, p 1344.)

D. Etiology. Hyperuricemia and gout may be primary or secondary.

1. **Primary hyperuricemia** and **gout** apparently result from an innate **defect in purine metabolism** or **uric acid excretion.** The exact cause of the defect usually is unknown.
   - a. Hyperuricemia may result from **uric acid overproduction, impaired renal clearance of uric acid,** or a **combination** of these.
   - b. Some patients with primary hyperuricemia and gout have a known enzymatic defect, such as hypoxanthine-guanine phosphoribosyltransferase (HGPRT) deficiency or phosphoribosyl-1-pyrophosphate (PRPP) synthetase excess (see Figure 50-1).
   - c. Principally for therapeutic purposes, patients with primary hyperuricemia and gout can be classified as **overproducers** or **underexcretors** of uric acid.
     - (1) **Overproducers** (about 10% of patients) synthesize abnormally large amounts of uric acid and excrete excessive amounts—more than 800–1000 mg daily on an unrestricted diet or more than 600 mg daily on a purine-restricted diet. These individuals generally have a markedly increased miscible urate pool (greater than 2.5 g).
     - (2) **Underexcretors** (about 90% of patients) generally produce normal or nearly normal amounts of uric acid but excrete less than 600 mg daily on a purine-restricted diet. They generally have only a slightly increased miscible urate pool. Some underexcretors also are overproducers.

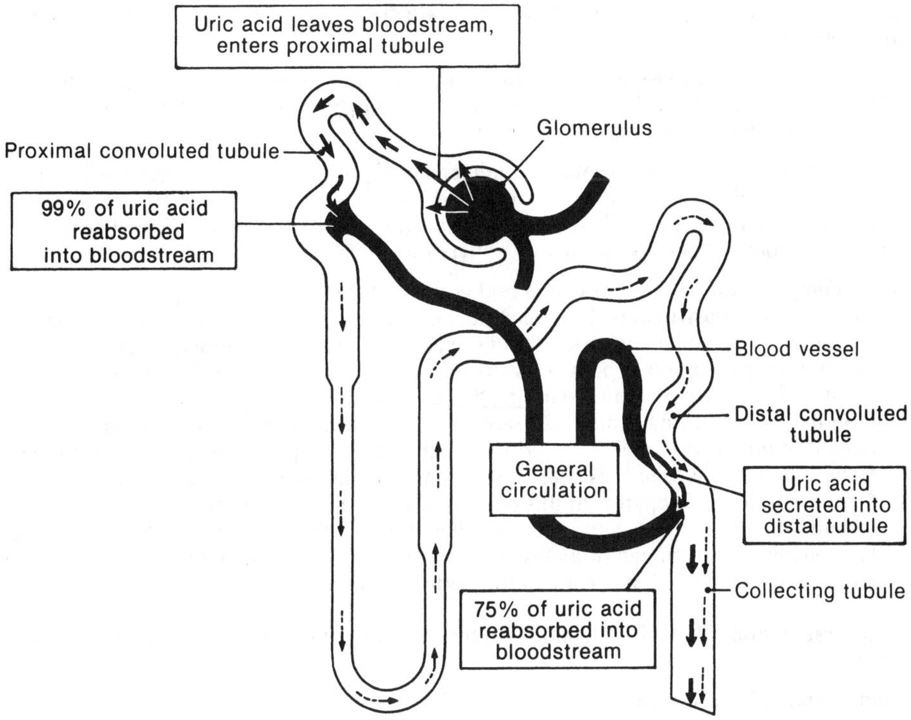

Figure 50-2. Uric acid filtration, reabsorption, and secretion sites. At the glomerulus, uric acid is filtered and enters the proximal tubule. Here, approximately 99% of uric acid is reabsorbed into the bloodstream. At the distal tubule, uric acid is secreted; subsequently, about 75% of the amount secreted is reabsorbed. Therefore, almost all urinary uric acid is excreted at the distal tubule.

2. **Secondary hyperuricemia** and **gout** develop during the course of another disease or as a result of drug therapy.
   a. **Hematologic causes** of hyperuricemia and gout (associated with increased nucleic acid turnover and breakdown to uric acid)
      (1) Lymphoproliferative disorders
      (2) Myeloproliferative disorders
      (3) Certain hemolytic anemias and hemoglobinopathies
   b. **Chronic renal failure.** In this condition, reduced renal clearance of uric acid can lead to hyperuricemia.
   c. **Drug-induced disease**
      (1) **Aspirin** and **other salicylates** inhibit tubular secretion of uric acid when given in low doses (e.g., less than 2 g/day of aspirin). At high doses, these substances frequently cause uricosuria.
      (2) **Cytotoxic drugs** increase uric acid concentrations by enhancing nucleic acid turnover and excretion.
      (3) **Diuretics** (except spironolactone) may cause hyperuricemia; most likely, this occurs either via volume depletion, which, in turn, increases proximal tubular reabsorption, or via impaired tubular secretion of uric acid.
      (4) **Ethambutol** and **nicotinic acid** increase uric acid concentrations by competing with urate for tubular secretion sites, thereby decreasing uric acid excretion.
      (5) **Cyclosporine** decreases renal urate clearance.
      (6) **Alcohol** alters uric acid metabolism both by **increasing uric acid production** through an increase in adenine nucleotide catabolism and by **suppressing renal uric acid excretion** as a result of lactate inhibition of renal tubular uric acid secretion.
   d. **Miscellaneous disorders.** Diabetic ketoacidosis, psoriasis, and chronic lead poisoning are examples of conditions that may cause hyperuricemia.

E. Pathophysiology

1. Gouty arthritis develops when **monosodium urate crystals** are deposited in the synovium of involved joints.

2. An **inflammatory response** to monosodium urate crystals leads to an attack of acute gouty arthritis; painful joint swelling is characterized by redness, warmth, and tenderness. A systemic reaction may accompany joint symptoms.

3. If gout progresses untreated, **tophi,** or **tophaceous deposits** (deposits of monosodium urate crystals) eventually lead to joint deformity and disability; kidney involvement may lead to renal impairment. However, these developments are uncommon in the general gout population and represent late complications of hyperuricemia.

4. **Renal complications** of hyperuricemia and gout can have serious consequences.
   a. **Acute tubular obstruction.** This complication may develop secondary to uric acid precipitation in the collecting tubules and ureters, with subsequent blockage and renal failure. It is most common in patients with gout secondary to myeloproliferative or lymphoproliferative disorders—particularly after chemotherapy.
   b. **Urolithiasis.** Occurring in about 20% of gout patients, urolithiasis is characterized by formation of uric acid stones in the urinary tract. Low urine pH seems to be a contributing factor. The risk of urolithiasis rises as serum and urinary uric acid levels increase.
   c. **Chronic urate nephropathy.** In this complication, urate deposits arise in the renal interstitium. Most clinicians agree, however, that chronic hyperuricemia rarely, if ever, leads to clinically significant nephropathy. The presence of concomitant disease (e.g., diabetes mellitus, hypertension) may explain the finding of nephropathy in gout patients.

F. **Clinical presentation.** Clinical evaluation and the need for intervention depend on the clinical presentation.

1. **Asymptomatic hyperuricemia**

2. **Acute gouty arthritis**

3. **Intercritical gout**

4. **Chronic tophaceous gout**

II. ASYMPTOMATIC HYPERURICEMIA is characterized by an elevated serum uric acid level but has no signs or symptoms of deposition disease (arthritis, tophi, or urolithiasis).

A. **Clinical presentation.** No definitive evidence indicates that asymptomatic hyperuricemia is harmful. Clinicians cannot predict which asymptomatic patients will develop gout symptoms or hyperuricemia-related complications. However, the risk of symptom development and complications increases as the serum uric acid level rises.

B. **Therapy.** Asymptomatic hyperuricemia does not have any adverse effects before the development of gout. Therefore, **drug treatment is not required,** although it is prudent to determine the causes of the hyperuricemia and correct them, if possible. **Supportive interventions** may include maintenance of adequate urine output (to prevent uric acid stone formation), avoidance of high purine foods, and regular medical appointments to monitor the serum uric acid level and check for clinical evidence of deposition disease.

III. ACUTE GOUTY ARTHRITIS. This clinical presentation of gout is characterized by **painful arthritic attacks** of sudden onset.

A. **Pathogenesis.** Monosodium urate crystals form in articular tissues; this process sets off an inflammatory reaction. Trauma, exposure to cold, or another triggering event may be involved in the development of the acute attack.

B. **Signs and symptoms**

1. The **initial attack** is abrupt, usually occurring at night or in the early morning as synovial fluid is reabsorbed. This severe arthritic pain progressively worsens and generally involves only one or a few joints.

a. The **affected joints** typically become hot, swollen, and extremely tender. Seventeenth-century British physician Thomas Sydenham described his personal experience with gout this way: "Now it is a violent stretching and tearing of the ligaments—now, it is a gnawing pain and now a pressure and tightening. So exquisite and lively . . . is the feeling of the part affected, that it cannot bear the weight of bedclothes nor the jar of a person walking in the room."

b. The **most common site** of the initial attack is the first metatarsophalangeal joint; an attack there is known as **podagra.** Other sites that may be affected include the instep, ankle, heel, knee, wrist, elbow, and fingers.

2. The first few untreated attacks typically last 3–14 days. Later attacks may affect more joints and take several weeks to resolve.

3. During recovery, as edema subsides, local desquamation and pruritus may occur.

4. **Systemic symptoms** during an acute attack may include fever, chills, and malaise.

C. Diagnostic criteria

1. **Definitive diagnosis** of gouty arthritis can be made by demonstration of **monosodium urate crystals** in the synovial fluid of affected joints. These needle-shaped crystals are termed negatively birefringent when viewed through a polarized light microscope.

2. **Serum analysis** usually reveals an above-normal uric acid level: however, this finding is not specific for acute gout. Other **common serum findings** include leukocytosis and a moderately elevated erythrocyte sedimentation rate.

3. A **dramatic therapeutic response to colchicine** may be helpful in establishing the diagnosis, but this is not absolute because other causes of acute arthritis may respond as well.

4. When fluid cannot be aspirated from the affected joint, a **diagnosis of gout is supported by:**
   a. A prior history of **acute monarticular arthritis** (especially of the big toe) followed by a **symptom-free period**
   b. The presence of **hyperuricemia**
   c. Rapid **resolution of symptoms after colchicine** therapy

5. **Other conditions** that may **mimic** gout may include pseudogout (calcium pyrophosphate dihydrate crystal disease) or septic arthritis.

D. Treatment goals

1. To relieve pain and inflammation

2. To terminate the acute attack

3. To restore normal function to the affected joints

E. Therapy

1. **General therapeutic principles**
   a. The affected joint (or joints) should be immobilized.
   b. Anti-inflammatory drug therapy should begin immediately. For maximal therapeutic effectiveness, these drugs should be kept on hand so that the patient may begin therapy as soon as a subsequent attack begins.
   c. Urate-lowering drugs should not be given until the acute attack is controlled, as these drugs may prolong the attack by causing a change in uric acid equilibrium.

2. **Specific drugs.** Any of the following agents may be used:
   a. **Colchicine.** The traditional drug of choice for relieving pain and inflammation and ending the acute attack, colchicine is most effective when initiated 12–36 hours after symptoms begin (the period of maximal leukocyte migration).
      (1) **Mechanism of action.** Colchicine apparently **impairs leukocyte migration** to inflamed areas and disrupts urate deposition and the subsequent inflammatory response.
      (2) **Dosage and administration**
         (a) **Oral regimen**
            (i) The effective dose of colchicine in patients with acute gout is close to that which causes GI symptoms. The drug usually is administered orally in a

dose of 1 mg initially, followed by 0.5 mg every 2 hours until pain relief occurs or abdominal discomfort or diarrhea develops or a total dose of 8 mg has been administered. Except in patients who have renal or hepatic dysfunction or are elderly and frail, colchicine given in this way is safe, although it entails some discomfort for the patient.

(ii) Most patients have some pain relief by 18 hours and diarrhea by 24 hours; joint inflammation subsides gradually within 48 hours for 75%–80% of patients.

(iii) During **subsequent attacks,** patients may receive half of the total dose administered for the initial attack, then receive the remaining half as 0.5 mg every 1–2 hours.

(b) Intravenous (IV) regimen. This route is used rarely now but has advantages when NSAIDs are contraindicated or when patients cannot take oral medications.

(i) A single dose of 2 mg usually is given in 30 ml of normal saline solution and infused slowly over 5 minutes. Two additional doses of 1 mg each may be given at 6-hour intervals, but the total dose should never exceed 4 mg. The doses should be reduced by at least 50% in patients with hepatic or renal disease or in elderly patients. Because it causes tissue irritation, colchicine should **never be given intramuscularly or subcutaneously.**

(ii) IV administration may relieve acute gouty arthritis more rapidly than oral administration. However, severe toxicity may occur without warning because the early signs of toxicity (e.g., GI hypermobility) may not occur.

(3) Precautions and monitoring effects

(a) GI distress (e.g., nausea, abdominal cramps, diarrhea) occurs in up to 80% of patients receiving oral colchicine. This dosage form should be avoided in patients with peptic ulcer disease and other GI disorders.

(b) Local extravasation (causing local pain and necrosis) can occur with administration of IV colchicine. This risk can be reduced by use of a secure IV line.

(c) Colchicine therapy may cause bone marrow depression. This rare effect develops mainly in patients who receive excessive doses or who have underlying renal or hepatic disease. Excessively high acute doses (especially given intravenously) or long-term therapy may result in neurologic, renal, hepatic, or other toxicity.

b. Nonsteroidal anti-inflammatory drugs (NSAIDs)

(1) Indications. Some physicians consider these drugs the agents of choice, especially the newer NSAIDs. These drugs may be preferred when treatment is delayed significantly after symptom onset or when the patient cannot tolerate the adverse GI effects of colchicine.

(a) Indomethacin (Indocin) is usually given in a dose of 50 mg three times daily until pain is tolerable; then rapidly reduce the dose to complete cessation of the drug. Definite relief of pain usually occurs within 2–4 hours. Tenderness and heat usually subside in 24–36 hours, and swelling gradually disappears in 3–5 days. Do not use the sustained-release dosage form.

(b) Other NSAIDs, such as **naproxen** (Naprosyn) 750 mg followed by 250 mg every 8 hours until the attack subsides or **sulindac** (Clinoril) 200 mg twice a day to start and reducing dose with satisfactory response (7 days of therapy usually adequate), are specifically approved for this indication, but many other NSAIDs have been used successfully.

(2) Precautions and monitoring effects

(a) Adverse effects of indomethacin usually are dose-related. These effects occur in 10%–60% of patients and may warrant drug discontinuation. They primarily include GI complaints of nausea and abdominal discomfort and central nervous system (CNS) effects of headaches and dizziness. Indomethacin should be taken with food or milk to minimize gastric mucosal irritation.

(b) Precautions. NSAIDs, in general, require cautious use in patients with a history of hypertension, CHF, peptic ulcer disease, or mild-to-moderate renal failure.

c. Corticosteroids

(1) Intraarticular injections of a corticosteroid are usually very effective in patients with acute monarticular gout, and their use is becoming more widespread as experience with the diagnostic aspiration of joints increases. Aspiration alone can sometimes greatly reduce the pain of gout. The appropriate dose of corticosteroids is related to the size of the joint: an intraarticular dose of **methylprednisolone acetate** (e.g., Depo-Medrol) ranges from 5–10 mg (for a small joint) to 20–60 mg (for a large joint such as the knee), depending on the volume of the effusion.

(2) **Systemic corticosteroid therapy** is administered usually only when NSAIDs and colchicine have been ineffective or are contraindicated. There are reports of good responses, without a rebound effect, to **oral prednisone** (30–50 mg per day initially, with the dose tapered during a period of 7–10 days), **intramuscular corticotropin** (40 U) or **triamcinolone acetonide** (60 mg), or **IV methylprednisolone** (a daily dose of 50–150 mg administered during a 30-minute period, with the dose tapered over 5 days).

IV. INTERCRITICAL GOUT

IV. INTERCRITICAL GOUT is the symptom-free period after the first attack. This phase may be interrupted by the recurrence of acute attacks.

A. Onset of subsequent attacks varies. In most patients, the second attack occurs within 1 year of the first, but in some it may be delayed for 5–10 years. A small percentage of patients never experience a second attack. If hyperuricemia is insufficiently treated, subsequent attacks may become progressively longer and more severe and may involve more than one joint.

B. Treatment goals

1. To reduce the frequency and severity of recurrent attacks
2. To minimize urate deposition in body tissues, thereby preventing progression to chronic tophaceous gout

C. Therapy. Gout can be prevented by identifying and correcting the cause of hyperuricemia or by administering drugs that inhibit the synthesis of urate or increase its excretion.

1. **Nondrug urate-reducing measures.** Potentially reversible factors that contribute to increased urate production include a high-purine diet (e.g., all meats, including organ meats, seafood, beans, peas, asparagus), obesity, and regular alcohol consumption. The purine content of the diet does not usually contribute more than 1.0 mg/dl to the serum urate concentration, but moderation in dietary purine consumption should be considered. Weight reduction sometimes reduces the serum uric acid level slightly; however, "crash diets" should be avoided.

2. **Prophylaxis** after resolution of an acute gout attack may consist of **low-dose colchicine,** 0.5–1.5 mg daily. **Adverse effects** from colchicine at these doses are uncommon. **Low-dose NSAIDs** may also be used, but the incidence of side effects is typically higher than with low doses of colchicine.

3. **Urate-reducing drug therapy.** Gout may be prevented by reducing serum urate concentrations to values less than 6.0 mg/dl. A reduction to less than 5.0 mg/dl may be required for the resorption of tophi. The decision to begin drug therapy should be carefully considered, as urate-lowering drug treatment should be lifelong. Urate-reducing drugs include **uricosurics,** which increase renal uric acid excretion, and the xanthine oxidase inhibitor, **allopurinol,** which reduces uric acid production.

   a. Indications for therapy with a drug that lowers serum urate concentrations should be considered when **all** of the following criteria are met:

   (1) The cause of the hyperuricemia cannot be corrected or, if corrected, does not lower the serum urate concentration to less than 7.0 mg/dl.

   (2) The patient has had two or three definite attacks of gout or has tophi.

   (3) The patient is convinced of the need to take medication regularly and permanently.

   b. Specific drugs

   (1) Uricosurics include **probenecid** (Benemid) and **sulfinpyrazone** (Anturane). These drugs are preferred for underexcretors. Long-term uricosuric therapy reduces the incidence of gouty arthritis attacks, prevents formation of new tophi, and helps resolve existing tophi.

   (a) Mechanism of action. Probenecid and sulfinpyrazone block uric acid reabsorption at the proximal convoluted tubule, thereby increasing the rate of uric acid excretion (see Figure 50-2).

(b) **Indications.** Uricosurics generally are used to reduce hyperuricemia in patients who excrete less than 600 mg of uric acid per day.

(c) **Dosage and administration**

(i) **Probenecid** is given initially in two daily oral doses of 250 mg for 1 week, then increased to 500 mg twice daily every 1–2 weeks until the serum uric acid level drops below 6 mg/dl. Most patients respond to a dose of 1.5 g/day or less.

(ii) **Sulfinpyrazone** is given initially in two daily oral doses of 50 mg, then increased by 100 mg weekly. Most patients respond to a dose of 200 mg/day or less.

(d) **Precautions and monitoring effects**

(i) Uricosuric therapy should not be initiated during an acute gout attack. During the first 6–12 months of therapy, these drugs may increase the frequency, severity, and duration of acute attacks (by changing the equilibrium of body urate). Therefore, some clinicians administer prophylactic colchicine concomitantly during the early months of uricosuric therapy.

(ii) The **risk** is **minimized** by concurrently administering prophylactic drugs (see IV C 2), delaying urate-lowering therapy until several weeks after the last attack of gout, and starting therapy with a low dose of the drug that is chosen. When used concurrently with urate-lowering drugs, colchicine may be discontinued after the serum urate level becomes normal and is stable for 2 or 3 months.

(iii) Patients should maintain a **high fluid intake** (at least 2 L/day) and a high urine output during uricosuric therapy to decrease renal urate precipitation. The **greatest potential risks** of therapy with uricosuric drugs are the formation of **uric acid crystals** in urine and the deposition of **uric acid** in the **renal tubules, pelvis,** or **ureter,** causing renal colic or the deterioration of renal function. These risks can be reduced by initiating therapy with a low dose and increasing the dose slowly and by maintaining a high urine volume (preferably of alkaline urine, which can be achieved with 1 g of sodium bicarbonate taken 3–4 daily; plus a high fluid intake of at least 2 L/day), particularly during the early weeks of therapy.

(iv) Uricosurics are **contraindicated** in patients with urinary tract stones.

(v) These drugs generally are ineffective in patients with creatinine clearances below 50–60 ml/min.

(vi) **Aspirin** and **other salicylates** antagonize the action of uricosurics.

(vii) **Probenecid** is well tolerated by most patients, but it occasionally causes **adverse effects** [e.g., GI distress (8%), hypersensitivity reactions (5%)].

(viii) **Sulfinpyrazone** causes GI distress in 10%–15% of patients. Hypersensitivity reactions occur rarely. Sulfinpyrazone reduces platelet adhesiveness and may cause blood dyscrasias; periodic blood counts should be done.

(2) The only **xanthine oxidase inhibitor** available is **allopurinol.**

(a) **Mechanism of action.** Allopurinol and its long-acting metabolite, oxypurinol, block the final steps in uric acid synthesis by inhibiting xanthine oxidase, an enzyme that converts xanthine to uric acid. Thus the drug reduces the serum uric acid level while increasing the renal excretion of the more soluble oxypurine precursors; this decreases the risk of uric acid stones and nephropathy.

(b) **Indications.** Allopurinol is considered by many to be the drug of choice for lowering uric acid levels because of its effectiveness in both underexcretors and overproducers, but it is specifically the preferred urate-reducing agent for patients in the following categories:

(i) Patients who are clearly overproducers (overexcretors) of uric acid

(ii) Patients with recurrent tophaceous deposits or uric acid stones

(iii) Patients with renal impairment (but dose needs to be decreased)

(c) **Dosage and administration.** Allopurinol is given initially in a daily dose of 100–300 mg (preferably as a single dose), then increased in weekly increments if needed. Typically, the uric acid level starts to fall after 1–2 days with maximal effect for a given dose in 7–10 days. A dose of 300 mg/day reduces serum urate concentrations to normal values in 85% of patients with gout. A normal dose of 300 mg/day for a patient with normal renal function should be decreased to 200 mg/day for a patient with a CrCl of 60 ml/min and decreased to 100 mg/day for a patient with a CrCl of 30 ml/min.

(d) Precautions and monitoring effects. Allopurinol is generally well tolerated.

(i) A **rash** develops in approximately 2% of patients treated with allopurinol and in approximately 20% of those receiving both allopurinol and ampicillin. The rash usually subsides after the allopurinol has been discontinued and may not recur if therapy is resumed with a lower dose.

(ii) The most serious side effect of allopurinol, which occurs in less than 1 in 1000 cases, is **exfoliative dermatitis,** often with vasculitis, fever, liver dysfunction, eosinophilia, and acute interstitial nephritis. Up to 20% of patients with this type of reaction become very sick. It is more likely to occur in patients with renal disease or those receiving diuretic therapy. Prednisone seems to be effective in such patients, but the discontinuation of allopurinol and the use of supportive therapy may be sufficient in cases that are not severe.

(iii) Allopurinol may induce more frequent acute gout attacks. This risk can be minimized by administration of low doses and concurrent colchicine therapy.

V. CHRONIC TOPHACEOUS GOUT.

This rare clinical presentation may develop if hyperuricemia and gout remain untreated for many years.

A. Pathogenesis. Persistent hyperuricemia leads to the development of tophi in the synovia, olecranon bursae, and various periarticular locations. Eventually, articular cartilage may be destroyed, resulting in joint deformities, bone erosions, deposition of tophi within tissues, and renal disease.

B. Clinical evaluation

1. Patients may develop large subcutaneous tophi in the pinna of the external ear (the classic site) as well as in other locations.
2. Typically, the urate pool is many times the normal size.

C. Therapy. Allopurinol and probenecid may be given in combination to treat severe cases.

STUDY QUESTIONS

Directions: Each of the numbered items or incomplete statements in this section is followed by answers or by completions of the statement. Select the **one** lettered answer or completion that is **best** in each case.

1. All of the following statements concerning an acute gouty attack are correct EXCEPT

(A) the diagnosis of gout is assured by a good therapeutic response to colchicine because no other form of arthritis responds to this drug
(B) to be assured of the diagnosis, monosodium urate crystals must be identified in the synovial fluid of the affected joint
(C) attacks frequently occur in the middle of the night
(D) an untreated attack may last up to 2 weeks
(E) the first attack usually involves only one joint, most frequently the big toe (first metatarsophalangeal joint)

2. A 42-year-old obese man has been diagnosed with gout. He has had three acute attacks this year, and his uric acid level is presently 11.5 mg/dl (upper limit of normal is 7 mg/dl). He has no other diseases. Rational treatment of this patient during the interval period between gouty attacks might include any of the following EXCEPT

(A) acetaminophen or aspirin 650 mg as needed for joint pain
(B) probenecid
(C) colchicine
(D) allopurinol
(E) a decrease in caloric intake

3. A 45-year-old man is admitted to the hospital with the diagnosis of an acute attack of gout. His serum uric acid is 10.5 mg/dl (normal is 3–7 mg/dl). Which of the following would be the most effective initial treatment plan?

(A) Before treating this patient, immobilize the affected joint and obtain a 24-hour urinary uric acid level to determine which drug, either allopurinol or probenecid, would be the best agent to initiate therapy
(B) Begin oral colchicine 1 mg initially, followed by 0.5 mg every 2 hours until relief is obtained, gastrointestinal distress occurs, or a maximum of 8 mg has been taken; also, begin probenecid 250 mg twice a day concurrently
(C) Administer oral indomethacin 50 mg three times a day for 2 days; then gradually taper the dose over the next few days
(D) Administer oral naproxen 750 mg followed by 250 mg every 8 hours for 3 weeks
(E) Give colchicine 0.5 mg intramuscularly followed by 1 mg intravenously piggyback every 12 hours for 2 weeks

Directions: The question below contains three suggested answers, of which **one or more** is correct. Choose the answer

A if **I only** is correct
B if **III only** is correct
C if **I and II** are correct
D if **II and III** are correct
E if **I, II, and III** are correct

4. Allopurinol is recommended rather than probenecid in the treatment of hyperuricemia in which of the following situations?

I. When the patient has several large tophi on the elbows and knees
II. When the patient has an estimated creatinine clearance of 15 ml/min
III. When the patient has leukemia and there is concern regarding renal precipitation of urate

ANSWERS AND EXPLANATIONS

1. The answer is A *[III B 1, 2, C 1, 3].*
Other forms of acute arthritis may respond to colchicine, so that the diagnosis of gout cannot be established unequivocally by a good response to this agent. A definitive diagnosis requires the presence of urate crystals in the affected joint, although the presence of other symptoms or laboratory findings may suggest a probable diagnosis of gout.

2. The answer is A *[I D 2 c (1); III E 2 a; IV C].*
Aspirin in doses less than 2 g/day can inhibit uric acid secretion. Weight reduction, allopurinol, or probenecid to lower the serum uric acid levels, and prophylactic colchicine are all appropriate interventions in the interval phase to reduce the incidence of acute gouty attacks.

3. The answer is C *[III E 1 c, 2 a, b (1) (a); IV C].*
The most effective initial plan in treating an acute attack of gout is to administer indomethacin orally, giving 50 mg three times a day for 2–3 days, then gradually tapering the dosage over the next few days. Even though joint immobilization is an appropriate initial step, drugs for pain relief should be administered as soon as possible. Uric acid modification therapy (allopurinol or probenecid) should not be initiated until the acute attack is under control. Initiating therapy with probenecid at this point may prolong the resolution of an acute attack of gouty arthritis, which can usually be accomplished within 7 days of NSAID therapy. Colchicine should never be given intramuscularly because it causes tissue irritation.

4. The answer is E (all) *[IV C].*
In the treatment of hyperuricemia, allopurinol is indicated rather than probenecid when large tophi are present, when the creatinine clearance is less than 50–60 ml/min (probenecid would be ineffective, but allopurinol dosage would have to be decreased), when the patient is an overproducer of uric acid, and when there is a need to prevent the formation of large amounts of uric acid (e.g., when conditions such as leukemia are present).

51
Peptic Ulcer Disease

Paul F. Souney
Cheryl Stoukides

I. INTRODUCTION

A. Definition

1. **Peptic ulcer disease** refers to a group of disorders characterized by circumscribed lesions of the mucosa of the upper gastrointestinal (GI) tract (particularly the stomach and duodenum). The lesions occur in regions exposed to gastric juices.
2. **Gastroesophageal reflux disease (GERD)** refers to the retrograde movement of gastric contents from the stomach into the esophagus. Reflux may occur without consequences and thus be considered a normal physiologic process, or it may lead to profound symptomatic or histologic conditions (GERD). When reflux leads to inflammation (with or without erosions or ulcerations) of the esophagus, it is called **reflux (erosive) esophagitis.**

B. Manifestations

1. **Duodenal ulcers** almost always develop in the duodenal bulb (the first few centimeters of the duodenum). A few, however, arise between the bulb and the ampulla.
2. **Gastric ulcers** form most commonly in the antrum or at the antral–fundal junction.
3. **Less common forms of peptic ulcer disease**
   a. **Stress ulcers** result from serious trauma or illness, major burns, or ongoing sepsis. The **most common site** of stress ulcer formation is the proximal portion of the stomach.
   b. **Zollinger-Ellison syndrome** is a severe form of peptic ulcer disease in which intractable ulcers are accompanied by extreme gastric hyperacidity and at least one gastrinoma (a non–β-islet cell tumor of the pancreas or another site).
   c. **Stomal ulcers** (also called marginal ulcers) may arise at the anastomosis or immediately distal to it in the small intestine in patients who have undergone ulcer surgery and have experienced subsequent ulcer recurrence after a symptom-free period.
   d. **Drug-associated ulcers** occur in patients who chronically ingest substances that damage the gastric mucosa, such as nonsteroidal anti-inflammatory drugs (NSAIDs).
4. **Reflux esophagitis** is most often recognized by the presence of recurrent symptoms (e.g., heartburn) or altered epithelial morphology visualized radiologically, endoscopically, or histologically. Heartburn is substernal burning or regurgitation that may radiate to the neck. Other symptoms include belching, water brash, chest pain, asthma, chronic cough, hoarseness, and laryngitis.

C. Epidemiology

1. **Incidence.** Peptic ulcer disease is the most common disorder of the upper GI tract.
   a. **Duodenal ulcers** affect approximately 4%–10% of the United States population; **gastric ulcers** occur in approximately 0.03%–0.05% of the population.
   b. Nearly 80% of peptic ulcers are duodenal; the others are gastric ulcers.
   c. Most duodenal ulcers appear in people between age 20 and 50; onset of gastric ulcers usually occurs between age 45 and 55.
   d. The 1-year point prevalence of active gastric or duodenal ulcer in the United States in men and women is about 1.8%; the lifetime prevalence of peptic ulcer ranges from 11%–14% for men and 8%–11% for women.
   e. Approximately 10%–20% of gastric ulcer patients also have a concurrent duodenal ulcer.
   f. In the United States, 44% of the adult population experience **heartburn** at least once a month; 14% take some type of "indigestion" medication at least twice a week. Of pa-

tients with GERD symptoms who have undergone endoscopy, 50%–65% have apparent esophagitis.

2. **Hospitalization**
   a. Hospitalization rates in the United States for peptic ulcers have been declining; these rates dropped from 25.2 per 10,000 in 1965 to 16.5 per 10,000 in 1981. This reflects a decrease in hospitalization for uncomplicated cases due to increased outpatient diagnosis and treatment.
   b. There has been little or no decrease in duodenal ulcer perforations and only a slight decrease in hemorrhages.

3. **Mortality**
   a. The mortality rate for gastric ulcers declined between 1962 and 1979 from 3.5 per 100,000 to 1.1 per 100,000.
   b. For duodenal ulcer, the mortality rate declined from 3.1 per 100,000 to 0.9 per 100,000.
   c. Although death from GERD is uncommon, morbidity is not, because of the prevalence of the well-recognized complications such as esophageal ulceration (5%), stricture formation (4%–20%), and the development of Barrett's columnar-lined esophagus (8%–20%).

D. Description

1. **Ulcer size.** The average duodenal ulcer typically has a diameter of less than 1 cm; most gastric ulcers are somewhat larger (1–2.5 cm in diameter).
2. Most ulcers are sharply demarcated and have a round, oval, or elliptical shape.
3. The mucosa surrounding the ulcer typically is inflamed and edematous.
4. Ulcers penetrate the **muscularis propria** and, in some cases, extend into the serosa or even into the pancreas.
5. Fibrous tissue, granulation tissue, and necrotic debris form the ulcer base. During ulcer healing, a scar forms as epithelium from the edges covers the ulcer surface.
6. Nearly all duodenal ulcers are benign; up to 10% of gastric ulcers are malignant.

E. Etiology. The two major observations regarding peptic ulcer disease are the causal relationship among NSAID intake, gastroduodenal mucosal injury, the pathogenesis of gastric ulcer and, to a lesser extent, duodenal ulcer, and the association of ***Helicobacter pylori*** infection in the pathogenesis of duodenal ulcer (and to a lesser extent, gastric ulcer).

1. ***H. pylori*** (formerly *Campylobacter pylori*) is a gram-negative microaerophilic, spiral bacterium with multiple flagella that lives and infects the gastric mucosa. This bacterium is able to survive in the acidic gastric environment by its ability to produce urease, which hydrolyzes urea into ammonia. Ammonia neutralizes gastric HCl, creating a neutral cloud surrounding the organism.
   a. In the United States, the **prevalence** of *H. pylori* increases with age from approximately 10% at 20 years of age to approximately 50% at 60 years of age; approximately 17% of *H. pylori*-positive individuals will develop a duodenal ulcer. Prevalence is higher in developing countries.
   b. *H. pylori* is associated with several common GI disorders.
      (1) Always present in the setting of active chronic gastritis
      (2) Present in the vast majority of duodenal (more than 90%) and gastric (60%–90%) ulcers
      (3) Sometimes present with nonulcer dyspepsia (probably in 50% of cases)
      (4) In gastric cancer, 85%–95% (Although the association is strong, no causal relationship has yet been proven in gastric cancer. The World Health Organization has classified *H. pylori* as a Group 1 carcinogen.)
   c. *H. pylori* **eradication** can cure peptic ulcers and reduce ulcer recurrence; it can eliminate the need for maintenance therapy in many ulcer patients.

2. **Genetic factors**
   a. The lifetime prevalence of developing an ulcer in **first-degree relatives** of ulcer patients is about threefold greater than in the general population. This may be secondary to clustering of *H. pylori* within families.
   b. People with **blood type O** have an above-normal incidence of duodenal ulcers.

3. **Smoking.** Smokers have an increased risk of developing peptic ulcer disease. In addition, cigarette smoking delays ulcer healing and increases the risk and rapidity of relapse after the ulcer heals. Nicotine decreases biliary and pancreatic bicarbonate secretion. Smoking also accelerates the emptying of stomach acid into the duodenum.
4. **NSAIDs.** When ingested chronically, aspirin, indomethacin, and other NSAIDs promote gastric ulcer formation.
   a. These drugs may injure the gastric mucosa by allowing back-diffusion of hydrogen ions into the mucosa.
   b. NSAIDs also inhibit the synthesis of prostaglandins, which are substances with a cytoprotective effect on the mucosa.
5. **Alcohol.** A known mucosal irritant, alcohol causes marked irritation of the gastric mucosa if ingested in large quantities at concentrations of 20% or greater. The only association between ethanol intake and ulcer disease exists in patients with portal cirrhosis.
6. **Coffee.** Both regular and decaffeinated coffee contain peptides that stimulate release of gastrin, a hormone that triggers the flow of gastric juice. However, a direct link between coffee and peptic ulcer disease has not been proven.
7. **Corticosteroids.** A review of 42 randomized trials concluded that adrenocorticosteroids can be incriminated in ulcer pathogenesis in patients who receive daily corticosteroids for more than 1 month, in those that receive more than a total dose equivalent to 1 gram of prednisone, and in those with prior ulcers. No other associations between corticosteroid intake and ulcers have been found.
8. **Associated disorders.** Peptic ulcer disease is more common in patients with hyperparathyroidism, emphysema, rheumatoid arthritis, and alcoholic cirrhosis.
9. **Advanced age.** Degeneration of the pylorus permits bile reflux into the stomach, creating an environment that favors ulcer formation.
10. **Psychologic factors.** Once assigned key roles in the pathogenesis of peptic ulcer disease, stress and personality type now are viewed as relatively minor influences.

F. Pathophysiology. Ulcers develop when an imbalance exists between factors that protect gastric mucosa and factors that promote mucosal corrosion. Approximately 90% of patients with duodenal ulcer and 70% of patients with gastric ulcer have *H. pylori* infection.

1. **Protective factors**
   a. Normally, the mucosa secretes a thick mucus that serves as a barrier between luminal acid and epithelial cells. This barrier slows the inward movement of hydrogen ions and allows their neutralization by bicarbonate ions in fluids secreted by the stomach and duodenum.
   b. Alkaline and neutral pancreatic biliary juices also help buffer acid entering the duodenum from the stomach.
   c. An **intact mucosal barrier** prevents back-diffusion of gastric acids into mucosal cells. It also has the capacity to stimulate local blood flow, which brings nutrients and other substances to the area and removes toxic substances (e.g., hydrogen ions). Mucosal integrity also promotes cell growth and repair after local trauma.
2. **Corrosive factors.** Peptic ulcer disease reflects the inability of the gastric mucosa to resist corrosion by irritants, such as pepsin, hydrochloric acid (HCl), and other gastric secretions.
   a. **Exposure to gastric acid** and **pepsin** is necessary for ulcer development.
   b. **Disrupted mucosal barrier integrity** allows gastric acids to diffuse from the lumen back into mucosal cells, where they cause injury.
3. **Physiologic defects associated with peptic ulcer disease.** Researchers have identified various physiologic defects in patients with duodenal and gastric ulcers.
   a. **Duodenal ulcer patients** may have the following defects:
      (1) Increased capacity for gastric acid secretion
         (a) Some duodenal ulcer patients have up to twice the normal number of parietal cells (which produce HCl).
         (b) Nearly 70% of duodenal ulcer patients have elevated serum levels of **pepsinogen I** and a corresponding increase in pepsin-secreting capacity.
      (2) Increased parietal cell responsiveness to gastrin

(3) Above-normal postprandial gastrin secretion
(4) Defective inhibition of gastrin release at low pH, possibly leading to failure to suppress postprandial acid secretion
(5) Above-normal rate of gastric emptying, resulting in delivery of a greater acid load to the duodenum

b. **Gastric ulcer patients** typically exhibit the following characteristics:
(1) Deficient gastric mucosal resistance, direct mucosal injury, or both
(2) Elevated serum gastrin levels (in acid hyposecretors)
(3) Decreased pyloric pressure at rest and in response to acid or fat in the duodenum
(4) Delayed gastric emptying
(5) Increased reflux of bile and other duodenal contents
(6) Subnormal mucosal levels of prostaglandins (these levels normalize once the ulcer heals)

4. **GERD** requires both initiation and perpetuation of the reflux of gastric contents. Esophagitis develops when noxious substances in the refluxate (i.e., acid, pepsin) are in contact with the esophageal mucosa long enough to cause irritation and inflammation.

a. In patients with GERD, 65% of reflux events occur via transient lower esophageal sphincter (LES) relaxation (TLESR). The main difference between normal individuals and those with GERD is the frequency of TLESR. GERD patients have more frequent and prolonged TLESR. TLESR represents a decrease in LES pressure that is not associated with swallowing or peristalsis.

b. Other mechanisms of LES incompetence are increased abdominal pressure and spontaneous reflux during periods of very low LES pressure.

c. Such motility problems are permissive; that is, they allow reflux of acid and other noxious substances.

G. **Clinical presentation.** Signs and symptoms of peptic ulcer disease vary with the patient's age and the location of the lesion. Only about 50% of patients experience classic ulcer symptoms. The remainder are asymptomatic or report vague or atypical symptoms.

1. **Pain.** Patients typically describe heartburn or a gnawing, burning, aching, or cramp-like pain. Some patients report abdominal soreness or hunger sensations. It is unclear whether peptic ulcer pain results from chemical stimulation or from spasm.

a. **Duodenal ulcer pain** usually is restricted to a small, midepigastric area near the xiphoid. Pain may radiate below the costal margins into the back or the right shoulder. Pain from a duodenal ulcer frequently awakens the patient between midnight and 2 A.M.; it is almost never present before breakfast.

b. **Gastric ulcer pain** is less localized. It may be referred to the left subcostal region. Gastric ulcer rarely produces nocturnal pain.

c. **GERD** patients most commonly present with heartburn, belching, regurgitation, or water brash; **atypical presentations** include chest pain, hoarseness/laryngitis, loss of dental enamel, asthma, chronic cough or dyspepsia.

d. **Food** usually relieves duodenal ulcer pain but may cause gastric ulcer pain. This finding may explain why duodenal ulcer patients tend to gain weight, whereas gastric ulcer patients may lose weight. Pain characteristically occurs 90 minutes to 3 hours after meals in duodenal ulcer patients, while pain in gastric ulcer patients is usually present 45–60 minutes after a meal. Food aggravates reflux disease.

2. **Nausea** and **vomiting** may occur with either ulcer type.

3. **Disease course.** Both duodenal and gastric ulcers tend to be chronic, with spontaneous remissions and exacerbations. Within a year of the initial symptoms, most patients experience a relapse.

a. In many cases, relapse is seasonal, occurring more often in the spring and autumn.

b. All patients with a confirmed duodenal or gastric ulcer should be tested for *H. pylori* infection. If the patient is *H. pylori*-positive, eradication therapy will reduce recurrence rate significantly and preclude the need for maintenance medication.

c. GERD is also a chronic disease; most patients with reflux esophagitis who are healed with antisecretory drug therapy will experience a recurrence within 6 months of discontinuation of the healing regimen. Maintenance therapy reduces the recurrence of esophagitis.

H. **Clinical evaluation**

1. **Physical findings.** Patients with peptic ulcer disease may exhibit superficial and deep epigastric tenderness and voluntary muscle guarding. With duodenal ulcer, patients also may show unilateral spasm over the duodenal bulb. Gastric ulcer patients may have weight loss.
2. **Diagnostic test result**
   a. **Blood tests** may show hypochromic anemia.
   b. **Stool tests** may detect occult blood if the ulcer is chronic.
   c. **Gastric secretion tests** may reveal hypersecretion of HCl in duodenal ulcer patients and normal or subnormal HCl secretion in gastric ulcer patients.
   d. **Upper GI series** (barium x-ray) reveals the ulcer crater in up to 80% of cases. Duodenal bulb deformity suggests a duodenal ulcer.
   e. **Upper GI endoscopy,** the most specific test, may be done if barium x-ray yields inconclusive results. This procedure confirms an ulcer in at least 95% of cases and may detect ulcers not demonstrable by radiography.
   f. **Biopsy** might be necessary to determine whether a gastric ulcer is malignant.
   g. *H. pylori* status is determined by noninvasive tests (not requiring endoscopy) or invasive methods (requiring endoscopy).
      (1) **Noninvasive.** Serology, the test of choice when endoscopy is not indicated, is inexpensive. Several office tests are available.
      (2) **Invasive.** These methods include histologic visualization of *H. pylori* or measurement of urease activity, which require biopsy.

I. Treatment objectives

1. Relieve pain and other symptoms and promote healing
2. Prevent complications of peptic ulcer disease
3. Minimize recurrence
4. Maintain adequate nutrition
5. Teach the patient about the disease to improve therapeutic compliance

II. THERAPY

A. Drug therapy. Peptic ulcer patients usually are treated with antacids, histamine$_2$ (H_2)-receptor antagonists, or both; other drugs are added as necessary. Drug regimens that suppress nocturnal acid secretion are found to result in the highest duodenal ulcer healing rates. Drug therapy typically provides prompt symptomatic relief and promotes ulcer healing within 4–6 weeks (Figure 51-1). GERD management requires more aggressive acid suppression regimens; the pharmacodynamic endpoint is to maintain the pH in the esophagus at 4 or more (Figure 51-2).

1. **Antacids.** These compounds, which neutralize gastric acid, are used to treat ulcer pain and heal the ulcer. Studies show antacids and H_2-receptor antagonists to be equally effective. Antacids are available as **magnesium, aluminum, calcium,** or **sodium salts.** The most widely used antacids are mixtures of aluminum hydroxide and magnesium hydroxide (Table 51-1). Duodenal ulcers rarely occur in the absence of acid or when the hourly maximum acid output is less than 10 mEq. Peptic activity decreases as acidity decreases; experimental ulcer formation is inhibited by antacids; and acid-reducing operations cure ulcers.
   a. **Mechanism of action and therapeutic effects.** Antacids reduce the concentration and total load of acid in the gastric contents. By increasing gastric pH, antacids also inhibit pepsin activity. In addition, they strengthen the gastric mucosal barrier.
   b. **Choice of agent**
      (1) **Nonsystemic antacids** (e.g., magnesium or aluminum substances) are preferred to systemic antacids (e.g., sodium bicarbonate) for intensive ulcer therapy because they avoid the risk of alkalosis.
      (2) **Liquid antacid forms** have a greater buffering capacity than tablets. However, tablets are more convenient to carry. With either dosage form, the size and frequency of doses may limit patient compliance.
      (3) **Antacid mixtures** (e.g., aluminum hydroxide with magnesium hydroxide) provide more even, sustained action than single-agent antacids and permit a lower dosage of each compound. In addition, compounds in a mixture may interact so as to

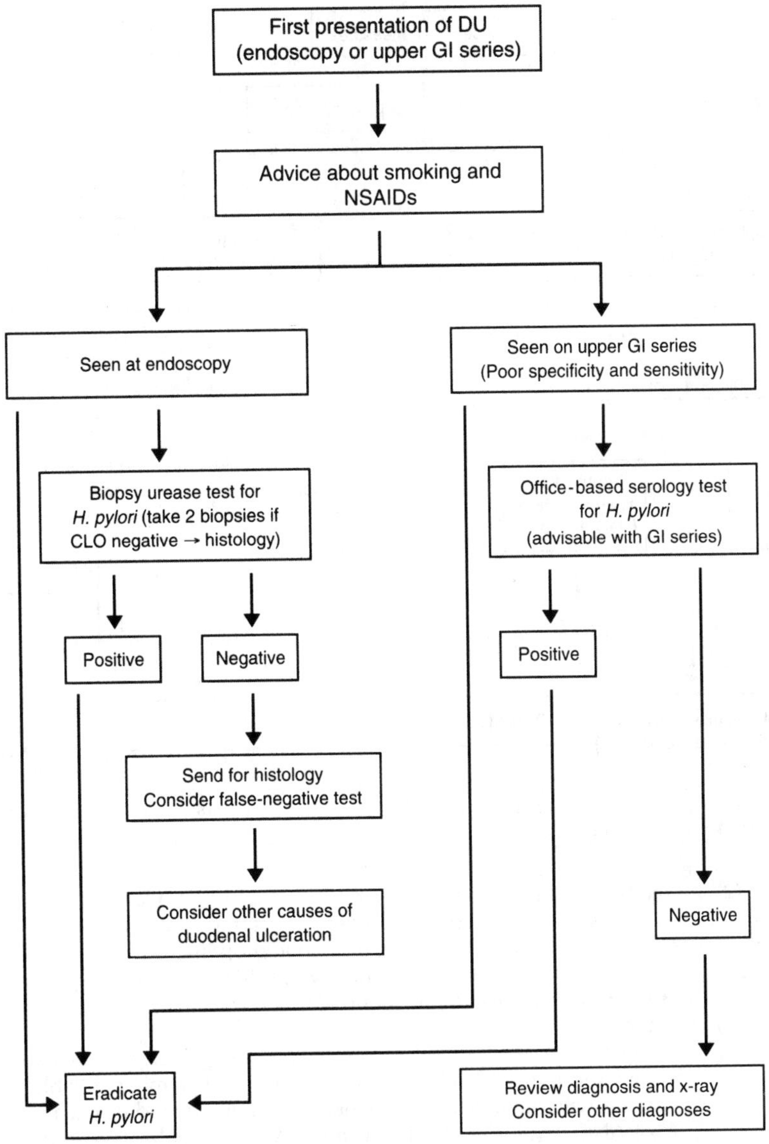

Figure 51-1. Treatment strategy for management of duodenal ulcer. *CLO* = test to measure presence of urease (*H. pylori*)

negate each other's untoward effects. For instance, the constipating effect of aluminum hydroxide may counter the diarrhea that magnesium hydroxide frequently produces.

(4) Calcium carbonate usually is avoided because it causes acid rebound, may delay pain relief and ulcer healing, and induces constipation. Another potential adverse effect of this compound is hypercalcemia; the risk is increased if calcium carbonate is taken with milk or another alkaline substance. The milk-alkali syndrome (i.e., hypercalcemia, alkalosis, azotemia, nephrocalcinosis) can also occur.

c. Administration and dosage

(1) Antacids differ greatly in acid-neutralizing capacity (ANC), defined as the number of milliequivalents (mEq) of a 1 N solution of HCl that can be brought to a pH of 3.5 in 15 minutes. With most duodenal ulcer patients, approximately 50 mEq/hr of available antacid is needed for ongoing neutralization of gastric contents. Therefore, the required dosage depends on the ANC of the specific antacid.

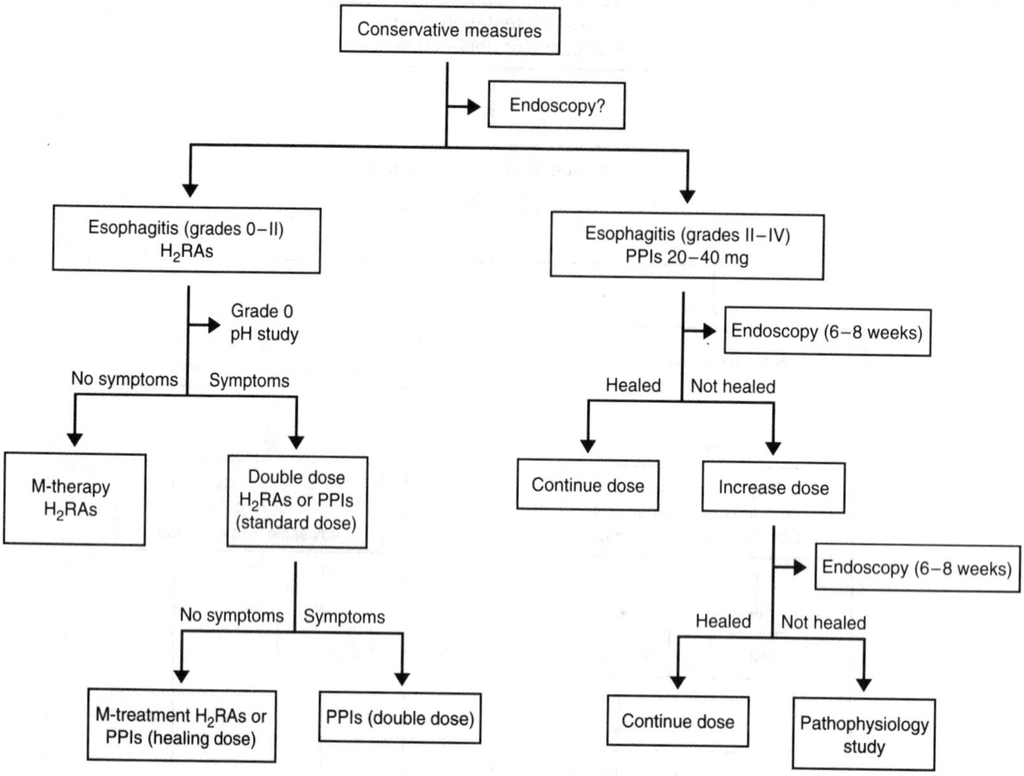

Figure 51-2. Treatment strategy for management of GERD. *H_2RAs* = histamine H_2-receptor antagonist; *PPI* = proton pump inhibitor; *M* = maintenance

(2) In the fasting state, antacids have only a transient intragastric buffering effect (15–20 minutes). When ingested 1 hour after a meal, they have a much more prolonged effect, about 3–4 hours; therefore, they should optimally be taken 1 and 3 hours after meals and before sleep. Consequently, the typical antacid regimen calls for doses 1–3 hours after meals and at bedtime.

(3) Dosage

(a) Because the ANC of antacid products varies widely, no standard dosage can be given in terms of milliliters of suspension or number of tablets. However, patients with duodenal ulcers generally require individual dosages of 80–160 mEq of ANC (equivalent to 30–60 ml of Mylanta or Maalox). Thus, the total daily dosage may be as much as 420 ml of Mylanta or Maalox if the standard seven-times–daily dosing regimen is used. Because of the large doses and the need for frequent administration, compliance with antacid treatment regimens has been low.

(b) Antacid therapy usually continues for 6–8 weeks.

d. Precautions and monitoring effects

(1) Calcium carbonate and magnesium-containing antacids should be used cautiously in patients with severe renal disease.

(2) Sodium bicarbonate is contraindicated in patients with hypertension, congestive heart failure (CHF), severe renal disease, and edema. It should not be used for ulcer therapy.

(3) All antacids should be used cautiously in elderly patients (particularly those with decreased GI motility) and renally impaired patients.

(4) Aluminum-containing antacids should be used cautiously in patients who suffer from dehydration or intestinal obstruction.

(5) The combination of calcium carbonate with an alkaline substance (e.g., sodium bicarbonate) and milk may cause the milk-alkali syndrome.

Table 51-1. Comparison of Antacids at a Dose of 140 mEq/hr

Brand Name	Neutralizing Capacity (mEq H+/ml antacid)	Therapeutic Dose (140 mEq) (ml or no. of tablets)	Composition	Sodium Ion Content (mg/day)
		Liquids (Concentrated)		
Maalox TC	4.2	33	$Al(OH)_3$ $Mg(OH)_3$	55
Titralac	4.2	33	$CaCO_3$ Glycerine	508
Delcid	4.1	34	$Al(OH)_3$ $Mg(OH)_3$	71
Mylanta II	3.6	39	$Al(OH)_3$ $Mg(OH)_3$ Simethicone	60
		Liquids (Regular)		
Camalox	3.2	44	$Al(OH)_3$ $Mg(OH)_3$ $CaCO_3$	154
Gelusil II	3.0	47	$Al(OH)_3$ $Mg(OH)_3$ Simethicone	86
Maalox Plus	2.3	61	$Al(OH)_3$ $Mg(OH)_3$ Simethicone	214
Gelusil	2.2	64	$Al(OH)_3$ $Mg(OH)_3$ Simethicone	63
Riopan Plus	1.8	78	$Al(OH)_3$ $Mg(OH)_3$ Simethicone	76
Amphojel	1.4	100	$Al(OH)_3$	980
		Tablets		
Camalox	16.7	8	$Al(OH)_3$ $Mg(OH)_3$	84
Mylanta II	11.0	13	$Al(OH)_3$ $Mg(OH)_3$ Simethicone	126
Tums	10.5	13	$CaCO_3$ $Al(OH)_3$ $Mg(OH)_3$	246
Riopan Plus	10.0	14	$Al(OH)_3$ $Mg(OH)_3$ Simethicone	29
Titralac	9.5	9.5	$CaCO_3$ Glycerine	32
Rolaids	6.9	6.9	$Al_2(CO_3)_3$	7420
Maalox Plus	5.7	5.7	$Al(OH)_3$ $Mg(OH)_3$ Simethicone	245
Amphojel	2.0	2.0	$Al(OH)_3$	3430

Reprinted from Sleisenger MH, Fordtran JS (eds): *Gastrointestinal Disease: Pathophysiology, Diagnosis and Management*. Philadelphia, WB Saunders, 1983, p 718.

(6) Low-sodium antacids obviate the problem of fluid retention in hypertension and heart disease.
(7) Chronic administration of calcium carbonate–containing antacids should be avoided because of hypercalcemia and calcium ion stimulation of acid secretion.
(8) Aluminum or magnesium toxicity is unlikely in patients with normal renal function. The encephalopathy of tissue deposition of aluminum occurs only in dialysis patients receiving aluminum hydroxide for control of hyperphosphatemia. Chronic use of magnesium-containing antacids is not advisable in patients with renal insufficiency.
(9) Constipation can occur in patients using calcium carbonate and aluminum-containing antacids.
(10) Diarrhea is a common adverse effect of magnesium-containing antacids. If diarrhea occurs, the patient may alternate the antacid mixture with aluminum hydroxide.
(11) Hypophosphatemia and osteomalacia can occur with long-term use of aluminum hydroxide, but these conditions can also occur with short-term use in severely malnourished patients, such as alcoholics.

e. **Significant interactions.** Because antacids alter gastric pH and affect absorption of ingested substances, they have a high potential for drug interactions. To ensure consistent absorption and therapeutic efficacy, orally administered drugs should be given 30–60 minutes before antacids.
(1) Antacids bind with **tetracycline,** inhibiting its absorption and reducing its therapeutic efficacy.
(2) Antacids may destroy the coating of **enteric-coated drugs,** leading to premature drug dissolution in the stomach.
(3) Antacids may interfere with the absorption of many drugs, including **cimetidine, ranitidine, digoxin, isoniazid, anticholinergics, iron products,** and **phenothiazines** [see II A 2 e (3)].
(4) Antacids may reduce the therapeutic effects of **sucralfate** (see II A 3 d).

2. **H_2-receptor antagonists.** These drugs may be preferred to other antiulcer agents because of their convenience and lack of effect on GI motility. Although reasonably effective in treating mild-to-moderate GERD symptoms, H_2-receptor antagonists are less reliable for healing erosive esophagitis. All current choices require multiple, divided doses for GERD management.

a. **Mechanism of action and therapeutic effects.** H_2-receptor antagonists (Table 51-2) competitively inhibit the action of histamine at parietal cell receptor sites, reducing the vol-

Table 51-2. Histamine H_2-Receptor Antagonsits

	Cimetidine (Tagamet)	Ranitidine (Zantac)	Famotidine (Pepcid)	Nizatidine (Axid)
Ring structure	Imidazole	Furan	Thiazole	Thiazole
Relative potency	1	4–10	4–10	20–50
Evening dose (mg)				
Active ulcer	800	300	40	300
Maintenance	400	150	20	150
Bioavailability (F)	60%–70%	50%–60%	40%–45%	90%–100%
Peak time (t_{max}) (hr)	1–3	1–3	1–3.5	0.5–3
Volume of distribution (L/kg)	1	1.4	1.1–1.4	0.8–1.6
Protein binding	20%	15%	15%–22%	32%–35%
Renal elimination	60%–75%	30% oral 70% intravenous	65%–70%	65%–75%
Half-life (hr)				
Normal	2	2–3	2.5–4	1.6
Anuric	4–5	4–10	20+	6–8/5
Clearance (L/h)	30–48	46	19–29	40–60

Reprinted from Hurwitz A: Clinical pharmacology of agents for the treatment of acid-related disorders. In *Peptic Ulcer Disease and Other Acid-Related Disorders.* Edited by Zakim D, Dannenberg AJ. New York, Academic Research Associates, 1991, p 343.

ume and hydrogen ion concentration of gastric acid secretions (Figure 51-3). These agonists accelerate the healing of most ulcers.

b. Choice of agent. Cimetidine, ranitidine, famotidine, or **nizatidine** may be administered to treat peptic ulcers or hypersecretory states (e.g., Zollinger-Ellison syndrome).

(1) **Cimetidine,** the first H_2-receptor antagonist approved for clinical use, reduces gastric acid secretion by approximately 50% (at a total daily dosage of 1000 mg).

(2) **Ranitidine,** a more potent drug, causes a 70% reduction in gastric acid secretion (at a total daily dosage of 300 mg).

(3) **Famotidine** is the most potent H_2-receptor antagonist. After a 40-mg dose, mean nocturnal gastric acid secretion is reduced by 94% for up to 10 hours.

(4) **Nizatidine,** the newest H_2-receptor agonist, may be used to treat and prevent recurrence of duodenal ulcers. This agent seems similar to ranitidine, but its clinical place in therapy has not been thoroughly elucidated.

c. Administration and dosage

(1) **Cimetidine** usually is administered orally in a dosage of 300 mg four times daily (with meals and at bedtime) for up to 8 weeks.

(a) Alternatively, duodenal ulcer patients may receive 400 mg twice daily or 800 mg at bedtime. An 800-mg bedtime dose is also effective in treating gastric ulcers.

(b) Hospitalized patients may receive parenteral doses of 300 mg intravenously every 6 hours.

(c) For duodenal ulcer prophylaxis, 400 mg may be given orally at bedtime. (However, in 20%–40% of patients, the ulcer recurs despite cimetidine prophylaxis.)

(2) **Ranitidine** usually is given orally in a dosage of 150 mg twice daily. Duodenal ulcer patients may receive 300 mg at bedtime, alternatively. Therapy continues for up to 8 weeks.

(a) Hospitalized patients may receive ranitidine by the intravenous (IV) or intramuscular route (50 mg every 6–8 hours).

(b) Prophylactic therapy may be administered to reduce the risk of ulcer recurrence. The approved prophylactic dosage is 150 mg at bedtime.

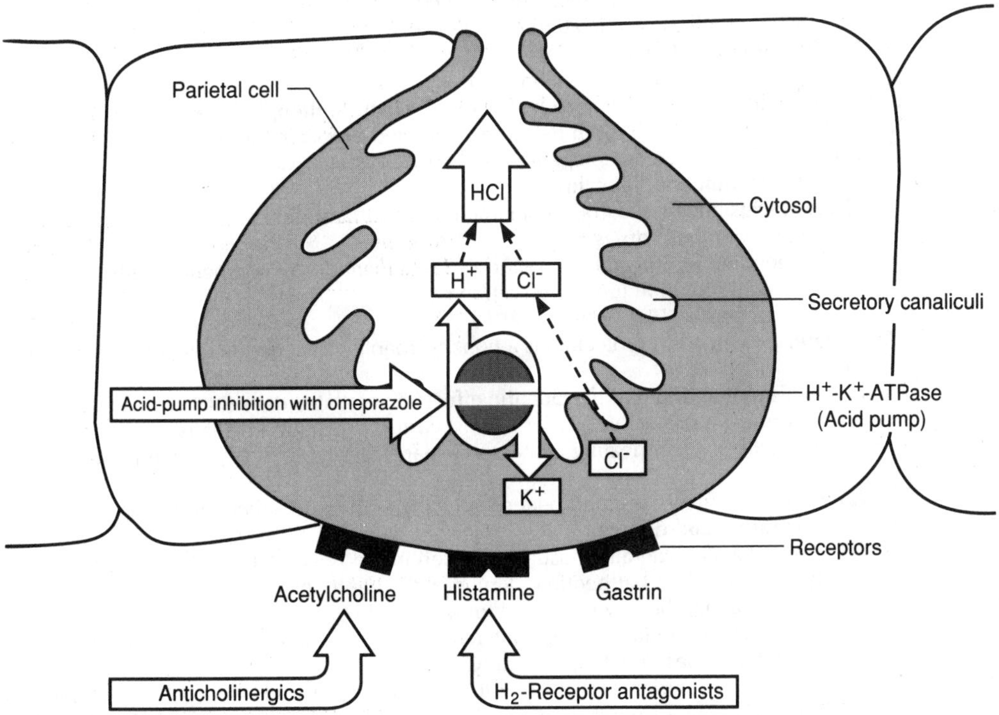

Figure 51-3. Schematic representation of parietal cell depicting sites of drug action.

(c) Ranitidine 150 mg twice daily can be administered to maintain healing of erosive esophagitis; for this purpose it is better than placebo, but less effective than omeprazole.

(d) Ranitidine bismuth citrate (RBC), combined with antibiotics such as clarithromycin, is indicated for eradication of *H. pylori* in patients with duodenal ulcer.

(3) **Famotidine,** administered to duodenal ulcer patients, is given in an oral dosage of 40 mg at bedtime for acute therapy for a maximum of 8 weeks. For prophylactic therapy, the dosage is 20 mg at bedtime.

(a) Hospitalized patients may receive an IV injection of 20 mg every 12 hours.

(b) As with cimetidine and ranitidine, the ulcer may recur after drug discontinuation.

(4) **Nizatidine,** for the treatment of duodenal ulcers, is given orally in a dosage of 300 mg once daily at bedtime or 150 mg twice daily for up to 8 weeks. For prophylactic therapy, the dosage is 150 mg at bedtime.

d. Precautions and monitoring effects

(1) Ranitidine must be used cautiously in patients with hepatic impairment. Hepatotoxicity is unusual and occurs most often during IV administration. Cimetidine has also been associated with hepatotoxicity.

(2) Cimetidine may cause such hematologic disorders as thrombocytopenia, agranulocytosis, and aplastic anemia.

(3) All of these agents may cause headache and dizziness. Cimetidine additionally may lead to confusion, particularly if patients are over age 60 years or if the dosage is not adjusted for patients with decreased kidney or liver function.

(4) Cimetidine has a weak androgenic effect, possibly resulting in male gynecomastia and impotence.

(5) Cimetidine and ranitidine rarely can cause bradycardia, which is reversible on discontinuation of therapy.

(6) Evaluate *H. pylori* status in any patient with confirmed ulcer disease; eradication of *H. pylori* reduces the need for maintenance therapy in patients with duodenal or gastric ulcers. Patients with complicated ulcer disease should continue maintenance therapy until the eradication of *H. pylori*.

e. Significant interactions

(1) Cimetidine binds the cytochrome P-450 system of the liver and, thus, may interfere with the metabolism of such drugs as **phenytoin, theophylline, phenobarbital, lidocaine, warfarin, imipramine, diazepam,** and **propranolol.**

(2) Cimetidine decreases hepatic blood flow, possibly resulting in reduced clearance of **propranolol** and **lidocaine**.

(3) **Antacids** impair absorption of cimetidine and ranitidine and should be given 1 hour apart from these drugs.

(4) Cimetidine inhibits the excretion of procainamide by competing with the drug for the renal proximal tubular secretion site.

3. **Sucralfate.** This mucosal protectant is a nonabsorbable disaccharide containing sucrose and aluminum.

a. Mechanism of action and therapeutic effects. Sucralfate adheres to the base of the ulcer crater, forming a protective barrier against gastric acids and bile salts.

(1) Sucralfate's ulcer-healing efficacy compares favorably to that of the H_2-receptor antagonists.

(2) Duodenal ulcers respond better than gastric ulcers to sucralfate therapy.

b. Administration and dosage

(1) An oral agent, sucralfate usually is given in a dosage of 1 g four times daily (1 hour before meals) and at bedtime. Unless radiography or endoscopy documents earlier ulcer healing, therapy continues for 4–8 weeks.

(2) Continued sucralfate therapy after remission postpones ulcer relapse more effectively than does cimetidine therapy.

(3) There is no evidence that combining sucralfate with H_2-receptor antagonists improves healing or reduces recurrence rates.

c. Precautions and monitoring effects. Constipation is the most common adverse effect of sucralfate.

d. Significant interactions

(1) **Antacids** may reduce mucosal binding of sucralfate, decreasing its therapeutic efficacy and, thus, should be given 30–60 minutes apart from sucralfate if used in combination ulcer therapy.
(2) Sucralfate may interfere with the absorption of orally administered **digoxin, tetracycline, phenytoin, iron, ciprofloxacin,** and **cimetidine** if doses are given simultaneously.

4. **GI anticholinergics** (e.g., belladonna leaf, atropine, propantheline) sometimes are used as adjunctive agents for relief of refractory duodenal ulcer pain. However, these agents have no proven value in ulcer healing.
   a. **Mechanism of action.** Anticholinergics decrease basal and stimulated gastric acid and pepsin secretion.
      (1) Given in combination with antacids, anticholinergics delay gastric emptying, thereby prolonging antacid retention. They are most effective when taken at night and in large doses.
      (2) Anticholinergics occasionally are used in patients who do not respond to H_2-receptor antagonists alone.
   b. **Administration and dosage**
      (1) Taken 30 minutes before food, anticholinergics inhibit meal-stimulated acid secretion by 30%–50% with a duration of 4–5 hours.
      (2) An optimal effective dose varies from patient to patient.
   c. **Precautions and monitoring effects**
      (1) All anticholinergics have side effects to varying degrees, such as dry mouth, blurred vision, tachycardia, urinary retention, and constipation.
      (2) These drugs are contraindicated in patients with gastric ulcers because they prolong gastric emptying. They also are contraindicated in patients with narrow-angle glaucoma and urinary retention.

5. **Prostaglandins** may prove valuable in ulcer therapy. These agents suppress gastric acid secretion and may guard the gastric mucosa against damage from NSAIDs. **Misoprostol** has been approved for use in the prevention of gastric ulcers caused by NSAIDs.
   a. **Mechanism of action.** Misoprostol has both antisecretory (inhibiting gastric acid secretion) and mucosal protective properties. NSAIDs inhibit prostaglandin synthesis, and a deficiency of prostaglandin within the gastric mucosa may lead to diminishing bicarbonate and mucus secretion, contributing to the mucosal damage caused by NSAIDs. Misoprostol increases bicarbonate and mucus production at doses of 200 μg and above—doses that can also be antisecretory. Misoprostol also maintains mucosal blood flow.
   b. **Administration and dosage**
      (1) Misoprostol is indicated for the prevention of NSAID-induced gastric ulcers in patients at high risk for complications from gastric ulcers (e.g., patients over 60 years of age, patients with concomitant debilitating disease, patients with a history of ulcers).
      (2) Misoprostol has not been shown to prevent duodenal ulcers in patients taking NSAIDs.
      (3) The recommended adult dosage is 200 μg four times daily with food; it must be taken for the duration of NSAID therapy; if this dose cannot be tolerated, 100 μg four times daily can be used.)
      (4) Adjustment of dosage in renally impaired patients is not routinely needed.
   c. **Precautions and monitoring effects**
      (1) Misoprostol is contraindicated in women who are pregnant because of its abortifacient property. Patients must be advised of the abortifacient property and warned not to give the drug to others.
      (2) Misoprostol should not be used in women with childbearing potential unless the patient requires NSAID therapy and is at high risk of complications from gastric ulcers associated with use of the NSAIDs or is at high risk of developing gastric ulceration. In such a patient, misoprostol may be prescribed if the patient:
         (a) Is capable of complying with effective contraceptive measures
         (b) Has received both oral and written warnings of the hazards of misoprostol, the risk of possible contraception failure, and the danger to other women of childbearing potential should the drug be taken by mistake
         (c) Had a negative serum pregnancy test within 2 weeks before beginning therapy

(d) Will begin misoprostol only on the second or third day of the next normal menstrual period

(3) The most frequent adverse effects are diarrhea (14%–40%) and abdominal pain (13%–20%). Diarrhea is dose-related, usually develops early in the course (more than 2 weeks), and is often self-limiting. Discontinuation of misoprostol is necessary in about 2% of patients. Administration with food minimizes the diarrhea.

d. **Significant interactions.** None has been reported.

6. **Proton Pump inhibitors (PPIs). Omeprazole** is the first PPI available in the United States; **lansoprazole** has been approved recently in the United States for more limited indications; **pantoprazole** is currently under investigation.

a. **Mechanism of action and therapeutic effects.** The gastric proton pump H^+, K^+-ATPase has a sulfhydryl group near the potassium-binding site on the luminal side of the canalicular membrane. Omeprazole sulfonamide (the active form) forms a stable disulfide bond with this specific sulfhydryl, thereby inactivating the ATPase and shutting off acid secretion.

(1) Because of the potency and marked reduction in gastric acidity, omeprazole is more rapidly effective than other approved agents in treating peptic ulcer disease (i.e., it tends to control symptoms and heal ulcers more rapidly than other antiulcer drugs). PPIs provide effective healing of duodenal ulcers; healing rates at 4 weeks are similar to those reported for H_2RA therapy at 8 weeks.

(2) PPIs are effective in healing erosive esophagitis; provide more rapid symptom relief and more consistent healing than H_2-receptor antagonists; omeprazole is also effective in maintenance of healing of erosive esophagitis.

(3) Omeprazole 40 mg daily and clarithromycin 500 mg three times daily are approved for eradication of *H. pylori* (14-day treatment regimen).

(4) Omeprazole has resulted in significant improvement in patients with pathologic hypersecretory conditions (e.g., Zollinger-Ellison syndrome) and GERD compared to H_2-receptor antagonists.

(5) Lansoprazole is currently approved for healing of duodenal ulcers, short-term management of erosive esophagitis, and management of pathologic hypersecretory conditions (Zollinger-Ellison syndrome).

b. **Administration and dosage**

(1) Omeprazole is more potent than H_2-blockers. In the usual dosage (20 mg daily), this agent inhibits over 90% of 24-hour acid secretion in most patients, infrequently producing achlorhydria. Lansoprazole 30 mg provides comparable acid inhibition to omeprazole 20 mg.

(2) **Recommended adult dosages**

(a) Erosive esophagitis initially is healed with 20 mg omeprazole for 8–12 weeks; omeprazole may be administered for as long as medically necessary to maintain healing of erosive esophagitis; maintenance therapy significantly reduces recurrence rates.

(b) Omeprazole 20 mg may be used to manage GERD symptoms in patients who have failed previous therapy with H_2RA therapy.

(c) The recommended dosage to maintain healing of erosive esophagitis is omeprazole 20 mg daily for as long as medically necessary.

(d) Duodenal ulcer requires 20 mg daily. Most patients heal within 4 weeks.

(3) Omeprazole is a delayed-release capsule and should be taken before eating. It can be used concomitantly with antacids. It should not be opened, chewed, or crushed.

(4) No dosing adjustments are necessary in patients with impaired renal or hepatic function or in the elderly.

c. **Precautions and monitoring effects**

(1) Headache, diarrhea, abdominal pain, nausea and vomiting, and flatulence have been reported in more than 1% of patients.

(2) Fever, fatigue, malaise, elevated liver enzymes, dizziness, vertigo, skin rash, and itching have been reported in less than 1% of patients.

d. **Significant interactions**

(1) Omeprazole interferes with the hepatic microsomal enzyme metabolism (cytochrome P-450) of **diazepam, warfarin,** and **phenytoin.**

(2) Although metabolized by the cytochrome P-450 enzyme system, no evidence of an interaction with **theophylline** and **propranolol** to date exists. Lansoprazole may increase clearance of theophylline by approximately 10%.

(3) Because gastric pH plays a role in the bioavailability of **ketoconazole, ampicillin esters,** and **iron salts,** prolonged gastric acid inhibition with PPIs may decrease the absorption of these agents.
(4) Antacids may be used concomitantly with omeprazole lansoprazole.
(5) Increased cyclosporin levels have been reported after omeprazole administration.
(6) Food may reduce the bioavailability of lansoprazole by 50%; food does not reduce the bioavailability of omeprazole.

7. **Bismuth compounds (investigational);** colloidal bismuth subcitrate (CBS, tripotassium dicitratobismuthate, TDB). In the United States, bismuth subsalicylate (Pepto-Bismol) is the only available bismuth product.
   a. **Mechanism of action.** CBS blocks pepsin activity, binds mucus to retard hydrogen back-diffusion, stimulates prostaglandin synthesis, and suppresses *H. pylori.*
   b. **Administration and dosage**
      (1) CBS has been used since 1971 to treat gastric and duodenal ulcers. Efficacy rates are as follows:
         (a) **Duodenal ulcer:** 80% were healed at 4 weeks and 95% at 8 weeks.
         (b) **Gastric ulcer:** 68% were healed at 4 weeks and 81% at 8 weeks.
      (2) After healing by CBS, mucosal morphology is described as more normal in appearance than after H_2-blocker therapy; recurrence rates are also lower.
      (3) CBS precipitates at about pH 3.5, binding to ulcer craters. Animal studies have shown that this binding is unique to CBS among the bismuth compounds studied and does not occur with bismuth subsalicylate (Pepto-Bismol).
      (4) Bismuth subsalicylate has been combined with antibiotics and antisecretory drugs for *H. pylori* eradication regimens. Bismuth subsalicylate (2 tabs four times a day) + tetracycline 500 mg qid + metronidazole 250 mg qid. When this combination is administered for 14 days, *H. pylori* eradication rates are approximately 90%. In patients with active ulcer disease, add either omeprazole 20 mg daily or ranitidine 300 mg daily.
   c. **Precautions and monitoring effects**
      (1) Headache, abdominal pain, diarrhea, rash, and dark stool are a few of the adverse effects.
      (2) Absorbed bismuth has caused encephalopathy (not CBS).
      (3) Salicylism with tinnitus may result from high doses of bismuth subsalicylate.

8. **Prokinetic agents.** Cisapride is currently the only approved agent in this class.
   a. **Mechanism of action.** Cisapride produces release of acetylcholine from the myenteric plexus and thereby may increase gastric emptying and LES pressure; cisapride does not affect TLESR. It does not increase or decrease gastric acid secretion.
   b. **Administration and dosage.** Cisapride is indicated for the relief of nocturnal symptoms of reflux; it is administered in doses of 10–20 mg four times a day.
   c. **Precautions and monitoring**
      (1) The **most common** side effects are diarrhea and abdominal pain.
      (2) Rare cases of cardiac arrhythmias have been reported.
   d. **Significant interactions**
      (1) Ketoconazole potently inhibits the metabolism of cisapride, resulting in an eightfold increase in the area under the curve (AUC) of cisapride. Coadministration of cisapride and ketoconazole can result in prolongation of the QT interval on the ECG. Coadministration of itraconazole, miconazole IV, or troleandomycin is similarly contraindicated.
      (2) The acceleration of gastric emptying by cisapride could affect the rate of absorption of other drugs. Patients receiving narrow therapeutic drugs or other drugs that require careful titration should be monitored closely.
      (3) Coagulation times in patients receiving oral anticoagulants have increased in some cases.
      (4) Cimetidine may increase peak plasma concentration and AUC of cimetidine.

9. **Sedatives** are useful adjuncts in promoting rest for highly anxious ulcer patients.

B. Other therapeutic measures

1. **Modification of diet and social habits**
   a. Previously emphasized in ulcer therapy, strict dietary limitations now are considered largely unnecessary.

(1) Bland or milk-based diets formerly were recommended; however, research indicates that these diets do not speed ulcer healing. In fact, most experts now advise ulcer patients to **avoid milk** because recent studies show that milk increases gastric acid secretion. Also, because milk leaves the stomach quickly, it lacks an extended buffering action.

(2) Small, frequent meals, also previously recommended, can worsen ulcer pain by causing acid rebound 2–4 hours after eating.

b. **Current dietary guidelines** emphasize avoiding foods and beverages known to exacerbate gastric discomfort or to promote acid secretion. This category typically includes coffee, caffeinated beverages, and alcohol.

c. **Smoking.** Patients who smoke should be encouraged to quit because smoking markedly slows ulcer healing, even during optimal ulcer therapy.

d. **NSAIDs** should be avoided by ulcer patients.

2. **Surgery.** An ulcer patient who develops complications may require surgery—sometimes on an emergency basis (see III). Incapacitating recurrent ulcers also may warrant surgery.

a. **Types of surgical procedures** for ulcer disease include antrectomy and truncal vagotomy (Billroth I procedure), partial gastrectomy and truncal vagotomy (Billroth II procedure), highly selective (proximal gastric) vagotomy, and total gastrectomy (the treatment of choice for Zollinger-Ellison syndrome that is unresponsive to medical management).

b. A **vagotomy** severs a branch of the vagus nerve, thereby decreasing HCl secretion. An **antrectomy,** by removing the antrum, eliminates some acid-secreting mucosa as well as the major source of gastrin.

C. The general indications for antireflux surgery are failure of medical therapy to heal or prevent relapse of erosive esophagitis, inability of medical therapy to prevent recurrence of stricture, or a patient whose lifestyle is adversely affected by need for medical therapy. **Fundoplication** successfully relieves symptoms and heals lesions in approximately 85% of patients.

III. COMPLICATIONS.

Complications of peptic ulcer disease cause approximately 7000 deaths in the United States annually.

A. Hemorrhage.

This life-threatening condition develops from widespread gastric mucosal irritation or ulceration with acute bleeding.

1. **Clinical features.** The patient may vomit fresh blood or a coffee-grounds–like substance. Other signs include passage of bloody or tarry stools, diaphoresis, and syncope. With major blood loss, manifestations of **hypovolemic shock** may appear: The pulse rate may exceed 110, or systolic blood pressure may drop below 100.

2. **Management**

a. Patient stabilization, bleeding cessation, and measures to prevent further bleeding are crucial.

(1) Airway, breathing, and circulation must be ensured.

(2) IV crystalloids and colloids (e.g., hetastarch) should be infused as needed.

(3) The patient's electrolyte status must be monitored and any imbalances corrected promptly.

b. **Gastric lavage** may be performed via a nasogastric or orogastric tube; iced saline solution is instilled until the aspirate returns free of blood.

c. Vasoconstrictors, antacids, or H_2-receptor antagonists may be administered. **Vasopressin,** an agent that causes contraction of the GI smooth muscle, may be given to constrict vessels and control bleeding.

d. **Emergency surgery** usually is indicated if the patient does not respond to medical management.

B. Perforation.

Penetration of a peptic ulcer through the gastric or duodenal wall results in this acute emergency. Perforation most commonly occurs with ulcers located in the anterior duodenal wall.

1. **Clinical features.** Sudden acute upper abdominal pain, rigidity, guarding, rebound tenderness, and absent or diminished bowel sounds are typical manifestations. Several hours after

onset, symptoms may abate somewhat; this apparent remission is dangerously misleading because peritonitis and shock may ensue.

2. **Management.** Emergency surgery is almost always necessary.

C. **Obstruction.** Inflammatory edema, spasm, and scarring may lead to obstruction of the duodenal or gastric outlet. The pylorus and proximal duodenum are the most common obstruction sites.

1. **Clinical features.** Typical patient complaints include postprandial vomiting or bloating, appetite and weight loss, and abdominal distention. Tympany and a succussion splash may be audible on physical examination. Gastric aspiration after an overnight fast typically yields more than 200 ml of food residue or clear fluid contents. (Gastric cancer must be ruled out as the cause of obstruction.)

2. **Management**
   a. **Conservative measures** (as in routine ulcer therapy) are indicated in most cases of obstruction.
   b. Patients with marked obstruction may require **continuous gastric suction** with careful monitoring of fluid and electrolyte status. A **saline load test** may be performed after 72 hours of continuous suction to test the degree of residual obstruction.
   c. If less than 200 ml of gastric contents are aspirated, liquid feedings can begin. **Aspiration** is performed at least daily for the next few days to monitor for retention and to guide dietary modifications as the patient progresses to a full regular diet.
   d. **Surgery** is indicated if medical management fails.

D. **Postsurgical complications**

1. **Dumping syndrome.** Affecting about 10% of patients who have undergone partial gastrectomy, this disorder is characterized by rapid gastric emptying.
   a. **Causes.** The mechanism underlying dumping syndrome is poorly defined. However, intestinal exposure to hypertonic chyme may play a key role by triggering rapid shifts of fluid from the plasma to the intestinal lumen.
   b. **Clinical features.** The patient may experience weakness, dizziness, anxiety, tachycardia, flushing, sweating, abdominal cramps, nausea, vomiting, and diarrhea.
      (1) Manifestations may develop 15–30 minutes after a meal (early dumping syndrome) or 90–120 minutes after a meal (late dumping syndrome).
      (2) Reactive hypoglycemia may partly account for some cases of late dumping syndrome.
   c. **Management.** The patient usually is advised to eat six small meals of high protein and fat content and low carbohydrate content. Fluids should be ingested 1 hour before or after a meal but never with a meal. **Anticholinergics** may be given to slow food passage into the intestine.

2. **Other postsurgical complications** include reflux gastritis, afferent blind loop syndrome, stomal ulceration, diarrhea, malabsorption, early satiety, and iron deficiency anemia.

E. **Refractory ulcers.** Ulcers that fail to heal on a prolonged course of drug treatment should not be confused with ulcers that recur after therapy is stopped. It is difficult to predict which patients will have a refractory ulcer.

1. **Differential diagnosis.** Any compliant patient who continues to have dyspeptic symptoms after 8 weeks of therapy should have gastroscopy and biopsy to exclude rare causes of ulceration in the duodenum, such as Crohn's disease, tuberculosis, lymphoma, pulmonary or secondary carcinoma, and cytomegalovirus (CMV) infection in immunodeficient patients. Fasting plasma gastrin concentration should be measured to exclude the Zollinger-Ellison syndrome.

2. **Treatment**
   a. Available data indicate that only maximum acid inhibition, with a regimen such as omeprazole (20 mg bid), offers advantage over continued therapy with standard antiulcer regimens.
   b. Eradication of *H. pylori* infection, when present, is likely to facilitate healing and alter the natural history of refractory ulcers.

c. Every effort should be made to discover and reduce or eliminate NSAID use.
d. Perform surgery.

F. Maintenance regimens

1. Despite healing after withdrawal of therapy, 70% of ulcers recur in 1 year, and 90% in 2 years. Similarly, erosive esophagitis will recur in more than 80% of individuals within 1 year after discontinuation of antisecretory therapy.

2. Candidates for long-term maintenance therapy include patients with serious concomitant diseases; four relapses per year; or a combination of risk factors, producing a more severe natural history of peptic disease (e.g., old age, male sex, a long history of aspirin or NSAID use, heavy alcohol intake, cigarette smoking, a history of peptic ulcer disease in an immediate relative, high maximal acid output, and a history of ulcer complications).

3. Patients with confirmed ulcer disease should be evaluated for presence of *H. pylori.* Eradication of *H. pylori* minimizes the recurrence of ulcer disease. Patients with a history of complicated ulcer disease should have *H. pylori* eradication confirmed.

STUDY QUESTIONS

Directions: Each of the numbered items or incomplete statements in this section is followed by answers or by completions of the statement. Select the **one** lettered answer or completion that is **best** in each case.

1. Which of the following organisms has been implicated as a possible cause of chronic gastritis and peptic ulcer disease?

(A) *Campylobacter jejuni*
(B) *Escherichia coli*
(C) *Helicobacter pylori*
(D) *Calymmatobacterium granulomatis*
(E) *Giardia lamblia*

2. All of the following statements concerning antacid therapy used in the treatment of duodenal or gastric ulcers are correct EXCEPT

(A) antacids may be used to heal the ulcer but are ineffective in controlling ulcer pain
(B) antacids neutralize acid and decrease the activity of pepsin
(C) if used alone for ulcer therapy, antacids should be administered 1 hour and 3 hours after meals and at bedtime
(D) if diarrhea occurs, the patient may alternate the antacid product with aluminum hydroxide
(E) calcium carbonate should be avoided because it causes acid rebound and induces constipation

3. As part of a comprehensive management strategy to treat peptic ulcer disease, patients should be encouraged to do all of the following EXCEPT

(A) decrease caffeine ingestion
(B) eat only bland foods
(C) stop smoking
(D) avoid alcohol
(E) avoid the use of milk as a treatment modality

4. A gastric ulcer patient requires close follow-up to document complete ulcer healing because

(A) perforation into the intestine is common
(B) spontaneous healing of the ulcer may occur in 30%–50% of cases
(C) there is the risk of the ulcer being cancerous
(D) symptoms tend to be chronic and recur
(E) weight loss may be severe in gastric ulcer patients

Directions: Each item below contains three suggested answers, of which **one or more** is correct. Choose the answer

A if **I only** is correct
B if **III only** is correct
C if **I and II** are correct
D if **II and III** are correct
E if **I, II, and III** are correct

5. Correct statements concerning cigarette smoking and ulcer disease include which of the following?

I. Smoking delays healing of gastric and duodenal ulcers
II. Nicotine decreases biliary and pancreatic bicarbonate secretion
III. Smoking accelerates the emptying of stomach acid into the duodenum

6. When administered at the same time, antacids can decrease the therapeutic efficacy of which of the following drugs?

I. Sucralfate
II. Ranitidine
III. Cimetidine

Directions: The group of items in this section consists of lettered options followed by a set of numbered items. For each item, select the **one** lettered option that is most closely associated with it. Each lettered option may be selected once, more than once, or not at all.

Questions 7–11

For each effect, select the agent that is most likely associated with it.

(A) Sodium bicarbonate
(B) Aluminum hydroxide
(C) Calcium carbonate
(D) Magnesium hydroxide
(E) Propantheline

7. May cause diarrhea

8. Cannot be used by patients with heart failure

9. Use with milk and an alkaline substance can cause milk-alkali syndrome

10. May cause dry mouth

11. Can be alternated with an antacid mixture to control diarrhea

ANSWERS AND EXPLANATIONS

1. The answer is C *[I E 1].*
Helicobacter pylori commonly is found in patients with peptic ulcer disease and always in association with chronic gastritis. Elimination of the organism has resulted in healing of the gastritis and the duodenal ulcer. More data, however, are needed before a definitive cause-and-effect relationship can be established.

2. The answer is A *[II A 1].*
Antacids have been shown to heal peptic ulcers, and their main use in modern therapy is to control ulcer pain. Antacids should be taken 1 hour and 3 hours after meals because the meal prolongs the acid-buffering effect of the antacid. If diarrhea becomes a problem with antacid use, an aluminum hydroxide product can be alternated with the antacid mixture; this takes advantage of the constipating property of aluminum. Because calcium carbonate causes acid rebound and constipation, its use should be avoided.

3. The answer is B *[II B 1 a (1)].*
Bland food diets are no longer recommended in the treatment of ulcer disease because research indicates that bland or milk-based diets do not accelerate ulcer healing. Studies show that patients can eat almost anything; however, they should avoid foods that aggravate their ulcer symptoms.

4. The answer is C *[I D 6].*
Five percent to ten percent of gastric ulcers may be due to cancer. The ulcer may respond to therapy; however, failure of the ulcer to decrease satisfactorily in size and to heal with therapy may suggest cancer. Close follow-up is necessary to document complete ulcer healing.

5. The answer is E (all) *[I E 3; II B 1 c].*
Clinical studies have shown that smoking increases susceptibility to ulcer disease, impairs spontaneous and drug-induced healing, and increases the risk and rapidity of recurrence of the ulcer. These findings may result in part from nicotine's ability to decrease biliary and pancreatic bicarbonate secretion, thus decreasing the body's ability to neutralize acid in the duodenum. Also, the accelerated emptying of stomach acid into the duodenum may predispose to duodenal ulcer and may decrease healing rates.

6. The answer is E (all) *[II A 1 e (3), 3 d].*
The mean peak blood concentration of cimetidine and the area under the 4-hour cimetidine blood concentration curve were both reduced significantly when cimetidine was administered at the same time as an antacid. The absorption of ranitidine is also reduced when it is taken concurrently with an aluminum magnesium hydroxide antacid mixture. To avoid this interaction, the antacid should be administered 1 hour before or 2 hours after the administration of cimetidine or ranitidine. Antacids may reduce mucosal binding of sucralfate, decreasing its therapeutic efficacy. Antacids should, therefore, be given 30–60 minutes before or after sucralfate.

7–11. The answers are: 7-D *[II A 1 b (3)],* **8-A** *[II A 1 d (2)],* **9-C** *[II A 1 d (5)],* **10-E** *[II A 4 c (1)],* **11-B** *[II A 1 b (3)].*
Magnesium-containing products tend to cause diarrhea, possibly because of magnesium's ability to stimulate the secretion of bile acids by the gallbladder. Because of its sodium content, sodium bicarbonate is contraindicated in patients with congestive heart failure (CHF), hypertension, severe renal disease, and edema. Sodium bicarbonate is no longer used in peptic ulcer therapy. In addition to causing acid rebound, calcium carbonate, if taken with milk and an alkaline substance for long periods, may cause the milk-alkali syndrome. It also may cause adverse effects such as hypercalcemia, alkalosis, azotemia, and nephrocalcinosis. Propantheline, like other anticholinergic agents, may cause dry mouth, blurred vision, urinary retention, and constipation. These agents sometimes are used as adjuncts to relieve duodenal ulcer pain. They are contraindicated in gastric ulcer because they delay gastric emptying. Aluminum hydroxide is constipating and can be alternated with the patient's current antacid when that antacid product is causing diarrhea.

52
Diabetes Mellitus

Helen L. Figge

I. INTRODUCTION

A. Definition. Diabetes mellitus (DM) refers to a group of disorders characterized by absent or deficient insulin secretion or peripheral insulin resistance, resulting in hyperglycemia and impaired metabolism.

B. Classification. DM occurs in two major forms.

1. **Type I: Insulin-dependent DM** (IDDM, formerly known as juvenile-onset or ketosis-prone diabetes)
   a. This form is most common in children and in adults up to age 30 years but may occur at any age.
   b. Type I diabetic patients are predisposed to **ketoacidosis**—accumulation of ketone bodies in body tissues and fluids.
   c. Disease onset is sudden.
   d. Beta cells, insulin-producing cells of the pancreatic islets of Langerhans, are destroyed, causing **absolute insulin deficiency.**
   e. All type I diabetic patients require insulin replacement therapy.

2. **Type II: Non–insulin-dependent DM** (formerly called adult-onset diabetes; may be insulin requiring)
   a. Most type II diabetic patients are over 40 years old and obese.
   b. Disease onset typically is gradual.
   c. In most cases, type II DM is characterized by **insensitivity to insulin in the target tissues, deficient response of pancreatic beta cells to glucose,** or both.
   d. Because some insulin is secreted, ketoacidosis is prevented.
   e. Only a minority of type II diabetic patients require insulin replacement therapy.

C. Incidence. In the United States, DM affects an estimated 1%–5% of the population. Type I DM accounts for approximately 10% of cases; type II, for about 90% of cases.

D. Etiology. Various factors are thought to contribute to the development of DM.

1. **Type I DM.** Genetic predisposition, environmental factors, and autoimmunity have been proposed.
   a. **Genetics.** Certain genetic markers in the human leukocyte antigen (HLA) system have been strongly linked with type I DM. In addition, many patients have a family history of the disease; that is, 50% of individuals having an identical twin with type I DM also have diabetes.
   b. **Environment.** Viruses (e.g., rubella) and toxic chemicals are among the environmental factors that researchers believe may affect the pancreas and cause beta cell destruction in individuals who are genetically predisposed to DM.
   c. **Autoimmunity.** An autoimmune component is suggested by the presence of antibodies to islet-cell antigens in most new-onset type I diabetic patients. Much evidence has accumulated to support the autoimmune hypothesis. Both humoral and cell-mediated abnormalities have been described. An abnormal immune response could cause the body to destroy beta cells because it has misidentified them as foreign.

2. **Type II DM.** Genetic factors and a beta cell or peripheral site defect have been implicated.
   a. **Genetics.** Nearly all identical twins of patients with type II DM also have the disease. A high percentage of other type II diabetic patients have a strong family history of the disease.

b. A **beta cell defect** is postulated to cause abnormalities in insulin secretion resulting in a relative deficiency of insulin.

c. A **peripheral site defect** is postulated to lead to insulin resistance—tissue insensitivity to the action of insulin. This condition is thought to result from a post-receptor defect.

3. Secondary diabetes may arise from such conditions as endocrine disorders (e.g., Cushing's syndrome), pregnancy, pancreatic disease, and use of drugs that antagonize insulin (e.g., thiazide diuretics, adrenocorticosteroids).

E. Pathophysiology. In untreated type I and type II DM, the disease follows a typical progression.

1. Without adequate insulin, which stimulates glucose transports across cell membranes, glucose transport to most cells diminishes. Also, the conversion of glucose to glycogen diminishes. As a result, glucose is trapped in the bloodstream and **hyperglycemia** occurs. Some glucose also spills into the urine.

2. Hyperglycemia leads to **osmotic diuresis** and subsequent **dehydration** and **electrolyte abnormalities.**

3. In type I DM, without insulin to stimulate glucose uptake, cells must use protein and fat as energy sources.

a. Fat is broken down into **free fatty acids** and **glycerol.**

b. In the liver, free fatty acids are further broken down into **ketone bodies.**

c. Breakdown is so rapid that excessive ketone bodies spill into the bloodstream. (In type II DM, however, the presence of some insulin prevents ketonemia.)

d. Increased amounts of glycerol, another by-product of fat metabolism, worsen hyperglycemia.

F. Clinical evaluation

1. Physical findings. Type I DM has an abrupt onset and, in some cases, an acute presentation. With type II DM, symptoms develop gradually; some patients are asymptomatic or have only mild symptoms.

a. Classic signs and symptoms of untreated DM include polydipsia (excessive thirst), polyuria (excessive urination), and polyphagia (excessive hunger). Other common findings are dry, itchy skin; frequent skin and vaginal infections; and visual disturbances.

b. In addition to the above, the person with type I DM may present with fatigue, weakness, and unintentional weight loss, with or without signs and symptoms of ketoacidosis (see III A 1).

c. The person with type II DM may present with hyperosmolar coma.

d. Symptom severity and onset help differentiate type I and type II DM.

e. Long-standing DM causes typical progressive changes in the retina, kidneys, nervous system, cardiovascular system, and integumentary system. For physical findings reflecting these changes, see III B.

2. Laboratory findings

a. The diagnosis of DM is confirmed by a **fasting blood glucose level of 140 mg/dl or more** on at least two occasions.

b. If the fasting blood glucose level is normal (below 140 mg/dl) but the patient has suggestive signs and symptoms, an **oral glucose tolerance test (OGTT)** should be done.

(1) Glucose (75 g), dissolved in 300 ml of water, is given after a 12-hour fast.

(2) A blood glucose level of 200 mg/dl or more at 2 hours and in at least one earlier sample after the glucose dose is administered confirms DM.

c. A **random blood glucose level of 200 mg/dl** or more also confirms DM.

d. Reversible factors that promote hyperglycemia (e.g., increased calorie intake, pregnancy, certain medications) should be ruled out before a diagnosis of DM is established.

G. Treatment objectives

1. To maintain optimal health, thus permitting a productive life

2. To equalize the supply of and demand for insulin to prevent symptomatic hyperglycemia and hypoglycemia

3. To avoid acute disease complications (e.g., ketosis)

4. To prevent or minimize complications of long-standing disease
5. To teach the patient about the disease and ensure therapeutic compliance

II. THERAPY. Diet, drug therapy, exercise, glucose monitoring, patient education, and self-care are crucial in the management of DM.

A. Diet. All people with diabetes must eat a well-balanced diet to regulate blood glucose. **People with type I DM** must **eat at properly spaced intervals. Those with type II DM**—most of whom are obese—should follow a **weight-reduction diet** (increased weight is associated with more pronounced hyperglycemia). Dietary therapy alone is sufficient to control hyperglycemia in many type II patients.

1. Intake of **carbohydrates, proteins,** and **fats** should be regulated, with carbohydrates accounting for 45%–50% of total caloric intake, proteins accounting for 15%–20%, and fats accounting for 35%–40%.
2. **Refined** and **simple sugars** should be avoided.
3. High intake of **fiber** (e.g., bran, beans, fruits, vegetables) seems to improve blood glucose control.
4. **Cholesterol** intake is limited to less than 300 mg/day.
5. The **food exchange system** increases flexibility in meal planning. This system lists equivalent carbohydrate, protein, and fat values for foods in six basic groups.
6. The glycemic index, another meal planning aid, categorizes carbohydrates according to the blood glucose level they produce after ingestion; the lower the level, the lower a given carbohydrate's glycemic index. Although this system may allow the patient with diabetes to select carbohydrates more carefully, researchers debate its value because the glycemic index of carbohydrates may change when they are consumed along with proteins or fats.
7. Factors that change the blood glucose level (e.g., stress, exercise) necessitate dietary adjustment. For example, before vigorous exercise, the diabetic should consume 30–40 g of a complex carbohydrate, plus protein.

B. Drug therapy. Insulin, sulfonylureas, and metformin are used in the treatment of DM.

1. **Insulin**
   a. **Indications.** Insulin replacement therapy is indicated for all patients with type I DM and for those with type II DM whose hyperglycemia does not respond to dietary or oral antihyperglycemic drug therapy.
   b. **Mechanism of action.** Insulin lowers the blood glucose level by increasing glucose transport across cell membranes, enhancing glucose conversion to glycogen, inhibiting release of free fatty acids from adipose tissue, and inhibiting lipolysis and glycogenolysis.
   c. **Choice of agent**
      (1) **Source.** Commercial insulin is derived from three principal sources: beef, pork, and biosynthetic human insulin (produced by recombinant DNA techniques). Use of human insulin in the majority of patients with diabetes is preferred because of its reduced antigenicity.
      (2) **Concentration.** Most insulins come in a concentration of 100 units/ml (U100), dispensed in 10-ml vials.
         (a) Concentrated insulin preparations (U500) are available for patients with insulin resistance.
         (b) Children and adults requiring small insulin quantities may use U40 insulin.
      (3) **Preparations**
         (a) **Three major types of insulin** differ in onset and duration of action (Table 52-1).
            (i) **Fast-acting insulin products** include **regular** and **semilente insulin** (insulin zinc suspension).
            (ii) **Intermediate-acting insulin products** include **lente** and **NPH** (isophane insulin suspension).
            (iii) **Long-acting insulin products** include **PZI** (protamine zinc insulin) and **ultralente** (extended insulin zinc suspension).

Table 52-1. Major Characteristics of Insulin Preparations

Preparation	Onset of Action (Hours)	Peak Effect (Hours)	Duration of Action (Hours)
Fast-acting insulins			
Regular	0.25–1	2–6	4–12
Semilente	0.5–1	3–6	8–16
Intermediate-acting insulins			
Lente	1–4	6–16	12–28
NPH	1.5–4	6–16	12–24
Long-acting insulins			
PZI	3–8	14–24	24–48
Ultralente	4	18–24	36

NPH = isophane insulin suspension; *PZI* = protamine zinc insulin.

(b) Insulin mixtures. Some patients with diabetes need a mixture of insulin types (e.g., a rapid-acting insulin to control morning hyperglycemia and an intermediate-acting insulin to control later hyperglycemia).

(i) Insulin may be mixed by the patient or bought in a premixed form (e.g., Novolin 70/30, consisting of 70% NPH insulin and 30% regular insulin).

(ii) Insulins mixed together should be of the same concentration.

d. Administration and dosage. For routine use, insulin is administered by **subcutaneous injection.**

(1) The subcutaneous injection site should be rotated to avoid lipohypertrophy and fibrosis. However, to prevent variations in drug absorption, injections should be given within the same region (e.g., the abdomen).

(2) Patients with acute hyperglycemia or ketoacidosis may require continuous intravenous administration with regular insulin (insulin drip).

(3) Insulin pump. This delivery method, which provides tighter glycemic control, is indicated for selected diabetic patients who need long-term therapy, who have widely fluctuating blood glucose levels, or whose life-styles preclude regular meals. However, there is a risk of developing serious hypoglycemia when using a pump.

(a) The **closed-loop pump** senses and responds to changing blood glucose levels. Through a subcutaneous needle in the thigh or abdominal wall, the pump administers appropriate amounts of insulin continuously. Because it requires blood aspiration, it can be used only in a hospital setting.

(b) The **open-loop pump** does not have a glucose sensor. It infuses insulin in small continuous doses and in large doses that the patient releases when appropriate (e.g., before meals).

e. Precautions and monitoring effects

(1) Improper insulin therapy may induce **hypoglycemia,** especially in patients with unpredictable changes in insulin requirements. Other causes of hypoglycemia include skipping meals, vigorous exercise, and accidental insulin overdose.

(a) To reverse insulin hypoglycemia in an **unresponsive patient,** glucose may be injected intravenously or honey or a glucose product (e.g., Glutose) may be inserted into the patient's buccal pouch. In addition, glucagon may be given subcutaneously, intramuscularly, or intravenously at a dose of 0.5–1 unit (0.5–1 mg).

(b) A **conscious patient** may be given a food or a beverage containing a simple, fast-acting carbohydrate (e.g., candy, fruit juice) to raise the blood glucose level. Patients should be counseled not to use diet beverages to treat a reaction.

(2) Two types of **insulin reactions** may occur—reactions with **adrenergic symptoms** (e.g., diaphoresis, tachycardia) or reactions with **neuroglycopenia** (e.g., confusion, irritability, loss of consciousness, weakness).

(a) Patients with adrenergic symptoms are usually aware of the fact that they are having a reaction.

(b) Patients with neuroglycopenia may have hypoglycemic unawareness and are at risk for loss of consciousness and seizures. These patients should never be tightly controlled.

(3) Local or systemic **insulin allergy** may occur, particularly after the first dose. Manifestations include allergic urticaria, anaphylaxis, and angioedema.

(4) **Lipoatrophy** (subcutaneous fat loss triggered by an immune reaction) may occur at the injection site. Pure insulin forms have reduced the incidence of this adverse reaction.

(5) **Lipohypertrophy** and **fibrosis** may develop in patients who do not rotate injection sites.

(6) **Insulin resistance** is defined as the need for more than 200 units/day of insulin (in the absence of ketoacidosis). This condition may result from obesity, infection, glucocorticoid excess, or a high concentration of circulating immunoglobulin G (IgG) anti-insulin antibodies.

(a) Nearly all patients receiving insulin develop such antibodies; however, in cases of insulin resistance, serum insulin-binding capacity usually exceeds 30 units/L.

(b) The condition may resolve spontaneously. In some cases, though, it necessitates a switch to a less antigenic insulin (e.g., to pork or human insulin), use of multiple injections of regular insulin rather than an intermediate-acting product, or prednisone therapy (60 mg/day) to suppress the immune response.

(7) Too much insulin can cause the **Somogyi effect** (insulin rebound syndrome). In this syndrome, nocturnal hypoglycemia stimulates a surge of counterregulatory hormones, triggering morning hyperglycemia.

(8) Various factors may change a diabetic patient's insulin requirements. Regular glucose self-monitoring is needed to evaluate changing insulin requirements and therapeutic efficacy (see II D, E).

(a) Infection, weight gain, puberty, inactivity, hyperthyroidism, and Cushing's disease tend to increase insulin needs.

(b) Renal failure, adrenal insufficiency, malabsorption, hypopituitarism, weight loss, and increased exercise tend to reduce insulin needs.

(9) PZI and regular insulin must not be mixed together in the same syringe.

f. Significant interactions

(1) A decreased response to insulin may occur when **corticosteroids, nicotinic acid,** or **thiazide diuretics** are administered concomitantly.

(2) Hypoglycemic effects may increase, leading to prolonged hypoglycemia, with concomitant use of insulin and **monoamine oxidase (MAO) inhibitors, β-blockers, salicylates, oxytetracycline, fenfluramine,** alcohol, **sulfonylureas,** or **pentamidine.**

2. **Sulfonylureas (oral hypoglycemics)** are used to control hyperglycemia in selected patients with type II diabetes.

a. **Indications.** These drugs help to reduce blood glucose levels in type II DM that does not respond to diet alone. Because the action of sulfonylureas seems to depend on functioning beta cells, these drugs should never be used in people with type I DM.

b. **Mechanism of action.** As an acute action, sulfonylureas stimulate beta cell tissue to secrete insulin. In the long term, these drugs appear to reduce cellular insulin resistance.

c. **Choice of agent. First-generation sulfonylureas** include **acetohexamide, chlorpropamide, tolbutamide,** and **tolazamide. Second-generation agents,** considerably more potent, include **glipizide** and **glyburide.** The most clinically significant difference among sulfonylureas is duration of action (Table 52-2).

(1) **Tolbutamide,** with the shortest duration, is administered mainly to elderly patients with type II DM for whom hypoglycemia is a more serious complication.

(2) **Acetohexamide, tolazamide, glipizide,** and **glyburide** have intermediate durations of action. (The duration of acetohexamide is prolonged in renal disease.)

(3) **Chlorpropamide** has the longest duration of action and poses a risk to patients with renal or hepatic impairment. It also causes more severe and frequent side effects (including hypoglycemia and hyponatremia) than the other sulfonylureas.

d. **Administration and dosage** (see Table 52-2)

e. **Precautions and monitoring effects**

(1) Sulfonylureas are contraindicated in patients without functioning beta cells, children, pregnant and lactating women, and patients with allergy to sulfa agents. They also are contraindicated during stressful conditions that increase the risk of hyper- or hypoglycemia.

(2) These agents should not be used in patients with severe renal or hepatic impairment.

(3) Sulfonylurea therapy has been associated with a possible increased risk of cardiovascular mortality and morbidity.

Table 52-2. Dosages and Other Characteristics of Sulfonylureas

Agent	Usual Daily Dosage (mg)	Number of Daily Doses	Duration of Action (Hours)	Activity of Hepatic Metabolites
First-generation agents				
Acetohexamide	250–1500	1–2	12–18	Two and a half times more active than original
Chlorpropamide	100–500	1	60	Active
Tolazamide	100–1000	1–2	12–14	Three inactive, three weak
Tolbutamide	500–3000	2–3	6–12	Inactive
Second-generation agents				
Glipizide	2.5–40	1–2	24	Inactive
Glyburide	1.25–20	1–2	24	Mostly inactive

(4) Hypoglycemia and alcohol intolerance may occur during sulfonylurea therapy. Alcohol tolerance is less common with second-generation agents.

(5) Sulfonylureas should not be discontinued without a physician's approval.

(6) Untoward reactions to sulfonylureas include gastrointestinal (GI) disturbances (e.g., nausea, gastric discomfort, vomiting, constipation), tachycardia, headache, skin rash, and hematologic problems (e.g., agranulocytosis, pancytopenia, hemolytic anemia).

(7) Sulfonylureas pose a risk of cholestatic jaundice.

(8) Sulfonylurea therapy has a relatively **high failure rate** (25%–40%).

(a) **Primary therapeutic failure.** The agent fails to control hyperglycemia within the first 4 weeks after initiation.

(b) **Secondary therapeutic failure.** The drug controls hyperglycemia initially but fails to maintain control. Approximately 5%–30% of initial responders experience secondary therapeutic failure. There is generally no reason to continue sulfonylurea therapy once insulin therapy has been initiated in such patients.

f. Significant interactions

(1) Prolonged hypoglycemia and masking of hypoglycemia symptoms may occur with concomitant use of **β-blockers** and **clonidine.**

(2) **Alcohol, salicylates, nonsteroidal anti-inflammatory drugs (NSAIDs), methyldopa, chloramphenicol, warfarin, MAO inhibitors, probenecid,** and **ranitidine** may intensify the hypoglycemic effects of sulfonylureas.

(3) A decreased hypoglycemic response may occur with concomitant use of **corticosteroids, aminophylline, bleomycin, thiazide diuretics, ethacrynic acid, levodopa, rifampin, phenytoin,** and **oral contraceptives.**

3. Metformin HCl is used to control hyperglycemia in selected type II diabetic patients.

a. Indications. Use as monotherapy when diet alone does not control type II DM. Can be used in combination with a sulfonylurea when diet plus a single agent do not control hyperglycemia.

b. Mechanism of action. Metformin is a biguanide and is not related to the sulfonylureas. The drug decreases hepatic glucose production, decreases intestinal absorption of glucose, and increases peripheral glucose uptake and utilization. Combination therapy with metformin and a sulfonylurea agent may have a synergistic effect.

c. Administration and dosage. Dosage ranges from 500 mg orally twice a day to 850 mg orally three times a day (maximum recommended dose of 2550 mg total per day).

d. Precautions and monitoring effects

(1) Contraindicated in cases of renal dysfunction or in patients receiving iodinated contrast agents for radiologic studies which can cause transient renal dysfunction.

(2) Lactic acidosis is a rare but serious complication and is fatal in 50% of cases.

(3) Avoid metformin in patients with clinical or laboratory evidence of impaired hepatic function.

(4) Should not be used in patients with type I diabetes.

(5) Use with caution in the elderly.

(6) Safety in pregnancy and lactation has not been established.

(7) Renal function should be monitored periodically.

(8) Untoward reactions include GI symptoms, which are most common with initiation of treatment. Serum B12 levels may decline.

e. **Significant interactions.** Alcohol, cationic drugs, cimetidine, furosemide, nifedipine, and iodinated contrast material can result in increased activity.

C. **Exercise.** A carefully planned and religiously followed exercise program enhances glucose uptake to cells, thereby reducing the blood glucose level. Patients with severe retinopathy must consult an ophthalmologist before starting to exercise.

1. **Aerobic exercise** (e.g., swimming, walking, running) has a desirable hypoglycemic effect because it uses glucose as fuel; aerobic exercise also promotes cardiovascular health.

2. **Anaerobic exercise** (e.g., weight-lifting) should be avoided by people with diabetes because it induces stress that leads to increased blood glucose levels. Also, anaerobic exercise may cause deleterious cardiovascular effects (e.g., increased blood pressure).

D. **Glucose monitoring.** Frequent measurement of the blood glucose level is a key aspect of DM therapy. It helps determine therapeutic efficacy, guides and refines any adjustments to drug therapy, and, when performed by the patient at home, permits better understanding of the glycemic effects of specific foods.

1. **Urine glucose testing** is generally no longer recommended; it has been replaced by blood glucose testing.

2. **Blood glucose testing.** This type of testing is generally indicated for all people with diabetes. Blood glucose tests are more reliable than urine glucose tests.

a. Some patients (especially those with type I diabetes) need to measure their blood glucose level several times daily—typically before or after meals.

b. Well-controlled type II diabetic patients may require monitoring once or twice a week.

c. **Test methods and products**

(1) **Reagent strips** (e.g., Chemstrip bG, Dextrostix, Visidex II) are visual tests in which a blood droplet is applied to the test strip.

(2) **Glucose meters** (multiple brands) are more accurate and convenient to use than reagent strips because they give a numerical blood glucose value.

(3) The **hemoglobin A_{1c} test** (also known as the **glycohemoglobin** or **glycosylated hemoglobin test**) shows long-term glycemic control and serves as an index of therapeutic efficacy or compliance.

(a) A hemoglobin variant produced by glycosylation or hemoglobin A, hemoglobin A_{1c} is more abundant in diabetic patients than in nondiabetic ones.

(b) The hemoglobin A_{1c} level reflects the average blood glucose level over the preceding 6–8 weeks.

(c) A hemoglobin A_{1c} level of 7.5% or lower indicates good glycemic control; a level of 9.0% or higher reflects poor control.

(d) Patients with underlying hemoglobinopathies will have anomalous values.

3. Urine ketone monitoring should be performed if blood sugars are high or if the patient is acutely ill.

E. **Patient education and self-care.** Patient education about the disease and patient participation in medical care are important aspects of DM management.

1. **Patient education** improves understanding of the disease, thereby promoting compliance with dietary, drug, and exercise regimens and glucose self-monitoring. Patients also must be taught how to prevent, recognize, and treat hypoglycemia and hyperglycemia.

2. **Self-care measures** are necessary to avoid the potentially dire consequences of trauma and skin abrasions, resulting from disease complications, such as neuropathy and peripheral vascular compromise.

a. The patient must inspect the skin daily for abrasions, pain, or swelling, and see a physician promptly for treatment. Injuries should be covered immediately with sterile gauze.

b. Even minor trauma, especially to the legs and feet, should be avoided.

c. Daily foot cleansing should be performed using only soap and water (with a thermometer to check water temperature if the patient has neuropathy-induced sensation loss). Skin should be dried gently and vegetable oil applied.

d. Corns and calluses should be removed by a podiatrist.
e. Only properly fitting, low-heeled shoes should be worn.
f. Routine ophthalmology followup is essential for all diabetic patients.

F. **Pancreas and islet cell transplantation.** These experimental procedures may be performed to treat some cases of DM.

G. **Disease management in pregnancy.** Approximately 2%–3% of pregnant women with no history of DM develop diabetes or impaired glucose tolerance—presumably from the increased insulin requirements of pregnancy.

1. DM in pregnancy carries an increased risk of neonatal morbidity.
2. Tight glycemic control is especially important during pregnancy to avoid neonatal complications. Continuous insulin infusion (via an insulin pump) or multiple insulin injections may be required.
3. Sulfonylureas are contraindicated in pregnant women.
4. Weight reduction is not recommended because this could compromise fetal development.
5. Some experts advise inducing labor or performing a cesarean section at 37–38 weeks gestation.
6. Glucose tolerance usually normalizes within a few weeks after delivery.

III. COMPLICATIONS

A. **Acute complications.** Life-threatening complications of DM include diabetic ketoacidosis and hyperglycemic hyperosmolar nonketotic coma. Hypoglycemia, another acute complication, usually stems from drug therapy [see II B 1 e (1)].

1. **Diabetic ketoacidosis (DKA).** Usually affecting only patients with type I DM, this disorder typically arises after a short period (hours or days) of deteriorating glycemic control. Hyperglycemia and ketonemia trigger osmotic diuresis, electrolyte loss, hypovolemia, and metabolic acidosis. DKA is often the presenting disorder in children with previously undiagnosed type I DM.
   a. **Precipitating factors** include stress, infection, exercise, excessive alcohol consumption, improper insulin therapy, and dietary noncompliance—conditions that lead to an absence or deficiency of insulin.
   b. **Physical findings** include Kussmaul's respirations, acetone breath odor, dehydration, dry skin, poor skin turgor, reduced level of consciousness (ranging from confusion to coma), and abdominal pain. Without treatment, death ensues.
   c. **Laboratory findings** include elevated levels of blood glucose and ketone bodies (e.g., acetone, acetoacetate), low arterial pH and carbon dioxide partial pressure (Pco_2) values, and abnormal serum electrolyte values.
   d. **Therapy** involves fluid, intravenous insulin by continuous infusion, and electrolyte replacement.

2. **Hyperglycemic hyperosmolar nonketotic coma (HHNC),** which occurs in patients with type II DM, has a higher mortality rate than DKA.
   a. **Precipitating factors** include various illnesses and conditions that increase insulin requirements [e.g., severe burns, GI bleeding, central nervous system (CNS) injury, acute myocardial infarction].
      (1) Use of certain drugs (e.g., steroids, glucagon, thiazide diuretics, cimetidine, propranolol) also can trigger HHNC.
      (2) Such medical procedures as intravenous hyperalimentation and peritoneal dialysis increase the risk of HHNC.
   b. **Physical findings** include polyuria, polydipsia, dehydration, hypotension, rapid respirations, abdominal discomfort, nausea, vomiting, tachycardia, palpitations, focal neurologic signs, and reduced level of consciousness.
   c. **Laboratory findings** include an extremely elevated blood glucose level (800 mg/dl or higher) and a serum osmolarity of 280 mOsm/kg or more.
   d. **Therapy** involves fluid, insulin, and electrolyte replacement.

B. Chronic complications. DM is associated with a high risk for a number of chronic illnesses.

1. **Cardiovascular disease**
   a. Atherosclerosis and peripheral vascular disease are more severe and more common in diabetic patients than in nondiabetic ones; also, disease onset typically is earlier.
   b. Microvascular changes, characterized by thickening of the capillary basement membrane, may lead to retinopathy and skin changes.
   c. Diabetic patients with insulin resistance have a higher incidence of hypertension than nondiabetic ones.

2. **Ocular complications**
   a. Premature cataracts are most common in people with diabetes who have severe chronic hyperglycemia.
   b. Diabetic retinopathy, a consequence of microvascular changes, affects approximately 50% of diabetic patients within 10 years of disease onset.
      (1) This syndrome is the leading cause of new blindness in the United States.
      (2) Retinal microaneurysm, the earliest sign of retinopathy, may progress to punctate hemorrhage, exudation, and proliferative retinopathy.
      (3) Retinal detachment, secondary glaucoma, and vision loss may ensue.

3. **Diabetic nephropathy,** another manifestation of microvascular pathology, ultimately may lead to renal insufficiency or failure.
   a. Diabetic nephropathy is characterized by proteinuria, microalbuminuria, glomerular lesions, and renal arteriosclerosis.
   b. People with diabetes account for approximately 25% of patients with end-stage renal failure.

4. **Diabetic neuropathies** typically involve both the autonomic and peripheral nervous systems.
   a. Gastric atony, incontinence, diarrhea, and impotence reflect autonomic involvement.
   b. Peripheral neuropathy may give rise to impaired perception of pain and temperature (particularly in the lower extremities).
   c. Ischemia may cause skeletal muscle atrophy and motor abnormalities.

5. **Skin and mucous membrane complications** stem from vascular changes and neuropathy.
   a. Diabetic patients have an increased risk for infection, such as *Candida* infections of the skin and vagina. Erythema commonly develops beneath the breasts and between fingers; eruptive xanthomas occur most often in long-standing, poorly controlled DM.
   b. Atrophic lesions (round painless lesions) and diabetic dermopathy (reddish-brown papular spots) are common, especially on the lower extremities.
   c. An ulcerating necrotic lesion called **necrobiosis lipoidica diabeticorum** may develop on the anterior leg surface or the dorsum of the ankle.
   d. Injury, infection, neuropathy, vascular disease, or ischemia may lead to gangrene, which is 20 times more common in people with diabetes than in those who are not diabetic.

C. Prevention of chronic complications. The diabetes control and complications trial (DCCT) showed that the risk of retinopathy is significantly reduced in type I diabetic patients who achieve tight glucose control.

STUDY QUESTIONS

Directions: Each of the numbered items or incomplete statements in this section is followed by answers or by completions of the statement. Select the **one** lettered answer or completion that is **best** in each case.

1. Current criteria used in the diagnosis of diabetes mellitus (DM) include all of the following symptoms EXCEPT

(A) fasting hyperglycemia
(B) polyuria
(C) polydipsia
(D) tinnitus
(E) weight loss

2. The most useful glucose test used in monitoring diabetes mellitus (DM) therapy is

(A) urine monitoring
(B) blood monitoring
(C) renal function monitoring
(D) cardiovascular monitoring
(E) vascular monitoring

3. Which of the following statements concerning insulin replacement therapy is most likely true?

(A) Most commercial insulin products vary little with respect to time, course, and duration of hypoglycemic activity
(B) Regular insulins cannot be mixed with NPH (isophane insulin suspension)
(C) Regular insulin cannot be given intravenously
(D) Cutting down on carbohydrate consumption is a necessity for all diabetic patients
(E) Insulin therapy does not have to be monitored closely

4. A mass of adipose tissue that develops at the injection site is usually due to the patient's neglect in rotating the insulin injection site. This is known as

(A) lipoatrophy
(B) hypertrophic degenerative adiposity
(C) lipohypertrophy
(D) atrophic skin lesion
(E) dermatitis

5. Sulfonylureas are a primary mode of therapy in the treatment of

(A) insulin-dependent (type I) diabetes mellitus (IDDM) patients
(B) diabetic patients experiencing severe hepatic or renal dysfunction
(C) diabetic pregnant women
(D) patients with diabetic ketoacidosis
(E) non–insulin-dependent (type II) DM patients

6. Patients taking chlorpropamide should avoid products containing

(A) acetaminophen
(B) ethanol
(C) vitamin A
(D) penicillins
(E) milk products

7. The standard recommended dose of glyburide is

(A) 0.5–2 mg/day
(B) 1.25–20 mg/day
(C) 50–100 mg/day
(D) 200 mg/day
(E) 200–1000 mg/day

Questions 8–12

A 20-year-old previously healthy man presents to the emergency room with a 2-week history of polyuria, polydipsia, and a 20-lb unintentional weight loss. He complains of weakness, fatigue, nausea, and abdominal pain. Physical examination reveals dry, parched mucous membranes. Blood pressure is 110/70 and pulse is 90 supine; blood pressure is 90/60, and pulse is 120 upright. Temperature is 100°F (axillary); respiratory rate is 24. General examination of the heart and lungs is unremarkable. No retinopathy is present. The abdomen is soft with mild tenderness but no rebound. Laboratory values are as follows:

Blood glucose 420 mg/dl
Sodium (Na) 130 mEq/L(A)
Potassium (K) 3.7 mEq/L
Chloride (Cl) 97 mEq/L
Bicarbonate (HCO_3^-) 10 mEq/L
Arterial blood gas 7.20 (pH)
Urinalysis 3 + glucose and 3 + ketones
Chest radiograph Unremarkable
Abdominal radiograph (KUB) Unremarkable

8. What is the most likely diagnosis in this patient?

(A) Type II diabetes mellitus (DM) with hyperosmolar state
(B) Type I DM with diabetic ketoacidosis
(C) Type II DM without hyperosmolar state
(D) Type I DM without diabetic ketoacidosis

9. Initial appropriate therapy includes

(A) intravenous fluids and a sulfonylurea agent
(B) intravenous fluids alone
(C) intravenous fluids, 10 units of subcutaneous regular insulin, and discharge to home
(D) intravenous fluids, intravenous regular insulin by continuous drip at 6 units/hr, and hospital admission

10. After the acute illness has resolved, what further therapy would be appropriate?

(A) None, observe only
(B) Start a second-generation sulfonylurea
(C) Daily administration of a regimen of NPH (isophane insulin suspension) and regular insulin plus dietary modification
(D) Dietary modification alone

11. Appropriate follow-up of the patient once discharged to home includes all of the following EXCEPT

(A) periodic monitoring of hemoglobin A_{1c} levels
(B) periodic opthalmologic examinations
(C) home glucose monitoring with a glucose meter
(D) weight loss diet and an attempt to wean from insulin

12. The patient is at risk for developing all of the following complications EXCEPT

(A) hypoglycemia
(B) coronary artery disease
(C) retinopathy
(D) nonketotic hyperglycemia hyperosmolar state

ANSWERS AND EXPLANATIONS

1. The answer is D *[I E, F 1 a].*
Frequent urination (polyuria), thirst (polydipsia), and weight loss are all common signs of diabetes. When these symptoms are present, it is necessary to have a fasting blood glucose level drawn to determine a diabetic state. A fasting blood glucose level of 140 mg/dl or greater on more than one occasion is diagnostic of a diabetic state.

2. The answer is B *[II D 1, 2].*
Blood glucose monitoring is the most useful form of monitoring glucose levels. Urine monitoring provides only gross estimates of the current status and cannot rule out hypoglycemia. Renal function and cardiovascular functions provide evidence of long-standing disease and are not useful for monitoring daily progress.

3. The answer is D *[II A 1, B 1 c (3) (a)].*
Many commercial insulin preparations vary with respect to duration of activity and time for peak plasma level. Regular insulin can be mixed with NPH (isophane insulin suspension) and can be given intravenously. All insulin therapies should be monitored closely and on a daily basis. Careful regulation of carbohydrate intake is very important for all diabetic patients—carbohydrate consumption plays a major role in the balance of glucose metabolism and antagonizes the effects of insulin therapy.

4. The answer is C *[II B 1 e (5)].*
Lipohypertrophy consists of masses of adipose tissue that develop at the injection site, usually in patients who do not rotate the injection sites properly. The masses gradually disappear if injection in these sites is avoided.

5. The answer is E *[II B 2 a].*
Sulfonylureas should not be used as primary therapy in insulin-dependent (type I) diabetes mellitus (IDDM) patients, in those who have severe hepatic or renal dysfunction, or in those patients who are pregnant. Diabetic ketoacidosis (DKA) should never be treated with sulfonylureas; this condition must be treated with insulin, fluids, and electrolyte replacement. However, sulfonylureas help to reduce blood glucose levels in type II DM that does not respond to diet alone.

6. The answer is B *[II B 2 c (3), e (4), f (2)].*
Acute ingestion of ethanol (alcohol) by patients who are taking any antidiabetic agent carries the risk of severe hypoglycemia especially due to the potential hypoglycemic effects of ethanol (especially if consumed in the fasting state).

7. The answer is B *[II B 2 c; Table 52-2].*
The standard recommended dose of glyburide is 1.25–20 mg/day. Doses greater than 20 mg are not recommended by the manufacturer. Patients may be started on a low dose (e.g., 1.25 mg/day) and titrated up to an effective oral dose, as clinically indicated.

8–12. The answers are: 8-B *[I F 1],* **9-D** *[II B 1 d (2)],* **10-C** *[II A, B 1 a, 2 a],* **11-D** *[II D 2 c (2), (3)],* **12-D** *[III A 2].*
Type I diabetes mellitus (DM) with diabetic ketoacidosis (DKA) is the most likely diagnosis in the patient described in the question. The patient presented with high blood sugar, weight loss, acidosis, and positive urine ketones (high level). This is a typical presentation of DKA.

Type I DM always requires insulin therapy; it can never be left untreated or treated with diet or liquids alone and can never be treated with sulfonylurea agents. DKA requires hospitalization and should be treated with an insulin drip until the acidosis clears. Patients with DKA are dehydrated and must be given intravenous fluids.

All diabetic patients should be followed with periodic hemoglobin A_{1c} measurements and ophthalmologic examination annually. Home glucose monitoring is the optimal way to follow a patient's level of control. Weight loss and an attempt to wean from insulin are appropriate only for type II DM. Those patients with type I diabetes cannot be weaned from insulin therapy.

Hypoglycemia is a possible complication of insulin therapy. All diabetic patients are at risk for coronary artery disease and retinopathy. Nonketotic hyperglycemic hyperosmolar coma is typically a complication of type II DM.

53
Thyroid Disease

John E. Janosik

I. PHYSIOLOGY

A. Thyroid hormone regulation

1. The thyroid gland synthesizes, stores, and secretes hormones that are important to growth, development, and the metabolic rate. These hormones are **thyroxine (T_4)** and **triiodothyronine (T_3)**.
2. The thyroid gland also secretes **calcitonin,** which reduces blood calcium ion concentration.
3. Thyroid hormone secretion and transport are controlled by **thyroid-stimulating hormone (thyrotropin; TSH).** TSH is released by the anterior pituitary gland, which is triggered by **thyrotropin-releasing hormone (TRH),** secreted from the hypothalamus.
   a. The process produces increased levels of thyroid hormone (circulating free T_4 and free T_3), which, in turn, signals the pituitary to stop releasing TSH **(negative feedback).**
   b. Conversely, low blood levels of free hormone trigger pituitary release of TSH, which stimulates the thyroid gland to secrete T_4 and T_3 until free hormone levels return to normal. At this point, the pituitary gland ceases to release TSH, which completes the feedback loop (Figure 53-1).
   c. This homeostatic mechanism attempts to maintain the level of circulating thyroid hormone within a very narrow range.

B. Biosynthesis (Figure 53-2)

1. Essential to synthesis of thyroid hormones is dietary iodine, reduced to **inorganic iodide,** which the thyroid actively extracts from the plasma through iodide trapping **(iodide pump).**

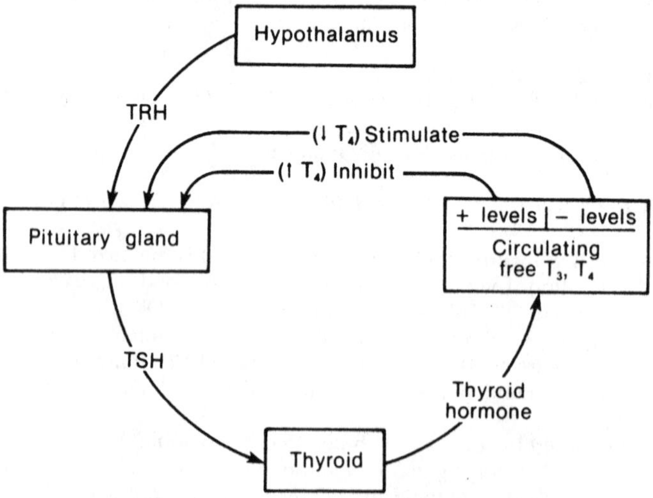

Figure 53-1. Thyroid hormone regulation loop. This carefully balanced hormone regulation system uses both positive (stimulating) and negative (inhibiting) feedback to maintain homeostasis. Disruption of any of these elements can produce serious consequences, such as myxedema crisis (underavailability of thyroid hormone) or thyroid storm (over-abundance of thyroid hormone). *TRH* = thyroid-releasing hormone; *TSH* = thyroid-stimulating hormone; T_4 = thyroxine; T_3 = triiodothyronine.

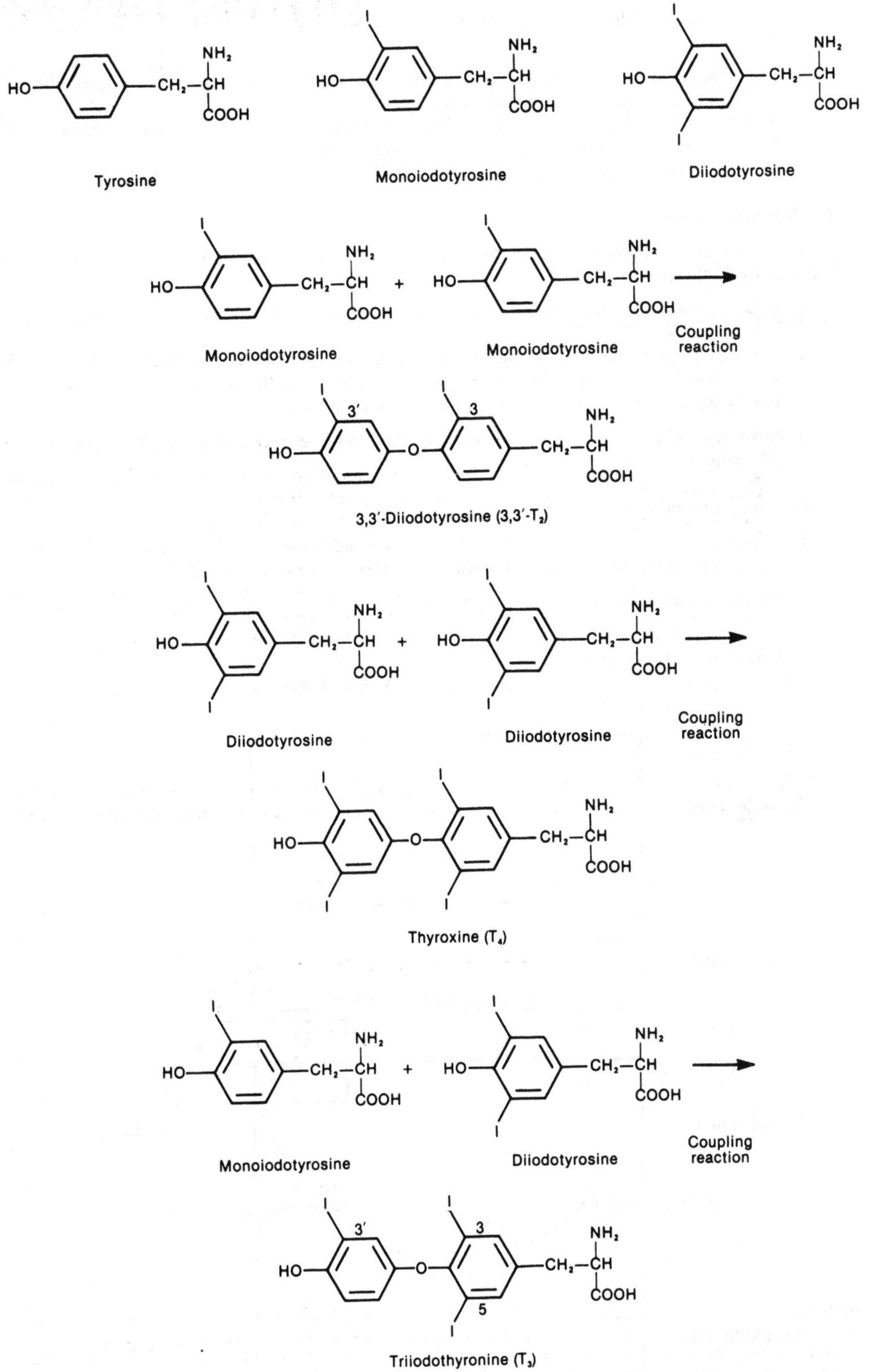

Figure 53-2. Biosynthesis of thyroid hormones. The major products are thyroxine (T_4) and triiodothyronine (T_3). These are formed in the follicle cells of the thyroid gland by iodination of tyrosine residues. Monoiodo- and diiodotyrosine residues are formed first. These then react to form T_3 and T_4.

Some of this iodide is stored within the colloid; some diffuses into the lumen of thyroid follicles.

2. Iodide is oxidized by peroxidase and bound to tyrosyl residues within the thyroglobulin molecule in a process called **organification.**
   a. The synthesis begins with iodide binding to tyrosine, forming **monoiodotyrosine (MIT).**
   b. MIT then binds another iodide to form **diiodotyrosine (DIT).**
   c. Then, slowly, a coupling reaction binds MIT and DIT, producing T_3 and T_4.

C. Hormone transport

1. After TSH stimulation of the thyroid gland, T_3 and T_4 are cleaved from thyroglobulin and released into the circulation.
2. When in the circulation, thyroid hormone is transported bound to several plasma proteins, a process that:
   a. Helps to protect the hormone from premature metabolism and excretion
   b. Prolongs its half-life in the circulation
   c. Allows the thyroid hormone to reach its site of action
3. Most thyroid hormone is transported by **thyroxine-binding globulin (TBG). Prealbumin** and **albumin** also serve as carriers.

D. Hormone metabolism

1. Peripheral conversion of T_4 to T_3 occurs in the pituitary gland, liver, and kidneys and accounts for about 80% of T_3 generation.
2. **Deiodination** accounts for most hormone degradation. The major steps in this process are shown in Figure 53-3.
3. Deiodinated hormones are excreted in feces and urine.

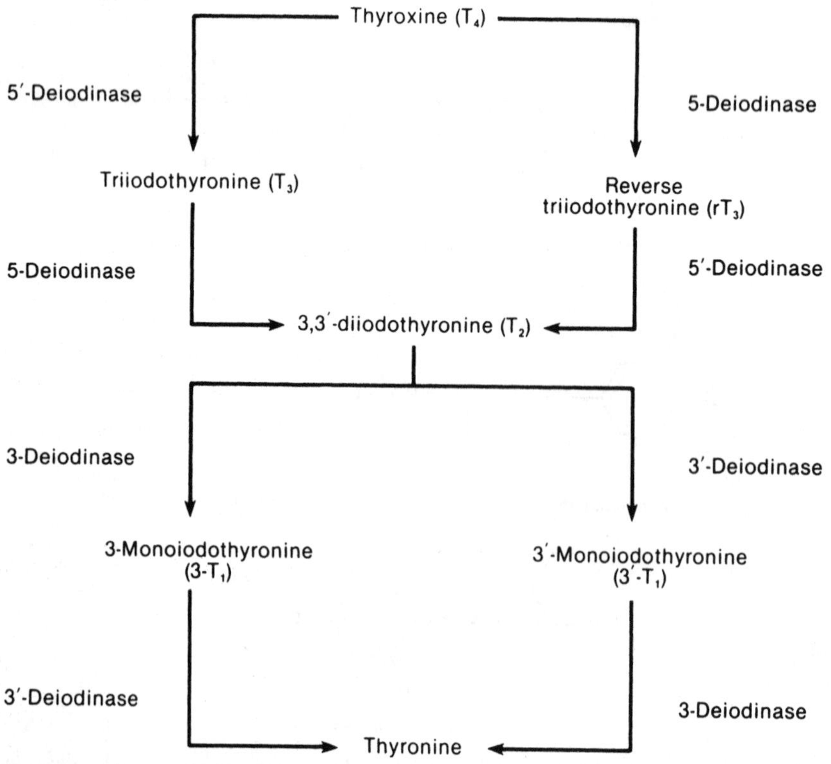

Figure 53-3. Thyroxine metabolism: major steps in the primary and alternative deiodination pathways.

4. Minor nondeiodination pathways of metabolism include conjugation with sulfate and glucuronide, deamination, and decarboxylation.

E. Hormone function. Although the effects of thyroid hormones are known, the basic mechanisms producing these effects elude precise definition; however, they seem to activate the messenger RNA (mRNA) transcription process and can promote protein synthesis or (in excessive amounts) protein catabolism. **Thyroid hormones** affect the following:

1. Growth and development
2. Calorigenics by increasing the rate of basal metabolism
3. Cardiovascular system by increasing the metabolic rate, which increases blood flow, cardiac output, and heart rate (may be related in part to an increased tissue sensitivity to catecholamines)
4. The central nervous system (CNS) by increasing or diminishing cerebration
5. Musculature by causing a fine tremor
6. Sleep by inducing fatigued wakefulness with hyperthyroidism or somnolence with hypothyroidism
7. Lipid metabolism by stimulating lipid mobilization and degradation

F. Thyroid function studies (Table 53-1)

1. **Serum total thyroxine (TT_4)**
   a. This test provides the most direct reflection of thyroid function by indicating hormone availability to tissues. Total (free and bound) T_4 is determined by radioimmunoassay, which is sensitive and rapid.
   b. Changes in thyroid globulin concentration, particularly TBG, which increases during pregnancy, alter the total concentration of T_4 and may produce a misleading high or low test result.
   c. However, these changes in TBG do not affect the concentration of free T_4. Therefore, to clarify thyroid function, either protein-binding (T_3 uptake test) or free T_4 must be measured.
   d. An elevated TT_4 level indicates hyperthyroidism; a decreased TT_4 level, hypothyroidism. However, the TT_4 level in a euthyroid patient can be altered by other factors, such as pregnancy or febrile illnesses (which elevate the TT_4), nephrotic syndrome or cirrhosis (which lower it), and various drugs (Table 53-2).

2. **Serum total triiodothyronine (TT_3)**
   a. This sensitive and highly specific test measures total (free and bound) T_3.
   b. Serum T_3 and T_4 usually rise and fall together; however, hyperthyroidism commonly causes a disproportionate rise in T_3, and the TT_3 can rise before the TT_4 level. Therefore, TT_3 is useful for early detection or to rule out hyperthyroidism. Many of the symptoms associated with hyperthyroidism are due to elevated TT_3.
   c. This test may not be diagnostically significant for hypothyroidism, in which TT_3 levels may fall but stay within the normal range. The TT_3 may be low in only 50% of patients with hypothyroidism.
   d. If there is an abnormality in binding proteins, this test can yield the same misleading results as the TT_4 readings. Other factors affecting test results include pregnancy (which

Table 53-1. Test Results in Thyroid Disorders

Thyroid Function Test	Hypothyroidism	Hyperthyroidism
Serum resin triiodothyronine uptake (RT_3U)	↓ (< 35%)	↑ (> 45%)
Serum total thyroxine (TT_4)	↓ (< 5 μg/dl)	↑ (> 12 μg/dl)
Serum total triiodothyronine (TT_3)	↓ (< 80 ng/dl)	↑ (> 180 ng/dl)
Free thyroxine index (FTI)	↓ (< 5.5)	↑ (< 10.5)
Serum thyrotropin (TSH)	↑ (> 6 μU/ml)	↓ (< 0.5 μU/ml)
Sensitive thyrotropin (TSH) assay	↑ (> 5 μU/ml)	↓ (< 0.2 μU/ml)

↑ = increased levels; ↓ = decreased levels.

Table 53-2. Effects of Drugs on Thyroid Function Tests

Drug	Serum T_4	Resin T_3 Uptake	Free Thyroxine Index (FTI)	Serum T_3	Serum TSH	Comment
p-Aminosalicylic acid (PAS)	↓	(nd)	↓	(nd)	↑ *	Antithyroid effect, rarely, with long-term use
Aminoglutethimide (*Cytadren*)	↓	(nd)	(nd)	(nd)	↑	
Amiodarone[1]	↑	(nd)	(nd)	↓	(nd)	Inhibits peripheral conversion of T4 to T3.
Anabolic steroids and androgens	↓	↑	0	↓ *	(nd)	Decreased serum TBG
Antithyroid drugs: Propylthiouracil (PTU) or methimazole (*Tapazole*)	↓	↓	↓	↓	0 or ↑	TSH may increase if patient becomes hypothyroid
Asparaginase (*Elspar*)	↓	↑	(nd)	↓ *	↑ *	Decreased serum TBG
Barbiturates	↓ [a]	(nd)	↓	(nd)	(nd)	Stimulates T_4 metabolism
Contraceptives, oral	↑	↓	0	↑	0	TBG usually increased
Corticosteroids	0 or ↓	0 or ↑	0 or ↓	↓	↓	Usual doses decrease TBG; high doses may increase TBG
Danazol (*Danocrine*)	↓	↑	0[b]	↓	0 or ↓	Decreased serum TBG
Estrogens	↑	↓	0	↑	0	Increased serum TBG
Ethionamide (*Trecator*)	↓	(nd)	↓ *	(nd)	↑ *	Antithyroid effect
Fluorouracil (*Adrucil*)	↑	↓	(nd)	↑	0	Patients clinically euthyroid; TBG increased
Heparin, intravenous	↑ [c]	0 or ↑	↑ *	0	(nd)	FTI is increased with some measures
Hypoglycemics (sulfonylureas)	0[d]	0[d]	0[d]	(nd)	(nd)	
Iodides, inorganic	0	0	0	(nd)	(nd)	
Iodides, organic	0	0	0	(nd)	(nd)	
Levodopa and levodopa-carbidopa (*Sinemet*)	0	0	0	0	↓ [e]	
Levothyroxine (*Levothroid*)	↑ (s)[f,g]	↑ or 0 or ↓ [f,g]	0 or ↑ [f,g]	↑ or 0[f,g]	↑ or 0[f]	
Liothyronine (*Cytomel*)	↓ [f]	0 or ↓ [f]	↓ [f]	↑ or ↓ [f,g]	0[f]	
Liotrix (*Thyrolar*)	0[f] or ↓ (s)	0[f]	0[f]	0[f,g]	0[f]	
Lithium carbonate (*Eskalith*)	0 or ↓	0 or ↓	0 or ↓	0 or ↓	0 or ↑	
Methadone (*Dolophine*)	↑ (s)	↓	0	↑	0	Increased serum TBG
Mitotane (*Lysodren*)	↓	0	0*	(nd)	(nd)	
Nitroprusside (*Nipride*)	↓	(nd)	(nd)	(nd)	(nd)	Clinical hypothyroidism
Oxyphenbutazone (*Oxalid*) and phenylbutazone (*Butazolidin*)	0 or ↓	↑	↓	(nd)	↑ *	May compete with T_4 for TBG binding. Rarely, overt hypothyroidism and goiter may occur

Perphenazine (*Trilafon*)	↑	↓	↓	↑	0*	
Phenytoin (*Dilantin*)	↓	0 or ↑ (s)	0 or ↓ (s)	↓	0	Stimulates T_4 metabolism and may compete with T_4 for TBG binding
Propranolol (*Inderal*)	0 or ↑ [h]	0[i]	(nd)	↓ [j]	0	
Resorcinol (excessive topical use)	↓	↓	↓	↓	↑	
Salicylates (large doses)	↓	↑ (s)	↓ *	↓	0*	Compete with T_4 for TBG binding

↑ = increased; ↓ = decreased; 0 = no effect; (s) = slight effect; (nd) = no data (Adapted from *The Medical Letter* 23:31, 1981).

*Effect deduced rather than based on reported clinical evidence.

[a]Patients requiring thyroid replacement therapy have decreased serum thyroxine when barbiturates are given.

[b]Free thyroxine index may increase slightly but usually remains in the normal range.

[c]T_4 assay by competitive protein binding is spuriously increased, but T_4-RIA is probably not affected. Free thyroxine measured by dialysis may be increased.

[d]May occasionally decrease serum T_4 and increase resin T_3 uptake.

[e]Slight decrease in euthyroid patients; but in long-standing hypothyroid patients, levodopa considerably decreases the elevated TSH.

[f]In a patient on adequate doses for thyroid replacement.

[g]Increased T_4, FTI, and T_3 tend to return to normal after several months of therapy with levothyroxine. After liothyronine, T_3 may be elevated 2 hours after a dose and depressed 24 hours after a dose.

[h]Increased T_4 levels are reported in one study, but not in others.

[i]With short-term propranolol in hyperthyroid patients.

[j]In euthyroid subjects, the decreased serum T_3 returns to normal with continued propranolol therapy.

[1]Taken from Rae P, Farrar J, Beckett G, Toft A. *Assessment of thyroid status in elderly people.* BMJ 1993;307:177-80.

increases TT_3 levels), malnutrition or hepatic or renal disease (which lower TT_3 levels), or various drugs (see Table 53-2).

3. Resin triiodothyronine uptake (RT_3U)

a. This test clarifies whether abnormal T_4 levels are due to a thyroid disorder or to abnormalities in the binding proteins because it evaluates the binding capacity of TBG.

b. If an abnormal amount (high or low) of thyroid hormone is present in the blood, the RT_3U results **change in the same direction** as the altered level—elevated in hyperthyroidism, decreased in hypothyroidism.

c. However, if abnormalities in binding proteins underlie the abnormal levels of TT_4, TT_3, or both, the RT_3U results **change in the opposite direction**—decreasing as TBG increases; increasing as TBG decreases.

d. Various drugs can cause spurious changes in the RT_3U (see Table 53-2).

4. Serum thyrotropin (TSH) and sensitive TSH assays

a. Serum TSH assay

(1) This test is the **most sensitive** test for detecting the hypothyroid state because the hypothalamic–pituitary axis compensates very quickly for even slight decreases in circulating free hormone by releasing more TSH. The TSH levels may be elevated even before low circulating levels of TT_4 are detectable by diagnostic testing.

(2) Serum TSH is not a reliable test for hyperthyroidism (in which TSH is suppressed) because low levels and low–normal levels of TSH may be indistinguishable with the current technology.

(3) Effects of drugs on the serum TSH are shown in Table 53-2.

b. Sensitive TSH assay

(1) The sensitive TSH assay uses immunoradiometric methodology or other new methods of analysis instead of the older radioimmunoassay techniques and demonstrates greater sensitivity in the detection of thyroid disease than older tests.

(2) This assay is usually **more expensive** and **more commonly used** to monitor patients receiving replacement therapy to control overtreatment. (Overtreatment may contribute to excessive bone demineralization, ECG changes, or elevation of liver function tests).

5. Free thyroxine index (FTI)

a. This is not a separate test but rather an estimation of the free T_4 level through a mathematical interpretation of the relationship between RT_3U and serum T_4 levels:

$$\text{FTI} = \frac{TT_4 \times RT_3U}{\text{mean serum } RT_3U}$$

b. FTI values are elevated in hyperthyroidism, when TBG is low and decreased in hypothyroidism, or when TBG is elevated.

c. Effects of drugs on FTI are shown in Table 53-2.

G. Strategies and cost considerations for testing

1. The **most frequently** used and **least expensive** tests for screening are the TT_4 and the RT_3U, which are used to calculate the FTI. A serum TSH assay may also be used but at an additional cost.

2. Thyroid disease screening for the otherwise generally healthy population is **not cost-effective** based on the rate of detection and cost associated with massive screening.

3. The most appropriate **target population** for screening includes elderly patients hospitalized for exacerbations of chronic diseases or who are coincidentally diagnosed with a chronic disease [e.g., congestive heart failure (CHF), rheumatoid arthritis], mental status changes, or psychosocial problems.

4. The American Thyroid Association recommends a FTI and a sensitive TSH assay as the primary laboratory tests to diagnose thyroid disease. The sensitive TSH assay is useful in detecting patients at risk of receiving an excess amount of thyroxine as replacement therapy.

II. HYPOTHYROIDISM.

The inability of the thyroid gland to supply sufficient thyroid hormone results in varying degrees of hypothyroidism from mild, clinically insignificant forms to the life-threatening extreme, myxedema coma.

A. Classification

1. **Primary hypothyroidism** is due to:
   a. Gland destruction or dysfunction caused by disease or medical therapies (e.g., radiation, surgical procedures)
   b. Failure of the gland to develop or congenital incompetence (i.e., **cretinism**)

2. **Secondary hypothyroidism** is due to a pituitary disorder that inhibits TSH secretion. The thyroid gland is normal but lacks appropriate stimulation by TSH.

3. **Tertiary hypothyroidism** refers to a condition in which the pituitary–thyroid axis is intact, but the hypothalamus lacks the ability to secrete TRH to stimulate the pituitary.

B. Causes

1. **Hashimoto's thyroiditis,** which is a chronic lymphocytic thyroiditis that is considered to be an autoimmune disorder

2. **Treatment of hyperthyroidism,** such as radioactive iodine therapy, subtotal thyroidectomy, or administration of antithyroid agents

3. **Surgical excision**

4. **Goiter** (enlargement of the thyroid gland)
   a. **Endemic goiter** results from inadequate intake of dietary iodine. This is common in regions with iodine-depleted soil and in areas of endemic malnutrition.
   b. **Sporadic goiter** can follow ingestion of certain drugs or foods containing **progoitrin** (L-5-vinyl-2-thio-oxazolidone), which is inactive and converted by hydrolysis to goitrin. Goitrins inhibit oxidation of iodine to iodide and prevent iodide from binding to thyroglobulin, thereby decreasing thyroid hormone production. Progoitrin has been isolated in cabbage, kale, peanuts, brussels sprouts, mustard, rutabaga, kohlrabi, spinach, cauliflower, and horseradish. **Goitrogenic drugs** include propylthiouracil (PTU), iodides, phenylbutazone, cobalt, and lithium.
   c. **Less common causes** include acute (usually traumatic) and subacute thyroiditis, nodules, nodular goiter, and thyroid cancer.

C. Signs and symptoms

1. Early clinical features tend to be somewhat vague: lethargy, fatigue, forgetfulness, sensitivity to cold, unexplained weight gain, and constipation.

2. Progressively, the characteristic features of myxedema emerge: dry, flaky, inelastic skin; coarse hair; slowed speech and thought; hoarseness; puffy face, hands, and feet; eyelid droop; hearing loss; menorrhagia; decreased libido; slow return of deep tendon reflexes (especially in the Achilles tendon). If untreated, myxedema coma will develop.

D. Laboratory findings (see Table 53-1)

E. Treatment goal is replacement therapy using oral agents (Table 53-3).

F. Therapeutic agents

1. **Desiccated thyroid preparations**
   a. At one time the agent of choice, desiccated thyroid has fallen out of favor since standardized synthetic levothyroxine preparations have become available.
   b. Desiccated thyroid preparations are not considered bioequivalent; they have evidenced varying amounts of active substances. Although they met established *United States Pharmacopeia (USP)* criteria for iodine content, variation in activity was noted. The content assay, while specific for iodine, was unable to specify the ratio of T_3 to T_4, and this ratio varies with animal source. Porcine gland preparations have a higher T_3 to T_4 ratio than those from ovine or bovine sources.

2. **Fixed ratio (liotrix) preparations.** In an effort to standardize the T_3 to T_4 ratio, substances that mimic glandular content were developed. However, the T_3 component proved unnecessary (because T_4 is metabolized to T_3) and even disadvantageous because of T_3–induced **adverse effects** (e.g., tremor, headache, palpitations, diarrhea).

3. **Levothyroxine**

Table 53-3. Thyroid Replacement Preparations

Preparation	Trade Names	Advantage	Disadvantage	Comments	Source
Dessicated thyroid	Thyroid USP Enseals Thyroid Strong Armour Thyroid Thyrar	Low cost	Some preparations have unpredictable results Inconsistent T_3:T_4 ratio T_3 increases adverse effects	Contains T_3 Some brands are standardized by iodine content*	Porcine, bovine, or ovine thyroid glands
Liothyronine	Cytomel	Predictable results Useful for myxedema crisis	Lacks T_4	Usually reserved for myxedema crisis	Synthetic
Liotrix	Thyrolar	Standardized formulation	T_3 increases adverse effects Expensive	Fixed T_3:T_4 ratio of 1:4 Metabolism of T_4 to T_3 renders T_3 component unnecessary	Synthetic
Levothyroxine	Levothroid Synthroid Levoxyl	Predictable results Intravenous preparation available	Expensive	Agent of choice Does not contain T_3 All preparations are not interchangeable	Synthetic

*Iodine content, as well as T_3:T_4 ratio, varies with species.

T_3 = triiodotyronine; T_4 = thyroxine.

a. Predictable results and lack of T_3–induced side effects have made levothyroxine the agent of choice.
b. The **two major brands** of levothyroxine preparations (Levothroid, Synthroid) have been compared for bioequivalence and were shown to be equivalent in patients with hypothyroidism.
c. The **average adult maintenance** dose is 75–150 μg/day. The dose range has been shown to be 1.5–1.7 μg/kg/day or an average of 1.6 μg/kg/day for otherwise healthy adults.
d. **Elderly** or **chronically ill patients** require an average dose of 50–100 μg/day which is 25–50 μg/day less than otherwise healthy adults of the same height and weight.
e. Thyroxine levels return to normal within a few weeks. Clinical improvement begins in 2 weeks with full resolution of signs and symptoms of hypothyroidism by 3–6 months of therapy.

G. Precautions and monitoring effects

1. Adult patients with a history of cardiac disease and elderly patients should begin therapy with lower doses (e.g., 25 μg/day of levothyroxine). After 2–4 weeks, the dose should be increased gradually to an individually adjusted maintenance dose (usually less than 100 μg daily).

2. Patients should be observed on initiation of therapy for possible **cardiac complications,** such as angina, palpitations, or arrhythmias.

3. Serum thyroid levels should be monitored, particularly T_4, sensitive TSH and RT_3U levels, as well as the FTI. Serum thyroxine tests remain elevated during the first few months of treatment even with the presence of clinical symptoms. Serum thyroxine tests do not predict the clinical state. Testing is unnecessary unless non-compliance is suspected.

4. It is recommended to monitor the sensitive TSH test 2–6 months after the last dose change. However, this test continues to change for up to 1 year. Testing early may result in overtreatment.

5. Levothyroxine administration, particularly long-term therapy, can induce thyrotoxicosis; T_4 levels can rise even though the dosage remains unchanged. Monitor for clinical signs of thyroid disease.

6. **Accelerated bone loss** has been associated with over treatment. Patients receiving replacement therapy with low TSH values may have lower bone mineral density since excess hormone accelerates the rate of remodeling (rate of resorption > rate of formation) and may contribute to an increased incidence of nontraumatic fracture.

7. **Drug interactions. Cholestyramine,** a bile acid sequestrant, can contribute to a decrease in **thyroxine** bioavailability when administered concomitantly. Cholestyramine should be administered at least 6 hours after oral thyroxine to reduce the potential for this clinically significant drug interaction.

H. Myxedema coma is a life-threatening complication with a high mortality rate.

1. It is **most common** in elderly patients with preexisting, although usually undiagnosed, hypothyroidism.

2. **Precipitating factors** include alcohol, sedative, or narcotic use; overuse of antithyroid agents; abrupt discontinuation of thyroid hormone therapy; infection; exposure to cold temperatures; and iatrogenic insult due to radiation therapy or thyroid surgery.

3. The patient usually declines from profound lethargy to coma, hypothermia, and a significant decrease in respiratory rate, potentially leading to respiratory failure as the crisis progresses. Hypometabolism produces a fluid and electrolyte imbalance that leads to fluid retention and hyponatremia. **Cardiac effects** include decreased heart rate and contractility, decreasing cardiac output.

4. **Treatment** consists of rapid restoration of T_3 and T_4 levels to normal.
   a. A loading dose of levothyroxine 400–500 μg is given as an IV bolus. Liothyronine, 25 μg, is then given orally every 6 hours.
   b. Treatment is continued until improvement is noted. Then, liothyronine is discontinued, and levothyroxine is changed to the oral preparation. A maintenance dose is then determined (see II G).

III. HYPERTHYROIDISM is the overabundance of thyroid hormone. **Thyrotoxicosis** is the general term applied to overactivity of the thyroid gland.

A. Graves' disease (diffuse toxic goiter)

1. The **most common form** of hyperthyroidism, Graves' disease occurs primarily, but not exclusively, in **young women.**
2. The basis of this disease is an **autoimmune disorder** in which antibodies bind to and activate TSH receptors, resulting in the overproduction of thyroid hormone.
   a. These antibodies are termed **long-acting thyroid stimulators (LATS)** because their duration of action extends beyond that of TSH. As TSH is only mimicked, not overabundant, neither testing for TSH nor attempts to influence it are productive.
   b. Antibody titers often are elevated in patients with Graves' disease.
3. **Signs and symptoms** characteristic of Graves' disease include:
   a. Diffusely enlarged nontender goiter
   b. Nervousness, irritability, anxiety, insomnia
   c. Heat intolerance and profuse sweating
   d. Weight loss despite increased appetite
   e. Tremor, muscle weakness
   f. Palpitations and tachycardia
   g. Exophthalmos, stare, and lid lag (slow upper lid closing)
   h. Diarrhea
   i. Thrill or bruit over the thyroid
   j. Periorbital edema

B. Plummer's disease (toxic nodular goiter)

1. This **form of thyrotoxicosis** is less common than Graves' disease. Its underlying cause remains unknown, but its incidence is highest in patients over 50 years of age, and it arises usually from a long-standing nontoxic goiter.
2. The thyrotoxicosis is a result of one or more adenomatous nodules autonomously secreting excessive thyroid hormone, which suppresses the rest of the gland. Scanning confirms the diagnosis if it indicates that activity and iodine uptake are confined to the nodular mass unless TSH is introduced.
3. **Signs and symptoms** are essentially the same as for Graves' disease except that one or more nodular masses are found, rather than diffuse glandular enlargement, and ophthalmopathy is usually absent. **Cardiac abnormalities** (e.g., CHF, tachyarrhythmias) are commonly seen with Plummer's disease.

C. Less common forms of hyperthyroidism

1. **Jodbasedow phenomenon** is an overproduction of thyroid hormone following a sudden, large increase in iodine ingestion—through either a sudden reversal of an iodine-deficient diet or the introduction of iodide or iodine in contrast agents or drugs (e.g., the antiarrhythmic agent amiodarone).
2. **Factitious hyperthyroidism** occurs with abusive ingestion of thyroid replacement agents, usually in a misguided effort to lose weight. Diagnosis is aided by the absence of glandular swelling and of exophthalmos and the lack of autoimmune activity found in Graves' disease.

D. Laboratory findings (see Table 53-1)

E. Treatment goal. Symptomatic relief is provided until definitive treatment can be effected.

F. Therapeutic agents

1. **β-Adrenergic blocking agents—propranolol**
   a. Propranolol reduces some of the peripheral manifestations (e.g., tachycardia, sweating, severe tremor, nervousness) of hyperthyroidism.
   b. In addition to providing symptomatic relief, propranolol inhibits the peripheral conversion of T_4 to T_3.

2. **Antithyroid agents—propylthiouracil (PTU) and methimazole**
   a. **Action.** These agents may help attain remission through direct interference with thyroid hormone synthesis. Both agents inhibit iodide oxidation and iodothiouracil coupling. In addition, PTU (but not methimazole) diminishes peripheral deiodination of T_4 to T_3.
   b. **Therapeutic uses** of these drugs include:
      (1) **Definitive treatment** in which remission is achieved
      (2) **Adjunctive therapy** with radioactive iodine until the radiation takes effect
      (3) **Preoperative preparation** to establish and maintain a euthyroid state until definitive surgery can be performed
   c. **Dosages**
      (1) **Propylthiouracil**
         (a) For **adults,** the initial dose is 300–450 mg/day in three divided doses (i.e., 100–150 mg every 8 hours). Adult patients with severe disease may require as much as 600–1200 mg/day initially.
         (b) The initial dose is continued for about 2 months; then a maintenance dose of 100–150 mg/day is given, as a single dose or divided into two doses.
         (c) Maintenance therapy is continued for approximately 1 year, then gradually discontinued over 1–2 months while the patient is monitored for signs of recurrent hyperthyroidism. The patient may remain in remission for several years. A recurrent episode of hyperthyroidism is most likely to occur within 3–6 months of drug discontinuation.
         (d) If hyperthyroidism recurs after drug therapy is stopped, the agent should be restarted and alternative therapy should be considered (e.g., thyroid gland ablation or removal).
      (2) **Methimazole**
         (a) The initial dose range is 5–60 mg/day in three divided doses, depending on disease severity. After 2 months of therapy, a maintenance dose of 5–30 mg/day is initiated.
         (b) Maintenance therapy is continued for approximately 1 year at which time the drug is gradually discontinued, usually over 1–2 months.
   d. **Precautions and monitoring effects**
      (1) Serum thyroid levels and the FTI should be monitored for a return to normal.
      (2) Goiter size should decrease with reduced hormone output.
      (3) The incidence of **adverse effects** is less than 1% with PTU and less than 3% with methimazole. The adverse effects are similar for the two agents.
         (a) The most bothersome are **dermatologic reactions** (e.g., rash, urticaria, pruritus, hair loss, skin pigmentation). Others include headache, drowsiness, paresthesia, nausea, vomiting, vertigo, neuritis, loss of taste, arthralgia, and myalgia.
         (b) **Severe adverse effects**—agranulocytosis, granulocytopenia, thrombocytopenia, drug fever, hepatitis, and hypoprothrombinemia—occur less frequently. Patients receiving methimazole who are over 40 years old and are receiving doses above 40 mg/day are at increased risk of developing agranulocytosis. Patients receiving PTU who are over 40 years old are at increased risk of developing agranulocytosis, but no dose association has been established.

3. **Radioactive iodine (RAI)**
   a. **Action.** The thyroid gland picks up the radioactive element iodine-131 (^{131}I) as it would regular iodine. The radioactivity subsequently destroys some of the cells that would otherwise concentrate iodine and produce T_4, thus decreasing thyroid hormone production.
   b. **Advantages**
      (1) **High cure rate**—almost 100% for patients with Graves' disease and only slightly less for patients with Plummer's disease
      (2) **Avoids surgical risks**—such as adverse reaction to anesthetics, hypoparathyroidism, nerve palsy, bleeding, and hoarseness
      (3) **Less expensive**—avoids cost of hospitalization
   c. **Disadvantages**
      (1) Risk of delayed hypothyroidism
      (2) Slight, though undocumented, risk of genetic damage
      (3) Multiple doses, which may be required, may delay therapeutic efficacy for a long period (many months or a year)

d. **Dosage.** A dose of 80–100 mCi of ^{131}I per estimated gram of thyroid gland is recommended. Some protocols use lower dosages, but these may be less effective, requiring retreatment. When the dose is higher, there is a potential risk that hypothyroidism will develop.

e. **Precautions and monitoring effects**
   (1) Radioiodine therapy generally is reserved for patients past the childbearing years because effects on future offspring are not known.
   (2) Response to ^{131}I is hard to gauge, and patients must be monitored early for recurrence of hyperthyroidism, and later for hypothyroidism, which may develop even 20 years or more after therapy.

4. **Subtotal thyroidectomy.** Partial removal of the thyroid gland may be indicated if drug therapy fails or radioactive iodine is undesirable. This is a difficult procedure, but the success rate is high and the cure rapid. Risks include those mentioned in III F 3 b (2), precipitating thyroid storm, and permanent postoperative hypothyroidism. The risk of inducing thyroid storm can be minimized by obtaining a euthyroid state through use of antithyroid agents or propranolol (see III F 1).

G. Complications

1. **Hypothyroidism** may occur iatrogenically or, it has been proposed, as a natural sequel to Graves' disease.

2. **Thyroid storm (thyrotoxic crisis)** is a sudden exacerbation of hyperthyroidism caused by rapid release (leakage) of thyroid hormone. It is invariably fatal if not treated rapidly. In this crisis, unchecked hypermetabolism leads ultimately to dehydration, shock, and death.
   a. **Precipitating factors** include thyroid trauma or surgery, RAI therapy, infection, and sudden discontinuation of antithyroid therapy.
   b. **Characteristics.** It is characterized by a TT_4 level of 25–30 μg/dl, rapidly rising fever, tachycardia disproportionate to the fever, and unexplained, pronounced restlessness and tremor.
   c. **Treatment**
      (1) **PTU,** in doses of 150–250 mg orally every 6 hours, is the preferred agent because PTU blocks peripheral deiodination of T_4 to T_3, while methimazole does not. However, if necessary, **methimazole,** 15 mg orally every 6 hours, can be used instead.
      (2) **Propranolol,** in doses of 20–200 mg orally every 6 hours or 1–3 mg intravenously every 4–6 hours, should be administered unless contraindicated (e.g., if the patient has CHF).
      (3) **Potassium iodide,** in doses of 50–100 mg every 12 hours, is given (after PTU) to minimize intrathyroidal iodine uptake.
      (4) **Other supportive therapy** includes rehydration, cooling, antibiotics, rest, and sedation.

STUDY QUESTIONS

Directions: Each of the numbered items or incomplete statements in this section is followed by answers or by completions of the statement. Select the **one** lettered answer or completion that is **best** in each case.

1. What is the correct formula to use for calculating the free thyroxine index (FTI)?

(A) $T_4 \times RT_3U$/mean serum RT_3U
(B) $T_3 \times T_3$/mean serum RT_3U
(C) $T_3 \times RT_3U$/mean serum RT_3U
(D) $T_4 \times RT_3U \times$ mean serum RT_3U
(E) $T_3 \times RT_3U \times$ mean serum RT_3U

2. What precursor besides dietary iodine is required for thyroxine biosynthesis?

(A) Triiodothyronine (T_3)
(B) Threonine
(C) Tyrosine
(D) Thyrotropin (thyroid-stimulating hormone)
(E) Thyroxine-binding globulin (TBG)

3. All of the following conditions are causes of hyperthyroidism EXCEPT

(A) Graves' disease
(B) Hashimoto's thyroiditis
(C) toxic multinodular goiter
(D) triiodothyronine toxicosis
(E) Plummer's disease

4. Which of the following preparations is used to attain remission of thyrotoxicosis?

(A) Propranolol
(B) Liotrix
(C) Levothyroxine
(D) Propylthiouracil
(E) Desiccated thyroid

5. The thyroid gland normally secretes which of the following substances into the serum?

(A) Thyrotropin-releasing hormone (TRH)
(B) Thyrotropin (thyroid-stimulating hormone)
(C) Diiodothyronine (DIT)
(D) Thyroglobulin
(E) Thyroxine (T_4)

6. All of the following conditions are causes of hypothyroidism EXCEPT

(A) endemic goiter
(B) surgical excision
(C) Hashimoto's thyroiditis
(D) goitrin-induced iodine deficiency
(E) Graves' disease

7. Common tests to monitor patients receiving replacement therapy for hypothyroidism include all of the following EXCEPT

(A) thyrotropin (TSH) stimulation test
(B) sensitive TSH assay
(C) free thyroxine index (FTI)
(D) triiodothyronine resin uptake (RT_3U)
(E) total thyroxine (TT_4)

8. Which of the following pairs of preparations has been most studied for bioequivalence?

(A) Levoxyl—Thyrolar
(B) Thyroglobulin—Proloid
(C) Levothroid—Synthroid
(D) Cytomel—Synthroid
(E) Desiccated thyroid—Armour thyroid

9. The inhibition of pituitary thyrotropin secretion is controlled by which of the following?

(A) Free thyroxine (T_4)
(B) Thyroid-releasing hormone (TRH)
(C) Free thyroxine index (FTI)
(D) Reverse triiodothyronine (rT_3)
(E) Total thyroxine (TT_4)

10. Which of the following agents has been shown to interact with oral thyroxine (T_4) replacement therapy?

(A) Propylthiouracil
(B) Cholestyramine
(C) Thyrotropin
(D) Levothyroxine
(E) Lovastatin

11. What laboratory tests are currently recommended by the American Thyroid Association to diagnose thyroid disease?

(A) Triiodothyronine resin uptake (RT_3U) and total thyroxine (TT_4)
(B) Thyrotropin (TSH) and free thyroxine index (FTI)
(C) Total thyroxine (TT_4) and sensitive TSH assay
(D) Free T_4 and sensitive TSH assay
(E) Free T_4 and RT_3U

12. What patient population should be screened for thyroid disease?

(A) Hospitalized patients
(B) Elderly patients with chronic disease
(C) Elderly hospitalized patients
(D) College students
(E) Women over 20 years old

13. What is the average replacement dose of levothyroxine for an otherwise healthy adult?

(A) 25–50 μg/day
(B) 50–100 μg/day
(C) 75–150 μg/day
(D) 100–200 μg/day
(E) 200–400 μg/day

14. What factors affect the optimal replacement dose of levothyroxine?

(A) Age, height, and weight
(B) Duration of hypothyroidism
(C) Pretreatment TSH level
(D) Presence of chronic illness
(E) All of the above

ANSWERS AND EXPLANATIONS

1. The answer is A *[I F 5].*
The free thyroxine index (FTI) is a mathematical interpretation of the relationship between the resin triiodothyronine uptake (RT_3U) and serum thyroxine (T_4) levels, compared to the mean population value for RT_3U. The FTI is calculated using reported values for total thyroxine (TT_4) and RT_3U. The normal FTI value in euthyroid patients is 5.5–12.

2. The answer is C *[I B].*
Biosynthesis of thyroid hormones begins with iodide binding to tyrosine, which forms monoiodotyrosine (MIT). Monoiodotyrosine binds another iodide atom to form diiodotyrosine (DIT). When MIT and DIT are formed, a coupling reaction occurs, which produces triiodothyronine (T_3), thyroxine (T_4), reverse triiodothyronine (rT_3), and other byproducts.

3. The answer is B *[II B 1; III A, B]*
Hashimoto's thyroiditis (chronic lymphocytic thyroiditis) is a cause of hypothyroidism. The incidence of Hashimoto's thyroiditis is 1%–2%, and it increases with age. It is more common in women than in men and in whites than in blacks. There may be a familial tendency. Patients with Hashimoto's thyroiditis have elevated titers of antibodies to thyroglobulin: A titer of greater than 1:32 is seen in over 85% of patients. Two variants of Hashimoto's thyroiditis have been described: gland fibrosis and idiopathic thyroid atrophy, which is most likely an extension of Hashimoto's thyroiditis.

4. The answer is D *[III F 1, 2].*
In hyperthyroid patients, remission of thyrotoxicosis is achieved with propylthiouracil (PTU) by two mechanisms: (1) interference of iodination of the tyrosyl residues, ultimately reducing production of thyroxine (T_4); (2) inhibition of peripheral conversion of T_4 to triiodothyronine (T_3). Propranolol is commonly used as an adjunct to PTU for symptomatic management of hyperthyroidism.

5. The answer is E *[I A 1].*
The major compounds secreted by the thyroid gland, after its stimulation by thyrotropin, are triiodothyronine (T_3) and thyroxine (T_4). When released from the thyroid, T_3 and T_4 are transported by plasma proteins, namely thyroxine-binding globulin (TBG), thyroxine-binding prealbumin, and albumin.

6. The answer is E *[II B; III A 1].*
Graves' disease (diffuse toxic goiter) is the most common form of hyperthyroidism. It occurs most often in women in the third and fourth decades of life. There is a genetic and familial predisposition. The etiology is linked to an autoimmune reaction between immunoglobulin G (IgG) and the thyroid.

7. The answer is A *[II G 4].*
The thyrotropin (TSH) stimulation test measures thyroid tissue response to exogenous TSH. It is not commonly used to monitor thyroid replacement therapy. It may be useful in the initial diagnosis of hypothyroidism.

8. The answer is C *[II F 3 b].*
Many brands of levothyroxine are currently available. Both generic and trade-name preparations have been studied with an emphasis on Levothroid and Synthroid. The importance of bioequivalence becomes apparent when patients have received different brands of levothyroxine and have exhibited changes in therapeutic response to equivalent replacement doses.

9. The answer is A *[I A 3 a].*
An increase in the blood level of thyroid hormone [circulating free thyroxine (T_4) and free triiodothyronine (T_3)] signals the pituitary to stop releasing thyroid-stimulating hormone (thyrotropin; TSH). The free fraction of T_4 is available to bind at the pituitary receptors.

10. The answer is B *[II G].*
Euthyroid patients receiving oral replacement therapy have become hypothyroid after concomitant administration of bile acid sequestrant therapy. It appears that bioavailability is reduced as a result of administering these agents at close dosing intervals. It is recommended that at least 6 hours pass before administration of a bile acid sequestrant. It would be preferable to select another nonbile acid sequestrant when clinically possible.

11. The answer is D *[I G 4].*
The free thyroxine (free-T_4) and the sensitive thyrotropin (TSH) assay should be used only for the diagnosis of patients most likely to have thyroid disease based on clinical presentation, relative risk (e.g., age, sex, family history) not for population screening. The sensitive TSH assay is also useful to monitor replacement therapy and to minimize overtreatment and the corresponding risk of accelerated bone loss.

12. The answer is B *[I G 3].*
Cost versus benefit is critical to the decision of choosing to screen entire populations. Because the frequency of detection has been proven to be higher in elderly patients (2%–5%) with chronic disease, the relative minor costs associated to obtain resin triiodothyronine uptake (RT_3U) and serum total thyroxine (TT_4) to calculate a free thyroxine index (FTI) are worth the cost. A serum thyrotropin (TSH) assay can be reserved for patients with an abnormal FTI. Another consideration is to use the sensitive TSH assay for diagnosis in place of the serum TSH assay at a higher cost but without the necessity of retesting. If patients admitted to the hospital for an acute illness were screened, but the results are misleading, they may be prescribed inappropriate therapy because acute illness may be associated with the temporary effects causing abnormal test results.

13. The answer is C *[II F 3 c].*
The average adult maintenance dose is 75–150 μg/day, which has been shown to be 1.5–1.7 μg/kg/day. The dose is usually adjusted in increments of 25–50 μg/day every 4 weeks. The total daily dose used to be 100–200 μg/day, which resulted in overtreatment after the introduction of the sensitive TSH assay. Elderly or chronically ill patients require an average dose of 50–100 μg/day, which is 25–50 μg/day less than otherwise healthy adults of the same height and weight.

14. The answer is E *[II F 3 d].*
Elderly or chronically ill patients require an average dose of 50–100 μg/day, which is 25–50 μg/day less than otherwise healthy adults of the same height and weight. Because the average dose for replacement therapy is between 1.5 and 1.7 μg/kg/day, weight affects the total daily dose.

54
Renal Failure

Andrew L. Wilson

I. ACUTE RENAL FAILURE

A. Definition. Acute renal failure (ARF) is the sudden, potentially reversible interruption of kidney function, resulting in retention of nitrogenous waste products in body fluids.

B. Classification and etiology. ARF is classified according to its cause.

1. **Prerenal ARF** stems from impaired renal perfusion, which may result from:
   a. Reduced arterial blood volume [e.g., hemorrhage, vomiting, diarrhea, other gastrointestinal (GI) fluid loss]
   b. Urinary losses from excessive diuresis
   c. Decreased cardiac output [e.g., from congestive heart failure (CHF) or pericardial tamponade]
   d. Renal vascular obstruction (e.g., stenosis)
   e. Severe hypotension
2. **Intrarenal ARF (intrinsic or parenchymal ARF)** reflects structural kidney damage resulting from any of the following conditions.
   a. **Acute tubular necrosis (ATN),** the leading cause of ARF, may be associated with:
      (1) Exposure to nephrotoxic aminoglycosides, anesthetics, pesticides, organic metals, and radiopaque contrast materials
      (2) Ischemic injury (e.g., surgery, circulatory collapse, severe hypotension)
      (3) Pigment (e.g., hemolysis, myoglobinuria)
   b. Acute glomerulonephritis
   c. Tubular obstruction, as from hemolytic reactions or uric acid crystals
   d. Acute inflammation (e.g., acute tubulointerstitial nephritis, papillary necrosis)
   e. Renal vasculitis
   f. Malignant hypertension
   g. Radiation nephritis
3. **Postrenal ARF** results from obstruction of urine flow anywhere along the urinary tract. Causes of postrenal ARF include:
   a. Ureteral obstruction, as from calculi, uric acid crystals, or thrombi
   b. Bladder obstruction, as from calculi, thrombi, tumors, or infection
   c. Urethral obstruction, as from strictures, tumors, or prostatic hypertrophy
   d. Extrinsic obstruction, as from hematoma, inflammatory bowel disease, or accidental surgical ligation

C. Pathophysiology. ARF progresses in three phases.

1. **Initiating phase**
   a. The initiating phase is defined as the time between the renal insult and the point at which extrarenal factors no longer reverse the damage caused by the obstruction or other cause of ARF. This phase may not be well defined clinically and may escape notice or diagnosis.
   b. **Urine output** may drop markedly to 400 ml/day or less **(oliguria).** In some patients, urine output falls below 100 ml/day **(anuria).** Oliguria may last only hours or as long as 4–6 weeks. However, it has been shown that 40%–50% of ARF patients are not oliguric or anuric.
   c. **Nitrogenous waste products** accumulate in the blood.

(1) **Azotemia** reflects urea accumulation due to impaired glomerular filtration and concentrating capacity.
(2) Serum creatinine, sulfate, phosphate, and organic acid levels climb rapidly.

d. The **serum sodium concentration** falls below normal from intracellular fluid shifting and dilution.

e. **Hyperkalemia** occurs if potassium intake is not restricted or body potassium is not removed. Without treatment, hyperkalemia may lead to neuromuscular depression and paralysis, impaired cardiac conduction, arrhythmias, respiratory muscle paralysis, cardiac arrest, and ultimately death.

2. **Maintenance phase**

a. This phase begins when urine output rises above 500 ml/day—typically after several days of oliguria. A rise in urine output or a "diuretic response" may not be seen in nonoliguric patients.

b. Urine output rises in increments of several milliliters to 300–500 ml/day. Urine output may double from day to day in the initial recovery period.

c. Azotemia and associated laboratory findings may persist until urine output reaches 1000–2000 ml/day.

d. The maintenance phase carries a risk of fluid and electrolyte abnormalities, GI bleeding, infection, and respiratory failure.

3. **Recovery phase.** During the recovery phase, renal function gradually returns to normal. Most recovered renal function appears in the first 2 weeks; however, recovery of renal function may continue for a year. Residual impairment may persist indefinitely.

D. Clinical evaluation

1. **Physical findings.** Initially, ARF causes azotemia and, in 50%–60% of cases, oliguria. Later, electrolyte abnormalities and other severe systemic effects occur.

a. **Urine output** typically is **low,** from 20 to 500 ml/day. Complete anuria is rare.

b. **Signs** and **symptoms of hyperkalemia,** resulting from reduced potassium excretion by impaired kidneys, include:
(1) Neuromuscular depression (e.g., paresthesias, muscle weakness, paralysis)
(2) Diarrhea and abdominal distention
(3) Slow or irregular pulse
(4) Electrocardiographic changes with potential cardiac arrest

c. **Uremia,** caused by excessive nitrogenous waste retention, leads to nausea, vomiting, diarrhea, edema, confusion, fatigue, neuromuscular irritability, and coma.

d. **Metabolic acidosis,** a common complication of ARF, is evidenced by:
(1) Deterioration of mental status, obtundation, coma, and lethargy
(2) Depressed cardiac contractility and decreased vascular resistance, leading to hypotension, pulmonary edema, and ventricular fibrillation
(3) Nausea and vomiting
(4) Respiratory abnormalities (e.g., hyperventilation, Kussmaul's respiration)

e. **Hyperphosphatemia** arises from decreased phosphate excretion.
(1) As serum phosphate rises, hypocalcemia results from the formation of insoluble calcium phosphate complexes.
(2) The signs and symptoms relate to resultant hypocalcemia and metastatic soft tissue calcification.
(3) Manifestations of hypocalcemia include:
(a) Neuromuscular irritability, cramps, spasms, and tetany
(b) Hypotension
(c) Soft-tissue calcification
(d) Mental status changes (e.g., confusion, mood changes, loss of intellect and memory)
(e) Hyperactive deep tendon reflexes and Trousseau's and Chvostek's signs
(f) Abdominal cramps
(g) Stridor and dyspnea

f. **Hyponatremia** results from dilution and intracellular fluid shifts during the diuretic phase of ARF. Physical findings include lethargy, weakness, seizures, cognitive impairment, and possible reduction in level of consciousness.

g. **Intravascular volume depletion,** suggesting **prerenal failure,** may cause:

(1) Flat jugular venous pulses when the patient lies supine
(2) Orthostatic changes in blood pressure and pulse
(3) Poor skin turgor and dry mucous membranes

h. Other findings suggesting **prerenal failure** include:
(1) An abdominal bruit, possibly indicating renal artery stenosis
(2) Increased paradoxus, suggesting pericardial tamponade
(3) Increased jugular venous pressure, pulmonary rales, and a third heart sound, signaling CHF

i. Postrenal failure caused by obstructed urinary flow may manifest itself in:
(1) A suprapubic or flank mass
(2) Bladder distention
(3) Costovertebral angle tenderness
(4) Prostate enlargement

2. Diagnostic test results

a. Urinalysis includes an examination of sediment; identification of proteins, glucose, ketones, blood, and nitrites; and measurement of urinary pH and urine specific gravity (concentration) or osmolality (dilution). Prior administration of fluids, diuretics, and changes in urinary pH may confound accurate diagnosis, using urinalysis.

(1) **Urinary sediment examination**
(a) Few casts and formed elements are found in prerenal ARF.
(b) Pigmented cellular casts and renal tubular epithelial cells appear with ATN.
(c) Red blood cell and white blood cell casts generally reflect inflammatory disease.
(d) Large numbers of broad white cell casts suggest chronic renal failure.

(2) The presence of blood in the urine **(hematuria)** or proteins **(proteinuria)** indicates renal dysfunction.
(3) **Urine-specific gravity** ranges from 1.010 to 1.016 in ARF.
(4) **Urine osmolality** typically rises in prerenal ARF.

b. Measurement of urine sodium and **creatinine levels** can help classify ARF.
(1) In **prerenal** ARF, the urine creatinine level **increases,** and urine sodium level **decreases.**
(2) In **intrarenal** ARF resulting from ATN, the urine creatinine level **decreases,** and the urine sodium level **increases.**

c. Creatinine clearance, an index of the **glomerular filtration rate (GFR),** allows estimation of the number of functioning nephrons; decreased creatinine clearance indicates renal dysfunction.

d. Blood chemistry provides an index of renal excretory function and body chemistry status. Findings typical of ARF include:
(1) Increased blood urea nitrogen (BUN)
(2) Increased serum creatinine
(3) Possible increase in hemoglobin and hematocrit values
(4) Abnormal serum electrolyte values
(a) Serum potassium level above 5 mEq/L
(b) Serum phosphate level above 2.6 mEq/L (4.8 mg/dl)
(c) Serum calcium level below 4 mEq/L (8.5 mg/dl), reflecting hypocalcemia. (The serum calcium level must be correlated with the serum albumin level. Each rise or fall of 1 g/dl of serum albumin beyond its normal range is responsible for a corresponding increase or decrease in serum calcium of approximately 0.8 mg/dl. A below normal serum albumin level may result in a deceptively low serum calcium level.)
(d) Serum sodium level below 135 mEq/L, reflecting hyponatremia

(5) Abnormal arterial blood gas values [pH below 7.35, bicarbonate concentration (HCO^{-3}) below 22], reflecting metabolic acidosis

e. Renal failure index (RFI) is the ratio of urine sodium concentration to the urine-to-serum creatinine ratio. The RFI helps determine the etiology of ARF. Typically, the RFI is less than 1 in prerenal ARF or acute glomerulonephritis (a cause of intrarenal ARF). The RFI is greater than 2 in postrenal ARF and in other intrarenal causes of ARF.

f. Electrocardiography (ECG) may show evidence of hyperkalemia—that is, tall, peaked T waves; widening QRS complexes; prolonged PR interval, progressing to decreased amplitude and disappearing P waves; and, ultimately, ventricular fibrillation and cardiac arrest.

g. **Radiographic findings**
   (1) **Ultrasound** may detect upper urinary-tract obstruction.
   (2) **Kidney, ureter,** or **bladder radiography** may reveal:
      (a) Urinary tract calculi
      (b) Enlarged kidneys, suggesting ATN
      (c) Asymmetrical kidneys, suggesting unilateral renal artery disease, ureteral obstruction, or chronic pyelonephritis
   (3) **Radionuclide scan** may reveal:
      (a) Bilateral differences in renal perfusion, suggesting serious renal disease
      (b) Bilateral differences in dye excretion, suggesting parenchymal disease or obstruction as the cause of **ARF**
      (c) Diffuse, slow, dense radionuclide uptake, suggesting ATN
      (d) Patchy or absent radionuclide uptake, possibly indicating severe, acute glomerulonephritis
   (4) **Computerized tomography (CT) scan** may provide better visualization of an obstruction.

h. **Renal biopsy** may be performed in selected patients when other test results are inconclusive.

E. Treatment objectives

1. Correct reversible causes of ARF, preventing or minimizing further renal damage or complications.
   a. Discontinue nephrotoxic drugs; remove other nephrotoxins through dialysis or gastric lavage for poisonings.
   b. Treat underlying infection.
   c. Remove any urinary-tract obstructions.

2. Correct and maintain proper fluid and electrolyte balance. Match fluid, electrolyte, and nitrogen intakes to urine output.

3. Treat body chemistry alterations, especially hyperkalemia and metabolic acidosis when present. Treatment may include renal dialysis.

4. Improve urine output.

5. Treat systemic manifestations of ARF.

F. Therapy

1. **Conservative management** alone may suffice in uncomplicated ARF.
   a. **Fluid management**
      (1) Fluid intake should match fluid losses. **Sensible losses** (i.e., urine, stool, tube drainage) and **insensible losses** (i.e., skin, respiratory tract) should be included in fluid balance calculations.
      (2) Volume overload should minimize the risk of hypertension and CHF.
      (3) The patient should be weighed daily to determine fluid volume status.
   b. **Dietary measures**
      (1) Because catabolism accompanies renal failure, the patient should receive a **high-calorie, low-protein diet.** Such a diet helps to:
         (a) Reduce renal work load by decreasing production of end products of protein catabolism that the kidneys cannot excrete
         (b) Prevent ketoacidosis
         (c) Alleviate manifestations of uremia (e.g., nausea, vomiting, confusion, fatigue)
      (2) If edema or hypertension is present, sodium intake should be restricted.
      (3) Potassium intake must be limited in most patients.

2. **Management of body chemistry alterations**
   a. **Treatment of hyperkalemia**
      (1) **Dialysis** may be used to treat acute, life-threatening hyperkalemia (see II F 7).
      (2) **Calcium chloride**
         (a) **Mechanism of action and therapeutic effects.** Calcium chloride or calcium gluconate replaces and maintains body calcium, counteracting the cardiac effects of acute hyperkalemia.

(b) **Administration and dosage.** When used to reverse hyperkalemia-induced cardiotoxicity, calcium chloride is given intravenously, as 5–10 ml of a 10% solution (1.4 mEq Ca^{2+}/ml) administered over 2 minutes. Doses of up to 20 ml of a 10% solution are safe when given slowly. The initial dose may be followed by another 10–20 ml of a 10% solution placed in a larger fluid volume and administered slowly.

(c) **Precautions and monitoring effects**

(i) Intravenous (IV) calcium is contraindicated in patients with ventricular fibrillation or renal calculi.

(ii) The infusion rate should not exceed 0.5 ml/min. Patients should remain recumbent for about 15 minutes after infusion.

(iii) The ECG should be monitored during calcium gluconate therapy.

(iv) Calcium gluconate should not be mixed with solutions containing sodium bicarbonate because this can lead to precipitation.

(v) **Adverse effects** include tingling sensations and renal calculus formation.

(d) **Significant interactions.** Calcium may cause increased digitalis toxicity when administered concurrently with digitalis preparations.

(3) **Sodium bicarbonate** may be given as an emergency measure for severe hyperkalemia or metabolic acidosis.

(a) **Mechanism of action and therapeutic effect.** IV sodium bicarbonate restores bicarbonate that the renal tubules cannot reabsorb from the glomerular filtrate and increases arterial pH. This results in a shift of potassium into cells and reduces serum potassium.

(b) **Onset of action** is 15–30 minutes.

(c) **Administration and dosage**

(i) Sodium bicarbonate is administered intravenously.

(ii) The dosage is calculated as follows:

$$[50\% \text{ of body weight (kg)}] \times [\text{desired arterial bicarbonate } (HCO^{-3}) - \text{actual } HCO^{-3}]$$

(d) **Precautions and monitoring effects**

(i) To avoid sodium and fluid overload, sodium bicarbonate must be given cautiously. Half of the patient's bicarbonate deficit is replaced over the first 12 hours of therapy.

(ii) Sodium bicarbonate may precipitate calcium salts in IV solutions and should not be mixed in the same infusion fluid.

(iii) Arterial blood gas values and serum electrolyte levels should be monitored closely during sodium bicarbonate therapy.

(4) **Regular insulin with dextrose**

(a) **Mechanism of action and therapeutic effect.** The combination of insulin with dextrose deposits potassium with glycogen in the liver, reducing the serum potassium.

(b) **Onset of action** is 15–30 minutes.

(c) **Administration and dosage.** Regular insulin (20–30 U in 200–300 ml of 20% dextrose) is administered intravenously over 30 minutes.

(d) **Precautions and monitoring effects**

(i) The serum glucose level should be monitored during therapy.

(ii) The patient should be assessed for signs and symptoms of fluid overload.

(5) **Sodium polystyrene sulfonate (SPS)**

(a) **Mechanism of action.** SPS is a potassium-removing resin that exchanges sodium ions for potassium ions in the intestine (1 g of SPS exchanges 0.5–1 mEq/L of potassium). The SPS is distributed throughout the intestines and excreted in the feces.

(b) **Therapeutic effect.** Administered as an adjunctive treatment for hyperkalemia, SPS reduces potassium levels in the serum and other body fluids.

(c) **Onset of action** of orally administered SPS is 2 hours; effects are seen in 1 hour when SPS is administered as a retention enema.

(d) **Administration and dosage**

(i) SPS is usually administered orally, although it may be given through a nasogastric tube. The oral dose is 15–30 g in a suspension of 70% sorbitol, administered every 4–6 hours until the desired therapeutic effect is achieved.

(ii) When oral or nasogastric administration is not possible due to nausea, vomiting, or paralytic ileus, SPS may be given by retention enema. The rectal dose is 30–50 g in 100 ml of sorbitol as a warm emulsion, administered deep into the sigmoid colon every 6 hours. Administration may be done with a rubber tube that is taped in place or via a Foley catheter with a balloon inflated distal to the anal sphincter.

(e) Precautions and monitoring effects

(i) The patient's serum electrolyte levels should be monitored closely during SPS therapy. Sodium, chloride, bicarbonate and pH should be monitored in addition to potassium.

(ii) SPS therapy usually continues until the serum potassium level drops to between 4 and 5 mEq/L.

(iii) The patient should be assessed regularly for signs of potassium depletion, including irritability, confusion, cardiac arrhythmias, ECG changes, and muscle weakness.

(iv) SPS exchanges sodium for potassium, so sodium overload may occur during therapy.

(v) For oral administration, SPS should be mixed only with water or sorbitol. Orange juice, which has a high potassium content, should not be used because it decreases the effectiveness of the SPS. For rectal administration, SPS should be mixed only with water and sorbitol, never with mineral oil.

(vi) Adverse effects of SPS include constipation, fecal impaction with rectal administration, nausea, vomiting, and diarrhea.

(vii) SPS should not be used as the sole agent in the treatment of severe hyperkalemia; other agents or therapies should be used in conjunction with this agent.

(f) Significant interactions. Magnesium hydroxide and other nonabsorbable cation-donating laxatives and antacids may decrease the effectiveness of potassium exchange by SPS and may cause systemic alkalosis.

b. Treatment of metabolic acidosis. Sodium bicarbonate may be given if the arterial pH is below 7.35 [see I F 2 a (3)].

c. Treatment of hyperphosphatemia

(1) Dialysis may be used to treat acute, life-threatening hyperphosphatemia accompanied by acute hypocalcemia (see II F 7).

(2) Aluminum hydroxide (an aluminum-containing antacid)

(a) Mechanism of action and therapeutic effect. Aluminum binds excess phosphate in the intestine, thereby reducing phosphate concentration.

(b) Onset of action is 6–12 hours.

(c) Administration and dosage. Aluminum hydroxide is administered orally as a tablet or suspension. For the treatment of hyperphosphatemia, 0.5–2 or 15–30 ml of suspension are administered three or four times daily with meals.

(d) Precautions and monitoring effects

(i) Aluminum hydroxide may cause constipation and anorexia.

(ii) Serum phosphate levels should be monitored because aluminum hydroxide can cause phosphate depletion.

(iii) Aluminum hydroxide can cause calcium resorption and bone demineralization.

(3) Calcium carbonate may be given instead of aluminum hydroxide to treat hyperphosphatemia.

d. Treatment of hypocalcemia. Immediate treatment is necessary if the patient has severe hypocalcemia, as evidenced by tetany.

(1) Calcium gluconate [see I F 2 a (2)]

(a) Mechanism of action and therapeutic effect. This drug replaces and maintains body calcium, raising the serum calcium level immediately.

(b) Administration and dosage. When used to reverse hypocalcemia, calcium gluconate is administered intravenously in a dosage of 1–2 g over a period of 10 minutes, followed by a slow infusion (over 6–8 hours) of an additional 1 g.

(c) Precautions and monitoring effects and significant interactions [see I F 2 a (2) (c), (d)]

(2) **Oral calcium salts.** Calcium carbonate, chloride, gluconate, or lactate may be given by mouth when oral intake is permitted or if the patient has relatively mild hypocalcemia. The usual adult dosage is 4–6 g/day given in three or four divided doses.

e. **Treatment of hyponatremia**

(1) Moderate or asymptomatic hyponatremia may require only **fluid restriction.**

(2) **Sodium chloride** may be given for severe symptomatic hyponatremia (i.e., a serum sodium level below 120 mEq/L).

(a) **Mechanism of action and therapeutic effect.** Sodium chloride replaces and maintains sodium and chloride concentration, thereby increasing extracellular tonicity.

(b) **Administration and dosage**

(i) A 3% or 5% sodium chloride solution may be administered by slow IV infusion. The amount of solution needed is calculated from the following equation:

$$(\text{Normal serum sodium level} - \text{actual serum sodium level}) \times \text{total body water}$$

(ii) Typically, 400 ml or less are administered.

(c) **Precautions and monitoring effects**

(i) Hypertonic sodium chloride must be administered very slowly to avoid circulatory overload, pulmonary edema, or central pontine myelinolysis.

(ii) Serum electrolyte levels must be monitored frequently during therapy.

(iii) Excessive infusion may cause hypernatremia and other serious electrolyte abnormalities and may worsen existing acidosis.

3. **Management of systemic manifestations**

a. **Treatment of fluid overload and edema.** As water and sodium accumulate in extracellular fluid during ARF, fluid overload and edema may occur. **Diuretics** and dopamine may be given to reduce fluid volume excess and edema. Treatment should be initiated as soon as possible after oliguria begins. **Mannitol** or a **loop diuretic** may be used; thiazide diuretics are avoided in renal failure because they are ineffective when creatinine clearance is less than 25 ml/min, and they may worsen the patient's clinical status.

(1) **Step 1: Loop (high-ceiling) diuretics.** These agents include **furosemide, bumetanide,** and **ethacrynic acid.** Loop diuretics are more potent and faster-acting than thiazide diuretics.

(a) **Mechanism of action and therapeutic effects.** Loop diuretics inhibit sodium and chloride reabsorption at the loop of Henle, promoting water excretion.

(b) **Onset of action** for an oral dose is 1 hour; several minutes for an IV dose. Duration of action for an oral dose is 6–8 hours; 2–3 hours for an IV dose.

(c) **Administration and dosage**

(i) **Furosemide,** the **most commonly used** loop diuretic, usually is administered intravenously in patients with ARF to hasten the therapeutic effect. The dose is titrated to the patient's needs; the usual initial dose is 1–1.5 mg/kg. If the first dose does not produce a urine output of 10–15 ml within 20–30 minutes, a dose of 2–3 mg/kg is administered; if the desired response still does not occur, a dose of 3–6 mg/kg is administered 20–30 minutes after the second dose.

(ii) **Bumetanide** may be given to patients who are unresponsive or allergic to furosemide. The usual dosage, administered intravenously or intramuscularly in the treatment of ARF, is 0.5–1 mg/day; however, some patients may require up to 20 mg/day. A second or third dose may be given at intervals of 2–3 hours. When bumetanide is given orally, the dosage is 0.5–2 mg/day, repeated up to two times, if necessary, at intervals of 2–3 hours.

(iii) **Ethacrynic acid** is **less commonly used** to treat ARF because ototoxicity (sometimes irreversible) is associated with its use. It may be given intravenously (slowly over several minutes) in a dose of 50–100 mg. The usual oral dosage is 50–200 mg/day; some patients may require up to 200 mg twice daily.

(iv) Torsemide may also be given to patients unresponsive to or allergic to furosemide. The usual dose is 20 mg, administered intravenously. Doses may be increased by doubling up to 200 mg; 10–20 mg of torsemide is equipotent to 40 mg of furosemide, 1 mg bumetanide.

(d) Precautions and monitoring effects

(i) Loop diuretics must be used cautiously because they may cause orthostatic hypotension, fluid and electrolyte abnormalities, including volume depletion and dehydration, hypocalcemia, hypokalemia, hypochloremia, hyponatremia, hypomagnesemia, and transient ototoxicity, especially with rapid IV injection.

(ii) Serum electrolyte levels should be monitored frequently and the patient assessed regularly for signs and symptoms of electrolyte abnormalities.

(iii) Blood pressure and pulse rate should be assessed during diuretic therapy.

(iv) GI reactions include abdominal pain and discomfort, diarrhea (with furosemide and ethacrynic acid), and nausea (with bumetanide).

(v) Blood glucose levels should be monitored in diabetic patients receiving loop diuretics because these agents may cause hyperglycemia and impaired glucose tolerance.

(vi) Patients who are allergic to sulfonamides may be hypersensitive to bumetanide and furosemide.

(vii) Furosemide and ethacrynic acid may cause agranulocytosis.

(e) Significant interactions

(i) **Aminoglycoside antibiotics** may potentiate ototoxicity when administered with any loop diuretic.

(ii) **Indomethacin** may hamper the diuretic response to furosemide and bumetanide; **probenecid** may hamper the diuretic response to bumetanide.

(iii) Ethacrynic acid may potentiate the anticoagulant effects of **warfarin.**

(iv) Sweating and flushing may occur when chloral hydrate is administered to patients receiving IV furosemide.

(2) Step 2: Mannitol, an osmotic diuretic, is a non-reabsorbable polysaccharide.

(a) **Mechanism of action and therapeutic effect.** Mannitol increases the osmotic pressure of the glomerular filtrate; fluid from interstitial spaces is drawn into blood vessels expanding plasma volume and maintaining or increasing the urine flow. This drug may be given to prevent ARF in high-risk patients, such as those undergoing surgery or suffering from severe trauma or hemolytic transfusion reactions.

(b) **Onset of action** is 15–30 minutes. Duration of action is 3–4 hours.

(c) **Administration and dosage.** Mannitol is available in solutions, ranging from 5% to 25%. For the treatment of oliguric ARF or the prevention of ARF, the usual initial dose is 12.5–25 g, administered intravenously; the maximum daily dosage is 100 g, administered intravenously. The exact concentration of the solution is determined by the patient's fluid requirements.

(d) Precautions and monitoring effects

(i) Mannitol is contraindicated in patients with anuria, pulmonary edema or congestion, severe dehydration, and intracranial hemorrhage (except during craniotomy).

(ii) Mannitol may cause or worsen pulmonary edema and circulatory overload. If signs and symptoms of these problems develop, the infusion should be stopped.

(iii) Other adverse effects of mannitol include fluid and electrolyte abnormalities, water intoxication, headache, confusion, blurred vision, thirst, nausea, and vomiting.

(iv) Vital signs, urine output, daily weight, cardiopulmonary status, and serum and urine sodium and potassium levels should be monitored during mannitol therapy.

(v) Mannitol solutions with undissolved crystals should not be administered.

(3) Step 3: Dopamine. This vasopressor, an immediate metabolic precursor of epinephrine and norepinephrine, is a potent sympathomimetic agent.

(a) **Mechanism of action and therapeutic effect.** Given at doses between 1 and 5 μg/kg/min, dopamine dilates mesenteric and renal blood vessels, which leads to enhanced renal blood flow, increased GFR, sodium excretion, and urine output. Dopamine has been used as a means to prevent as well as treat ARF.

(b) **Administration and dosage.** Dopamine is given intravenously at 1–5 μg/kg/min. The dose is titrated to the desired response.

(c) **Precautions and monitoring effects**

(i) Dosages greater than 10 μg/kg/min stimulate α-receptors and produce peripheral vasoconstriction, raising systemic blood pressure. Dosages greater than 20 μg/kg/min may decrease renal blood flow as α-receptor stimulation overwhelms the dopaminergic vasodilation.

(ii) Dopamine may cause hypotension, tachycardia, arrhythmias, palpitations, anginal pain, ECG abnormalities, and vasoconstriction. These signs and symptoms may warrant slowing of the infusion rate.

(iii) Adverse GI effects include nausea and vomiting.

(iv) Extravasation may result in necrosis and tissue sloughing.

(v) Dopamine must be used cautiously in patients receiving monoamine oxidase (MAO) inhibitors.

(vi) During the infusion, the patient's blood pressure, pulse, cardiac function, urine output, and extremity temperature and color should be assessed.

(d) **Significant interactions**

(i) **Phenytoin** may cause reduced blood pressure.

(ii) **Ergot alkaloids** can lead to dangerously elevated blood pressure.

b. **Treatment of other systemic manifestations.** ARF typically causes hematologic, GI, and skin disturbances (see II F 5).

4. **Dialysis.** Hemodialysis or peritoneal dialysis may be necessary in ARF patients who develop anuria; acute fluid overload; severe hyperkalemia, metabolic acidosis, or hyperphosphatemia; GFR below 5 ml/min; BUN level above 100 mg/dl; or serum creatinine level above 10 mg/dl. For a discussion of dialysis, see II F 7.

II. CHRONIC RENAL FAILURE

A. **Definition.** Chronic renal failure (CRF) is the progressive, irreversible deterioration of renal function. Usually resulting from long-standing disease, CRF sometimes derives from ARF that does not respond to treatment.

B. Classification and pathophysiology

1. CRF typically progresses slowly through mild impairment to end-stage renal disease with a total loss of kidney function.
   a. **Mild-to-moderate CRF** is characterized by decreased renal reserve (GFR of 20–70 ml/min). Despite some loss of renal function at lower GFR, homeostasis is preserved.
   b. **Severe CRF,** where GFR is 5–10 ml/min, is characterized by some clinical evidence of renal failure. At this stage, slight azotemia occurs. Renal reserve has decreased so that the patient may have some trouble maintaining fluid and electrolyte status under stress. This is particularly true when cardiac function is also compromised.
   c. **End-stage renal disease,** when GFR is below 5 ml/min, is characterized by frank uremia. Fluid and electrolyte imbalances develop, azotemia worsens, and systemic manifestations appear.

2. As CRF progresses, nephron destruction worsens, leading to deterioration in the kidneys' filtration, reabsorption, and endocrine functions.

3. Renal function typically does not diminish until about 75% of kidney tissue is damaged. Ultimately, the kidneys become shrunken, fibrotic masses.

C. **Etiology.** Minor causes of CRF in adults include:

1. Diabetic nephropathy
2. Hypertension
3. Glomerulonephritis
4. Polycystic kidney disease
5. Long-standing vascular disease (e.g., renal artery stenosis)
6. Long-standing obstructive uropathy (e.g., renal calculi)

7. Exposure to nephrotoxic agents

D. Clinical evaluation

1. **Physical findings.** Signs and symptoms, which vary widely, do not appear until renal insufficiency progresses to renal failure.
   a. **Metabolic abnormalities** include loss of the ability to maintain sodium, potassium, and water homeostasis, leading to hyponatremia or hypernatremia, based on relative sodium or water intake. Hyperkalemia is uncommon until end-stage disease. Fluid overload, edema and CHF may become a problem unless fluid intake is closely managed. As renal failure progresses, the inability to excrete acid and maintain buffer capacity leads to metabolic acidosis (see I D 1 b, d, g, h).
   b. **Neurologic manifestations** include short attention span, loss of memory, and listlessness. As CRF progresses, these advance to confusion, stupor, seizures, and coma. Neuromuscular findings include peripheral neuropathy; pain, itching, and a burning sensation, particularly in the feet and legs. If dialysis is not started after these abnormalities occur, motor involvement begins, including loss of deep tendon reflexes, weakness, and finally, quadriplegia.
   c. **Cardiovascular problems** include arterial hypertension, peripheral edema, CHF, and pulmonary edema. Pericarditis is now increasingly infrequent as a result of early dialysis.
   d. **GI manifestations** include nausea, vomiting, constipation, stomatitis, and an unpleasant taste in the mouth. CRF patients have an increased incidence of ulcers, pancreatitis, and diverticulosis.
   e. **Respiratory problems** include dyspnea when CHF is present, pulmonary edema, pleuritic pain, and uremic pleuritis.
   f. **Integumentary findings** typically include pale yellowish, dry, scaly skin; severe itching; uremic frost; ecchymoses; purpura; and brittle nails and hair.
   g. **Musculoskeletal changes** range from muscle and bone pain to pathologic fractures and calcifications in the brain, heart, eyes, joints, and vessels.
   h. **Hematologic disturbances** include anemia. The signs and symptoms of anemia arise from lack of erythropoietin and reduced life span of red blood cells, including:
      (1) Pallor of the skin, nail beds, palms, conjunctivae, and mucosa
      (2) Abnormal bruising or ecchymoses
      (3) Dyspnea and angina pectoris
      (4) Extreme fatigue

2. **Diagnostic test results**
   a. **Creatinine clearance** may range from 0 to 70 ml/min, reflecting renal impairment.
   b. **Blood tests** typically show:
      (1) Elevated BUN and serum creatinine levels
      (2) Reduced arterial pH and bicarbonate concentration
      (3) Reduced serum calcium level
      (4) Increased serum potassium and phosphate levels
      (5) Possible reduction in the serum sodium level
      (6) Normochromic, normocytic anemia (hematocrit 20%–30%)
   c. **Urinalysis** may reveal glycosuria, proteinuria, erythrocytes, leukocytes, and casts. Specific gravity is fixed at 1.010.
   d. **Radiographic findings.** Kidney, ureter, and bladder radiography, IV pyelography, renal scan, renal arteriography, and nephrotomography may be performed. Typically, these tests reveal small kidneys (less than 8 cm in length).

E. Treatment objectives

1. Improve patient comfort and prolong life.

2. Treat systemic manifestations of CRF.

3. Correct body chemistry abnormalities.

F. Therapy. Management of the CRF patient is generally conservative. Dietary measures and fluid restriction relieve some symptoms of CRF and may increase patient comfort and prolong life until dialysis or renal transplantation is required or available (see I F 1 a, b).

1. **Treatment of edema and CHF. Digitalis preparations** and **diuretics** may be given to manage edema and CHF and to increase urine output.
   a. **Digitalis preparations.** These agents include **digoxin, digitoxin, digitalis leaf,** and **deslanoside.** See Chapter 42 for a discussion of these drugs.
   b. **Diuretics.** An osmotic diuretic, a loop diuretic, or a thiazide-like diuretic may be given.
      (1) **Osmotic and loop diuretics.** See I F 3 a (1), (2) for information on the use of these drugs in renal failure.
      (2) **Thiazide-like diuretics. Metolazone** is the most commonly used diuretic in CRF.
         (a) **Mechanism of action and therapeutic effect.** Metolazone reduces the body's fluid and sodium volume by increasing sodium reabsorption in the ascending limb of the loop of Henle, thereby increasing urinary excretion of fluid and sodium.
         (b) **Administration and dosage.** Metolazone is given orally at 5–20 mg/day; the dose is titrated to the patient's needs. Furosemide and metolazone act synergistically. Combination use is common.
         (c) **Precautions and monitoring effects**
            (i) Metolazone should not be given to patients with hypersensitivity to sulfonamide derivatives, including thiazides.
            (ii) To avoid nocturia, the daily dose should be given in the morning.
            (iii) Metolazone may cause hematologic reactions, such as agranulocytosis, aplastic anemia, and thrombocytopenia.
            (iv) Fluid volume depletion, hypokalemia, hyperuricemia, hyperglycemia, and impaired glucose tolerance may occur during metolazone therapy.
            (v) Metolazone may cause hypersensitivity reactions, including vasculitis and pneumonitis.
         (d) **Significant interactions**
            (i) **Diazoxide** may potentiate the antihypertensive, hyperglycemic, and hyperuricemic effects of metolazone.
            (ii) **Colestipol** and **cholestyramine** decrease the absorption of metolazone.

2. **Treatment of hypertension. Antihypertensive agents** may be needed if blood pressure becomes dangerously high as a result of edema and the high renin levels that occur in CRF. Antihypertensive therapy should be initiated in the lowest effective dose and titrated according to the patient's needs.
   a. **Angiotensin-converting enzyme (ACE) inhibitors-captopril, enalapril, lisinopril**—are widely used to treat CRF because they help preserve renal function and typically cause fewer adverse effects than other antihypertensive agents (see Chapter 41).
   b. **β-Adrenergic blockers,** including **propranolol** and **atenolol,** reduce blood pressure through various mechanisms (see Chapter 41).
   c. **Other antihypertensive agents** are sometimes used in the treatment of CRF, including α-adrenergic drugs, **clonidine, methyldopa,** and vasodilators, such as **hydralazine** (see Chapter 41).

3. **Treatment of hyperphosphatemia** involves administration of a phosphate binder, such as aluminum hydroxide or calcium carbonate (see I F 2 c).

4. **Treatment of hypocalcemia**
   a. **Oral calcium salts** [see I F 2 d (2)]
   b. **Vitamin D**
      (1) **Mechanism of action and therapeutic effect.** Vitamin D promotes intestinal calcium and phosphate absorption and utilization and, thus, increases the serum calcium concentration.
      (2) **Choice of agent.** For the treatment of hypocalcemia in CRF and other renal disorders, **calcitriol** (vitamin D_2, the active form of vitamin D) is the preferred vitamin D supplement because of its greater efficacy and relatively short duration of action. Other single-entity preparations include dihydrotachysterol, ergocalciferol, and calcifediol.
      (3) **Administration and dosage.** Calcitriol is given orally; the dose is titrated to the patient's needs (0.5–1 μg/day may be effective).
      (4) **Precautions and monitoring effects**
         (a) Vitamin D administration may be dangerous in patients with renal failure and must be used with extreme caution.

(b) Vitamin D toxicity may cause a wide range of signs and symptoms, including headache, dizziness, ataxia, convulsions, psychosis, soft-tissue calcification, conjunctivitis, photophobia, tinnitus, nausea, diarrhea, pruritus, and muscle and bone pain.
(c) Vitamin D has a narrow therapeutic index, necessitating frequent measurement of BUN and serum and urine calcium and potassium levels.
(d) Because hyperphosphatemia generally accompanies hypocalcemia in renal failure, dietary phosphate should be given during vitamin D therapy to prevent calcification and deterioration in renal function [see I F 2 c (2)].

5. Treatment of other systemic manifestations of CRF

a. Treatment of anemia includes administration of iron (e.g., ferrous sulfate), folate supplements, and erythropoietin.
(1) Severe anemia may warrant infusion of fresh frozen packed cells or washed packed cells.
(2) To increase red blood cell production, androgens may be given.
(3) Erythropoietin stimulates the production of red cell progenitors and the production of hemoglobin. It also accelerates the release of reticulocytes from the bone marrow.
(a) An initial dose of erythropoietin is 50–100 U/kg intravenously or subcutaneously three times a week. The dose may be adjusted upward to elicit the desired response.
(b) Erythropoietin works best in patients with a hematocrit below 30%. During the initial treatment, the hematocrit increases 1%–3.5 % in a 2-week period. The target hematocrit is 33%–35%. Maintenance doses are titrated based on hematocrit after this level is reached.
(c) Erythropoietin therapy should be temporarily stopped if hematocrit exceeds 36%. Additional side effects include hypertension in up to 25% of patients. Headache and malaise have been reported.
(d) The effects of erythropoietin are dependent on a ready supply of iron for hemoglobin synthesis. Patients who do not respond should have iron stores checked. This includes serum iron, total iron-binding capacity, transferrin saturation, and serum ferritin. Iron supplementation should be increased as indicated.

b. Treatment of GI disturbances
(1) Antiemetics help control nausea and vomiting.
(2) Cimetidine may be given to relieve gastric irritation.
(3) Docusate sodium or methylcellulose may be used to prevent constipation.
(4) Enemas may be given to remove blood from the GI tract.

c. Treatment of skin problems. An antipruritic agent, such as diphenhydramine, may be used to alleviate itching.

6. Management of body chemistry abnormalities (see I F 2)

7. Dialysis. When CRF progresses to end-stage renal disease and no longer responds to conservative measures, long-term dialysis or renal transplantation is necessary to prolong life.

a. Hemodialysis is the preferred dialysis method for patients with a reduced peritoneal membrane, hypercatabolism, or acute hyperkalemia.
(1) This technique involves shunting of the patient's blood through a dialysis membrane-containing unit for diffusion, osmosis, and ultrafiltration. The blood is then returned to the patient's circulation.
(2) Vascular access may be obtained via an arteriovenous fistula or an external shunt.
(3) The procedure takes only 3–8 hours; most patients need only two or three treatments a week. With proper training, patients can perform hemodialysis at home.
(4) The patient receives heparin during hemodialysis to prevent clotting.
(5) Various complications may arise, including hemorrhage, hepatitis, anemia, septicemia, cardiovascular problems, air embolism, rapid shifts in fluid and electrolyte balance, itching, nausea, vomiting, headache, seizures, and aluminum osteodystrophy.

b. Peritoneal dialysis is the preferred dialysis method for patients with bleeding disorders and cardiovascular disease.
(1) The peritoneum is used as a semipermeable membrane. A plastic catheter inserted into the peritoneum provides access for the dialysate, which draws excess fluids,

wastes, and electrolytes across the peritoneal membrane periodically by osmosis and diffusion.

(2) Peritoneal dialysis can be carried out in three different modes.

(a) **Intermittent peritoneal dialysis** is an automatic cycling mode lasting 8–10 hours, performed three times a week. This mode allows nighttime treatment and is appropriate for working patients.

(b) **Continuous ambulatory peritoneal dialysis** is performed daily for 24 hours with four exchanges daily. The patient can remain active during the treatment.

(c) **Continuous cyclic peritoneal dialysis** may be used if the other two modes fail to improve creatinine clearance. Dialysis takes place at night; the last exchange is retained in the peritoneal cavity during the day, then drained that evening.

(3) **Advantages** of peritoneal dialysis include a lack of serious complications, retention of normal fluid and electrolyte balance, simplicity, reduced cost, patient independence, and a reduced need (or no need) for heparin administration.

(4) **Complications** of peritoneal dialysis include hyperglycemia, constipation, and inflammation or infection at the catheter site. Also this method carries a high risk of peritonitis.

8. **Renal transplantation.** This surgical procedure allows some patients with end-stage renal disease to live normal and—in many cases—longer lives.

a. **Histocompatibility** must be tested to minimize the risk of transplant rejection and failure. Human leukocyte antigen (HLA) type, mixed lymphocyte reactivity, and blood group types are determined to assess histocompatibility.

b. Renal transplant material may be obtained from a living donor or a cadaver.

c. **Three types of graft rejection** can occur.

(1) **Hyperacute (immediate) rejection** results in graft loss within minutes to hours after transplantation.

(a) Acute urine flow cessation and bluish or mottled kidney discoloration are intraoperative signs of hyperacute rejection.

(b) Postoperative manifestations include kidney enlargement, fever, anuria, local pain, sodium retention, and hypertension.

(c) Treatment for hyperacute rejection is immediate nephrectomy.

(2) **Acute rejection** may occur 4–60 days after transplantation.

(3) Chronic rejection occurs more than 60 days after transplantation.

(a) Signs and symptoms include low-grade fever, increased proteinuria, azotemia, hypertension, oliguria, weight gain, and edema.

(b) Treatment may include alkylating agents, cyclosporine, antilymphocyte globulin, and corticosteroids. In some cases, nephrectomy is necessary.

d. Complications include:

(1) Infection, diabetes, hepatitis, and leukopenia, resulting from immunosuppressive therapy

(2) Hypertension, resulting from various causes

(3) Cancer (e.g., lymphoma, cutaneous malignancies, head and neck cancer, leukemia, colon cancer)

(4) Pancreatitis and mental and emotional disorders (e.g., suicidal tendencies, severe depression, brought on by steroid therapy)

STUDY QUESTIONS

Directions: Each of the numbered items or incomplete statements in this section is followed by answers or by completions of the statement. Select the **one** lettered answer or completion that is **best** in each case.

Questions 1–5

A 48-year-old black man has a history of mild to severe hypertension. His hypertension has been poorly controlled with enalapril and hydrochlorothiazide. On prior visits, his blood pressure control has varied and seems to correspond with a lack of compliance with his treatment regimen. The patient states that he occasionally forgets his pills or does not take them when he is feeling "okay." The patient's history does not include diabetes mellitus or heart disease. He completed a 14-day course of clarithromycin for an upper respiratory infection in the past month and has returned to the clinic for follow-up review of the infection and his hypertension therapy.

On this visit, the patient complains of dizziness, loss of energy, increased frequency of urination, and edema of the lower extremities. His physical examination reveals an overweight man with a standing blood pressure of 175/100, moderate edema of the ankles, and a slight third heart sound. Laboratory results include blood urea nitrogen (BUN) 45 mg/100 ml, serum creatinine 3.7 mg/100 ml, serum calcium 5.3 mg/ml, serum potassium of 6.3 mg/ml, and a hematocrit of 25. Serum iron, total iron-binding capacity, transferrin saturation, and serum ferritin are normal. Microscopic urine and chemical analyses reveal mild proteinuria and a specific gravity of 1.010.

1. The history, physical examination, laboratory values, and current signs and symptoms suggest that the patient has which of the following conditions?

(A) Acute renal failure brought on by a nephrotoxic drug (clarithromycin, enalapril)
(B) Acute renal failure resulting from renal obstruction by a kidney stone
(C) Acute renal failure precipitated by severe dehydration
(D) Chronic renal failure resulting from hypertension

2. Treatment of the patient's fluid retention and edema should begin with all of the following, EXCEPT

(A) restriction of fluid intake
(B) therapy with furosemide or metolazone
(C) treatment of hypertension using a β-blocker or angiotensin converting enzyme inhibitor
(D) digitalis glycoside therapy if congestive heart failure is present
(E) hemodialysis

3. The most likely cause of the anemia seen in this patient is

(A) urinary blood loss
(B) vitamin B_{12} deficiency
(C) iron deficiency
(D) decreased red cell life span and a deficiency of erythropoietin

4. This patient's symptoms seemed to appear suddenly and may result from his history of uncontrolled hypertension. Which statement best describes hypertension?

(A) A major cause of chronic renal failure
(B) A major cause of acute renal failure
(C) A major cause of both chronic and acute renal failure
(D) Only seen in patients whose renal failure has caused excessive fluid retention

5. When should peritoneal dialysis or hemodialysis be considered to treat this patient's renal failure?

(A) As soon as possible to prevent further complications resulting from decreased renal function
(B) Only when renal function has decreased to a point where fluid and electrolyte status cannot be maintained using conservative measures
(C) On an intermittent basis as the situation demands
(D) Only if the patient is a kidney transplant candidate

6. Acute renal failure (ARF) may be caused by all of the following EXCEPT

(A) acute tubular necrosis (ATN) due to drug therapy (e.g. aminoglycosides, contrast media)
(B) severe hypotension or circulatory collapse
(C) decreased cardiac output, as from congestive heart failure
(D) hemolysis, myoglobinuria
(E) hyperkalemia

7. Life-threatening cardiac arrhythmias due to hyperkalemia should be treated with

(A) calcium chloride or calcium gluconate intravenously
(B) digoxin or other digitalis preparations
(C) loop diuretics to rapidly eliminate potassium
(D) sodium polystyrene sulfonate (SPS)

8. Aluminum hydroxide is used to treat hyperphosphatemia associated with renal failure. Chronic use of aluminum hydroxide may cause all of the following conditions EXCEPT

(A) phosphate depletion
(B) calcium resorption and bone demineralization
(C) anorexia and constipation
(D) fluid retention

9. The diuretic of choice for the initial treatment of a patient with either acute or chronic renal failure (ARF, CRF) whose creatinine clearance is below 25 ml/min is

(A) hydrochlorothiazide
(B) bumetanide
(C) furosemide
(D) ethacrynic acid

10. Erythropoietin is used commonly to treat the anemia associated with chronic renal failure (CRF). The effectiveness of erythropoietin is limited by which of the following conditions?

(A) A patient's allergy to erythropoietin
(B) Depletion of iron stores, requiring oral or parenteral supplementation
(C) The ineffectiveness of erythropoietin, as 30% of patients do not respond
(D) The anemia of chronic renal failure is not due to a lack of erythropoietin, so erythropoietin will not ameliorate

ANSWERS AND EXPLANATIONS

1. The answer is D *[II D 1].*
The fluid and electrolyte status of the patient described in the case combined with the urine specific gravity, lack of crystals or casts in the urine, and the complaint of fatigue suggest chronic renal failure resulting from uncontrolled hypertension or an unknown cause. The antibiotic therapy (clarithromycin) and antihypertensive drug (enalapril) are not nephrotoxic, and the patient's blood pressure and fluid status do not indicate a prerenal cause.

2. The answer is E *[II F 1, 2].*
All of these measures are indicated as initial therapy for the treatment of edema and fluid retention due to chronic renal failure except hemodialysis, which should be reserved until more conservative measures are tried.

3. The answer is D *[II D 1 h].*
There is no evidence of frank blood loss. The decreased hematocrit and the clinical signs indicate the anemia of chronic renal failure due to the shortened red blood cell life span. Decreased erythropoietin is the cause.

4. The answer is A *[II C 2].*
Systemic long-standing high blood pressure is the second most common cause of chronic renal failure (CRF). Only malignant hypertension can cause acute renal failure (ARF), which is not common. High blood pressure is common after substantial renal damage has occurred in both CRF and ARF, but it does not occur as the first or only manifestation.

5. The answer is B *[II F 7].*
Dialysis should be considered when the patient's renal function has decreased to a point where conservative measures are ineffective. Peritoneal dialysis and hemodialysis have associated complications and morbidity, so intermittent or early use of these therapies is not indicated. Patients can be maintained on dialysis for extended periods, so eligibility for transplant is not required.

6. The answer is E *[I B 1–3].*
Hyperkalemia is a sign of acute and chronic renal failure, resulting from the decreased renal function and changes in acid–base balance

7. The answer is A *[I F 2 a].*
Intravenous calcium chloride or gluconate is used to treat potassium-induced arrhythmias. Digoxin is not indicated. Loop diuretics and sodium polystyrene sulfonate (SPS) do not have a significant effect on potassium in a short period to treat a life-threatening arrhythmia. SPS and loop diuretics, along with dialysis, may be considered to remove potassium in the short term, preventing the recurrence of arrhythmias.

8. The answer is D *[I F 2 c (2)]*
Common effects of the sustained use of aluminum-containing antacids include phosphate depletion, calcium resorption, bone demineralization, anorexia, and constipation. Fluid retention does not result from the use of antacids containing aluminum hydroxide.

9. The answer is C *[I F 3 a (1) (c)].*

Furosemide is the diuretic of choice for the initial treatment of a patient with either acute or chronic renal failure (ARF, CRF) whose creatinine clearance is below 25 ml/min. A thiazide diuretic has little effect at a creatinine clearance below 25 ml/min. Bumetanide, torsemide, and ethacrynic acid are appropriate only if the patient is allergic to furosemide or if repeated doses of furosemide are ineffective.

10. The answer is B *[II F 5 a].*

Erythropoietin is widely used and highly effective in treating the anemia associated with chronic renal failure (CRF). Few reports of patients refractory to erythropoietin therapy have appeared in medical literature. However, the depletion of iron stores will not allow the formation of red blood cells, even in the presence of appropriate amounts of erythropoietin. All CRF patients receiving erythropoietin require some iron supplementation, and most patients require parenteral iron to achieve sufficient supplies to continue developing hemoglobin over the term of their illness.

55
Principles of Cancer Chemotherapy

Amy J. Becker

I. PRINCIPLES OF ONCOLOGY. The term *cancer* refers to a heterogeneous group of diseases.

A. Characteristics of cancer cells. Tumors arise from a single abnormal cell, which continues to divide indefinitely. The lack of growth controls, ability to invade local tissues, and ability to spread, or **metastasize,** are characteristics of cancer cells. These properties are not present in normal cells.

B. Incidence. Cancer is the **second leading cause of death** in the United States. Approximately 30% of all people develop cancer at some point in their lives. Not all cancer patients die of their disease; some forms of cancer are considered curable if detected and treated early.

C. Etiology. Many factors have been implicated in the etiology of cancer. The **most common** of these factors are listed below.

1. **Viruses,** including Epstein-Barr virus (EBV), hepatitis B virus (HBV), and human papillomaviruses (HPV)
2. **Environmental and occupational exposures,** such as ionizing and ultraviolet radiation and exposure to chemicals, including vinyl chloride, benzene, and asbestos
3. **Life-style factors,** such as high-fat, low-fiber diets and tobacco and ethanol use
4. **Medications,** including alkylating agents and immunosuppressants
5. **Genetic factors,** including inherited mutations, cancer-causing genes (oncogenes), and tumor-suppressor genes

D. Detection and **diagnosis** are critical for the appropriate treatment of cancer.

1. **Warning signs** of cancer have been outlined by the American Cancer Society.
   - **a. C**hange in bowel or bladder habits
   - **b. A** sore that does not heal
   - **c. U**nusual bleeding or discharge
   - **d. T**hickening or lump in the breast or elsewhere
   - **e. I**ndigestion or difficulty swallowing
   - **f. O**bvious change in a wart or mole
   - **g. N**agging cough or hoarseness
2. **Guidelines for screening** asymptomatic people for the presence of cancer have been established by the National Cancer Institute, the American Cancer Society, and the United States Preventive Health Service Task Force. These screening tests include **mammography** for detection of breast cancer, **fecal occult blood tests** for detection of colon cancer, and **Papanicolaou (Pap) smears** for the detection of cervical cancer.
3. **Tumor markers** are biochemical indicators of the presence of neoplastic proliferation detected in serum, plasma, or other body fluids. These tumor markers may be used initially as screening tests, to reveal further information after abnormal test results or to monitor the efficacy of therapy. Elevated levels of these markers are not definitive for the presence of cancer; false positive results do occur.
   - **a.** Carcinoembryonic antigen (CEA)
   - **b.** Alpha-fetoprotein (AFP)
   - **c.** Prostate specific antigen (PSA)

4. **Tumor biopsy.** The definitive test for the presence of cancerous cells is a biopsy and pathologic examination of the biopsy specimen.

5. **Imaging studies,** such as x-rays, computerized tomography (CT) scans, magnetic resonance imaging (MRI), or positron emission tomography (PET) may be used to aid in the diagnosis or location of a suspected tumor.

6. **Other laboratory tests** commonly used for cancer diagnosis include complete blood counts (CBCs) and blood chemistries.

E. **Staging** is the categorizing of patients according to the extent of their disease. The stage of the disease is used to determine prognosis and treatment. Two different staging systems are widely employed for the staging of neoplasms.

1. **TNM classification**
   a. *T* indicates tumor size and is classified from 0 to 4, with 0 indicating the absence of tumor.
   b. *N* indicates the presence and extent of regional lymph node spread and is scaled from 0 to 3, with 0 indicating no regional lymph node involvement and 3 indicating extensive involvement.
   c. **M** indicates the presence or absence of distant metastases and can be classified as only 0 or 1.
   d. T2N1M0 thus indicates a moderate-size tumor with limited nodal disease and no distant metastases.

2. **AJC** staging, developed by the American Joint Committee on Staging, denotes cancers as stage 0 through IV. The high numbers indicate large tumors with extensive nodal involvement. Generally, high numbers also indicate a worse prognosis.

F. **Survival** depends on the tumor type, the extent of disease, and the therapy received.

1. Four of ten patients survive more than 5 years. Although some of these patients continue to be free of all detectable disease, not all patients who survive are cured. Oncologists prefer to use the term **complete response** or **remission** to indicate a patient with no evidence of disease after treatment. This is not a synonym for cure. For some slow-growing tumors, these disease-free periods may extend for 10–15 years after the initial remission. However, a number of patients who have achieved complete remission may have a relapse, possibly even dying of their cancer.

2. With the recent progress made in cancer research and treatment, more tumors are considered treatable than ever before.

II. CELL LIFE CYCLE.
Knowledge of the cell life cycle and cell cycle kinetics is essential to the understanding of the activity of chemotherapy agents in the treatment of cancer (Figure 55-1).

A. Phases of the cell cycle

1. **M phase,** or **mitosis,** is the phase in which the cell divides into two daughter cells.

2. **G_1 phase,** or **postmitotic gap,** is where RNA and the proteins required for the specialized functions of the cell are synthesized.

3. **S phase** (follows G_1) is the phase in which DNA synthesis occurs.

4. **G_2 phase,** or the **premitotic** or **postsynthetic gap,** is the phase in which RNA and the enzymes topoisomerase I and II are produced.

5. **G_0 phase,** or **resting phase,** is the phase in which the cell is not committed to division. Cells in this phase are generally not very sensitive to chemotherapy. Some of these cells may re-enter the actively dividing cell cycle. In a process called **recruitment,** some chemotherapy regimens are designed to enhance this re-entry by killing a large number of actively dividing cells.

B. Cell growth kinetics.
Several terms describe cell growth kinetics.

1. **Cell growth fraction** is the proportion of cells in the tumor dividing or preparing to divide. As the tumor enlarges, the cell growth fraction decreases because a larger proportion of cells may not be able to obtain adequate nutrients and blood supply for replication.

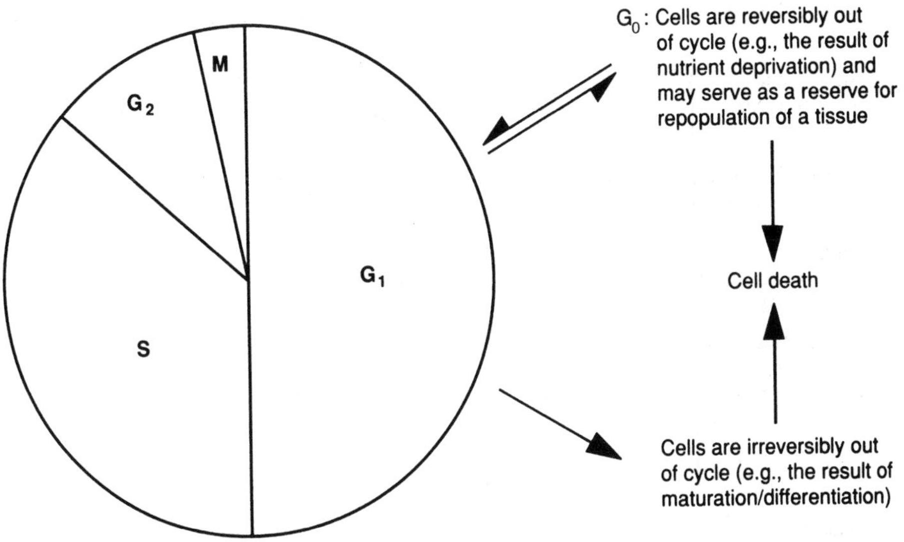

Figure 55-1. Diagrammatic representation of the cell growth cycle, emphasizing the relationship between proliferating cell populations. [Reprinted from Holleb AI, et al (eds): *American Cancer Society Textbook of Clinical Oncology.* Atlanta, American Cancer Society, 1991.]

2. **Cell cycle time** is the average time for a cell that has just completed mitosis to grow and again divide and again pass through mitosis. Cell cycle time is specific for each individual tumor.

3. **Tumor doubling time** is the time for the tumor to double in size. As the tumor gets larger, its doubling time gets longer because it contains a smaller proportion of actively dividing cells due to restrictions of space, nutrient availability, and blood supply.

4. The **Gompertzian growth curve** illustrates these cell growth concepts (Figure 55-2).

C. **Tumor Cell Burden** is the number of tumor cells in the body. Because of the large number of cells required to produce clinical symptoms (approximately 10^9 cells), the tumor may be in the plateau phase of the growth curve by the time it is detected. Each cycle of cancer chemotherapy kills a certain percentage of the tumor cells. As tumor cells are killed, cells in G_0 may be recruited into G_1, resulting in tumor regrowth. Thus, repeated cycles of chemotherapy are required to achieve a complete response or remission. The percentage of cells killed is dependent on the chemotherapy dose (Figure 55-3).

D. Chemotherapeutic agents may be classified according to their **reliance on cell cycle kinetics** for their cytotoxic effect. Combinations of chemotherapy agents that are active in different phases of the cell cycle may result in a greater cell kill. A cell cycle classification of some commonly used chemotherapeutic agents is listed below.

1. **Phase-specific agents** are most active against cells that are in a specific phase of the cell cycle. For example:

   a. M phase: vinca alkaloids, taxanes

   b. G_1 phase: asparaginase, prednisone

   c. S phase: antimetabolites

   d. G_2 phase: bleomycin, etoposide

2. **Phase-nonspecific agents** are effective while cells are in the active cycle but do not require that the cell be in a particular phase. Examples include alkylating agents, antitumor antibiotics, and cisplatin.

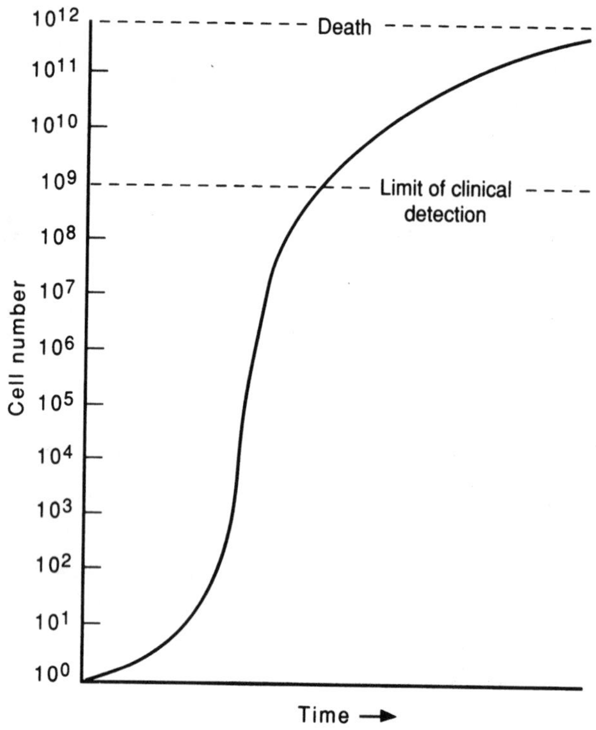

Figure 55-2. The gompertzian growth curve. During the early stages of its development a tumor's growth is exponential. But as a tumor enlarges, the growth slows. By the time a tumor becomes large enough to cause symptoms and be clinically detectable, the majority of its growth has already occurred and is no longer exponential. [Reprinted from Holleb AI, et al (eds): *American Cancer Society Textbook of Clinical Oncology.* Atlanta, American Cancer Society, 1991.]

3. **Cell cycle-nonspecific agents** are effective in all phases, including G_0. Examples include nitrosoureas and radiation.

III. CHEMOTHERAPY

A. Objectives of chemotherapy

1. A **cure** may be sought with aggressive therapy for a prolonged period of time to eradicate all disease. For leukemias, this curative approach may consist of remission induction, attempting the maximal cell kill, followed by consolidation therapy to eradicate all clinically undetectable disease and to lower the tumor cell burden below 10^3, where host immunologic defenses may keep the cells in control.
2. If the goal is **palliation,** chemotherapy may be given to control symptoms. Palliative therapy is usually given when complete eradication of the tumor is considered unlikely or the patient refuses aggressive therapy.
3. **Adjuvant** chemotherapy is given after more definitive therapy, such as surgery, to eliminate any remaining disease.
4. **Neoadjuvant** chemotherapy is given to decrease the tumor burden before surgery or radiation.

B. Chemotherapy dosing may be based on **body weight,** body surface area (**BSA**), or area under the concentration versus time curve (**AUC**). BSA is most frequently used because it provides an accurate comparison of activity and toxicity across species. In addition, BSA correlates with cardiac output, which determines renal and hepatic blood flow and, thus, affects drug elimination.

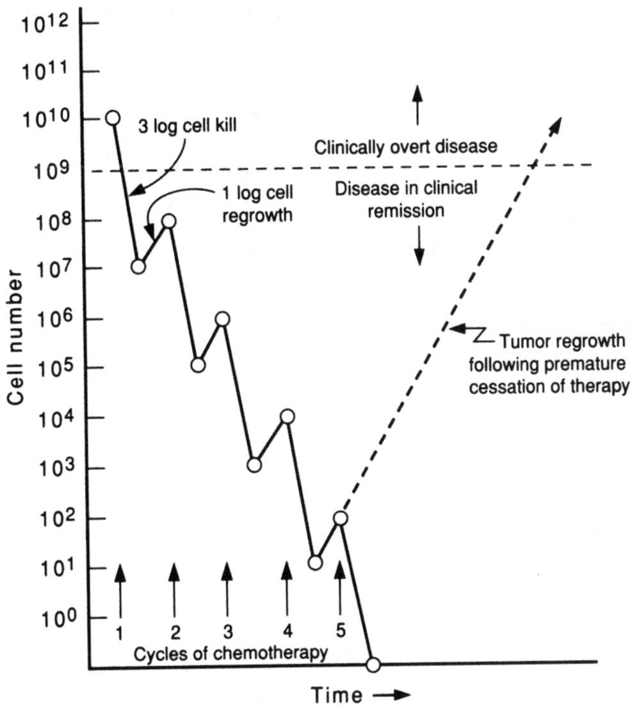

Figure 55-3. Relationship between tumor cell survival and chemotherapy administration. The exponential relationship between chemotherapy drug dose and tumor cell survival dictates that a constant proportion, not number, of tumor cells is killed with each cycle of treatment. In this example each cycle of drug administration results in 99.9% (3 log) cell kill, and 1 log of cell regrowth occurs between cycles. The broken line indicates what would occur if the last cycle of therapy was omitted: Despite complete clinical remission of disease, the tumor would ultimately recur. [Reprinted from Holleb AI, et al (eds): *American Cancer Society Textbook of Clinical Oncology.* Atlanta, American Cancer Society, 1991.]

C. Dosing adjustments may be required for kidney or liver dysfunction in order to prevent toxicity.

D. Combination chemotherapy is usually more effective than single-agent therapy.

1. The reasons for administering combination chemotherapy include:
   - **a.** Overcoming or preventing resistance
   - **b.** Cytotoxicity to resting and dividing cells
   - **c.** Biochemical enhancement of effect
   - **d.** Rescue of normal cells
2. **Dosing** and **scheduling** of combination regimens are important as they are designed to allow recovery of normal cells. These regimens generally are given as short courses of therapy in cycles.
3. **Acronyms** often are used to designate chemotherapy regimens. For example, CMF refers to a combination of cyclophosphamide, methotrexate, and fluorouracil used in the treatment of breast cancer.

E. Administration

1. **Routes** of administration vary, although intravenous (IV) bolus administration is employed most commonly.
2. Other administration techniques include oral, subcutaneous, intrathecal, intra-arterial, intraperitoneal, intravesical, continuous IV infusion, and hepatic artery infusion.
3. Drugs that may be given **intrathecally** are methotrexate, hydrocortisone, cytarabine, and thiotepa. Drugs should not be administered by the intrathecal route without specific information supporting intrathecal administration. Patients have died when vincristine and other

drugs have been administered by the intrathecal route. Caution should be used in the preparation and delivery of drugs to be used in this manner.

F. **Response to chemotherapy** is defined in a number of ways and does not always correlate with patient survival.

1. **Complete response (CR)** indicates disappearance of all disease–clinical, gross, and microscopic.
2. **Partial response (PR)** indicates a greater than 50% reduction in tumor size, lasting a reasonable period of time. Some evidence of disease remains after therapy.
3. **Response rate (RR)** is defined as CR plus PR.
4. **Progression** or **no response** after therapy is defined by a greater than 25% increase in tumor size or the appearance of new lesions.

IV. CLASSIFICATION OF CHEMOTHERAPEUTIC AGENTS

A. **Alkylating agents** were the first group of antineoplastic agents. The prototype of this class is mechlorethamine, or **nitrogen mustard,** which was researched as a chemical warfare agent. Alkylating agents cause cross-linking and abnormal base-pairing of DNA strands, which inhibit replication of the DNA. This mechanism is known as **alkylation.** The subclassifications of alkylating agents are listed below by chemical class. Examples of each are noted.

1. **Nitrogen mustards:** chlorambucil, cyclophosphamide, ifosfamide, mechlorethamine (nitrogen mustard), melphalan.
2. **Ethylenimines** and **methylmelamines:** thiotepa (triethylene thiophosphoramide), altretamine (hexamethylmelamine)
3. **Alkyl sulfonates:** busulfan
4. **Nitrosoureas:** carmustine (BCNU), lomustine (CCNU), semustine (methyl CCNU), streptozocin
5. **Triazenes:** dacarbazine (DTIC)
6. **Platinum coordination complexes:** carboplatin, cisplatin
7. **Substituted ureas:** hydroxyurea
8. Procarbazine

B. Most of the **antitumor antibiotics** are obtained from organisms of the *Streptomyces* genus. These agents may act by either alkylation (mitomycin) or **intercalation.** Intercalation is the process by which the drug slides between DNA base pairs and inhibits DNA synthesis. Examples of antitumor antibiotics and their synonyms are listed below.

1. **Anthracyclines:** daunorubicin (daunomycin), doxorubicin (adriamycin, hydroxydaunorubicin), idarubicin
2. **Anthracendiones** (synthetic): mitoxantrone
3. **Other agents:** bleomycin, dactinomycin (actinomycin D), mitomycin, plicamycin (mithramycin)

C. **Antimetabolites** are structural analogues of naturally occurring substrates for biochemical reactions. They inhibit DNA synthesis by acting as false substitutions in the production of nucleic acids. The classes of antimetabolites are listed below.

1. **Adenosine analogues:** cladribine (2CdA), fludarabine, pentostatin (deoxycoformycin)
2. **Folic acid analogues (folate antagonists):** edatrexate, methotrexate, trimetrexate
3. **Purine analogues (purine antagonists):** mercaptopurine, thioguanine
4. **Pyrimidine analogues (pyrimidine antagonists):** cytarabine (ARA-C, cytosine arabinoside), fluorouracil

D. Plant alkaloids are derived from plants. The vinca alkaloids arrest cell division by preventing formation of the mitotic spindle. The podophyllotoxins inhibit the enzyme topoisomerase II, which is necessary for DNA production. The taxanes promote microtubule assembly and stabilization, thus prohibiting cell division. Examples of plant alkaloids are listed below.

1. **Vinca alkaloids:** vinblastine, vincristine, vindesine, vinorelbine
2. **Podophyllotoxins:** etoposide (VP-16), teniposide (VM-26)
3. **Taxanes:** docetaxol (taxotere), paclitaxel (taxol)

E. Hormones are a class of heterogeneous compounds that have varying effects on cells. Below is a list of some of the **most commonly used agents** in cancer therapy.

1. **Androgens:** fluoxymesterone, testosterone
2. **Antiadrenals:** aminoglutethimide
3. **Antiandrogens:** flutamide
4. **Antiestrogens:** tamoxifen
5. **Corticosteroids:** dexamethasone, prednisone
6. **Estrogens:** diethylstilbestrol (DES), ethinyl estradiol
7. **Estrogen/nitrogen mustard:** estramustine
8. **Gonadotropin hormone-releasing analogues (LHRH analogues):** goserelin, leuprolide
9. **Progestins:** medroxyprogesterone, megestrol

F. Asparaginase is an **enzyme** that causes the degradation of asparagine to aspartic acid and ammonia. Unlike normal cells, tumor cells lack the ability to synthesize this amino acid.

G. Biologic response modifiers alter or enhance the patient's immunologic response to the tumor. Examples are listed below.

1. **Bacillus Calmette-Guerin (BCG)**
2. **Colony-stimulating factors:** filgrastim (G-CSF), sargramostim (GM-CSF)
3. **Interferons:** interferon-α, interferon-β, interferon-γ
4. **Interleukins:** aldesleukin (IL-2)
5. **Levamisole**
6. **Monoclonal antibodies**

V. TOXICITIES OF CHEMOTHERAPY AGENTS.

Chemotherapeutic agents are most toxic to rapidly proliferating cells. The tissues most commonly affected are those of the mucous membranes, skin, hair, gastrointestinal (GI) tract, and bone marrow. Of these, bone marrow toxicity can be the most life threatening.

A. Bone marrow suppression is the **most common** dose-limiting **side effect** of cancer therapy.

1. **Complications**
   - a. A significant decrease in the white blood cell count, particularly the neutrophils **(neutropenia),** predisposes the patient to development of serious infections. **Colony-stimulating factors** may be used to lessen the degree of neutropenia.
   - b. Platelet production may also be decreased **(thrombocytopenia),** which can lead to bleeding, and may require platelet transfusions.
   - c. **Anemia** secondary to cancer chemotherapy does not occur as frequently as other bone marrow toxicities because of the long half-life of red blood cells (about 120 days).
2. The **time course** of myelosuppression varies with the chemotherapy regimen. In general, the onset of myelosuppression is 7–10 days after the chemotherapy has been administered. The lowest point of the counts, called the **nadir,** is usually reached in 10–14 days. Recovery of counts usually occurs in 2–3 weeks.

3. The extent of myelosuppression is **dose-related.** Drugs that can cause severe myelosuppression include carmustine, cytarabine, daunorubicin, doxorubicin, and paclitaxel.

4. Some chemotherapy agents cause little or no myelosuppression. These include asparaginase, bleomycin, and vincristine.

B. Dermatologic toxicity

1. **Alopecia** is the loss of hair commonly observed in chemotherapy patients. Hair loss may be partial or complete. There are no safe and effective ways to prevent hair loss. Chemotherapy agents that commonly cause alopecia include cyclophosphamide, doxorubicin, mechlorethamine, and paclitaxel.

2. **Local necrosis** may result from **extravasation** of vesicant chemotherapy drugs during their administration. Vesicant agents include dactinomycin, daunorubicin, doxorubicin, idarubicin, mechlorethamine, mitomycin, paclitaxel, vinblastine, and vincristine.
   a. Most vesicant extravasations produce **immediate pain** or **burning.** However, a delayed reaction may occur hours or weeks later. Significant tissue injury, including ulceration or necrosis, may require plastic surgery intervention.
   b. The **treatment** of extravasations remains controversial. It is generally agreed that heat should be applied to extravasations of vinca alkaloids and taxanes, and that cold packs should be applied to all other extravasations.

3. Cancer chemotherapy can also cause **skin changes** such as dryness and sensitivity to sunlight. Examples are fluorouracil and methotrexate.

C. GI toxicities are frequently experienced by patients receiving chemotherapy.

1. **Nausea** and **vomiting** are often the most distressing toxicities from the patient's point of view.
   a. Severe vomiting can result in dehydration, electrolyte imbalances, and esophageal tears, and may cause the patient to discontinue therapy.
   b. Nausea and vomiting may be **acute, delayed,** or **anticipatory** in nature. Antiemetics should be used prophylactically to prevent the occurrence of nausea and vomiting, particularly with chemotherapeutic agents that have a high emetogenic risk.
   c. Table 55-1 lists **commonly used chemotherapeutic agents** and their emetogenic potential. The occurrence of nausea and vomiting is influenced by the emetogenicity of the chemotherapeutic agent, chemotherapeutic dose, method of administration, and individual patient characteristics.

2. **Stomatitis** is a generalized inflammation of the oral mucosa or other areas of the GI tract where there is rapid turnover of cells.
   a. **Signs** and **symptoms** include erythema, pain, dryness of the mouth, burning or tingling of the lips, ulcerations, and bleeding.
   b. Chemotherapy agents associated with stomatitis include fluorouracil and methotrexate.
   c. **Time course.** Stomatitis usually appears within a week after the offending agent is administered, and resolves in 10–14 days.
   d. **Consequences** of stomatitis include infection of the ulcerated areas, inability to eat, pain requiring opioid analgesics, and subsequent decreases in chemotherapy doses.

3. Other GI toxicities include **diarrhea** (e.g., fluorouracil), **constipation** (e.g., vincristine), **anorexia,** and **taste changes.**

D. Chills and **fever** may occur after the administration of some chemotherapy agents. This fever generally can be differentiated from fever due to infection because of its temporal relationship to chemotherapy administration. Bleomycin commonly is associated with this reaction.

E. Pulmonary toxicity is generally irreversible and may be fatal.

1. **Signs** and **symptoms** are shortness of breath, nonproductive cough, and low-grade fever. In some cases, the risk of pulmonary toxicity increases as the cumulative dose of the drug increases (e.g., bleomycin).

2. Chemotherapeutic agents associated with pulmonary toxicity include bleomycin, busulfan, carmustine, and mitomycin.

Table 55-1. Emetogenic Potential of Cancer Chemotherapeutic Agents

Very Highly Emetogenic	Highly Emetogenic	Moderately Emetogenic	Low Emetogenic Risk
Cisplatin	Carmustine	Carboplatin	Asparaginase
Cyclophosphamide (> 2 g/m^2)	Cyclophosphamide (1–2 g/m^2)	Cyclophosphamide (< 1 g/m^2)	BCG
Cytarabine (≥ 500 mg/m^2)	Dactinomycin	Cytarabine (200–500 mg/m^2)	Bleomycin
Dacarbazine	Etoposide (≥ 500 mg/m^2)	Daunorubicin	Busulfan
Ifosfamide	Lomustine	Doxorubicin	Chlorambucil
Mechlorethamine	Methotrexate (≥ 200 mg/m^2)	Idarubicin	Cladribine
Melphalan (intravenous)	Thiotepa (≥ 15 mg/m^2)	Mitomycin	Cytarabine (< 200 mg/m^2)
Streptozocin		Plicamycin	Etoposide (< 500 mg/m^2)
		Vinblastine	Fludarabine
			Fluorouracil
			Flutamide
			Hydroxyurea
			Interferon-α
			Leuprolide
			Levamisole
			Megestrol
			Melphalan (oral)
			Mercaptopurine
			Methotrexate (< 200 mg/m^2)
			Mitoxantrone
			Paclitaxel
			Tamoxifen
			Teniposide
			Thioguanine
			Thiotepa (< 15 mg/m^2)
			Vincristine
			Vinorelbine

F. **Cardiac toxicity** may manifest as an acute or chronic problem.

1. **Acute changes** are generally transient electrocardiograph abnormalities that may not be clinically significant.
2. **Chronic cardiac toxicity** is irreversible congestive heart failure. **Risk factors** include chest irradiation and high cumulative doses of cardiotoxic chemotherapy.
3. Chemotherapy agents that are associated with chronic cardiotoxicity include daunorubicin, doxorubicin, and idarubicin.

G. **Hypersensitivity reactions** may occur with any chemotherapy agent. Life-threatening reactions, including anaphylaxis, appear to be more common with asparaginase, carboplatin, cisplatin, etoposide, paclitaxel, and teniposide.

H. **Neurotoxicity** may occur with systemic or intrathecal chemotherapy.

1. Vincristine is associated with **autonomic** and **peripheral** neuropathies. Patients may experience gait disturbances, numbness and tingling of hands and feet, and loss of deep tendon reflexes. Intrathecal administration of vincristine results in fatal neurotoxicity.
2. **Peripheral neuropathy** and **ototoxicity** are common dose-limiting toxicities of cisplatin. Sensory neuropathies may be associated with paclitaxel.
3. High doses of cytarabine may produce **cerebellar toxicity** that manifests initially as loss of eye–hand coordination and may progress to coma.
4. **Arachnoiditis** has been associated with intrathecal administration of cytarabine and methotrexate.

I. **Hemorrhagic cystitis** is a bladder toxicity that is seen most commonly after administration of cyclophosphamide and ifosfamide. **Acrolein,** a metabolite of these agents, is thought to cause a chemical irritation of the bladder mucosa, resulting in bleeding. Preventive measures include aggressive hydration with subsequent frequent urination, and the administration of the uroprotectant mesna. **Mesna** acts by binding to acrolein and preventing it from contacting the bladder mucosa.

J. **Renal toxicity** may manifest by elevations in serum creatinine and blood urea nitrogen (BUN), as well as electrolyte abnormalities. Nephrotoxicity is associated with cisplatin, ifosfamide, methotrexate, and streptozocin.

K. **Hepatotoxicity** may manifest as elevated liver function tests, jaundice, or hepatitis. Asparaginase, cytarabine, mercaptopurine, and methotrexate are known to cause hepatic toxicity.

L. **Secondary malignancies,** such as solid tumors, lymphomas, and leukemias, may occur many years after chemotherapy or radiation. Antineoplastic agents known to possess a high carcinogenic risk include etoposide, melphalan, and mechlorethamine.

M. Chemotherapy may cause **infertility** which may be temporary or permanent. Cyclophosphamide, chlorambucil, mechlorethamine, melphalan, and procarbazine are associated with a significant incidence of infertility in males and females.

VI. OTHER THERAPEUTIC MODALITIES

A. **Surgery** may be diagnostic (biopsy, exploratory laparotomy, "second-look") or therapeutic (tumor debulking or removal). Surgery is often combined with chemotherapy and/or radiation.

B. **Radiation therapy** involves high doses of ionizing radiation directed at the cancerous tissue. Radiation may be combined with surgery and/or chemotherapy. Depending on the area of the body being irradiated, **adverse reactions** may include stomatitis, nausea and vomiting, diarrhea, and myelosuppression.

STUDY QUESTIONS

Directions: Each of the numbered items or incomplete statements in this section is followed by answers or completions of the statement. Select the **one** lettered answer or completion that is **best** in each case.

1. Which statement regarding phase-specific chemotherapeutic agents is correct? They

(A) are most effective in one phase of the cell cycle
(B) are effective in all phases of the cell cycle
(C) are only effective in G_0 phase
(D) include the alkylating agents
(E) include the antitumor antibiotics

2. Body surface area (BSA) is used in calculating chemotherapy doses because

(A) BSA is an indicator of tumor cell mass
(B) BSA correlates with cardiac output
(C) BSA correlates with gastrointestinal transit time
(D) the National Cancer Institute requires that BSA be used
(E) the FDA requires that BSA be used

3. The rationale for combination chemotherapy includes all of the following EXCEPT

(A) biochemical enhancement of effect
(B) rescue of normal cells
(C) overcoming or preventing resistance
(D) biochemical nullification of effect
(E) cytotoxic to both resting and dividing cells

4. All of the following chemotherapy agents can be administered intrathecally EXCEPT

(A) methotrexate
(B) cytarabine
(C) hydrocortisone
(D) thiotepa
(E) vincristine

5. Which of the following chemotherapeutic agents is classified as an alkylating agent?

(A) Cyclophosphamide
(B) Etoposide
(C) Mechlorethamine
(D) Paclitaxel
(E) Cyclophosphamide and mechlorethamine

6. Which of the following chemotherapy agents acts by intercalation?

(A) Vincristine
(B) Paclitaxel
(C) Doxorubicin
(D) Vincristine and paclitaxel

7. How do antimetabolites exert their cytotoxic effect?

(A) Inhibiting DNA synthesis by sliding between DNA base pairs
(B) Inhibiting RNA synthesis by sliding between RNA base pairs
(C) Acting as false metabolites in the microtubules
(D) Acting as false substitutions in the production of nucleic acids
(E) Promoting microtubule assembly and stabilization

8. Which of the following chemotherapy agents are correctly paired according to their mechanism of action?

(A) Vincristine and paclitaxel
(B) Etoposide and paclitaxel
(C) Docetaxol and paclitaxel
(D) Docetaxol and etoposide
(E) Vincristine and etoposide

9. Hormonal agents that are useful in the treatment of cancer include

(A) tamoxifen
(B) prednisone
(C) flutamide
(D) tamoxifen and flutamide
(E) tamoxifen, prednisone, and flutamide

10. When does the neutrophil nadir associated with chemotherapy agents generally occur?

(A) During administration of the chemotherapy
(B) 1–2 days after therapy
(C) 10–14 days after therapy
(D) 1 month after therapy
(E) When the platelet count begins to rise

11. Stomatitis is characterized by all of the following signs and symptoms EXCEPT

(A) headache
(B) erythema
(C) bleeding
(D) ulcerations
(E) dryness of mouth

12. Which of the following statements describes hemorrhagic cystitis? It

(A) is caused by excretion of tumor cell breakdown products
(B) is associated with ifosfamide administration
(C) is caused by the administration of mesna
(D) can be prevented or treated with acrolein
(E) can be treated with G-CSF

ANSWERS AND EXPLANATIONS

1. The answer is A *[I D 1,2,3].*
Phase-specific agents are most active in one specific phase of the cell cycle. These agents have no activity against cells in G_0, the resting phase. Examples of phase-specific agents include the vinca alkaloids, asparaginase, the antimetabolites, and etoposide.

2. The answer is B *[III B].*
BSA correlates with cardiac output, which determines renal and hepatic blood flow and, thus, affects drug elimination.

3. The answer is D *(III D 1).*
Combination chemotherapy has been developed to have maximal cytotoxicity to tumor cells and minimal toxicity to normal cells. The drugs are dosed and scheduled such that maximal cell kill occurs, while sparing normal cells as much as possible. Combination regimens often contain agents with different spectrums of toxicity.

4. The answer is E *[III E 3].*
Intrathecally administered vincristine is fatal. All syringes of vincristine must be labeled "Fatal if given intrathecally. For intravenous use only."

5. The answer is E *[IV A 1].*
Cyclophosphamide and mechlorethamine are nitrogen mustards, a subgroup of the alkylating agents. Etoposide and paclitaxel are plant alkaloids.

6. The answer is C *[IV B 1].*
Doxorubicin is an antitumor antibiotic that inhibits DNA synthesis by intercalation. Vincristine and paclitaxel are plant alkaloids that act on microtubule assembly.

7. The answer is D *[IV C].*
Antimetabolites are structural analogues of naturally occurring substrates for biochemical reactions. They inhibit DNA synthesis by acting as false substitutions in the production of DNA.

8. The answer is C *[IV D 3].*
Docetaxol and paclitaxel belong to the taxane subgroup of plant alkaloids. They act by promoting microtubule assembly and stabilization, resulting in inhibition of cell division.

9. The answer is E *[IV E 3,4,5].*
Tamoxifen is an antiestrogen used in the treatment of breast cancer. Prednisone is used for its antilymphocytic properties in the treatment of non-Hodgkins lymphoma. Flutamide is an antiandrogen used in the treatment of prostate cancer.

10. The answer is C *[V A 2].*
Bone marrow suppression, particularly of the neutrophils, usually is the most profound 10–14 days after chemotherapy. A few agents, such as the nitrosoureas, have delayed and prolonged marrow suppression.

11. The answer is A *[V C 2].*
Stomatitis, or mucositis, is an inflammation of the mucous membranes, particularly the oral mucosa. Although the symptoms generally are limited to the mouth and throat, stomatitis may affect any part of the gastrointestinal tract, potentially causing diarrhea and anal fissures.

12. The answer is B *[V I].*
Hemorrhagic cystitis results from irritation of the lining of the bladder by acrolein, a metabolite of ifosfamide and cyclophosphamide. Mesna may be used to inactivate the acrolein, thus preventing hemorrhagic cystitis.

56
Pain

David R. Platt

I. INTRODUCTION

A. Definition

1. **Pain** is an unpleasant sensory and emotional experience that usually is associated with structural or tissue damage. It is a subjective, individual experience that has physical, psychological, and social determinants. There is no objective measurement of pain.

2. **Acute pain** occurs following tissue injury, such as trauma or surgery. The pain is usually self-limiting, decreasing with time as the injury heals. It is described as a linear process with a beginning and an end. Increased autonomic nervous system activity often accompanies acute pain, causing tachycardia, tachypnea, hypertension, diaphoresis, and mydriasis. Increased anxiety also may occur.

3. **Chronic pain** is pain that lasts more than several months. **Chronic nonmalignant pain** is a complication of acute injury where the healing process does not occur as expected. The pain is constant and consumes the patient's existence. It does not improve with time and is described as a cyclic process (vicious cycle). Compared to acute pain, there is no longer autonomic nervous system stimulation so the patient may not "appear" in pain. Instead the patient may be depressed, suffer insomnia, weight loss, sexual dysfunction, and may not be able to cope with the normal activities of daily living, including family and job-related activities.

4. **Chronic cancer pain** occurs in 60%–90% of patients with cancer. Its characteristics are similar to those of chronic nonmalignant pain. In addition to depression, fear, anger, and agony may be prominent occurrences. The etiology of chronic cancer pain can be related to the tumor, cancer therapy, or be idiosyncratic. Tumor causes of pain include bone metastasis, compression of nerve structures, occlusion of blood vessels, obstruction of bowel, or infiltration of soft tissue.

5. **Breakthrough pain** is the intermittent, transitory increase in pain that occurs at a greater intensity over baseline chronic pain. It may have temporal characteristics, precipitating factors, and predictability.

B. Principles of management

1. **Comprehensive pain assessment** should determine the characteristics of the patient's pain complaint, clinical status, and pain management history.
   a. Assessment of the pain complaint should include location, quality, provocative factors, temporal qualities, severity, and pain history.
   b. Assessment of clinical status should include the extent of underlying trauma or disease. Also, the patient's physical, psychological, and social conditions should be determined.
   c. Assessment of pain management history includes drug allergies, analgesic response, onset, duration, and side effects.

2. **Appropriate pain management targets** should be established.
   a. The primary pain management goal is to improve patient comfort.
   b. For acute pain management, improved comfort can aid the healing and rehabilitation process.
   c. For chronic pain, the specific objectives are to break the pain cycle (i.e., erase pain memory) and minimize breakthrough pain.
   d. Other targets for chronic pain management include improvement of general well-being, sleep, outlook, self-esteem, activities of daily living, support, and mobility.

3. **Individualized pain management regimens** should be determined and initiated promptly.
   a. The optimal analgesic regimen, including dose, dosing interval, and mode of administration, should be selected.
   b. Additional pharmacologic adjuncts and nonpharmacologic therapies should be added if needed.
   c. The most common regimens for acute pain include intermittent (as needed) dosing, patient controlled analgesia (PCA), or epidural infusions with narcotic or non-narcotic agents.
   d. Although the practice is controversial, narcotic use usually is minimized or avoided for chronic nonmalignant pain. Non-narcotic analgesics and nonpharmacologic management usually are maximized.
   e. For chronic cancer pain, an individualized around-the-clock analgesic regimen is established, using a long-acting analgesic. An intermittent, as-needed regimen for breakthrough pain, using a short-acting analgesic, is also determined.
4. **Monitoring** the pain management regimen and **re-assessment** of the patient's pain should occur on a continuous, timely basis. Any changes in analgesic, dose, dosing interval, or method of administration should be carried out immediately.

II. ANALGESICS

A. **Peripherally-acting, non-narcotic analgesics** include aspirin, other salicylates, acetaminophen, and nonsteroidal anti-inflammatory drugs (NSAIDs) (Table 56-1). Aspirin products, acetaminophen, and low-dose ibuprofen and naproxen are available for use without a prescription.

Table 56-1. Some Commonly Used Peripherally-acting Non-narcotic Analgesics

Drug	Average Oral Dose (mg)*	Dosing Interval (hr)	Maximum Daily Adult Dose (mg)
Acetaminophen	500–1000	4–6	4000
Salicylates			
Aspirin	500–1000	4–6	4000
Choline magnesium trisalicylate	1000–1500	12	2000–3000
Diflunisal	1000 (load)		
	500 (maintenance)	8–12	1500
Nonsteroidal anti-inflammatory drugs (NSAIDs)			
Propionic acids			
Ibuprofen	200–400	4–6	2400
Naproxen	500 (load)		
	250 (maintenance)	6–8	1250
Naproxen sodium	550 (load)		
	275 (maintenance)	6–8	1375
Fenoprofen	200	4–6	800
Ketoprofen	25–50	6–8	300
Indoleacetic acid			
Indomethacin	25	8–12	100
Anthranilic acid			
Mefenamic acid	500 (load)		
	250 (maintenance)	6	1500
Pyranocarboxylic acid			
Etodolac	200–400	6–8	1200
Pyrrolopyrrole			
Ketorolac	10	6	40
	IM: 30–60 (load)		
	IM: 15–30 (maintenance)	6	120

IM = intramuscular

*Except where indicated

1. **Mechanism of action.** Salicylates and NSAIDs are prostaglandin inhibitors and prevent peripheral nociception by vasoactive substances such as prostaglandins and **bradykinins.** The exact mechanism of action of acetaminophen is not known.

2. **Therapeutic effects**
   a. The peripherally-acting, non-narcotic analgesics have several effects in common. These effects distinguish these agents from narcotic analgesics.
      (1) They are antipyretic.
      (2) They are anti-inflammatory (except acetaminophen).
      (3) There is a ceiling effect to the analgesia.
      (4) They do not cause tolerance.
      (5) They do not cause physical or psychologic dependence.
   b. The efficacy of non-narcotics is compared to aspirin. Most are comparable to aspirin; however several NSAIDs have shown a superior effect to 650 mg of aspirin.
      (1) Diflunisal (500 mg)
      (2) Ibuprofen (200–400 mg)
      (3) Naproxen sodium (550 mg)
      (4) Ketoprofen (25–50 mg)

3. **Clinical use**
   a. Generally, the non-narcotic analgesics are **used orally to manage mild-to-moderate pain.**
      (1) They are particularly suited for acute pain of skeletal muscle (orthopedic) or oral (dental) origin.
      (2) They are used in chronic malignant pain and can have an additive effect with narcotic analgesics.
      (3) They also may be effective in managing pain due to the bone metastases.
   b. The NSAID, ketorolac, is administered intramuscularly and is useful in moderate-to-severe pain, particularly in cases where narcotics are undesirable (e.g., with drug addicts, excessive narcotic sedation, respiratory depression).
   c. Patients may vary in their response and tolerance to non-narcotic analgesics. If a patient does not respond to the maximum therapeutic dose, then an alternate NSAID should be tried. Likewise, if a patient experiences side effects with one drug, then another agent should be tried.
   d. Several drugs (e.g, diflunisal, choline magnesium trisalicylate, naproxen) have long half-lives and, therefore, may be administered less frequently.
   e. The cost of non-narcotic analgesics is highly variable and should be considered when an agent is selected.

4. **Adverse effects**
   a. **Gastrointestinal (GI) effects.** Most non-narcotic analgesics cause GI symptoms secondary to prostaglandin inhibition. At normal doses, acetaminophen and choline magnesium trisalicylate produce minimal GI upset.
      (1) The most common GI symptom is dyspepsia, but ulceration, bleeding, or perforation can occur.
      (2) Patients most predisposed to severe GI effects include the elderly, patients with a history of ulcers or chronic disease, and those who smoke or use alcohol.
      (3) To minimize GI effects, the lowest possible analgesic dose should be used. Aspirin, available as enteric-coated products, may minimize GI upset. Combination therapy with a GI "protectant" (e.g., antacid, H_2-antagonist, sucralfate, misoprostol) may be needed.
      (4) Even in normal doses, acetaminophen can cause hepatotoxicity in patients with liver disease or chronic alcoholism.
   b. **Hematologic effects.** Most non-narcotic analgesics inhibit platelet aggregation. The effect is produced by reversible inhibition of prostaglandin synthetase. Aspirin is an irreversible inhibitor. Acetaminophen and choline magnesium trisalicylate lack antiplatelet effects.
      (1) The effect of the NSAIDs correlates to the presence of an effective serum concentration.
      (2) Use of anticoagulants (e.g., heparin, warfarin) is relatively contraindicated in combination with aspirin or NSAIDs.
   c. **Renal effects.** NSAIDs can produce renal dysfunction.
      (1) The mechanism of NSAID-induced renal dysfunction includes prostaglandin inhibition, interstitial nephritis, impaired renin secretion, and enhanced tubular water/sodium reabsorption.

(2) Many risk factors have been implicated including congestive heart failure (CHF), chronic renal failure (CRF), cirrhosis, dehydration, diuretic use, and atherosclerotic disease in elderly patients.

(3) The renal dysfunction is commonly manifested as abrupt onset oliguria with sodium/water retention. The effect reverses after discontinuation of the NSAID.

d. Miscellaneous effects

(1) Some patients exhibit acute hypersensitivity reactions to aspirin. Manifestations include either a rhinitis or asthma presentation or a true allergic reaction (e.g., urticaria, wheals, hypotension, shock, syncope). A cross-sensitivity to other NSAIDs may develop.

(2) Some NSAIDs produce central nervous system (CNS) effects, including impaired mentation and attention deficit disorder.

5. Drug interactions. Salicylates have two clinically significant drug interactions.

a. Oral anticoagulants. Aspirin should be avoided in anticoagulated patients. Aspirin inhibits platelet function and can cause gastric mucosal damage. This significantly increases the risk of bleeding in anticoagulated patients. Also, doses of more than 3 g/day of aspirin produce hypoprothrombinemia. Choline magnesium trisalicylate or acetaminophen should be used if a non-narcotic is needed in an anticoagulated patient.

b. Methotrexate. Salicylates may enhance the toxicity of methotrexate. The primary mechanism is blockage of methotrexate renal tubular secretion by salicylates. The resultant methotrexate toxicity has been reported as pancytopenia or hepatotoxicity. Salicylates should be avoided in patients receiving methotrexate.

B. Narcotic analgesics include the opiate agonists (Table 56-2). There is also a group of mixed agonist–antagonist drugs (Table 56-3). Because of their abuse potential, opiates are classified as controlled drugs and are placed in schedules II or III. Special regulations control their prescribing.

1. Mechanism of action

a. Endogenous opiates afford the body self-pain relieving mechanisms. These endogenous peptides include the endorphins, enkephalins, and dynorphins.

b. Exogenous opiates are classified as agonists (stimulate opiate receptors), antagonists (displace agonists from opiate receptors), and mixed opiates (agonist–antagonist or partial agonist actions).

c. Opiate receptors are located in the brain and spinal cord. Several types of opiate receptors have been identified, including mu, kappa, delta, sigma, and epsilon.

d. Stimulation of mu receptors produces the characteristic narcotic (morphine-like) effects:

(1) Analgesia
(2) Miosis
(3) Euphoria
(4) Respiratory depression
(5) Sedation

Table 56-2. Some Commonly Used Opiate Agonists

	Equivalent Dose (mg)*		
Drug	**Parenteral**	**Oral**	**Duration of Effect (hr)**
Codeine	75	130	3–4
Oxycodone	. . .	20–30	3–4
Morphine	10	20–30 (chronic dosing) 60 (single dose)	4–6†
Hydromorphone	1.5	7.5	3–4
Levorphanol	2	4	4–8
Meperidine	100	400	2–3
Methadone	10	20	6–8
Fentanyl	0.1	. . .	1–2‡

*These drugs produce analgesia equivalent to 10 mg intramuscular morphine.
†Controlled-release morphine has a duration of effect of about 8-12 hours.
‡Transdermal fentanyl has a duration of effect of about 72 hours.

Table 56-3. Mixed Agonist–Antagonists

Drug	Equivalent Dose (mg)*	Duration of Effect (hr)
Partial agonist		
Buprenorphine	0.4 (intramuscular)	6–8
Mixed agonists–antagonists		
Pentazocine	60 (intramuscular)	3–6
	180 (oral)	3–6
Nalbuphine	10 (intramuscular)	3–6
Butorphanol	2 (intramuscular)	3–4
Dezocine	10 (intramuscular)	3–4

*These drugs produce analgesia equivalent to 10 mg intramuscular morphine.

(6) Physical dependence
(7) Bradycardia

e. The specific mechanism (central and spinal) of opiate agonist is alteration of the effects of nociceptive neurotransmitters, possibly norepinephrine or serotonin.

2. Clinical use

a. Narcotics are used for the **management of moderate-to-severe pain** (acute or chronic pain) of somatic or visceral origin.

b. The use of narcotics should be individualized for each patient. The optimal analgesic dose varies from patient to patient. Each analgesic regimen should be titrated by increasing the dose up to the appearance of limiting adverse effects. Changing to another analgesic should only occur after an adequate therapeutic trial.

c. The appropriate route of administration should be selected for each patient.

(1) Oral administration is the preferred route, particularly for patients with chronic, stable pain.

(2) Intramuscular, subcutaneous administration is very commonly used in the post-operative period. Fluctuations in absorption may occur, particularly in elderly or cachectic patients.

(3) Intravenous (IV) bolus administration has the most rapid, predictable onset of effect.

(4) IV infusion is used to titrate pain relief rapidly, particularly in patients with unstable chronic pain. Morphine is most commonly used, often with supplemental IV bolus doses for breakthrough pain. A mechanical infusion device is necessary.

(5) IV patient-controlled analgesia (PCA) is most often used for acute post-operative pain. It produces prompt analgesia with minimal side-effects because small doses (e.g., 1–2 mg morphine) are delivered at frequent intervals (e.g., every 10 minutes). It allows patient control of pain management. Morphine and meperidine are the most commonly used agents. A mechanical infusion device and properly trained patient and staff are necessary.

(6) Epidural and **intrathecal administration** is used for acute postoperative pain and early management of chronic cancer pain.

(a) Low opiate doses stimulate spinal opiate receptors and reduce the amount of narcotic reaching the brain. This results in delayed or minimal effects such as sedation, nausea, and respiratory depression. The opiate distribution that causes such effects is dependent on the site of spinal injection, water solubility of the opiate, and volume infused. For example, after lumbar administration of a more water-soluble opiate (morphine), severe respiratory depression can be observed 12–24 hours after initial dosing.

(b) Local side effects of intraspinal opiate administration are itching and urinary retention. Depending on the opiate used and the type of pain being treated, intermittent doses or continuous infusions (via a mechanical infusion device) can be employed (Tables 56-4 and 56-5).

(7) Rectal administration is an alternative for patients unable to take oral narcotics. Generally, poor absorption results in available analgesic response. It is an unacceptable route of administration for many patients.

(8) Transdermal administration is an alternative for patients with chronic pain who are unable to take oral narcotics. A controlled-release patch is available for fentanyl.

Table 56-4. Epidurally Administered Narcotics (Intermittent Dosing)

Drug	Usual Dose (mg)	Onset of Action (min)	Time to Peak Effect (min)	Duration of Action (hr)
Morphine	5–10	25	60	12–24
Fentanyl	0.1	5–10	20	6
Meperidine	50–100	5–10	15–30	7
Hydromorphone	1	10–15	20	12
Buprenorphine	0.3	30	40–60	8–9

Table 56-5. Epidurally Administered Narcotics (Continuous Infusion)

Drug	Initial Bolus Dose (mg)	Infusion Concentration (mg/ml)	Infusion Rate (mg/hr)
Morphine	2	0.05-0.25	0.2–1.5
Fentanyl	0.05–0.1	0.005–0.025	0.02–0.15
Meperidine	50–100	10–20	5–20
Hydromorphone	0.5-1	0.02-0.05	0.15–0.3

Slow onset requires additional analgesia while starting treatment. The duration of analgesia is 72 hours per patch. A slow reduction of effect follows removal of the patch and requires 24–36 hours of monitoring.

d. Patients who have chronic pain or acute pain that is constant throughout the day should receive regularly scheduled (around-the-clock) doses of narcotics.

(1) Long-acting opiates (e.g., controlled-release morphine, methadone) are preferable.

(2) A supplement given as needed may be necessary to manage breakthrough pain, for which short-acting opiates (e.g., immediate-release morphine, hydromorphone) are preferable. If frequent supplements are required, then the around-the-clock regimen should be adjusted based on morphine equivalents (see Table 56-2).

e. Although the analgesia and side effects of opiates are qualitatively similar, individual patients may respond differently. Analgesic selection is based on:

(1) Patient's past analgesia experience

(2) Need for a rapid onset of effect

(3) Preference for a long (or short) duration of action

(4) Preference for a particular mode of delivery

(5) Preference for a particular dosage form

(a) Controlled-release morphine for a long duration of action (8–12 hours) may be preferable to opiates with long half-lives (e.g., methadone, levorphanol), which can accumulate and cause overdose symptoms (e.g., respiratory depression).

(b) Transdermal fentanyl can be used for patients who are unable to swallow.

(c) Rectal suppositories can be used for patients who are unable to swallow. They are available for morphine, hydromorphone, and oxymorphone.

(d) Concentrated hydromorphone injection (10 mg/ml) can be used for cachectic patients who require subcutaneous injections and in patients whose injection volumes must be minimized.

(6) Individual sensitivity to side effects includes nausea, euphoria, sedation, and respiratory depression.

(a) Partial agonists or mixed agonist-antagonists may be preferable for acute pain management in patients at risk for respiratory depression secondary to opiate agonists. These agents should not be used in patients who have received chronic doses of opiates because withdrawal symptoms will occur.

(b) Epidural administration may be preferable for critically ill patients at risk for respiratory depression secondary to systemic narcotic administration.

3. Adverse effects. All narcotics can produce a variety of side effects that range from bothersome to life-threatening.

a. Constipation occurs as a result of decreased intestinal tone and peristalsis. There is a patient variability, but generally most patients experience constipation after several days of therapy. Constipation may be more bothersome with certain types of opiates (e.g., codeine). It may occur sooner and be more problematic in hospitalized or bedridden patients or in patients who have received anesthesia or drugs with anticholinergic effects. Prophylaxis with a laxative/stool softener combination (e.g., bisacodyl/docusate) and dietary counseling are warranted in patients who need chronic opiate therapy.

b. **Nausea** and **vomiting** occur due to central stimulation of the chemoreceptor trigger zone. It is more problematic with one-time or intermittent parenteral dosing for acute pain. Occasionally, patients require concomitant therapy with an antiemetic (e.g., hydroxyzine, prochlorperazine); however these agents may add to the sedative effects of opiates.

c. **Sedation** is a dose-related effect but sometimes is enhanced by concomitant use of other drugs with sedating effects (e.g., benzodiazepines, antiemetics). Most chronic pain patients become tolerant to this effect, but occasionally the addition of a CNS stimulant, such as dextroamphetamine or methylphenidate, is needed. Patients starting therapy with narcotics should be warned about driving or operating machinery. Sedation may be a sign of excessive dosing or accumulation. However, sedation should not be confused with physiologic sleep in patients who have pain control difficulties. Patients in pain often develop insomnia. When pain is brought under control by appropriate narcotic titration, the patient initially may sleep for several hours.

d. **Respiratory depression** is the most serious adverse effect accompanying narcotic overdose. Respiratory depression may be a sign of an excessive dose, accumulation of long half-lived opiates (e.g., methadone, levorphanol), or accumulation of active morphine metabolites in renal failure patients.

   (1) Respiratory rate should be carefully monitored in patients receiving IV or epidural opiates, in neonates, in elderly patients, and in patients receiving other drugs that cause respiratory depression.

   (2) The opiate antagonist, naloxone, is administered intravenously to reverse life-threatening respiratory depression. Use of naloxone in an opiate-dependent patient (e.g., a chronic cancer pain patient) can precipitate opiate withdrawal.

e. **Anticholinergic effects,** such as dry mouth and urinary retention, can be bothersome for some patients.

f. **Hypersensitivity** reactions, such as itching due to histamine release, can occur secondary to opiate use, particularly with epidural or intrathecal administration. Wheals sometimes occur at the site of morphine injection. These reactions do not represent true allergy.

g. **CNS excitation,** such as myoclonus and other seizure-like activity, can be produced with the use of meperidine in renal failure. These symptoms have also been observed in patients with normal renal functions who receive high doses of meperidine (e.g., more than 800 mg/day of intramuscular meperidine). The accumulation of the metabolite normeperidine is the cause.

4. **Drug interactions**

   a. Narcotics have additive CNS depressant effects when used in combination with other drugs that also are CNS depressants (e.g., alcohol, anesthetics, antidepressants, antihistamines, barbiturates, benzodiazepines, phenothiazines).

   b. Narcotics, particularly meperidine, can cause severe reactions such as excitation, sweating, rigidity, and hypertension in patients receiving monoamine oxidase (MAO). Meperidine should be avoided and other narcotics started at lower doses in patients on MAO inhibitors.

5. **Tolerance** means that increasing doses of opiate are needed to maintain analgesia. This is usually observed as a decreasing duration of analgesia in chronic pain patients. The addition of a NSAID may help delay or provide adequate analgesia in tolerant patients.

6. **Dependence.** The use of opiates for chronic pain results in physical dependence, such that the abrupt discontinuation of the opiate results in the development of withdrawal symptoms.

   a. Withdrawal symptoms include anxiety, irritability, insomnia, chills, salivation, rhinorrhea, diaphoresis, nausea, vomiting, GI cramping, and piloerection.

      (1) The appearance and intensity of withdrawal symptoms vary according to the half-life of the opiate. For example, the withdrawal symptoms after discontinuation of chronic methadone may take several days to develop and be less intense as compared to withdrawal from morphine (shorter half-life).

      (2) The development of tolerance may be associated with withdrawal symptoms.

(3) The use of naloxone in a patient receiving chronic opiate therapy produces acute withdrawal.

b. The development of physical dependence seen in chronic pain patients is not the same as psychologic dependence or addiction. Also, the "drug-seeking" behavior observed in many acute pain patients (i.e, postoperative pain) is not a sign of addiction, but rather a need for adequate pain relief. The analgesic needs of this type of patient should be reassessed and usually necessitates increasing the dose of opiate, changing to a longer duration drug, changing to a PCA, or adding an analgesic adjunct.

C. Tramadol is an oral, centrally-acting analgesic with weak opiate activity. It has not been placed in a controlled drug schedule.

1. Mechanism of action

a. Tramadol is a synthetic aminocyclohexanol that binds to opiate receptors, inhibiting norepinephrine and serotonin.

b. The analgesic effects are partially antagonized by naloxone.

2. Clinical use

a. Tramadol is used for moderate to moderately severe pain.

b. The recommended dosage is 50–100 mg every 4–6 hours, up to a maximum of 400 mg/day.

c. At maximum dosage, tramadol appears no more effective than acetaminophen–codeine combinations.

3. Adverse effects

a. GI effects include nausea, constipation, and dry mouth.

b. CNS effects include dizziness, headache, sedation, and seizures (overdose).

c. Diaphoresis

4. Drug interactions

a. Tramadol can increase the sedative effect of alcohol and hypnotics.

b. Tramadol inhibits monamine uptake and should not be used with monamine oxidase inhibitors.

D. Analgesic adjuncts. Other classes of drugs affect nonopiate pain pathways and may be useful in certain types of pain (e.g., neurogenic pain). These drugs often are used with other analgesics and some may help manage narcotic side-effects (Table 56-6).

E. Nonpharmacologic pain management. Other therapeutic modalities for pain management include cognitive behavioral interventions and physical methods. These modalities are appropri-

Table 56-6. Analgesic Adjuncts

Class	Drugs	Indications
Tricyclic antidepressants	Amitriptyline Desipramine Doxepin Imipramine	Neurogenic pain; chronic pain complicated by depression or insomnia
Anticonvulsants	Carbamazepine Clonazepam Phenytoin Valproate	Lancinating neurogenic pain (e.g., trigeminal neuralgia, phantom limb pain, post-trauma neurogenic pain)
Neuroleptics	Fluphenazine Haloperidol Prochlorperazine	Refractory neurogenic pain; pain complicated by delirium or nausea (prochlorperazine)
Corticosteroid	Dexamethasone	Pain from neural infiltration
Antihistamine	Hydroxyzine	Pain complicated by anxiety or nausea
Benzodiazepines	Alprazolam Lorazepam	Pain complicated by anxiety or muscle spasm
Amphetamines	Dextroamphetamine Methylphenidate	For excessive opiate-induced sedation in chronic pain patients

ate for interested patients, patients experiencing anxiety with their pain, patients who have incomplete relief from analgesic therapy, and patients who need to avoid or reduce analgesic use (e.g., those with chronic nonmalignant pain).

1. **Cognitive behavioral interventions** include education and instruction, simple relaxation, biofeedback, and hypnosis.
2. **Physical methods** include heat and cold applications, massage, exercise, rest, immobilization, and transelectrode neurostimulation.

STUDY QUESTIONS

Directions: Each of the numbered items or incomplete statements in this section is followed by answers or by completions of the statement. Select the **one** lettered answer or completion that is **best** in each case.

1. An emaciated 69-year-old man with advanced inoperable throat cancer is hospitalized for pain management. He is receiving a morphine solution (40 mg orally) every 3 hours for pain. He complains of dysphagia and the frequency with which he must take morphine. An appropriate analgesic alternative for this patient would be

(A) changing to a controlled-release oral morphine
(B) increasing the dose of the oral morphine solution
(C) changing to intramuscular methadone
(D) changing to transdermal fentanyl
(E) decreasing the frequency of oral morphine administration

Questions 2 and 3

A 52-year-old woman with a diagnosis of ovarian cancer presents with complaints of pain. Her pain was reasonably well controlled with two capsules of oxycodone every 4 hours until 2 weeks ago at which point she was hospitalized for pain control. She was placed on meperidine (75 mg) every 3 hours but still complained about pain. Her meperidine dosage was increased to 100 mg every 2 hours.

2. At the dosage of meperidine, the patient is likely to experience

(A) excellent pain relief
(B) respiratory depression
(C) worsening renal function
(D) myoclonic seizures
(E) excessive sedation

3. An appropriate next step in this patient's therapy would be to

(A) add a nonsteroidal anti-inflammatory drug (NSAID)
(B) discontinue the meperidine and convert her to a controlled-release oral morphine
(C) continue the present meperidine dosage because she will eventually get relief
(D) decrease the meperidine dose to avoid side effects
(E) consider hypnosis or relaxation techniques

4. A 20-year-old victim of a motor vehicle accident is 3 days post surgery for orthopedic and internal injuries. He has been in severe pain on a regimen of intramuscular morphine (5–10 mg) every 4 hours as needed for pain. A pain consultant starts the patient with a 20-mg intravenous morphine loading dose and then begins a continuous intravenous morphine infusion with as-needed morphine boosters. Two hours after this regimen is started, the patient is asleep. The nurse is concerned and calls the physician. The physician should

(A) call for a psychiatric consult
(B) administer naloxone
(C) examine the patient and reconfirm the dosage and monitoring parameters
(D) add an injectable nonsteroidal anti-inflammatory drug (NSAID)
(E) add an amphetamine

5. Potential adverse effects associated with aspirin include all of the following EXCEPT

(A) gastrointestinal ulceration
(B) renal dysfunction
(C) enhanced methotrexate toxicity
(D) cardiac arrhythmias
(E) hypersensitivity asthma

6. All of the following facts are true about nonsteroidal anti-inflammatory drugs (NSAIDs) EXCEPT

(A) they are antipyretic
(B) there is a ceiling effect to their analgesia
(C) they can cause tolerance
(D) they do not cause dependence
(E) they are anti-inflammatory

7. Which of the following narcotics has the longest duration of effect?

(A) Methadone
(B) Controlled-release morphine
(C) Levorphanol
(D) Transdermal fentanyl
(E) Dihydromorphone

Directions: The item below contains three suggested answers of which one or more is correct. Choose the answer

A if **I only** is correct
B if **III only** is correct
C if **I and II** are correct
D if **II and III** are correct
E if **I, II, and III** are correct

8. Agents that are safe to use in a patient with bleeding problems include

I. choline magnesium trisalicylate
II. acetaminophen
III. ketorolac

ANSWERS AND EXPLANATIONS

1. The answer is D *[II B 2 c (8)].*
Patients with throat cancer often cannot take oral analgesics. The patient described in the question is also having pain difficulties with an every 3-hour regimen. Transdermal fentanyl is a good alternative because, after titration, excellent analgesia can be produced without using oral or parenteral agents. Also, the frequency of analgesic use may be decreased when titration has occurred.

2 and 3. The answers are: 2-D *[II B g],* **3-B** *[II B 2 c (1), d (1)].*
Myoclonic seizures can occur after frequent, high-dose meperidine due to the accumulation of the metabolite, normeperidine. Both oxycodone and meperidine have short durations of effect. In the chronic pain patient, an around-the-clock regimen, using a controlled-released oral morphine, would be an appropriate alternative. With titration, the patient should have good pain relief with an every 8- to 12-hour regimen.

4. The answer is C *[II B 3 c].*
A patient suffering from pain cannot sleep properly. When the pain is adequately controlled, the patient may sleep initially for many hours. This usually is not oversedation due to the narcotic. These patients should be monitored closely (e.g., respiratory rate), and other sedating drugs eliminated. Usually, no other intervention is needed.

5. The answer is D *[II A 4].*
Aspirin has several adverse effects and drug interactions. However, cardiac arrhythmias are not induced by aspirin.

6. The answer is C *[II A 2].*
Unlike the opiates, nonsteroidal anti-inflammatory drug (NSAID) use is not associated with the development of tolerance.

7. The answer is D *[Table 56-2].*
Transdermal fentanyl is a controlled-release dosage form that is effective for a 72-hour period. All of the other drugs listed in the question are effective for periods of 1–8 hours.

8. The answer is C (I,II) *[II A 4 b].*
Unlike aspirin and nonsteroidal anti-inflammatory drugs (NSAIDs), acetaminophen and choline magnesium trisalicylate lack antiplatelet effect. Therefore, they are safe to use for patients with bleeding problems.

57
Nutrition and the Hospitalized Patient

Robert A. Quercia
Kevin P. Keating

I. NUTRITIONAL PROBLEMS IN HOSPITALIZED PATIENTS

A. Incidence. It has been estimated that 30%–50% of patients admitted to hospitals have some degree of malnutrition. As many as 75% of patients undergo a deterioration of nutritional status while hospitalized.

B. Definitions

1. **Malnutrition** is a pathologic state, resulting from a relative or absolute deficiency or excess of one or more essential nutrients.

2. **Marasmus** is a chronic disease that develops over months or years as a result of a deficiency in total caloric intake. Depletion of fat stores and skeletal protein occurs to meet metabolic needs. Marasmic patients are generally not hypermetabolic and are able to preserve their visceral protein compartment as determined by measurements of serum albumin, prealbumin, and transferrin.
   - **a.** Marasmus is a well-adapted form of malnutrition, and despite a cachectic appearance, immunocompetence, wound healing and the ability to handle short-term stress are generally well preserved.
   - **b.** Nutritional support in these patients should be initiated cautiously because aggressive repletion can result in severe metabolic disturbances, such as hypokalemia and hypophosphatemia.

3. **Kwashiorkor** is an acute process that can develop within weeks and is associated with visceral protein depletion and impaired immune function. It is due to poor protein intake with adequate to slightly inadequate caloric intake; thus, patients usually appear well nourished. A hypermetabolic state (e.g., trauma, infection) combined with protein deprivation can rapidly develop into a severe kwashiorkor malnutrition characterized by hypoalbuminemia, edema, and impaired cellular immune function.
   - **a.** In hospitalized patients, the development of kwashiorkor has been implicated in poor wound healing, gastrointestinal (GI) bleeding, and sepsis.
   - **b.** Aggressive nutritional support to replete protein stores and decrease morbidity and mortality is indicated when the diagnosis of kwashiorkor is made.

4. **Mixed marasmic kwashiorkor** is a severe form of protein–calorie malnutrition that usually develops when a marasmic patient is subjected to an acute hypermetabolic stress, such as trauma, surgery, or infection.
   - **a.** This condition results in depletion of fat stores, skeletal muscle protein, and visceral protein.
   - **b.** Because of the marked immune dysfunction that develops in this state, vigorous nutritional support is indicated.

II. NUTRITIONAL ASSESSMENT AND METABOLIC REQUIREMENTS

A. Nutritional assessment. The two most commonly used tools for nutritional assessment are discussed below.

1. **Subjective global assessment (SGA)** relies heavily on the patient's history.
   - **a.** SGA takes into account:
     - **(1)** Recent weight change
     - **(2)** Diet history

(3) Type and length of symptoms impacting on nutritional status (e.g., nausea, vomiting, diarrhea)
(4) Functional status
(5) Metabolic demands of the current disease process
(6) Gross physical signs
(a) Status of subcutaneous fat
(b) Evidence of muscle wasting
(c) Presence or absence of edema and ascites

b. Patients are then classified as being well nourished or moderately or severely malnourished.

2. **Prognostic nutritional index (PNI)** is derived from a formula that attempts to quantify a patient's risk of developing operative complications based on a variety of markers of nutritional status.

PNI (%) = 158 − 16.6 (ALB) − 0.78 (TSF) − 0.20 (TFN) − 5.8 (DH), where ALB is the serum albumin (g/dl); TSF is the triceps skin fold thickness (mm); TFN is the serum transferrin (mg/dl); and DH is the delayed hypersensitivity skin-test reactivity graded 0 (nonreactive), 1 (< 5 mm induration), or 2 (≥ 5 mm induration).

a. **Predicted risk of complications.** Low risk (PNI < 40%); intermediate risk (PNI = 40 − 49%); high risk (PNI ≥ 50%).
b. **Serum markers** (i.e., albumin, transferrin) are indicators of visceral protein status.
c. **Delayed hypersensitivity reaction** is an indicator of immune competence.
d. **PNI** is of value in predicting complications of stable patients scheduled to undergo elective surgery.

3. **Body composition analysis** assesses nutritional status by measuring and comparing the ratios of various body compartments.
a. **Bioelectrical impedance.** The resistance to an electrical current is used to calculate lean body mass. The equipment is relatively inexpensive and easy to use. The results are inaccurate in critically ill patients and patients with fluid and electrolyte abnormalities.
b. **Dual energy x-ray absorptiometry.** The differential attenuation of x-rays is used to measure fat and lean body mass. The equipment is expensive and results are effected by hydration status.
c. **Total body potassium** estimates lean body mass by using a whole body counter to measure a potassium isotope concentrated in lean tissue. This method of body composition analysis is impractical and available at only a few centers.
d. **Total body water** estimates lean body mass from deuterium total body water measurements. This technique is clinically impractical.
e. **In-vivo neutron activation analysis.** Unlike other techniques, this analysis divides the body into several compartments. This technique requires a significant dose of radiation and is available only at a few research centers.

4. **Tests of physiologic function** attempt to quantitate malnutrition based on the decrease in muscle strength caused by amino acid mobilization.
a. **Maximum voluntary grip strength** is measured with isokinetic dynamometry. The results correlate well to total body protein. This test requires patient cooperation.
b. **Electrical stimulation of the ulnar nerve** measures contractile function of the adductor pollicis muscle. This technique does not require voluntary patient effort and is inexpensive and easy to do. Its prognostic reliability is still under evaluation.

B. Metabolic requirements

1. **Energy requirements** are determined as **nonprotein calories (NPC).** It is important to avoid excess calories to minimize complications of nutrient delivery and to optimize nutrient metabolism. Energy requirements can be determined by the following three methods:
a. **Indirect calorimetry** or **measured energy expenditure (MEE)** is the most accurate method of determining caloric requirements. Oxygen consumption and carbon dioxide production are measured directly. Energy expenditure is related directly to oxygen consumption and is calculated from these measurements.
b. **Estimated energy expenditure (EEE)** first requires the calculation of the **basal energy expenditure (BEE)** from the **Harris-Benedict equation;** the BEE is then multiplied by appropriate stress and activity factors.
(1) Men. BEE = 66.5 + [13.8 × wt (kg)] + [5 x ht (cm)] − [6.8 x age (years)]

(2) Women. BEE = 655 + [9.6 × wt (kg)] + [1.8 x ht (cm)] − [4.7 x age (years)]
(3) **Stress factors.** Uncomplicated surgery 1.00–1.05, peritonitis 1.05–1.25, and sepsis or multiple trauma 1.25–1.5
(4) **Activity factors.** Bed rest 0.95–1.10 and ambulation 1.10–1.30

c. **Simple nomogram.** The least accurate method of estimating caloric requirements, this technique is based on the patient's weight in kilograms. It is useful when the other methods cannot be used. Patients with mild-to-moderate degrees of stress require approximately 25–30 kcal/kg/day, whereas the severely stressed patient (e.g., a patient with major burns) may require 35 kcal/kg/day or more.

2. **Protein (nitrogen) requirements** can be determined by a number of techniques, but nitrogen balance determinations and nomograms appear to be the most practical.
   a. **Nitrogen balance techniques.** The practitioner determines the patient's nitrogen output and develops a nutritional support program in which the protein administered results in a nitrogen input that exceeds losses.
      (1) Nitrogen balance = 24-hour nitrogen intake − 24-hour nitrogen output.
      (2) A 24-hour nitrogen intake = 24-hour total protein intake, divided by 6.25 (approximately 16% of protein is comprised of nitrogen).
      (3) A 24-hour nitrogen output = [24-hour urine urea nitrogen (UUN) x 1.25] + 2, where 1.25 accounts for nonurea urine nitrogen losses (e.g., ammonia creatinine) and 2 accounts for nonurine nitrogen losses (e.g., skin, feces). Total urinary nitrogen (TUN) determinations are currently available in some centers. Because TUN is a more accurate method of assessing urinary nitrogen losses it should be used when available in place of a 24-hour UUN x 1.25 when calculating a nitrogen balance.
      (4) A positive nitrogen balance of 3–6 g is the goal.
      (5) This method cannot be used in renally impaired patients.
   b. **Nomogram method.** This method estimates protein needs based on lean body weight. Protein requirements are 1.5–2.0 g protein/kg/day for hospitalized patients.
   c. **Nonprotein calorie to nitrogen (NPC:N) ratio.** A NPC:N ratio of 125–150:1 generally has been recommended for the mildly to moderately stressed patient to achieve optimal nitrogen retention and protein synthesis. In the severely stressed patient, some studies indicate ratios as low as 85:1 may be effective.

3. **Essential fatty acids**
   a. **Linoleic acid** cannot be synthesized by humans. It is a primary component of cell membranes and is required for prostaglandin synthesis.
   b. Deficiency states are characterized by diarrhea, dermatitis, and hair loss.
   c. The currently available lipid emulsions have a high linoleic acid content.
   d. Providing 4%–7% of a patient's caloric requirements as linoleic acid from lipid emulsion prevents the development of essential fatty acid deficiency.

4. **Vitamins** are essential for proper substrate metabolism. Accepted daily allowances for oral administration have been established, but there is no consensus recommendations for intravenous (IV) administration.
   a. **Vitamin A** (fat soluble). Normal stores can last up to a year but are rapidly depleted by stress. Vitamin A has essential functions in vision, growth, and reproduction. Recommended oral intake is 2500–5000 IU/day. IV requirements are 2800–8000 IU/day secondary to binding of the IV form to glass and plastic.
   b. **Vitamin D** (fat soluble). In conjunction with parathormone and calcitonin, vitamin D helps to regulate calcium and phosphorous homeostasis. Recommended intake is 100–400 IU/day. IV requirements are 200–400 IU/day.
   c. **Vitamin E** (fat soluble) appears to function as an antioxidant, inhibiting the oxidation of free unsaturated fatty acids. Recommended daily oral allowances are 12–15 IU/day. Suggested IV requirements are 2.1–60 IU/day. The presence of polyunsaturated fatty acids increases the requirement for vitamin E, which needs to be considered with the use of lipid system parenteral nutrition (PN).
   d. **Vitamin K** (fat soluble) plays an essential role in the synthesis of clotting factors. The suggested oral intake is 0.7–2.0 mg/day.
   e. **Vitamin B_1 (thiamine)** [water soluble] functions as a coenzyme in the phosphogluconate pathway and as a structural component of nervous system membranes. The development of its deficiency state (i.e., acute pernicious beriberi with high output cardiac failure) is well described in patients on PN receiving inadequate thiamine replacement. A

prolonged deficiency state can cause Wernicke's encephalopathy. Recommended doses are 0.5 mg/1000 oral calories/day and 3–21 mg/day in PN.

f. **Vitamin B_2 (riboflavin)** [water soluble] functions as a coenzyme in oxidative phosphorylation. Essentially, no intracellular stores are maintained. Oral requirements are 1.3–1.7 mg/day. IV requirements are 3.6–7.5 mg/day.
g. **Vitamin B_3 (niacin)** [water soluble] functions as a coenzyme in oxidative phosphorylation and biosynthetic pathways. **Pellagra** is the well-described deficiency state. Oral requirements are 14.5–19.8 mg/day. IV requirements are 40–140 mg/day.
h. **Vitamin B_5 (pantothenic acid)** [water soluble]. The functional form of vitamin B_5 is coenzyme A, which is essential to all acylation reactions. Oral requirements are 5–10 mg/day. IV requirements are 10–29 mg/day.
i. **Vitamin B_6 (pyridoxine)** [water soluble] functions as a coenzyme in a variety of enzymatic pathways. Deficiency states are accentuated by some medications, including isoniazid, penicillamine, and cycloserine. Oral requirements are 1.5–2.0 mg/day. Intravenous requirements are 4.0–6.3 mg/day.
j. **Vitamin B_7 (biotin)** [water soluble] functions in carboxylation reactions. It is synthesized by intestinal flora; therefore, deficiency states are rare. IV requirements are 60 μg/day.
k. **Vitamin B_9 (folic acid)** [water soluble] is involved in a variety of biosynthetic reactions and amino acid conversions. Stores usually last 3–6 months; however, rapid depletion is seen with metabolic stress. Deficiency of vitamin B_{12} causes deficiency in folate. A megaloblastic anemia is classic in the deficiency state. Oral requirements are 200–400 μg/day. IV requirements are 0.4–1.0 mg/day.
l. **Vitamin B_{12} (cyanocobalamin)** [water soluble] has a variety of metabolic and biosynthetic functions. Because of large stores, deficiency states can take years to develop. Megaloblastic (pernicious) anemia is one manifestation of deficiency. Oral requirements are 2–3 μg/ day. IV requirements are 5.0–15 μg/day.
m. **Vitamin C (ascorbic acid)** [water soluble] has a variety of metabolic and biosynthetic functions, including collagen synthesis. Body stores are minimal. A deficiency state results in the clinical syndrome of scurvy. No specific requirement has been recommended. Recommended oral intake is 30–45 mg/day. IV requirements are 100–500 mg/day.

5. **Trace mineral deficiency** may develop during PN because of reduced intake, increased use, decreased plasma binding, or increased excretion.
   a. **Iron** is necessary for hemoglobin and myoglobin production and is a necessary cofactor in a variety of enzymatic reactions. Deficiency is classically demonstrated by a hypochromic, microcytic anemia as well as by the development of immune deficiency. Oral requirements are 16–18 mg/day. IV requirements are 0.5–1.0 mg/day.
   b. **Zinc** is necessary for DNA and RNA synthesis and is a necessary cofactor in a variety of enzymatic reactions. Zinc deficiency results in impaired wound healing, growth retardation, hair loss, dermatitis, diarrhea, anorexia, and glucose intolerance. Patients at high risk for developing zinc deficiency are those with long-term steroid therapy, malabsorption syndromes, fistulas, sepsis, and major surgery. Oral requirements are 10–15 mg/day. IV requirements are 2.5–4.0 mg/day.
   c. **Copper** is necessary for heme synthesis, electron transport, and wound healing. Deficiency that develops during PN usually manifests as anemia, leukopenia, and neutropenia. Oral requirements are 30 μg/kg/day. IV requirements are 20 μg/kg/day (0.5–1.5 mg/ day).
   d. **Manganese** is involved in protein synthesis and possibly glucose use. Oral requirements are 0.7–22 mg/day. Intravenous requirements are 2–10 μg/kg/day (0.1–0.8 mg/day).
   e. **Selenium** is important in antioxidant reactions. Deficiency during PN has been associated with muscle pain and cardiomyopathy. IV requirements are 20–40 μg/day.
   f. **Iodine** is a component of the thyroid hormones. Deficiency manifests as a goiter. Recommended intake is 1 μg/kg/day.
   g. **Chromium** is important in glucose use and potentiates the effect of insulin. Signs of deficiency include hyperglycemia and abnormal glucose tolerance. Oral requirements are 70–80 μg/day. IV requirements are 0.14–0.2 μg/kg/day (10–15 μg/day).
   h. **Molybdenum** is essential to xanthine oxidase. Oral requirements are 2.0 μg/kg/day.

III. METHODS OF SUPPORT

A. PN is also called **total parenteral nutrition (TPN)** and **hyperalimentation.** It is used to meet the patient's nutritional requirements when this cannot be accomplished by the enteral route.

1. **Indications.** When the enteral route cannot be used because of dysfunction or disease states (e.g., acute pancreatitis, inflammatory bowel disease, complete bowel obstruction), PN is instituted.

2. **Initiation** of PN should be undertaken within 1–3 days in moderately to severely malnourished patients when the inadequacy of enteral support is anticipated for more than 5–7 days. In healthy or mildly malnourished patients, PN should be initiated within 5–7 days if enteral support has not been initiated.

3. **Routes of administration**
   a. **Central venous route** is used with hypertonic PN formulations (i.e., dextrose concentrations greater than 10%). Most commonly, dextrose concentrations of 25% are used centrally, and the osmolarity exceeds 2000 mOsm/L. Such highly osmolar solutions must be infused into a large-diameter central vein (e.g., superior vena cava) where they are rapidly diluted by high flow rates.
   b. **Peripheral venous route** can be used when the dextrose concentration is 10% or less. However, solutions with 10% dextrose, amino acids, electrolytes, and trace minerals have a resulting osmolarity of 900–1000 mOsm/L. The hypertonicity of this solution can result in phlebitis and frequent IV site changes. Peripheral PN is better tolerated with a dextrose concentration of 5% administered concurrently with a lipid emulsion.

4. **NPC sources**
   a. **Dextrose monohydrate** is the form of dextrose used for parenteral administration. It yields 3.4 kcal/g. It is the component in PN formulas that contributes the most to osmolarity. It is available commercially in concentrations up to 70%.
   b. **IV lipids** are commercially available as 10% or 20% emulsions derived from soybean oil (Intralipid) or a combination of soybean oil and safflower oil (Liposyn II).
      (1) Both the 10% and 20% emulsions are isotonic (280 and 340 mOsm/L) and can be administered via the peripheral vein with a low incidence of phlebitis; these emulsions provide 1.1 and 2.0 kcal/ml, respectively. They contain 1.2% egg yolk phospholipids as the emulsifying agent and 2.25%–2.5% glycerol to make the emulsions isosmotic.
      (2) Lipid emulsions can be given as part of the daily NPC requirement or 2–3 times per week to prevent essential fatty acid deficiency. Both types of lipid emulsion contain particles of 0.4–0.5 μm, which prevents the use of 0.22 μm bacterial retention filters.

5. **Protein (nitrogen) source. Synthetic crystalline amino acids** are currently used as the nitrogen source in PN formulations.
   a. These formulations are available commercially in concentrations of 3.5%, 5.5%, 7%, 8.5%, 10%, 11.4%, and 15%.
   b. These formulations yield 4 kcal/g.
   c. These solutions generally contain a mixture of free essential and nonessential L-amino acids.
   d. Specialized amino acid formulations are available for specific disease states.

6. **Systems of PN**
   a. **Glucose system PN**
      (1) **Definitions.** The glucose system PN is a parenteral formulation in which dextrose is used exclusively as the NPC source. Nitrogen is provided as crystalline amino acids. Electrolytes, vitamins, and trace minerals are added to the formulation as needed.
      (2) **Administration.** The glucose system PN formulations usually have dextrose concentrations of 25% or greater and must be administered by the central venous route. These formulations are also referred to as two-in-one formulations because the dextrose and amino acids are usually mixed in one container with electrolytes, vitamins, and trace minerals.
         (a) Because of the high dextrose concentration, initial administration should be at low hourly rates (e.g., 50 ml/hr) and increased gradually over 24 hours to avoid hyperglycemia (> 200 mg/dl).
         (b) To avoid reactive hypoglycemia (< 70 mg/dl), discontinuation should be gradual over several hours.
         (c) Lipid emulsions should be administered for **essential fatty acid replacement** in a dose that provides 4%–7% of required calories as linoleic acid. This can be

accomplished by the administration of 250 ml of 20% or 500 ml of 10% emulsion, two to three times weekly.

b. Lipid system PN

(1) **Definition.** The lipid system PN is a parenteral formulation in which lipid is administered daily to provide a substantial proportion of the NPC. Nitrogen is provided as crystalline amino acids. Electrolytes, vitamins, and trace minerals are added to the formulation as needed.

(2) **Administration.** The lipid system PN is administered peripherally when the dextrose concentration is less than or equal to 10% and centrally when the dextrose concentration is more than 10%.

(a) **Piggyback method.** The solution with amino acids, dextrose, electrolytes, trace minerals, and vitamins is infused concurrently with a separate bottle of lipid emulsion through a Y site on the intravenous administration set.

(b) **Total nutrient admixture method** (TNA, three-in-one, all-in-one). Lipids, amino acids, dextrose, electrolytes, trace minerals, and vitamins are mixed in one container and administered by the central or peripheral route, depending on dextrose concentration.

(i) **Advantages** include simplification of administration and decreased training time for home PN patients.

(ii) **Disadvantages** include the inability to inspect for particulate matter in the opaque admixture, the inability to use 0.22 μm bacterial retention filters, and stability problems.

(iii) Because the presence of lipid emulsion in TNAs obscures the presence of a precipitate and may present a life-threatening hazard to patients, the FDA suggests that the piggyback method be used to administer lipid emulsion. If a TNA is deemed medically necessary, then specific admixture guidelines recommended by the FDA should be followed. Also, a particle filter (i.e., 1.2 micron) should be used with TNA administration.

(c) **Lipid dosage**

(i) Lipid calories should not exceed 60% of total daily calories, including protein calories.

(ii) Maximum dosage of lipids for adults is 2.5 g/kg/day.

(iii) Baseline and weekly serum triglycerides must be monitored in patients on lipid system PN.

(3) **Adverse effects** of lipids are uncommon. The most frequent adverse effects include fever, chills, sensation of warmth, chest pain, back pain, vomiting, and urticaria (overall incidence less than 1%). Severe hypoxemia has been reported with rapid infusion of lipid emulsion.

7. Additives

a. Electrolytes. PN formulations must include adequate amounts of sodium, magnesium, calcium, chloride, potassium, phosphorus, and acetate. The intracellular "anabolic" electrolytes–potassium, magnesium, and phosphate–are essential for protein synthesis. Requirements vary widely, depending on a patient's fluid and electrolyte losses; renal, hepatic, and endocrine status; acid–base balance; metabolic rate; and type of PN formula used. The electrolyte composition of the PN formula must be adjusted to meet the needs of the individual patient.

b. Vitamins and trace minerals. Vitamins are usually added to PN solutions in the form of commercially available multivitamin preparations containing the recommended daily allowances. Because of stability problems, these preparations usually consist of two vials or a dual chamber vial. One vial or chamber contains vitamins A, D, E, B_1, B_2, B_3, B_5, B_6, and C. The second vial or chamber contains vitamins B_{12}, biotin, and folic acid. Trace minerals may be added individually or as a commercially available multielement preparation. Precise requirements for trace minerals have yet to be determined.

c. Insulin may be required for patients receiving PN formulations (especially glucose system PN) to maintain blood glucose levels less than 200 mg/dl. If insulin is required, it is best provided by the addition of an appropriate amount of regular insulin to the PN formulation at the time of admixture. Although a small amount of insulin (5–10 units per bag) may be adsorbed to the container and tubing, such losses can be overcome by appropriate titration of the dose. The addition of insulin to the PN formulation has the advantage of changes in the rate of PN infusion being automatically accompanied by appropriate changes in the rate of insulin infusion.

d. **Miscellaneous drugs.** A number of medications have been successfully admixed with PN formulations for continuous infusion. The H_2-receptor antagonists are the most common drugs used in this way. The routine addition of medications to PN formulations remains controversial because of:
   (1) **Questions of stability** over the wide range of PN component concentrations
   (2) Possible **therapeutic inadequacy** or toxicity secondary to PN rate changes and loss of peak and trough levels
   (3) Increased **potential for waste** with dose changes

8. **Complications** with the use of PN can be serious and potentially life-threatening but can be avoided by careful management. Complications can be divided into mechanical, infectious, and metabolic.
   a. **Mechanical** complications generally relate to the central venous catheter or its placement and include pneumothorax, catheter occlusion, and venous thrombosis.
   b. **Infectious** complications usually are related to the central venous catheter. This line-related sepsis is secondary to multiple catheter manipulations, contamination during insertion, or contamination during routine maintenance. Hyperglycemia and IV lipids also have been implicated.
   c. **Metabolic** complications are the most common. These include hyperglycemia, hypoglycemia, hypokalemia, hypomagnesemia, hypophosphatemia, metabolic acidosis, respiratory acidosis, prerenal azotemia, and zinc deficiency.

B. **Enteral nutrition (EN).** Use of the GI tract to achieve total nutritional support or partial support in combination with the parenteral route should be attempted whenever possible in the face of inadequate oral intake. Theoretic advantages include maintenance of normal digestion, absorption, and gut mucosal barrier function.

1. **Contraindications** to EN include complete intestinal obstruction, high output intestinal fistulas, severe acute pancreatitis, severe acute inflammatory bowel disease, and severe diarrhea.

2. **Routes of administration.** Tube feedings can be administered via nasogastric, nasoduodenal, nasojejunal, gastrostomy, and jejunostomy tubes.

3. **EN formulations** can be classified as being standard (complete) or modular.
   a. **Standard formulas** generally contain carbohydrates, fats, vitamins, trace minerals, and a nitrogen source. They are further classified according to their nitrogen source.
      (1) **Monomeric** formulas contain crystalline amino acids as their nitrogen source. These formulas are usually marketed commercially for specific indications (e.g., ileus, pancreatitis, hepatic coma).
      (2) **Short-chain peptide** formulas contain di- and tripeptides from hydrolyzed protein or de novo synthesis as their nitrogen source. They are currently marketed for the metabolically stressed patient.
      (3) **Polymeric** formulas contain either intact proteins or protein hydrolysates as their nitrogen source. Most patients can be managed with these formulas.
   b. **Modular formulas** consist of separate modules of specific nutrients that can be combined or administered separately. They are used for supplemental use or to custom design an EN formula to meet a specific clinical situation.
      (1) **Carbohydrate modules** differ in the type of carbohydrate present (e.g., polysaccharides, disaccharides, monosaccharides).
      (2) **Protein modules** contain either intact protein, hydrolyzed protein, or crystalline amino acids.
      (3) **Fat modules** contain either long-chain triglycerides (LCT) prepared from vegetable oils or medium-chain triglycerides (MCT) prepared from coconut oil. MCT are more water soluble and more easily absorbed than LCT. (Bypassing the intestinal lacteal and lymphatic system, MCT are transported directly to the portal system.) MCT are, however, relatively expensive and contain no essential fatty acids.

4. **Complications.** The two **most common** complications of EN are diarrhea and improper tube placement.
   a. **Diarrhea** in patients receiving EN is usually secondary to concomitant administration of medication (e.g., antibiotics). Infectious etiologies should be eliminated (e.g., *Clostridium*

difficile), after which antidiarrheal medications may be beneficial. Reducing the rate or concentration may also be effective.

b. A **feeding tube improperly placed** into the tracheobronchial tree can have disastrous consequences. Tube feedings should never be initiated without radiologic verification of tube position.

c. **Aspiration**

IV. MONITORING SUPPORT

A. Parenteral nutrition (PN). In addition to appropriate general medical and nursing care, patients receiving PN initially require daily and weekly laboratory monitoring to assess nutritional progress and metabolic status.

1. **Electrolytes**
   a. Initially, **potassium, sodium,** and **chloride** should be determined daily. Potassium is used intracellularly; thus, hypokalemia is not an uncommon finding.
   b. **Calcium, magnesium,** and **phosphate** are primarily intracellular electrolytes, serum levels of which become depleted during protein synthesis. Serum levels generally do not fall as rapidly as potassium; therefore, monitoring two to three times a week is recommended initially until the patient is stabilized, then weekly thereafter.
   c. **Bicarbonate** should be monitored to assess acid–base balance. Hyperchloremic metabolic acidosis may develop in patients on PN. This imbalance can be corrected by providing the potassium and sodium as acetate (converted to bicarbonate in the serum) rather than as the chloride salt. After initial correction, provision of one-half the sodium and potassium requirements as the acetate salt and one-half as the chloride salt may be beneficial.

2. **Serum glucose** should be monitored daily, particularly in central glucose systems. Maintaining a blood glucose concentration between 100–200 mg/dl is generally recommended.

3. **Weights** obtained on a daily or every other day basis track optimum lean body weight gain of 1/4–1/2 lb/day. Weight gain in excess of 1/2 lb/day generally indicates fluid overload or fat deposition.

4. **Visceral proteins** (e.g., albumin, prealbumin, transferrin) are important indicators of the adequacy of nutritional support.
   a. **Albumin** is useful in the initial assessment of nutritional status, but its long half-life (18–21 days) limits its utility as a short-term marker of nutritional repletion.
   b. **Prealbumin** has a short half-life (2–3 days) and is a more sensitive and early indicator of the adequacy of nutritional support. Its serum value is falsely elevated in renal failure.
   c. **Transferrin** has an intermediate half-life (7–10 days), which makes weekly monitoring useful. Transferrin may be falsely elevated in iron-deficiency states.

5. **Serum creatinine** and **blood urea nitrogen (BUN)** should be obtained at least weekly. Evidence of renal impairment may require modification of the PN formula. Elevation of the BUN in the absence of renal impairment may be secondary to the PN formula (e.g., excess nitrogen, low NPC:N ratio) and appropriate adjustments need to be made.

6. **Liver function tests** [aspartate aminotransferase (AST), alanine aminotransferase (ALT), alkaline phosphatase, and lactate dehydrogenase (LDH), bilirubin] require weekly monitoring because of potential toxicity from the PN formulation (i.e., fatty infiltration of the liver). Abnormal liver function studies may necessitate changes in the PN formulation.

7. **Serum triglycerides** should be measured for a baseline and weekly thereafter for patients on lipid system PN. It is not necessary to monitor triglycerides on a weekly basis for patients receiving lipids two to three times per week for essential fatty acid replacement.

8. **Twenty-four hour UUN** should be obtained weekly to determine nitrogen balance for patients in whom nitrogen requirements are uncertain. These are usually highly stressed, severely ill, or injured patients in an intensive care unit (ICU) setting.

9. **Serum iron** levels should be obtained weekly to determine deficiency and to allow appropriate interpretation of serum transferrin levels.

B. EN generally requires less intense laboratory monitoring. Specific laboratory guidelines for monitoring EN support vary from institution to institution.

V. DISEASE-SPECIFIC SUPPORT

A. Nutritional support for renal failure. The goal of nutritional support in acute renal failure (ARF) is to meet the patient's NPC requirements while minimizing volume, protein load, and potential electrolyte imbalance.

1. **PN formulations** used in ARF are low-nitrogen, high-caloric density formulas (e.g., 2% amino acid/47% dextrose), resulting in NPC:N ratios of approximately 500:1.

2. **Commercial renal failure formulations** (e.g., Nephramine, RenAmin, Aminosyn RF), containing primarily essential amino acids, have shown no clinical advantage over less expensive, low-concentration standard amino acid formulations.

3. **Standard glucose system formulation** (4.25% amino acid/25% dextrose) can generally be used in renal failure patients who are being dialyzed on a regular basis. This formulation is particularly useful in severely malnourished patients because it can provide adequate protein to attain positive nitrogen balance, which is not possible with renal failure PN.

4. **Monitoring transferrin** is a more sensitive and accurate visceral protein marker compared to albumin and prealbumin for assessing nutritional progress in these patients.

5. **Enteral formulations** that are low in nitrogen and calorie dense (1.7–2.0 NPC/ml) are available for patients with renal failure.

B. Nutritional support for hepatic failure. Patients with hepatic failure have altered protein metabolism, resulting in decreased serum levels of branched-chain amino acids (i.e., leucine, isoleucine, valine) and increased levels of aromatic amino acids (i.e., phenylalanine, tyrosine, tryptophan), methionine, and glutamine. A similar amino acid profile can exist in the cerebrospinal fluid (CSF) and is thought to contribute to hepatic encephalopathy. Fluid and electrolyte disturbances are frequently associated with hepatic failure as well.

1. **PN formulations** enriched in branched-chain amino acids (36%) and low in aromatic amino acids (e.g., Hepatamine) improve mental status in patients with altered serum amino acid profiles and hepatic encephalopathy. However, studies have not demonstrated definitive clinical differences in morbidity and mortality with these expensive formulations compared to standard formulas.

2. **Adequate NPC** with a 20–40 g/day protein load (e.g., 2% amino acid/25% dextrose) is an alternative approach to the use of hepatic failure amino acid formulations. Protein load can be liberalized slowly as long as mental status does not deteriorate.

3. **EN formulations** (e.g., Hepatic-Aid II) enriched with branched-chain amino acids and low in aromatic amino acids are commercially available for patients with hepatic failure.

C. Nutritional support for respiratory failure. The type and amount of substrate administered as NPC can have an impact upon a patient's ventilatory status. Overfeeding results in lipogenesis, which produces eight times the amount of carbon dioxide produced by glycolysis. This increased carbon dioxide load requires an increase in minute ventilation or respiratory acidosis ensues. Even in the presence of appropriate amounts of NPC administered as carbohydrate, the carbon dioxide load generated by glycolysis may be excessive for the patient with underlying pulmonary dysfunction [e.g., chronic obstructive pulmonary disease (COPD)].

1. **PN lipid system formulations** (e.g., 4.25% amino acid/15% dextrose with daily lipid emulsion), where the lipid component constitutes 40%–50% of the total NPC, may be beneficial in reducing the ventilatory demands in respiratory failure patients because lipolysis generates less carbon dioxide than glycolysis.

2. **EN formulations** containing similar amounts of fat can be prepared from standard EN formulas with the use of lipid modules (i.e., MCT oil, corn oil). More expensive commercial pulmonary formulas are also available.

D. Nutritional support for cardiac failure. The goal in these patients is to meet metabolic needs while restricting fluid and sodium intake.

1. **PN formulations** that provide protein and calories in as high a concentration as possible is the goal of nutritional therapy. This can be accomplished with both central glucose or lipid

system PN formulations (e.g., 5% amino acid/35% dextrose; 7% amino acid/21% dextrose/20% lipid emulsion).

2. **Serum electrolyte monitoring** and **adjustment** are imperative in cardiac failure patients receiving PN, particularly when potent diuretics are used concurrently.

3. **EN formulations** with high nutrient density are available for oral supplementation or tube feedings. Infusion of enteral tube feedings should begin at one-third to one-half the strength, with a gradual increase in concentration, while maintaining a slow infusion rate (30–50 ml/hr) to avoid rapid increases in fluid load, cardiac output, heart rate, and myocardial oxygen consumption.

E. **Nutritional support in pancreatitis.** Severe acute pancreatitis is a hypercatabolic state that without nutritional support renders the patient a poor surgical candidate and at increased risk of infection. The goal of nutritional support in severe acute pancreatitis is to "rest" the pancreas by limiting exocrine stimulation while providing adequate nutrition.

1. **PN** is generally favored over EN to achieve this goal in the early phases of pancreatitis. Lipid system PN has been shown to be safe and effective when administered to these patients, provided there is no concurrent hyperlipidemia; in fact, it may be valuable in the patient with recalcitrant hyperglycemia.

2. **EN,** using chemically defined (elemental), low-fat formulas administered into the jejunum, results in minimal pancreatic stimulation and has been used safely in these patients.

VI. TECHNICAL ASPECTS OF PARENTERAL NUTRITION (PN) PREPARATIONS

A. PN formula preparation is performed **aseptically** in the pharmacy under a laminar flow hood that filters the air, removing airborne particles and microorganisms.

B. **Compatibility** of the various components of PN formulations is determined by several factors, including their concentration, solution pH, temperature, and the order of admixture. The **most common** compatibility concern regards the addition of calcium and phosphate salts to PN solutions.

C. Following admixture of the various components, the PN solution should be **visually inspected** for precipitate or particulate matter. After labeling and final checking, the PN solution should be refrigerated until delivery to the nursing unit.

D. A statistically valid, continuous **sterility testing program** should be an essential component of quality control in preparing PN solutions.

VII. HOME PARENTERAL NUTRITION (HPN).

HPN has become a widely accepted and useful technique for provision of complete nutritional requirements in the home setting. When used appropriately, this modality benefits the patient medically and psychologically with a decreased cost to the health care system.

A. **Indications** for HPN include short bowel syndrome, severe inflammatory bowel disease, radiation enteritis, enterocutaneous fistulae, and selected malignancies.

B. **Candidate selection** requires a multidisciplinary approach to determine if the patient and family can assume the responsibility and training needed for safe and successful HPN.

C. **Administration.** HPN is infused through a central venous Silastic catheter (e.g., Hickman, Broviac), which allows for prolonged PN with low clotting and infection rates. The PN solution is generally infused over a 12- to 15-hour period at night. This type of **cycling program** allows the patient to be free from the infusion pump during the day, allowing for a more normal lifestyle.

D. **Clinical monitoring** and follow-up are done periodically, depending on the needs of the individual patient. Long-term HPN patients generally are seen by the physician on a monthly basis after initial stabilization.

VIII. MISCELLANEOUS

A. Conditionally essential nutrients

1. **Glutamine.** Because of its instability, glutamine is currently not a component of commercially available PN amino acid solutions and is found in free form in relatively few EN formulas. It is known to be used as a primary fuel source by enterocytes and may exert a trophic effect on the gut mucosa. It is most widely used as a PN component for bone marrow transplant patients, where its use is associated with a significant decrease in infectious complications. Glutamine-containing dipeptides that are stable and highly soluble are being investigated as a source of glutamine in PN. At present, glutamine must be added to the PN solution at the time of compounding. Optimum PN dose, contraindications, and EN necessity in free form are controversial and require further investigation.

2. **Arginine** has been shown experimentally and clinically to enhance immune function. EN formulas enriched with arginine are available commercially. Optimum dose has yet to be determined.

3. **Anti-oxidant formulations.** Oxidant production occurs as part of the normal inflammatory response and has been implicated in reperfusion injury. The body also produces antioxidant defenses to limit oxidant damage to healthy tissue. These defenses rely on adequate intake of dietary nutrients, such as the sulfur-containing amino acids, vitamin E, vitamin C, selenium, and zinc. Several investigators believe provision of these nutrients should be an early priority in critically ill patients. Optimum doses remain controversial.

4. **Tyrosine, cysteine,** and **taurine** are either absent or present in low concentrations in commercially available PN formulas. They are believed to be conditionally essential amino acids by some investigators.

5. **Omega 3 polyunsaturated fatty acids** are derived from fish oils and are currently found in some EN formulations. These fatty acids have been shown experimentally to enhance immune response, protect against tumor growth, and inhibit some of the proinflammatory effects of omega-6 fatty acids. In addition, they have been shown to lower cardiovascular risk factors by decreasing platelet activation, lowering blood pressure, and reducing triglycerides. However, well-controlled clinical trials in humans are needed to confirm the beneficial effects seen in animal models.

B. Soluble fiber

Soluble fiber is present in some commercially available EN formulas. This fiber is fermented by normal large intestinal flora to short-chain fatty acids that are used by colonocytes as a fuel source. These short-chain fatty acids also seem to have a trophic effect on the large intestinal mucosa.

C. Growth factors

Growth factors. The use of recombinant human growth hormone, insulin-like growth factor, and anabolic steroids, in combination with nutritional support to improve nitrogen balance and reduce hospital length of stay in select patient populations, is currently under investigation.

STUDY QUESTIONS

Directions: Each of the numbered items or incomplete statements in this section is followed by answers or by completions of the statement. Select the **one** lettered answer or completion that is **best** in each case.

1. A hospitalized patient with low visceral proteins (albumin, 1.9; transferrin, 90), normal somatic proteins, and normal body weight is

(A) suffering from severe marasmic malnutrition
(B) at low risk for hospital-acquired infection and other complications
(C) suffering from severe kwashiorkor malnutrition
(D) suffering from mixed marasmic kwashiorkor
(E) suffering from chronic malnutrition

2. Which of the following methods would be the most accurate in assessing the calorie requirements of a critically ill patient in the intensive care unit?

(A) Estimated energy expenditure (EEE)
(B) Nomogram
(C) Measured energy expenditure (MEE)
(D) Prognostic nutritional index (PNI)
(E) Nitrogen balance

3. Which of the following statements concerning parenteral nutrition (PN) is true? PN

(A) is indicated after 7 days for patients with severe malnutrition who are unable to meet their needs by the enteral route
(B) is indicated within 5–7 days for patients who are well nourished on admission but unable to meet their needs by the enteral route
(C) should never be administered to patients who can take any food by mouth
(D) is contraindicated for use in the home setting
(E) is more effective than enteral nutrition (EN)

4. Which of the following statements concerning glucose system parenteral nutrition (PN) is true? It

(A) requires central venous administration
(B) should be discontinued without tapering
(C) requires the daily administration of lipid emulsion
(D) cannot provide adequate calories for the highly stressed patient
(E) requires daily serum triglyceride monitoring

5. Which of the following statements regarding the monitoring of patients on nutritional support is true?

(A) Albumin is the best marker to follow short-term nutritional progress
(B) Prealbumin is the best marker to follow in patients with renal failure
(C) Transferrin is falsely decreased in iron-deficiency states
(D) Optimal lean body weight gain is 1/4–1/2 lb/day
(E) Optimal positive nitrogen balance is greater than 8–10 g of nitrogen daily

6. A patient in acute renal failure (ARF) who is not on regular dialysis would benefit most from which of the following parenteral nutrition (PN) programs?

(A) 4.25% amino acid/25% dextrose
(B) 7% amino acid/21% dextrose/20% lipid emulsion
(C) 2% amino acid/47% dextrose
(D) 2% amino acid/5% dextrose
(E) 2% amino acid/25% dextrose

7. Which amino acid solution would be best tolerated in patients with liver disease and encephalopathy?

(A) Low-branched chain, high-aromatic amino acid solution
(B) Essential amino acid solution
(C) Low-aromatic, high-branched chain amino acid solution
(D) Glutamine-enriched amino acid solution
(E) Methionine- and cysteine-enriched amino acid solution

Questions 8–10

A 57-year-old man involved in a motor vehicle accident sustains severe chest and abdominal injuries. After resuscitation, he is brought to the operating room where he undergoes a splenectomy, partial hepatectomy, segmental small bowel resection, and insertion of a feeding jejunostomy. He is in the intensive care unit and on a ventilator. The attending surgeon would like him started on tube feedings beginning on the first postoperative day. His prior history is significant for tobacco abuse and moderate emphysema. He is 175 cm tall and weighs 100 kg. The indirect calorimeter is currently unavailable to ascertain his energy requirements.

8. The best estimate of this patient's nonprotein calorie (NPC) needs would be

(A) 2900–3400 NPC
(B) 2400–2900 NPC
(C) 1900–2400 NPC
(D) 1400–1900 NPC
(E) 900–1400 NPC

Six days after initiating enteral support, the patient develops a small bowel fistula at the site of his small bowel anastomosis. His 24-hour urine urea nitrogen (UUN) is 15. He is switched to parenteral nutrition (PN) using Aminosyn 4.25% (6.7 g of nitrogen per liter).

9. To meet the patient's previously calculated needs and put him in positive nitrogen balance, this patient would require

(A) 47% dextrose/4.25% amino acid at 150 ml/hr
(B) 25% dextrose/4.25% amino acid at 150 ml/hr
(C) 47% dextrose/4.25% amino acid at 135 ml/hr
(D) 25% dextrose/4.25% amino acid at 135 ml/hr
(E) 47% dextrose/4.25% amino acid at 75 ml/hr

10. Concerned about a persistent respiratory acidosis and a high minute ventilation, the physician obtains a measured energy expenditure (MEE), which indicates that the patient is not being overfed. He switches the patient to lipid system PN. The order calls for a 15% dextrose/4.25% amino acid/ insulin/cimetidine formulation at 135 ml/hr with 500 ml of 20% lipid emulsion daily. The physician is concerned about the order because

(A) the resultant NPC:N ratio is unacceptable
(B) the cimetidine is incompatible with the insulin in the formulation
(C) the lipid administration is excessive
(D) lipid system PN is contraindicated in patients on mechanical ventilation
(E) none of the above

ANSWERS AND EXPLANATIONS

1. The answer is C *[I B 3].*
Kwashiorkor is an acute process that can develop within weeks. It is associated with visceral protein depletion and impaired immune function.

2. The answer is C *[II B 1 a].*
Measured energy expenditure (MEE) is the most accurate method of determining caloric requirements. It is especially beneficial in severely ill patients in whom stress factors are variable.

3. The answer is B *[III A 2].*
Parenteral nutrition (PN) should be initiated within 5–7 days in healthy or mildly malnourished patients if enteral support is inadequate. In moderately to severely malnourished patients, PN should be undertaken within 1–3 days if enteral support is inadequate.

4. The answer is A *[III A 6 a (2)].*
Glucose system parenteral nutrition (PN) formulations usually have a dextrose concentration of 25% or greater and must be administered by the central venous route. These highly osmolar solutions (2000 mOsm/L) are rapidly diluted by high flow rates in large diameter central veins.

5. The answer is D *[IV A 3].*
Weights obtained on a daily or every other day basis are used to track the optimal lean body weight gain of 1/4–1/2 lb/day. Weight gain in excess of this amount generally indicates fluid overload or fat deposition.

6. The answer is C *[V A 1].*
Parenteral nutrition (PN) formulations for use in acute renal failure (ARF) are high-caloric density, low-nitrogen formulas that can meet caloric requirements in a small volume and with a small protein load. They are used until renal failure resolves or dialysis is undertaken.

7. The answer is C *[V B 1].*
Parenteral nutrition (PN) formulations enriched in branched chain amino acids and low in aromatic amino acids have been shown to improve mental status in hepatic failure patients with altered serum amino acid profiles and encephalopathy.

8–10. The answers are: 8-B *[II B 1 b],* **9-D** *[II B 2 a],* **10-E** *[II B 2 c; III A 4, 6 b, 7 d; V C].*
Use of the Harris-Benedict equation to determine basal energy expenditure (BEE) and multiplying that by a stress factor of 1.25–1.50 for multiple trauma is the most accurate way of determining this patient's nonprotein calorie (NPC) needs in the absence of indirect calorimetry.

A mixture of 25% dextrose/4.25% amino acid at 135 ml/hr yields 2754 NPC and 22 g of nitrogen (N) [3.24 L/day; 850 NPC/L; 6.7 g N/L]. The patient's 24-hour urine urea nitrogen (UUN) was 15 g N. Nitrogen in − nitrogen out = nitrogen balance. Thus, 22 g N − [(15 g N x 1.25) + 2 g N] = + 1 g N.

NPC:N is an acceptable 122:1. Cimetidine can be added to the parenteral nutrition (PN) to run as a continuous infusion. This patient is receiving 1 g fat/kg/day (31% of total calories as lipid). Lipid system PN is sometimes beneficial in patients with underlying pulmonary disease.

58 Immunosuppressive Agents in Organ Transplantation

David I. Min

I. ORGAN TRANSPLANTATION

A. **Definition.** Replacement of a diseased vital organ with a viable organ from a living or cadaver donor. Solid organ transplantation has become the therapy of choice for many patients with end-organ failure (i.e., heart, liver, lung, and kidney disease). However, it generally requires immunosuppression to overcome the immunologic barrier between donor and recipient, except in syngenic (i.e., twins) or autologous transplantation.

B. **Classification**

1. **Solid organ transplantation**
   a. **Life-saving transplantation** occurs when there is no alternative life-sustaining method available (e.g., heart, heart–lung, lung, and liver transplantation).
   b. **Non–life-saving transplantation** occurs when there are alternative life-sustaining methods available, such as dialysis or external insulin injection (e.g., kidney, pancreas, cornea transplantation). In these cases, transplantation improves a patient's quality of life or long-term survival significantly.

2. **Bone marrow transplantation** is used for mostly hematologic malignancy or aplastic anemia

II. GRAFT REJECTION

A. **Transplant immunology** (see Chapter 10)

1. **Graft rejection.** The body immune system recognizes the allograft (transplanted organ) as a foreign antigen and initiates the immune response to remove or destroy transplanted graft. This reaction is called "rejection." The degree of this reaction depends on the genetic similarities or differences between the organ of the donor and the immune system of the recipient.

2. **Histocompatibility.** The antigens that determine the compatibility between the donor and the recipient are called **histocompatibility antigens,** the gene being located on chromosome 6. In many transplants (i.e., bone marrow or kidney transplant), this histocompatibility matching is an important factor for determining the long-term survival of the graft. However, more selective, potent immunosuppression may alleviate the importance of tissue matching between donor and recipient. An exception is in bone marrow transplantations; the tissue matching is still important in these cases.

3. **Other factors.** Another group of substances that plays an important role is the **ABO blood group system** of red blood cells. The donor and recipient must be ABO-compatible; otherwise, immediate graft destruction occurs. Some patients may have a preformed antibody for unspecified donors through multiple blood transfusions or other reasons. In this case, patients may destroy the transplanted organ immediately. To detect the preformed antibody, the recipient's serum is tested immediately before the transplantation (cross-match).

B. **Type of graft rejection**

1. **Time course rejections**
   a. **Hyperacute.** In this type of rejection, the transplant organ is destroyed immediately (within minutes or hours) by a preformed antibody or complement system. Today, this is extremely rare. Hyperacute rejection occurs only in an ABO-mismatched organ or a

cross-match positive (preformed antibody) organ. There is no adequate treatment available.

b. **Acute.** This type of rejection occurs within a few days to several months after transplantation. It is mediated by T-lymphocyte (cell-mediated immunity) and can be reversed by steroids or antibody therapy, such as muromonab-CD3 or antithymocyte globulin.

c. **Chronic.** This type of rejection occurs several months to several years after transplantation. This reaction is mediated by B-lymphocyte (antibody) and there is no adequate treatment available.

2. **Graft versus host, host versus graft**

In most solid organ transplants, rejection occurs as the host immune system rejects or attacks the transplant organ (host versus graft). However, in bone marrow transplant, the host is generally immune deficient and the transplanted graft is immune competent, which attracts host tissues (graft versus host).

III. PROPHYLAXIS AND TREATMENT OF GRAFT REJECTION (Table 58-1)

A. Calcineurin inhibitors

1. **Cyclosporine (Sandimmune)**

a. **Mechanism of action.** Cyclosporine binds intracellular receptor, cyclophiline. The resulting complex inhibits calcineurin, an intracellular phosphatase, which activates the promoter region for the gene-encoding cytokine (e.g., interleukin-2). Consequently, T-cell

Table 58-1. Current Immunosuppressive Agents Used in Organ Transplantation

Classification	Drug	Usual Initial Dose	Major Side Effects	Monitoring
Calcineurin inhibitor	Cyclosporine Tacrolimus (FK506)	10 mg/kg/day 0.1–0.3 mg/kg/day	Nephrotoxicity Neurotoxicity	Blood concentrations and serum creatinine concentrations monitoring
Antimetabolites	Azathioprine	1.5–3 mg/kg/day	Bone marrow suppression	WBC count monitoring
	Mycophenolate mofetil	1 g twice daily	Same as above	Same as above
	Methotrexate	15 mg/m² on day 1, 10 mg/m²/day on days 3, 6, and 11	Same as above	Same as above
Alkylating agent	Cyclophosphamide	3–4 mg/kg/day for 4 days followed by a reduction to 1 mg/kg/day for treatment of rejection	Hemorrhagic cystitis	WBC count
Antibody products	Muromonoab CD3 (OKT3)	5 mg daily for 7–14 days	Cytokine release syndromes (flu-like syndrome)	Signs and symptoms, CD3+ cell count
	Antithymocyte globulin	15–30 mg/kg/day for 7 to 14 days	Leukopenia and thrombocytopenia	T-cell count
Corticosteroids	Prednisone or methylprednisolone	500 mg IV on the day of surgery and rapidly tapering to 10 mg daily at 1 month	Fluid retention, psychosis, cataracts, osteonecrosis	Signs and symptoms

activation is inhibited in the early stage of immune response to foreign antigen, such as a graft.

b. **Dosage and monitoring.** The pharmacokinetics of cyclosporine are unpredictable and affected by many factors, such as age, time after transplant, different oral formulation (Neoral, Sandimmune), or drugs. Oral bioavailability is about 30%. Generally, 10 mg/kg/day of oral cyclosporine is used in solid organ transplantation and adjusted according to the blood levels. Serum creatinine should be monitored with the blood levels of cyclosporine. The blood levels are useful in the clinical monitoring.

c. **Side effects. Nephrotoxicity** is the major side effect. Neurotoxicity and hepatotoxicity are also common. Numerous **drug interactions** have been reported (Table 58-2).

2. **Tacrolimus (Prograf)**

a. **Mechanism of action.** Tacrolimus works in a similar way to cyclosporine (III A 1).

b. **Dosage and monitoring.** The pharmacokinetics of tacrolimus are variable, and oral bioavailability is about 25%. Blood levels are useful in clinical monitoring.

c. **Side effects. Nephrotoxicity** is the major side effect. Neurotoxicity and gastrointestinal (GI) toxicity are more common than with cyclosporine.

B. Antimetabolites

1. **Azathioprine (Imuran)**

a. **Mechanism of action.** Azathioprine is converted to 6-mercaptopurine in the body and is a non-specific purine synthesis inhibitor. It interferes with DNA and RNA synthesis so that it may reduce both cell-mediated and humoral immune responses.

b. **Dosage and monitoring.** An initial dose of 3–5 mg/kg/day is administered preoperatively. Immediately after transplantation, the dose is usually tapered to a maintenance dose of 1–3 mg/kg/day or titrated to the patient's white blood cell (WBC) count. The WBC count is generally maintained greater than 3000/mm^3.

c. **Side effects.** Bone marrow suppression (leukopenia, thrombocytopenia) is the **major** side effect. In addition, xanthine oxidase inhibitor allopurinol inhibits azathioprine metabolism. When these drugs are used concurrently, the azathioprine dose should be reduced by 80%. Otherwise, the patient may develop severe leukopenia due to azathioprine overdose.

2. **Mycophenolate mofetil (CellCept)**

a. **Mechanism of action.** In the body, mycophenolate mofetil is converted to mycophenolic acid, which inhibits *de novo* purine synthesis pathway by inhibiting inosine dehydrogenase. As a result, it inhibits DNA and RNA synthesis in the immune cells.

Table 58-2. Major Drug Interactions of Cyclosporine and Tacrolimus with Other Drugs

Drugs	Mechanism	Effects	Management
Antiepileptic drugs Phenytoin Phenobarbital Carbamazepine	Increased metabolism by inducing cytochrome p-450 enzyme	Cyclosporine or tacrolimus trough levels drop within 48 hrs after initiation of these drugs	Increase cyclosporine dose or tacrolimus with frequent monitoring of blood levels
Rifampin or isoniazid	Same as above	Same as above	Same as above
Azole antifungal agents Ketoconazole Fluconazole Itraconazole	Inhibition of liver cytochrome p-450 enzyme by these drugs	Significant increase of cyclosporine or tacrolimus levels	Reduce cyclosporine or tacrolimus dose with frequent monitoring of levels
Macrolide antibiotics Erythromycin Josamycin	Inhibition of liver and GI cytochrome p-450 enzyme	Increase AUC (×2) and cyclosporine or tacrolimus trough levels (×2–3)	Same as above
Calcium channel blockers Verapamil Diltiazem Nicardipine	Same as above	Same as above	Reduce cyclosporine or tacrolimus dose or use nifedipine, isradipine

b. **Dosage and monitoring.** A dosage of 2 g/day is administered as two divided doses.
c. **Side effects.** Bone marrow suppression (leukopenia, thrombocytopenia) is the **major** side effect, as in azathioprine. In addition, GI side effects are more common than with azathioprine.

3. **Methotrexate.** This agent is used mainly in autoimmune disease and preventing graft versus host disease in bone marrow transplant (BMT) patients.
   a. **Mechanism of action.** Methotrexate prevents dihydrofolic acid from converting to tetrahydrofolic acid by inhibiting the enzyme dihydrofolate reductase. As a result, DNA and protein synthesis are inhibited.
   b. **Dosage and monitoring.** Dosage regimens in the BMT patients usually consist of 15 mg/m^2/day on day 1 after transplant, 10 mg/m^2/day on days 3, 6, and 11 with other agents such as cyclosporine.
   c. **Side effects.** Bone marrow suppression (leukopenia, thrombocytopenia) is the **major** side effect, as in azathioprine. In addition, diarrhea and mucositis are common.

C. **Alkylating agent. Cyclophosphamide** is the alkylating agent mainly used for BMT patients. Rarely is it used as a substitute agent for azathioprine in solid organ transplantation.

1. **Mechanism of action.** Cyclophosphamide is converted to the active metabolite, phosphoramide mustard in the liver, which inhibits the cross-linking of DNA, leading to cell death.

2. **Dosage and monitoring.** The recommended dosage of cyclophosphamide up to 3–4 mg/kg/day for 4 days followed by a reduction to 1 mg/kg/day to treat graft rejection. The dosage should be titrated to maintain a WBC count greater than 4000/mm^3.

3. **Side effects.** Hemorrhagic cystitis and bone marrow suppression (leukopenia, thrombocytopenia) are the **major** side effects. In addition, nausea, vomiting, and diarrhea are common.

D. **Antibody products**

1. **Muromonab CD3 (Orthoclone OKT3)** is the first therapeutic mouse monoclonal antibody produced for use in humans.
   a. **Mechanism of action. OKT3** is a mouse IgG2a immunoglobulin that binds to the CD3 structure on T lymphocytes. When OKT3 is bound to the CD3 region of T cells, these T cells lose the antigen-recognition function and cannot initiate rejection process.
   b. **Dosage and monitoring.** The dosage is 5 mg/day intravenous (IV) for 7–14 days to prevent or treat rejection. The CD3+ lymphocyte counts are monitored, and it is desirable that the CD+ cell be maintained at less than 30/mm^3.
   c. **Side effects.** With the first few doses, the patient develops severe flu-like symptoms, such as fever, chills, nausea, vomiting, and headache. The OKT3 stimulates T cells, and these symptoms are caused by abrupt release of cytokines such as interleukin-1, tumor necrosis factor-a, and interleukin-6 from opsonized T cells (cytokine-release syndrome).

2. **Antithymocyte globulin (Atgam)**
   a. **Mechanism of action.** Antithymocyte globulin is a purified polyclonal immunoglobulin from horses that binds to the human T cells. However, it may have cross reactivity against the red blood cells, platelets, and granulocytes.
   b. **Dosage and monitoring.** The dosage is 15–20 mg/day IV infusion through a central line for 7–14 days for prevention or treatment of rejection. The T-lymphocyte counts are monitored and maintained at less than 100/mm^3.
   c. **Side effects.** Antithymocyte globulin may cause fever, chills, erythema, leukopenia, thrombocytopenia, and anaphylactic reaction or serum sickness.

E. **Corticosteroids. Prednisone** and **methylprednisolone** are the major corticosteroid products used for transplant patients.

1. **Mechanisms of action.** Corticosteroids have multiple pharmacologic effects in various cells. Corticosteroids bind with intracellular glucocorticoid receptors, which results in altering DNA and RNA translation. As a result, corticosteroids cause a rapid and profound drop in circulating T lymphocytes. They have potent anti-inflammatory effects by inhibiting arachidonic acid release and macrophage phagocytosis.

2. **Dosage and monitoring.** Prednisone and methylprednisolone are used in both preventing and treating graft rejection and acute graft versus host disease. In general, prophylactic

dosage in solid organ transplantation is 1–2 mg/kg/day tapered over months to 0.1–0.3 mg/kg/day. In the case of treatment, the dosage is 500 mg of methylprednisolone IV for 3–5 days or 1–2 mg/kg/day of oral prednisone and taper rapidly.

3. **Side effects.** The long-term side effects are more troubling than the short-term effects. These include psychologic disturbance (i.e., euphoria, depression), adrenal axis suppression, hypertension, sodium and water retention, myopathy, impaired wound healing, increased appetite, osteoporosis, hyperglycemia, and cataracts.

IV. COMPLICATIONS OF IMMUNOSUPPRESSION

A. Infections

1. **Risk.** Transplant patients have a high risk of acquiring an infection due to patient factors such as diabetes mellitus, hepatitis, or uremia. In addition, immunosuppressive agents can cause various effects, such as leukopenia, lymphopenia or T-cell dysfunction, which inhibit adequate immune response to the infection.
2. **Time course.** The risk of infection is greatest during the first 3 months after transplantation, when higher doses of immunosuppression are used and again after a rejection episode is treated. This risk correlates with the overall level of immunosuppression.
3. **Types of infections** include bacterial, fungal, viral, and protozoan.
4. **Prevention**
   a. **Trimethoprim-sulfa.** One single- or double-strength tablet daily for 6 months significantly reduces the *Pneumocystis carnii* pneumonia and bacterial urinary tract infection. After 6 months, three times a week is effective.
   b. **Cytomegalovirus (CMV) infection.** High doses of acyclovir (800 mg qid for normal renal function; doses should be adjusted according to renal function) or high titer cytomegalovirus immunoglobulin is effective in reducing the incidence of CMV infection.
   c. **Nystatin solution** or **clotrimazole troche** reduce oral candidiasis.

B. Increased risk of malignancy

1. **Cause.** Continuous immunosuppression interferes with normal immune surveillance and function for malignancy. In addition, some of the immunosuppressive drugs may be directly carcinogenic or may activate oncogenic virus, such as the Epstein-Barr virus.
2. **Characteristics.** Cancers that occur most frequently in the general population (e.g., lung, breast, colon) are not more evident among transplant patients. However, various cancers uncommon in the general population are often more prevalent in transplant patients (e.g., lymphomas, squamous cell carcinomas of the lip and skin, Kaposi's sarcoma, other sarcoma).
3. **Post-transplant lymphoproliferative diseases (PTLD).** The incidence of lymphoma appears to correlate with the intensity of immunosuppression. It is well documented that T-cell specific agents, including OKT3, cyclosporine, and tacrolimus, increase the incidence of lymphoproliferative diseases.
4. **Treatment.** In the case of non-vital organ transplant, immunosuppression should be reduced or stopped. If the lymphoma is related to the Epstein-Barr virus, acyclovir therapy appears to be effective.

C. Hypertension.

Many immunosuppressive agents cause hypertension. Cyclosporine and tacrolimus increase the arterial blood pressure, and steroids may exacerbate hypertension after transplantation by fluid and sodium retention. Treatment usually requires the use of multiple agents, including diuretics and calcium channel blockers.

STUDY QUESTIONS

Directions: Each of the numbered items or incomplete statements in this section is followed by answers or by completion of the statement. Select the **one** lettered answer or completion that is **best** in each case.

1. A 45-year-old patient with diabetes mellitus received the cadaveric renal transplant 2 years ago. She was maintaining cyclosporine 200 mg twice daily, azathioprine 100 mg daily, and prednisolone 20 mg daily; her serum creatinine was 1.5 mg/ml. One week ago, she developed a respiratory infection and her physician started erythromycin 500 mg three times a day. Three days later, her creatinine level rose to 2.6 mg/day with a cyclosporine trough level of 450 ng/ml (therapeutic range 100–200 ng/ml). What is the likely cause of her recent renal function deterioration?

(A) Azathioprine is a nephrotoxic drug
(B) Erythromycin has synergistic nephrotoxicity with cyclosporine
(C) She may have an acute graft rejection
(D) Erythromycin inhibits cyclosporine metabolism and increases cyclosporine blood concentrations, resulting in renal toxicity
(E) Prednisone is a nephrotoxic drug

2. The patient in question 1 had severe joint pain with a serum uric acid level of 15 mg/dl. Her physician prescribed allopurinol 300 mg daily for treatment of gout. What is the pharmacist's appropriate response to this prescription? The pharmacist should

(A) advise her physician to reduce her azathioprine dose by 80%
(B) advise her physician to reduce her cyclosporine dose by 80%
(C) advise her physician to increase her azathioprine dose by 80%
(D) advise her physician to stop prednisone
(E) dispense the prescription as it is written

3. All of the following descriptions regarding muromonab CD3 (OKT3) are correct EXCEPT

(A) it is a mouse antibody
(B) it is a monoclonal antibody directing to CD3 receptor complex in T cell
(C) its most common side effect is cytokine release syndrome upon the first few doses
(D) it increases risk of cancer
(E) it is a human immunoglobulin product

4. All of the following are side effects of long-term steroid use EXCEPT

(A) osteonecrosis
(B) hyperglycemia
(C) leukopenia
(D) fluid retention
(E) cataracts

5. All of the following statements are complications of antimetabolites, such as azathioprine or mycophenolate, EXCEPT

(A) leukopenia
(B) increased risk of cytomegalovirus infection
(C) increased risk of polycythemia
(D) thrombocytopenia
(E) increased risk of lymphoma

ANSWERS AND EXPLANATIONS

1. The answer is D *[III A; see Table 58-2].*
This patient's renal dysfunction is caused most likely by cyclosporine toxicity due to drug interaction. Erythromycin is a cytochrome p-450 enzyme inhibitor, which inhibits various drug metabolism, including cyclosporine, tacrolimus, and theophylline. When erythromycin is started in the patient taking cyclosporine or tacrolimus, cyclosporine or tacrolimus blood levels should be monitored carefully with serum creatinine concentrations, and the dosage of cyclosporine or tacrolimus should be adjusted according to the blood concentrations. Because she had a good renal function for 2 years and high cyclosporine levels, it is unlikely that she has acute graft rejection.

2. The answer is A *[III B 1].*
Azathioprine is metabolized by xanthine oxidase, and allopurinol is a xanthine oxidase inhibitor, which inhibits azathioprine metabolism. When these two drugs are used concurrently, the azathioprine dose should be reduced by 80%. Otherwise, the patient may develop severe leukopenia due to overdose of azathioprine.

3. The answer is E *[III D 1 c].*
The OKT3 is a monoclonal antibody from mouse that directs to the CD3 receptor complex on the T-cell membrane. This CD3 receptor complex recognizes the antigen and initiates immune response. The OKT3 opsonizes this CD3 receptor complex, which prevents or reverses the rejection process. The most common side effect of OKT3 is cytokine-release syndrome, which occurs at the first few doses and manifests as severe flu-like symptoms.

4. The answer is C *[III E 3].*
Osteonecrosis, hyperglycemia, fluid retention, and cataracts are long-term complications of steroid therapy. The steroid therapy generally increases WBC count.

5. The answer is C *[II B].* .
Azathioprine or mycophenolate may cause bone marrow suppression, which manifests as leukopenia and thrombocytopenia. These also cause general immunosuppression, which increases the risk of opportunistic infections such as cytomegalovirus infection and cancer.

APPENDIX A

PRESCRIPTION DISPENSING INFORMATION AND METROLOGY

Prescriptions

PARTS OF PRESCRIPTION

A prescription is an order for medication issued by a physician, dentist, veterinarian, or other licensed practitioner authorized to prescribe medication to be used by a patient. It is usually written on a single sheet of paper commonly imprinted with the prescriber's name, address and telephone number. Medication orders are similar to prescriptions but are written on the chart of and intended for the use by inpatients in an Institutional setting. Although all prescriptions should contain accurate and appropriate information regarding the patient and medication being prescribed, a prescription order for a **controlled substance** must contain the following information:

1. The date of issue
2. The full name and address of the patient
3. The drug name, strength, dosage form and quantity prescribed
4. Directions for use
5. The name, address and DEA number of the prescriber
6. Signature of the prescriber

A written prescription order is required for substances in **Schedule II**. Prescriptions for **Schedule II** controlled substances are **never** refillable. Any other prescription with no indication of refills is not refillable. Prescriptions for medications in **Schedules III, IV** and **V** may be issued either in writing or orally to the pharmacist and may be refilled up to five times within 6 months of the date of issue, **if so authorized by the prescriber.** If the prescriber wishes the patient to continue with the medication after 6 months or five refills, a **new** prescription order is required.

THE PRESCRIPTION LABEL

In addition to containing the patient's, pharmacy's and prescriber's names, the prescription label should also accurately identify the medication and proper directions for use. The label for a prescription order for a **controlled substance** must contain the following information:

1. The pharmacy name and address
2. The serial number assigned to the prescription by the pharmacy
3. The date of initial filling
4. The name of the patient
5. The name of the prescriber
6. The directions for use
7. Cautionary statements as required by law*

AUXILIARY LABELS

Auxiliary or cautionary labels may be useful in providing additional important information to patients regarding proper use of the medication. "Shake Well" for suspensions or emulsions, "For External Use

---

*The label of any drug listed as a Controlled Substance in Schedules II, III or IV of the Controlled Substances Act must contain the following warning:
CAUTION: Federal law prohibits the transfer of this drug to any person other than the patient for whom it was prescribed.

Only" for topical lotions, solutions or creams. "May Cause Drowsiness," or "Alcohol may Intensify this effect" would be useful for many of the medications which cause CNS depression. The information contained on auxiliary labels should be brought to the attention of the patient as the medication is being dispensed. Only appropriate auxiliary labels should be placed on the prescription container because too many labels may be confusing to the patient.

Following is an example of a prescription for a common generic medication:

Harold Williams M.D.
214 Main Street
Boston, MA 02115
(617) 123-4567

Name: John Smith Date: 1/23/96
Address: 100 Washington Street Boston, MA 02115 Age: 28

Rx

Penicillin VK 250mg #40

Sig: one tablet po q.i.d. × 10 days

Refills 1 ______________ M.D.
DEA# AW1234567

Following is an example of a prescription that requires extemporaneous compounding:

Harold Williams M.D.
214 Main Street
Boston, MA 02115
(617) 123-4567

Name: John Smith Date: 1/23/96
Address: 100 Washington Street Boston, MA 02115 Age: 28

Rx

Precipitated Sulfur	2%
Salicylic Acid	2%
Petrolatum qs ad	30 g

M/ft oint

Sig: Apply to rash t.i.d.

Refills 1 ______________ M.D.
DEA# AW1234567

Common Abbreviations

There is considerable variation in the use of capitalization, italicization, and punctuation in abbreviations. The forms of abbreviation in this list are those most often encountered by pharmacists.

A, aa., or $\overline{aa}$	of each
a.c.	before meals
ad	to, up to
a.d.	right ear
ad lib.	at pleasure, freely
a.m.	morning
amp.	ampule
ante	before
aq.	water
a.s.	left ear
asa	aspirin
a.u.	each ear, both ears
b.i.d.	twice a day
BP	British Pharmacopoeia
BSA	body surface area
c. or $\bar{c}$	with
cap. or caps.	capsule
cp	chest pain
D.A.W.	dispense as written
cc or cc.	cubic centimeter
comp.	compound, compounded
dil.	dilute
D.C., dc, or disc.	discontinue
disp.	dispense
div.	divide, to be divided
dl or dL	deciliter
d.t.d.	give of such doses
DW	distilled water
D_5W	dextrose 5% in water
elix.	elixir
e.m.p.	as directed
et	and
ex aq.	in water
fl or fld	fluid
fl oz	fluid ounce
ft.	make
g or Gm	gram
gal.	gallon
GI	gastrointestinal
gr or gr.	grain
gtt or gtt.	drop, drops
H	hypodermic
h. or hr.	hour
h.s.	at bedtime
IM	intramuscular
inj.	injection
IV	intravenous
IVP	intravenous push
IVPB	intravenous piggyback
K	potassium
l or L	liter
lb.	pound
M	mix
m^2 or M^2	square meter
mcg, mcg., or µg	microgram
mEq	milliequivalent
mg or mg.	milligram
ml or mL	milliliter
µl or µL	microliter
♏	minim
N&V	nausea and vomiting
Na	sodium
N.F.	National Formulary
No.	number
noct.	night, in the night
non rep.	do not repeat
NPO	nothing by mouth
N.S., NS, or N/S	normal saline
1/2 NS	half strength normal saline
O	pint
o.d.	right eye, every day
o.l. or o.s.	left eye
OTC	over the counter
o.u.	each eye, both eyes
o_2	both eyes
oz.	ounce
p.c.	after meals
PDR	*Physicians' Desk Reference*
p.m.	afternoon; evening
p.o.	by mouth
Ppt	precipitated
pr	for the rectum
prn or p.r.n.	as needed
pt.	pint
pulv.	powder
pv	for vaginal use
q.	every
q.d.	every day
q.h.	every hour
q. 4 hr.	every four hours
q.i.d.	four times a day
q.o.d.	every other day
q.s.	a sufficient quantity
q.s. ad	a sufficient quantity to make
R	rectal
R.L. or R/L	Ringer's lactate
℞	prescription
s. or $\bar{s}$	without
Sig.	write on label
sol.	solution
S.O.B.	shortness of breath
s.o.s.	if there is need (once only)
ss. or $\overline{ss}$	one half
stat.	immediately
subc, subq, or s.c.	subcutaneously
sup. or supp	suppository
susp.	suspension
syr.	syrup
tab.	tablet
tal.	such, such a one

tal. dos.	such doses
tbsp. or T	tablespoonful
t.i.d.	three times a day
tr. or tinct.	tincture
tsp. or t.	teaspoonful
TT	tablet triturates
U or u.	unit
u.d. or ut dict.	as directed
ung.	ointment
U.S.P. or USP	United States Pharmacopoeia
w/v	weight/volume

Metrology

METRIC, APOTHECARY, AND AVOIRDUPOIS SYSTEMS

Metric system

1. Basic units

Mass = g or gram
Length = m or meter
Volume = L or liter
1 cc (cubic centimeter) of water is approximately equal to 1 ml and weighs 1 g.

2. Prefixes

kilo-	10^3 or 1000 times the basic unit
hekto-	10^2 or 100 times the basic unit
deka-	10 or 10 times the basic unit
deci-	10^{-1} or 0.1 times the basic unit
centi-	10^{-2} or 0.01 times the basic unit
milli-	10^{-3} or 0.001 times the basic unit
micro-	10^{-6} or one-millionth of the basic unit
nano-	10^{-9} or one-billionth of the basic unit
pico-	10^{-12} or one-trillionth of the basic unit

Examples of these prefixes include milligram (mg), which equals one-thousandth of a gram, and deciliter (dl), which equals 100 ml or 0.1 L.

Apothecary system

1. Volume (fluids or liquid)

60 minims (♏) = 1 fluidrachm or fluidram (f ʒ) or (ʒ)
8 fluidrachms (480 minims) = 1 fluid ounce (f ℥ or ℥)
16 fluidounces = 1 pint (pt or 0)
2 pints (32 fluidounces) = 1 quart (qt)
4 quarts (8 pints) = 1 gallon (gal or C)

2. Mass (weight)

20 grains (gr) = 1 scruple (℈)
3 scruples (60 grains) = 1 drachm or dram (ʒ)
8 drachms (480 grains) = 1 ounce (℥)
12 ounces (5760 grains) = 1 pound (lb)

Avoirdupois system

1. Volume

1 fluidrachm = 60 min.
1 fluid ounce = 8 fl. dr.
= 480 min.
1 pint = 16 fl. oz.
= 7680 min.
1 quart = 2 pt.
= 32 fl. oz.
1 gallon = 4 qt.
= 128 fl. oz.

2. Mass (weight)

The *grain* is common to both the apothecary and avoirdupois systems.
437.5 grains (gr) = 1 ounce (oz)
16 ounces (7000 grains) = 1 pound (lb)

CONVERSION

Exact equivalents

Exact equivalents are used for the conversion of specific quantities in pharmaceutical formulas and prescription compounding.

1. Length

1 meter (m) = 39.37 in.
1 inch (in) = 2.54 cm.

2. Volume

1 ml = 16.23 minims (♏)
1 ♏ = 0.06 ml
1 f ʒ = 3.69 ml
1 f ℥ = 29.57 ml
1 pt = 473 ml
1 gal (U.S.) = 3785 ml

3. Mass

1 g = 15.432 gr
1 kg = 2.20 lb (avoir.)
1 gr = 0.065 g or 65 mg
1 oz (avoir.) = 28.35 g
1 ℥ (apoth.) = 31.1 g
1 lb (avoir.) = 454 g
1 lb (apoth.) = 373.2 g

4. Other equivalents

1 oz (avoir.) = 437.5 gr
1 ℥ (apoth.) = 480 gr
1 gal (U.S.) = 128 fl ℥
1 fl ℥ (water) = 455 gr
1 gr (apoth.) = 1 gr (avoir.)

Approximate equivalents

Approximate equivalents may be used by physicians in prescribing the dose quantities using the metric and apothecary systems of weights and measures, respectively.

Household units are often used to inform the patient of the size of the dose. In view of the almost universal practice of employing the *teaspoon* ordinarily available in the household for the administration of medicine, the teaspoon may be regarded to represent 5 ml. When accurate measurement of a liquid dose is required, the USP recommends that a calibrated oral syringe or dropper is used.

1 fluid dram	= 1 teaspoonful
	= 5 ml
4 fluidounces	= 120 ml
8 fluidounces	= 1 cup
	= 240 ml
1 grain	= 65 mg
1 kg	= 2.2 pounds (lbs)

Surface Area Nomograms
Body Surface Area of Adults and Children[a]

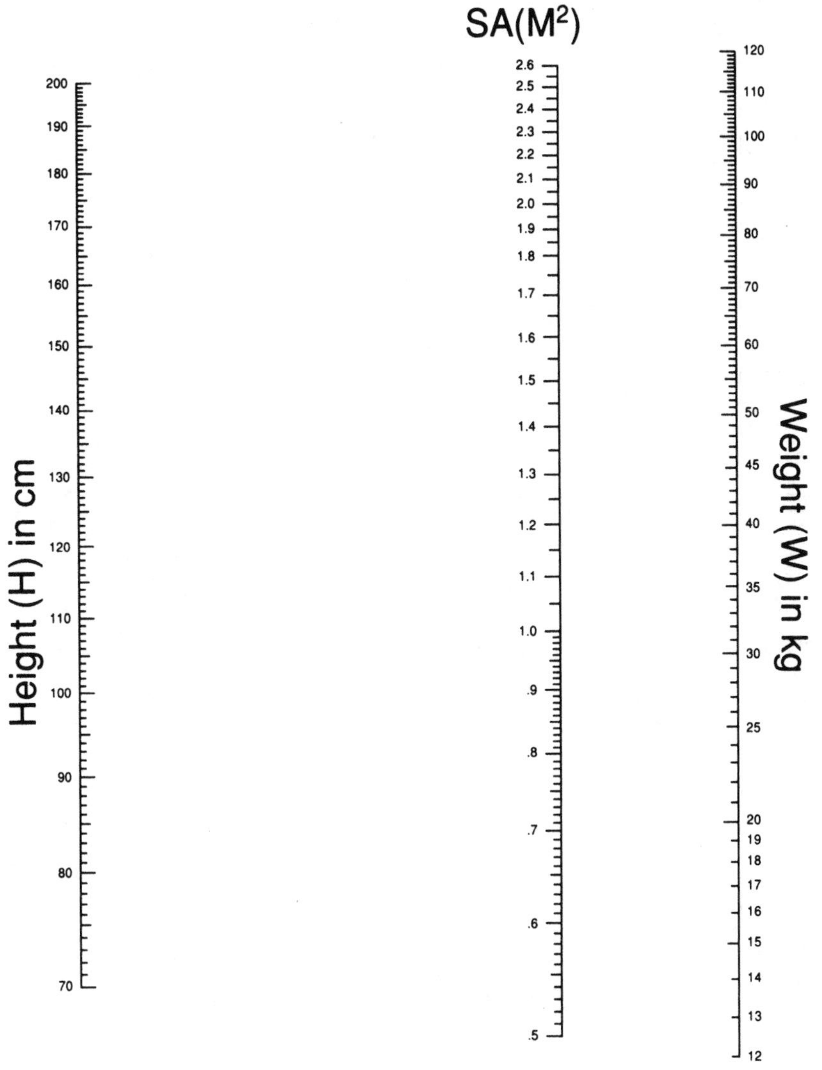

$$SA = W^{.5378} \times H^{.3964} \times .024265$$

Nomogram representing the relationship among height, weight, and surface area in adults and children. To use the nomogram, a ruler is aligned with the height and weight on the two lateral axes. The point at which the center line is intersected gives the corresponding value for surface area. Reprinted with permission.

[a] From Haycock GB, Schwartz GJ, Wisotsky DH: Geometric method for measuring body surface area: a height-weight formula validated in infants, children, and adults. *J. Pediatr,* 93:62–66, 1978.

Body Surface Area of Infants*

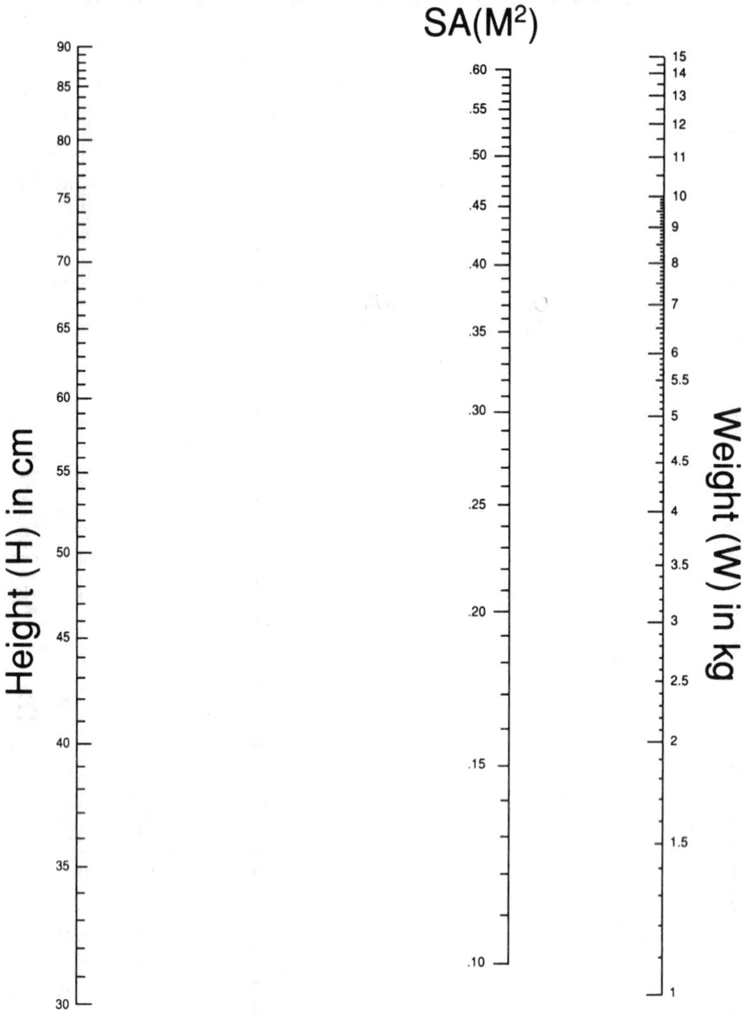

$$SA = W^{.5378} \times H^{.3964} \times .024265$$

Nomogram representing the relationship among height, weight, and surface area in infants. To use the nomogram, a ruler is aligned with the height and weight on the two lateral axes. The point at which the center line is intersected gives the corresponding value for surface area. Reprinted with permission.

*From Haycock GB, Schwartz GJ, Wisotsky DH: Geometric method for measuring body surface area: a height–weight formula validated in infants, children, and adults. *J. Pediatr,* 93:62–66, 1978.

APPENDIX **B**

COMMON PRESCRIPTION DRUGS AND OVER-THE-COUNTER PRODUCTS

How to crack the *Orange Book* drug codes*

Drug product selection can be a complicated matter. The Food and Drug Administration (FDA) publishes a guide entitled *Approved Drug Products with Therapeutic Equivalence Evaluations* to help you choose alternatives to prescribed drugs, but pharmacists often find the material difficult to decipher. So, here is a simplified explanation of what is going on.

More commonly known as the GI *Orange Book,* the compilation offers a detailed description (pared-down definitions appear below) of each of the two-letter drug ratings. It also provides a listing of all approved products and their equivalency ratings if they are multiple-source drugs.

The first letter of the rating—either an "A" or a "B"—is most pertinent to you. Products receiving an "A" rating are considered by the FDA to be "therapeutically equivalent" to other "pharmaceutically equivalent" products. That means, among other things, that the product is deemed bioequivalent to something else containing identical amounts of the same active ingredient manufactured in the same dosage form.

A "B" rating, on the other hand, is a signal that, for one reason or another, the FDA has not judged that product to be bioequivalent. That does not, however, mean that the product has been deemed inequivalent or that it will not work. It may, for instance, simply be that nobody has ever performed the necessary bioequivalence testing.

The second letter of the code gives you a bit more information. In many cases, it refers to product category. Each drug type has its own subset of rules. For instance, a label of "AT" refers to a topical considered to be therapeutically equivalent to another product with the same active ingredient in the same strength and dosage form.

Or take a "BS" rating. The "S," or second letter, tells you the drug has been stamped inequivalent because of "drug standard deficiencies." In other words, the standards used to judge a particular product's equivalency are not up to doing the job.

The "BX" rating indicates that a product is not bioequivalent ("B") because the agency did not have enough data to prove that a product was equivalent ("X"). There are probably fewer than 100 drugs that fall into this category.

Finally, pharmacists will find that an estimated 20% of drugs on today's market receive no rating at all and thus do not appear in the *Orange Book.* Such products were in existence before 1938 and have received a "grandfathered" FDA approval. They predate the approval process and are simply assumed to be safe and effective because they have been in use for so long (e.g., digoxin tablets and phenobarbital).

If a prescription is written generically, you can essentially choose whatever appropriate product you wish to use. Although you have to look to your state's laws when it comes to a substitutable prescription for a brand-name product, keep in mind that you are guaranteed therapeutic equivalence only with an "A" rated product.

WHAT THEY MEAN

The following codes and descriptions are taken from the Food and Drug Administration's (FDA's) *Approved Drug Products with Therapeutic Equivalence Evaluations,* also known as the *Orange Book.*

AA: Products not presenting bioequivalence problems in conventional dosage forms
AB: Products meeting necessary bioequivalence requirements
AN: Solutions and powders for aerosolization

*Reprinted from *1993 Red Book.* Montvale, NJ, Medical Economics Inc., 1993.

AO: Injectable oil solutions
AP: Injectable aqueous solutions
AT: Topical products
BC: Controlled-release tablets, capsules, and injectables
BD: Active ingredients and dosage forms with documented bioequivalence problems
BE: Enteric-coated oral dosage forms
BN: Products in aerosol—nebulizer drug-delivery systems
BP: Active ingredients and dosage forms with potential bioequivalence problems
BR: Suppositories or enemas for systemic use
BS: Products having drug standard deficiencies
BT: Topical products with bioequivalence issues
BX: Insufficient data

Prescription Drugs Listed by Trade Name

Trade Name	Generic Name	Trade Name	Generic Name
Accupril	Quinapril HCl	Coumadin	Warfarin
Adalat CC	Nifedipine	Cycrin	Medroxyprogesterone
Altace	Ramipril	Darvocet-N	Propoxyphene/ acetaminophen
Alupent	Metaproterenol sulfate	Daypro	Oxaprozin
Amaryl	Glimepiride	Deltasone	Prednisone
Ambien	Zolpidem tartrate	Demulen 1/35 28	Ethinyl estradiol/ ethynodiol
Amoxil	Amoxicillin	Depakote	Divallproax sodium
Ansaid	Flubiprofen	Desogen	Desogestrel/ ethinyl estradiol
Antivert	Hydroxyzine HCl	Diabeta	Gylburide
Ativan	Lorazepam	Dilacor XR	Diltiazem HCl
Atrovent	Ipratropium bromide	Dilantin	Phenytoin
Augmentin	Amoxicillin/clavulanate potassium	Duricef	Cefadroxil monohydrate
Axid	Nizatidine	Dyazide	Triamterene/ hydrochlorothiazide
Azmacort	Triamcinolone acetonide	DynaCirc	Isradipine
Bactrim DS	Trimethoprim/ sulfamethoxazole	E-Mycin	Erythromycin
Bactroban	Mupirocin	E.E.S.	Erythromycin ethyl succi-nate
Beconase AQ	Beclomethasone dipropi-onate	ERYC	Erythromycin
Bentyl	Dicyclomine HCl	Elavil	Amitriptyline HCl
Betoptic	Betaxolol HCl	Elocon	Mometasone furoate
Bleph-10	Prednisone acetate/sod. Sulfacetamide	Entex LA	Phenylpropanolamine HCl/guaifenesin
BuSpar	Buspirone HCl	Ery-Tab	Erythromycin
Bumex	Bumetanide	Erythrocin Sterate	Erythromycin stearate
Calan SR	Verapamil HCl	Estrace	Estradiol
Capoten	Captopril	Estraderm	Estradiol
Carafate	Sucralfate	Feldene	Piroxicam
Cardizem CD	Diltiazem HCl	Fioricet	Butalbital/aspirin/ caffeine
Cardura	Doxazosin mesylate	Fiorinal w/ Codeine	Butalbital/aspirin/ caffeine/codeine
Catapres	Clonidine HCL	Flagyl	Metronidazole
Ceclor	Cefaclor	Flexeril	Cyclobenzaprine HCl
Ceftin	Cefuroxime axetil	Floxin	Ofloxacin
Cefzil	Cefprozil	Glucophage	Metformin HCl
Centrax	Prazepam	Glucotrol	Glipizide
Cipro	Ciprofloxacin	Glynase Prestab	Glyburide
Claritin	Loratidine	Haldol	Haloperidol
Cleocin T	Clindamycin phosphate	Hismanal	Astemizole
Clinoril	Sulindac		
Compazine	Prochlorperazine		
Corgard	Nadolol		
Cortisporin Otic HC	Polymyxin B/neomycin/ hydrocortisone		

Humulin 70/30	Isophane insulin suspension/regular insulin (human synthetic)
Humulin N	Isophane insulin suspension (human synthetic)
Humulin R	Regular insulin (human synthetic)
Hydrodiuril	Hydrochlorothiazide
Hygroton	Chlorthalidone
Hytrin	Terazosin HCl
Imitrex	Sumatriptan succinate
Inderal	Propranolol
Intal	Cromolyn sodium
Invirase	Saquinavir mesylate
Isoptin SR	Verapamil
K-Dur	Potassium chloride
Keflex	Cephalexin
Klonopin	Clonazepam
Klor-Con 10	Potassium chloride
Lanoxin	Digoxin
Lasix	Furosemide
Levoxyl	Levothyroxine
Lo/Ovral-28	Norgestrel/ethinyl estradiol
Lodine	Etodolac
Loestrin-Fe 1.5/30	Norethindrone/ethinyl estradiol
Lopressor	Metoprolol
Lorabid	Loracarbef
Lorcet Plus	Hydrocodone/acetaminophen
Lotensin	Benazepril
Lotrisone	Clotrimazole/betamethasone
Lozol	Indapamide
Macrobid	Nitrofurantoin macrocrystals
Maxzide	Triamterene/hydrochlorothiazide
Medrol	Methylprednisolone
Mellaril	Thioridazine HCl
Mevacor	Lovastatin
Miacalcin	Calcitonin-salmon
Micro-K 10	Potassium chloride
Micronase	Glyburide
Minipres	Prazosin HCl
Minocin	Minocycline HCl
Motrin	Ibuprofen
Naprosyn	Naproxen
Nasacort	Triamcinolone
Nasalcrom	Cromolyn sodium
Navane	Thiothixene HCl
Nitro-Dur	Nitroglycerine
Nitrostat	Nitroglycerine
Nizoral Cream	Ketoconazole
Nolvadex	Tamoxifen
Norpramin	Desipramin HCl
Norvasc	Amlodipine
Novolin 70/30	Isophane insulin suspension/regular insulin
Ogen	Estropipate
Ortho-Cept 28	Desogestrel/ethinyl estradiol
Ortho-Novum 1/35 28	Norethindrone/ethinyl estradiol
Ortho-Novum 777	Norethindrone/ethinyl estradiol
PCE	Erythromycin
Pamelor	Nortriptyline HCl
Parafon Forte DSC	Chlorzoxazone
Paxil	Paroxetine
Pediazole	EES/sulfisoxazole acetyl
Pepcid	Famotidine
Peridex	Chlorhexidine
Phenergan	Promethazine
Pravachol	Pravastatin
Premarin	Estrogen, conjugated
Prilosec	Omeprazole
Prinivil	Lisinopril
Procardia XL	Nifedipine
Propulsid	Cisapride
Proventil	Albuterol
Provera	Medroxyprogesterone acetate
Prozac	Fluoxetine HCl
Reglan	Metoclopramide HCl
Relafen	Nabumetone
Restoril	Temazepam
Retin-A	Tretinoin
Risperdal	Risperidone
Ritalin	Methylphenidate
Rufen	Ibuprofen
Seldane	Terfenadine
Seldane-D	Terfenadine/
Septra DS	Trimethoprim/sulfamethoxazole
Serax	Oxazepam
Sinequan	Doxepin HCl
Slo-Bid	Theophylline anhydrous
Soma	Carisoprodol
Sporanox	Itraconazole
Sumycin	Tetracycline HCl
Suprax	Cefixime
Synthroid	Levothyroxine
Tagamet	Cimetidine
Talwin NX	Pentazocine HCl/naloxone HCl
Tegretol	Carbamazepine
Tenoretic	Atenolol/chlorthalidone
Tenormin	Atenolol
Terazol 7	Terconazole
Theo-Dur	Theophylline anhydrous
Timoptic	Timolal maleate
Toradol	Ketorolac
Tranxene	Chlorazepate dipotassium
Trental	Pentoxifylline
Tri-Levien 28	Levonorgestrel/ethinyl estradiol
Trimox	Amoxicillin

Continued on next page

Prescription Drugs Listed by Trade Name

Trade Name	Generic Name	Trade Name	Generic Name
Triphasil-28	Levonorgestrel/ethinyl estradiol	Vibramycin	Doxycycline HCl
Triphasil-28	Levonorgestrel/ethinyl estradiol	Vicodin	Hydrocodone bitartrate/ acetaminophen
Trusopt	Dorzolamide HCl	Vicoden ES	Hydrocodone/ acetaminophen
Tylenol w/ Codeine	Acetaminophen w/ codeine	Voltaren	Diclofenac
Ultram	Tramadol HCl	Xanax	Alprazolam
Valium	Diazepam	Z-PAK	Azithromycin
Vancenase AQ	Beclomethasone	Zantac	Ranitidine HCl
Vanceril	Beclomethasone	Zestril	Lisinopril
Vasotec	Enalapril maleate	Zocor	Simvastatin
Veetids	Penicillin VK potassium	Zoloft	Sertraline
Ventolin	Albuterol	Zovirax	Acyclovir
Verelan	Verapamil	Zyloprim	Allopurinol

Prescription Drugs Listed by Generic Name

Generic Name	Trade Name	Generic Name	Trade Name
Acetaminophen w/ Codeine	Tylenol w/ Codeine	Cefixime	Suprax
Acyclovir	Zovirax	Cefprozil	Cefzil
Albuterol	Proventil	Cefuroxime Axetil	Ceftin
Albuterol	Ventolin	Cephalexin	Keflex
Allopurinol	Zyloprim	Chlorazepate Dipotassium	Tranxene
Alprazolam	Xanax	Chlorhexidine	Peridex
Amitriptyline HCl	Elavil	Chlorthalidone	Hygroton
Amlodipine	Norvasc	Chlorzoxazone	Parafon Forte DSC
Amoxicillin	Trimox	Cimetidine	Tagamet
Amoxicillin	Amoxil	Ciprofloxacin	Cipro
Amoxicillin/Clavulanate Potassium	Augmentin	Cisapride	Propulsid
Astemizole	Hismanal	Clindamycin Phosphate	Cleocin T
Atenolol	Tenormin	Clonazepam	Klonopin
Atenolol/Chlorthalidone	Tenoretic	Clonidine HCl	Catapres
Azithromycin	Z-PAK	Clotrimazol/ Betamethasone	Lotrisone
Beclomethasone	Vanceril	Cromolyn Sodium	Intal
Beclomethasone	Vancenase AQ	Cromolyn Sodium	Nasalcrom
Beclomethasone dipropionate	Beconase AQ	Cyclobenzaprine HCl	Flexeril
Benazepril	Lotensin	Desipramin HCl	Norpramin
Betaxolol HCl	Betoptic	Desogestrel/ethinyl estradiol	Ortho-Cept 28
Bumetanide	Bumex	Desogestrel/ethinyl estradiol	Desogen
Buspirone HCl	BuSpar	Diazepam	Valium
Butalbital/ acetaminophen/ caffeine	Fioricet	Diclofenac	Voltaren
		Dicyclomine HCl	Bentyl
Butalbital/ aspirin/caffeine/ codeine	Florinal w/ Codeine	Digoxin	Lanoxin
		Diltiazem HCl	Cardizem CD
		Diltiazem HCl	Dilacor XR
Calcitonin-salmon	Miacalcin	Divalproax sodium	Depakote
Captopril	Capoten	Dorzolamide HCl	Trusopt
Carbamazepine	Tegretol	Doxazosin mesylate	Cardura
Carisoprodol	Soma	Doxepin HCl	Sinequan
Cefaclor	Ceclor	Doxycycline HCl	Vibramycin
Cefadroxil Monohydrate	Duricef	EES/Sulfisoxazole Acetyl	Pediazole
		Enalapril Maleate	Vasotec

Erythromycin	PCE
Erythromycin	Ery-Tab
Erythromycin	ERYC
Erythromycin	E-Mycin
Erythromycin Ethyl Succinate	E.E.S.
Erythromycin Stearate	Erythrocin Sterate
Estradiol	Estrace
Estradiol	Estraderm
Estrogen, conjugated	Premarin
Estropipate	Ogen
Ethinyl estradiol/ ethynodiol	Demulen 1/35 28
Etodolac	Lodine
Famotidine	Pepcid
Flubiprofen	Ansaid
Fluoxetine HCl	Prozac
Furosemide	Lasix
Glimepiride	Amaryl
Glipizide	Glucotrol
Glyburide	Micronase
Glyburide	Diabeta
Glyburide	Glynase Prestab
Haloperidol	Haldol
Hydrochlorothiazide	Hydrodiuril
Hydrocodone Bitartrate	Vicodin
Hydrocodone/ Acetaminophen	Lorcet Plus
Hydrocodone/ Acetaminophen	Vicodin ES
Hydroxyzine HCl	Antivert
Ibuprofen	Rufen
Ibuprofen	Motrin
Indapamide	Lozol
Ipratropium Bromide	Atrovent
Isophane insulin suspension (human synthetic)	Humulin N
Isophane insulin suspension/regular insulin	Novolin 70/30
Isophane insulin suspension/regular insulin (human synthetic)	Humulin 70/30
Isradipine	DynaCirc
Itraconazole	Sporanox
Ketoconazole	Nizoral Cream
Ketorolac	Toradol
Laratidine	Claritin
Levonorgestrel/Ethinyl Estradiol	Triphasil-28
Levonorgestrel/ethinyl estradiol	Triphasil 28
Levonorgestrel/ethinyl estradiol	Tri-Levien 28
Levothyroxine	Levoxyl
Levothyroxine	Synthroid
Lisinopril	Prinivil
Lisinopril	Zestril
Loracarbef	Lorabid
Lorazepam	Ativan
Lovastatin	Mevacor
Medroxyprogesterone	Cycrin
Medroxyprogesterone Acetate	Provera
Memetasone furoate	Elocon
Metaproterenol sulfate	Alupent
Metformin HCl	Glucophage
Methylphenidate	Ritalin
Methylprednisolone	Medrol
Metoclopramide HCl	Reglan
Metoprolol	Lopressor
Metronidazole	Flagyl
Minocycline HCl	Minocin
Mupirocin	Bactroban
Nabumetone	Relafen
Nadolol	Corgard
Naproxen	Naprosyn
Nifedipine	Adalat CC
Nifedipine	Procardia XL
Nitrofurantoin Macrocrystals	Macrobid
Nitroglycerine	Nitrostat
Nitroglycerine	Nitro-Dur
Nizatidine	Axid
Norethindrone/ Ethinyl Estradiol	Ortho-Novum 1/35 28
Norethindrone/ Ethinyl Estradiol	Ortho-Novum 777
Norethindrone/ ethinyl estradiol	Loestrin-Fe 1.5/30
Norgestrel/ Ethinyl Estradiol	Lo/Ovral-28
Nortriptyline HCL	Pamelor
Ofloxacin	Floxin
Omeprazole	Prilosec
Oxaprozin	Daypro
Oxazepam	Serax
Paroxetine	Paxil
Penicillin VK Potassium	Veetids
Pentazocine HCL/ Naloxone HCL	Talwin NX
Pentoxifylline	Trental
Phenylpropanolamine HCL/guaifenesin	Entex LA
Phenytoin	Dilantin
Piroxicam	Feldene
Polymyxin B/ Neomycin/ Hydrocortisone	Cortisporin Otic HC
Potassium Chloride	Klor-Con 10
Potassium Chloride	Micro-K 10
Potassium Chloride	K-Dur
Pravastatin	Pravachol
Prazepam	Centrax
Prazosin HCL	Minipres
Prednisone	Deltasone

Continued on next page

Prescription Drugs Listed by Generic Name

Generic Name	Trade Name
Prednisone Acetate/ Sod. Sulfacetamide	Bleph-10
Prochlorperazine	Compazine
Promethazine	Phenergan
Propoxyphene/ acetaminophen	Darvocet-N
Propranolol	Inderal
Quinapril HCl	Accupril
Ramipril	Altace
Ranitidine HCl	Zantac
Regular insulin (human synthetic)	Humulin R
Risperidone	Risperdal
Saquinavir mesylate	Invirase
Sertraline	Zoloft
Simvastatin	Zocor
Sucralfate	Carafate
Sulindac	Clinoril
Sumatriptan succinate	Imitrex
Tamoxifen	Nolvadex
Temazepam	Restoril
Terazosin HCl	Hytrin
Terconazole	Terazol 7
Terfenadine	Seldane
Terfenadine/	Seldane-D
Tetracycline HCL	Sumycin
Theophylline Anhydrous	Theo-Dur
Theophylline Anhydrous	Slo-Bid
Thioridazine HCL	Mellaril
Thiothixene HCL	Navane
Timolal Maleate	Timoptic
Tramadol HCl	Ultram
Tretinoin	Retin-A
Triamcinolone	Nasacort
Triamcinolone acetonide	Azmacort
Triamterene/ Hydrochlorothiazide	Dyazide
Triamterene/ Hydrochlorothiazide	Maxzide
Trimethoprim/ Sulfamethoxazole	Bactrim DS
Trimethoprim/ Sulfamethoxazole	Septra DS
Verapamil	Isoptin SR
Verapamil	Verelan
Verapamil HCl	Calan SR
Warfarin	Coumadin
Zolpidem tartrate	Ambien

Top 200 OTC Products

The following list contains the top 200 over-the-counter (OTC) products distributed through retail channels based on measurement of dollar volume for the 12-month period ending October 31, 1994.

Rank	Product	Manufacturer
1	Lifescan 1-Touch Test Strips 50ct #198	Lifescan, Inc. (Div of J&J)
2	Tylenol Extra Strength Gelcaps 50	McNeil Consumer Prods Co.
3	Gillette Sensor Cartridge Refills 5ct	Gillette Co.-Shaving Div.
4	Centrum Vitamins 130	Laderle
5	Gillette Sensor Cartridge Refills 10ct	Gillette Co.-Shaving Div.
6	Advil Tablets 24	Whitehall Laboratories
7	Bausch&Lomb Renu Disinfecting Sol. 12	Bausch & Lomb
8	Advil Tablets 50	Whitehall Laboratories
9	Advil Tablets 100	Whitehall Laboratories
10	Opti-Free Disinfectant Solution 12 oz.	Alcon
11	Tylenol Extra Strength Caplets 100	McNeil Consumer Prods Co.
12	Ensure Plus Vanilla 8 oz. 6pk	Ross Laboratories
13	Ensure Vanilla 8 oz. 6pk	Ross Laboratories
14	Tylenol Extra Strength Caplets 50	McNeil Consumer Prods Co.
15	Aosept Disinfection & Neutral Sol. 12 oz.	Ciba Vision Corp.
16	Tylenol Extra Strength Gelcaps 100	McNeil Consumer Prods Co.
17	Tampax Oel Super 32	Tambrands Inc.
18	Q-Tips Swabs 300	Chesebrough-Ponds, USA
19	Tylenol Extra Strength Gelcaps 24	McNeil Consumer Prods Co.
20	Monistat 7 Cream 1.59 oz.	Advanced Care Prods Div. of Ortho

Rank	Product	Manufacturer
21	Advil Caplets 50	Whitehall Laboratories
22	Robitussin DM Syrup 4	A.H. Robins Consumer Prods. Div.
23	Advil Caplets 24	Whitehall Laboratories
24	Early Pregnancy Test Stick Single	Warner-Wellcome
25	Monistat 7 Disposable 1.59 oz.	Advanced Care Prods Div. of Ortho
26	Nyquil Night Time Cold Medicine 6 oz.	The Procter & Gamble Co.
27	Ibuprofen Tablets 200mg 100ct	Private Label
28	Revlon Super Luster Cream Lipstick #6863	Revlon Inc.
29	Fixodent Adhesive 2.4 0 oz.	The Procter & Gamble Co.
30	Gillette Sensor Cartridge Refills 15	Gillette Co.-Shaving Div.
31	Tampax Oel Regular 32	Tambrands Inc.
32	Tylenol Extra Strength Caplets 24	McNeil Consumer Prods Co.
33	Colgate Toothpaste 7	Colgate-Palmolive Co.
34	Ensure Plus Chocolate 8 oz. 6pk	Ross Laboratories
35	Tavial-D 12-Hr Relief Decongestant Tab 8	Sanchez Consumer Prods
36	Tavial-D 12-Hr Relief Decongestant Tab 16	Sanchez Consumer Prods
37	Ibuprofen Tablets 200mg 50ct	Private Label
38	Advil Caplets 100	Whitehall Laboratories
39	Imodium Anti-Diarrheal Caplets 12ct	McNeil Consumer Prods Co.
40	Alka-Selzer Plus Tablets 20	Miles Laboratories, Inc.
41	Monistant 7 Suppositories	Advanced Care Prods Div. of Ortho
42	Swabs 300	Private Label
43	Gillette Sensor Woman Cartridges 5ct	Gillette Co.-Shaving Div.
44	O B Tampon Super 27	Personal Prods Corporation
45	Crest Tartar Control Toothpaste Tube 6.4	The Procter & Gamble Co.
46	Always Plus Long Super/Wings 20	The Procter & Gamble Co.
47	Benadryl 25mg. 24	Warner-Wellcome
48	Kotex Overnight Pads 14	Kimberly-Clark
49	Charmstrip Bg II Strips 50	Boehringer Mannheim
50	Gillette Good News Regular 10ct	Gillette Co.-Shaving Div.
51	Pantene Pro-Vitamin Shampoo+Cond Dry 13 oz.	The Procter & Gamble Co.
52	Tampax Oel Super Plus 32	Tambrands Inc.
53	Tylenol Extra Strength Tablets 100	McNeil Consumer Prods Co.
54	Nyquil Cherry Night Time Cold Medicine	The Procter & Gamble Co.
55	First Choice One Touch Test Strip50	Polymer Technology Corp.
56	Afrin Nasal Spray 5	Scharing Healthcare
57	Cover Girl Pressed Powder	Novell Corporation
58	Robitussin DM Syrup 8	A.H. Robins Consumer Prods. Div.
59	Theragran M 130	E.R. Squibb & Sons
60	Listerine Mouthwash 32	Warner-Wellcome
61	Ensure Chocolate 8 oz. 6pk	Ross Laboratories
62	Tylenol p.m. Caplets 24	McNeil Consumer Prods Co.
63	Benadryl 4	Warner-Wellcome
64	Sudafed 30mg. Tablets 24	Warner-Wellcome
65	Gillette Atra Plus Refill	Gillette Co.-Shaving Div.
66	Monistat 7 Suppository 7/Cream 9gm Combo	Advanced Care Prods Div. of Ortho
67	Tylenol Extra Strength Tablets 60	McNeil Consumer Prods Co.
68	Pantene Pro-Vitamin Shampoo+Cond Perm 13	The Procter & Gamble Co.
69	Pantene Pro-Vitamin Shampoo+Cond Nor 13 oz.	The Procter & Gamble Co.
70	Stay Free Super Maxi Pads 24	Personal Prods Corporation
71	Tylenol Extra Strength Tablets 30	McNeil Consumer Prods Co.
72	Centrum Silver Multi Vitamins 100	Lederle
73	Dimetapp Elixir 4	A.H. Robins Consumer Prods. Div.
74	Tylenol Infant Drops .5 oz.	McNeil Consumer Prods Co.
75	O B Tampon Super Plus 27	Personal Prods Corporation
76	Ensure Plus Strawberry 6-Pack 8 oz.	Ross Laboratories
77	Playtex Deodorant Tampons Super 22	Playtex Inc.

Continued on next page

Rank	Product	Manufacturer
78	Always Regular Maxi 24	The Procter & Gamble Co.
79	Imodium Anti-Diarrheal Caplets 18ct	McNeil Consumer Prods Co.
80	Imodium Anti-Diarrheal Caplets 6ct	McNeil Consumer Prods Co.
81	Neosporin Ointment .5 oz.	Warner-Wellcome
82	Ginsana Diet Supplement Vitamins 30	Sunsource Health Prods Inc.
83	Always Plus Extra Long Super/Wings 16	The Procter & Gamble Co.
84	Mentadent Fresh Mint Paste Pump 3.5 oz.	Chesebrough-Ponds, USA
85	Equal Packets 200	Nutrasweet Co.
86	Kotex Maxi Pads 24ct	Kimberly-Clark
87	Alka-Seltzer Plus Tablets 36	Miles Laboratories, Inc.
88	Always Plus Regular Maxi/Wings 20	The Procter & Gamble Co.
89	Depend Undergarment Elast-Leg Xub Poly 30	Kimberly-Clark
90	Tylenol P.M. Caplets 50	McNeil Consumer Prods Co.
91	Tylenol Extra Strength Geltabs 50ct	McNeil Consumer Prods Co.
92	Benadryl Tablets 24	Warner-Wellcome
93	Fact Plus Pregnancy Kit	Advanced Care Prods Div. of Ortho
94	Crest Toothpaste Tube 6.4	The Procter & Gamble Co.
95	Depend Fitted Briefs Medium 24ct	Kimberly-Clark
96	Scope Mouthwash 24	The Procter & Gamble Co.
97	Maniadant Cool Mint Paste Pump 3.5 oz.	Chesebrough-Ponds, USA
98	Equal Packets 100	Nutrasweet Co.
99	Lotrimin Anti-Fungal Cream 24gm	Schering Healthcare
100	Advil Tablets 250	Whitehall Laboratories
101	Visine Original Eye Drops .5 oz.	Pitzer Consumer Health Care
102	Pantene Pro-Vitamin Shampoo + Cond Xbd 13 oz.	The Procter & Gamble Co.
103	Colgate Tartar Paste Tube 6.4	Colgate-Palmolive Co.
104	Nyquil Liqui Caps 12ct	The Procter & Gamble Co.
105	Scope Mouthwash 12	The Procter & Gamble Co.
106	Excodria Extra Strength Tablets 100	Bristol Myers Prods
107	Advil Tablets 165	Whitehall Laboratories
108	Rev Super Luster Frost Lipstick #6954	Revlon Inc.
109	Stay Free Regular Maxi Pads 24	Personal Prods Corporation
110	Clear Blue Easy Pregnancy Kit Single	Whitehall Laboratories
111	Tylenol Child Suspension Grape Drops .5 oz.	McNeil Consumer Prods Co.
112	Listerine Mouthwash 18	Warner-Wellcome
113	Miconazole 7 Cream 1.59 oz.	Private Label
114	Neosporin Ointment Max. Strength Plus .5 oz.	Warner-Wellcome
115	Tylenol Extra Strength Geltabs 24ct	McNeil Consumer Prods Co.
116	Ensure Strawberry 8 oz. 6pk	Ross Laboratories
117	Robitussin CF-Syrup 4	A.H. Robins Consumer Prods. Div.
118	Colgate Toothpaste 9	Colgate-Palmolive Co.
119	Nyquil Night Time Cold Medicine 10 oz.	The Procter & Gamble Co.
120	Aracin Tablets 100	A.H. Robins Consumer Prods. Div.
121	Listerine Cool Mint 32 oz.	Warner-Wellcome
122	Advil Cold & Sinus Caplets 20ct.	Whitehall Laboratories
123	Bayer Aspirin 100	Starling Health USA
124	Primalene Mint/Mouthpiece 15 Ml.	Whitehall Laboratories
125	Ultra Slim Fast Chocolate R-T-D Can 11 oz.	Slim Fast Foods
126	Ibuprofen Caplets 100	Private Label
127	Alka-Seltzer Foil 36	Miles Laboratories, Inc.
128	Tampax Oel Slender Regular 32	Tambrands Inc.
129	Crest Tartar Gel Tube 6.4	The Procter & Gamble Co.
130	Thermoscan Hm-1 Instant Thermometer	Thermoscan, Inc.
131	Mytasia Liquid 12	McNeil Consumer Prods Co.
132	Lotrimin Anti-Fungal Cream 12gm.	Schering Healthcare
133	Tylenol Allergy Sinus Caplets 24	McNeil Consumer Prods Co.
134	Primalene Mist Refill 15 Ml. #91030	Whitehall Laboratories
135	Tylenol Extra Strength Gelcaps 150	McNeil Consumer Prods Co.

Rank	Product	Manufacturer
136	Halls Cough Drops Mentho-Lyptus Bag 30	American Chicle Co.
137	Maybelline Moisture Whip Lipstick	The Maybelline Co.
138	Correctol Tablets 30	Schering Healthcare
139	Playtex Deodorant Tampons Regular 22	Playtex Inc.
140	Maybelline Great Lash Mascara	The Maybelline Co.
141	Efidac/24 24-Hr Cold Relief Tablets 6ct	Ciba Consumer Pharmaceutical Co.
142	Oil of Olay Lotion 4 oz.	The Procter & Gamble Co.
143	Mint Mouthwash 24 oz.	Private Label
144	Glucofilm Test Strips 50	Miles Laboratories, Inc.
145	Aquafresh Toothpaste 6.4	SmithKline-Beecham
146	Gillette Good News Plus 10ct	Gillette Co.-Shaving Div.
147	Pepto-Bismol Liquid 8	The Procter & Gamble Co.
148	Huggies Baby Wipes 80	Kimberly-Clark
149	Easy Strips 50ct #560	Boehringer Mannheim
150	Kolex Security Tampons Super 22	Kimberly-Clark
151	Early Pregnancy Test Stick Double	Warner-Wellcome
152	Scope Mouthwash 36	The Procter & Gamble Co.
153	Rembrandt Toothpaste Mint 3 oz.	Den-Mal Corporation
154	Tylenol Extra Strength Caplets 175	McNeil Consumer Prods Co.
155	First Response 1 Step Single Pregnancy Kt	Carter Prods
156	Pert Plus Shampoo Normal 15	The Procter & Gamble Co.
157	Preparation H Suppositories 12	Whitehall Laboratories
158	Playtex Tampons Regular 22	Playtex Inc.
159	Always Ultra Maxi w/Wings 20	The Procter & Gamble Co.
160	Cover Girl Continuous Color Lipstick	Novell Corporation
161	Fixodent Adhesive 1.4 oz.	The Procter & Gamble Co.
162	Motrin Ibuprofen Tablets 24	The Upjohn Co.
163	Rev Moon Drop Moist Cream Lipstick	Revlon Inc.
164	Listerine Cool Mint 18 oz.	Warner-Wellcome
165	Revlon Moon Drop Luminesse Lipfrost	Revlon Inc.
166	Neosporin Maximum Strength Plus Cream .5 oz.	Warner-Wellcome
167	Tylenol Child Cough & Cold Liquid 4 oz.	McNeil Consumer Prods Co.
168	Vitamin E 400iu 100ct	Private Label
169	Maxi Pads Super 24	Private Label
170	Vicks Vaporub 1.5 oz.	The Procter & Gamble Co.
171	Stay Free Ultra Plus Maxi Pads 20ct	Personal Prods Corporation
172	Preparation H Ointment 1	Whitehall Laboratories
173	Tylenol Extra Strength Geltabs 100ct	McNeil Consumer Prods Co.
174	Sanitary Guards Super Plus 24ct	Personal Prods Corporation
175	Tylenol Elixir 4	McNeil Consumer Prods Co.
176	Ibuprofen Caplets 50	Private Label
177	Gillette Good News Regular 5ct	Gillette Co.-Shaving Div.
178	Halls Cough Drops Cherry Bag 30	American Chicle Co.
179	Tracer Bg Strips 50	Boehringer Mannheim
180	Gillette Trac II Plus 10	Gillette Co.-Shaving Div.
181	Chapstick Regular	A.H. Robins Consumer Prods. Div.
182	Sensodyne Toothpaste Mint Tube 4 oz.	Block Drug Co. Inc.
183	Rembrandt Whitening Toothpaste Tube 3 oz.	Den-Mat Corporation
184	Lifescan One Touch Basic Glucose System	Lifescan, Inc. (Div of J&J)
185	Mentadent Freshmint Pads Pump 5.2 oz.	Chesebrough-Ponds, USA
186	Motrin Ibuprofen Caplets 24	The Upjohn Co.
187	Chemstrip Bg Strips 100	Boehringer Mannheim
188	Always Ultra Long Maxi W/Wings 18	The Procter & Gamble Co.
189	Huggies Baby Wipes Unscented 80	Kimberly-Clark
190	Always Regular Thin Maxi 24	The Procter & Gamble Co.
191	Ultra Brite Toothpaste 6	Colgate-Palmolive Co.
192	Baby Fresh Wipes 84ct Refill	Scott Paper Co.

Continued on next page

Rank	Product	Manufacturer
193	Tylenol Maximum Sinus Caplets 24	McNeil Consumer Prods Co.
194	Crest Tartar Control Toothpaste Tube 4.6	The Procter & Gamble Co.
195	Gillette Trac II Refill 10	Gillette Co.-Shaving Div.
196	Kotex Super Maxi Pads 24	Kimberly-Clark
197	Schick Tracer Refills 5ct	Warner-Lambert spg.
198	Edge Protect Gel Aloe Sensitive 7 oz.	S.C. Johnson & Son, Inc.
199	Tums Assorted Flavor 150	SmithKline-Beecham
200	Depend Fitted Briefs Large 18ct	Kimberly-Clark

APPENDIX C

REFERENCE CHARTS USEFUL FOR PATIENT COUNSELING

Drugs That Should Not Be Crushed

Pharmacists may frequently encounter patients who, for one reason or another, cannot swallow tablets or capsules. When an alternative liquid formulation is not available, pulverizing the solid dosage form before administration may serve as a quick, safe solution to the problem.

However, not all pharmaceutical products may be crushed before administration. A variety of slow-release formulations can deliver dangerous immediate doses of their active ingredients if the integrity of the delivery system is destroyed and enteric-coated products must remain intact in order to prevent their dissolution in the stomach.

Listed below are various slow-release as well as enteric-coated products which should not be crushed or chewed. Slow-release (sr) represents products that are controlled-release, extended-release, long-acting, and timed release. Enteric-coated (ec) represents products that are delayed-release.

In general, capsules containing slow-release or enteric-coated particles may be opened and their contents administered on a spoonful of soft food. Instruct patients not to chew the particles, though. (Patients should, in fact, be discouraged from chewing any medication unless it is specifically formulated for that purpose.)

This list should not be considered all-inclusive. Generic and alternate brands of some products may exist. Tablets intended for sublingual or buccal administration (not included in this list) should also be administered only as intended, in an intact form.

Enteric-coated = ec Other = or Slow-release = sr

Accutane	Roche	sr
Acutrim tablets	Ciba	sr
Adalat CC	Miles	sr
Adipost capsules	JMI	sr
Aerolate III	Fleming	sr
Aerolate JR	Fleming	sr
Aerolate SR	Fleming	sr
Allerest tablets	Ciba	sr
Arthritis Foundation Aspirin tablets	McNeil	ec
Asacol tablets	Procter & Gamble	ec
Atrohist Plus tablets	Adams	sr
Atrohist Sprinkle capsules	Adams	sr
Azulfidine EN-tab tablets	Pharmacia	ec
Bayer 8-Hour tablets	Sterling Health	sr
Bayer Enteric	Sterling Health	ec
Bellergal-S tablets	Sandoz	sr
Bisacodyl tablets	various manufacturers	ec
Bontril Slow-Release capsules	Carnick	sr
Brexin LA	Savage	sr
Bromfed capsules	Muro	sr
Bromfed-PD capsules	Muro	sr
Calan SR	Searle	sr
Carbiset-TR	Nutripharm	sr
Cardene SR capsules	Syntex	sr
Cardizem CD	Marion Merrell Dow	sr
Cardizem SR capsules	Marion Merrell Dow	sr
Charcoal Plus	Kramer	ec
Choledyl tablets	Parke-Davis	ec
Choledyl SA tablets	Parke-Davis	sr
ChlorTrimeton tablets	Schering	sr
Codimal LA capsules	Central	sr
Codimal LA Half capsules	Central	sr
Colestid tablets	Upjohn	or
Comhist LA capsules	Roberts	sr
Compazine Spansule capsules	SKB	sr
Congess JR capsules	Fleming	sr
Congess SR capsules	Fleming	sr
Contac 12 Hour capsules	SKB	sr
Contac Maximum Strength 12 Hour caplets	SKB	sr
Control capsules	Thompson	sr
Cotazym-S capsules	Organon	ec
Creon 5, 10, 20	Solvay	ec
Cystospaz-M capsules	Polymedica	sr
Dallergy-Jr capsules	Laser	sr
Deconamine SR capsules	Berlex	sr

Enteric-coated = ec Other = or Slow-release = sr

Deconsal II	Adams	sr
Deconsal LA	Adams	sr
Deconsal Pediatric	Adams	sr
Depakote tablets	Abbott	ec
Desoxyn Gradumet tablets	Abbott	sr
Dexatrim capsules	Thompson	sr
Dexedrine Spansule	SKB	sr
Diamox Sequel capsules	Lederle	sr
Dilacor XR capsules	RPR	sr
Dilatrate-SR capsules	Reed & Camrick	sr
Dimetane Extentab tablets	Robins	sr
Dimetapp Extentab tablets	Robins	sr
Disobrom tablets	Geneva	sr
Disophrol Chronotab tablets	Schering-	sr
Donnatal Extentab tablets	Robins	sr
Donnazyme tablets	Robins	ec
Doryx capsules	Parke-Davis	ec
Drixoral tablets	Schering	sr
Drize capsules	Ascher	sr
Dulcolax tablets	Ciba	ec
Duotrate-45 capsules	JMI	sr
Duratuss tablets	Whitby	sr
Easprin tablets	Parke-Davis	ec
Ecotrin tablets	SKB	ec
Ecotrin Maximum Strength	SKB	ec
Endal tablets	Forest	sr
Entex-LA tablets	Procter & Gamble	sr
Entex PSE tablets	Procter & Gamble	sr
ERYC capsules	Parke-Davis	ec
ERY-TAB tablets	Abbott	ec
Erythromycin capsules	various manufacturers	ec
Erythromycin tablets	various manufacturers	ec
Eskalith-CR tablets	SKB	sr
Eudal SR tablets	Forest	sr
Exgest LA tablets	Camrick	sr
Extendryl JR capsules	Fleming	sr
Extendryl SR capsules	Fleming	sr
Fedahist Gyrocaps capsules	Schwarz Pharma	sr
Fedahist Timecaps	Schwarz Pharma	sr
Feosol capsules	SKB	sr
Fero-Folic 500	Abbott	sr
Fero-Grad-500 tablets	Abbott	sr
Fero-Gradumet tablets	Abbott	sr
Ferro-Sequel capsules	Lederle	sr
Fumatinic capsules	Laser	sr
Glucotrol XL tablets	Roerig	sr
Guaifed capsules	Muro	sr
Guaifed-PD capsules	Muro	sr
GuaiMAX-D	Central	sr
Halfprin tablets	Kramer	ec
Hemaspan caplet	Bock Pharmacal	sr
Histafed-LA capsules	Geriatric	sr
Humibid DM Sprinkle capsules	Adams	sr
Humibid DM tablets	Adams	sr
Humibid LA tablets	Adams	sr
Humibid Sprinkle	Adams	sr
Iberet-500 tablets	Abbott	sr
Iberet-Folic-500 tablets	Abbott	sr
Imdur	Key	sr
Inderal LA capsules	Wyeth-Ayerst	sr
Inderide LA capsules	Wyeth-Ayerst	sr
Indocin-SR capsules	Merck	sr
Indomethacin	Inwood	sr
Ionamin	Fisons	sr
Isoclor Timesule	Ciba	sr
Isoptin SR	Knoll	sr
Isordil Tembid capsules	Wyeth-Ayerst	sr
Isordil Tembid tablets	Wyeth-Ayerst	sr
Isosorbide Dinitrate SR	various manufacturers	sr
Kaon-CL tablets	Adria	sr
Kaon-CL-10 tablets	Adria	sr
K-Dur 10 tablets	Key	sr
K-Dur 20 tablets	Key	sr
K-Tab tablets	Abbott	sr
Klor-Con 8/Klor-Con 10 tablets	Upsher-Smith	sr
Klotrix tablets	Apothecon	sr
Levsinex capsules	Schwarz Pharma	sr
Lithobid tablets	Solvay	sr
Mag-Tab SR	Niche	sr
Meprospan-200 capsules	Wallace	sr
Meprospan-400 capsules	Wallace	sr
Mestinon tablets	ICN	sr
Minocin capsules	Lederle Labs	ec
Micro-K Extencap capsules	Robins	sr
MS Contin tablets	Purdue Frederick	sr
Naldecon tablets	Bristol	sr
Nasatab LA	ECR Pharm.	sr
Nico-400	JMI	sr
Nicobid Tempule capsules	RPR	sr
Nitroglyn capsules	Kenwood	sr
Nitrong tablets	RPR	sr
Nolamine tablets	Camrick	sr
Norflex tablets	3M	sr
Norpace-CR capsules	Searle	sr
Novafed capsules	Marion Merill Dow	sr
Novafed-A capsules	Marion Merrill Dow	sr
Optilets 500 filmtab	Abbott	or
Optilets M 500 filmtab	Abbott	or
Oramorph SR	Roxane	sr
Ornade Spansule capsules	SKB	sr
Oruvail capsules	Wyeth-Ayerst	sr
Pancrease capsules	McNeil	ec
Pancrease MT 10, 16, 20 capsules	McNeil	ec
Papaverine capsules	various manufacturers	sr

Enteric-coated = ec　Other = or　Slow-release = sr

Product	Manufacturer	Type
Pavabid Plateau Cap capsules	Marion Merrill Dow	sr
PBZ-SR tablets	Geigy	sr
Pentasa	Marion Merrill Dow	sr
Phyllocontin tablets	Purdue Frederick	sr
Plendil	Astra Merck	sr
Pneumomist	ECR Pharm.	sr
Polaramine Repetab tablets	Schering	sr
Poly-Histine-D capsules	Bock	sr
Poly-Histine-D Ped Caps	Bock	sr
Prelu-2 capsules	Boehringer Ingelheim	sr
Prilosec	Astra Merck	ec
Procainamide HCl	various manufacturers	sr
Procan-SR tablets	Parke-Davis	sr
Procardia XL tablets	Pfizer	sr
Pronestyl-SR tablets	Apothecon	sr
Proventil Repetabs	Schering	sr
Quibron-T/SR tablets	Roberts	sr
Quinaglute Dura-Tab tablets	Berlex	sr
Quinidex Extentab tablets	Robins	sr
Respbid tablets	Boehringer Ingelheim	sr
Ritalin-SR tablets	Ciba	sr
Robimycin Robitab tablets	Robins	ec
Rondec-TR tablets	Ross	sr
Ru-Tuss tablets	Boots	sr
Seldane-D tablets	Marion Merrell Dow	sr
Sinemet CR	DuPont	sr
Slo-bid Gyrocaps capsules	RPR	sr
Slo-Niacin	Upsher Smith	sr
Slo-Phyllin 125, 250 capsules	RPR	sr
Slow-Fe tablets	Ciba	sr
Slow-K tablets	Summit	sr
SLOW-Mag	Searle	sr
Sudafed 12-Hour tablets	Burroughs Wellcome	sr
Tamine SR tablets	Geneva	sr
Tavist-D tablets	Sandoz	sr
Teldrin Spansules capsules	SKB	sr
Temaril capsules	Allergan	sr
Tenuate Dospan tablets	Marion Merrill Dow	sr
Tessalon Pearies	Forest	or
Theo-24 capsules	Whitby	sr
Theobid capsules	Whitby	sr
Theoclear-LA capsules	Central	sr
Theochron tablets	various manufacturers	sr
Theo-Dur tablets	Key	sr
Theolair-SR tablets	3M	sr
Theo-Time capsules	Major	sr
Theovent capsules	Schering	sr
Theox tablets	Carnick	sr
Thorazine capsules	SKB	sr
Toprol XL tablets	Astra	sr
Touro A&H capsules	Dartmouth	sr
Touro EX tablets	Dartmouth	sr
T-Phyl tablets	Purdue Frederick	sr
Tranxene-SD tablets	Abbott	or
Trental tablets	Hoechst	sr
Triaminic-12 tablets	Sandoz	sr
Triaminic TR tablets	Sandoz	sr
Trinalin Repetabs tablets	Schering	sr
Tylenol Extended Relief caplets	McNeil	sr
Uniphyl tablets	Purdue Frederick	sr
Ultrase	Scandipharm	ec
Valrelease capsules	Roche	sr
Vanex Forte caplets	Abana	sr
Vanex-LA tablets	Abana	sr
Verelan capsules	Lederle	sr
Volmax tablets	Allen & Hanburys	sr
Voltaren tablets	Geigy	ec
Zephrex-LA tablets	Bock Pharmacal	sr
Zorprin tablets	Boots	sr
Zymase capsules	Organon	ec

Sugar-Free Products

Listed below, by therapeutic category, is a selection of drug products that contain no sugar. When recommending these products to diabetic patients, keep in mind that many may contain sorbitol, alcohol, or other sources of carbohydrates. This list should not be considered all-inclusive. Generics and alternate brands of some products may be available. Always check product labeling for a current listing of inactive ingredients.

ANALGESICS

Product	Manufacturer
Children's Myapap Elixir	My-K
Children's Panadol Drops	Sterling Health
Children's Panadol Liquid	Sterling Health
Children's Panadol Tablets, Chewable	Sterling Health
Children's Tylenol Tablets, Chewable	McNeil
Children's Tylenol Suspension Liquid	McNeil
Dolanex Elixir	Lannett
Feverall Sprinkle Caps	Upsher-Smith

Infant's Tylenol Drops	McNeil
Infant's Tylenol Suspension Drops	McNeil
Junior Strength Tylenol Chewable Tablets	McNeil
Methadone HCl	Roxane
Myapap Drops	My-K
St. Joseph Aspirin-Free Drops	Plough
St. Joseph Aspirin-Free Liquid	Plough
Tempra 1 Drops	Mead Johnson
Tempra 2 Syrup	Mead Johnson
Tempra 3 Tablets, Chewable	Mead Johnson
Tempra Tablets, Chewable	Mead Johnson

ANTACIDS/ANTIFLATULENTS

Alka-Seltzer Lemon Lime Effervescent Tablets	Moles
Aluminum Hydroxide Concentrated Suspension	Roxane
Caiglycine Tablets	Rugby
Citrocarbonate Granules	Upjohn
Di-Gel Liquid	Plough
Dimacid	Otis Clapp
Eno Powder	Beecham
Extra Strength Maalox Suspension	RPR
Gaviscon Liquid	Marion
Gelusil Liquid	Parke-Davis
Galusil II Suspension	Parke-Davis
Maalox HRF Suspension	RPR
Maalox Suspension	Rorer
Magnesia and Alumina Oral Suspension USP	various
Mallamint Tablets, Chewable	Mallard
Marblen Suspension	Fleming
Milk of Magnesia USP	various
Nephrox Suspension	Fleming
Pepto-Bismol Liquid	Procter & Gamble
Pepto-Bismol Tablets	Procter & Gamble
Phosphadjel Suspension	Wyeth-Ayerst
Riopan Plus Suspension	Whitehall
Riopan Suspension	Whitehall
Tetralac Plus Liquid	3M
Tetralac Plus Tablets	3M
Tetralac Tablets	3M

ANTIASTHMATIC/RESPIRATORY AGENTS

Elixophyllin-GG Liquid	Forest
Mudrane-GG Elixir	Poythress
Organidin Solution	Wallace
Potassium Iodide Solution	Roxane
Slo-Phyllin Syrup	RPR
Theoclear-80 Syrup	Central

ANTIDIARRHEALS

Dissorb Liquid	Schering
Kaolin with Pectin Suspension	various
Konsyl Powder	Lafayette
Peplo-Blemol Liquid	Procter & Gamble
Peplo-Blemol Tablets	Procter & Gamble
Peplo Diarrhea Control Liquid	Procter & Gamble

ANTIHISTAMINES/DECONGESTANTS

Dimetane D-C	Robins
Hay-Febrol Liquid	Scot-Tussin
Novahistine Elfxir	Lakeside
Ryna Liquid	Wallace
Trind Liquid	Mead Johnson

ANTIMANIC AGENTS

Cibalith-S Syrup	Ciba
Lithium Citrate Syrup	Roxane

BLOOD MODIFIERS/IRON PREPARATIONS

Geritol Complete Tablets	Beecham
Incremin with Iron Syrup	Lederle
Kovitonic Liquid	Freeda
Niferex Elixir	Central
Nu-Iron Elixir	Mayrand

CORTICOSTEROIDS

Dexamethasone Solution	Roxane
Pediapred Oral Liquid	Fisons

COUGH/COLD/ALLERGY PREPARATIONS

Anatuss Syrup	Mayrand
Cerose-DM Liquid	Wyeth-Ayerst
Chlorgest HD	Great Southern
Codegest Expectorant	Great Southern
Codiclear DH Syrup	Central
Codimal-DM Syrup	Central
Dexafed Cough Syrup	Hauck
Diabetic Tussin DM	Health Care Prods.
Diabetic Tussin EX Liquid	Health Care Prods.
Dimetane-DC Cough Syrup	Robins
Dimetane-DX Cough Syrup	Robins
Entuss-D Liquid	Roberts Hauck
Hayfebrol Liquid	Scot-Tussin
Hytuss 2X Capsules	Hyrex
Hytuss Tablets	Hyrex
Naldecon CX Adult Liquid	Apothecon
Naldecon DX Adult Liquid	Apothecon
Naldecon DX Children's Syrup	Apothecon
Naldecon DX Pediatric Drops	Apothecon
Naldecon EX Children's Syrup	Apothecon
Naldecon EX Pediatric Drops	Apothecon
Naldecon Senior DX Liquid	Apothecon
Naldecon Senior EX Liquid	Apothecon
Organidin NR Liquid/Tablets	Wallace
Robitussin Pediatric Cough and Cold Liquid	Robins
Robitussin Pediatric Cough Suppressant Liquid	Robins
Rondec-DM Syrup	Ross
Ryna Liquid	Wallace
Ryna-C Liquid	Wallace
Ryna-CX Liquid	Wallace
Safe Tussin 30 Liquid	Kramer
S-T Forte 2 Liquid	Scot-Tussin
S-T Forte SF Liquid	Scot-Tussin
Scot-Tussin DM Cough Chasers	Scot-Tussin
Scot-Tussin DM Liquid	Scot-Tussin
Scot-Tussin Expectorant	Scot-Tussin

Scot-Tussin Original Liquid	Scot-Tussin
Tolu-Sed Cough Syrup	Scherer
Tolu-Sed DM Liquid	Scherer
Trind-DM Liquid	Mead Johnson
Trind Liquid	Mead-Johnson
Tussar SF Syrup	RPR
Tuss-DM Tablets	Hyrex
Tuss-LA Tablets	Hyrex
Tussi-Organidin DM NR Liquid	Wallace
Tussi-Organidin Liquid	Wallace
Tussi-Organidin NR Liquid	Wallace
Tussirex Sugar-Free Liquid	Scot-Tussin
Vicondin-Tuss Syrup	Knoll
GASTROINTESTINAL DRUGS	
Reglan Syrup	Robins
LAXATIVES	
Agoral Marshmallow Emulsion	Parke-Davis
Agoral Plain Emulsion	Parke-Davis
Agoral Raspberry Emulsion	Parke-Davis
Citrucel Sugar Free Powder	SKB
Emulsoll	Paddock
Fiberall Powder	Ciba
Haley's M-O	Winthrop
Hydrocil Instant Powder	Reid-Rowell
Kondremul Plain Emulsion	Ciba
Konsyl D Powder	Konsyl Pharm
Konsyl Powder	Konsyl Pharm
Metamucil Sugar Free Powder	Procter & Gamble
MISCELLANEOUS	
Bicitra Solution	Willen
Nicorette Chewing Gum	SKB
Nicorette DS Chewing Gum	SKB
Polycitra-K Solution/Crystals	Willen
Polycitra-LC Solution	Willen
MOUTH/THROAT PREPARATIONS	
Anbesol Gel	Whitehall
Babee Teething Lotion	Pfeiffer
Baby Orajel	Del Pharm
Chloraseptic Mouthwash/Gargle	Proctor & Gamble
Moi-Stir Solution	Kingswood
Mycinettes Lozenges	Pfeiffer
Mycinette Spray	Pfeiffer
N'ice Lozenges	SKB
Orajel Brace-Aid Gel	Del Pharm
Orajel/d Gel	Del Pharm
Orajel Mouth Aid Liquid	Del Pharm
Rid-A-Pain Drops	Pfeiffer
Rid-A-Pain Gel	Pfeiffer
Salivart Solution	Gebauer
Sucrets Maximum Strength Mouthwash/Gargle	SKB
Sucrets Throat Spray	SKB
Tanac Liquid	Del Pharm
Tanac Roll-On Liquid	Del Pharm
POTASSIUM SUPPLEMENTS	
Cena-K Liquid	Century
Kaochlor-S-F Liquid	Adria
Kaon-Cl 20% Liquid	Adria
Kaon Elixir	Adria
Kay Ciel Elixir	Forest
Kay Ciel Powder	Forest
Klor-Con Powder	Upsher-Smith
Klor-Con/25 Powder	Upsher-Smith
Klor-Con/EF Tablets	Upsher-Smith
Klorvess Effervescent Granules	Sandoz
Kolyum Liquid	Pennwalt
PSYCHOTROPICS/SEDATIVES	
Serentil Concentrate	Boehringer Ingelheim
VITAMINS/MINERALS	
Bugs Bunny Complete Chewable Tablets	Miles
Bugs Bunny Plus Iron Chewable Tabs	Miles
Bugs Bunny with Extra C Chewable Tabs	Miles
Caltrate 600 Tablets	Lederle
Decagen Tablets	Goldline
Luride Drops	Colgate/Hoyt
Luride Lozi-tabs	Colgate/Hoyt
Luride-SF Lozi-tabs	Colgate/Hoyt
One-A-Day Essential Tablets	Miles
One-A-Day Maximum Formula Tablets	Miles
One-A-Day Women's Formula Tablets	Miles
Oyst-Cal 500 Tablets	Goldline
Pediaftor Drops	Ross
Phos-Flur Rinse/Supplement	Colgate-Hoyt
Posture Tablets	Whitehall
Tri-Vi-Sol Drops	Mead Johnson
Vi-Daylin ADC Drops	Ross
Vi-Daylin Drops	Ross
Vi-Daylin/F ADC Drops	Ross
Vi-Daylin/F Drops	Ross
Vi-Daylin/F Plus Iron Drops	Ross
Vi-Daylin Plus Iron ADC Drops	Ross
Vi-Daylin Plus Iron Drops	Ross
Vitalize SF Liquid	Scot-Tussin

Alcohol-Free Products

The following is a selection of alcohol-free products grouped by therapeutic category. The list is not comprehensive. Generic and alternate brands may exist. Always check product labeling for definitive information on specific ingredients.

ANALGESICS

Demerol Syrup	Sanofi/Winthrop
Halenol Children's Liquid	Halsey
Liquiprin Infant's Drops	Menley & James
Motrin Children's	McNeil
Panadol Children's Liquid	Sterling Health
Panadol Infant's Drops	Sterling Health
Tempra 1 Drops	Mead Johnson
Tempra 2 Syrup	Mead Johnson
Tylenol Children's Elixir	McNeil
Tylenol Children's Suspension	McNeil
Tylenol Infant's Drops	McNeil
Tylenol Infant's Suspension Drops	McNeil

ANTIASTHMATIC AGENTS

Alupent Syrup	Boehringer Ingelheim
Aquaphyllin Syrup	Femdale
Dilor G Liquid	Savage
Dyline-GG Liquid	Seatrace
Elixophyllin-GG Liquid	Forest
Metaprel Syrup	Sandoz
Slo-Phyllin GG Syrup	RPR
Slo-Phyllin 80 Syrup	RPR
Theoclear-80 Liquid	Central
Theolair Liquid	3M

ANTICONVULSANTS

Mysoline Suspension	Wyeth-Ayerst
Tridione Solution	Abbott
Zarontin Syrup	Parke-Davis

ANTIDIARRHEALS

Kaodene Non-Narcotic Liquid	Pfeiffer
Kaopectate Advanced Formula	Upjohn
Kaopectate Children's Liquid	Upjohn
Pepto-Bismol Suspension	Procter & Gamble

ANTIEMETICS

Emetrol Solution	Bock

COUGH/COLD/ALLERGY PREPARATIONS

Actifed Syrup	Burroughs Wellcome
Anaplex HD Syrup	Medi-Plex Pharm.
Anaplex Liquid	Medi-Plex Pharm.
Chlorgest HD	Great Southern
Codegest Expectorant	Great Southern
Dallergy-D Syrup	Laser
Deconamine Syrup	Kenwood
Delsym Liquid	McNeil
Diabetic Tussin DM Liquid	Health Care Products
Diabetic Tussin EX Liquid	Health Care Products
Donatussin DC Syrup	Laser
Donatussin Drops	Laser
Donatussin Pediatric Syrup	Laser
Dorcol Children's Cold Formula Liquid	Sandoz
Dorcol Children's Cough Syrup	Sandoz
Dorcol Children's Decongestant Liquid	Sandoz
Drixoral Syrup	Schering-Plough
Hayfebrol Liquid	Scot-Tussin
Hycodan Syrup	Du Pont
Hycomine Pediatric Syrup	Du Pont
Hycomine Syrup	Du Pont
Ipsatol Cough Formula Liquid	Kenwood
Kolephrin GG/DM Liquid	Pfeiffer
Naldecon CX Adult Liquid	Apothecon
Naldecon DX Children's Syrup	Apothecon
Naldecon DX Pediatric Drops	Apothecon
Naldecon EX Children's Syrup	Apothecon
Naldecon EX Pediatric Drops	Apothecon
Naldecon Senior DX Liquid	Apothecon
Naldecon Senior EX Liquid	Apothecon
Organidin NR Liquid	Wallace
PediaCare Cough-Cold Formula Liquid	McNeil
PediaCare Infants' Decongestant Drops	McNeil
PediaCare Night Rest Cough-Cold Formula	McNeil
Pneumotussin HC Syrup	EC Pharm
Poly-Histine CS Syrup	Bock
Poly-Histine DM Syrup	Bock
Robitussin Pediatric Cough & Cold Formula	A. H. Robins
Robitussin Pediatric Cough Suppressant	A. H. Robins
Rondec Oral Drops	Ross
Rondec Syrup	Ross
Ryna-C Liquid	Wallace
Ryna-CX Liquid	Wallace
Ryna Liquid	Wallace
Rynatuss Pediatric Suspension	Wallace
Safe Tussin 30 Liquid	Kramer
Scot-Tussin DM Liquid	Scot-Tussin
Scot-Tussin Original 5-Action Cold Formula	Scot-Tussin
Scot-Tussin Original 5-Action Liquid	Scot-Tussin
Sudafed Children's Liquid	Burroughs Wellcome
Triaminic DM Syrup	Sandoz
Triaminic Expectorant Liquid	Sandoz
Triaminic Nite Lite Liquid	Sandoz

Triaminic Oral Infant Drops	Sandoz
Triaminic Syrup	Sandoz
Triaminicol Multi-Symptom Relief Syrup	Sandoz
Tussar DM Cough Syrup	RPR
Tussi Organidin DM NR Liquid	Wallace
Tussi Organidin NR Liquid	Wallace
Tussirex Sugar Free Liquid	Scot-Tussin
Tussirex Syrup	Scot-Tussin
Tylenol Children's Cold Multi-Symptom Liquid	McNeil
Tylenol Children's Cold Plus Cough Multi-Symptom Liquid	McNeil
Vicks Children's NyQuil Liquid	Procter & Gamble
Vicks Pediatric Formula 44D Liquid	Procter & Gamble
Vicks Pediatric Formula 44E Liquid	Procter & Gamble
Vicks Pediatric Formula 44M Liquid	Procter & Gamble
Vicodin Tuss Syrup	Knoll Pharm.
MOUTH/THROAT PRODUCTS	
Baby Orajel	Del Pharm.
Baby Orajel Nighttime	Del Pharm.
Chloraseptic Spray/Gargle	Vicks
Fluorinse	Oral-B
Gly-Oxide Liquid	SKB
ELECTROLYTES	
Kolyum Liquid	Fisons
HEMATINICS	
Feostat Drops	Forest
Feostat Suspension	Forest
Troph-Iron Liquid	SKB
LAXATIVES	
Agoral Emulsion	Parke-Davis
Colace Liquid	Johnson
Haley's M-O Liquid	Sterling Health
Kondremul Plain Liquid	Ciba
Liqui-doss	Ferndale
Milkinol Emulsion	Schwarz Pharma
Neoloid Emulsion	Kenwood
Phillip's Milk of Magnesia Liquid	Sterling Health
MISCELLANEOUS	
Glandosane	Kenwood
PSYCHOTROPICS	
Haldol Concentrate	McNeil
Stelazine Concentrate	SKB
Thorazine Syrup	SKB
VITAMINS	
Poly-Vi-Sol Drops	Mead Johnson
Poly-Vi-Sol Drops w/ Iron	Mead Johnson
Theragran Liquid	Bristol-Meyers Squibb
Tri-Vi-Sol ADC Drops	Mead Johnson
Tri-Vi-Sol ADC Drops w/ Iron	Mead Johnson
Vitalize SF Liquid	Scot-Tussin

Drugs That May Cause Photosensitivity

The drugs in this table are known to cause photosensitivity in some individuals. Effects can range from itching, scaling, rash, and swelling to skin cancer, premature skin aging, skin and eye burns, cataracts, reduced immunity, blood vessel damage, and allergic reactions.

The list is not all-inclusive, and shows only representative brands of each generic. When in doubt, always check specific product labeling. Individuals should be advised to wear protective clothing and to apply sunscreens while taking the medications listed below.

Generic name	Representative Brands
Acetazolamide	Diamox
Amantadine	Symmetrel
Amiloride/hydrochlorothiazide	Moduretic
Amiodarone	Cordarone
Amitriptyline	Elavil, Endep
Amoxapine	Asendin
Astemizole	Hismanal
Atenolol/chlorthalidone	Tenoretic
Auranofin	Ridaura
Azatadine	Optimine
Azatadine/pseudoephedrine	Trinalin Repetabs
Azithromycin	Zithromax
Benazepril	Lotensin
Benazepril/hydrochlorothiazide	Lotensin HCT
Bendroflumethiazide	Naturetin
Benzthiazide	Exna
Bisoprolol/hydrochlorothiazide	Ziac
Bromodiphenhydramine/codeine	Ambenyl
Brompheniramine/phenylpropanolamine/codeine	Dimetane-DC
Brompheniramine/pseudoaphadrine/dextromethorphan	Dimetane-DX
Captopril	Capoten
Captopril/hydrochlorothiazide	Capozide
Carbamazepine	Tegretol
Chlordiazepoxide/amitriptyline	Limbitrol
Chlorhexidine gluconate	Hibistat
Chlorothiazide	Dluril
Chlorpheniramine	Chlorpheniramine
Chlorpheniramine/D-pseudoephedrine	Deconamine
Chlorpheniramine/phenylpropanolamine	Ru-Tuss II, Ornade
Chlorpromazine	Thorazine

Generic name	Representative Brands
Chlorpropamide	Diabinese
Chlorprothixene	Taractan
Chlorthalidone	Hygroton, Thalitone
Chlorthalidone/ reserpine	Demi-Regroton, Regroton
Cinoxacin	Cinobac
Ciprofloxacin	Cipro
Clemastine	Tavist
Clemastine/ phenylpropanolamine	Tavist-D
Clofazime	Lamprene
Clomipramine	Anafranil
Clonidine/ chlorthalidone	Combipres
Coal tar	Estar Gel, PsoriGel
Contraceptive, oral	see Estrogen/Progestin
Cyclobenzaprine	Flexeril
Cromolyn sodium	Intal
Cyproheptadine	Periactin
Dacarbazine	DTIC-Dome
Dantrolene sodium	Dantrium
Dapsone	Dapsone
Demeclocycline	Declomycin
Desipramine	Norpramin, Pertofrane
Dexchlorpheniramine	Polaramine
Diclofenac	Voltaren, Cataflam
Diflunisal NSAID	Dolobid
Diltiazem	Cardizem
Diphenhydramine	Benadryl
Diphenylpyraline	Hispril
Divalproex Sodium	Depakote
Doxepin	Sinequan
Doxycycline	Vibramycin, Doryx
Enalapril	Vasotec
Enalapril/ hydrochlorothiazide	Vaseretic
Enoxacin	Penetrex
Erythromycin ethylsuccinate/ sulfisoxazole	Pediazole
Estazotam	Prosom
Estrogen	Premarin
Estrogen/progestin	Ortho-Novum, Ovral
Ethionamide	Trecator-SC
Etodolac	Lodine
Etretinate	Tegison
Felbarnate	Felbatol
Floxuridine	FUDR Injectable
Flucytosine	Ancobon
Fluorouracil	Adrucil, Efudex
Fluphenazine	Prolixin, Permitil
Flurbiprofen	Ansaid
Flutamide	Eulexin
Fluvastatin	Lescol
Fosinopril	Monopril
Furosemide	Lasix
Glipizide	Glucotrol
Glyburide	Diabeta, Micronase
Gold Glynase compounds	Solganal
Gold sodium	Myochrysine thiomalate
Griseofulvin	Fulvicin, Gris-PEG
Guanethidine/ hydrochlorothiazide	Esimil
Haloperidol	Haldol
Hexachlorophene	Phisohex
Hydralazine/ hydrochlorothiazide	Apresazide, Apresoline-Esidrix
Hydrochlorothiazide	Esidrix, Hydrodiuril, Oretic
Hydrochlorothiazide/ deserpidine	Oreticyl
Hydrochlorothiazide/ triamterene	Dyazide, Maxzide
Hydroflumethiazide	Diucardin, Saluron
Hydroflumethiazide/ reserpine	Salutensin/ Salutensin-Deml
Ibuprofen	Advil, Motrin, Nuprin
Imipramine	Tofranil
Indapamide	Lozol
Interferon ALFA-2B	Intron A
Interferon ALFA-N3	Alferon N
Interferon BETA-18	Betaseron
Isocarboxazid	Marplan
Isotretinoin	Accutane
Ketoprofan	Orudis, Oruvail
Levamisole	Ergamisol
Lisinopril	Prinivil, Zestril
Lisinopril/ hydrochlorothiazide	Prinzide, Zestoretic
Lomefloxacin	Maxaquin
Loratadine	Claritin
Lovastatin	Mevacor
Maprotiline	Ludlomil
Meperidine/ promethazine	Mepergan
Mesalamine	Pentasa
Mesoridazine	Serentil
Methacycline	Rondomycin
Methazolamide	Neptazane
Methdilazine	Tacaryl
Methotrexate	Folex, Mexate, Mexate-AQ
Methotrimeprazine	Levoprome
Methyclothiazide	Aquatensen, Enduron
Methyclothiazide/ deserpidine	Enduronyl
Methyclothiazide/ reserpine	Diutensin-R
Methyldopa/ chlorothiazide	Aldoclor
Methyldopa/ hydrochlorothiazide	Aldoril
Metolazone	Diulo, Mykrox, Zaroxolyn
Metoprolol/ hydrochlorothiazide	Lopressor HCT
Minocycline	Minocin
Nabilone	Cesamet
Nabumetone	Relafen
Nadolol/ bendroflumethiazide	Corzide
Nalidixic acid	NegGram
Naproxen	Aleve, Anaprox, Naprosyn
Norfloxacin	Noroxin, Chibroxin

Generic name	Representative Brands
Nortriptyline	Pamelor
Oflaxacin	Floxin
Olsalazine	Dipentum
Oxaprozin	Daypro
Oxytetracycline	Terramycin
Oxytetracycline/ sulfamethizole/ phenazopyridine	Urobiotic-250
Paroxetine	Paxil
Pentostatin	Nipent
Perphenazine	Trilafon
Perphenazine/ amitriptyline	Etrafon, Triavil
Phenelzine	Nardil
Phenylbutazone	Butazolidin
Phenylpropanolamine/ pheniramine/ pyrilamine	Triaminic TR
Piroxicam	Feldene
Polythiazide	Renese
Pravastatin	Pravachol
Prazosin/polythiazide	Minizide
Prochlorperazine	Compazine
Promethazine	Phenergan
Propranolol/ hydrochlorothiazide	Inderide
Protriptyline	Vivactil
Pyrazinamide	Pyrazinamide
Quinapril	Accupril
Quinethazone	Hydromox
Quinidine gluconate	Quinaglute Dura-Tabs
Quinidine sulfate	Quindex Extentabs, Quinora
Ramipril	Altace
Rauwolfla Serpentina/ bendroflumethiazide	Rauzide
Reserpine/ chlorothiazide	Diupres
Reserpine/hydralazine/ hydrochlorothiazide	Ser-Ap-Es
Reserpine/ hydrochlorothiazide	Hydropres, Serpasil-Esidrix
Risperidone	Risperdal
Selegline	Eldepryl
Sertraline	Zoloft
Simvastatin	Zocor
Sotalol	Betapace
Spironolactone/ hydrochlorothiazide	Aldactazide
Sulfacetamide sodium/ phenylephrine	Vasosulf

Generic name	Representative Brands
Sulfadoxine/ pyrimethamine	Fansidar
Sulfamethizole	Thiosulfil Forte
Sulfamethizole/ phenazopyridine	Thiosulfil-A
Sulfamethoxazole	Gantanol
Sulfamethoxazole/ phenazopyridine	Azo Gantanol
Sulfamethoxazole/ trimethoprim	Bactrim, Septra
Sulfasalazine	Azulfidine
Sulfasoxazole	Gantrisin
Sulfasoxazole/ phenazopyridine	Azo Gantrisin
Sulfone	Dapsone
Sulindac	Clinoril
Terfenadine	Seldane
Terfenadine/ pseudoaphedrine	Seldane-D
Tetracycline	Achromycin, Sumycin
Thioridazine	Mellaril
Thiothixene	Navane
Timolol/ hydrochlorothiazide	Timolide
Tolazamide	Tolinasa
Tolbutamide	Orinase
Tranylcypromine	Pamate
Tretinoin	Retin-A
Triamterene	Dyrenium
Trichlormethiazide	Metahydrin, Naqua
Trifluoperazine	Stelazine
Triflupromazine	Vesprin
Trimeprazine	Temaril
Trimethoprim	Trimpex
Trimethoprim sulfate/ polymyxin B sulfate	Polytrim
Trimipramine	Surmontil
Tripelennamine	PBZ
Triprolifine	Actidil
Triprolidine/ pseudoephedrine	Actifed
Triprolidine/ pseudoephedrine/ codeine	Actifed with codeine
Valproic acid	Depakene
Venlafaxine	Effexor
Vinblastine	Velban
Zolpidem	Ambien

Drug–Alcohol Interactions

The following information has been extracted from PharmaCIS™, the new *Clinical Integration System for Drug Utilization Review™* from Red Book® Database Services. PharmaCIS database modules cover the full range of OBRA requirements for DUR, including production of leaflets for patient education and screening for drug/drug interactions, previous allergies, therapeutic duplication and improper dosing.

For further information on how PharmaCIS can be integrated into your pharmacy system, contact your system vendor or Red Book Database Services at 800-722-3062.

Listings are presented in alphabetical order by product with summary warning statements for each interaction. Degrees of onset and severity are indicated by numbers as outlined at the bottom of the page.

Product	Interaction	Onset	Severity
Acetaminophen	Concurrent use of acetaminophen and alcohol may result in increased hepatotoxicity.	2	2
Acetohexamide	Concurrent use of acetohexamide and alcohol may result in altered serum glucose levels.	1	2
Alfentanil	Concurrent use of alfentanil and alcohol may result in decreased therapeutic effects for alfentanil.	2	2
Alprazolam	Concurrent use of alprazolam and alcohol may result in increased sedation.	1	2
Amobarbital	Concurrent use of amobarbital and alcohol may result in increased sedation.	1	2
Aspirin	Concurrent use of aspirin and alcohol may result in increased gastrointestinal blood loss.	1	2
Cefamandole	Concurrent use of cefamandole and alcohol may result in disulfiram-like reactions.	2	2
Cefmenoxime	Concurrent use of cefmenoxime and alcohol may result in disulfiram-like reactions.	1	2
Cefoperazone	Concurrent use of cefoperazone and alcohol may result in disulfiram-like reactions.	2	2
Cefotetan	Concurrent use of cefotetan and alcohol may result in disulfiram-like reactions.	2	2
Chloral hydrate	Concurrent use of chloral hydrate and alcohol may result in increased sedation.	1	3
Chlordiazepoxide	Concurrent use of chlordiazepoxide and alcohol may result in increased sedation.	1	2
Chlorpromazine	Concurrent use of chlorpromazine and alcohol may result in increased sedation.	1	2
Chlorpropamide	Concurrent use of chlorpropamide and alcohol may result in disulfiram-like reactions.	1	2
Cimetidine	Concurrent use of cimetidine and alcohol may result in increased ethanol concentrations.	1	3
Clorazepate	Concurrent use of clorazepate and alcohol may result in increased sedation.	1	2
Cocaine	Concurrent use of cocaine and alcohol may result in increased heart rate and blood pressure.	1	1
Codeine	Concurrent use of codeine and alcohol may result in increased sedation.	1	2
Diazepam	Concurrent use of diazepam and alcohol may result in increased sedation.	1	2
Dimethimdene	Concurrent use of dimethimdene and alcohol may result in increased sedation.	1	2
Diphenhydramine	Concurrent use of diphenydramine and alcohol may result in increased sedation.	1	2
Disulfiram	Concurrent use of disulfiram and alcohol may result in ethanol intolerance.	1	1
Furazolidone	Concurrent use of furazolidone and alcohol may result in disulfiram-like reactions.	1	2
Glutethimide	Concurrent use of glutethimide and alcohol may result in increased sedation.	1	2
Hydrocodone	Concurrent use of hydrocodone and alcohol may result in increased sedation.	1	2
Hydromorphone	Concurrent use of hydromorphone and alcohol may result in increased sedation.	1	2
Insulin	Concurrent use of insulin and alcohol may result in increased hypoglycemia.	1	1
Isoniazid	Concurrent use of isoniazid and alcohol may result in decreased isoniazid concentrations and disulfiram-like reactions.	2	2
Isotretinoin	Concurrent use of isotretinoin and alcohol may result in disulfiram-like reactions.	1	2
Ketoconazole	Concurrent use of ketoconazole and alcohol may result in disulfiram-like reactions.	1	2
Lorazepam	Concurrent use of lorazepam and alcohol may result in increased sedation.	1	2

Onset: 1 = Rapid (within 24 hours)
2 = Delayed (after 24 hours)

Severity: 1 = Major (Possibly life threatening or potential permanent damage.)
2 = Moderate (May exacerbate patient's condition.)
3 = Minor (Little if any clinical effect.)

Product	Interaction	Onset	Severity
Meperidine	Concurrent use of meperidine and alcohol may result in increased sedation.	1	2
Meprobamate	Concurrent use of meprobamate and alcohol may result in increased sedation.	1	2
Methadone	Concurrent use of methadone and alcohol may result in increased sedation.	1	2
Methotrexate	Concurrent use of methotrexate and alcohol may result in increased hepatotoxicity.	2	2
Metronidazole	Concurrent use of metronidazole and alcohol may result in disulfiram-like reactions.	1	2
Morphine	Concurrent use of morphine and alcohol may result in increased sedation.	1	2
Moxalactam	Concurrent use of moxalactam and alcohol may result in disulfiram-like reactions.	2	2
Nitroglycerin	Concurrent use of nitroglycerin and alcohol may result in hypotension.	1	2
Oxycodone	Concurrent use of oxycodone and alcohol may result in increased sedation.	1	2
Pentazocine	Concurrent use of pentazocine and alcohol may result in increased sedation.	1	2
Pentobarbital	Concurrent use of pentobarbital and alcohol may result in increased sedation.	1	2
Phenobarbital	Concurrent use of phenobarbital and alcohol may result in increased sedation.	1	2
Procarbazine	Concurrent use of procarbazine and alcohol may result in disulfiram-like reactions and increased sedation.	1	2
Tolbutamide	Concurrent use of tolbutamide and alcohol may result in altered serum glucose concentrations.	1	2
Triazolam	Concurrent use of triazolam and alcohol may result in increased sedation.	1	2

Onset: 1 = Rapid (within 24 hours)
2 = Delayed (after 24 hours)

Severity: 1 = Major (Possibly life threatening or potential permanent damage.)
2 = Moderate (May exacerbate patient's condition.)
3 = Minor (Little if any clinical effect.)

Drug–Tobacco Interactions

Product	Interaction	Onset	Severity
Amphetamine	Concurrent use of amphetamine and tobacco may result in increased smoking behavior.	1	3
Codeine	Concurrent use of codeine and tobacco may result in decreased pain tolerance.	1	3
Dextroamphetamine	Concurrent use of dextroamphetamine and tobacco may result in increased smoking behavior.	1	3
Imipramine	Concurrent use of imipramine and tobacco may result in decreased imipramine concentrations.	2	2
Lidocaine	Concurrent use of lidocaine and tobacco may result in decreased lidocaine concentrations.	2	3
Nortriptyline	Concurrent use of nortriptyline and tobacco may result in decreased nortriptyline concentrations.	2	2
Oral contraceptives (Combination-type)	Concurrent use of oral contraceptives (combination-type) and tobacco may result in increased cardiovascular disease.	2	3
Pentazocine	Concurrent use of pentazocine and tobacco may result in decreased pentazocine concentrations.	2	2
Propoxyphene	Concurrent use of proproxyphene and tobacco may result in decreased propoxyphene concentrations.	2	2
Theophylline	Concurrent use of theophylline and tobacco may result in decreased theophylline concentrations.	2	2
Tolbutamide	Concurrent use of tolbutamide and tobacco may result in decreased tolbutamide concentrations.	2	2

Onset: 1 = Rapid (within 24 hours)
2 = Delayed (after 24 hours)

Severity: 1 = Major (Possibly life threatening or potential permanent damage.)
2 = Moderate (May exacerbate patient's condition.)
3 = Minor (Little if any clinical effect.)

Use-in-Pregnancy Ratings

The U.S. Food and Drug Administration's Use-in-Pregnancy rating system weighs the degree to which available information has ruled out risk to the fetus against the drug's potential benefit to the patient. The following is a listing of drugs (by generic name) for which ratings are available. Since a number of drugs have never received a formal rating, the lists are not all-inclusive. If a drug you're researching doesn't appear in these listings, be sure to check its prescribing information. Precautions do need to be taken with many of the unrated drugs.

X

CONTRAINDICATED IN PREGNANCY

Studies in animals or humans, or investigational or post-marketing reports, have demonstrated fatal risk which clearly outweighs any possible benefit to the patient.

Acetohydroxamic Acid
Anisindione
Belladonna Alkaloids/Ergotamine Tartrate/ Phenobarbital
Benzphetamine Hydrochloride
Chlorotrianisene
Clomiphene Citrate
Danazol
Demecarium Bromide
Desogestrel and Ethinyl Estradiol
Dienestrol
Diethylstilbestrol
Dihydroergotamine Mesylate
Ephedrine Hydrochloride/ Phenobarbital/ Potassium Iodide/Theophylline
Ergotamine Tartrate
Ergotamine Tartrate with Caffeine
Estazolam
Estradiol
Estradiol Cypionate and Testosterone Cyplonate
Estradiol, Injectable
Estramustine Phosphate Sodium
Estrogens, Conjugated
Estrogens, Conjugated and Meprobamate
Estrogens, Conjugated and Methyltestosterone
Estrogens, Esterified
Estrogens, Esterified and Methyltestosterone
Estrone
Estropipate
Ethinyl Estradiol
Ethinyl Estradiol and Norethindrone
Ethinyl Estradiol and Norgestimate
Ethinyl Estradiol and Norgestrel
Ethinyl Estradiol with Ethynodiol Diacetate
Etretinate
Finastaride
Fluoxymesterone
Fluvastatin Sodium
Goserelin Acetate
Histrelin Acetate
Isoflurophate
Isotretinoin
Leuprolide Acetate
Levonorgestrel
Lovastatin
Medroxyprogesterone Acetate, Contraceptive
Megestrol Acetate
Menotropins
Mestranol and Norethindrone
Methotrexate
Methyltestosterone
Misoprostol
Nafarelin Acetate
Nandrolone
Norethindrone
Norethindrone Acetate
Norgestrel
Oxandrolone
Oxymetholone
Oxytocin
Plicamycin
Pravastatin Sodium
Quazepam
Quinestrol
Quinine Sulfate
Ribavirin
Simvastatin
Stanozolol
Temazepam
Testosterone, Injectable
Testosterone, Transdermal
Triazolam
Urofollitropin
Vitamin A
Warfarin Sodium

D

POSITIVE EVIDENCE OF RISK

Investigational or post-marketing data show risk to the fetus. Nevertheless, potential benefits may outweigh the potential risk.

Alprazolam
Altretamine
Amikacin Sulfate
Aminoglutethimide
Amiodarone Hydrochloride
Amitriptyline Hydrochloride
Amobarbital Sodium
Amobarbital Sodium and Secobarbital Sodium
Aspirin
Atenolol
Atenolol with Chlorthalidone
Azathioprine
Benazepril Hydrochloride
Benazepril Hydrochloride with Hydrochlorothiazide
Busulfan
Butabarbital Sodium
Calcium Iodide and Codeine
Calcium Iodide and Isoproterenol Sulfate
Captopril
Captopril with Hydrochlorothiazide
Carboplatin
Carmustine
Chlorambucil
Chlordiazepoxide
Cisplatin
Cladribine
Colchicine
Cortisone Acetate
Cyclophosphamide
Cytarabine
Daunorubicin Hydrochloride
Dicumarol
Divalproex Sodium
Doxorubicin Hydrochloride
Doxycycline
Enalapril
Enalapril Maleate with Hydrochlorothiazide
Etoposide
Floxuridine
Fludarabine Phosphate
Fluorouracil, Systemic
Fluorouracil, Topical
Flutamide
Fosinopril Sodium
Halazepam
Hydroxyprogesterone Caproate
Idarubicin Hydrochloride
Ifosfamide
Kanamycin Sulfate
Lisinopril
Lithium Carbonate
Lithium Citrate
Lomustine
Lorazepam
Mechlorethamine Hydrochloride
Melphalan
Mephobarbita
Meprobamate
Mercaptopurine
Metaraminol Bitartrate
Methimazole
Midazolam Hydrochloride
Minocycline Hydrochloride
Mitoxantrone Hydrochloride
Nalbuphine Hydrochloride
Neomycin Sulfate
Neomycin Sulfate and Polymyxin B Sulfate
Neomycin Sulfate and Polymyxin B Sulfate, Irrigant
Netilmicin Sulfate
Nicotine
Nortriptyline Hydrochloride
Oxazepam
Oxytetracycline Hydrochloride
Oxytetracycline Hydrochloride/ Phenazopyridine/ Sulfamethizole
Paclitaxel
Paramethadione
Pentobarbital Sodium
Pentostatin
Phenacemide
Phenobarbital
Phensuximide
Pipobroman
Polythiazide
Potassium Iodide
Primidone
Procarbazine Hydrochloride
Progesterone
Propylthiouracil
Quinapril Hydrochloride
Quinethazone
Ramipril
Reserpine and Trichlormethiazide
Secobarbital Sodium
Streptomycin Sulfate
Strontium-89 Chloride
Tamoxifen Citrate
Teniposide
Thioguanine
Tobramycin Sulfate, Injectable
Trimethaphan Camsylate
Trimetrexate Glucuronate
Valproic Acid
Vinblastine Sulfate
Vincristine Sulfate

C

RISK CANNOT BE RULED OUT

Human studies are lacking, and animal studies are either positive for risk or are lacking as well. However, potential benefits may outweigh the potential risk.

Acetaminophen and Oxycodone Hydrochloride
Acetaminophen and Pentazocine Hydrochloride
Acetaminophen with Butalbital
Acetaminophen with Codeine Phosphate
Acetaminophen with Hydrocodone Bitartrate
Acetaminophen/ Butalbital/Caffeine
Acetaminophen/ Butalbital/Caffeine/ Codeine Phosphate
Acetaminophen/ Caffeine/ Chlorpheniramine/ Hydrocodone/ Phenylephrine
Acetaminophen/ Caffeine/ Dihydrocodeine Bitartrate
Acetaminophen/ Chlorpheniramine Maleate/Phenylpropanolamine Hydrochloride/ Phenyltoloxamine Citrate
Acetazolamide
Acetic Acid and Desonide

Acetohexamide
Acetylcholine Chloride
Acyclovir
Adenosine
Albumin, Normal Serum, Human
Albuterol
Alclometasone Dipropionate
Alcohol, Dehydrated
Aldesleukin
Alfentanil Hydrochloride
Alglucerase
Allergenic Extracts
Allopurinol
Alteplase, Recombinant
Aluminum Chloride (Hexahydrate)
Amantadine Hydrochloride
Amcinonide
Amino Acids with Electrolytes, Injectable
Amino Acids, Injectable
Amino Acids/Calcium Chloride/Dextrose/Electrolytes
Aminocaproic Acid
Aminohippurate Sodium
Aminophylline
Aminosalicylic Acid
Amiodipine Besylate
Ammonium Chloride
Ammonium Lactate
Ammonium Molybdate
Amoxapine
Amphetamine
Amrinone Lactate
Amyl Nitrite
Amyl Nitrite/Sodium Nitrite/Sodium Thiosulfate
Amylase/Cellulase/Lipase/Protease
Anistreplase
Antazoline Phosphate and Naphazoline Hydrochloride
Anthralin
Anti-Inhibitor Coagulant Complex
Anticoagulant Citrate Phosphate Dextrose
Antihemophilic Factor
Antihemophilic Factor, Human
Antihemophilic Factor, Porcine
Antipyrine and Benzocaine
Antipyrine/Benzocaine/Phenylephrine Hydrochloride
Antithrombin III (Human)
Antivenin (Crotalidae) Polyvalent
Antivenin (Latrodectus Mactans)
Asparaginase
Aspirin and Carisoprodol
Aspirin and Methocarbamol
Aspirin with Butalbital
Aspirin with Codeine Phosphate
Aspirin with Hydrocodone Bitartrate
Aspirin/Butalbital/Caffeine
Aspirin/Butalbital/Caffeine/Codeine Phosphate
Aspirin/Caffeine/Orphenadrine Citrate
Aspirin/Carisoprodol/Codeine Phosphate
Asternizole
Atovaquone
Atracurium Besylate
Atropine Sulfate and Difenoxin Hydrochloride
Atropine Sulfate and Diphenoxylate Hydrochloride
Atropine Sulfate and Edrophonium Chloride
Atropine Sulfate, Injectable
Atropine Sulfate, Ophthalmic
Atropine Sulfate, Oral
Atropine Sulfate/Benzoic Acid/Hyposcyamine/Methenamine/Methylene Blue/Phenylsalicylate
Auranofin
Aurothioglucose
Azatadine Maleate with Pseudoephedrine Sulfate
BCG
Bacitracin, Ophthalmic
Baclofen
Balanced Salt Solution
Beclomethasone Dipropionate
Belladonna Alkaloids and Butabarbital Sodium
Belladonna Alkaloids and Opium
Belladonna Alkaloids/Chlorpheniramine Maleate/Phenylephrine Hydrochloride/Phenylpropanolamine Hydrochloride
Belladonna and Phenobarbital
Benazepril Hydrochloride
Benazepril Hydrochloride with Hydrochlorothiazide
Bendroflumethiazide
Bendroflumethiazide and Nadolol
Bendroflumethiazide and Rauwolfia Serpentina
Benzocaine
Benzonatate
Benzoyl Peroxide
Benzoyl Peroxide with Sulfur
Benzthiazide
Benzylpenicilloyl Polylysine
Bepridil Hydrochloride
Beta Carotene
Betamethasone Dipropionate with Clotrimazole
Betamethasone Sodium Phosphate
Betamethasone, Topical
Betaxolol Hydrochloride, Ophthalmic
Betaxolol Hydrochloride, Oral
Bethanechol Chloride
Bile Salts/Pancreatin/Pepsin
Biperiden
Bisoprolol Fumarate
Bisoprolol Fumarate with Hydrochlorothiazide
Bitolterol Mesytate
Botulinum Toxin type A
Bretylium Tosylate
Bromodiphenhydramine Hydrochloride and Codeine Phosphate
Brompheniramine Maleate and Pseudoephedrine Hydrochloride
Brompheniramine Maleate/Codeine Phosphate/ Phenylpropanolamine Hydrochloride
Brompheniramine/Dextromethorphan/Pseudoephedrine
Bucilzine Hydrochloride
Budesonide
Bumetanide
Buprenorphine Hydrochloride
Butoconazole Nitrate
Butorphanol Tartrate
Caffeine with Sodium Benzoate
Calcifediol
Calcipotriene
Calcitonin
Calcitriol
Calcium Acetate
Calcium, Injectable
Capreomycin Sulfate
Captopril
Captopril with Hydrochlorothiazide
Carbachol
Carbamazepine
Carbetapentane/Chlorpheniramine/Ephedrine/Phenylephrine
Carbidopa and Levodopa
Carbinoxamine Maleate with Pseudoephedrine Hydrochloride
Carbinoxamine Maleate/Dextromethorphan Hydrobromide/Pseudoephedrine Hydrochloride
Carboprost Tromethamine
Cardioplegic Solution
Carisoprodol
Carteolol Hydrochloride, Ophthalmic
Carteolol Hydrochloride, Oral
Cellulose Sodium Phosphate
Chloral Hydrate
Chloramphenicol
Chlorcyclizine Hydrochloride and Hydrocortisone Acetate
Chloroprocaine Hydrochloride
Chloroquine
Chlorothiazide
Chlorothiazide with Reserpine
Chloroxine
Chloroxylenol/Hydrocortisone/Pramoxine Hydrochloride
Chlorpheniramine Maleate and Epinephrine Hydrochloride
Chlorpheniramine Maleate and Pseudoephedrine Hydrochloride
Chlorpheniramine Maleate with Phenylpropanolamine Hydrochloride
Chlorpheniramine Maleate/Dextromethorphan Hydrobromide/Guaifenesin/Phenylephrine Hydrochloride
Chlorpheniramine Maleate/Ephedrine Sulfate/Guaifenesin/Hydriodic Acid
Chlorpheniramine Maleate/Hydrocodone Bitartrate/Phenylephrine Hydrochloride
Chlorpheniramine Maleate/Hydrocodone Bitartrate/Pseudoephedrine Hydrochloride
Chlorpheniramine Maleate/Phenylephrine Hydrochloride/Phenylpropanolamine Hydrochloride/Phenyltoloxamine Citrate
Chlorpheniramine Maleate/Phenylephrine Hydrochloride/Phenylpropanolamine Hydrochloride/Pyrilamine Maleate
Chlorpheniramine Maleate/Phenylephrine Hydrochloride/Phenyltoloxamine Citrate
Chlorpheniramine Polistirex with Hydrocodone Pollstirex
Chlorpheniramine Tannate with Pseudoephedrine Tannate
Chlorpheniramine Tannate/Phenylephrine Tannate/Pyrilamine Tannate
Chlorpromazine
Chlorpropamide
Chlorthalidone with Clonidine Hydrochloride
Chlorzoxazone
Cholera Vaccine
Cholestyramine
Choline Bitartrate and Dexpanthenol
Choline Magnesium Trisalicylate
Chromic Chloride
Chymopapain
Cilastatin Sodium and Imipenem
Cinoxacin
Ciprofloxacin Hydrochloride, Ophthalmic
Ciprofloxacin, Systemic
Cisapride
Citric Acid and Potassium Bicarbonate
Citric Acid/Glucono-delta-lactone/Magnesium Carbonate
Citric Acid/Magnesium Oxide/Sodium Carbonate
Clarithromycin
Clidinium Bromide

Clobetasol Propionate
Clocortolone Pivalate
Clofazimine
Clofibrate
Clomipramine Hydrochloride
Clonazepam
Clonidine
Clotrimazole
Cocaine Hydrochloride
Codeine
Codeine Phosphate and Promethazine Hydrochloride
Codeine Phosphate with Pseudoephedrine Hydrochloride
Codeine Phosphate/Guaifenesin/Phenylpropanolamine Hydrochloride
Codeine Phosphate/Guaifenesin/Pseudoephedrine Hydrochloride
Codeine Phosphate/Phenylephrine Hydrochloride/Promethazine Hydrochloride
Codeine Phosphate/Pseudoephedrine Hydrochloride/Triprolidine Hydrochloride
Corticotropin
Cosyntropin
Crotamiton
Cyclopentolate Hydrochloride
Cycloserine
Cyclosporine
Cyclothiazide
Cysteine Hydrochloride
Dacarbazine
Dactinomycin
Dantrolene Sodium
Dapsone
Deferoxamine Mesylate
Deserpidine
Desipramine Hydrochloride
Desonide
Desoximetasone
Dexamethasone Sodium Phosphate and Neomycin Sulfate, Topical
Dexamethasone Sodium Phosphate with Neomycin Sulfate, Ophthalmic
Dexamethasone Sodium Phosphate, Inhalation
Dexamethasone and Tobramycin
Dexamethasone, Ophthalmic
Dexamethasone, Oral
Dexamethasone, Topical
Dexchlorpheniramine Maleate/Guaifenesin/Pseudoephedrine Sulfate
Dexpanthenol
Dextran 40
Dextran and Dextrose
Dextroamphetamine Sulfate
Dextromethorphan Hydrobromide and Guaifenesin
Dextromethorphan Hydrobromide and Promethazine Hydrochloride
Dextrose
Dextrose and Electrolytes
Dextrose and Electrolytes, Intraperitoneal
Dextrose and Potassium Chloride
Dextrose and Ringer's solution
Dextrose and Sodium Chloride
Dextrose/Electrolytes/Fructose/Invert Sugar
Dextrose/Lactated Ringer's solution/Potassium Chloride
Dextrose/Potassium Chloride/Sodium Chloride
Dezocine
Diatrizoate Meglumine
Diatrizoate Sodium
Diazoxide
Diazoxide, Injectable
Dichlorphenamide
Diflorasone Diacetate
Diflunisal
Digestive Enzymes/Hyposcyamine Sulfate/Phenyltoloxamine Citrate
Digitoxin
Digoxin
Digoxin Immune Fab (Ovine)
Dihydrotachysterol
Ditiazem Hydrochloride
Dimethyl Sulfoxide
Dinoprostone, Cervical
Dinoprostone, Vaginal
Diphtheria and Tetanus Toxoids
Diphtheria/Haemophilus b/Pertussis/Tetanus Vaccine
Diphtheria/Pertussis/Tetanus
Disopyramide Phosphate
Disulfiram
Dopamine Hydrochloride
Doxacurium Chloride
Doxazosin Mesylate
Doxepin Hydrochloride
Dronabinol
Droperidol
Droperidol and Fentanyl Citrate
Dyclonine Hydrochloride
Dyphylline
Dyphylline and Guaifenesin
Echothiophate Iodide
Econazole Nitrate
Edetate Disodium
Edrophonium Chloride
Electrolytes and Polyethylene Glycol
Electrolytes, Injectable
Enalapril
Enalapril Maleate with Hydrochlorothiazide
Enoxacin
Ephedrine Sulfate
Epinephrine Bitartrate and Pilocarpine Hydrochloride
Epinephrine, Ophthalmic
Epinephrine, Systemic
Epoetin Alfa
Ergocalciferol
Erythrityl Tetranitrate
Erythromycin Ethylsuccinate with Sulfisoxazole Acetyl
Esmolol Hydrochloride
Ethanolamine Oleate
Ethchlorvynol
Ethiodized Oil
Ethionamide
Ethosuximide
Ethotoin
Etidronate Disodium, Injectable
Etidronate Disodium, Oral
Etodolac
Etomidate
Factor IX (Human)
Factor IX Complex, Human
Fat Emulsion
Felbamate
Felodipine
Fenfluramine Hydrochloride
Fentanyl
Ferrous Fumarate/Folic Acid/Minerals/Vitamins, Multi
Ferrous Fumarate/Vitamin B12/Vitamin C
Ferrous Gluconate/Liver Extract/Vitamins, Multi
Filgrastim
Flecainide Acetate
Fluconazole
Flucytosine
Fludrocortisone Acetate
Flumazenil
Flunisolide
Fluocinolone Acetonide
Fluocinonide
Fluorescein Sodium and Proparacaine Hydrochloride
Fluorometholone
Fluphenazine
Flurandrenolide
Flurbiprofen Sodium, Ophthalmic
Fluticasone Propionate
Folic Acid/Polysaccharide-Iron Complex/Vitamin B12
Foscarnet Sodium
Fosinopril Sodium
Furazolidone
Furosemide
Gabapentin
Gadodlamide
Gadopentetate Dimeglumine
Gadoteridol
Gallium Nitrate
Ganciclovir Sodium
Gemfibrozil
Gentamicin Sulfate and Prednisolone Acetate
Gentamicin Sulfate, Ophthalmic
Glipizide
Globulin, Immune
Globulin, Immune Rho (D)
Glycerin
Gold Sodium Thiomalate
Gonadotropin, Chorionic
Griseofulvin
Guaifenesin
Guaifenesin and Hydrocodone Bitartrate
Guaifenesin and Hydromorphone Hydrochloride
Guaifenesin and Phenylephrine Hydrochloride
Guaifenesin and Phenylpropanolamine Hydrochloride
Guaifenesin and Pseudoephedrine Hydrochloride
Guaifenesin and Theophylline
Guaifenesin and Theophylline Sodium Glycinate
Guaifenesin/Hydrocodone Bitartrate/Pheniramine Maleate/Phenylephrine Hydrochloride/Phenylpropanolamine Hydrochloride
Guaifenesin/Hydrocodone Bitartrate/Pheniramine Maleate/Phenylpropanolamine Hydrochloride/Pyritamine Maleate
Guaifenesin/Hydrocodone Bitartrate/Phenylephrine Hydrochloride
Guaifenesin/Hydrocodone Bitartrate/Pseudoephedrine Hydrochloride
Guaifenesin/Phenylephrine Hydrochloride/Phenylpropanolamine Hydrochloride
Guanabenz Acetate
Guanethidine Monosulfate
Haemophilus B Conjugate Vaccine
Haemophilus B Conjugate Vaccine (Tetanus Toxoid Conjugate)
Halcinonide
Halobetasol Propionate
Haloperidol
Halothane
Hemin
Heparin
Hepatitis B Vaccine, Recombinant
Hepatitis B Immune Globulin (Human)
Hetastarch
Hexachlorophene
Histamine Phosphate
Homatropine Hydrobromide
Homatropine Methylbromide and Hydrocodone Bitartrate
Hyaluronidase
Hydralazine Hydrochloride
Hydralazine Hydrochloride with Hydrochlorothiazide
Hydralazine Hydrochloride/Hydrochlorothiazide/Reserpine
Hydrochlorothiazide and Lisinopril
Hydrochlorothiazide and Methyldopa
Hydrochlorothiazide and Propranolol Hydrochloride
Hydrochlorothiazide and Timolol Maleate
Hydrochlorothiazide and Triamterene
Hydrochlorothiazide with Metoprolol Tartrate
Hydrochlorothiazide with Reserpine
Hydrocodone Bitartrate with Phenylephrine Hydrochloride
Hydrocodone Bitartrate with Phenylpropanolamine Hydrochloride
Hydrocodone Bitartrate with Pseudoephedrine Hydrochloride

Hydrocodone Bitartrate/ Pheniramine Maleate/ Phenylephrine Hydrochloride/ Phenylpropanolamine Hydrochloride/ Pyrilamine Maleate
Hydrocodone Bitartrate/ Phenylephrine Hydrochloride/ Pyrilamine Maleate
Hydrocodone/ Pheniramine/ Phenylephrine/ Phenylpropanolamine/Pyrilamine
Hydrocortisone Acetate and Pramoxine Hydrochloride
Hydrocortisone Acetate with Lidocaine
Hydrocortisone Acetate with Neomycin Sulfate
Hydrocortisone Cypionate
Hydrocortisone with Iodoquinol
Hydrocortisone, Rectal
Hydrocortisone, Topical
Hydrocortisone/ Neomycin Sulfate/Polymyxin B Sulfate
Hydroflumethiazide
Hydroflumethiazide with Reserpine
Hydromorphone Hydrochloride
Hydroquinone
Hydroxyamphetamine Hydrobromide with Tropicamide
Hydroxyzine
Hyoscyamine Sulfate
Idoxuridine
Imiglucerase
Imiipramine
Indigotindisulfonate Sodium
Indium in-111 Pentetreotide
Indocyanine Green
Influenza Virus Vaccine
Interferon Alfa-2A
Interferon Alfa-2B
Interferon Alfa-N3
Interferon Beta-1B
Interferon Gamma-1B
Iodoquinol
Iopanoic Acid
Iron Dextran
Isoetharine Hydrochloride
Isoflurane
Isoniazid
Isoniazid and Rifampin
Isoniazid/Pyrazinamide/Rifampin
Isoproterenol
Isoproterenol Hydrochloride with Phenylephrine Bitartrate
Isosorbide Dinitrate
Isosulfan Blue
Isoxsuprine Hydrochloride
Isradipine
Itraconazole
Japanese Encephalitis Virus Vaccine
Ketoconazole, Oral
Ketoconazole, Topical
Ketorolac Tromethamine, Ophthalmic
Ketorolac Tromethamine, Systemic
Labetalol Hydrochloride
Lactated Ringer's
Leucovorin Calcium
Levamisole Hydrochloride
Levobunolol Hydrochloride, Ophthalmic
Levocabastine Hydrochloride
Levodopa
Lisinopril
Liver Derivative Complex
Lomefloxacin Hydrochloride
Loxapine
Lymphocyte Immune Globulin
Lypressin
Lysine Hydrochloride/ Potassium Bicarbonate/ Potassium Chloride
Mafenide Acetate
Magnesium Chloride, Injectable
Magnesium Salicylate
Magnesium Salicylate and Phenyltoloxamine Dihydrogen Citrate
Manganese Chloride
Mannitol and Sorbitol
Mannitol, Injectable
Mazindol
Measles Virus Vaccine
Measles and Rubella Virus Vaccine Live
Measles/Mumps/ Rubella Virus Vaccine Live
Mebendazole
Mecamylamine Hydrochloride
Medrysone
Mefenamic Acid
Mefloquine Hydrochloride
Meningococcal Polysaccharide Vaccine
Mepenzolate Bromide
Mephentermine Sulfate
Mephenytoin
Mepivacaine Hydrochloride
Mesoridazine Besylate
Metaproterenol Sulfate
Methacholine Chloride
Methamphetamine Hydrochloride
Methazolamide
Methenamine Hippurate
Methenamine Mandelate
Methenamine Mandelate and Sodium Acid Phosphate
Methocarbamol
Methoxamine Hydrochloride
Methoxsalen
Methoxyflurane
Methscopolamine Bromide
Methyclothiazide with Reserpine
Methyldopa
Methylene Blue
Methylergonovine Maleate
Methylprednisolone Acetate and Neomycin Sulfate
Metipranolol
Metocurine Iodide
Metoprolol
Metyrosine
Mexiletine Hydrochloride
Miconazole Nitrate
Miconazole, Injectable
Milrinone Lactate
Minoxidil, Oral
Minoxidil, Topical
Mitotane
Mivacurium Chloride
Mometasone Furoate
Monobenzone
Monoctanoin
Morphine Sulfate
Mumps Skin Test Antigen
Mumps Virus Vaccine Live
Muromonab-CD3
Nabumetone
Nadolol
Naloxone Hydrochloride and Pentazocine Hydrochloride
Naltrexone Hydrochloride
Naphazoline Hydrochloride
Naphazoline Hydrochloride and Pheniramine Maleate
Natamycin
Neostigmine
Niacin
Nicardipine Hydrochloride
Nicotine Polacrilex
Nifedipine
Nimodipine
Nitrofurazone, Topical
Nitroglycerin
Nizatidine
Norepinephrine Bitartrate
Norfloxacin, Ophthalmic
Norfloxacin, Oral
Novobiocin Sodium
Nystatin and Triamcinolone Acetonide
Nystatin, Oral
Ofloxacin, Ophthalmic
Ofloxacin, Systemic
Olsalazine Sodium
Omeprazole
Opium Tincture
Orphenadrine Citrate
Oxamniquine
Oxaprozin
Oxtriphylline
Oxytetracycline Hydrochloride/ Phenazopyridine/ Sulfamethizole
Pamidronate Disodium
Pancrelipase
Pancuronium Bromide
Paraldehyde
Paregoric
Pegademase Bovine
Pegaspargase
Penbutolol Sulfate
Pentagastrin
Pentamidine Isethionate
Pentastarch
Pentazocine Lactate
Pentoxifylline
Perphenazine
Phenazopyridine Hydrochloride and Sulfisoxazole
Phendimetrazine Tartrate
Phenelzine Sulfate
Pheniramine Maleate/Phenylpropanolamine Hydrochloride/ Pyrilamine Maleate
Phenoxybenzamine Hydrochloride
Phentermine
Phentolamine Mesylate
Phenylephrine Hydrochloride
Phenylephrine Hydrochloride and Promethazine Hydrochloride
Phenylephrine Hydrochloride and Scopolamine Hydrobromide
Phenylephrine Hydrochloride and Sulfacetamide Sodium
Physostigmine Salicylate
Physostigmine Sulfate
Phytonadione
Pilocarpine Hydrochloride, Oral
Pilocarpine, Ophthalmic
Pimozide
Pipecuronium Bromide
Pirbuterol Acetate
Plasma Protein Fraction (Human)
Pneumococcal Vaccine, Polyvalent
Podofilox
Polio Vaccine
Polymyxin B Sulfate and Trimethoprim Sulfate
Polythiazide and Prazosin Hydrochloride
Polythiazide and Reserpine
Potassium Acetate
Potassium Acid Phosphate
Potassium Acid Phosphate and Sodium Acid Phosphate
Potassium Bicarbonate
Potassium Chloride and Potassium Gluconate
Potassium Chloride and Sodium Chloride
Potassium Chloride, Injectable
Potassium Chloride, Oral
Potassium Citrate
Potassium Iodide and Theophylline
Potassium Phosphate
Potassium Phosphate, Monobasic and Sodium Phosphate, Dibasic
Povidone-Iodine
Pralidoxime Chloride
Prazosin Hydrochloride
Prednicarbate
Prednisolone Acetate, Ophthalmic
Prednisolone and Sulfacetamide Sodium
Procainamide Hydrochloride
Procaine Hydrochloride
Prochlorperazine
Procyclidine Hydrochloride
Promethazine Hydrochloride
Propafenone Hydrochloride
Propantheline Bromide
Proparacaine Hydrochloride
Propranolol Hydrochloride
Protamine Sulfate
Proteinase Inhibitor (Human), Alpha 1
Protirelin
Protriptyline Hydrochloride

Pseudoephedrine Hydrochloride
Pseudoephedrine Hydrochloride and Terfenadine
Pyrazinamide
Pyridostigmine Bromide
Pyrimethamine
Pyrimethamine and Sulfadoxine
Quinapril Hydrochloride
Quinidine Gluconate
Quinidine Polygalacturonate
Quinidine Sulfate
Rabies Immune Globulin (Human)
Rabies Vaccine
Rabies Vaccine Adsorbed
Ramipril
Reserpine
Reserpine and Trichlormethiazide
Respiratory Vaccine, Mixed
Rho (D) Immune Globulin
Rifampin
Rimantadine Hydrochloride
Ringer's Solution, Irrigation
Ringer's Solution, Injectable
Risperidone
Rubella Virus Vaccine
Rubella and Mumps Vaccine
Salmeterol Xinafoate
Salsalate
Sargramostim
Scopolamine
Secretin
Selegiline Hydrochloride
Selenious Acid
Selenium Sulfide
Sermoretin Acetate
Skin Test Antigens, Multiple
Sodium Benzoate and Sodium Phenylacetate
Sodium Bicarbonate
Sodium Chloride, Injectable
Sodium Lactate
Sodium Nitroprusside
Sodium Phosphate
Sodium Polystyrene Sulfonate
Sodium Tetradecyl Sulfate
Sodium Thiosulfate
Somatrem
Somatropin
Sorbitol
Stavudine
Streptokinase
Streptozocin
Succimer
Succinylcholine Chloride
Sufentanil Citrate
Sulconazole Nitrate
Sullabenzamide/ Sulfacetamide/ Sulfathiazole
Sulfacetamide Sodium and Sulfur
Sulfacetamide Sodium, Ophthalmic
Sulfacetamide Sodium, Topical
Sulfadiazine
Sulfamethizole
Sulfamethoxazole
Sulfamethoxazole and Trimethoprim
Sulfanilamide
Sulfaoxazole Diolamine, Ophthalmic
Sulfaoxazole, Oral
Sumatriptan Succinate
Suprofan
Tacrine Hydrochloride
Tacrolimus
Terazosin Hydrochloride
Terconazole
Terfenadine
Teriparatide Acetate
Testolactone
Tetanus Immune Globulin
Tetanus Toxoid Adsorbed
Tetracaine Hydrochloride, Injectable
Tetrahydrozoline Hydrochloride
Theophylline
Thiabendazole
Thiopental Sodium
Thioridazine Hydrochloride
Thiothixene
Thrombin
Thyrotropin
Timolol Maleate, Ophthalmic
Timolol Maleate, Oral
Tioconazole
Tiopronin
Tocainide Hydrochloride
Tolazamide
Tolazoline Hydrochloride
Tolbutamide
Tolbutamide Sodium
Tolmetin Sodium
Tranylcypromine Sulfate
Trazodone Hydrochloride
Tretinoin
Triamcinolone Acetonide, Inhalation
Triamcinolone Acetonide, Topical
Triamcinolone Diacetate
Triamcinolone Hexacetonide
Trientine Hydrochloride
Triethanolamine Polypeptide Oleate-Condensate
Trifluoperazine Hydrochloride
Triflupromazine Hydrochloride
Trifluridine
Trimethoprim
Trimipramine Maleate
Troleandomycin
Tromethamine
Tuberculin
Tubocurarine Chloride
Typhoid Vaccine
Vancomycin Hydrochloride
Vasopressin
Vecuronium Bromide
Venlafaxine Hydrochloride
Verapamil Hydrochloride
Vidarabine
Vitamin B12
Vitamin C
Vitamin K
Yellow Fever Vaccine
Zalcitabine
Zidovudine

B

NO EVIDENCE OF RISK IN HUMANS

Either animal findings show risk while human findings do not, or, if no adequate human studies have been done, animal findings are negative.

Acebutolol Hydrochloride
Acetylcysteine
Acrivastine and Pseudoephedrine Hydrochloride
Amiloride Hydrochloride
Amiloride Hydrochloride with Hydrochlorothiazide
Amoxicillin
Amoxicillin with Clavulanate Potassium
Amphotericin B, Injectable
Ampicillin
Ampicillin Sodium and Sulbactam Sodium
Aprotinin
Arginine Hydrochloride
Aspirin/Oxycodone Hydrochloride/ Oxycodone Terephthalate
Azatadine Maleate
Azithromycin
Aztreonam
Bacampicillin Hydrochloride
Bentiromide
Brompheniramine Maleate, Injectable
Bupropion Hydrochloride
Buspirone Hydrochloride
Carbenicillin Indanyl Sodium
Cefaclor
Cefadroxil Monohydrate
Cefamandole Nafate
Cefazolin Sodium
Cefixime
Cefmetazole Sodium
Cefonicid Sodium
Cefoperazone Sodium
Cefotaxime Sodium
Cefotetan Disodium
Cefoxitin Sodium
Cefpodoxime Proxetil
Cefprozil
Ceftazidime
Ceftizoxime Sodium
Ceftriaxone Sodium
Cefuroxime Axetil
Cefuroxime Sodium
Cephalexin
Cephalothin Sodium
Cephapirin Sodium
Cephradine
Chlorhexidine Gluconate
Chlorothiazide and Methyldopa
Chlorpheniramine Maleate with Phenylpropanol-amine Hydrochloride
Chlorpheniramine Maleate, Injectable
Chlorpheniramine Maleate/ Dextromethorphan Hydrobromide/ Guaifenesin/Phenyl-propanolamine Hydrochloride
Chlorthalidone
Ciclopirox Olamine
Cimetidine
Clavulanate Potassium with Ticarcillin Disodium
Clemastine Fumarate
Clindamycin, Systemic
Clindamycin, Topical
Clindamycin, Vaginal
Clotrimazole
Cloxacillin Sodium
Clozapine
Cromolyn Sodium
Cromolyn Sodium, Oral
Cyclobenzaprine Hydrochloride
Cyproheptadine Hydrochloride
Dapiprazole Hydrochloride
Desflurane
Desmopressin Acetate
Dexchlorpheniramine Maleate
Dextran-1
Dextrothyroxine Sodium
Diclofenac, Ophthalmic
Diclofenac, Oral
Dicyclomine Hydrochloride
Didanosine
Diethylpropion Hydrochloride
Dimenhydrinate, Injectable
Diphenhydramine Hydrochloride
Dipivefrin Hydrochloride
Dipyridamole, Injectable
Dipyridamole, Oral
Dornase Alfa
Doxapram Hydrochloride
Edetate Calcium Disodium
Enflurane
Enoxaparin
Erythromycin, Injectable
Erythromycin, Ophthalmic
Erythromycin, Oral
Erythromycin, Topical
Ethacrynic Acid
Ethambutol Hydrochloride
Etidocaine Hydrochloride
Famciclovir
Famotidine
Flavoxate Hydrochloride
Fluoxetine Hydrochloride
Flurbiprofen, Oral
Glucagon
Glyburide
Glycopyrrolate
Gonadorelin Acetate
Gonadorelin Hydrochloride
Granisetron Hydrochloride
Guanadrel Sulfate
Guanethidine Monosulfate with Hydrochlorothiazide
Guanfacine Hydrochloride
Haloprogin
Hydrochlorothiazide
Indapamide
Indomethacin
Insulin-Pork, Concentrated
Iodamide Meglumine
Iohexol
Iopamidol
Iothalamate
Iothalamate Meglumine
Iothalamate Meglumine and Iothalamate Sodium
Ioversol

Ioxaglate Meglumine and Ioxaglate Sodium
Ipratropium Bromide
Isosorbide
Isosorbide Mononitrate
Ketoprofen
Lactulose
Levocamiline
Lidocaine Hydrochloride, Injectable
Lidocaine Hydrochloride, Local Anesthesia
Lidocaine with Prilocaine
Lidocaine, Topical
Lincomycin Hydrochloride
Lindane
Lodoxamide Tromethamine
Loperamide Hydrochloride
Loracarbef
Loratadine
Malathion
Maprotiline Hydrochloride
Masoprocol
Meclizine Hydrochloride
Meclocycline Sulfosalicytate
Meclofenamate Sodium
Mesalamine
Mesna
Methdilazine Hydrochloride
Methicillin Sodium
Methohexital Sodium
Methyclothiazide
Methyldopa
Metoclopramide Hydrochloride
Metolazone
Metrizamide
Metronidazole, Systemic
Metronidazole, Topical
Metronidazole, Vaginal
Mezlocillin Sodium
Molindone Hydrochloride
Moricizine Hydrochloride
Mupirocin
Nafcillin Sodium
Naftifine Hydrochloride
Nalbuphine Hydrochloride
Naloxone Hydrochloride
Naproxen
Nedocromil Sodium
Niclosamide
Nitrofurantoin
Nystatin, Topical
Octreotide Acetate
Ondansetron Hydrochloride
Oxacillin Sodium
Oxiconazole Nitrate
Oxybutynin Chloride
Oxycodone Hydrochloride
Oxytetracycline Hydrochloride/ Phenazopyridine/ Sulfamethizole
Paroxetine Hydrochloride
Pemoline
Penicillin G Benzathine
Penicillin G Benzathine and Penicillin G Procaine
Penicillin G Potassium
Penicillin G Procaine
Penicillin G Sodium
Penicillin V Potassium
Pergolide Mesylate
Permethrin
Phenazopyridine Hydrochloride
Phenazopyridine Hydrochloride and Sulfamethoxazole
Phenazopyridine Hydrochloride and Sulfisoxazole
Pindolol
Piperacillin Sodium
Piperacillin Sodium and Tazobactam Sodium
Praziquantel
Prednisolone Tebutate
Prednisone
Prilocaine Hydrochloride and Prilocaine with Epinephrine
Probenecid
Probucol
Propofol
Ranitidine Hydrochloride
Rifabutin
Ritodrine Hydrochloride
Rocuronium Bromide
Sertraline Hydrochloride
Silver Sulfadiazine
Sincalide
Sotalol Hydrochloride
Spectinomycin Hydrochloride
Spironolactone
Staphage Lysate (SPL)
Sucralfate
Sulfasalazine
Sutilains
Terbinafine Hydrochloride
Terbutaline Sulfate
Tetracycline Hydrochloride, Topical
Ticarcillin Disodium
Ticlopidine Hydrochloride
Tobramycin
Torsemide
Tranexamic Acid
Triamterene
Trichlormethiazide
Urokinase
Ursodiol
Zolpidem Tartrate

A

CONTROLLED STUDIES SHOW NO RISK

Adequate, well-controlled studies in pregnant women have failed to demonstrate risk to the fetus.

Ferrous Sulfate/ Folic Acid/ Vitamins, Multi
Levothyroxine Sodium
Liothyronine Sodium
Liotrix
Lysine/Vitamin B Complex/Zinc Sulfate
Magnesium Sulfate, Injectable
Thyroid
Vitamin B1
Vitamin B6, Injectable

Drugs Excreted in Breast Milk

The following is a selection of drug products, listed in alphabetical order, that can be excreted in breast milk. The list is not comprehensive. Generics and alternate brands of some products may exist. When recommending to pregnant or nursing patients, always check product labeling for specific precautions for taking any drug product.

Actifed with Codeine
Adalat
Adapin
Aldactazide
Aldactone
Aldoclor
Aldomet
Aldoril
Alfenta
Ambien
Amen
Anatuss LA
Ansaid
Asacol
Asendin
Astramorph/PF
Atretol
Atromid-S
Augmentin
Axid
Azactam
Azo Gantanol
Azo Gantrisin
Azulfidine
Bactrim
Bentyl
Biavax II
Bicillin C-R
Bicillin L-A
Biltricide
Biocadren
Bricanyl
Butisol Sodium
Cafergot
Calan
Capoten
Capozide
Cardioquin
Cardizem
Cataflam
Catapres
Cefizox
Cefotan
Cellin
Centrax
Ceptaz
Choledyl
Cinobac
Cipro
Claforan
Claritin
Cleocin
Clozaril
Combipres
Compazine
Cordarone
Corgard
Cortisporin
Cortone Acetate
Corzide
Coumadin
Cycrin
Cystospaz
Cytotec
Cytoxan
Damason-P
Dapsone
Daraprim
Decadron
Demerol Hydrochloride
Demulen
Depakene
Depakote
Depo-Provera
Deprol
Desogen
Desoxyn
Desyrel
Dexedrine
Diabinese
Didrex
Diflucan
Dilacor XR
Dilantin
Dilaudid
Diprivan
Disalcid
Diucardin
Diupres
Diuril
Diuril Sodium
Dolobid
Doral
Doryx
Duragesic
Duramorph
Duratuss HD
Dyazide
Dyrenium
E-Mycin
E.E.S.
Elavil
Empirin with Codeine
Endep
Enduron
Equagesic
Ergomar
Ery-Tab
ERYC
EryPed
Erythrocin Stearate
Esgic
Esidrix
Esimil
Eskalith
Ethmozine
Fansidar
Fedahist
Felbatol
Fioricet
Fioricet with Codeine
Fiorinal
Fiorinal with Codeine
Flagyl
Florinef Acetate
Floxin
Fluorescite
Fortaz
Gantanol
Gantrisin
Halcion
Haldol
Hydeltra-T.B.A.
Hydeltrasol
Hydrocortone
HydroDIURIL
Hydromox
Hydropres
Hylorel
Ilosone
Imitrex
Imuran
Inderal
Inderide

Indocin
INH
Inversine
Isoptin
Keflex
Kefurox
Kefzol
Kerlone
Konaklon
Kutrase
Lamprene
Lanoxicaps
Lanoxin
Lariam
Lasix
Lescol
Levothroid
Levsin
Levsinex
Lincocin
Lindane
Lioresal
Lithium Carbonate
Lithobid
Lo/Ovral
Lomotil
Loniten
Lopressor
Lopressor HCT
Lortab ASA
Lotensin
Ludiomil
Lufyllin
Lufyllin-GG
Macrobid
Macrodantin
Marinol
Maxzide
Mefoxin
Mepergan
Meruvax II
Methergine
Methotrexate Sodium
MetroGel
Mezlin
Midamor
Miltown
Minizide
Minocin
Moduretic
Mono-Gesic
Monocid
Monodox
Monopril
MS Contin
MSIR
Mykrox
Myochrysine
Mysoline
Naprosyn
Nembutal Sodium
Neosar
Nicorette
Nizoral
Nordette
Norlutate
Normodyne
Norpace
Novahistine DH
Novahistine Expectorant
Nucofed
Nucofed Expectorant
Nydrazid
Obetrol
Ogen
Oramorph SR
Oretic
Ortho-Cept
Ortho-Cyclen
Ortho-Est
Ortho Tri-Cyclen
Ovcon
Ovral
Ovrette
Oxistat
Paxil
PCE
Pediazole
PediOtic
Pentasa
Persantine
Pfizerpen
Pfizerpen-AS
Phenergan with Codeine
Phenergan VC with Codeine
Phenobarbital
Phrenilin
Phrenilin Forte
PMB
Pravachol
Prinzide
Procan SR
Proloprim
Propulsid
Prostep
Protostat
Provera
Prozac
Psorcon
Pyrazinamide
Quadrinal
Quarzan
Quibron
Quibron-T
Quinaglute
Quinamm
Quinidex
Reglan
Rescudose
Reserpine
Ridaura
Rifamate
Rimactane
Robaxisal
Rocaltrol
Rocephin
Rogaine
Roxanol
Salflex
Sandimmune
Sectral
Sedapap
Semprex-D
Septra
Ser-Ap-Es
Seromycin
Slo-bid
Solganal
Soma
Soma Compound
Soma Compound with Codeine
Spectrobid
Sporanox
Stadol NS
Stelazine
Synthroid
Syntocinon
T-PHYL
Tagamet
Tambocor
Tavist
Tazicef
Tegretol
Tenoretic
Tenormin
Tenuate
Testoderm
Thalitone
Theo-24
Theo-Dur
Theo-X
Theolair
Thiosulfil Forte
Thorazine
Ticlid
Timolide
Timoptic
Tolectin
Toprol-XL
Trandate
Tranxene
Trental
Trillsate
Trimpex
Triostat
Triphasil
Tylenol with Codeine
Unasyn
Uniphyl
Vancaril
Vancocin Hydrochloride
Vantin
Vascor
Vaseretic
Vasotac
Versed
Vibra-Tabs
Vibramycin Hyctate
Vibramycin Monohydrate
Vicodin ES
Visken
Voltaren
Wygesic
Xanax
Zantac
Zaroxolyn
Zefazone
Zestoratic
Ziac
Zinacef
Zosyn
Zovirax
Zyloprim

Drug Product Abbreviations and Dosage Forms

Drug Product	Example	Company	Description/Comment
Caplet	Advil Caplet	Whitehall	Ibuprofen in a capsule-shaped compressed tablet (caplet)
Chronotab	Disophrol Chronotab	Schering	Dexbrompheniramine maleate/pseudoephedrine sulfate controlled release tablet
CR	Norspace CR	Searle	Disopyramide phosphate (controlled release) capsule
Depo	Depo-Medrol	Upjohn	Sterile methylprednisolone acetate suspension
Dispertabs	PCE	Abbott	Erythromycin enteric coated particles in a tablet
Dividose	Desyrel	Mead Johnson	Trazodone in a bisected/trisected tablet
Dospan	Tenuate Dospan	Marion Merrell Dow	Diethylproprion hydrochloride controlled release tablet
DS	Septra DS	Burroughs Wellcome	Trimethoprim/Sulfamethoxazole (Double Strength)
Dura-tab	Quinaglute	Berlex	Quinidine gluconate sustained release tablet
Enduret	Preludine Enduret	Boehringer-Ingelheim	Phenmetrazine hydrochloride prolonged action tablets
Enseal	DES Enseals	Lilly	Enteric coated
Extencaps	Micro-K Extencaps	Robins	Microencapsulated potassium chloride controlled release capsule
Extentab	Dimetane Extentabs	Robins	Brompheniramine maleate extended (controlled) release tablets
Filmtab	Erythrocin Stearate Filmtab	Abbott	Erythromycin stearate film coated compressed tablet
Forte	Thiosulfil Forte	Wyeth-Ayerst	Higher dose (0.5 g) sulfamethizole (Forte = stronger)
GITS	Procardia XL	Pfizer	Nifedipine gastrointestinal therapeutic system
Gradumet	Desoxyn Gradumet	Abbott Pharmaceuticals	Methamphetamine hydrochloride sustained release tablet
Gyrocap	Slo-Bid Gyrocaps	Rhone-Poulenc	Theophylline anhydrous controlled release capsule
Infatab	Dilantin Infatabs	Parke-Davis	Phenytoin tablets, USP
Kapseals	Dilantin Kapseals	Parke-Davis	Extended phenytoin sodium capsule (Kapseal = sealed hard gelatin capsule)
LA	Inderal LA	Wyeth-Ayerst	Propranolol hydrochloride (long acting) capsule
Ocumeter	Timoptic	Merck Sharp & Dohme	Ophthalmic drop dispenser
Oros	Acutrim	CIBA Geigy	Phenylpropanolamine HCl controlled release osmotic tablet
Pennkinetic	Tussionex	Pennwalt	Hydrocodone polistirex/chlorpheniramine polistirex extended release ion exchange suspension
Perles	Tessalon Perles	Du Pont	Benzonatate in a soft gelatin capsule (Perle)
Plateau Caps	Nitro-Bid Plateau Caps	Marion Merrell Dow	Nitroglycerin controlled release capsules
Progestasert	Progestasert	Alza	Intrauterine progesterone contraceptive system
Pulvule	Darvon Compound	Lilly	Propoxyphene hydrochloride/aspirin/caffeine capsule (Pulvule)
Repetabs	Polaramine Repetabs	Schering	Dexchlorpheniramine maleate repeat action tablets
RTU	Flagyl I.V. RTU	Searle	Metroidazole injection ready-to-use (RTU)
SA	Sudafed SA	Burroughs Wellcome	Pseudoephedrine hydrochloride sustained release (sustained action) tablet

Continued on next page

Drug Product Abbreviations and Dosage Forms—*continued*

Drug Product	Example	Company	Description/Comment
Sequels	Ferro-Sequels	Lederle	Ferrous (iron) fumarate sustained release capsule
Softab	Bucladin-S	Stuart	Buclizine chewable tablet
Spansule	Dexedrine Spansule	SmithKline Beecham	Dextroamphetamine sulfate controlled release capsule
Spinhaler	Intal Inhaler	Fisons	Cromolyn sodium inhalation aerosol for delivery of powder from capsule
Sprinkle	Theo-Dur Sprinkle	Key	Microencapsulated theophylline granules contained in capsule which may be swallowed whole or sprinkled on food
SR	Elixophyllin SR	Berlex	(Sustained release) theophylline
Tabloid	Empirin Aspirin tablets	Burroughs Wellcome	Compressed tablet (Tabloid) containing 325 mg aspirin
Tembids	Isordil Tembids capsules	Wyeth-Ayerst	Isosorbide dinitrate controlled release capsule
Tempules	Nicobid Tempules	Rhone-Poulenc	Niacin timed release capsule
Ten-tab	Tepanil Ten-tab	3M Riker Laboratories	Diethylpropion hydrochloride sustained release tablets
Timesule	Isoclor Timesul	Fisons	Chlorpheniramine maleate/pseudoephedrine sulfate controlled release capsule
Tubex	Closed injection system	Wyeth-Ayerst	Injection system for delivering premeasured doses of medication
-Dur	Theo-Dur	Key	Theophylline anhydrous sustained release

Dietary Considerations

Potassium and Tyramine Content of Foods and Beverages

Potassium Content of Selected Foods, Beverages, and Salt Substitutes*†

Beverages [8 fl ℥]	mg	mEq
Apple juice, bottled/canned	296	7.6
Apricot juice, nectar, canned	286	7.3
Grape juice, bottled/canned	334	8.5
Grapefruit juice, canned	378	9.7
Milk, whole, 3.5% fat (high in sodium)	351	9.0
Milk, lowfat, 2% fat (high in sodium)	377	9.6
Milk, skim (high in sodium)	406	10.4
Orange juice, fresh	496	12.7
Orange juice, canned	436	11.2
Pineapple juice, canned	334	8.5
Pruce juice, canned	706	18.1
Tangerine juice, canned	443	11.3
Tomato juice, canned (high in sodium)	598	15.3

Fruits	mg	mEq
Apricots, raw, 3 medium	313	8.0
Banana, raw, 1 medium	451	11.5
Cantaloupe, raw, 1 cup pieces	494	12.6
Dates, dried, 10	541	13.8
Figs, dried, 10	1332	34.1
Fruit cocktail, canned, 1 cup	230	5.9
Grapefruit, pink, raw, ½ medium	158	4.0
Orange, navel, raw, 1 medium	250	6.4
Peach, raw, 1 medium	171	4.4
Pear, raw, 1 medium	208	5.3
Pineapple, raw, 1 cup pieces	175	4.5
Prunes, dried, 10	626	16.0
Raisins, seedless, ⅔ cup	751	19.2
Strawberries, raw, 1 cup	247	6.3
Watermelon, raw, 1 cup	186	4.8

Vegetables	mg	mEq
Avocado, raw, 1 medium (California)	1097	28.1
Avocado, raw, 1 medium (Florida)	1484	38.0
Beans, green lima, cooked, ½ cup	338	8.6
Beans, red kidney, cooked, ½ cup	425	10.9
Broccoli, cooked, ⅔ cup	267	6.8
Brussels sprouts, cooked 6—8 medium	273	7.0
Carrot, raw, 1 large	341	8.7
Corn, yellow, canned, ½ cup	138	3.5
Mushrooms, raw, 10 small	414	10.6
Potato, baked, 1 medium	503	12.9
Spinach, cooked, ½ cup	291	7.4
Squash, winter, baked, ½ cup	461	11.8
Tomato, raw, 1 medium	366	9.4

Salt Substitutes	mg	mEq
Adolph's, 1 g	485	12.4
Co-Salt, 1 g	469	12.0
Diasal, 1 g	442	11.3
Featherweight K, 1 g	465	11.9
Lite-Salt, 1 g (high in sodium)	293	7.4
Morton, 1 g	504	12.9
Neocurtasal, 1 g	470	12.1
NoSalt (Regular), 1 g	500	12.8
NoSalt (Seasoned), 1 g	266	6.8
Nu-Salt, 1 g	434	11.1
Salfree, 1 g	548	14.1

*Food values adaped from Pennington JAT, Church HN: *Bowes and Church's Food Values of Portions Commonly Used,* 14th ed. Philadelphia, JB Lippincott, 1985.

†Potassium content amounts are approximations. Salt substitute formulations, and hence potassium content, are subject to change by manufacturer. Salt substitute values from: Pearson RE, Fish KH: Potassium content of selected medicines, foods and salt substitutes. *Hosp Pharm* 1971;6:6–9; Sopko JA, Freeman RM: Salt substitutes as a source of potassium. *JAMA* 1977; 238:608–10; and product information.

Tyramine Content of Foods and Beverages*†

Alcoholic Beverages	Estimated Levels‡
Beer and ale§	Low
Chartreuse‖	Unknown
Drambuie‖	Unknown
Sherry‖	Low
Wine, red#	Low
Wine, white**	Little or none

Cheese	Estimated Levels‡
American, processed	Low
Blue	Moderate to high
Boursault	Very high
Brick, natural	Moderage to high
Brie	Moderate to high
Camembert	Very high
Cheddar	Very high
Cottage cheese	Little or none
Cream cheese	Little or none
Emmenthaler	Very high
Gruyere	Moderate to high
Mozzarella	Moderate to high
Parmesan	Moderate to high
Romano	Moderate to high
Roquefort	Moderate to high
Stilton	Very high

Fruits	Estimated Levels‡
Bananas	Low
Figs, canned, particularly if overripe	Low to moderate

Meat and Fish	Estimated Levels‡
Beef liver, unrefrigerated, fermented	Moderate
Caviar	High
Chicken, liver, unrefrigerated, fermented	Moderate
Fish, unrefrigerated, fermented	Moderate
Fish, dried	Moderate
Herring, dried, salted	Moderate to high
Herring, pickled, if spoiled	Highest levels found
Sausages, fermented: Bologna, Pepperoni, Salami, Summer sausage	Very high
Other unrefrigerated, fermented meats	Moderate

Vegetables	Estimated Levels‡
Avocado, particularly if overripe	Low to moderate
Broad bean pods	Probably contain dopamine
Fava beans, particularly if overripe	Contain dopamine

Other Foods and Beverages	Estimated Levels‡
Caffeine, very large amounts	A weak pressor agent
Chocolate, very large amounts	Contains phenylethylamine, a weak pressor agent
Yeast extracts such as Marmete††	Very high

*Anon: Monoamine oxidase inhibitors for depression. *Med Lett Drugs Ther* 1980;22:58–60.

†For more detailed information, consult McCabe B, Tsuang MT: Dietary consideration in MAO inhibitor regimens. *J Clin Psychiatry* 1982;43:178–81.

‡The tyramine content of most foods is not entirely predictable. These estimates are taken from isolated reports, some based on small samples. The amount of tyramine in food and beverages could vary with different conditions, different samples, and different manufacturers.

§Fermentation of beer does not ordinarily involve processes that produce tyramine. However, the amount can vary greatly, and some imported beers have caused reactions in patients taking MAO inhibitors. McCabe and Tsuang (footnote †) state that beer is among the most important food restrictions and should be avoided.

‖Some patients have had reactions.

#Fermentation of wine does not ordinarily produce tyramine. However, contamination with other than the usual fermenting organisms and production of appreciable amounts of tyramine have occurred in Chianti and could occur in any red wine.

**White wine is free of tyramine because it is made without the grape pulp and seeds, which may be the source of amino acids in red wine.

††Baked goods do not contain appreciable amounts of tyramine.

APPENDIX D

STATE AND NATIONAL PHARMACY ORGANIZATIONS

Colleges and Schools of Pharmacy

UNITED STATES

Alabama

School of Pharmacy
Auburn University
Alabama 36849-5501
334-844-8351

School of Pharmacy
Samford University
800 Lakeshore Drive
Birmingham, AL 35229
205-870-2820

Arizona

College of Pharmacy
The University of Arizona
Tuscon, AZ 85721
520-626-1427

Arkansas

College of Pharmacy
University of Arkansas for Medical Sciences
4301 West Markham Slot 522
Little Rock, AR 72205-7122
501-686-5557

California

School of Pharmacy
University of California S-926
San Francisco, CA 94143-0446
415-476-1225

School of Pharmacy
University of the Pacific
3601 Pacific Avenue
Stockton, CA 95211
209-946-2561

School of Pharmacy
University of Southern California
1985 Zonal Avenue
Los Angeles, CA 90033-1086
213-342-1369

Colorado

School of Pharmacy
University of Colorado
Health Sciences Center C238
4200 East Ninth Avenue
Denver, CO 80262-0238
303-270-5055

Connecticut

School of Pharmacy
The University of Connecticut
Box U-92/372 Fairfield Roac
Storrs, CT 06269-2092
860-486-2129

District of Columbia

College of Pharmacy & Pharmaceutical Sciences
Howard University
2300 4th Street N.W.
Washington, DC 20059
202-806-6530

Florida

College of Pharmacy & Pharmaceutical Sciences
Florida Agricultural and Mechanical University
Tallahassee, FL 32307-3800
904-599-3593

College of Pharmacy
Nova Southeastern University
1750 NE 167th Street
N. Miami Beach, FL 33162-3097
305-949-4000

College of Pharmacy
University of Florida
Box 100484
Health Science Center
Gainesville, FL 32610-0484
904-392-9713

Georgia

Southern School of Pharmacy
Mercer University
3001 Mercer University Drive
Atlanta, GA 30341-4155
770-986-3300

College of Pharmacy
University of Georgia
Athens, GA 30602-2351
706-542-1911

Idaho

College of Pharmacy
Idaho State University
Pocatello, ID 83209-0009
208-236-2175

Illinois

Chicago College of Pharmacy
Midwestern University
555 31st Street
Downers Grove, IL 60515-1235
708-971-6417

College of Pharmacy
University of Illinois at Chicago
833 South Wood Street
Chicago, IL 60515-1235
312-996-7240

Indiana

College of Pharmacy and Health Sciences
Butler University
4600 Sunset Avenue
Indianapolis, IN 46208
317-940-9322

School of Pharmacy and Pharmaceutical Sciences
1330 Heine Pharmacy Building
Purdue University
West Lafayette, IN 47907-1330
317-494-1357

Iowa

College of Pharmacy
Drake University
2507 University Avenue
Des Moines, IA 50311-4505
515-271-2172

College of Pharmacy
The University of Iowa
Iowa City, IA 52242
319-335-8794

Kansas

School of Pharmacy
University of Kansas
2056 Malott
Lawrence, KS 66045-2500
913-864-3591

Kentucky

College of Pharmacy
University of Kentucky
Rose Street—Pharmacy Building
Lexington, KY 40536-0082
606-247-2737

Louisiana

School of Pharmacy
Northeast Louisiana University
700 University Avenue
Monreo, LA 71209-0470
318-342-1600

College of Pharmacy
Xavier University of Louisiana
7325 Palmetto Street
New Orleans, LA 70125
504-483-7424

Maryland

School of Pharmacy
University of Maryland
20 North Pine Street
Baltimore, MD 21201-1180
410-706-7650

Massachusetts

Massachusetts College of Pharmacy and Allied Health Sciences
179 Longwood Avenue
Boston, MA 02115-5896
617-732-2800

Bouve College of Pharmacy and Health Sciences
Northeastern University
360 Huntington Avenue
Boston, MA 02115
617-373-3321

Michigan

College of Pharmacy
Ferris State University
220 Ferris Drive
Big Rapids, MI 49307-2740
616-592-2254

College of Pharmacy
The University of Michigan
Ann Arbor, MI 48109-1065
313-764-7312

College of Pharmacy and Allied Health Professions
Wayne State University
105 Shapero Hall
Detroit, MI 48202-3489
313-577-1574

Minnesota

College of Pharmacy
University of Minnesota
5-130 Health Sciences Unit F
308 Harvard Street SE
Minneapolis, MN 55455-0343
612-624-1900

Mississippi

School of Pharmacy
The University of Mississippi
University, MS 38677-9814
601-232-7265

Missouri

St. Louis College of Pharmacy
4588 Parkview Place
St. Louis, MO 63110-1088
314-367-8700

School of Pharmacy
University of Missouri—Kansas City
5005 Rockhill Road
Kansas City, MO 64110-2499
816-235-1609

Montana

School of Pharmacy and Allied Health Professions
University of Montana
Missoula, MT 59812-1075
406-243-4621

Nebraska

School of Pharmacy and Allied Health Professions
Creighton University
2500 California Plaza
Omaha, NE 68178
402-280-2950

College of Pharmacy
University of Nebraska
600 S. 42nd Street
Omaha, NE 68198-6000
402-559-4333

New Jersey

College of Pharmacy
Rutgers University
The State University of New Jersey
PO Box 789
Piscataway, NJ 08855-0789
908-445-2666

New Mexico

College of Pharmacy
Health Sciences Center
The University of New Mexico
Albuquerque, NM 87131-6749
505-277-6749

New York

Arnold & Marie Schwartz
College of Pharmacy and
Health Sciences
Long Island University
75 DeKalb Avenue at
University Plaza
Brooklyn, NY 11201
718-488-1060

College of Pharmacy and Allied
Health Professions
St. John's University
Grand Central and Utopia
Parkways
Jamaica, NY 11439
718-990-6275

School of Pharmacy
University at Buffalo
C126 Cooke-Hochstetter
Complex
Buffalo, NY 14260-1200
716-645-2823

Albany College of Pharmacy
Union University
106 New Scotland
Albany, NY 12208
518-445-7200

North Carolina

School of Pharmacy
Campbell University
PO Box 1090
Bules Creek, NC 27506
910-893-1200

School of Pharmacy
University of North Carolina
Beard Hall CB#7360
Chapel Hill, NC 27599-7360
919-966-1121

North Dakota

College of Pharmacy
Box 5055
North Dakota State University
Fargo, ND 58105
701-231-7456

Ohio

College of Pharmacy
Ohio Northern University
Ada, OH 45810
419-772-2275

College of Pharmacy
The Ohio State University
500 West 12th Avenue
Columbus, OH 43210-1291
614-292-2266

College of Pharmacy
University of Cincinnati—
Medical Center
PO Box 670004
Cincinnati, OH 45267-0004
513-558-3784

College of Pharmacy
The University of Toledo
2801 West Bancroft Street
Toledo, OH 43606-3390
419-530-2019

Oklahoma

School of Pharmacy
Southwestern Oklahoma State
University
100 Campus Drive
Weatherford, OK 73096
405-774-3105

College of Pharmacy
University of Oklahoma
PO Box 26901
Oklahoma City, OK
73190-5040
405-271-6484

Oregon

College of Pharmacy
Oregon State University
Pharmacy Building 203
Corvallis, OR 97331-3999
503-737-3424

Pennsylvania

Mylan School of Pharmacy
Duquesne University
Pittsburgh, PA 15282
412-396-6380

School of Pharmacy
Philadelphia College of
Pharmacy and Science
600 South Forty-Third Street
Philadelphia, PA 19104-4495
215-596-8870

School of Pharmacy
Temple University of the
Commonwealth System of
Higher Education
3307 North Broad Street
Philadelphia, PA 19140
215-707-4990

School of Pharmacy
University of Pittsburgh
1106 Salk Hall
Pittsburgh, PA 15261
412-648-8579

Puerto Rico

School of Pharmacy
University of Puerto Rico
PO Box 365067
San Juan, PR 00936-5067
809-758-2525

Rhode Island

College of Pharmacy
University of Rhode Island
Kingston, RI 02881-0809
401-874-2761

South Carolina

College of Pharmacy
Medical University of South
Carolina
171 Ashley Avenue
Charleston, SC 29425-2301
803-792-3115

College of Pharmacy
University of South Carolina
Columbia, SC 29208
803-777-4151

South Dakota

College of Pharmacy
South Dakota State University
Box 2202C
Brookings, SD 57007-0099
605-688-6197

Tennessee

College of Pharmacy
University of Tennessee
847 Monroe Avenue, Suite 200
Memphis, TN 38163
901-448-6036

Texas

College of Pharmacy and Health Sciences
Texas Southern University
3100 Cleburne
Houston, TX 77004
713-313-7164

College of Pharmacy
University of Houston
4800 Calhoun
Houston, TX 77204-5511
713-743-1300

College of Pharmacy
University of Texas at Austin
Austin, TX 78712-1074
512-471-1737

Utah

College of Pharmacy
University of Utah
Salt Lake City, UT 84112
801-581-6731

Virginia

School of Pharmacy
Virginia Commonwealth University
MCV Campus—Box 980581
410 North 12th Street
Richmond, VA 23928-7436
804-828-3000

Shenandoah University
1460 University Drive
Winchester, VA 22601
540-665-1282

Washington

School of Pharmacy
University of Washington
H-364 Health Science Center
Box 357631
Seattle, WA 98195
206-543-2453

College of Pharmacy
Washington State University
Pullman, WA 99164-6510
509-335-8664

West Virginia

School of Pharmacy
WVU HSC 1136 HSN
PO Box 9500
Morgantown, WV 26506-9500
304-293-5101

Wisconsin

School of Pharmacy
University of Wisconsin—Madison
425 North Charter Street
Madison, WI 53706
608-262-1416

Wyoming

School of Pharmacy
University of Wyoming
PO Box 3375
Laramie, WY 82071-3375
307-766-6120

NEW SCHOOLS

California

College of Osteopathic Medicine of the Pacific
School of Pharmacy
College Plaza, 309 E. Second Street
Pomona, CA 91766-1889
909-469-5500

Texas

School of Pharmacy
Texas Tech University
Regional Academic Health Center
1400 Wallace Boulevard
Amarillo, TX 79106
806-354-5411

Pennsylvania

School of Pharmacy
Wilkes University
Wilkes-Barre, PA 18766
717-831-4280

SCHOOLS AND COLLEGES OF CANADA

Alberta

Faculty of Pharmacy and Pharmaceutical Sciences
The University of Alberta
Edmonton, AB
Canada T6G 2N8
403-492-3362

British Columbia

Faculty of Pharmaceutical Sciences
University of British Columbia
2146 East Mall
Vancouver, BC
Canada V6T 1Z3
604-822-2343

Manitoba

The Faculty of Pharmacy
The University of Manitoba
Winnipeg, MB
Canada R3T 2N2
204-474-8794

Newfoundland

Memorial University of Newfoundland
Health Science Centre
St. John's, NF
Canada A1B 3V6
709-737-6571

Nova Scotia

College of Pharmacy
Dalhousie University
5698 College Street
Halifax, NS
Canada B3H 3J5
902-494-2378

Ontario

Faculty of Pharmacy
University of Toronto
19 Russell Street
Toronto, ON
Canada M5S 2S2
416-978-2889

Quebec

Ecole de Pharmacie
Universite Laval
Quebec, PO
Canada G1K 7P4
418-656-3211

Faculte de Pharmacie
Universite de Montreal
C.P. 6126 Succursale
Centre-Ville
Montreal, PO
Canada H3C 3J7
514-343-6422

Saskatchewan

College of Pharmacy and
Nutrition
University of Saskatchewan
110 Science Place
Saskatoon, SK
Canada S7N 5C9
306-966-6327

PHARMACY OUTSIDE THE UNITED STATES

MALAYSIA

School of Pharmaceutical
Sciences
Universiti Sains Malaysia
Minden, Penang, 11800
Malaysia
011-60-4-657-7888

PHILIPPINES

University of the Philippines
Manila
Padre Faura
Manila, Philippines
011-632-58-58-80

THAILAND

Faculty of Pharmaceutical
Sciences
Chulalongkorn University
Phayathai Road
Bangkok 10330, Thailand
011-66-2-2528973

Faculty of Pharmacy
Mahidol University
Sri Ayutthaya Road
Bangkok 10400, Thailand
011-66-2-2474696

Faculty of Pharmacy
Chiang Mai University
Chiang Mai 50200, Thailand
011-66-53-222955

Faculty of Pharmaceutical
Sciences
Khon Kaen University
Khon Kaen, 40002, Thailand
011-66-43-236907

Faculty of Pharmacy
Slipakorn University
Sanamchan Palace Campus
Nakhon Pathom, 73000,
Thailand
011-66-34-255803

Faculty of Pharmaceutical
Sciences
Prince of Songkla University
Hat Yai Campus—Hat Yai
Songkla, 90110, Thailand
011-66-74-212824

Faculty of Pharmaceutical
Science
Ubon Ratchathani University
Ubon Ratchathani, Thailand
011-66-45-323209

UNITED KINGDOM

The Welsh School of Pharmacy
University of Wales, Cardiff
PO Box 13
King Edward VII Avenue
Cardiff, Wales CF1 3XF
011-44-1222-874781

National Pharmacy Organizations

Academy of Managed Care Pharmacy
William N. Tindali, Ph.D., R.Ph.
Executive Director
1321 Duke St., Suite 305
Alexandria, VA 22314
703-683-8416, Fax: 703-683-8417

American Association of Colleges of Pharmacy
Carl E. Trinca, Ph.D.
Executive Director
1426 Prince St.
Alexandria, VA 22314-2641
703-739-2330, Fax: 703-836-8962

American Association of Pharmaceutical Scientists
Lorraine L. Hurlbutt
Executive Director
1660 King St.
Alexandria, VA 22314-2747
703-548-3000, Fax: 703-684-7349

American College of Apothecaries
D. C. Huffman, Jr., Ph.D.
Executive Vice President
205 Daingerfield Rd.
Alexandria, VA 22314
703-684-8603, Fax: 703-683-3619

American College of Clinical Pharmacy
Robert Elenbass, Pharm.D.
Executive Director
3101 Broadway, Suite 380
Kansas City, MO 64111
816-531-2177, Fax: 816-531-4990

American Council on Pharmaceutical Education
Daniel A. Nona
Executive Director
311 W. Superior St., Suite 512
Chicago, IL 80610
312-664-3575, Fax: 312-664-4652

American Foundation for Pharmaceutical Education
Richard E. Faust, Ph.D.
President
618 Somerset St.
P.O. Box 7126
North Plainfield, NJ 07060
908-581-8077, Fax: 906-561-8169

American Institute of the History of Pharmacy
Gregory J. Higby, Ph.D.
Executive Director
425 North Charter St.
Madison, WI 53706-1508
606-262-5378

American Pharmaceutical Association
John A. Gans, Pharm.D.
Executive Vice President
2215 Constitution Ave., NW
Washington, DC. 20037
202-628-4410, Fax: 202-783-2351

American Society for Automation in Pharmacy
William A. Lockwood, Jr.
Executive Director
482 Norristown, Suite 112
Blue Bell, PA 19422
610-825-7783, Fax: 610-825-7641

American Society for Pharmacy Law
Donald A. Dee
Executive Vice President
P.O. Box 2184
Vienna, VA 22183
703-281-0107, Fax: 703-281-2897

American Society of Consultant Pharmacists
R. Timothy Webster
Executive Director
1321 Duke St.
Alexandria, VA 22314-3563
703-739-1300, Fax: 703-739-1321

American Society of Health Systems Pharmacists
Joseph A. Oddis, Sc.D.
Executive Vice President
7272 Wisconsin Ave.
Bethesda, MD 20614
301-657-3000, Fax: 301-657-1251

American Society of Pharmacognosy
Alice Clark
President
School of Pharmacy
University of Mississippi
University, MS 38677
601-232-7265, Fax: 601-232-5118

The Drug, Chemical & Allied Trades Association, Inc.
Richard J. Lerman, CCM
Executive Director
Two Roosevelt Ave., Suite 301
Syossel, NY 11791
516-496-3317, Fax: 516-496-2231

The Food and Drug Law Institute
John C. Villforth
President
1000 Vermont Ave., NW
Suite 1200
Washington, DC 20005
202-371-1420, Fax: 202-371-0649

Generic Pharmaceutical Industry Association
Lew A. Engman
President
1620 "I" St., NW., Suite 600
Washington, DC 20006
202-833-9070, Fax: 202-833-9612

National Association of Boards of Pharmacy
Carmen A. Catizone
Executive Director
700 Busse Highway
Park Ridge, IL 60068-2402
708-696-6227, Fax: 706-696-0124

National Association of Chain Drug Stores Inc.
Ronald L. Ziegier
President/CEO
413 North Lee St.
P.O. Box 1417-D49
Alexandria, VA 22313
703-549-3001, Fax: 703-836-4889

National Association of Pharmaceutical Manufacturers
Robert S. Milanese
President
320 Old Country Rd.
Garden City, L.I., NY 11530
New York, NY 10017
516-741-3699, Fax: 516-741-3696

National Association of Retail Druggists
Charles M. West
Executive Vice President
205 Daingerfield Rd.
Alexandria, VA 22314
703-683-8200, Fax: 703-683-3619

National Council for Prescription Drug Programs
Lee Ann Cleverly-Stember
President
4201 N. 24th St., Suite 365
Phoenix, AZ 85016-6266
602-957-9105, Fax: 602-955-0749

National Council of State Pharmaceutical Association Executives
A.H. Mebane, III, R.Ph.
Executive Director
P.O. Box 151
Chapel Hill, NC 27514-0151
919-967-2237, Fax: 919-968-9430

National Council on Patient Information and Education
Robert M. Bachman
Executive Director
686 11th St., NW, Suite 810
Washington, DC 20001
202-347-6711, Fax: 202-638-0773

National Managed Healthcare Congress
1000 Winter St., Suite 4000
Waltham, MA 02154
617-487-6700, Fax: 617-487-6709

National Pharmaceutical Council
Mark R. Knowles
President
1894 Preston White Dr.
Reston, VA 22091
703-620-6390, Fax: 703-476-0904

National Wholesale Druggists' Association
Ronald J. Streck
President
1621 Michael Faraday Dr., Ste. 400
Reston, VA 22090
703-767-0000, Fax: 703-767-6830

Nonprescription Drug Manufacturers Association
James D. Cope
President
1150 Connecticut Ave., NW
Washington, DC 20036
202-429-9260, Fax: 202-223-6835

Parenteral Drug Association Inc.
Edmund M. Fry
Executive Vice President
7500 Old Georgetown Rd.
Suite 620
Bethesda, MD 20614
301-966-0293, Fax: 301-966-0298

Pharmaceutical Research and Manufacturers of America
Gerald J. Mossinghoff
President
1100 15th St., NW
Washington, DC 20005
202-835-3400, Fax: 202-835-3429

State Pharmaceutical Editorial Association
Mark A. Pilkington
Secretary-Treasurer
223 W. Jackson Blvd.
Suite 1000
Chicago, IL 60606
312-939-7663, Fax: 312-939-7220

The U.S. Pharmacopeial Convention Inc.
Jarome A. Halperin
Executive Director
12601 Twinbrock Pkwy.
Rockville, MD 20652
301-881-0666, Fax: 301-816-8299

U.S. Adopted Names (USAN) Council
Fluta Freimanis, Pharm. D.
Secretariat
American Medical Association
515 N. State St.
Chicago, IL 60610
312-464-4045, Fax: 312-464-4184

State Pharmacy Organizations

Alabama
Sharon Taylor
Asst. Executive Director
1211 Carmichael Way
Montgomery, AL 36106-3672
205-271-4222, Fax: 205-271-5423

Alaska
Linda C. Hamm
Executive Director
P.O. Box 101185
Anchorage, AK 99510
907-563-8880, Fax: 907-563-8880

Arizona
Kim Roberson, R.Ph.
1845 E. Southern Ave.
Tempe, AZ 85282-5831
602-638-3365, Fax: 502-836-3557

Arkansas
Richard Back
Executive Vice President
417 S. Victory
Little Rock, AR 72201
501-372-5250, Fax: 501-372-0546

California
Robert Marshall
Chief Executive Officer
1112 "T" St. Suite 300
Sacramento, CA 95514
916-444-7811, Fax: 916-444-7929

Colorado
Val Kalnins R. Ph.
Executive Director
7853 E. Anapahoe CT., Ste. 1500
Englewood, CO 80112-1360
303-843-0326, Fax: 303-843-0786

Connecticut
Daniel C. Leone
Executive Vice President
35 Cold Spring Rd., Suite 125
Rocky Hill, CT 08067
203-583-4619, Fax: 203-257-8241

District of Columbia
James F. Harris
Executive Director
6406 Georgia Ave., NW, Ste. 202
Washington DC 20012
202-829-1515, Fax: 202-829-1515

Delaware
Maryenne Uricheck Hotzapfel, R. Ph.
Executive Director
1601 Milltown Road, Suite #8
Wilmington, DE 19808
302-892-2880, Fax: 302-892-2881

Florida
C. Rod Presnell
Executive Vice President
610 N. Adams St.
Tallahassee, FL 32301
904-222-2400, Fax: 904-561-6758

Georgia
Larry L. Braden, R. Ph.
Executive Vice President
P.O. Box 95527
Atlanta, GA 30347
404-231-5074, Fax: 404-237-8435

Hawaii
Edmund E. Ehlka
Executive Director
P.O. Box 1196
Honolulu, HI 96807
606-632-5782

Idaho
JoAnn Condie
Executive Director
1365 N. Orchard St., Suite 316
Boise, ID 83706-2250
208-376-2273, Fax: 208-376-5814

Illinois
Mark A. Pilkington
Executive Director
223 W. Jackson Blvd. Suite 1000
Chicago, IL 60606-6906
312-939-7300, Fax: 312-939-7220

Indiana
Lawrence J. Sage
Executive Vice President
729 N. Pennsylvania St.
Indianapolis, IN 46204-1171
317-634-4968, Fax: 317-632-1219

Iowa
Thomas R. Temple
Executive Vice President
8515 Douglas, Suite 16
Des Moines, IA 50322
515-270-0713, Fax: 515-270-2979

Kansas
Robert R. Williams
Executive Director
1308 W. 10th St.
Topeka, KS 66804
913-232-0439, Fax: 913-232-3764

Kentucky
Robert L. Barnett, Jr.
Executive Director
1228 U.S. Hwy. 127 S.
Frankfort, KY 40601
502-227-2303, Fax: 502-227-2258

Louisiana
Mona J. Davis
Executive Director
P.O. Box 14446
Baton Rouge, LA 70898-4446
504-926-2668, Fax: 504-926-1020

Maine
Stanley Stewart, R.Ph.
Executive Director
P.O. Box 817
Bangor, ME 04402-0817
207-947-0885, Fax: 207-947-1946

Maryland
David G. Miller
Executive Director
650 W. Lombard St.
Baltimore, MD 21201-1572
410-727-0746, Fax: 410-727-2253

Massachusetts
Linda E. Barry
Executive Vice President
5 Lexington Street, Suite 5
Waltham, MA 02154
617-736-0101

Michigan
Larry D. Wagenknecht
Executive Director
815 N. Washington Ave.
Lansing, MI 48906
517-484-1466, Fax: 517-484-4893

Minnesota
William E. Bond
Executive Director
International Court–North
2550 University Ave. W.
Suite 320N
St. Paul, MN 55114
800-451-8349 (non-metro MN)
612-644-3566, Fax: 612-644-3965

Mississippi
Sam Daniel
Executive Director
341 Edgewood Terrace Dr.
Jackson, MI 39206-6299
601-981-0416, Fax: 801-981-0451

Missouri
George L. Oestrich
Chief Executive Officer
410 Madison St.
Jefferson City, MO 65101-3189
314-636-7522, Fax: 314-636-7485

Montana
Jim Smith
Executive Director
P.O. Box 4718
Helena, MT 59604
406-449-3843, Fax: 406-443-1592

Nebraska
Tom R. Dolan, R. Ph.
Executive Director
6221 S. 58th St., Suite A
Lincoln, NE 68516
402-420-1500, Fax: 402-420-1406

Nevada
Karen Peska
Executive Director
3660 Baker Lane, Suite 204
Reno, NV 89509
702-826-3981, Fax: 702-825-0785

New Hampshire
Robert Lolley
President
2 Eagle Square, Suite 400
Concord, NH 03301-4956
603-229-0292, Fax: 603-224-7769

New Jersey
Alvin N. Gaser
Executive Officer
120 W. State St.
Trenton, NJ 06608
609-384-5596, Fax: 609-394-7806

New Mexico
R. Dale Tinker
Executive Director
4800 Zuni SE
Albuquerque, NM 57106-2896
505-265-8729, Fax: 505-255-8478

New York
Craig M. Burridge
Pine West Plaza IV
Washington Ave. Extension
Albany, NY 12205
518-669-6595, Fax: 518-454-0518

North Carolina
A.H. Mebane, III
P.O. Box 151
Chapel Hill, NC 27514-0151
919-967-2337, 800-652-7343
Fax: 919-988-9430

North Dakota
Howard C. Anderson, Jr., R.Ph.
Executive Secretary/Treasurer
P.O. Box 5006
Bismarck, ND 58502-5008
701-258-4968, Fax: 701-258-9312

Ohio
Ernest E. Boyd, Pharmacist
Executive Director
6037 Frantz Rd., Suite 106
Dublin, OH 43017
614-796-0037, Fax: 614-796-0978

Oklahoma
John D. Donner
Executive Director
45 NE 52nd St.
Box 18731
Oklahoma City, OK 73154
405-528-3338, Fax: 405-528-1417

Oregon
Chuck Gress
Executive Director
1460 State St.
Salem, OR 97301-4296
503-585-4887, Fax: 503-378-9067

Pennsylvania
Carmen A. DiCello, R.Ph.
Executive Director
508 N. Third St.
Harrisburg, PA 17101-1199
717-234-6151, Fax: 717-236-1618

Puerto Rico
LCDA Luciano Cano
President
G.P.O. Box 360206
San Juan, PR 00936-0206
809-753-7157, Fax: 809-759-9793

Rhode Island
Donald H. Fowler
Executive Director
500 Prospect St.
Pawtucket, RI 02860
401-725-4141, Fax: 401-725-9960

South Carolina
Jim Bracewell
Executive Vice President
1405 Calhoun St.
Columbia, SC 29201
803-254-1065, Fax: 803-254-9379

South Dakota
Galen Jordre
Executive Director
Box 518
Pierre, SD 57501-0518
605-224-2336, Fax: 605-224-1280

Tennessee
Baeteena Black
Executive Director
226 Capitol Blvd., Suite 810
Nashville, TN 37219
615-256-3023, Fax: 615-255-3526

Texas
Paul F. Davis
Executive Director
P.O. Box 14709
Austin, TX 78761
512-836-8350, Fax: 512-836-0308

Utah
C. Neil Jensen
Executive Director
1062 E. 21st St. S., Suite 212
Salt Lake City, UT 84106
801-484-9141, Fax: 801-484-8090

Vermont
Frederick H. Dobson, III, R.Ph.
P.O. Box 790
Richmond, VT 05477
802-434-3001, Fax: 802-434-4803

Virginia
Randall W. Wampler
Executive Director
3119 W. Clay St.
Richmond, VA 23230
804-355-7941, Fax: 804-355-7991

Washington
Raymond A. Olson
Executive Vice President
1420 Maple Ave. SW, Suite 101
Renton, WA 96055-3196
206-228-7171, Fax: 206-277-3897

West Virginia
Richard D. Stevens
Executive Director
Kanawha Valley Bldg.
300 Capitol St., Suite 1002
Charleston, WV 25301
304-344-5302, Fax: 304-344-5316

Wisconsin
Christopher J. Decker, R.Ph.
Executive Vice President
202 Price Place
Madison, WI 53705
608-238-5515, Fax: 608-238-5646

Wyoming
Keith Sande, R.Ph.
Executive Director
P.O. Box 541
Powell, WY 82435
307-754-4285

State Boards of Pharmacy

Alabama
Jerry Moore, R.Ph.
Executive Secretary
1 Perimeter Park S., Suite 425 S
Birmingham, AL 35243
205-967-0130, Fax: 205-967-1009

Alaska
Clay Kent
Licensing Examiner
Dept. of Commerce and
Economic Development
Division of Occupational Licensing
P.O. Box 110806
Juneau, AK 99811-0806
907-465-2589, Fax: 907-465-2974

Arizona
L. A. Lloyd, R.Ph.
Executive Director
5060 N. 19th Ave., Suite 101
Phoenix, AZ 85015
602-256-5125, Fax: 602-255-5740

Arkansas
Lester Hosto P.D.
Executive Director
101 E. Capitol Ave., Suite 218
Little Rock, AR 72201
501-662-0190, Fax: 501-662-0195

California
Patricia Harris
Executive Officer
400 "R" St., Suite 4070
Sacramento, CA 95814
916-445-5014, Fax: 916-327-6308

Colorado
D.L. Simmons
Program Administrator
1560 Broadway, Suite 1310
Denver, CO 80202-5146
303-894-7790, Fax: 303-894-7764

Connecticut
Margaret Soracchi, R.Ph.
Board Administrator
State Office Bldg., Room G-3A
165 Capitol Ave.
Hartford, CT 06106
203-686-3290, Fax: 203-566-7630

Delaware
Bonnie Wallner, R.Ph.
Executive Secretary
P.O. Box 637
Dover, DE 19903
302-739-4798, Fax: 302-739-3071

District of Columbia
Barbara Hagans
Contact Representative
614 "H" St. NW, Room 923
Washington, DC 20001
202-727-7832, Fax: 202-727-7662

Florida
John D. Taylor, R.Ph.
Executive Director
Health Care Administration
Board of Pharmacy
1940 N. Monroe St.
Northwood Center
Tallahassee, FL 32399-0775
904-488-7546, Fax: 904-922-7865

Georgia
Gregg W. Schuder
Executive Director
166 Pryor St. SW
Atlanta, GA 30303
404-656-3912, Fax: 404-651-9532

Hawaii
Charlene Tamanaha
Executive Officer
P.O. Box 3469
Honolulu, HI 96801
808-586-2698

Idaho
R. K. Markuson, R.Ph.
Director
P.O. Box 83720
Boise, ID 83720-0067
206-334-2356, Fax: 208-334-3536

Illinois
Ed Duffy, R.Ph.
Executive Administrator
Drug Compliance
Illinois Dept. of Professional Regulation
100 W. Randolph, Suite 9-300
Chicago, IL 60601
312-814-4573, Fax: 312-814-3145

Indiana
Frances L. Kelly
Director
402 W. Washington St., Room 041
Indianapolis, IN 45204
317-233-4403, Fax: 317-233-4236

Iowa
Lloyd K. Jessen, R.Ph., J.D.
1209 East Court Ave.
Executive Hills West
Des Moines, IA 50319
515-281-5944, Fax: 515-281-4609

Kansas
Tom Hitchcock
Executive Secretary
900 Jackson St., Room 513
Topeka, KS 66612-1231
913-296-4056, Fax: 913-296-8420

Kentucky
Ralph E. Bouvella, R.Ph. Phd., J.D.
Executive Director
1226 U.S. Hwy. 127 S.
Frankfort, KY 40601
502-564-3833, Fax: 502-564-2032

Louisiana
Howard B. Bolton, R.Ph.
Executive Director
5615 Corporate Blvd., 8th Floor
Baton Rouge, LA 70808
504-925-6496, Fax: 504-925-6499

Maine
Susan Greenlaw
Board Clerk
Dept. of Professional and
Financial Regulations
Board of Commissioners of the
Profession of Pharmacy
State House Station #35
Augusta, ME 04333
207-582-6723, Fax: 207-624-8637

Maryland
Tamara Banks
Administrative Officer
4201 Patterson Ave.
Baltimore, MD 21215
410-764-4755, Fax: 410-358-6207

Massachusetts
Charles R. Young, R.Ph.
Acting Executive Director
100 Cambridge St., Room 1514
Boston, MA 02202
617-727-9955, Fax: 617-727-2197

Michigan
Patrick Gaven, R.Ph.
Chairman
611 W. Ottawa St.
P.O. Box 30018
Lansing, MI 48909
517-373-9102, Fax: 517-373-2179

Minnesota
David E. Holmstrom, R.Ph., J.D.
Executive Director
2700 University Ave. W., Rm. 107
St. Paul. MN 55114-1079
612-642-0541, Fax: 612-643-3530

Mississippi
William L. Stevens
Executive Director
2310 Highway 80 W.
C & F Plaza, Suite D
Jackson, MS 39204
601-354-6750, Fax: 601-354-6071

Missouri
Kevin E. Kinkade, R.Ph.
Executive Director
P.O. Box 625
Jefferson City, MO 65102
314-751-0091, Fax: 314-526-3464

Montana
Warren R. Amole, Jr., R.Ph.
Executive Director
111 N. Last Chance Gulch
Helena, MT 59620-0513
406-444-1698, Fax: 406-444-1667

Nebraska
Katherine A. Brown
Executive Secretary
Board of Examiners in Pharmacy
P.O. Box 95007
301 Centennial Mall S.
Lincoln, NE 68509
402-471-2115, Fax: 402-471-0383

Nevada
Keith W. MacDonald, R.Ph.
Executive Secretary
1201 Terminal Way, Suite 212
Reno, NV 89502-3257
702-322-0691, Fax: 702-322-0895

New Hampshire
Paul G. Boisseau, R.Ph.
Executive Director
57 Regional Dr.
Concord, NH 03301
603-271-2350, Fax: 603-271-2856

New Jersey
H. Lee Gladstein, R.Ph.
Executive Director
124 Halsey St., 6th Fl.
P.O. Box 45013
Newark, NJ 07102
201-504-6450, Fax: 201-648-3355

New Mexico
Richard W. Thompson
Executive Director
1650 University Blvd. NE
Suite 400-B
Albuquerque, NM 87102
505-841-9102, Fax: 505-841-9113

New York
Lawrence H. Mokhiber, R.Ph.
Executive Secretary
Cultural Education Center
Room 3035
Albany, NY 12230
518-474-3848, Fax: 518-473-6995

North Carolina
David R. Work, R.Ph.
Executive Director
P.O. Box 459
Carrboro, NC 27510-0459
919-942-4454, Fax: 919-967-5757

North Dakota
William J. Grosz, Sc.D., R.Ph.
Executive Director
P.O. Box 1354
Bismarck, ND 58502-1354
701-258-1535, Fax: 701-258-9312

Ohio
Franklin Z. Wickham, R.Ph.
Executive Director
77 S. High St., 17th Floor
Columbus, OH 43255-0320
614-466-4143, Fax: 614-752-4838

Oklahoma
Bryan Potter, R.Ph.
Executive Secretary
4545 N. Lincoln Blvd., Suite 112
Oklahoma City, OK 73105
405-521-3815, Fax: 405-521-3758

Oregon
Ruth Vandever, R.Ph.
Executive Director
State Office Bldg., Suite 425
800 NE Oregon St., #9
Portland, OR 97232
503-731-4032, Fax: 503-731-4067

Pennsylvania
Richard Marshman, R.Ph.
Executive Secretary
P.O. Box 2649
Harrisburg, PA 17105-2849
717-783-7157, Fax: 717-783-4853

Puerto Rico
Amalo LaLuc
President
Call Box 10200
Santurce, PR 00908-5026
809-725-6161 Ext. 2245
Fax: 809-725-7903

Rhode Island
Mario Casinelli, Jr., R.Ph.
Chairman of the Board
Department of Health
Division of Drug Control
Three Capitol Hill, Room 304
Providence, RI 02906-5097
401-277-2837, Fax: 401-277-2490

South Carolina
Joseph L. Mullinax, R.Ph.
Administrator
S.C.L.L.R./Board of Pharmacy
1026 Sumter St., Room 209
P.O. Box 11927
Columbia, SC 29211
803-734-1010, Fax: 803-734-1552

South Dakota
Galen Jordre, R.Ph.
Secretary
P.O. Box 518
Pierre, SD 57501-0518
605-224-2336, Fax: 805-224-1280

Tennessee
J. Floyd Ferrell, Jr., R.Ph.
Director
500 James Robertson Pkwy.
Nashville, TN 37243-1149
615-741-2718, Fax: 615-741-6470

Texas
Fred S. Brinkley, Jr., R.Ph.
Executive Director
8505 Cross Park Dr., Suite 110
Austin, TX 78754
512-832-0661, Fax: 512-832-0855

Utah
David E. Robinson
Director
Utah Dept. of Commerce
Division of Occupational and Professional Licensing
160 E. 300 S.
P.O. Box 45605
Salt Lake City, UT 84145-0805
801-530-6628, Fax: 801-630-8511

Vermont
Carla Preston
Staff Assistant
109 State St.
Montpelier, VT 05809-1106
802-828-2875, Fax: 802-828-2496

Virginia
Scotti W. Milley, R.Ph.
Executive Director
6606 W. Broad St.
Richmond, VA 23230
804-662-9911, Fax: 804-662-9313

Washington
Donald H. Williams, R.Ph.
Executive Director
P.O. Box 47863
Olympia, WA 98504-7863
206-753-8834, Fax: 206-586-4359

West Virginia
Sam Kapourales, R.Ph.
President
236 Capitol St.
Charleston, WV 25301
304-556-0556, Fax: 304-558-0572

Wisconsin
Pat Schenck
Program Assistant
Wisconsin Dept. of Registration and Licensing
P.O. Box 8935
1400 E. Washington Ave.
Madison, WI 53708
606-288-2811, Fax: 606-267-0844

Wyoming
Marilynn H. Mitchell, R.Ph.
Executive Director
1720 S. Poplar St., Suite 5
Camper, WY 82601
307-234-0294, Fax: 307-234-7226

State Licensure Requirements

All states require candidates for pharmacist licensures to have graduated from an accredited college of pharmacy and to be of good moral character. All states except California use the National Association of Boards of Pharmacy Licensure Examination (NABPLEX). Virtually every state allows students to retake the exam in case of failure. A few states also require students to take the Federal Drug Law Exam or a practical exam. (Contact the appropriate state board about additional examinations.) Some states require full citizenship, and many states require a candidate to be at least 18 years old.

Most states will grant you a license on the basis of your having been licensed in another state. Check with individual state boards for special requirements and fees. There are two states that do not reciprocate licensure at all: Florida and California.

	Internship Requirements		CE Requirements	
State	**Total Hours**	**Postgrad Hours**	**Hours**	**Industry Intern Credit**
Albama	1,500	400	15/1 yr.	No
Alaska	1,500	160	15/1 yr.	No
Arizona	1,500	None	30/2 yrs.	500 hours
Arkansas	2,000	1,000	15/1 yr.	May be allowed
California	1,500	1,000	30/2 yrs.	Under 600 hours
Colorado	1,800	—	No	Case by case
Connecticut	1,500	None	15/1 yr.	Varies
Delaware	1,500	None	30/2 yrs.	N.A.
District of Columbia	1,500/1,000	None	30/2 yrs.	No
Florida	2,080 (varies)	N.A.	15/1 yr.	Case by case
Georgia	1,500	None	30/2 yrs.	Case by case
Hawaii	2,000	None	No	Yes
Idaho	1,500	None	5/1 yr.	One-half credit
Illinois	400	None	30/2 yrs.	No
Indiana	1,040	520	30/2 yrs.	No
Iowa	1,500	None	30/2 yrs.	May be allowed
Kansas	1,500	None	15/1 yr.	May be allowed
Kentucky	1,500	None	15/1 yr.	400 hours
Louisiana	1,500/1 yr.	500	5/1 yr.	No
Maine	1,500	None	15/1 yr.	May be allowed
Maryland	1,560	None	30/2 yrs.	Yes
Massachusetts	1,500	None	30/2 yrs.	Up to 400 hours
Michigan	1,000	None	30/2 yrs.	Up to 400 hours
Minnesota	1,500	None	30/2 yrs.	Varies
Mississippi	1,500	None	20/2 yrs.	300 hours
Missouri	1,500	None	10/1 yr.	200 hours
Montana	1,500	None	15/1 yr.	May be allowed
Nebraska	1,500	None	30/2 yrs.	May be allowed
Nevada	1,500	None	30/2 yrs.	No
New Hampshire	1,500	None	15/1 yr.	May be allowed
New Jersey	1,000	Varies	30/2 yrs.	No
New Mexico	1 yr/1500	None	15/1 yr.	Yes
New York	6 mos	None	No	No

State	Internship Requirements		CE Requirements	
	Total Hours	Postgrad Hours	Hours	Industry Intern Credit
North Carolina	1,500	None	10/1 yr.	Up to 500 hours
North Dakota	1,500	None	30/2 yrs.	400 hours
Ohio	1,500	None	45/3 yrs.	Up to 300 hours
Oklahoma	2,000	None	15/1 yr.	Yes
Oregon	1,500	400	15/1 yr.	Varies
Pennsylvania	1,500	None	30/2 yrs.	Case by case
Puerto Rico	1,500	None	35/3 yrs.	300 hours
Rhode Island	1,500	None	15/1 yr.	One-half credit
South Carolina	1,500	None	15/1 yr.	500 hours max.
South Dakota	1,500	None	12/1 yr.	400 hours
Tennessee	1,500	None	15/1 yr.	Up to 400 hours
Texas	1,500	None	12/1 yr.	Varies
Utah	1,500	None	No	Varies
Vermont	1,500	None	15/1 yr.	Up to 750 hours
Virginia	6 mos	None	No	Yes
Washington	1,500	None	15/1 yr.	300 hours
West Virginia	1,500	None	15/1 yr.	520 hours
Wisconsin	1,500	500	No	500 hours max.
Wyoming	1,500	None	6/1 yr.	500 hours max.

Reprinted from National Association of Boards of Pharmacy: *1992 NABP Survey of Pharmacy Law,* Park Ridge, IL, 1992.

APPENDIX E

BUDGETING FOR DRUG INFORMATION RESOURCES

A. Basic Library

References	Update	Cost*
American Hospital Formulary Service (AHFS) Drug Information	Quarterly	$145.00
Drug Facts and Comparisons	Monthly	$180.00
Drug Interaction Facts (disk available)	Quarterly	$ 83.00
Remington's Pharmaceutical Sciences		$125.00
Physicians' Desk Reference	Biannually	$ 67.00
Martindale: The Extra Pharmacopoeia		$205.00
Handbook of Non-prescription Drugs		$ 91.00
Handbook of Injectable Drugs		$135.00
USP DI (three-volume set)		$269.00

B. Additional Resources

References	Cost*
Therapeutics	
• *Pharmacotherapy: A Pathophysiologic Approach*	$110.00
• *Applied Therapeutics: The Clinical Use of Drugs*	$117.00
• *Textbook of Therapeutics: Drug and Disease Management*	$105.00
Internal Medicine	
• *Harrison's Principles of Internal Medicine*	$107.00
• *Cecil Textbook of Medicine*	$105.00
Pharmacokinetics	
• *Basic Clinical Pharmacokinetics*	$ 38.00
• *Applied Pharmacokinetics: Principles of Therapeutic Drug Monitoring*	$ 77.50
• *Basic Clinical Pharmacokinetics Handbook*	$ 25.00
Pharmacology	
• *Goodman and Gilman's The Pharmacological Basis of Therapeutics*	$ 85.00
Pregnancy/Breast-feeding	
• *Drugs in Pregnancy and Lactation*	$ 80.00
Pediatrics	
• *The Harriet Lane Handbook*	$ 30.00
• *Pediatric Dosage Handbook*	$ 31.75
Drug–Drug Interaction	
• *Drug Interactions & Updates Quarterly*	$ 77.80
• *Evaluations of Drug Interactions*	$199.00

C. Microfiche Systems

References	Update	Cost*
Iowa Drug Information System	Monthly	$1,750.00
Paul DeHaen Drug Data Information System		
Drugs in Prospect (DIP)		$1,300.00
Drugs in Research (DIR)		$ 800.00
Drugs in Use (DIU)		$1,000.00
Adverse Drug Reactions and Interactions Data (ADRID)		

D. CD-ROM Computer Systems/Programs	Cost*
Iowa Drug Information System	$ 4,000.00
Medline (SilverPlatter®)	$ 1,600.00
IPA (Knight-Ridder®)	$ 1,600.00
Facts & Comparisons	$ 450.00
Micromedex (POISINDEX, DRUGDEX, EMERGINDEX plus IDENTIDEX) > 200 licensed bed facility	
(any one) database plus Identidex	$12,926.00
(any two) databases plus Identidex	$25,336.00
(any three) databases plus Identidex	$32,961.00
Other Micromedex Databases	
Aftercare™: USP-DI and Injury & Illness	$ 2,808.00
Martindale: The Extra Pharmacopoeia	$ 1,195.00
Reprorisk®	$ 2,066.00
Drug-Reax™	$ 1,232.00
Inpharma	$ 1,920.00
Reactions	$ 1,200.00
PDR®	$ 4,616.00
Kinetidex™	$ 2,850.00
P&T Quik®	$ 485.00
Physicians' Desk Reference: Electronic Library (PDR & supplements, PDR for Nonprescription drugs, PDR for Ophthalmology, PDR Guide to Drug Interactions, Side Effects, Indications)	$ 595.00
Clinical Reference Library (Lexi-Comp)	$ 395.00
Clinical Pharmacology	$ 295.00
RX Triage™ Software	$ 480.00
Drug Information Fulltext	$ 895.00
AHFS Drug Information	$ 995.00
MedTeach™ Software	$ 350.00
DataKinetics Software	$ 495.00
CliniTrend™ Software	$ 495.00

E. Major On-Line Vendors
Ovid Technologies, Inc.
Knight-Ridder Information
Medlars Management System
PaperChase
System Development Corporation Search Service (SDC)

*Costs are approximate and are based on 1996 figures.

Index

NOTE: Page numbers in *italic* denote illustrations; those followed by *t* denote tables; those followed by Q denote questions; and those followed by E denote explanations.

D

G

I

O

P

Q

R

S